How to Practice Evidence-Based Psychiatry

Basic Principles and Case Studies

Edited by

C. Barr Taylor, M.D.

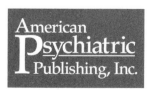

American Psychiatric Publishing, Inc.

Washington, DC
London, England

Note: The authors have worked to ensure that all information in this book is accurate at the time of publication and consistent with general psychiatric and medical standards, and that information concerning drug dosages, schedules, and routes of administration is accurate at the time of publication and consistent with standards set by the U.S. Food and Drug Administration and the general medical community. As medical research and practice continue to advance, however, therapeutic standards may change. Moreover, specific situations may require a specific therapeutic response not included in this book. For these reasons and because human and mechanical errors sometimes occur, we recommend that readers follow the advice of physicians directly involved in their care or the care of a member of their family.

Books published by American Psychiatric Publishing, Inc., represent the views and opinions of the individual authors and do not necessarily represent the policies and opinions of APPI or the American Psychiatric Association.

If you would like to buy between 25 and 99 copies of this or any other APPI title, you are eligible for a 20% discount; please contact APPI Customer Service at appi@psych.org or 800-368-5777. If you wish to buy 100 or more copies of the same title, please e-mail us at bulksales@psych.org for a price quote.

Copyright © 2010 American Psychiatric Publishing, Inc.
ALL RIGHTS RESERVED

Manufactured in the United States of America on acid-free paper
13 12 11 10 09   5 4 3 2 1
First Edition

Typeset in Adobe's Janson and Berthold's Poppl-Laudatio.

American Psychiatric Publishing, Inc.
1000 Wilson Boulevard
Arlington, VA 22209–3901
www.appi.org

Library of Congress Cataloging-in-Publication Data
How to practice evidence-based psychiatry : basic principles and case studies / edited by C. Barr Taylor. — 1st ed.
    p. ; cm.
  Includes bibliographical references and index.
  ISBN 978-1-58562-365-5 (alk. paper)
  1. Evidence-based psychiatry. 2. Evidence-based psychiatry—Case studies. I. Taylor, C. Barr (Craig Barr)
  [DNLM: 1. Psychiatry—methods. 2. Evidence-Based Medicine—methods. 3. Mental Disorders—therapy.
WM 140 H847 2010]
  RC455.2.E94H69 2010

  616.89—dc22

                                                                        2009028112

British Library Cataloguing in Publication Data
A CIP record is available from the British Library.

Contents

PART I
Basic Principles of Evidence-Based Psychiatry

PART II
Case Studies:
Evidence-Based Medicine Applied to Major DSM-IV Disorders

PART III
Case Studies:
Evidence-Based Psychiatric Practice in Different Settings

Contributors

Bibi Das, M.D.
Staff Psychiatrist and Clinical Educator, Stanford University School of Medicine, Stanford, California

Ira D. Glick, M.D.
Professor of Psychiatry and Behavioral Sciences, Stanford University School of Medicine, Stanford, California

Gregory E. Gray, M.D., Ph.D.
Clinical Professor of Psychiatry and the Behavioral Sciences, Keck School of Medicine, University of Southern California, Los Angeles, California; and private practice, Pasadena, California

Keith Humphreys, Ph.D.
Research Professor, Department of Psychiatry and Behavioral Sciences, Stanford University School of Medicine, Stanford, California

Terence A. Ketter, M.D.
Professor of Psychiatry and Behavioral Sciences, Stanford University School of Medicine, Stanford, California

Lorrin M. Koran, M.D.
Clinical Professor of Psychiatry and Behavioral Sciences, Emeritus, Stanford University School of Medicine, Stanford, California

Ben Kurian, M.D., M.P.H.
Assistant Professor, Department of Psychiatry, University of Texas Southwestern Medical Center, Dallas, Texas

Anna Lembke, M.D.
Instructor, Department of Psychiatry and Behavioral Sciences, Stanford University School of Medicine, Stanford, California

Steven E. Lindley, M.D. Ph.D.
Assistant Professor, Department of Psychiatry and Behavioral Sciences, Stanford University School of Medicine, Stanford, California; Director of Outpatient Mental Health, VA Palo Alto Health Care System, Menlo Park, California

Gretchen Lindner, Ph.D.
Staff Psychologist, PTSD Clinical Team, VA Palo Alto Health Care System, Menlo Park, California

Joanna M. Marino, M.A.
Psychology Intern, University of Florida Department of Public Health; University of Florida, Gainesville, Florida

Anthony J. Mascola, M.D.
Assistant Clinical Professor, Department of Psychiatry and Behavioral Sciences, Stanford University Medical Center, Stanford, California

Matthew H. May, M.D.
Private Practice and Adjunct Clinical Faculty, Department of Psychiatry and Behavioral Sciences, Stanford University School of Medicine, Stanford, California

James E. Mitchell, M.D.
Christoferson Professor and Chair, Department of Clinical Neuroscience; Chester Fritz Distinguished University Professor, University of North Dakota School of Medicine and Health Sciences; and President, Neuropsychiatric Research Institute, Fargo, North Dakota

Douglas S. Rait, Ph.D.
Chief, Couples and Family Therapy Clinic, Stanford Medical Center, and Clinical Professor of Psychiatry and Behavioral Sciences, Stanford University School of Medicine, Stanford, California; Director, Family Therapy Program, VA Palo Alto Health Care System, Menlo Park, California

James Reich, M.D.
Adjunct Associate Professor of Psychiatry, Stanford University School of Medicine, Stanford, California; Clinical Professor of Psychiatry, University of California, San Francisco Medical School, San Francisco, California

Margaret F. Reynolds-May, B.A.
M.D. Candidate and Office of Student Affairs, Yale University School of Medicine, New Haven, Connecticut

Anthony J. Rothschild, M.D.
Irving S. and Betty Brudnick Endowed Chair and Professor of Psychiatry, Department of Psychiatry, and Director, Senior Scholars Program, University of Massachusetts Medical School, Worcester, Massachusetts

Richard E. Shanteau, M.D.
Staff Psychiatrist, Kaiser Foundation Hospitals, South San Francisco, California

Caroline Spiranovic, Ph.D.
Research and Development Associate, Sentiens Pty Ltd, West Perth, Australia

Violeta Tan, M.D.
Psychiatry Resident, Department of Psychiatry and Behavioral Sciences, Stanford University School of Medicine, Stanford, California

Dennis Tannenbaum, M.B.Ch.B., FRANZCP
Chief Executive Officer and Consultant Psychiatrist, Sentiens Pty Ltd, West Perth, Australia

C. Barr Taylor, M.D.
Professor of Psychiatry and Behavioral Sciences, Stanford University School of Medicine, Stanford, California

Madhukar H. Trivedi, M.D.
Professor of Psychiatry, Betty Jo Hay Distinguished Chair in Mental Health, and Chief, Division of Mood Disorders, University of Texas Southwestern Medical School, Dallas, Texas

Po W. Wang, M.D.
Clinical Associate Professor, Department of Psychiatry and Behavioral Sciences, Stanford University School of Medicine, Stanford, California

Disclosure of Interests

Ira D. Glick, M.D.—*Grant/research support:* Astra-Zeneca, Bristol-Myers Squibb/Otsuka, GlaxoSmithKline, National Institute of Mental Health, Solvay, Shire, Pfizer, Eli Lilly and Company; *Consult/advisory board:* Impax, Bristol-Myers Squibb, Janssen, Eli Lilly and Company, Lunkbeck, Organon BioSciences, Pfizer, Shire, Solvay, Vanda; *Speakers' bureau:* AstraZeneca, Bristol-Myers Squibb/Otsuka, Janssen, Pfizer, Shire.

Terence A. Ketter, M.D.—*Grant/research support:* Abbott Laboratories, AstraZeneca, Bristol-Myers Squibb, Cephalon, Eli Lilly and Company, GlaxoSmithKline, Pfizer, Repligen Corporation, Wyeth. *Consultant:* Abbott Laboratories, AstraZeneca, Bristol-Myers Squibb, Dainip-pon Sumitomo Pharma, Eli Lilly and Company, Glaxo-SmithKline, Janssen, Jazz Pharmaceuticals, Novartis, Organon International, Solvay, Valeant Pharmaceuticals, Vanda Pharmaceuticals, Wyeth, Xenoport. *Lecture hono-raria:* Abbott Laboratories, AstraZeneca, Bristol-Myers Squibb, Eli Lilly and Company, GlaxoSmithKline, Noven Pharmaceuticals, Pfizer. *Employee* (Nzeera Ketter, M.D., spouse): Johnson & Johnson.

Lorrin M. Koran, M.D.—*Grant/research support:* Eli Lilly and Company, Somaxon, Sepacor. *Consultant:* Jazz Pharmaceuticals. *Speakers' bureau:* Forest Laboratories.

Ben Kurian, M.D., M.P.H.—*Grant/research support:* Agency for Healthcare Research and Quality, National Institute of Mental Health, Targacept.

Anthony J. Rothschild, M.D.—*Grant/research support:* Cyberonics, National Institute of Mental Health, Novar-tis, Takeda, Wyeth. *Consultant:* Eli Lilly and Company, GlaxoSmithKline, Forest Laboratories, Pfizer. *Trademarks:* The Rothschild Scale for Antidepressant Tachyphylaxis (RSAT). *Other:* Eli Lilly and Company and Pfizer provided study medication free of charge for the National Institute of Mental Health Study of the Pharmacotherapy of Psy-chotic Depression (STOP-PD).

Alan F. Schatzberg, M.D.—*Consultant:* BrainCells, CeNeRx, Corcept (Co-Founder), Eli Lilly and Company, Forest Laboratories, Merck, Neuronetics, Novartis, Path-ways Diagnostics, Pfizer, PharmaNeuroBoost, Quintlies, Synosis, Xytis, Wyeth. *Honorarium:* GlaxoSmithKline, Roche. *Patents:* Named inventor on pharmacogenetic use patents on prediction of antidepressant response.

Dennis Tannenbaum, M.B.Ch.B., F.R.A.N.Z.C.P.—CEO of Sentiens Pty, Ltd.

C. Barr Taylor, M.D.—*Grant/research support:* Na-tional Institute of Mental Health, National Institute on Aging, National Cancer Institute, Schweizerische Anor-exia Nervosa Stiflung (Switzerland), Commonwealth De-partment of Health and Ageing (Australia), Department of Veterans Affairs.

Madhukar H. Trivedi, M.D.—*Grant/research support:* Agency for Healthcare Research and Quality, Corcept Therapeutics, Cyberonics, Merck, National Alliance for Research in Schizophrenia and Depression, National In-stitute of Mental Health, National Institute on Drug Abuse, Novartis, Pharmacia and Upjohn, Predix Pharma-ceuticals, Solvay, Targacept. *Consultant/speaker:* Abbott Laboratories, Abdi Brahim, Akzo, AstraZeneca, Bristol-Myers Squibb, Cephalon, Fabre-Kramer Pharmaceuticals, Forest Laboratories, GlaxoSmithKline, Janssen, Johnson & Johnson, Eli Lilly and Company, Meade-Johnson In-ternational, Neuronetics, Parke-Davis Pharmaceuticals, Pfizer, Sepraco, VantagePoint, Wyeth-Ayerst Laborato-ries.

Po W. Wang, M.D.—*Grant/research support:* Abbott Laboratories, AstraZeneca, Bristol-Myers Squibb, Eisai, Elan Pharmaceuticals, Eli Lilly and Company, Glaxo-SmithKline, Janssen, Novartis, Repligen Corporation, Shire, Solvay, Wyeth. *Consultant:* Abbott Laboratories, Corcept Therapeutics, Pfizer, Sanofi-Aventis. *Lecture honoraria:* AstraZeneca, Bristol-Myers Squibb, Eli Lilly and Company, GlaxoSmithKline, Pfizer, Sanofi-Aventis.

The following contributors stated that they had no competing interests during the year preceding manuscript submittal:

Bibi Das, M.D.
Gregory E. Gray, M.D., Ph.D.
Keith Humphreys, Ph.D.
Anna Lembke, M.D.
Steven E. Lindley, M.D., Ph.D.
Gretchen Lindner, Ph.D.
Joanna M. Marino, M.A.

Anthony J. Mascola, M.D.
Matthew H. May, M.D.
James E. Mitchell, M.D.
Douglas S. Rait, Ph.D.
James Reich, M.D.
Margaret F. Reynolds-May, B.A.
Richard E. Shanteau, M.D.
Caroline Spiranovic, Ph.D.
Violeta Tan, M.D.

Foreword

We are in a great practice era in psychiatry. Advances in both psychotherapy and psychopharmacology have led to several effective approaches to many mental health problems. And the knowledge base on which we base psychiatric practice only continues to grow. Thus, I am delighted with the publication of *How to Practice Evidence-Based Psychiatry: Basic Principles and Case Studies*. This valuable new book will help residents, practicing psychiatrists, and mental health workers find the most useful and relevant information to inform and improve their practices.

In this text, C. Barr Taylor, M.D., has approached expounding on evidence-based practice in two ways. First, he has done a masterful job in revising and updating a splendid book, the *Concise Guide to Evidence-Based Psychiatry*, by Gregory E. Gray, M.D., Ph.D., which provides details on how to obtain and interpret medical evidence. The revisions include new chapters on how to consider other sources of information, including guidelines and measurements, and how to provide effective long-term treatment to patients with complicated, comorbid problems. Second, Dr. Taylor has recruited experts from a variety of specialty areas and practice settings to describe how they incorporate the latest evidence and outcome studies into their practice. These cases are both interesting and inspiring. I trust you will find them relevant and helpful to your everyday practice.

Over the last few years, the American Psychiatric Association has developed tools to facilitate aspects of evidence-based psychiatric practice, including the publication of practice guidelines and performance measures. One example, the *Handbook of Psychiatric Measures*, provides information about and ready access to many measures relevant to diagnosis, treatment, and evidence-based psychiatric practice. American Psychiatric Publishing, Inc., also has published a variety of resource books that provide the latest evidence and information on available and developing treatments, including basic textbooks and practitioner guides to the core psychotherapy competencies. Still, as Dr. Taylor notes, the major challenge for the modern practitioner is to apply and incorporate into his or her practice the most effective psychosocial and biological interventions that are based on the latest evidence.

How to Practice Evidence-Based Psychiatry: Basic Principles and Case Studies is an invaluable tool in helping you become a better practitioner. My congratulations to Dr. Taylor and his colleagues.

Alan F. Schatzberg, M.D.

Preface

In recent years, there has been an increased emphasis on evidence-based psychiatric practice. Many practice settings encourage clinicians to follow evidence-based guidelines and algorithms, medical students and residents are expected to develop and retain skills in evidence-based practice, and clinicians are encouraged to follow procedures to carefully evaluate the quality of the evidence they use in their practice. Despite this emphasis, many psychiatrists and other mental health professionals remain unfamiliar with methods and philosophy of evidence-based medicine (EBM) and, even more important, have little experience or guidance as to how to use evidence and the products developed from evidence (guidelines, algorithms) in clinical practice. The purpose of this book is to address the latter issue. The application of evidence to real clinical cases is difficult. Much of the evidence comes from patients who are less impaired and complicated than those we see in practice, focuses on immediate rather than long-term issues, and fails to address the need for integrated treatment.

I start with the assumption that guidelines, algorithms, and other sources of evidence and the interpretation of evidence need to be adapted to the individual patient by the clinician. I also believe that the best way to practice evidence-based psychiatry is to set measurable treatment goals and then to monitor progress toward those goals.

This book was written with two major goals in mind. The first goal is to discuss the methods and philosophy of evidence-based psychiatry. To achieve this goal, I updated and expanded the *Concise Guide to Evidence-Based Psychiatry*, by Gregory E. Gray, M.D., Ph.D., a popular, well-written, and easily understandable book on this topic. I was fortunate to have Dr. Gray's help with this process. The second goal is to discuss how the psychiatrist and other mental health specialists can incorporate evidence-based psychiatry into their clinical practice. To do so requires clinicians to use various tools—some of which may not be strictly evidence based, such as guidelines, expert opinion, and their own clinical experience and expertise. I invited experienced clinicians, many of whom are experts in their own right, to discuss cases in which they followed aspects of evidence-based care. I also decided that it would be useful to discuss the use of evidence-based practice when American Psychiatric Association guidelines are available and in various settings, including private practice. As the reader will see, the case presenters approached this task in various ways.

This book was written with three audiences in mind. The first audience consists of psychiatrists and other mental health professionals who wish to learn about evidence-based psychiatry on their own and who wish to incorporate evidence-based psychiatry into their busy practice. The first section (the updated *Concise Guide*) can be used both as an introduction to the topic and as a ready reference for researching the literature and appraising evidence.

The second audience is psychiatry residents and other mental health trainees. Several textbooks on the topic of EBM are available, including the *Concise Guide to Evidence-Based Psychiatry*. The first section of this book, the updated *Concise Guide*, focuses on the needs of psychiatry residents and of other mental health trainees by emphasizing the information resources of most use in finding answers to clinical questions in clinical practice. In addition, examples are drawn from the psychiatric literature rather than from general medicine or surgery. The second and third sections include cases that may be useful for residents. I have used these cases in my lectures on evidence-based psychiatry. I also invited a resident to discuss a patient she treated.

The third audience is residency program directors and faculty who are looking for a brief introduction to evidence-based psychiatry and examples of how evidence-based psychiatry can be practiced. The Accreditation Council for Graduate Medical Education requires that all residents develop EBM skills as part of the "practice-based learning and improvement" core competency, and the program directors and faculty need to be more aware of these practices. Chapter 15 includes updated suggestions from the *Concise Guide to Evidence-Based Psychiatry* for teaching EBM in psychiatry residency training programs.

It is my hope that the information and examples in this book can help achieve the goal of evidence-based psychiatry, which is to provide the best care to our patients.

C. Barr Taylor, M.D.

Cautionary Statement

The cases presented in this volume are meant to illustrate how experienced clinicians have approached various clinical issues. However, they are not meant to be recommendations as to how other clinicians should treat similar cases, and other clinicians might have equally useful approaches to their patients. The cases are not meant, either, to be recommendations of measures that should be used or dosages of medications that should be given unless their status as such is clearly stated by the authors.

Readers should note that Internet addresses change frequently. If a link provided is no longer current, a search from the referenced homepage by title or keyword may locate the cited document.

Acknowledgments

The development of *How to Practice Evidence-Based Psychiatry: Basic Principles and Case Studies* has relied on the help of many individuals. The first section of the book is primarily an update of the excellent *Concise Guide to Evidence-Based Psychiatry*, by Gregory E. Gray, M.D., Ph.D., with new chapters added to expand the focus to evidence-based psychiatry practice. I am deeply grateful for the chance to update this material. Dr. Gray was also very willing and available to review and revise updates.

I also would like to thank all the contributors to this book. All prepared interesting and important cases and responded to any suggestions for changes. I appreciate their willingness to be forthright in discussing how they approach cases with evidence-based medicine procedures.

Many individuals from American Psychiatric Publishing contributed in many important ways to this project. I particularly want to thank Bob Hales, Editor-in-Chief, and John McDuffie, Editorial Director, who provided much support and advice for this project, and Roxanne Rhodes, Senior Editor, and the Books Department staff for their careful work in editing and preparing the manuscript.

I want to thank the many individuals who read drafts of various chapters and provided important feedback and recommendations, including Vickie Chang, Darby Cunning, Debra Safer, Violeta Tan, and Mickey Trockel. This project began with discussions in the Behavioral Medicine Clinic in the Stanford Medical School Department of Psychiatry about how to practice evidence-based medicine. I want to thank Bruce Arnow, Chris Hayward, Elias Aboujaoude, Debra Safer, Anthony Mascola, and Kim Bullock for their suggestions about how to think about and present these difficult ideas. Smita Das helped me develop some of the original forms and procedures that eventually became central to the cases I present. Nicole DeBias was incredibly helpful in preparing, editing, and assembling the many pieces for submission to American Psychiatric Publishing.

Basic Principles of Evidence-Based Psychiatry

I

What Is Evidence-Based Psychiatric Practice?

C. Barr Taylor, M.D.
Gregory E. Gray, M.D., Ph.D.

Evidence-based psychiatric practice (EBPP) is a broad term referring to clinical practice that is informed by evidence about interventions and considers patient needs, values, and preferences and their integration in determining individual care (Kazdin 2008). EBPP uses evidence-based medicine (EBM) to assess the quality of evidence relevant to the risks and benefits of treatments (including lack of benefit). According to the Centre for Evidence-Based Medicine, "Evidence-based medicine is the conscientious, explicit and judicious use of current best evidence in making decisions about the care of individual patients" (Sackett et al. 1996).

Gray (2004), in *Concise Guide to Evidence-Based Psychiatry*, noted that EBM focuses on the use of clinical expertise to integrate research evidence, patient preferences, and clinical state in making decisions about patient care (Guyatt et al. 2000; Haynes et al. 2002a, 2002b; Straus and McAlister 2000). Usually, EBM addresses a particular issue (e.g., "What is the evidence that a particular treatment is effective for a particular problem?"). EBPP refers to the more complicated problem of integrating various sources of evidence, including experience, in treating patients in real-world settings and over long periods. The challenge of EBPP is to determine how "the evidence" fits a particular patient with multiple problems.

Over the last decade, the data from innumerable studies have been massaged by experts into guidelines, algorithms, consensus statements, reviews, textbooks, meta-analyses, and other documents.

These are important sources for EBPP. In psychiatry, we also need to consider psychosocial, psychotherapeutic, and psychopharmacological sources of expertise and evidence. Thus, we think it is better to take a broad perspective and focus on both the *evidence* and the *expertise*. The goal of EBPP is to improve patient care, and we need to consider a set of practices relevant to achieving that aim.

Gray (2004) has noted that all practice guidelines involve some degree of judgment and bias in their development (Browman 2001; Drake et al. 2001; Greenhalgh 2001), the extent of which is often unstated. In addition, clinical practice guidelines are often introduced as part of a "top-down" approach to changing clinician behavior, which may lead to clinician resistance. Ideally, EBM and EBPP are "bottom-up" approaches, in which clinicians make decisions based on ability to search and appraise the medical literature and use this information in their practice situation. Yet in practice, few clinicians have the time to find and read systematic reviews and thus rely on guidelines and algorithms. What remains most important is that patients are provided the best treatment available, and the best way to determine that is to monitor progress against some standard. Taking these considerations together, EBPP includes

- Accurate evaluation and treatment planning
- Consideration of treatment algorithms, guidelines, and best practices when planning and providing treatment

- Use of measures to determine progress of an individual patient
- Review of a patient's progress against personal and published standards
- Consideration of "evidence and experts" in clinical decisions
- Expertise in providing a range of therapies or in making them available through other resources or providers
- Periodic review of general practice outcomes

The cases in Parts II and III of the book illustrate how various clinicians have considered treatment algorithms, guidelines, and best practices and measures when planning and delivering treatment. In Chapter 4, we discuss the many resources available to find evidence relevant to your clinical questions. Yet even with the availability of these many resources for facilitating EBPP, new knowledge will continue to be added, and the practitioner will be faced with the need to interpret the summary sources and to search for new information. In addition, the process an individual goes through in evaluating a source is similar to that used by many experts. For this reason, we have updated the *Concise Guide to Evidence-Based Psychiatry* (Gray 2004). Part I of the book can be used to learn the principles and practices of EBM and EBPP.

The Development of Evidence-Based Medicine and Psychiatry

EBM arose for a variety of reasons, but perhaps the main one was the need to find ways to use the vast knowledge accumulating from clinical trials in ways that might improve or provide more cost-effective care. A search (conducted 4/06/08) of the term "depression treatment" in PubMed identified more than 100,000 articles, with more than 10,000 published in the last few years. Many of the scientific practices of EBM are designed to find ways to systematically sort through such evidence to find information that might improve care.

EBM had its origin in the Department of Clinical Epidemiology and Biostatistics at McMaster University in Canada (Guyatt 2002). In 1981, members of that department began publishing a series of articles in the *Canadian Medical Association Journal* that were intended to teach clinicians how to critically appraise the medical literature. In 1990, they began to move

beyond teaching critical appraisal skills and started developing a new philosophy of medical education, which they termed *evidence-based medicine*. In this new model, physicians would rely heavily on the medical research literature, rather than on textbooks or tradition, when approaching patient care problems. From 1993 to 2000, the McMaster group published a series of 25 articles in *JAMA* that defined many aspects of EBM. These articles have been revised and published in book form (Guyatt and Rennie 2002); they are also available, in their original form, at the Centre for Health Evidence (2007) Web site.

Although EBM was developed in Canada and described in *JAMA*, it has probably had its greatest effect in Britain. In part, this was because of the support of the National Health Service (NHS) (Baker and Kleijnen 2000; Ferguson and Russell 2000; Reynolds 2000; Trinder 2000). The NHS viewed EBM as a way both to improve the quality of care and to control costs by identifying and promoting therapies that worked and by eliminating therapies that were ineffective or harmful. The NHS funds university-based centers for EBM, surgery, child health, general practice, pathology, pharmacotherapy, nursing, dentistry, and mental health, as well as the NHS Centre for Reviews and Dissemination (1999) and the United Kingdom's Cochrane Centre (Baker and Kleijnen 2000; Sackett et al. 1996). In addition, the BMJ Publishing Group publishes several evidence-based journals and the semiannual publication *Clinical Evidence*, which is distributed to general practitioners by the NHS (Baker and Kleijnen 2000; Barton 2001).

In 1999, the Special Health Authority of the NHS in England and Wales established the National Institute for Clinical Excellence (NICE). In 2005, it joined with the Health Development Agency to become the new National Institute for Health and Clinical Excellence (still abbreviated NICE).

NICE publishes clinical appraisals of treatments with a consideration of cost-effectiveness. Since 2005, the NHS in England and Wales has been legally obliged to provide funding for medicines and treatments recommended by NICE's technology appraisal board. (Details as to how NICE develops guidelines can be found at www.nice.org.uk.)

NICE is not without its critics. As mentioned, it began with the goal of increasing access to effective treatments. It has been criticized, however, for the slow release of its appraisals; some of its assessments have seemed unfair, and the institute has been vilified for recommendations to limit or deny coverage for some high-profile medicines for cancer and other life-threatening diseases. The most controversial decisions seem to be related to refusal to pay for expensive treatments assessed to have marginal benefit of extending life or improving quality of life. Some believe that one of the greatest threats of EBM is its use to determine what services will be reimbursed (Steinbrook 2008).

According to Gray (2002), the uptake of EBM has been slower in the United States than overseas. He noted that the slow incorporation of EBM into psychiatry practice may be related to mental health professionals' belief that their patients' individuality and the nonquantifiable aspects of psychotherapy preclude the application of EBM to psychotherapeutic interventions (Geddes 2000; Geddes et al. 1997; Goss and Rowland 2000; Kazdin 2008; Mace et al. 2001; Parry 2000). We hope the cases presented later in this book dispel this myth.

In recent years, however, EBPP has achieved wide influence in many systems. In the United States, the Agency for Healthcare Research and Quality (2008) has established the National Guideline Clearinghouse (NGC; www.guideline.gov). This important resource is a comprehensive database of evidence-based clinical practice guidelines and related documents. NGC was originally created by the Agency for Healthcare Research and Quality in partnership with the American Medical Association (AMA) and the American Association of Health Plans (now America's Health Insurance Plans). The NGC mission is to provide physicians, nurses, other health professionals, health care providers, health plans, integrated delivery systems, purchasers, and others an accessible mechanism for obtaining objective, detailed information on clinical practice guidelines and to further their dissemination, implementation, and use.

The Veterans Health Administration (VHA) of the U.S. Department of Veterans Affairs (VA) may be in the forefront of providing evidence-based mental health practice. The recent VHA Handbook lays out minimum requirements for VHA mental health services (U.S. Department of Veterans Affairs 2008). In the section on evidence-based psychotherapies, the VHA notes that all veterans with posttraumatic stress disorder (PTSD) must have access to cognitive processing therapy or prolonged exposure therapy and that medical centers and very large community-based outpatient clinics must provide adequate staff capacity to allow the delivery of evidence-based psychotherapy to their patients. In addition, all veterans with depression or anxiety disorders must have access to three evidence-based treatments, as appropriate: cognitive-behavioral therapy (CBT), acceptance and commitment therapy, or interpersonal therapy. In addition, all care sites need to provide evidence-based pharmacotherapy for mood disorders, anxiety disorders including PTSD, psychotic disorders, substance use disorders, dementia, and other cognitive disorders. The VHA noted, "Such care is to be consistent with current VA clinical practice guidelines and informed by current scientific literature." The VA has restricted internal Web sites providing access to VA clinical practice guidelines (vaww.oqp.med.va.gov/CPGintra/cpg/cpg.htm) and VHA clinical practice guidelines (vaww.national.cmop.va.gov/PBM/Clinical%20 Guidance/Forms/AllItems.aspx).

EBPP also has become important in some large health maintenance organizations, such as the Kaiser Permanente Health Care System, and in many preferred provider organizations.

The Accreditation Council for Graduate Medical Education (2008), the body that sets standards for training residents in psychiatry and other specialties, requires training programs to show how they are teaching competence in the methods of EBM.

EBM has had a major influence on psychiatric practice in the United Kingdom because of the role of the NHS, as well as the efforts of the Centre for Evidence-Based Mental Health at the University of Oxford (Baker and Kleijnen 2000; Ferguson and Russell 2000; Geddes 2000). These efforts have been aided by the journal *Evidence-Based Mental Health*, which is published jointly by the BMJ Publishing Group, the Royal College of Psychiatrists, and the British Psychological Society (Geddes et al. 1997). In addition, skill in applying EBM is tested in the critical appraisal paper that is now included in part II of the membership examination of the Royal College of Psychiatrists (Dhar 2001; Geddes 2000).

In 2006, the United Kingdom established the Improving Access to Psychological Therapies program to provide evidence-based mental health treatment for patients with anxiety and depressive disorders (Department of Health and Care Services Improvement Partnership 2006). The ambitious goal of this program is to improve services to 900,000 or more depressed people over the next few years, with half of those completing therapy recovering. The program uses a stepped-care model with the expectation that data will be obtained on all participants.

The American Psychological Association (2005) has been slow to promote evidence-based interventions, although they encourage evidence-based psychological practice. The Task Force on Evidence-Based Practice has a very nonspecific recommendation about evidence-based psychological practice:

> Clinical decisions should be made in collaboration with the patient, based on the best clinically relevant evidence, and with consideration for the probable costs, benefits, and available resources and options. It is the treating psychologist who makes the ultimate judgment regarding a particular intervention or treatment plan. The involvement of an active, informed patient is generally crucial to the success of psychological services. Treatment decisions should never be made by untrained persons unfamiliar with the specifics of the case. The treating psychologist determines the applicability of research conclusions to a particular patient. Individual patients may require decisions and interventions not directly addressed by the available research. The application of research evidence to a given patient always involves probabilistic inferences. Therefore, ongoing monitoring of patient progress and adjustment of treatment as needed are essential to EBPP [evidence-based psychological practice]. (p. 3)

Clinicians need to be aware of the many resources available to evaluate the effectiveness of psychological interventions. Several textbooks have recently been published on evidence-based psychological practice (e.g., Fisher and O'Donogue 2006; Freeman and Power 2007; Goodheart et al. 2006; Levy and Ablon 2009; Rubin 2007). The Oxford University Press has a division related to publishing detailed manuals for patients and therapists on how to apply evidence-based practices (www.us.oup.com/us/catalog/general/series/TreatmentsThatWork). One Web site (http://ucoll.fdu.edu/apa/lnksinter.html) provides links to more than 30 other Web sites providing data on evidence-based psychological interventions. The Substance Abuse and Mental Health Services Administration (SAMHSA) has created the National Registry of Evidence-Based Programs and Practices, a searchable database of interventions for the prevention and treatment of mental and substance use disorders (www.nationalregistry.samhsa.gov/).

Does Evidence-Based Medicine Improve Outcomes?

One should ask, however, whether the use of evidence improves outcomes. This is actually a difficult question to answer. It would not be ethical to conduct a controlled trial to determine whether the use of EBM guidelines, compared with nonuse, improved outcomes because the patients randomly assigned to the nonuse condition would be offered a treatment that other evidence would suggest to be inferior. One procedure is to estimate the benefit if guidelines were applied in a particular population or setting. For instance, some EBM guidelines have been identified to provide the "best care" for post–myocardial infarction (MI) patients, such as prescribing aspirin and beta-blockers. Following these guidelines has been shown to improve outcome compared with previous practice (Krumholz et al. 1998). For instance, Gemell et al. (2005) estimated that following the United Kingdom's National Service Framework guidelines for adopting the National Service Framework recommendations for pharmacological interventions would prevent an extra 1,027 deaths (95% confidence interval [CI] 418–1,994) in post–acute MI patients and an extra 37,899 (95% CI 25,690–52,503) deaths in heart failure patients in the first year after diagnosis. Lifestyle-based interventions would prevent an extra 848 (95% CI 71–1,614) deaths in post–acute MI patients and an extra 7,249 (95% CI 995–16,696) deaths in heart failure patients.

Collaborative care for depression treatment in populations is another example of an evidence-based quality improvement intervention. This model has been developed by Katon and others over many years (Katon and Seelig 2008). In a total of 37 randomized trials of collaborative care compared with usual primary care, collaborative care was associated with twofold increases in antidepressant adherence, improvements in depressive outcomes that last up to 5 years, increased patient satisfaction with depression care, and improved primary care satisfaction with treating depression (Katon and Seelig 2008). As another example, better adherence to guidelines developed to treat opioid-dependent patients in Veterans Affairs opioid substitution clinics resulted in greater reductions in heroin and cocaine use and greater improvement in mental health (Trafton et al. 2007).

Does Evidence-Based Psychiatric Practice Improve Outcomes?

Examining the effects of EBM-specific practices on carefully defined populations and problems is different from studying EBPP (Kazdin 2008). Again, EBM focuses on discrete conditions and issues, and EBPP focuses on the broader care of patients. EBPP is not what researchers study (Kazdin 2008), and doing so is difficult. The parameters of EBPP have not been clearly defined. We gave examples in the previous section of how following guidelines can improve care, but following guidelines is only one aspect of EBPP as previously defined. The systematic application of the Sequenced Treatment Alternatives to Relieve Depression (STAR*D) study guidelines, as illustrated in Trivedi and Kurian, Chapter 21 of this volume, is likely to improve treatment of depression.

Psychiatric Clinical Practice Is Not Always Evidence Based

Over the past few years, evidence has accumulated to suggest that there is a significant gap between the knowledge obtained from clinical trials regarding effective treatments for mental disorders and the actual treatment received by patients in clinical practice (Drake et al. 2001; Lehman and Steinwachs 1998; U.S. Department of Health and Human Services 1999; Young et al. 2001). Similar discrepancies have been noted in other fields of medicine, in which practice often lags years behind research findings (Egger et al. 2001; Geyman 2000; Haines and Donald 1998; Haines and Jones 1994). Other examples are that only about half of patients with diabetes have hemoglobin A1c levels below the recommended level of 8.0%; only one-third of patients with hypertension receive adequate treatment to lower blood pressure below guideline-recommended levels. According to a recent review, among patients in the community and primary care settings, more than 50% of those with depression do not receive accurate diagnoses or any prescription of depression treatment. Of those who are prescribed treatment, more than 50% do not

receive adequate dosages of antidepressants, and fewer than 10% receive evidence-based psychotherapy (Katon and Seelig 2008). Estimates suggest that about 40% of primary care patients drop out of depression treatment within 6 weeks, and fewer than half are taking antidepressants at 6 months (Simon 2002). Similar low levels of adherence to evidence-based guidelines have been found for other disorders such as substance abuse.

Wide variations are also seen in the way psychiatry and other medical specialties are practiced (Geddes and Harrison 1997; Geyman 2000). Clearly, some methods of treatment must be more effective than others and have more research to support their use, yet surveys conducted in academic medical centers have found that up to 40% of clinical decisions are unsupported by evidence from the research literature (Geddes et al. 1996; Greenhalgh 2001).

Why the Gap?

Two general types of information problems contribute to patients receiving less than optimal care (Gray 2002; Haynes et al. 1997). The first problem is one of "information overload," which creates difficulties for clinicians who want to determine which treatments are truly most effective. There are thousands of medical journals and millions of articles; therefore, no psychiatrist or other clinician should expect to keep up with all of the developments in his or her field. Furthermore, when one looks at the results of various studies, they often appear to be contradictory. In part, this is caused by false-positive and false-negative results, which often arise from small samples (Collins and MacMahon 2001; see also Gray and Taylor, Chapter 5 in this volume). One could consult review articles to summarize the literature, but most such reviews are "journalistic" or "narrative" reviews, not systematic reviews (see Gray, Chapter 6 in this volume). As a result, such articles are subject to the biases of the review's author(s), both in terms of studies cited and in the method of summarizing conflicting results (Cook et al. 1998; Egger et al. 2001; Greenhalgh 2001). Textbook chapters have the added problem of rapidly becoming out of date. All of this contributes to the lag before advances in treatment are recognized and find their way into practice.

The second type of information problem causes ineffective treatments to be adopted or maintained.

The problem is not a lack of information but rather the uncritical acceptance of available information. This may occur for a variety of reasons, such as over-reliance on one's own clinical experiences or on expert opinion, the uncritical acceptance of results of single studies, and the excessive influence of pharmaceutical companies through advertising and sponsorship of speakers (Greenhalgh 2001; Sackett et al. 2000). At the same time, one's own clinical experiences and expert opinions are important sources of information on how to provide patient care.

Problems With Evidence-Based Medicine

There are also many good reasons to question evidence-based medicine. A common complaint we hear from clinicians is that randomized studies enroll patients very unlike "my patients." This statement has some truth to it. First, patients in clinical studies tend to be younger *or* older than many patients in clinical practice. In medicine (less so in psychiatry), women have been underrepresented in clinical trials. Minorities are often absent or present in such small numbers as to make subanalyses meaningless. Many clinical trials exclude 90% or more of potentially interested subjects. For instance, Yastrubetskaya et al. (1997) found that only 4% of 186 elderly patients with elevated Hamilton Rating Scale for Depression scores were eligible for a Phase III trial of a new antidepressant. Taylor et al. (2007) compared patients used in meta-analyses of cardiac rehabilitation programs with two large samples of patients actually in such programs. Compared with patients in actual practice, patients presented in the meta-analyses were younger (54 vs. 64 years), more likely to be males (90% vs. 74%), more likely to have had an MI (86% vs. 53%) and not a coronary artery bypass graft (6% vs. 24%), and more likely to be in the program longer (18 vs. 8 weeks).

Randomized studies often exclude comorbid problems, whereas most patients seen in clinical practice have one or more comorbidities. To determine whether the results from placebo-controlled studies conducted in patients with manic episode can be generalized to a routine population of hospitalized acute manic patients, Storosum et al. (2004) examined the baseline characteristics of 68 patients with 74 episodes of acute mania who had been referred for routine treatment. In this study only 16% of the manic episodes would have qualified for the hypothetical trial.

Exclusion criteria do not necessarily bias the study in terms of a favorable outcome, although they may limit the external validity of the study. For instance, in the Storosum et al. (2004) sample, the most common exclusion criterion was the use of contraceptives. Excluding such patients reduces the external validity of the trial. In contrast, some other exclusion criteria (e.g., comorbid alcohol and drug use disorders) may have resulted in an overestimation of the efficacy of antimanic medications. Another limitation is that many clinical trials are very short—lasting less than a few months—and do not deal with the many patients who do not improve. A notable exception, among others, is the STAR*D trial, which has attempted to apply evidence-based care to real clinical populations as mentioned earlier.

Faced with these issues, clinicians need to consider the evidence of a treatment's efficacy as a "source" of information. From our standpoint, the challenge of the clinician is to view all evidence with a keen eye to its limitations but a possibility for its usefulness. In the cases provided later in this book, we include examples of how clinicians have used—and struggled with—sources of evidence as they try to provide effective care. The evidence needs to fit the realities of the patient. Because of the clinical challenges of integrated evidence with real cases, we favor a focus on "how the patient is doing."

Evidence Is Often Not Available

EBM assumes that treatments proven to be efficacious should be used over those lacking in evidence. Unfortunately, depending on the criteria for effectiveness, very few treatments have been shown to be beneficial. For instance, the BMJ *Clinical Evidence* base has evaluated more than 2,500 treatments (www.clinicalevidence.bmj.com/ceweb/about/knowledge.jsp). According to their criteria, only 13% were rated as beneficial, 23% were rated as likely to be beneficial, 8% were rated as a trade-off between beneficial and harmful, 6% were rated as unlikely to be beneficial, and 4% were rated as likely to be ineffective or harmful. Of the treatments, 46%—the largest proportion—were of unknown effectiveness. Use of only clearly beneficial treatments would severely limit options in patient care. Furthermore, the evidence for such beneficial treatments is likely to have been derived from studies that, as mentioned earlier, may have limited applicability to patients seen in clinical practice. A reasonable approach is first to consider treatments shown to be effective with similar patients and then to retain a healthy skepticism about other treatments.

Two particular situations in which lack of evidence is especially problematic are the head-to-head comparison of new pharmacological treatments and situations involving treatment-resistant patients. The first situation is problematic because new drugs are evaluated relative to placebos or older medications—not newer medications—in the Phase III trials conducted to obtain U.S. Food and Drug Administration approval. The second situation is problematic because few studies other than the STAR*D trial have systematically evaluated treatment approaches to treatment-resistant patients.

Problems in Practicing Evidence-Based Psychiatry

In addition to concerns about EBM and evidence-based treatments, several practical problems arise in practicing evidence-based psychiatry.

Limited Time to Look for Answers

The first problem is time. Finding new information relevant to a case can be time-consuming, and clinicians often have very tight schedules. It is important to consider that some general guidelines to help direct care can be easily obtained. The practitioner should periodically update guidelines and even customize them, as discussed in Taylor, Chapter 18 of this volume, if he or she believes that the evidence justifies doing so. Guidelines are also frequently updated and revised. Guidelines are available to cover most common conditions, and once they have been selected, using them requires less time.

A more complicated problem is how to build on these guidelines and algorithms, particularly to find evidence of therapies useful across procedures, and to evaluate *new* information.

Although many sources of evidence about treatments have been developed to aid the busy practitioner, such sources can be out of date. First, most EBM procedures rely on large data sets, and many meta-analyses may be focused on results from older studies and interventions. Thus, it is a challenge for

the practitioner to evaluate a potentially useful new intervention. The procedures for doing so require following EBM procedures, as discussed in the chapters in Part I of this book, but can be time consuming. Many other sources of more easily obtained current information, such as industry-sponsored continuing medical education courses, information from pharmaceutical representatives, and industry-sponsored reviews and seminars, may be biased.

Lack of Incentives for Evidence-Based Psychiatric Practice

Some practice settings now incorporate best practices as one form of EBPP, and clinicians are held accountable to these standards. However, in most settings, clinicians are free to practice EBPP as they wish. EBPP, particularly because it involves some of the more structured psychotherapies, may feel more demanding than do less-structured, nondirected approaches. As noted earlier, indications are that reimbursement may become more related to EBPP. The main reason that one should practice EBPP is the belief that doing so will improve patient care.

No Resources for Assessment

EBPP requires assessment of progress. Although simple assessment procedures are available, more routine assessments and data management may seem too much of an encumbrance for many practitioners. We discuss some simple procedures that can help overcome some of these problems (Chapters 8, 14, 16, 17) and also provide models in which electronic systems can support EBPP (Chapters 21 and 33).

Summary

The goal of mental health professionals should be to provide the most effective treatments to their patients. Doing so requires that they can determine which treatment approaches are more likely to be effective for a given patient, and this is, in essence, what EBPP is all about. Over the last decade, the data from innumerable studies have been massaged by experts into guidelines, algorithms, consensus statements, reviews, textbooks, meta-analyses, and other documents. These resources and the general principles developed for EBM have the potential to improve psychiatric practice significantly.

References

Accreditation Council for Graduate Medical Education: General competencies. Available at: www.acgme.org/outcome/comp/compfull.asp. Accessed June 25, 2009

Agency for Healthcare Research and Quality: Evidence-based practice centers (AHRQ). Available at: http://www.ahrq. gov/clinic/epc. Accessed June 25, 2009

American Psychological Association: APA Policy Statement on Evidence-Based Practice. August 2005. Available at: http://www2.apa.org/practice/ebpstatement.pdf. Accessed December 2, 2008

Baker M, Kleijnen J: The drive towards evidence-based health care, in Evidence-Based Counseling and Psychological Therapies: Research and Applications. Edited by Rowland N, Goss S. Philadelphia, PA, Routledge, 2000, pp 13–29

Barton S: Using clinical evidence. BMJ 322:503–504, 2001

Browman GP: Development and aftercare of clinical guidelines: the balance between rigor and pragmatism. JAMA 286:1509–1511, 2001

Centre for Health Evidence: Users' Guides to Evidence-Based Practice. 2007. Available at: http://www.cche.net/usersguides/main.asp. Accessed June 20, 2008

Collins R, MacMahon S: Reliable assessment of the effects of treatment on mortality and major morbidity, I: clinical trials. Lancet 357:373–380, 2001

Cook DJ, Mulrow CD, Haynes RB: Synthesis of best evidence for clinical decisions, in Systematic Reviews: Synthesis of Best Evidence for Health Care Decisions. Edited by Mulrow C, Cook D. Philadelphia, PA, American College of Physicians, 1998, pp 5–12

Department of Health and Care Services Improvement Partnership. Available at: http://www.iapt.nhs.uk. Accessed December 2, 2008

Dhar R: Evidence-based journal clubs and the critical review paper. Psychiatr Bull 25:67–68, 2001

Drake RE, Goldman HH, Leff HS, et al: Implementing evidence-based practices in routine mental health settings. Psychiatr Serv 52:179–182, 2001

Egger M, Smith GD, O'Rourke K: Rationale, potentials, and promise of systematic reviews, in Systematic Reviews in Health Care: Meta-Analysis in Context. Edited by Egger M, Smith GD, Altman DG. London, BMJ Books, 2001, pp 3–19

Ferguson B, Russell I: Towards evidence-based health care, in Evidence-Based Counseling and Psychological Therapies: Research and Applications. Edited by Rowland N, Goss S. Philadelphia, PA, Routledge, 2000, pp 30–43

Fisher JE, O'Donogue WE (eds): Practitioner's Guide of Evidence-Based Psychotherapy. New York, Springer, 2006

Freeman C, Power M (eds): Handbook of Evidence-Based Psychotherapies: A Guide for Research and Practice. New York, Wiley, 2007

Geddes J: Evidence-based practice in mental health, in Evidence-Based Practice: A Critical Appraisal. Edited by Trinder L, Reynolds S. Oxford, UK, Blackwell Scientific, 2000, pp 66–88

Geddes JR, Harrison PJ: Closing the gap between research and practice. Br J Psychiatry 171:220–225, 1997

Geddes JR, Game D, Jenkins NE, et al: What proportion of primary psychiatric interventions are based on evidence from randomised controlled trials? Qual Health Care 5:215–217, 1996

Geddes J, Reynolds S, Streiner D, et al: Evidence based practice in mental health. BMJ 315:1483–1484, 1997

Geyman JP: Evidence-based medicine in primary care: an overview, in Evidence-Based Clinical Practice: Concepts and Approaches. Edited by Geyman JP, Deyo RA, Ramsey SD. Boston, MA, Butterworth-Heinemann, 2000, pp 1–12

Goodheart CD, Kazdin AE, Sternberg RJ (eds): Evidence-Based Psychotherapy: Where Practice and Research Meet. Washington, DC, American Psychological Association, 2006

Goss S, Rowland N: Getting evidence into practice, in Evidence-Based Counseling and Psychological Therapies: Research and Applications. Edited by Rowland N, Goss S. Philadelphia, PA, Routledge, 2000, pp 191–205

Gray GE: Evidence-based medicine: an introduction for psychiatrists. J Psychiatr Pract 8:5–13, 2002

Gray GE: Concise Guide to Evidence-Based Psychiatry. Washington, DC, American Psychiatric Publishing, 2004

Greenhalgh T: How to Read a Paper: The Basics of Evidence Based Medicine, 2nd Edition. London, BMJ Books, 2001

Guyatt G: Preface, in Users' Guides to the Medical Literature: A Manual for Evidence-Based Clinical Practice. Edited by Guyatt G, Rennie D. Chicago, IL, AMA Press, 2002, pp xiii–xvi

Guyatt G, Rennie D (eds): Users' Guides to the Medical Literature: A Manual for Evidence-Based Clinical Practice. Chicago, IL, AMA Press, 2002

Guyatt GH, Haynes RB, Jaeschke RZ, et al: Users' guides to the medical literature, XXV: evidence-based medicine: principles for applying the users' guides to patient care. JAMA 284:1290–1296, 2000

Haines A, Donald A: Making better use of research findings. BMJ 317:72–75, 1998

Haines A, Jones R: Implementing findings of research. BMJ 308:1488–1492, 1994

Haynes RB, Sackett DL, Gray JA, et al: Transferring evidence from research into practice, II: getting the evidence straight. ACP J Club 126:A14–A16, 1997

Haynes RB, Devereaux PJ, Guyatt GH: Clinical expertise in the era of evidence-based medicine and patient choice. ACP J Club 136:A11–A14, 2002a

Haynes RB, Devereaux PJ, Guyatt GH: Physicians' and patients' choices in evidence based practice. BMJ 324:1350, 2002b

Katon WJ, Seelig M: Population-based care of depression: team care approaches to improving outcomes. J Occup Environ Med 50:459–467, 2008

Kazdin AE: Evidence-based treatment and practice: new opportunities to bridge clinical research and practice, enhance the knowledge base, and improve patient care. Am Psychol 63:146–159, 2008

Krumholz HM, Philbin DM Jr, Wang Y, et al: Trends in the quality of care for Medicare beneficiaries admitted to the hospital with unstable angina. J Am Coll Cardiol 31:957–963, 1998

Lehman AF, Steinwachs DM: Patterns of usual care for schizophrenia: initial results from the Schizophrenia Patient Outcomes Research Team (PORT) client survey. Schizophr Bull 24:11–20, 1998

Levy R, Ablon JS: Handbook of Evidenced-Based Psychodynamic Psychotherapy: Bridging the Gap Between Science and Practice. New York, Humana Press, 2009

Mace C, Moorey S, Roberts B (eds): Evidence in the Psychological Therapies: A Critical Guide for Practitioners. Philadelphia, PA, Brunner Routledge, 2001

National Health Service Centre for Reviews and Dissemination: Getting evidence into practice. Eff Health Care 5(1):1–16, 1999

Parry G: Evidence-based psychotherapy: an overview, in Evidence-Based Counseling and Psychological Therapies: Research and Applications. Edited by Rowland N, Goss S. Philadelphia, PA, Routledge, 2000, pp 57–75

Reynolds S: The anatomy of evidence-based practice: principles and methods, in Evidence-Based Practice: A Critical Appraisal. Edited by Trinder L, Reynolds S. Oxford, UK, Blackwell Scientific, 2000, pp 17–34

Rubin A: Practitioner's Guide to Using Research for Evidence-Based Practice. New York, Wiley, 2007

Sackett DL, Rosenberg WMC, Gray JAM, et al: Evidence-based medicine: what it is and what it isn't. BMJ 312:71–72, 1996

Sackett DL, Straus SE, Richardson WS, et al: Evidence-Based Medicine: How to Practice and Teach EBM, 2nd Edition. New York, Churchill Livingstone, 2000

Simon GE: Evidence review: efficacy and effectiveness of antidepressant treatment in primary care. Gen Hosp Psychiatry 24:213–222, 2002

Steinbrook R: Saying no isn't NICE—the travails of Britain's National Institute for Health and Clinical Excellence. N Engl J Med 359:1977–1981, 2008

Storosum JG, Fouwels A, Gispen-de Wied CC, et al: How real are patients in placebo-controlled studies of acute manic episode? Eur Neuropsychopharmacol 14:319–323, 2004

Straus SE, McAlister FA: Evidence-based medicine: a commentary on common criticisms. CMAJ 163:837–841, 2000

Taylor RS, Bethell HN, Brodie DA: Clinical trials versus the real world: the example of cardiac rehabilitation. British Journal of Cardiology 14:175–178, 2007

Trafton JA, Humphreys K, Harris AH, et al: Consistent adherence to guidelines improves opioid dependent patients' first year outcomes. J Behav Health Serv Res 4:260–271, 2007

Trinder L: Introduction: the context of evidence-based practice, in Evidence-Based Practice: A Critical Appraisal. Edited by Trinder L, Reynolds S. Oxford, UK, Blackwell Scientific, 2000, pp 1–16

U.S. Department of Health and Human Services: Mental health: a report of the Surgeon General. Washington, DC, U.S. Department of Health and Human Services, 1999

U.S. Department of Veterans Affairs: Uniform mental health services in VA medical centers and clinics. Available at: http://www.va.gov/vhapublications/ViewPublication.asp?pub_ID=1762 (p 31). Accessed June 25, 2009

Yastrubetskaya O, Chiu E, O'Connell S: Is good clinical research practice for clinical trials good clinical practice? Int J Geriatr Psychiatry 12:227–231, 1997

Young AS, Klap R, Sherbourne C, et al: The quality of care for depressive and anxiety disorders in the United States. Arch Gen Psychiatry 58:55–63, 2001

The 5-Step Evidence-Based Medicine Model

Gregory E. Gray, M.D., Ph.D.

An important aspect of evidence-based medicine (EBM) is being able to efficiently find accurate information and evidence relevant to clinical questions. The method and urgency of finding information vary from one setting to another. Evidence related to direct care of inpatients needs to be obtained quickly; clinicians usually have more time to obtain information relevant to outpatient practice. In this chapter, we focus on one approach to help clinicians answer clinical questions with primary evidence sources.

One EBM approach involves the application of a 5-step model (Table 2–1) to apply evidence from the medical literature to patient care problems (Gray 2002; Sackett et al. 2000). Details of this model are provided in Chapters 3–12. An example of the use of the technique in practice can be found in Chapter 18, "Major Depressive Disorder and Bulimia Nervosa," in this volume.

TABLE 2–1. The 5-step evidence-based medicine process

Step 1: Formulate the question
Step 2: Search for answers
Step 3: Appraise the evidence
Step 4: Apply the results
Step 5: Assess the outcome

Step 1: Formulate the Question

The EBM process begins with a clinical question, which may involve issues related to the diagnosis, treatment, prognosis, or etiology of a patient's illness. As I describe in Chapter 3, the question is formatted to include a patient problem or diagnosis; the treatment, diagnostic test, risk factor, or prognostic factor of interest, as well as any comparison; and the outcome of interest.

Step 2: Search for Answers

After formulating the question, the next step is to try to find an answer in the literature. This step involves an assessment of the type of evidence that is most appropriate for answering the question as well as the actual search for the evidence. Details of both processes can be found in Gray and Taylor, Chapter 4 in this volume.

Step 3: Appraise the Evidence

After an article has been located, it is necessary to appraise its validity and importance before applying the results. The specific questions to ask about validity and importance depend on the type of study design and the nature of the question. In addition, clinicians must decide whether the results can be applied to their particular patients and in their setting. The appraisal process is discussed in detail in Chapters 5–7 and 9–13.

Step 4: Apply the Results to Your Patient

Assuming that the evidence that the clinician has found is valid, important, applicable to his or her patient, and feasible in the practice setting, the next step is to apply it to the care of the patient, which is where clinical expertise is most important.

Step 5: Assess the Outcome

Step 5 includes an evaluation of the clinician's performance in searching the literature and in finding an answer to the clinical question posed, as well as an assessment of the patient's response to treatment.

Some Shortcuts

Studies in academic settings have found that the full 5-step model can be incorporated into routine practice (Ball 1998; Del Mar and Glasziou 2001; Sackett et al. 2000). In nonacademic settings, however, practitioners frequently voice concerns that are related to lack of time and information resources, as well as to an inadequate knowledge of the EBM process (Ely et al. 2002; Haines and Donald 1998; Lipman 2000; McColl et al. 1998; Straus and McAlister 2000; Trinder 2000; Young and Ward 2001).

Several shortcuts can be taken to streamline the process and to make it more practical in everyday clinical practice. First, it is important to recognize that a clinician does not have to go through the 5-step process for every patient encounter. After a question has been researched for one patient with a particular diagnosis, the answer can be applied to similar patients with the same diagnosis. In addition, because most patients of most clinicians fall into relatively few diagnostic categories, it soon becomes the exceptional patient who triggers the application of the full 5-step process. However, we believe it is important for the practitioner to set aside some time on a routine basis to search the literature and review evidence.

One way to keep up with the literature is to use preappraised information resources. Reviews, synopses, and summaries are available that address many issues raised by clinicians. The *BMJ* group has developed a whole set of tools to foster EBM (http://ebmh.bmj.com.). Some of these are available for free on the Internet, and others can be purchased. Most

practitioners now have access to important databases through the Internet. In Chapter 4, we discuss how to assess these resources.

The use of structured approaches to asking and answering questions can be an excellent approach to teaching EBM.

For instance, the Chairman's Rounds at the Department of Psychiatry at Duke University has residents use the QUEST model (QUestion, Evaluate, and SynThesize) to address a clinical issue. For instance, one of the grand rounds addressed the following issues: How do long-term medication and behavioral treatments compare with each other? Are there additional benefits when they are used together? What is the effectiveness of systematic, carefully delivered treatments compared with routine community care? The resident then provided a critical review of a randomized trial that addressed that issue, which included a review of the study design, with an assessment of validity, a discussion of strengths and weaknesses, and the bottom line. The grand rounds topics, indexed by diagnosis, can be found at http://psychiatry.mc.duke.edu/Residents/Quest.html. Despite these shortcuts, there still will be questions that cannot be readily answered by the results of a previous search (or by the use of preappraised information resources). It is important, therefore, that psychiatrists and other clinicians be able to carry out the full 5-step EBM process when necessary (Evans 2001; Gray 2002; Guyatt et al. 2000; R.B. Haynes 2001; Straus et al. 2002).

References

Ball C: Evidence-based medicine on the wards: report from an evidence-based minion. Evid Based Med 3:101–103, 1998

Del Mar CB, Glasziou PP: Ways of using evidence-based medicine in general practice. Med J Aust 174:347–350, 2001

Ely JW, Osheroff JA, Ebell MH, et al: Obstacles to answering doctors' questions about patient care with evidence: qualitative study. BMJ 324:710–713, 2002

Evans M: Creating knowledge management skills in primary care residents: a description of a new pathway to evidence-based practice in the community. Evid Based Med 6:133–134, 2001

Gray GE: Evidence-based medicine: an introduction for psychiatrists. J Psychiatr Pract 8:5–13, 2002

Guyatt GH, Meade MO, Jaeschke RZ, et al: Practitioners of evidence based care. BMJ 320:954–955, 2000

Haines A, Donald A: Getting research findings into practice: making better use of research findings. BMJ 317:72–75, 1998

Haynes RB: Of studies, summaries, synopses, and systems: the "4S" evolution of services for finding current best evidence. Evid Based Ment Health 4:37–39, 2001

Lipman T: Evidence-based practice in general practice and primary care, in Evidence-Based Practice: A Critical Appraisal. Edited by Trinder L, Reynolds S. Oxford, UK, Blackwell Scientific, 2000, pp 35–65

McColl A, Smith H, White P, et al: General practitioners' perception of the route to evidence based medicine: a questionnaire study. BMJ 316:361–365, 1998

Sackett DL, Straus SE, Richardson WS, et al: Evidence-Based Medicine: How to Practice and Teach EBM, 2nd Edition. New York, Churchill Livingstone, 2000

Straus SE, McAlister FA: Evidence-based medicine: a commentary on common criticisms. CMAJ 163:837–841, 2000

Straus S, McAlister F, Cook D, et al: Expanded philosophy of evidence-based medicine: criticisms of evidence-based medicine, in Users' Guides to the Medical Literature: A Manual for Evidence-Based Clinical Practice. Edited by Guyatt G, Rennie D. Chicago, IL, AMA Press, 2002, pp 211–222

Trinder L: A critical appraisal of evidence-based practice, in Evidence-Based Practice: A Critical Appraisal. Edited by Trinder L, Reynolds S. Oxford, UK, Blackwell Scientific, 2000, pp 212–241

Young JM, Ward JE: Evidence-based medicine in general practice: beliefs and barriers among Australian GPs. J Eval Clin Pract 7:201–210, 2001

Asking Answerable Questions

Gregory E. Gray, M.D., Ph.D.

Every clinical encounter generates questions. Some of these require information that can be obtained only from the patient or from a collateral source, such as a friend or family member. Answers to such questions are unique to the particular patient and concern that patient's illness or situation. These types of questions form the basis of a psychiatric interview and are not the subject of this chapter.

Background Questions Versus Foreground Questions

In this chapter, I focus on questions about a patient's illness that are more general and hence answerable in the psychiatric literature. Such questions are often divided into two categories: background and foreground questions (McKibbon et al. 2002; Sackett et al. 2000).

Background questions concern relatively well-established facts. These are the sorts of questions that are best answered by reference books or textbooks. Examples of background questions are:

- What are the DSM-IV-TR diagnostic criteria for panic disorder?
- What are the dosage forms for olanzapine?
- What is cognitive-behavioral therapy?

Such questions typically have two parts: the journalistic "who, what, when, where, why, and how" and the name of a disorder or therapy. Background questions are the types of questions that medical students and beginning residents most frequently ask.

Foreground questions, in contrast, concern the current best information on diagnosis, treatment, or prognosis of a disorder. Such questions are best answered by the research literature, not by textbooks, because they involve information that is still in a state of flux as new knowledge is accumulated. Foreground questions are the most frequent type of questions generated by senior residents or by practicing clinicians.

The 4-Part PICO Question

Foreground questions are best framed as a 4-part question (Table 3–1). The question should include the patient(s) or problem of interest; the intervention of interest, including any comparison group; and the outcomes of interest (Badenoch and Heneghan 2002; Dawes 1999; Geddes 1999; McKibbon et al. 2002; Sackett et al. 2000). Such questions are sometimes referred to as PICO questions (i.e., questions that use the mnemonic aid "**p**atient/problem, **i**ntervention, **c**omparison, and **o**utcome") (Gray 2002). A question formulated in this way provides the parameters needed to conduct an efficient literature search because it makes the type of information required very clear.

Patients or Problem

The first part of the question involves the patients or problem of interest. The degree of specificity has an influence on the ability to find an answer, as well as on the applicability of that answer to the particular patient of interest. Because the 4-part question is

TABLE 3–1. The 4-part PICO question

P:	Patient or problem of interest
I:	Intervention of interest
	Treatment
	Diagnostic test
	Risk factor
	Prognostic factor
C:	Comparison
	Implicit or explicit
O:	Outcome of interest
	Positive or negative

used as the starting point for the literature search, the patient or problem should be defined with a degree of specificity consistent with the way that study populations are defined. For example, if the clinician is interested in the treatment of depression in preadolescents, specifying that population as "preadolescents with major depression" is preferable to "patients with major depression" because there are reasons to believe that the response to treatment might be different. However, if the clinician becomes overly specific and specifies "9-year-old Latino girls with a first episode of major depression and with a paternal but not maternal history of recurrent major depression," he or she may not be able to find evidence that is specific to such a narrowly defined population.

Intervention and Comparison

Intervention can be a treatment or a diagnostic test. Loosely defined, it can also refer to a risk factor or prognostic factor. In most cases, the intervention of interest will be compared with another intervention; in some cases, the comparison is explicit.

For questions related to treatment, the intervention can be either a specific medication or a psychosocial intervention. The comparison can be another active treatment, a placebo, or "usual care."

Diagnostic questions are usually questions related to the performance of a diagnostic test, screening instrument, or rating scale. The performance is usually compared with either a diagnostic "gold standard" or outcome on a commonly used instrument. Details of such comparisons are given in Chapter 9, "Diagnostic Tests," in this volume.

For questions related to etiology, the "intervention" is actually a risk factor. Here the comparison is often implicit (i.e., the absence of that risk factor).

Questions related to prognosis may be either 3- or 4-part questions. A 3-part question might ask the prognosis of patients with first-episode schizophrenia in general, whereas a 4-part question might ask whether a particular patient characteristic (prognostic factor) alters the prognosis. Here, as in questions related to etiology, the comparison can be implicit (i.e., the absence of the particular prognostic factor).

Outcome(s)

The fourth part of the question relates to the outcome or outcomes of interest. Such outcomes can be either positive (clinical improvement, remission, or survival) or negative (relapse, self-injury, or death). For questions involving diagnosis, the outcome is a measure of agreement between the two diagnostic methods.

Examples of 4-Part PICO Questions

Treatment

Example of a 4-part question related to treatment:

> In adult patients with schizophrenia, does the addition of cognitive-behavioral therapy to usual care, compared with usual care alone, prevent relapse?

In this example, the patients are "adult patients with schizophrenia," the intervention is the "addition of cognitive-behavioral therapy to usual care," the comparison is "usual care alone," and the outcome is "relapse."

Diagnosis

Example of a 4-part question related to diagnosis:

> In a primary care clinic population, is the self-administration of a brief screening instrument as effective in identifying patients with major depression as is a structured brief clinical interview by a psychiatrist?

In this example, the patients are "a primary care clinic population," the intervention (diagnostic test) is a self-administered "brief screening instrument," the comparison (i.e., the "gold standard") is "a structured brief clinical interview by a psychiatrist," and the outcome is "a diagnosis of major depression."

Etiology/Harm

Example of a 4-part question related to etiology:

> Among rescue workers at the site of the World Trade Center disaster, does the amount of time working at the disaster site influence the risk of developing posttraumatic stress disorder?

In this example, the population of interest is "rescue workers at the site of the World Trade Center disaster," the intervention (risk factor) is "the amount of time working at the disaster site," the comparison is implicit (i.e., less time vs. more time), and the outcome is the onset of "posttraumatic stress disorder."

A different type of question related to harm, this time with an explicit comparison group:

> In elderly patients (age 65 years and older) with schizophrenia receiving maintenance therapy with an antipsychotic medication, are patients receiving olanzapine at less risk for developing tardive dyskinesia than are patients receiving risperidone?

In this example, the patients are "elderly patients (age 65 years and older) with schizophrenia," the treatment of interest is "olanzapine," the comparison treatment is "risperidone," and the outcome of interest is the "development of tardive dyskinesia."

Prognosis

Example of a 4-part question related to prognosis:

> In patients ages 15–45 years, do female patients have better social and vocational functioning than do male patients after experiencing their first episode of schizophrenia?

In this example, the patients are persons "ages 15–45 years…after experiencing their first episode of schizophrenia," the intervention (prognostic factor) is being "female," the comparison group is "male patients," and the outcome is "social and vocational functioning." Had the question not explicitly asked about differences between male and female patients, it would have been an equally acceptable 3-part prognostic question.

References

Badenoch D, Heneghan C: Evidence-Based Medicine Toolkit. London, BMJ Books, 2002

Dawes M: Formulating a question, in Evidence-Based Practice: A Primer for Health Professionals. Edited by Dawes M, Davies P, Gray A, et al. New York, Churchill Livingstone, 1999, pp 9–13

Geddes J: Asking structured and focused clinical questions: essential first step of evidence-based practice. Evid Based Ment Health 2:35–36, 1999

Gray GE: Evidence-based medicine: an introduction for psychiatrists. J Psychiatr Pract 8:5–13, 2002

McKibbon A, Hunt D, Richardson WS, et al: Finding the evidence, in Users' Guides to the Medical Literature: A Manual for Evidence-Based Clinical Practice. Edited by Guyatt G, Rennie D. Chicago, IL, AMA Press, 2002, pp 13–47

Sackett DL, Straus SE, Richardson WS, et al: Evidence-Based Medicine: How to Practice and Teach EBM, 2nd Edition. New York, Churchill Livingstone, 2000

Searching for Answers

Gregory E. Gray, M.D., Ph.D.
C. Barr Taylor, M.D.

After formulating a question, the next step in the evidence-based medicine (EBM) process is to search for the best evidence to answer it. However, before beginning a search for an answer to a clinical question, it is important to understand the nature of the question and the type of evidence that would best address it.

What Type of Evidence Is Best?

Some experts propose that certain types of research results should be given more weight than other types (Badenoch and Heneghan 2002; Phillips et al. 2001). In this model, types of evidence are put on a hierarchy with systematic reviews of randomized controlled trials (RCTs) being the best source of evidence and expert opinion the worst (see Table 4–1). The specific hierarchy depends on the type of clinical question being asked. Table 4–1 presents the evidence hierarchy for studies of therapy or harm. Types of evidence higher in the hierarchy are more apt to give a valid and unbiased estimate of the effect of an intervention than are those lower in the hierarchy. When attempting to answer a clinical question, the clinician should always rely on the evidence found that is highest in the hierarchy or in other ways determined to be the best evidence available.

These hierarchies of evidence have been validated by comparing results obtained from studies that addressed the same question but used different designs. In studies of a variety of therapies, for example, it has repeatedly been shown that observational studies may give misleading results compared with RCTs (Lacchetti and Guyatt 2002). Whether the observational studies over- or underestimate the effectiveness of a particular treatment or preventive practice depends on the specific intervention being considered (Reeves et al. 2001).

As an example of the use of an evidence hierarchy for questions related to treatment (Table 4–1), results from a systematic review of RCTs should be given more weight than the results from a single RCT, and results from an RCT should be given more weight than results from uncontrolled or nonexperimental studies. Thus, if a literature search produces a systematic review of RCTs, several individual RCTs, case reports, and an editorial, the clinician should rely on the systematic review because it is likely to be highest in the evidence hierarchy. However, one well-designed and conducted clinical trial with an adequate number of subjects followed up for a long time might very well provide much better evidence than that provided by analyzing results from many poorly conducted, short-term trials.

Expert Opinion

In the original publication (Gray 2004), expert opinion was listed, in Table 4–1, below case series as the worst source of evidence on the basis that some studies have suggested that expert opinion does not necessarily reflect the best evidence found in the literature (Antman et al. 1992) and *may* be influenced by personal gain or benefit from the recommendations. On the other hand, experts are often

TABLE 4–1. Hierarchy of evidence for studies of therapy or harm

Quality	Type of evidence
1a (best)	Systematic review of RCTs
1b	Individual RCT with narrow confidence interval
1c	"All-or-none" case series
2a	Systematic review of cohort studies
2b	Individual cohort study
	RCT with <80% follow-up
2c	Outcomes research
	Ecological study
3a	Systematic review of case-control studies
3b	Individual case-control study
4 (worst)	Case series

Note.   RCT=randomized controlled trial.
Source.   Adapted from Gray 2004; Phillips et al. 2001; Sackett et al. 2000.

used to write systematic reviews, perform meta-analyses, construct guidelines, and recommend best practices. Thus, expert opinion influences all sources of information and is a valuable and necessary source of information on how to choose treatments. Expert opinion should not, however, be considered fact unless the expert has provided strong evidence for that opinion. Furthermore, the expertise and bias of the experts should be considered in judging their recommendations in all sources of evidence-based psychiatry practice (EBPP).

Experts are considered to be individuals with considerable knowledge about a subject. Experts are called on to write guidelines, reviews, and synopses and to provide opinions about treatments. In judging expert opinion, one must consider both the person's level of expertise and how biased his or her judgment is likely to be about the issue at hand. A biased opinion is not necessarily bad. An expert's strong conviction about a treatment he or she has studied or developed may be appropriate. However, the expert must reassure the reader that his or her interpretation of the evidence base is influenced by this bias.

In medical publishing, journals now require authors to declare any conflicts of interest they might have. A conflict of interest is often defined as an actual or a perceived interest by an expert in an action

that results in, or has the appearance of resulting in, personal, organizational, or professional gain (www.icmje.org/#conflicts). The assumption is that the declaration of conflict of interest allows the reader to be aware that the expert's judgment may be clouded and makes the expert less likely to be affected by whatever conflict he or she has. This assumption has never been proven and is likely to be incorrect.

Conflicts of interest can exist in all aspects of evaluating evidence. Let's assume that Dr. T and three colleagues submit a review of the early effect of selective serotonin reuptake inhibitors on depression to the *Archives of General Psychiatry*. Before the article is accepted, each author is required to "disclose all potential conflicts of interest, including specific financial interests and relationships and affiliations (other than those affiliations listed on the title page of the manuscript) relevant to the subject of their manuscript" (http://archpsyc.ama-assn.org). Authors are instructed to "err on the side of full disclosure and should contact the editorial office if they have questions or concerns. All such disclosures should be listed in the Acknowledgments section at the end of the manuscript. Authors without conflicts of interest, including specific financial interests and relationships and affiliations relevant to the subject of their manuscript, should include a statement of no such interest in the Acknowledgments section of the manuscript." In addition, "authors are expected to provide detailed information about all relevant financial interests and relationships or financial conflicts within the past 5 years and for the foreseeable future (e.g., employment/affiliation; grants or funding; consultancies; honoraria; stock ownership or options; expert testimony; royalties; patents filed, received, or pending; or donation of medical equipment), particularly those present at the time the research was conducted and through publication, as well as other financial interests (such as patent applications in preparation) that represent potential future financial gain" (http://archpsyc.ama-assn.org).

Now suppose that the lead author, a well-known depression researcher, has received honoraria from several pharmaceutical companies and attended meetings sponsored by drug companies. The second author, also a well-known researcher, has received funding for research and consulting, speaker's fees, and travel expenses from a variety of companies that manufacture antidepressant drugs. The third author has received grants from pharmaceutical companies and from the government. The fourth author is an adviser to several pharmaceutical companies.

Now suppose that the same authors report no financial conflicts of interest. Which publication would one have more confidence in and why? Would you trust a positive outcome from the second group more than from the first and a negative outcome from the first more than from the second? In practice, this information about conflict of interests is not very helpful in judging an article. The first set of authors might have a level of expertise that allows them to interpret the database more accurately than does the second. The second group may have many conflicts but of a different nature. For instance, they may have a bias against the pharmaceutical industry or the use of medications. It is necessary to report such conflicts, but the mere reporting does not really help the reader determine whether the analysis is unbiased. (The example is derived from an actual article: see Taylor et al. 2006.)

The same issues apply to reviewers of articles. A reviewer is just as likely as an author to have conflicts of interest. For instance, reviewers are sometimes selected by looking at the publications at the end of an article. Are reviewers likely to accept papers that support their own ideas or support the "conventional" wisdom and to reject ideas that go against their own ideas or conventional wisdom? Is this bias less serious than that of an investigator who might have some financial gain in a product because he or she holds some shares of the company that produces it? Coyle, the editor of the *Archives of General Psychiatry*, notes: "It would not be reasonable to banish from the ARCHIVES all authors and reviewers who have perceived financial conflicts of interest. This strategy would exclude important clinical research and scientific expertise from these pages" (Coyle and Heckers 2006).

The American Heart Association attempts to address the issue of conflict of interest quite broadly. For instance, members of writing groups are asked to identify "all relationships within the last 2 years that are relevant to the topic of the manuscript." A relationship is "relevant" if the relationship or interest relates to the topic of the manuscript in terms of any of the following: the same or similar subject matter or topic; the same, similar, or competing drug or device, product or service, intellectual property or asset; a drug or device company or its competitor; or has the reasonable potential to result in

financial, professional, or other personal gain or loss for you, members of your household, or employer. The author or reviewer needs to answer this in relation to employment, research grants, other research support, speakers' bureau, honoraria, ownership interest, consultation/advisory board, or other. The instructions note that "A relationship is considered to be 'Significant' if (a) the person receives $10,000 or more during any 12 month period, or 5% or more of the person's gross income; or (b) the person owns 5% or more of the voting stock or share of the entity, or owns $10,000 or more of the fair market value of the entity. A relationship is considered to be 'Modest' if it is less than 'Significant' from the preceding definition." Such relationships are important to disclose, but more importantly, the authors or reviewers should be asked to note that their opinions are based on an "unbiased assessment of the facts." In practice, it is often very difficult to evaluate the expertise of the expert.

The "5S" Approach to Searching for Answers

Although many clinicians begin their search with MEDLINE, this is a relatively inefficient strategy because it typically identifies numerous articles that must then be individually reviewed for validity. A more efficient approach is the hierarchical "5S" strategy developed by Haynes (2001a, 2001b, 2006), which involves *systems, summaries, synopses, syntheses,* and *studies* (Table 4–2). At the top of the list are *systems,* by which Haynes means very detailed, often patient-specific data sources, which link the patient's conditions to current best practices. *Summaries* integrate the best available evidence to provide a full range of evidence addressing *all* management options for a given health problem, not just one aspect of the problem as found in single-study resources that make up the lower three categories in the 5S model. *Synopses* are very brief descriptions of original articles and reviews. They can be found under search terms such as *meta-analyses. Syntheses* are usually called "systematic reviews" in the research literature. Some databases allow you to limit search results by using that term in the search strategy. Single *studies* are the original journal articles that present the entire report of one study on one aspect or management of a health problem. The distinctions between these categories are somewhat arbi-

TABLE 4–2. The 5S approach to searching for answers

Type of information resource	Examples	Web site
Systems	Electronic records linked to patient guidelines and other evidence	
Summaries	American Psychiatric Association Practice Guidelines	http://www.psychiatryonline.com
	National Guideline Clearinghouse	http://www.guideline.gov
	Clinical Evidence	http://clinicalevidence.bmj.com
	PIER (Physicians' Information and Education Resource)	http://pier.acponline.org/index.html
	National electronic Library for Mental Health	http://www.library.nhs.uk/mentalhealth
	TRIP	http://www.tripdatabase.com
	PubMed	http://www.ncbi.nlm.nih.gov/sites/entrez?db=pubmed
	Google Scholar	http://scholar.google.com
	Evidence-based textbooks and journals	
Synopses (abstracts/summaries)	*Evidence-Based Mental Health*	http://ebmh.bmj.com
	ACP Journal Club	http://www.acpjc.org
	PubMed	http://www.ncbi.nlm.nih.gov/sites/entrez?db=pubmed
	Database of Abstracts of Reviews of Effects (DARE)	http://www.crd.york.ac.uk/crdweb
Syntheses (systematic reviews)	Cochrane Database of Systematic Reviews	http://www.cochrane.org/reviews
	DARE	http://www.crd.york.ac.uk/crdweb
Studies	PubMed	http://www.ncbi.nlm.nih.gov/sites/entrez?db=pubmed
	Google Scholar	http://scholar.google.com
	Cochrane Central Register of Controlled Trials	http://www.mrw.interscience.wiley.com
	National Institutes of Health clinical trials	http://www.clinicaltrials.gov

Source. Adapted from Gray 2004; Haynes 2001a, 2000b, 2006.

trary, and searches in any one category often result in finding articles or outcomes in all of the categories listed in Table 4–2.

In the 5S strategy, priority is given to sources of high-quality, preappraised information so that the clinician can omit the appraisal step (step 3) in the EBM process. Haynes (2006) noted that clinicians practicing in settings with an electronic medical record system may be able to link their patient's characteristics with current evidence-based guidelines for care within that system. If such a system is not available, he recommends that the clinicians then begin to look for summaries. Table 4–2 lists many sources of summaries, discussed later in this chapter.

If no summaries, guidelines, algorithms, or other more comprehensive and systematic reviews are available, Haynes recommends that the clinician then look for brief summaries and synopses over lengthier reviews, assuming that a busy clinician wants an answer as quickly and effortlessly as possible. Although this strategy is appropriate for quickly answering clinical questions in a practice setting, it is not necessarily the most appropriate strategy for performing a comprehensive search of the clinical literature.

Systems

The starting point for the search should be what Haynes (2006) has termed a *system*, an information source that covers a variety of diagnoses, provides a summary of the results of high-quality systematic reviews, and is frequently updated. Such a system would provide the user with a concise summary of the evidence, linked to the original studies. Some clinicians have access to electronic medical record systems with a computerized decision support system that can link a patient's characteristics to current evidence-based guidelines for care. For instance, the Clinical Research Information System (CRIS) used at Duke University, according to their Web site, provides all of the tools to seamlessly allow clinicians to use standard measures to assess patients. This information can be used "to establish and enforce clinical practices and guidelines." Many systems are developing quality assessment metrics that monitor aggregate outcomes related to preestablished standards. In theory, the standards and the practices that lead to them are evidence based.

Summaries (Including Guidelines, Algorithms, and Best Practices)

Many resources are available to help clinicians rapidly find evidence-based information. We have arbitrarily divided these into resources of clinical evidence, clinical guidelines, and algorithms.

Clinical Evidence

The *BMJ* Publishing Group has several publications, products, and activities to promote evidence medicine. *BMJ*'s *Clinical Evidence* is an international peer-reviewed journal that publishes systematic reviews of important clinical conditions. The reviews are frequently updated with the goal of providing busy clinicians with access to the very latest and most relevant medical knowledge for treatment decisions (http://clinicalevidence.bmj.com). *Clinical Evidence* attempts to provide clinically useful information by also including a comments section with recommended options, allowing for interactions among users. *Clinical Evidence* uses Cochrane reviews as a source of high-quality, systematic reviews but also uses reviews of primary studies and reviews of reviews. Reviews are updated annually with a new planned systematic search of databases and include frequent updating through *Clinical Evidence Updates* (www.bmjupdates.com). *BMJ* provides online access, a printed handbook, and a version for a personal digital assistant (PDA). The reviews may cover issues related to an intervention or condition. For instance, the review of smoking cessation ("Putting Evidence Into Practice: Smoking Cessation"; available as a PDF file at: www.clinicalevidence.bmj .com/ceweb/ resources/index.jsp) provides information on smoking rates, the disease burden from smoking and health benefits of cessation, predictors of quitting and maintained cessation, public policy on smoking, and interventions.

Another emerging and important source of EBM is PIER (the Physicians' Information and Education Resource). Unfortunately, PIER is only available to American College of Physicians (2009; ACP) members, although some reviews can be accessed online through the *ACP Journal Club* (www.acpjc.org). The *ACP Journal Club* (Haynes 2008) is designed to keep clinicians up to date, but articles may be relevant to an issue a clinician is researching.

The United Kingdom's National Health Service offers an online evidence-based mental health library (NeLMH 2009). This library is collaboratively produced by a core team working for the library with assistance from core groups, including the Centre for Evidence-Based Medicine (www .cebm.net), the Centre for Evidence-Based Mental Health (www.cebmh.com), the Royal College of Psychiatrists, the University of Oxford Department of Psychiatry, and the World Health Organization United Kingdom Collaborating Centre. For instance, the *Schizophrenia Annual Evidence Update 2008* (Mental Health Specialist Library 2008) brings together evidence-based guidelines, systematic reviews, important primary research, service development literature, and patient information.

The TRIP Database (www.tripdatabase.com) began in 1997 with the goal of answering "real" clinical questions using the principles of EBM. The TRIP Database includes a variety of resources that can be easily searched. The results can be filtered by systematic reviews, evidence-based synopses, guidelines, clinical questions, core-primary research, e-textbooks, and others.

Clinical Practice Guidelines and Algorithms

Table 4–3 lists major guidelines and algorithms available to practitioners. Online access to these may require registration and payment. The most useful starting point in searching for these guidelines is the National Guideline Clearinghouse (www.guideline.gov). This database of clinical practice guidelines is operated by the Agency for Healthcare Research and Quality (AHRQ), in association with the American Medical Association (AMA) and the American Association of Health Plans (AAHP). All guidelines must meet explicit quality criteria for inclusion (Agency for Healthcare Research and Quality 2000). Searching the database yields a structured abstract that is linked to the actual guideline. The database also allows several guidelines to be compared side by side. (General information about clin-

ical practice guidelines and algorithms can be found in Gray and Taylor, Chapter 7 in this volume.)

Most American psychiatrists are familiar with the practice guidelines developed by the American Psychiatric Association (APA). These guidelines cover the major psychiatric disorders and are available both in print form (American Psychiatric Association 2006) and online (www.psychiatryonline.com).

Synopses

If you have no access to a system and found no results from the summaries, the next step is to search for what Haynes (2001a, 2001b, 2006) has termed *synopses*, structured abstracts of high-quality systematic reviews or original articles. The advantages of these resources are that they have already been appraised for quality and are summarized; therefore, busy clinicians can quickly get to the bottom line without reading a lengthy article. Furthermore, these synopses can be accessed through online databases that can be searched quickly. Because these databases contain summaries of only those articles that meet certain quality criteria, they are much smaller than MEDLINE and yield fewer references.

TABLE 4–3. Sources of high-quality clinical practice guidelines and algorithms

Organization	Web site
American Psychiatric Association	http://www.psychiatryonline.com
British Association for Psychopharmacology Consensus Guidelines	http://www.bap.org.uk
Canadian Medical Association	http://www.cma.ca
Clinical Knowledge Summaries (United Kingdom National Health Service)	http://www.cks.library.nhs.uk/home
Expert Consensus Guidelines	http://www.psychguides.com
Harvard South Shore, Psychopharmacology Algorithm Project	http://mhc.com/Algorithms
International Psychopharmacology Algorithm Project (IPAP)	http://www.ipap.org
National Guideline Clearinghouse	http://www.guideline.gov
National Institute for Health and Clinical Excellence (NICE)	http://www.nice.org.uk
New Zealand Guidelines Group	http://www.nzgg.org.nz/index.cfm?
Scottish Intercollegiate Guidelines Network (SIGN)	http://www.sign.ac.uk/guidelines/index.html
Texas Medication Algorithm Project (TMAP)	http://www.dshs.state.tx.us/mhprograms/tmap.shtm
U.S. Department of Veterans Affairs	http://www.va.gov

Evidence-Based Mental Health

For psychiatry, the best source of synopses is *Evidence-Based Mental Health*, published quarterly by the BMJ Publishing Group with the Royal College of Psychiatrists and the British Psychological Society. The online version (http://ebmh.bmjjournals.com) is particularly useful in searching for answers to clinical questions related to common psychiatric disorders.

The staff at *Evidence-Based Mental Health* reviews the major medical and psychiatric journals to identify both original research articles and literature reviews that meet explicit quality criteria. They then prepare structured abstracts, sometimes reanalyzing the data to present it in a uniform format. An outside reviewer supplies a commentary. Finally, a declarative title summarizes the article's "clinical bottom line."

ACP Journal Club

ACP Journal Club, a publication that is similar to *Evidence-Based Mental Health*, is published bimonthly by the American College of Physicians–American Society of Internal Medicine and is available online (www.acpjc.org). Although the intended audience is internists, *ACP Journal Club* does include summaries of articles of psychiatric interest that are related primarily to disorders seen in primary care settings (e.g., depression, anxiety disorders, dementia, delirium, and substance abuse). If you do not have access to *Evidence-Based Mental Health*, then searching the (free) *ACP Journal Club* database may prove useful.

Syntheses

If a relevant synopsis cannot be found, the next step is to search for what Haynes (2001a, 2001b, 2006) has termed a *synthesis*, a high-quality systematic review. A detailed discussion of systematic reviews and how they are appraised for quality is given in Gray, Chapter 6 in this volume. The following discussion concentrates on the methods used for locating systematic reviews. A common method for systematic reviews is to define a protocol at the outset of the study. Greenhalgh and Peacock (2005) found that in a review of diffusion of service-level innovations in health care organizations, only 30% of the sources were obtained from the protocol defined at the outset of the study, 50% were identified by "snowballing" (such as pursuing references of references), and 24% were obtained by personal knowledge or personal contacts. They concluded that systematic reviews of complex evidence cannot rely solely on protocol-driven search strategies; however, "snowballing," personal knowledge, and personal contacts all influence the final database.

Cochrane Database of Systematic Reviews

The single best source of systematic reviews is the Cochrane Database of Systematic Reviews (Glanville and Lefebvre 2000; McKibbon et al. 2002). This database contains high-quality systematic reviews specially prepared by the Cochrane Collaboration, a multisite international workgroup (Antes and Oxman 2001; Cochrane Collaboration 2003). The full-text version of the reviews is available through medical libraries as part of their Ovid database subscription. Abstracts of the reviews are available online without charge (www.cochrane.org/reviews/index .htm).

Database of Abstracts of Reviews of Effectiveness

The Database of Abstracts of Reviews of Effectiveness (DARE) consists of structured abstracts of systematic reviews that meet certain quality criteria (National Health Service Centre for Reviews and Dissemination [NHS CRD] 2000). DARE is maintained by the NHS CRD at the University of York and can be accessed through their Web site (www.crd.york.ac.uk/crdweb). DARE is also available through medical libraries as part of Ovid's Evidence-Based Medicine Reviews, a database that combines Best Evidence, the Cochrane Database of Systematic Reviews, and DARE (Etchells 2000; Ovid 2002b). Because DARE provides only abstracts of reviews, the actual review must be obtained separately if further detail is required.

Health Technology Assessment Database

The Health Technology Assessment database is also maintained by the NHS CRD at the University of York, in collaboration with the International Network of Agencies for Health Technology Assessment (INAHTA; National Health Service Centre for Reviews and Dissemination 2002). It contains abstracts of critical reviews of health technologies, including treatments for psychiatric conditions. Most of the abstracts are linked to the Web site of the agency that produces the report, from which the full text of the document can be obtained. The Health Technology Assessment and DARE databases may be searched simultaneously from the NHS CRD Web site (www.crd.york.ac.uk/crdweb).

Other Sources of Systematic Reviews

Systematic reviews published in journals also may be identified through MEDLINE and similar databases or searched with Google Scholar. This can be accomplished most efficiently with the assistance of "filters" that attempt to limit the search results to systematic reviews or meta-analyses (Glanville and Lefebvre 2000; McKibbon et al. 1999; National Health Service Centre for Reviews and Dissemination 2002; Shojania and Berg 2001). This process is described in more detail in the next section.

Bandolier (www.medicine.ox.ac.uk/bandolier) is an online version of an evidence-based health care journal written by two Oxford scientists. The Web site uses a variety of sources to publish reviews and synopses. If the question being asked happens to fit into an area covered by the service, the information can be useful. For instance, *Bandolier* updated their systematic reviews related to addiction in August 2008. The review was actually a brief synopsis of findings from "three reviews and meta-analyses" of abstinence rates for alcohol addiction for acamprosate, naloxone, and opioid antagonists. The synopsis includes a "clinical bottom line": "Information on interventions for alcohol addictions is sparse. Without any drug intervention, about 1 user in 5 will be abstinent between 3 and 24 months." (Curiously, this conclusion is not supported by the data presented in the rest of the synopses.)

Studies

MEDLINE or similar databases should be used only if the above-mentioned other sources have proved unsuccessful. This is because such a search is apt to yield multiple studies requiring appraisal. In contrast, the resources described in the first three categories are sources of high-quality evidence that have generally already been preappraised for validity, thus sparing the need to go through the critical appraisal step before using the evidence.

Multiple databases can be useful in locating answers to mental health–related questions. However, much of the focus of this section is placed on MEDLINE, partly because psychiatrists are generally most familiar with this resource and can access it most readily.

MEDLINE

MEDLINE is a database maintained by the U.S. National Library of Medicine (NLM). It includes more than 12 million citations, both clinical and preclinical. MEDLINE may be accessed through a variety of different services. Libraries usually obtain the MEDLINE database through a commercial vendor, such as Ovid or SilverPlatter. MEDLINE access is available free of charge through the NLM's PubMed Web site (www.ncbi.nlm.nih.gov/sites/entrez?db=pubmed).

For most psychiatrists, the simplest starting point for a MEDLINE search (using PubMed) is the Clinical Queries interface. The Clinical Queries interface allows one to search by a clinical study category and to limit the scope of the search by category (etiology, diagnosis, therapy, prognosis, or clinical prediction guides) and scope (narrow or broad). PubMed then applies search filters to limit the search to particular types of articles. This filtering is achieved by addition of specific terms to the search, in addition to the terms that the user entered. For instance, Table 4–4 shows how to conduct a search with various filters. In this table, the clinician is interested in articles published since 2002 on the effect of trazodone on sleep but only wants to look at RCTs with a placebo.

TABLE 4–4.　Example of a PubMed search

Search: PubMed for the effects of trazodone on sleep

Go to: http://www.ncbi.nlm.nih.gov/sites/entrez?db=pubmed

Enter: "trazodone and sleep"

Select: Advanced Search

In the field "Search by Author, Journal, Publication Date, and more," type in the Publication Date Search, "2002 to present."

In the field "Limit by Topics, Languages, and Journal Groups," select "Randomized Controlled Trial."

In the "Index of Fields and Field Values," type in "placebo" and select "and."

If you scroll to the top of the page, you will see that you will be searching for randomized controlled trials published since 2002 using the terms (trazodone and sleep) AND (placebo).

The search results in seven studies.

Note.　Search performed on June 25, 2009.

The search strategies developed by Haynes et al. (2005) have been embedded in PubMed. For the busy clinician, the Limits function is likely to be more efficient than the Advanced Search mechanism. PubMed now includes several brief tutorials to teach the user about the system.

Other Databases

Although MEDLINE is usually the best starting point for a search, various other specialized databases may be useful in searching for particular types of evidence.

EMBASE, the *Excerpta Medica* Database. EMBASE is an international medical and pharmaceutical database that covers more than 7,000 journals from 70 countries (www.embase.com). EMBASE requires subscribing to the service.

Cumulative Index to Nursing and Allied Health Literature. The Cumulative Index to Nursing and Allied Health Literature (CINAHL) covers 1,000 English-language nursing and allied health journals (www.cinahl.com/library/library.htm). CINAHL requires a subscription.

ClinPSYC and PsycINFO. ClinPSYC and PsycINFO are databases produced by the American Psychological Association. PsycINFO covers 2,150 journals in more than 25 languages. It also includes books, dissertations, and other secondary publications. ClinPSYC is a clinically oriented subset of the PsycINFO database. PsycINFO and ClinPSYC are available through Ovid and many institutions.

Google Scholar. Google Scholar (http://scholar.google.com) is a search engine that searches articles available in the vast Google database. Selecting "Advanced Scholar Search" allows for some search restrictions (e.g., by dates published).

Alternatives to the 5S Approach

The 5S approach by Haynes (2001a, 2001b, 2006) is a stepwise search strategy, beginning with systems and progressing until an answer to the clinical question is found. An alternative strategy is to search several databases simultaneously that include two or more levels in the hierarchy. Two search engines that perform this function are the TRIP Database and SUMSearch.

TRIP Database

The TRIP Database (www.tripdatabase.com) was created in 1997 and is currently the search engine for the National electronic Library for Mental Health. Updated monthly, it is an attempt to link all of the high-quality evidence-based resources available on the Internet. A search that uses the TRIP Database will search the Cochrane Library, DARE, other collections of systematic reviews and guidelines, and even some online journals. It also has links to the PubMed Clinical Queries search interface.

SUMSearch

SUMSearch (http://sumsearch.uthscsa.edu) was developed at the University of Texas Health Science Center at San Antonio. SUMSearch is designed to query only Internet sites that contain evidence written by qualified professionals. Most of the links provided by SUMSearch come from three Internet sites: the NLM, DARE, and the National Guideline Clearinghouse. When querying MEDLINE at the NLM, SUMSearch uses search filters that have been developed by various researchers to search optimally for certain types of articles (Wilczynski et al. 2004). For example, when the clinician clicks the "treatment" focus, SUMSearch includes a search of MEDLINE using a filter validated to find randomized controlled clinical trials. Haase et al. (2007) compared the retrieval efficiency of SUMSearch and Google Scholar. The searches were limited by various terms, "clinical guidelines," and "specific diseases." The performance pattern between search engines was similar: search strategies including the term *guideline* yielded the highest sensitivity (SUMSearch: 81.5%; Google Scholar: 31.9%), and search strategies including the term *practice guideline* yielded the highest specificity (SUMSearch: 89.5%; Google Scholar: 95.7%) and the lowest number needed to read (SUMSearch: 7.0; Google Scholar: 9.3). Thus, SUMSearch was superior to Google Scholar in the retrieval of relevant information (Haase et al. 2007).

Examples of Searching for Evidence With Various Approaches

To explain and compare various approaches, two examples of clinical questions and their resulting search results are given. Of interest, we searched the same question used by Gray in 2004 to determine whether any new findings were available.

Example 1: Cognitive-Behavioral Therapy in Schizophrenia

In patients with schizophrenia, does the addition of cognitive-behavioral therapy (CBT) to usual treatment, compared with usual treatment alone, prevent relapse?

5S Approach

The starting point for this search was a summary, *Clinical Evidence*. We began by searching with the terms *schizophrenia*, *CBT*, and *relapse*. This resulted in a synopsis of a review (Jones et al. 2004), which concluded that CBT compared with standard care does not reduce relapse rates at up to 60 months compared with standard care alone. Evidence was graded as "high-quality." This conclusion differs from the conclusion reached from Gray's search in 2004, which also began with *Clinical Evidence*. In that search, the conclusion was that there is limited evidence from RCTs that CBT may reduce relapse rates. These somewhat contradictory findings point to the need for the practitioner to reassess treatment practices periodically because new evidence may change recommendations.

We then looked at the American Psychiatric Association (2006) "Practice Guideline for the Treatment of Patients With Schizophrenia," which noted that "Overall, the data support the efficacy of cognitive behavior therapy for reducing the frequency and severity of positive symptoms and the distress associated with these symptoms. Furthermore, these gains appear to continue over time. The benefits do not appear to extend to relapse, rehospitalization, or social functioning" (p. 669). With the search terms *schizophrenia* and *CBT*, the NeLMH produced another set of documents, including a 2003 review from the NHSCRD, a 2004 systematic review from the Cochrane database, and the same critical appraisal from the *Evidence-Based Mental Health* database. All three of these searches led to the same conclusion—that CBT is not effective in reducing relapse in patients with schizophrenia compared with usual treatment.

TRIP Database

The terms *cognitive-behavior therapy AND schizophrenia* were searched in the TRIP Database. Several MEDLINE articles were identified, but we then filtered the search by systematic reviews, evidence-based synopses, guidelines, clinical questions, and others. None yielded any useful information. The MEDLINE search, included in the search results, listed some articles that also could have been found by searching MEDLINE directly. We then took a "higher" order approach, first looking for general guidelines, and found that we could search to find specific issues about CBT and schizophrenia. Several articles were returned.

SUMSearch

The terms *cognitive-behavioral therapy AND schizophrenia* were searched in SUMSearch. The search, which took about 90 seconds, produced 112 documents, including one in Wikipedia. (The PubMed Full Text original-research search function did not respond in time; the page suggested searching PubMed directly or trying this search again later.) The search produced three guidelines, including the APA guideline. Under PubMed (possible guidelines), it produced several relevant articles, including a recent review of CBT for medication-resistant schizophrenia (Rathod et al. 2008) and several other guidelines not listed in the TRIP Database. Under PubMed (possible systematic reviews), it also produced some useful articles.

Google Scholar

Google Scholar was searched using the terms *cognitive-behavioral therapy AND schizophrenia*. The search, which took 0.21 seconds, retrieved about 4,400 citations, including reviews and summaries. The material probably included most of the articles listed under SUMSearch.

Example 2: Kava in Generalized Anxiety Disorder

In patients with generalized anxiety disorder, is kava extract more effective than a placebo in relieving symptoms of anxiety?

5S Approach

The search started with a summary (*Clinical Evidence*), but the section on generalized anxiety disorder did not mention kava as a treatment. An online search of *Evidence-Based Mental Health* with the terms *kava AND anxiety* failed to yield any articles. We also looked at clinical guidelines and found no useful information. We then searched the Cochrane

Library, which provided a November 18, 2002, review that concluded the following:

> Systematic literature database. Twenty-two potentially relevant double-blind, placebo-controlled RCTs were identified. Twelve trials met the inclusion criteria. The meta-analysis of seven trials suggests a significant treatment effect for the total score on the Hamilton Anxiety Scale in favor of kava extract. Few adverse events were reported in the reviewed trials, which were all mild, transient and infrequent. These data imply that, compared with placebo, kava extract might be an effective symptomatic treatment for anxiety although, at present, the size of the effect seems to be small. Rigorous trials with large sample sizes are needed to clarify the existing uncertainties. Particularly long-term safety studies of kava are needed.

The DARE database yielded 10 articles but none more recent or relevant than Pittler and Ernst (2003). No articles were retrieved from two other linked databases.

TRIP Database

The terms *kava AND anxiety* were searched in the TRIP Database. Nineteen systematic reviews were found, including Pittler and Ernst (2003). A meta-analysis by Saeed et al. (2007) concluded, "There is substantial evidence that kava has a positive effect on the symptoms of anxiety disorders." This meta-analysis included a Cochrane review, several recent small RCTs and an RCT on safety, and case reports on safety. We then ran a search of the Saeed et al. (2007) article in PubMed to examine "related articles." Doing so can identify articles citing Saeed et al. (2007). One published in 2008 concluded, with regard to herbal treatments, that "kava is effective in reducing anxiety symptoms....The association of kava with hepatotoxicity, however, is a significant concern" (van der Watt et al. 2008). We had our answer. Kava may be more effective than placebo in relieving symptoms of anxiety, but the risk exceeds the benefit. This search also illustrated that it is worthwhile to look at both benefits and risks.

SUMSearch

The terms *kava AND anxiety* were searched in SUM-Search. The search resulted in two guidelines (but not relevant ones); three PubMed possible guidelines; three DARE articles, one providing information on possible hepatotoxicity; and 22 possible systematic reviews, including those mentioned earlier. SUM-Search also included several articles from Wikipedia that seemed irrelevant to the issue of efficacy and safety. However, we found this ready reference to things such as kava production rather interesting.

Google Scholar

The Google Scholar search produced 3,210 articles in 0.09 seconds. However, it included (at the top) many older and nonrelevant articles.

PubMed

Finally, we ran a search on PubMed. It produced many of the same articles but also some that we had not seen in other searches.

Comparison and Recommendations

After performing several similar searches using different methods, we found that each of the approaches has certain advantages and disadvantages. The 5S approach was most tedious, and much of the material appeared in the other reviews. However, it is a worthwhile place to start for a summary that might be relevant. SUMSearch and the TRIP Database are both slower than a direct search of a database but provide a more comprehensive source of information. Google Scholar is very quick, but PubMed is wonderful in presenting the most recent (but not necessarily most relevant) information first.

On the basis of these admittedly unsystematic and undoubtedly biased observations, we would recommend a somewhat modified 5S approach. We would suggest beginning the search with *Clinical Evidence* because many questions can be answered easily and quickly with this resource. Furthermore, it has the advantage of being available online and in print, and it can be downloaded to a PDA. An alternative is to begin with one's favorite clinical guideline to determine whether information on the topic is available. Reviewing the guideline also allows one to examine the whole treatment approach to a problem.

If online access to *Evidence-Based Mental Health* is available, we recommend searching this database next. It includes synopses of original research that have not yet been incorporated into a systematic review, and the information is presented in a format that will provide an answer quickly.

TABLE 4–5. Suggested search strategy

Step	Resource	Web site
1	*Clinical Evidence*	http://clinicalevidence.com
2	*Evidence-Based Mental Health*	http://ebmh.bmjjournals.com
3	TRIP Database	http://www.tripdatabase.com
4	PubMed Clinical Queries	http://www.ncbi.nlm.nih.gov/corehtml/query/static/clinical.shtml

The third step is to go to clinical guidelines. However, these higher-level approaches may not answer more specific questions. The guidelines had to be reviewed to find statements about kava, for instance.

A quick look at SUMSearch and/or TRIP is worthwhile. The final step in our search would be PubMed. This allows for a very quick perusal of information. Table 4–5 outlines this approach.

Inability to Find an Answer

There are three general reasons for not finding an answer to a clinical question. The first reason has to do with the mechanics of the search process. Changing the search terms, searching by MeSH heading as well as text words, and other techniques described in more detail elsewhere (Greenhalgh 1997, 2001; McKibbon et al. 1999, 2002) may be of value if this is the case.

The second reason has to do with the nature of the question itself. Perhaps the patient population specified in the question is overly specific. Broadening the patient population in the question may result in the search yielding a possible answer. The problem then becomes one of deciding whether that answer can be generalized to a particular patient. This is a topic discussed in more detail in subsequent chapters.

The third reason for not finding an answer is either that the evidence does not exist or that the only evidence is relatively unreliable. The search strategies outlined earlier tend to find evidence that is high in the evidence hierarchy (Table 4–1). If such high-quality evidence does not exist, it is necessary to search for evidence lower in the hierarchy. This can be done through PubMed, by changing the search filters in the Clinical Queries interface from "specificity" to "sensitivity," or by doing a MEDLINE search without filters. Such strategies may result in lower-quality evidence, such as case series or case reports. In some cases, this may represent the best available evidence. Obtaining consultation is

another option. Although expert opinion is at the bottom of the evidence hierarchy, it is still better than nothing. Finally, EBM retains a place for clinical judgment (Haynes et al. 2002a, 2002b). In the absence of evidence from the literature, clinical judgment becomes even more important.

References

Agency for Healthcare Research and Quality: The National Guideline Clearinghouse fact sheet [Agency for Healthcare Research and Quality Web site]. July 2000. Available at: http://www.ahcpr.gov/clinic/ngcfact.htm. Accessed June 18, 2002

American College of Physicians: PIER: Physicians' Information and Education Resource. 2009. Available at: http://pier.acponline.org/index.html. Accessed June 25, 2009

American Psychiatric Association: Practice guideline for the treatment of patients with schizophrenia, 2nd edition, in Practice Guidelines for the Treatment of Psychiatric Disorders, Compendium. Washington, DC, American Psychiatric Association, 2006, pp 565–746

American Psychiatric Association: Practice Guidelines for the Treatment of Psychiatric Disorders, Compendium. Washington, DC, American Psychiatric Association, 2006

Antes G, Oxman AD: The Cochrane Collaboration in the 20th century, in Systematic Reviews in Health Care: Meta-Analysis in Context. Edited by Egger M, Smith GD, Altman DG. London, BMJ Books, 2001, pp 447–458

Antman EM, Lau J, Kupelnick B, et al: A comparison of results of meta-analyses of randomized control trials and recommendations of clinical experts: treatments for myocardial infarction. JAMA 268:240–248, 1992

Badenoch D, Heneghan C: Evidence-Based Medicine Toolkit. London, BMJ Books, 2002

CINAHL [Edward G. Miner Library Web site]. 2002a. Available at: http://www.urmc.rochester.edu/Miner/Educ/ebnfilt.htm. Accessed June 27, 2003

Clinical Research Information System (CRIS). Available at: http://psychiatry.mc.duke.edu/CMRIS/CMRIndex.htm. Accessed December 2, 2008

Cochrane Collaboration: Introductory leaflets. Available at: http://www.cochrane.org/cochrane/leaflet.htm. May 15, 2003. Accessed June 25, 2008

Coyle JT, Heckers S: Update on the conflict of interest policy for the ARCHIVES. Arch Gen Psychiatry 63:1178, 2006

Davidoff F, Haynes B, Sackett D, et al: Evidence based medicine. BMJ 310:1085–1086, 1995

Etchells E: Ovid. ACP J Club 132:A15, 2000

Glanville J, Lefebvre C: Identifying systematic reviews: key resources. Evid Based Ment Health 3:68–69, 2000

Gray GE: Concise Guide to Evidence-Based Psychiatry. Washington, DC, American Psychiatric Publishing, 2004

Greenhalgh T: How to read a paper: the Medline database. BMJ 315:180–183, 1997

Greenhalgh T: How to Read a Paper: The Basics of Evidence Based Medicine, 2nd Edition. London, BMJ Books, 2001

Greenhalgh T, Peacock R: Effectiveness and efficiency of search methods in systematic reviews of complex evidence: audit of primary sources. BMJ 331(7524):1064–1065, 2005

Haase A, Follmann M, Skipka G, et al: Developing search strategies for clinical practice guidelines in SUMSearch and Google Scholar and assessing their retrieval performance. BMC Med Res Methodol 7:28, 2007

Haynes RB: Of studies, summaries, synopses, and systems: the "4S" evolution of services for finding current best evidence. Evid Based Ment Health 4:37–39, 2001a

Haynes RB: Of studies, syntheses, synopses, and systems: the "4S" evolution of services for finding current best evidence. ACP J Club 134:A11–A13, 2001b

Haynes RB: Of studies, syntheses, synopses, summaries, and systems: the "5S" evolution of information services for evidence-based healthcare decisions. Evid Based Med 11:162–164, 2006

Haynes RB: ACP Journal Club: the best new evidence for patient care. ACP J Club 148:2, 2008

Haynes RB, Devereaux PJ, Guyatt GH: Clinical expertise in the era of evidence-based medicine and patient choice. ACP J Club 136:A11–A14, 2002a

Haynes RB, Devereaux PJ, Guyatt GH: Physicians' and patients' choices in evidence based practice. BMJ 324:1350, 2002b

Haynes RB, McKibbon KA, Wilczynski NL, et al: Optimal search strategies for retrieving scientifically strong studies of treatment from Medline: analytical survey. BMJ 330(7501):1179, 2005

Jones C, Cormac I, Silveira da Mota Neto JI, et al: Cognitive behaviour therapy for schizophrenia. Cochrane Database Syst Rev 2004 Oct 18;(4):CD000524

Lacchetti C, Guyatt G: Therapy and validity: surprising results of randomized controlled trials, in Users' Guides to the Medical Literature: A Manual for Evidence-Based Clinical Practice. Edited by Guyatt G, Rennie D. Chicago, IL, AMA Press, 2002, pp 13–47

McKibbon A, Eady A, Marks S: PDQ Evidence-Based Principles and Practice. Hamilton, ON, Canada, BC Decker, 1999

McKibbon A, Hunt D, Richardson WS, et al: Finding the evidence, in Users' Guides to the Medical Literature: A Manual for Evidence-Based Clinical Practice. Edited by Guyatt G, Rennie D. Chicago, IL, AMA Press, 2002, pp 247–265

National electronic Library for Health (NeLMH): NHS Evidence—mental health. July 2002. Available at: http://www.library.nhs.uk/MentalHealth. Accessed June 25, 2009

National Health Service Centre for Reviews and Dissemination (DARE): Available at: http://www.crd.york.ac.uk/crdweb. Accessed June 25, 2009

National Library for Health: The Mental Health Specialist Library. 2008. Available at: http://www.library.nhs.uk/mentalhealth. Accessed June 25, 2009

Phillips B, Ball C, Sackett D, et al: Levels of evidence [Centre for Evidence-Based Medicine Web site]. May 2001. Available at: http://www.cebm.net/levels_of_evidence.asp. Accessed June 27, 2003

Pittler MH, Ernst E: Kava extract for treating anxiety. Cochrane Database Syst Rev (1):CD003383, 2003

Rathod S, Kingdon D, Weiden P, et al: Cognitive-behavioral therapy for medication-resistant schizophrenia: a review. J Psychiatr Pract 14:22–33, 2008

Reeves BC, MacLehose RR, Harvey IM, et al: A review of observational, quasi-experimental and randomised study designs for the evaluation of the effectiveness of healthcare interventions, in The Advanced Handbook of Methods in Evidence Based Healthcare. Edited by Stevens A, Abrams K, Brazier J, et al. London, Sage, 2001, pp 116–135

Sackett DL, Straus SE, Richardson WS, et al: Evidence-Based Medicine: How to Practice and Teach EBM, 2nd Edition. New York, Churchill Livingstone, 2000

Saeed SA, Bloch RM, Antonacci DJ: Herbal and dietary supplements for treatment of anxiety disorders. Am Fam Physician 76:549–556, 2007

Shojania KG, Berg LA: Taking advantage of the explosion of systematic reviews: an efficient MEDLINE search strategy. Eff Clin Pract 4:157–162, 2001

Taylor MJ, Freemantle N, Geddes JR, et al: Early onset of selective serotonin reuptake inhibitor antidepressant action: systematic review and meta-analysis. Arch Gen Psychiatry 63:1217–1223, 2006

van der Watt G, Laugharne J, Janca A: Complementary and alternative medicine in the treatment of anxiety and depression. Curr Opin Psychiatry 21:37–42, 2008

Wilczynski NL, Haynes RB, Lavis JN, et al: Optimal search strategies for detecting health services research studies in MEDLINE. CMAJ 171:1179–1185, 2004

Clinical Trials

Gregory E. Gray, M.D., Ph.D.
C. Barr Taylor, M.D.

After identifying one or more articles or other resources to answer a clinical question, the next step in the evidence-based medicine (EBM) process is to appraise the evidence. In this chapter and in Chapters 6, 7, and 9–12 in this volume, guidance on appraising a variety of different types of evidence is provided.

Because questions about therapy are among those most frequently asked by clinicians, we begin with a discussion of individual studies of therapies. In Chapter 6, Gray focuses on the appraisal of systematic reviews of therapies, whereas in Chapter 7, Gray and Taylor focus on the appraisal of treatment guidelines.

Controlled Versus Uncontrolled Trials

Evidence about the effectiveness of a therapy can come from a variety of sources (Table 5–1). However, evidence from some types of studies is apt to be more biased and misleading than evidence from more rigorous study designs (Greenhalgh 2001; Guyatt 2002; Guyatt et al. 2002b; Lacchetti and Guyatt 2002), as explained in this section.

Single Case Reports

The least rigorous and potentially most biased type of evidence is that arising from a single case (Fletcher et al. 1996; Sackett et al. 1991). As clinicians, we like to believe that patients improve as a result of our efforts. We sometimes attribute patient improvement

to a therapy when it was, in fact, the result of spontaneous improvement. Published single case reports have the added problem of publication bias: clinicians are more apt to report their successes with a novel treatment than they are their failures (Easterbrook et al. 1991; Fletcher et al. 1996; Montori and Guyatt 2002; Song et al. 2001). Although a single case report might result in a hypothesis that is later tested in a clinical trial, such reports cannot be relied on to guide treatment (Fletcher et al. 1996; Hennekens et al. 1987; Sackett et al. 1991). Single case reports may be more useful, however, in alerting a clinician to possible adverse effects of a treatment, although even here the adverse event may be unrelated to the treatment (i.e., coincidental). In the psychological literature, single case studies (different from reports) have been used to generate hypotheses about potentially useful treatments. One model for a single case design is to use an ABAB approach, in which a baseline is obtained (A), followed by an intervention period (B), a return to baseline (A), and then a reintroduction of the intervention (B).

Case Series

A case series is only slightly better than a single case report (Fletcher et al. 1996). Here the author reports on a series of patients treated for a particular condition. Because patients are not enrolled in a formal study, it is difficult to know whether the results reflect all patients receiving a particular therapy or whether they reflect only the successes. As with single case reports, publication bias is a significant

TABLE 5–1.   Types of studies used to address treatment effectiveness

Uncontrolled studies

Single case reports

Case series

All-or-none case series[a]

Uncontrolled clinical trials

Controlled studies

Studies with historical controls

Studies with concurrent nonrandomized controls

    Patients of other physicians or clinical sites

    Patient or physician choice of treatment

    Systematic allocation

Randomized controlled trials[a]

With blinding[a]

Without blinding (open-label study)

[a]Strongest study designs.

problem in case series, and they are best regarded as a source of ideas for further study.

A particular type of case series, however, does rank high in the evidence hierarchy: the "all-or-none" case series (Badenoch and Heneghan 2002) (Table 4–1, Chapter 4). An all-or-none case series refers to a series of patients who receive treatment for a disease with a universally bad (usually fatal) outcome. If a new treatment leads to a better outcome in all of the patients treated, there is strong evidence of treatment effectiveness. Examples of such an all-or-none case series are some of the earliest reports of the effectiveness of antibiotics in treating infections, which were performed 6 decades ago. It is difficult, however, to think of a psychiatric disorder for which an all-or-none case series would be an appropriate study design.

Uncontrolled Clinical Trials

An uncontrolled clinical trial is a step up from a case series. In this study design, patients enrolled in the study receive the new treatment, but there is no control group. Unlike in a case series, there is a study protocol in an uncontrolled clinical trial that specifies the nature of the subjects, treatment, and outcome measures. Because no control group is used,

various factors can bias the results. These factors include the Hawthorne, experimenter expectancy (Pygmalion), and placebo effects; observer bias; regression toward the mean (Yudkin and Stratton 1996); and the natural history of the illness (Fletcher et al. 1996).

Historical Controls

Because improvement can occur spontaneously, as well as being a result of treatment, more convincing evidence about the effectiveness of a therapy comes from controlled trials. However, various control groups are sometimes used in clinical trials (Altman 1991; Bland 2000; Fletcher et al. 1996). The first type is a historical control. In this situation, the outcomes of the patients receiving the experimental therapy in the trial are compared with the outcomes of the patients with the same disorder and in the same treatment setting but who have received another therapy in the past. An example is the comparison of the lengths of stay of inpatients with schizophrenia treated with atypical antipsychotic medications with those of inpatients with schizophrenia treated in the same institution a decade earlier, prior to the introduction of atypical antipsychotic medications. Although the use of historical controls might be convenient, the results can be biased by changes in diagnostic criteria, patient acuity and demographics, and other aspects of care that may have occurred over time (Fletcher et al. 1996; Hennekens et al. 1987). Furthermore, information about the historical control group typically comes from medical records recorded for purposes other than research, whereas the information about patients receiving the experimental therapy is collected with the purpose of the study in mind. This difference in the type of information collected is a form of observer bias (Daly and Bourke 2000). As a result, clinical trials using historical controls often may provide misleading answers and generally overestimate the true treatment effectiveness (Altman 1991; Bland 2000; Everitt 1989; Fletcher et al. 1996).

Nonrandomized Clinical Trials

In other types of nonrandomized clinical trials, subjects are nonrandomly assigned to one or more therapies (Altman 1991; Bland 2000; Fletcher et al. 1996). Examples include studies comparing treatments at one clinic with treatments at another clinic or treatments by one set of providers with treatments by another set of providers. Other examples include studies in which patients volunteer for the treatment they are to receive or in which they are systematically allocated to a treatment group (e.g., every other patient is assigned to a particular treatment). However, the key characteristic of such studies is that the subjects are not randomly assigned to the clinic, provider, or therapy. As a result, the various groups of subjects may differ at the outset of the study in ways that affect their prognosis, which is referred to as "selection bias" or "allocation bias" (Daly and Bourke 2000; Fletcher et al. 1996). Such studies are not true experiments but are instead a type of observational study known as a *cohort study*.

Randomized Controlled Trials

The preferred study design to assess the effectiveness of a therapy is a randomized controlled trial (RCT) (Altman et al. 2001). In this study design, subjects are randomly assigned to either the control treatment or one or more experimental treatments at the onset of the trial. Such randomization serves to make the control and experimental groups comparable in characteristics that may influence prognosis (confounding factors) (Altman 1991; Altman et al. 2001; Daly and Bourke 2000; Fletcher et al. 1996). In addition, conventional tests of statistical significance are all based on the assumption of random assignment of subjects (Altman 1991; Cummings et al. 2001; Daly and Bourke 2000). The blinding of subjects, clinicians, and raters is an additional attempt to reduce sources of bias in RCTs (see next section).

Controlled usually refers to comparing an active treatment with no treatment or a placebo treatment. However, if one treatment is considered the standard, a common type of pharmaceutical study is to compare the active treatment with the new treatment, with the assumption that the new treatment needs to perform as well as the older treatment. In this model, the investigators may be satisfied if the new treatment performs "as well" as the older treatment. Such studies usually need to have a very large number of subjects to be meaningful; that is, to have sufficient power to detect small differences. Otherwise it may appear that the new and old treatments are the same, but mainly because the study did not have adequate power to detect differences, leading to a type II error.

Sources of Bias

The clinician interested in a particular therapy wants an unbiased estimate of how it compares with another therapy or placebo. The results of a particular study may over- or underestimate the true difference in effectiveness of the two therapies. One reason for this is chance (random error), discussed further in the next section. The other reason is bias (defined as a systematic deviation from the true results), which results in either a systematic overestimation or a systematic underestimation of treatment effectiveness (Guyatt 2002; Sitthi-amorn and Poshyachinda 1993). One goal, therefore, in study design is to minimize bias (Altman 1991).

Confounding

One source of bias in a clinical trial is having experimental and control groups that differ at the onset of the study in characteristics that affect outcome (Guyatt 2002). This is a form of selection bias, and the subject characteristics that affect outcome are known as *confounding factors* (Altman et al. 2001; Daly and Bourke 2000; Jadad 1998). Confounding factors can include variables such as age, sex, ethnicity, illness severity, and comorbid illnesses. Adjustment for known confounding factors can occur in the statistical analysis of a study (Daly and Bourke 2000). Such statistical techniques cannot, however, adjust for unknown confounding factors. Randomization will, however, automatically adjust for such confounding factors by tending to make the treatment and control groups similar (Altman 1991; Altman et al. 2001; Daly and Bourke 2000; Fletcher et al. 1996; Guyatt 2002). Even with randomization, there will still be some differences between the experimental and control groups, but the statistical techniques that are used to analyze studies assume a certain amount of chance variation and take it into account (Daly and Bourke 2000). Indeed, if some form of matching is used to attempt to further minimize differences in known confounding factors between the experimental and control groups, this must be taken into account in the statistical analysis; if it is not, tests of statistical significance will be overly conservative (Daly and Bourke 2000; Peto et al. 1976).

Hawthorne Effect

Several nonspecific effects also can bias the results, including Hawthorne, Pygmalion, and placebo effects. The Hawthorne effect was first observed in studies of worker productivity at the Hawthorne Western Electric plant in Illinois in 1924 and refers to the tendency of subjects to do better solely because they are being studied (Fletcher et al. 1996; Holden 2001). Some of this may involve subject expectations, but it can also be the result of nonspecific effects of the study situation, such as the increased attention received. The Hawthorne effect is one reason that studies involving historical controls will produce biased results: experimental subjects know that they are part of a study, and they therefore show the Hawthorne effect, whereas historical control subjects were not originally experimental subjects and hence did not show such an effect. The Hawthorne effect affects both the experimental and the control groups in an RCT and thus is eliminated as a source of bias in this study design.

Pygmalion Effect and Co-interventions

The Pygmalion effect, also called the *experimenter expectancy effect*, was first described in educational research, in which it was found that teacher expectations affect pupil performance (Rosenthal and Jacobson 1968). Subsequent research has indicated that experimenter expectations regarding treatment effect may result in differential attention or interactions with some subjects, which results in a change in subject behavior in the direction of experimenter hypothesis (Rosenthal and Rosnow 1991). A related effect is that of a clinician involved in a trial providing additional care (e.g., time, support) to patients in one treatment group but not to those in the other treatment group. This effect is known as *co-intervention* or *performance bias* (Altman et al. 2001; Fletcher et al. 1996; Guyatt 2002; Jüni et al. 2001). In clinical trials, this effect can be minimized by blinding clinicians to the treatment being provided. Such blinding can occur in drug trials; however, such blinding is obviously impossible in trials of psychotherapy. It can, however, be minimized by documenting adherence to treatment protocols (Guyatt 2002).

Placebo Effect

The third nonspecific effect is the placebo effect (Crow et al. 2001; Kaptchuk 1998; Laporte and Figueras 1994). In this effect, it is the subject's expectation of improvement, combined with other nonspecific psychotherapeutic effects, that leads to improvement (Chaput de Saintonge and Herxheimer 1994; Crow et al. 2001). The magnitude of the placebo response rate varies by disorder; it is greater in depression and anxiety disorders than in schizophrenia, but even in acute mania, there is a sizable placebo response (Charney et al. 2002) (Table 5–2). To separate the specific effects of a therapy from the nonspecific placebo effects, it is necessary to have a control group. Blinding the patient to the therapy being administered further reduces the placebo effect (Altman et al. 2001; Guyatt 2002), although this is far more difficult with psychosocial interventions than with drug therapies.

Observer, Detection, or Ascertainment Bias

The final important source of bias in a clinical trial is observer, detection, or ascertainment bias (Altman et al. 2001; Jadad 1998; Jüni et al. 2001). If an interviewer or rater knows which treatment a patient is receiving, he or she may differentially inquire about certain symptoms or see improvement where none exists. Blinding the interviewer or rater to the treatment is an important way of minimizing observer bias (Altman et al. 2001; Guyatt 2002; Jüni et al. 2001); however, it is difficult to do this entirely because the treatment received sometimes may be discerned from treatment side effects or from a patient's comments.

Minimizing Bias Through Blinding

To minimize sources of bias, the optimal study design is an RCT in which the subjects, clinicians, and raters are all blind to the treatment being administered. This is possible in drug trials; however, in many trials involving psychosocial interventions, only the rater can be blinded. The terms *single blind*, *double blind*, and *triple blind* are often used to describe the design type of a study, but there is little agreement about the meaning of the terms (Devereaux et al. 2001; Montori et al. 2002). Consequently, it is preferable to simply specify which of the various participants in a study are blinded to the treatment (Altman et al. 2001; Devereaux et al. 2002; Fletcher et al. 1996).

Basic Statistical Concepts

In reviewing the results of a clinical trial, it is important to have at least a basic understanding of biosta-

TABLE 5–2.   Placebo response rates in psychiatric disorders

Disorder	Outcome measure	Study duration	Placebo response rate (%)
Schizophrenia, acute episode	40% reduction in BPRS	6 weeks	8–32
Schizophrenia, maintenance	No relapse	9 months	34
Bipolar disorder, acute mania	50% reduction in YMRS	3 weeks	24
Bipolar disorder, maintenance	No relapse	2 years	19
Major depression	50% reduction in Ham-D	4–24 weeks (average 6 weeks)	30
Panic disorder	50% decrease in attacks	12 weeks	50
Social phobia	Much or very much improved	8–14 weeks	17–32
Obsessive-compulsive disorder	35% reduction in Y-BOCS	9–13 weeks	8–60

Note.   BPRS=Brief Psychiatric Rating Scale; Ham-D=Hamilton Rating Scale for Depression; Y-BOCS=Yale-Brown Obsessive Compulsive Scale; YMRS=Young Mania Rating Scale.
Source.   Data from Cookson et al. 2002; Walsh et al. 2002; Woods et al. 2001.

tistics. The following qualitative discussion does not discuss specific methods of statistical analysis or calculations; for such topics, the reader is referred to several excellent texts (Altman 1991; Bland 2000; Daly and Bourke 2000).

Hypothesis Testing

We begin with a hypothetical clinical trial comparing an experimental therapy with a control therapy. In this trial, participants are randomly assigned to one of two treatment groups. At the end of the trial, we assess the outcome in the two groups and find a difference. How do we know whether this difference is because the treatments differ in effectiveness or whether it is the result of chance? We know that even if the two treatments are identical, by chance alone there could be some difference in outcome. We therefore need to set a threshold, with differences in outcome greater than that threshold unlikely to be the result of chance alone. Conventionally, this threshold is set so that there is a 5% chance that a difference of that magnitude (or greater) will be the result of chance alone. In practice, an appropriate test statistic (e.g., t, F, or χ^2) is computed, from which a P value is derived. If $P<0.05$, the difference is considered *statistically significant*. This approach to data analysis is referred to as *hypothesis testing*, in that a difference in treatment effect that exceeds a threshold leads us to reject the null hypothesis that there is no difference between treatments.

The results of this clinical trial also can be conceptualized as falling into one of three categories: uncontrolled studies, controlled but not randomized studies, and randomized controlled trials (Table 5–3). In reality, the experimental and control treatments are either equivalent or different. In our experiment, either the difference exceeds the preset threshold and is considered "statistically significant" or it does not. Let us now consider some of the various combinations.

Type I Errors

If there is truly no difference between the experimental and the control treatments, our experiment, by chance alone, might find a difference large enough to be called "statistically significant." This is the equivalent of a *false-positive* result on a diagnostic test. In statistical terms, it is considered a type I error. In the example in the previous subsection, the threshold has been set so that a type I error occurs less than 5% of the time. In statistical terms, it is represented as $\alpha=0.05$, where α is the probability of a type I error.

Type II Errors

Now suppose that a difference truly exists between the two treatments. In our experiment, sometimes we find a large difference between the treatment groups, and sometimes, by chance alone, we may find only a small difference. Because we have set a threshold such that only differences that exceed the

TABLE 5–3. Possible outcomes of a clinical trial

	True difference between treatments	
Study outcome	No true difference	True difference exists
Difference found	False-positive result Type I error Probability = α	True-positive result Power = 1 − β
No difference found	True-negative result	False-negative result Type II error Probability = β

threshold are considered *statistically significant*, some of the results may not be considered *significant*, even though there is truly an underlying difference in the effectiveness of the two treatments. This is considered a type II error and is the equivalent of a *false-negative* result from a diagnostic test. The probability of a type II error occurring is represented by β.

Power

Ideally, we would like to have a high probability of detecting a difference when such a difference truly exists. This is the equivalent of a *true-positive* test result. Such a probability is given the term *power* and is represented by 1 minus β.

The magnitude of the treatment effect needed for it to be considered statistically significant is determined by the variability of the results and by the number of subjects studied. The more variable the data, the larger the difference that must be obtained; the larger the number of subjects, the smaller the treatment difference needed for statistical significance. The same is true regarding the power of the experiment to detect a real treatment effect: the more variable the data, the larger the number of subjects required. In general, small studies often lack the power to detect clinically significant differences in treatment effectiveness; for that reason, such studies are considered by some to be unethical (Collins and MacMahon 2001; Halpern et al. 2002).

Confidence Intervals

The approach to data analysis that has been summarized thus far is the classical approach of *hypothesis testing*, in which a difference in treatment effect that

exceeds a threshold is said to reject the null hypothesis that there is no difference between treatments. Such an approach focuses on *P* values and statistical significance, but it largely ignores the magnitude of any difference found (Sterne and Smith 2001).

An alternative approach that has become popular in recent years involves *confidence intervals* (CIs) (Gardner and Altman 2000). In this approach, the difference in treatment effectiveness between groups in the clinical trial is used to construct a CI. If a 95% CI is constructed, it implies that there is a 95% chance that the true difference in effectiveness lies within that interval. An interval that does not include zero is the equivalent of rejecting the null hypothesis (i.e., the equivalent of a statistically significant result).

There are several advantages to using CIs instead of hypothesis testing (Gardner and Altman 2000; Guyatt et al. 2002c). First, CIs provide a range in which the true treatment effectiveness is expected, with a narrow CI implying a precise estimate of treatment effectiveness. Second, in negative studies in which the null hypothesis is not rejected, CIs may suggest that a clinically important difference is present but that the power of the study to detect it was too low. There is a difference, for example, between a wide CI that barely overlaps zero and a narrow CI that centers on zero. In the first case, the width suggests that the study was too small to provide a precise estimate and that a large treatment difference cannot be excluded. In the second case, the estimate is quite precise and implies that any difference that exists is too small to be clinically important. Finally, CIs are useful in systematic reviews and meta-analyses (see Gray, Chapter 6 in this volume).

Measures of Treatment Effectiveness

There are many different approaches for describing the effectiveness of a treatment (Jaeschke et al. 2002; Sackett et al. 1991). A drug company promoting a new medication may choose the measure that puts the drug in the best light. However, for a clinician choosing a therapy or advising a patient, there is a need for measures that accurately reflect how one treatment compares with either a placebo or another active treatment.

In psychiatric research, especially drug trials, investigators frequently use a variety of rating scales. In reporting the results of a study, they may compare the differences in rating scale scores of patients in the experimental and control groups. Although the use of such rating scales may be necessary for U.S. Food and Drug Administration (FDA) approval and may generate data that can be easily analyzed, they also have limitations. For example, clinicians and patients cannot easily appreciate the practical implications of a small difference on a particular scale.

In contrast, dichotomous outcome measures are more clinically useful than rating scales. Examples of such outcome measures include dying, being readmitted to the hospital, achieving full remission, being rated as "improved" or "much improved," or having at least a 50% decrease in score on a rating scale. These are all measures that most clinicians and patients consider clinically significant and that can be more readily understood than continuous rating scales that yield a numerical score. In addition, the use of such dichotomous outcome measures allows for the calculation of several useful measures of clinical importance. In illustrating these various measures and their calculation, we have used the results of a hypothetical RCT, comparing an antidepressant drug with a placebo for the treatment of major depression; the outcome measure was "remission" (see Table 5–4).

Percentage Response

In our hypothetical experiment, 60% of the patients receiving the antidepressant drug responded. This is the simplest way of expressing the effectiveness of the antidepressant drug; however, it fails to take into account the high percentage of patients who responded to the placebo. To do so, a better measure of treatment response is thus necessary.

TABLE 5–4. Results of hypothetical experiment used to illustrate measures of treatment effect size

Treatment	Not responding (%)	Responding (%)
Placebo	60	40
Antidepressant	40	60

Control event rate (CER)=60%
Experimental event rate (EER)=40%
Relative risk=EER/CER=40/60=0.67
Relative risk reduction=(CER−EER)/CER=20/60=0.33
Odds ratio=[EER/(1−EER)]/[CER(1−CER)]=[(40/60)/(60/40)]=0.45
Absolute risk reduction (ARR)=CER−EER=60%−40%=20%
Number needed to treat=1/ARR=1/(0.2)=5

Relative Risk

In our example, 40% of the patients receiving the placebo responded and 60% of the patients receiving the placebo did not respond. By convention, when relative risk (RR) is used as a measure of treatment effectiveness, results are expressed in terms of a bad outcome (e.g., nonresponse). An effective treatment is therefore one that reduces bad outcomes. With this convention, the percentage of control subjects *not* responding is called the *control event rate* (CER), which in this example is 60%.

For those receiving the antidepressant, 60% of the patients responded, whereas 40% of the patients did not respond. The percentage of experimental subjects *not* responding is called the *experimental event rate* (EER), which in this example is 40%.

Relative risk is the ratio of EER to CER. In this case, RR=0.4/0.6=0.67, which means that patients receiving medication had only two-thirds the nonresponse rate of the placebo group. More effective treatments provide greater reductions in the risk of a negative outcome. RR values for effective treatments vary between 0 and 1, with smaller values indicating more effective treatments.

RR provides a comparison of the experimental and control treatments, but it can be misleading. For example, reducing the nonresponse rate from 90% to 45% yields the same RR as reducing it from 2% to 1%. In the first example, the treatment causes a much greater percentage of patients to respond than in the second example; however, both examples yield the same RR.

Relative Risk Reduction

Relative risk reduction (RRR) is calculated with the formulas (CER–EER)/CER or RRR=1–RR. Using the data in Table 5–4, RRR=0.2/0.6=0.33, which means that the nonresponse rate was decreased by one-third. Like RR, RRR varies between 0 and 1 for effective treatments; however, in this case, larger values (i.e., values closer to 1) indicate a more effective treatment. RRR has the same limitations as RR.

Odds Ratio

The odds ratio (OR) is a measure of treatment effect that is similar to RR. The odds of an event occurring are expressed as the ratio of the probability of the event occurring to the probability of the event not occurring. In our example, the odds of nonresponse are 1.5 (or 60 to 40) in the placebo group and 0.67 (or 40 to 60) in an experimental group. The OR is simply the ratio of the odds of a bad outcome in the experimental group divided by the odds of a bad outcome in a control group: 0.67/1.5=0.45. As with RR, for effective treatments, the OR varies between 0 and 1, smaller values being associated with a greater treatment effect. The OR is often used as an effect measure in meta-analyses because of its statistical properties (Deeks and Altman 2001).

Absolute Risk Reduction

Absolute risk reduction (ARR) is simply the difference between the CER and the EER. Using the data from Table 5–4, ARR=60% –40%=20%, which means that 20% fewer patients taking medication failed to respond; conversely, 20% more patients taking medication responded. Because this is an absolute (not relative) measure, it can be used to estimate the percentage of patients undergoing treatment who will benefit more from the experimental treatment than from the control treatment. ARR for effective treatments varies from 0% to 100% (or 0 and 1, if not expressed as a percentage), with larger values indicating more effective treatments. Unlike RR and RRR, ARR provides a measure of how many patients receiving treatment will benefit from it and thus avoids some of the limitations of these prior measures.

Number Needed to Treat

The measure believed by many to be the best expression of relative treatment effectiveness is number needed to treat (NNT) (Cook and Sackett 1995; Jaeschke et al. 2002; Laupacis et al. 1988; Sackett et al. 1991, 2000; Szatmari 1998). NNT is simply the reciprocal of the ARR. In our example, NNT= 1/0.2=5, which means that for every five patients treated with medication, there will be one less case of nonresponse than if all patients had received the control treatment. Put another way, for every five patients treated with medication, there will be one additional patient who responds to medication who would not have responded to the placebo. The calculation of CIs for NNT is given by Altman (1998) and can be found in Appendix B.

NNT is believed by most clinical epidemiologists to be the least misleading and the most clinically useful measure of treatment effectiveness, although patients sometimes have difficulty understanding the concept (Kristiansen et al. 2002). Inclusion of NNT in the reporting of the results of clinical trials is recommended in the Consolidated Standards of Reporting Trials (CONSORT) guidelines (Altman et al. 2001; Begg et al. 1996) (statement available at www.consort-statement.org). Despite this recommendation, relatively few trials report NNTs (Nuovo et al. 2002), so it is often necessary for the reader to go through the calculations himself or herself with the data presented in a published article.

Examples of NNTs for common therapies for psychiatric disorders are given in Table 5–5. As can be seen, most psychiatric therapies have NNTs in the range of 3 to 6, which means that for every three to six patients treated, there is one good outcome that would not otherwise have occurred. For comparative purposes, in a 5-week follow-up of patients with acute myocardial infusion, using death as an outcome measure, streptokinase infusion had an NNT of 15; in a 5.5-year follow-up of patients with moderate hypertension (diastolic blood pressures of 90–109 mm Hg), using death, stroke, and myocardial infarction as outcomes, antihypertensive drugs had an NNT of 128 (Sackett et al. 2000). Hence psychotropic medications are relatively effective when compared with other classes of drugs used in medicine. As another example, Citrome (2008) used NNT to compare new treatments for depression, schizophrenia, and bipolar disorder.

TABLE 5–5.   Examples of number needed to treat (NNT) for common psychiatric disorders and treatments

Disorder	Treatment comparison	Outcome measure	NNT
Major depression	Antidepressant vs. placebo	50% reduction in Ham-D	3
	IPT vs. clinical management	Recovery	5
	CBT plus antidepressant vs. monotherapy	50% reduction in Ham-D	5
Acute mania	Valproate or lithium vs. placebo	50% reduction in SADS-M	5
Bipolar disorder	Lithium vs. placebo	Relapse	3
Schizophrenia	Antipsychotic vs. placebo	40% reduction in BPRS or "much improved" CGI Scale	2–5
	Family intervention vs. usual care	Relapse	7
Panic disorder	SSRI vs. placebo	Panic free	3–6
Social phobia	Paroxetine vs. placebo	"Much improved" CGI Scale	3
	Group CBT vs. placebo	"Much improved" CGI Scale	3
Obsessive-compulsive disorder	SSRI vs. placebo	35% reduction in Y-BOCS	4–5
Bulimia nervosa	Antidepressant vs. placebo	Remission	9

Note.   BPRS=Brief Psychiatric Rating Scale; CBT=cognitive-behavioral therapy; CGI=Clinical Global Impressions; Ham-D=Hamilton Rating Scale for Depression; IPT=interpersonal psychotherapy; SADS-M=Schedule for Affective Disorders and Schizophrenia, mania component; SSRI=selective serotonin reuptake inhibitor; Y-BOCS=Yale-Brown Obsessive Compulsive Scale.
Source.   Data from Cookson et al. 2002; Geddes and Butler 2001; Hay and Bacaltchuk 2001; McIntosh and Lawrie 2001.

Critical Appraisal Guide for Therapy Studies

In this section of the chapter, we introduce a structured approach to the critical appraisal of therapy studies, which is mirrored in subsequent chapters that deal with other types of studies. The guidelines for appraisal of therapy studies are found in Table 5–6.

Is the Study Valid?

Before considering the results of a study, one must first focus on its "Methods" section to assess the study's validity. The first question to ask is whether the study was randomized with a concealed randomization list. Randomization minimizes bias that might result from patients with different prognoses being enrolled in either the experimental or the control treatment group (Altman et al. 2001; Collins and MacMahon 2001; Fletcher et al. 1996; Jüni et al. 2001; Lacchetti and Guyatt 2002; Sackett et al. 1991, 2000). Studies comparing randomized and nonrandomized trials of the same therapies have noted several instances of therapies that seemed

effective in nonrandomized trials being much less effective or ineffective in randomized studies, although this is not always the case (Ioannidis et al. 2001; Kunz and Oxman 1998; Lacchetti and Guyatt 2002). Of equal importance, however, is that the allocation list is concealed. There have been some instances in which investigators have been able to determine the assignment of the next patient to be enrolled and have used that information to systematically enroll sicker patients into one treatment group (Altman and Schulz 2001). In addition, studies comparing trials in which allocation was concealed with those in which it was not concealed have found important differences in the size of the treatment effect (Altman and Schulz 2001; Jüni et al. 2001; Kunz and Oxman 1998; Lacchetti and Guyatt 2002; Schulz 2000).

The next question to ask is whether subjects and clinicians were blinded to the treatment that was administered. As noted earlier, blinding represents an attempt to prevent observer bias, placebo effects, and experimenter expectancy effects from being responsible for any observed difference between the

TABLE 5–6. Critical appraisal guide for therapy studies

Is the study valid?

Is it a randomized controlled trial?

Was the randomization list concealed?

Were subjects and clinicians blinded to treatment being administered?

Were all subjects enrolled in the trial accounted for?

Were subjects analyzed in the groups to which they were assigned?

Despite randomization, were there clinically important differences between groups at the start of the trial?

Aside from the experimental treatment, were the groups treated equally?

Are the results important?

How large was the treatment effect (e.g., the number needed to treat)?

How precise were the results (e.g., the width of confidence intervals)?

Can the results be applied to my patient?

Is my patient too different from those in the study?

Is the treatment consistent with my patient's values and preferences?

Is the treatment feasible in this setting?

Source.   Adapted from Gray 2002, 2004; Guyatt et al. 2002a; Sackett et al. 2000.

experimental and the control groups. In general, nonblinded studies overestimate the true treatment effect size (Jüni et al. 2001; Schulz 2000). Third, one should check whether all subjects who entered the trial were accounted for at its conclusion and whether they were analyzed in the groups to which they had been randomly assigned.

In 1993, 30 experts, including medical journal editors, clinical trialists, epidemiologists, and methodologists, met with the aim of developing a new scale to assess the quality of RCT reports. However, during preliminary discussions, participants thought that many of the suggested scale items were irrelevant because they were not regularly reported by authors. In fact, accumulating evidence indicated that the quality of reports of RCTs was unsatisfactory (Altman and Doré 1990; Pocock et al. 1987). Therefore, the group began to focus on ways to improve the reporting of RCTs, which resulted in recommendations for the standardized reporting of clinical trials (Working Group on Recommendations for Reporting of Clinical Trials in the Biomedical Literature 1994). In 2001, the group created the CONSORT Statement (www.consort-statement.org) to help authors improve reporting of two parallel-design RCTs by using a checklist and flow diagram (Altman et al. 2001).

Accounting for all subjects is made easier when a flow diagram of subject progress through the phases of a randomized trial is included in the article, as suggested by the CONSORT guidelines (Altman et al. 2001; Moher et al. 2001). This is important because substantial loss of subjects to follow-up can seriously bias the results, an effect referred to as *attrition bias* (Guyatt and Devereaux 2002; Jüni et al. 2001). It is sometimes stated that at least 80% follow-up is sufficient for the results to be valid (Streiner and Geddes 2001), although other authors argue that this rule of thumb is misleading (Guyatt et al. 2002a). Intention-to-treat analysis, which includes data on patients who did not complete the trial in their assigned group, is the preferred method of analyzing the data, although the method has limitations (Altman et al. 2001; Collins and MacMahon 2001; Guyatt and Devereaux 2002; Guyatt et al. 2002a; Jüni et al. 2001; Streiner and Geddes 2001).

Many journals now require clinical trials to include a CONSORT flowchart (available at www .consort-statement.org/index.aspx?o=1031) and to provide evidence that issues raised in the CONSORT statement have been followed.

Many clinical trials are now available through www.clinicaltrials.gov, which includes more than 62,000 trials from 157 countries. To be registered, the trial sponsor needs to complete a detailed description of the study. The interested reader can find how to register a trial at http://prsinfo.clinicaltrials.gov. Trial registries acceptable to the *Archives of General Psychiatry* include www.clinicaltrials.gov, http://isrctn.org, http://actr.org.au, http://trialregister.nl, and www.umin.ac.jp/ctr.

Finally, clinicians should determine whether other differences between the control and the experimental groups could bias the results. For example: Despite randomization, were there significant differences between the two groups at the start of the trial that could have affected the outcome (i.e., confounding)? Aside from the experimental treatment, were the groups treated equally (i.e., no co-intervention)?

Only after the validity has been appraised should one turn to the results. After all, if the results are not valid, it does not matter what they show.

Are the Results Important?

When reviewing the results of a study, clinicians should give some thought as to what would be considered a clinically significant outcome measurement. As noted earlier, these are often dichotomous outcome measures, and NNT should be calculated if it is not given in the results.

Can the Results Be Applied to Other Patients?

The final step in the appraisal process is to assess whether the study results can be applied to other patients. Several considerations enter into this assessment. First, is the patient so different from the patients in the studies that the results do not apply? The question here can be reframed as: "Is the pathobiology of this patient so different from that of the study patients that the results cannot apply?" In general, the answer to this question is "no" (Sackett et al. 1991, 2000; Straus and McAlister 2001). However, quantitative differences may apply. In particular, if a patient's likelihood of improving *without* the experimental treatment is greater than that of the patients in the study, then the patient will receive less benefit from the treatment than expected, according to the calculated NNT (Sackett et al. 2000). Methods of calculating NNT related to outcomes can be found in Appendix B. Furukawa et al. (2002) confirmed the validity of this approach.

Two additional questions must be asked before the clinician applies the treatment to his or her patient. The first is whether the treatment is consistent with the patient's values and preferences. The second is whether the treatment is feasible in the clinician's setting. Assuming that the clinician has identified a valid study which has found an effective treatment that can be applied to his or her patient, the next steps in the EBM process (Table 2–1, Chapter 2) are to apply the treatment and then to evaluate the outcome.

Industry-Sponsored Trials

Industry-sponsored trials are a major source of information about the effectiveness of new medications. A recent review of 397 articles published over 3 years in four psychiatric journals found that 60% were industry supported (Perlis et al. 2005). Astonishingly, a systematic review of drug treatments of insomnia by the Agency for Healthcare Research and Quality found that all but 5 of 56 RCTs were apparently funded by the industry (Buscemi et al. 2007). Industry-sponsored trials accounted for most of the results used in the meta-analysis, and results from the meta-analysis were used to make evidence-based treatment recommendations.

From a marketing standpoint, pharmaceutical companies are interested in showing that their product is equally as effective as competing medications or may have advantages, such as fewer side effects (M. Angell 2004; Safer 2002). New medications also must be shown to be safe. The long-standing concerns about the role of industry in sponsoring trials and presenting biased results were fueled by two articles that showed that many publications related to a new cyclooxygenase (COX) inhibitor attributed primarily or solely to academic investigators were actually written by the sponsoring pharmaceutical company or medical publishing companies hired by the company (Ross et al. 2008) and that the sponsoring pharmaceutical company manipulated the data analysis in two clinical trials to minimize the increased mortality associated with the drug (Psaty and Kronmal 2008). According to several authors, bias in the way industry-sponsored research is conducted and reported is not unusual (Angell 2004, 2008; DeAngelis and Fontanarosa 2008). Because of the importance of the role of industry-sponsored research in establishing the database often used to generate evidence-based guidelines, we review this issue in detail in this chapter.

Safer (2002) identified several ways that pharmaceutical companies can bias the interpretation of the effects of their medication (see Table 5–7).

Using Doses Outside the Usual Range for Competitive Advantage

If a new medication is compared with an older medication prescribed at a higher-than-usual dose and a dose associated with more side effects, then patients taking the older medication will be less likely to continue taking it. For instance, Safer (2002) noted that at least eight industry-sponsored trials have compared a second-generation neuroleptic drug to a fixed high dose of haloperidol (20 mg) or to a haloperidol dose averaging >20 mg/day. Doses of haloperidol exceeding the customary levels of 4–10 mg/day may not produce better clinical results than do doses greater than that range, but they induce more extrapyramidal side effects (EPS) and lead to far more treatment dropouts. Comparing a newer neuroleptic with an older one used at a very high dose also can make the newer medication appear to have lower rates of EPS. However, one might argue that a high dose of the medication used for comparison may ensure that patients receive an adequate dose.

Substantially Altering the Dose Schedule of the Comparison Drug for Competitive Advantage

Industry-sponsored studies comparing two antidepressant drugs may schedule an unusually rapid and substantial dose increase in the one not manufactured by the sponsoring company (Safer 2002). Doses and dose schedules beyond the usual range, particularly early in treatment, may bring an increased rate of side effects. In studies comparing side effects of a new medication with those of an older one, use of a relatively low dose of the new medication may minimize the side effects of the new medication compared with the older one. In judging any industry-sponsored trial, the reader should assess whether the protocol follows standard dosing and if not, why not.

Using Self-Serving Measurement Scales and Making Misleading Conclusions From Measurement Findings

In early studies of risperidone, the investigations used a measure of the "worst extrapyramidal symptoms score," which Safer (2002) argued creates the

TABLE 5–7. Study design issues that can bias the outcome of a study comparing two medications

Using a dose of the comparable drug that is outside of the standard clinical range

Altering the usual dosing schedule of the competing drug

Using misleading research measurement scales

Selecting end points post hoc

Masking unfavorable side effects

Repeatedly publishing the same or similar findings

Selectively highlighting findings favorable to the sponsor

Editorializing in the abstract

Publishing the obvious

Engaging in statistical obfuscation

Selecting subjects and a time frame designed to achieve a favorable outcome

Withholding unfavorable results

Using masked sponsorship

Source. Adapted from Safer 2002.

impression that the medication was not associated with EPS. Alternatively, a nonstandard criterion for interpreting the outcome from a measurement can be misleading.

Selecting the Major Findings and End Points Post Hoc

Safer (2002) noted that some industry-sponsored trials select the end points post hoc. Doing so opens the door to "fishing" for results favorable to the medication. For instance, Jureidini and Tonkin (2003) argued that in a study of the effects of paroxetine on reducing depression, the authors changed the predetermined criteria to a criterion that seemed to favor the medication. However, Keller et al. (2003) responded to Jureidini and Tonkin's criticism by arguing that the field had since considered some of the secondary measures as better than those initially proposed. The CONSORT guidelines require that the primary analyses be specified in advance and followed up in part to avoid such problems. Nevertheless, secondary, exploratory analyses can provide important clues that need to be confirmed with randomized studies.

Masking Unfavorable Side Effects

Safer (2002) reported that sexual side effects from selective serotonin reuptake inhibitor (SSRI) antidepressants ranged from 2% to 73%, depending primarily on whether side effects were elicited merely by open-ended questioning or by a detailed inquiry. Reports by sponsoring pharmaceutical companies may downplay sexual side effects of SSRIs by using open-ended or nonspecific questions about side effects (Zajecka et al. 1999). In one instance, a drug company–sponsored review including more than 3,000 patients receiving SSRIs simply did not list any sexual side effects on its 23-item side-effect table (Preskorn 1997).

Publishing the Same or Similar Results

Safer (2002) noted that pharmaceutical manufacturers may publish the same or similar positive study results, perhaps to increase the visibility of their product. Such practices can be misleading and even have a detrimental effect on one of the key evidence-based medicine practices, the use of meta-analyses. For instance, Huston and Moher (1996) performed a meta-analysis of the effects of the antipsychotic agent risperidone. They identified 20 articles and several unpublished reports describing randomized, double-blind trials, but after a search they described as "vexing," "bewildering," and "intolerably time-consuming," they concluded that there were probably only 7 small trials and 2 large trials, one of the latter being reported "in part, transparently, and not so transparently in six different publications…the authorship was different for each." They wrote: "Multiple renditions of the same information is self-serving, wasteful, abuses the volunteer time of peer reviewers, and can be profoundly misleading; it brings into question the integrity of medical research." An editorial in *JAMA* by Rennie (1999) discussed in depth this problem of publication duplication.

Other Biases

Other biases in industry-sponsored trials include, as noted by Safer (2002), editorializing in the abstract, publishing the obvious, not following standard statistical procedures, including "borderline" significant findings, designing studies that select subjects and a time frame to achieve a favorable outcome, and withholding unfavorable results. The role of masked sponsorship was noted earlier.

Systematic Reviews of Industry-Sponsored Studies

Several reviews of industry-sponsored trials have suggested that there is a systematic bias favoring products that are made by the company funding the research. In one recent review, the authors did not find that studies funded by industry were of poorer quality than those funded by other sources of support, but studies sponsored by pharmaceutical companies were more likely to have outcomes favoring the company's product than were studies with other sponsors (OR=4.05, 95% CI 2.98–5.51; 18 comparisons) (Lexchin et al. 2003). Montgomery et al. (2004) examined randomized clinical trials of second-generation antipsychotics for treating schizophrenia. They noted that "within the industry-funded studies, outcomes of trials involving first authors employed by industry sponsors demonstrated a trend toward second generation over first generation antipsychotic to a greater degree than did trials involving first authors employed outside the industry ($P=0.05$)" (Montgomery et al. 2004).

Reporting study bias is not limited, of course, to the pharmaceutical industry. In the above-mentioned study by Montgomery et al. (2004) questioning industry-sponsored trials, the authors committed several of the errors noted by Safer (2002). They say, for instance, "Non-industry-funded studies showed a trend toward higher quality than industry-funded studies; however, the difference between the two was not significant."

In another analysis of the effects of funding source on outcome, Heres et al. (2006) identified 42 reports of head-to-head comparisons of second-generation antipsychotics. Of these, 33 were sponsored by a pharmaceutical company. In 90% of the studies, the reported overall outcome was in favor of the sponsor's drug. The authors noted that "This pattern resulted in contradictory conclusions across studies when the findings of studies of the same drugs but with different sponsors were compared." Heres and colleagues recommended that peer reviewers should verify whether the abstract really summarizes the overall results of the trial. They noted that in a study sponsored by the manufacturer of olanzapine that compared olanzapine with risperidone, the two medications were not different on 21 of 25 efficacy measures, yet the abstract emphasized the greater efficacy of olanzapine. In contrast, in a study sponsored by the manufacturer of risperidone that compared the same set of agents (risperidone and olanzapine), the two medications were found to be not different on 33 of 37 efficacy measures, including the a priori primary end points of the study, yet the abstract emphasized the greater efficacy of risperidone (Tandon 2006).

Caveat Emptor

In recent years, the rise of clinical trial registries, the requirement that studies meet prespecified standards to be included in medical reviews, the adoption of the CONSORT standards, and the emphasis by medical publishers to address issues like those raised earlier may have reduced potential bias in trials, including those sponsored by the pharmaceutical industry. Nevertheless, the practitioner should be very alert to the potential for bias, particularly given the influence of pharmaceutical representatives in medical education. Dr. Daniel Carlat (2007) described how he had been recruited, as a respected practitioner, to give drug talks and how difficult he found it to question the evidence he had been given to present.

Antidepressants and Suicide Risk

The recent controversy about the potential risk of antidepressants increasing suicidal ideation or risk in adolescents illustrates some of the complex issues related to evaluating evidence. We include it here, in part because the role of the pharmaceutical industry has been highlighted, but also to illustrate many of the limitations of the knowledge base used in evidence-based psychiatry practice.

The possibility that antidepressant medications, especially SSRIs, increase the risk of suicidal behavior was first raised in several case reports of children and adults during the early 1990s (King et al. 1991; Rothschild and Locke 1991; Teicher et al. 1990). In 2003, the U.K. Department of Health warned physicians against prescribing any SSRI antidepressant drug except fluoxetine for depressed youths younger than 18 years. In 2003, the FDA was also concerned about this risk and announced that it was reviewing "a possible increased rate" of suicidal behavior in youths taking paroxetine hydrochloride (U.S. Food and Drug Administration 2003). The FDA recommended that paroxetine not be used in children and adolescents for the treatment of major depressive disorder. On October 15, 2004, the FDA issued a so-

called black-box warning that all antidepressants pose significant risks of suicidality in children and adolescents and that children and adults taking antidepressants should be watched closely for increased suicidal thinking or behavior (U.S. Food and Drug Administration 2004). The warning immediately generated controversy in addition to opening discussion on more general issues of the FDA's role in drug safety.

One researcher believed that the focus for reporting should be on the pharmaceutical industry:

> Why was it left to regulatory bodies to publicize the lack of effectiveness of paroxetine and venlafaxine? The single published placebo controlled trial concluded that paroxetine was effective and safe in adolescent depression. But none of the large negative trials (2 each for paroxetine and venlafaxine) were published, a phenomenon that undermines evidence-based medicine. Pharmaceutical companies seeking regulatory approval are obliged to make the results of all clinical trials they sponsor available to regulatory agencies. However, there is no requirement for these results to be published or even made available to investigators. Those researchers, including myself, who *did* see results of negative paroxetine industry trials were prohibited by nondisclosure contracts from discussing them. (Garland 2004)

The black-box warning was controversial from the outset. Several organizations and researchers began to re-review both the efficacy and the risk of antidepressants used in children and adolescents. In 2003, the American College of Neuropharmacology (ACNP) convened a task force to evaluate the evidence for safety of SSRIs in youths, including reviewing published clinical trials and data from the U.K. Medicines and Healthcare Products Regulatory Agency (MHRA), as well as FDA analyses and reports made public online (Hammad 2004). The review by the ACNP concluded that "fluoxetine is effective in treating depression in children and adolescents" (Mann et al. 2006). The task force also addressed the relation between SSRIs and suicidal behavior in youths. The FDA's meta-analyses of the adverse event report data pooled across all drugs indicated that there was a statistically significant elevation (about twofold) in risk of suicidality for antidepressants relative to placebo (Hammad 2004). However, the ACNP report did not find convincing evidence that SSRIs increased the suicide rate in youths. The World Psychiatric Association (Möller et al. 2008) undertook an extensive review of the database and concluded that "antidepressants, including SSRIs, carry a small risk of inducing suicidal thoughts and suicide attempts, in age groups below 25 years."

Klein (2006) argued that the FDA relied on a poorly defined "surrogate measure" of completed suicide and noted that the validation of surrogate measures is very difficult when used to predict very rare events. He also noted that a major potential source of information of medications—that is, of their use "postmarketing"—is deeply flawed because it can rely on a few events (such as completed suicides) without considering the more complicated epidemiologic issues that would provide a more accurate position of risk (e.g., what is the relative risk in the population).

Posner et al. (2007) have developed the Columbia Classification Algorithm of Suicide Assessment (C-CASA) to classify "suicidal events" in terms of suicidal ideation, preparation toward suicide attempt, or completed suicide. In an analysis of 25 pediatric antidepressant trials, they found that the system was reliable. The FDA safety analysis of the risk of suicidality in a depressed pediatric sample that used these C-CASA ratings (Hammad et al. 2006) found reduced risk estimates when compared with earlier FDA estimates that relied on the pharmaceutical label. The practitioner faced with the "evidence" encounters a very complicated and confusing issue.

The warnings had an effect on reducing antidepressant use (Olfson et al. 2008). During the prewarning study period, a 36.0% per year ($P<0.001$) increase in total youth (ages 6–17 years) antidepressant use was reported, which was followed by decreases of 0.8% per year ($P=0.85$) and 9.6% per year ($P=0.21$) during the paroxetine and black-box warning study periods, respectively. The difference in trends between the prewarning and the paroxetine warning periods was significant ($P<0.001$). Paroxetine use in young people also significantly increased during the prewarning study period (30.0% per year; $P<0.001$) before significantly declining during the paroxetine warning study period (–44.2% per year; $P<0.001$) (Olfson et al. 2008).

There has been a more recent concern about raised suicide rates in adolescents (Bridge et al. 2008). For males and females, ages 10–19, rates of suicide increased from 2003 to 2004. Although for males, the suicide rate decreased by 1.8% between 2004 and 2005 (7.13 to 7.00 per 100,000), rates of suicide in 2004 and 2005 were still significantly greater than predicted by the 1996–2003 trend (2004 95% prediction interval [PI] 5.90–6.90; 2005 95% PI 5.63–6.66). The rate of suicide for females ages 10–19 years decreased by 16.7% between 2004 and 2005 (2.22 to 1.85 per 100,000); both 2004 and 2005 rates were significantly greater than the expected rates (2004 95% PI 1.18–1.67; 2005 95% PI 1.11–1.62). Although a reduction in antidepressant use needs to be considered as one factor, Bridge et al. (2008) note:

> Studies to identify causal agents are important next steps. These studies should involve comprehensive assessment of individual-level exposure and outcome data, as aggregate data alone cannot establish causal links. Possible factors to consider include changes in the prevalence of known risk factors (e.g., alcohol use, access to firearms), the influence of Internet social networks, higher rates of untreated depression in the wake of recent boxed warnings on antidepressants and increases in suicide among US troops, some being older adolescents.

The ACNP task force recommended the continued use of fluoxetine as an effective and readily available treatment for major depression in youth suicide, suicidal thinking, and plans for suicide. They also recommended that ongoing monitoring of suicidal thoughts in patients taking antidepressants is necessary.

The American Academy of Child and Adolescent Psychiatry (AACAP) urged the FDA not to issue a black-box warning against the use of all antidepressants for the treatment of depression in children and adolescents, noting that "Efficacy and safety data on pediatric antidepressant use has been the subject of ongoing review. The research and its reviews show efficacy, while the signal for the risks of increased suicidal thinking and self-harm events is not strong and can be monitored" (Sarles 2004). AACAP and the American Psychiatric Association (n.d.) also issued guidelines for physicians related to this recommendation.

What is the truth about the risk-benefit ratio of antidepressant use in depressed children and adolescents? Are antidepressants beyond fluoxetine effective in reducing depressive symptoms in children? In adolescents? Do they increase suicidal thoughts?

Behaviors? Completed events? Is the reduction in antidepressant use responsible for the rise in suicide rates in recent years? The uncertainty of the answers to these questions reflects the limits of evidence-based practice and the challenges to the practitioner in using evidence-based recommendations.

References

Altman DG: Practical Statistics for Medical Research. Boca Raton, FL, Chapman & Hall, 1991

Altman DG: Confidence intervals for the number needed to treat. BMJ 317:1309–1312, 1998

Altman DG, Doré CJ: Randomisation and baseline comparisons in clinical trials. Lancet 335:149–153, 1990

Altman DG, Schulz KF: Statistics notes: concealing treatment allocation in randomised trials. BMJ 323:446–447, 2001

Altman DG, Schulz KF, Moher D, et al: The revised CONSORT statement for reporting randomized trials: explanation and elaboration. Ann Intern Med 134:663–694, 2001

American Psychiatric Association (APA), American Academy of Child and Adolescent Psychiatry (AACAP): The use of medication in treating childhood and adolescent depression: information for physicians. n.d. Available at: http://www.parentsmedguide.org/physiciansmedguide.pdf. Accessed June 8, 2009

Angell A: The Truth About the Drug Companies: How They Deceive Us and What to Do About It. New York, Random House, 2004

Angell A: Industry-sponsored clinical research: a broken system. JAMA 300:1069–1071, 2008

Badenoch D, Heneghan C: Evidence-Based Medicine Toolkit. London, BMJ Books, 2002

Begg C, Cho M, Eastwood S, et al: Improving the quality of reporting of randomized controlled trials: the CONSORT statement. JAMA 276:637–639, 1996

Bland M: An Introduction to Medical Statistics, 3rd Edition. Oxford, UK, Oxford University Press, 2000

Bridge JA, Greenhouse JB, Weldon AH, et al: Suicide trends among youths aged 10 to 19 years in the United States, 1996–2005. JAMA 300:1025–1026, 2008

Buscemi N, Vandermeer B, Friesen C, et al: The efficacy and safety of drug treatments for chronic insomnia in adults: a meta-analysis of RCTs. J Gen Intern Med 22:1335–1350, 2007

Carlat D: Dr. Drug Rep. The New York Times Magazine, November 25, 2007

Chaput de Saintonge DM, Herxheimer A: Harnessing placebo effects in health care. Lancet 344:995–998, 1994

Charney DS, Nemeroff CB, Lewis L, et al: National Depressive and Manic-Depressive Association consensus statement on the use of placebo in clinical trials of mood disorders. Arch Gen Psychiatry 59:262–270, 2002

Citrome L: Compelling or irrelevant? Using number needed to treat can help decide. Acta Psychiatr Scand 117:412–419, 2008

Collins R, MacMahon S: Reliable assessment of the effects of treatment on mortality and major morbidity, I: clinical trials. Lancet 357:373–380, 2001

Cook RJ, Sackett DL: The number needed to treat: a clinically useful measure of treatment effect. BMJ 310:452–454, 1995

Cookson J, Taylor D, Katona C: The Use of Drugs in Psychiatry: The Evidence From Psychopharmacology, 5th Edition. London, Gaskell, 2002

Crow R, Gage H, Hampson S, et al: The placebo effect: methodological process and implications of a structured review, in The Advanced Handbook of Methods in Evidence Based Healthcare. Edited by Stevens A, Abrams K, Brazier J, et al. London, Sage, 2001, pp 73–89

Cummings SR, Grady D, Hulley SB: Designing an experiment: clinical trials I, in Designing Clinical Research, 2nd Edition. Edited by Hulley SB, Cummings SR, Browner WS, et al. Philadelphia, PA, Lippincott Williams & Wilkins, 2001, pp 143–155

Daly LE, Bourke GJ: Interpretation and Uses of Medical Statistics, 5th Edition. Oxford, UK, Blackwell Scientific, 2000

DeAngelis CD, Fontanarosa PB: Impugning the integrity of medical science: the adverse effects of industry influence. JAMA 299:1833–1835, 2008

Deeks JJ, Altman DG: Effect measures for meta-analysis of trials with binary outcomes, in Systematic Reviews in Health Care: Meta-Analyses in Context, 2nd Edition. Edited by Egger M, Smith GD, Altman DG. London, BMJ Books, 2001, pp 313–335

Devereaux PJ, Manns BJ, Ghali WA, et al: Physician interpretations and textbook definitions of blinding terminology in randomized controlled trials. JAMA 285:2000–2003, 2001

Devereaux PJ, Bhandari M, Montori VM, et al: Double blind, you have been voted off the island! Evid Based Ment Health 5:36–37, 2002

Easterbrook PJ, Berlin JA, Gopalan R, et al: Publication bias in clinical research. Lancet 337:867–872, 1991

Everitt BS: Statistical Methods for Medical Investigations. New York, Oxford University Press, 1989

Fletcher RH, Fletcher SW, Wagner EH: Clinical Epidemiology: The Essentials, 3rd Edition. Baltimore, MD, Williams & Wilkins, 1996

Furukawa TA, Guyatt GA, Griffith LE: Can we individualize the "number needed to treat"? An empirical study of summary effect measures in meta-analyses. Int J Epidemiol 31:72–76, 2002

Gardner MJ, Altman DG: Confidence intervals rather than P values, in Statistics With Confidence, 2nd Edition. Edited by Altman DG, Machin D, Bryant TN, et al. London, BMJ Books, 2000, pp 15–27

Garland EJ: Facing the evidence: antidepressant treatment in children and adolescents. CMAJ 170:489–491, 2004

Geddes J, Butler R: Depressive disorders. Clin Evid 6:726–742, 2001

Gray GE: Evidence-based medicine: an introduction for psychiatrists. J Psychiatr Pract 8:5–13, 2002

Gray GE: Concise Guide to Evidence-Based Psychiatry. Washington, DC, American Psychiatric Publishing, 2004

Greenhalgh T: How to Read a Paper: The Basics of Evidence Based Medicine, 2nd Edition. London, BMJ Books, 2001

Guyatt G: Therapy and harm: why study results mislead—bias and random error, in Users' Guides to the Medical Literature: A Manual for Evidence-Based Clinical Practice. Edited by Guyatt G, Rennie D. Chicago, IL, AMA Press, 2002, pp 223–231

Guyatt G, Devereaux PJ: Therapy and validity: the principle of intention-to-treat, in Users' Guides to the Medical Literature: A Manual for Evidence-Based Clinical Practice. Edited by Guyatt G, Rennie D. Chicago, IL, AMA Press, 2002, pp 267–273

Guyatt G, Cook D, Devereaux PJ, et al: Therapy, in Users' Guides to the Medical Literature: A Manual for Evidence-Based Clinical Practice. Edited by Guyatt G, Rennie D. Chicago, IL, AMA Press, 2002a, pp 55–79

Guyatt G, Haynes B, Jaeschke R, et al: Introduction: the philosophy of evidence-based medicine, in Users' Guides to the Medical Literature: A Manual for Evidence-Based Clinical Practice. Edited by Guyatt G, Rennie D. Chicago, IL, AMA Press, 2002b, pp 3–12

Guyatt G, Walter S, Cook D, et al: Therapy and understanding the results: confidence intervals, in Users' Guides to the Medical Literature: A Manual for Evidence-Based Clinical Practice. Edited by Guyatt G, Rennie D. Chicago, IL, AMA Press, 2002c, pp 339–349

Halpern SD, Karlawish JHT, Berlin JA: The continuing unethical conduct of underpowered clinical trials. JAMA 288:358–362, 2002

Hammad TA: Review and evaluation of clinical data. August 16, 2004. Available at: http://www.fda.gov/ohrms/dockets/ac/04/briefing/2004-4065b1-10-TAB08-Hammads-Review.pdf. Accessed June 9, 2009

Hammad TA, Laughren T, Racoosin J: Suicidality in pediatric patients treated with antidepressant drugs. Arch Gen Psychiatry 63:332–333, 2006

Hay P, Bacaltchuk J: Bulimia nervosa. Clin Evid 6:715–725, 2001

Hennekens CH, Buring JE, Mayrent SL: Epidemiology in Medicine. Boston, MA, Little, Brown, 1987

Heres S, Davis J, Maino K, et al: Why olanzapine beats risperidone, risperidone beats quetiapine, and quetiapine beats olanzapine: an exploratory analysis of head-to-head comparison studies of second-generation antipsychotics. Am J Psychiatry 163:185–194, 2006

Holden JD: Hawthorne effects and research into professional practice. J Eval Clin Pract 7:65–70, 2001

Huston P, Moher D: Redundancy, disaggregation, and the integrity of medical research. Lancet 347:1024–1026, 1996

Ioannidis JPA, Haidich A-B, Pappa M, et al: Comparison of evidence of treatment effects in randomized and nonrandomized studies. JAMA 286:821–830, 2001

Jadad A: Randomised Controlled Trials. London, BMJ Books, 1998

Jaeschke R, Guyatt G, Barratt A: Therapy and understanding the results: measures of association, in Users' Guides to the Medical Literature: A Manual for Evidence-Based Clinical Practice. Edited by Guyatt G, Rennie D. Chicago, IL, AMA Press, 2002, pp 351–368

Jüni P, Altman DG, Egger M: Systematic reviews in health care: assessing the quality of controlled clinical trials. BMJ 323:42–46, 2001

Jureidini J, Tonkin A: Paroxetine in major depression (letter). J Am Acad Child Adolesc Psychiatry 42:514, 2003

Kaptchuk TJ: Powerful placebo: the dark side of the randomised clinical trial. Lancet 351:1722–1725, 1998

Keller MB, Ryan R, Strober M, et al: Paroxetine in major depression: Dr. Keller et al reply. J Am Acad Child Adolesc Psychiatry 42:514–515, 2003

King RA, Riddle MA, Chappell PB, et al: Emergence of self-destructive phenomena in children and adolescents during fluoxetine treatment. J Am Acad Child Adolesc Psychiatry 30:179–186, 1991

Klein DF: The flawed basis for FDA post-marketing safety decisions: the example of anti-depressants and children. Neuropsychopharmacology 31:689–699, 2006

Kristiansen IS, Gyrd-Hansen D, Nexoe J, et al: Number needed to treat: easily understood and intuitively meaningful? Theoretical considerations and a randomized trial. J Clin Epidemiol 55:888–892, 2002

Kunz R, Oxman AD: The unpredictability paradox: review of empirical comparisons of randomised and non-randomised clinical trials. BMJ 317:1185–1190, 1998

Lacchetti C, Guyatt G: Therapy and validity: surprising results of randomized controlled trials, in Users' Guides to the Medical Literature: A Manual for Evidence-Based Clinical Practice. Edited by Guyatt G, Rennie D. Chicago, IL, AMA Press, 2002, pp 247–265

Laporte J-R, Figueras A: Placebo effects in psychiatry. Lancet 344:1206–1209, 1994

Laupacis A, Sackett DL, Roberts RS: An assessment of clinically useful measures of the consequences of treatment. N Engl J Med 318:1728–1733, 1988

Lexchin J, Bro LA, Djulbegovic B, et al: Pharmaceutical industry sponsorship and research outcome and quality: systematic review. BMJ 326:1167–1170, 2003

Mann JJ, Emslie G, Baldessarini R, et al: ACNP Task Force report on SSRIs and suicidal behavior in youth. Neuropsychopharmacology 31:473–492, 2006

McIntosh A, Lawrie S: Schizophrenia. Clin Evid 6:776–797, 2001

Moher D, Schulz KF, Altman D: The CONSORT statement: revised recommendation for improving the quality of reports of parallel-group randomized trials. JAMA 285:1987–1991, 2001

Möller HJ, Baldwin DS, Goodwin G, et al: Do SSRIs or antidepressants in general increase suicidality? WPA Section on Pharmacopsychiatry: consensus statement. Eur Arch Psychiatry Clin Neurosci 258 (suppl 3):3–23, 2008

Montgomery JH, Byerly M, Carmody T, et al: An analysis of the effect of funding source in randomized clinical trials of second generation antipsychotics for the treatment of schizophrenia. Control Clin Trials 25:598–612, 2004

Montori V, Guyatt G: Summarizing the evidence: publication bias, in Users' Guides to the Medical Literature: A Manual for Evidence-Based Clinical Practice. Edited by Guyatt G, Rennie D. Chicago, IL, AMA Press, 2002, pp 529–538

Montori VM, Bhandari M, Devereaux PJ, et al: In the dark: the reporting of blinding status in randomized controlled trials. J Clin Epidemiol 55:787–790, 2002

Nuovo J, Melnikow J, Chang D: Reporting number needed to treat and absolute risk reduction in randomized controlled trials. JAMA 287:2813–2814, 2002

Olfson M, Marcus SC, Druss BG: Effects of Food and Drug Administration warnings on antidepressant use in a national sample. Arch Gen Psychiatry 65:94–101, 2008

Perlis RH, Perlis CS, Wu Y, et al: Industry sponsorship and financial conflict of interest in the reporting of clinical trials in psychiatry. Am J Psychiatry 162:1957–1960, 2005

Peto R, Pike MC, Armitage P, et al: Design and analysis of randomized clinical trials requiring prolonged observation of each patient, I: introduction and design. Br J Cancer 34:585–612, 1976

Pocock SJ, Hughes MD, Lee RJ: Statistical problems in the reporting of clinical trials: a survey of three medical journals. N Engl J Med 317:426–432, 1987

Posner K, Oquendo MA, Gould M, et al: Columbia Classification Algorithm of Suicide Assessment (C-CASA): classification of suicidal events in the FDA's pediatric suicidal risk analysis of antidepressants. Am J Psychiatry 164:1035–1043, 2007

Preskorn SH: Clinically relevant pharmacology of selective serotonin reuptake inhibitors: an overview with emphasis on pharmacokinetics and effects on oxidative drug metabolism. Clin Pharmacokinet 32 (suppl 1):1–21, 1997

Psaty BM, Kronmal RA: Reporting mortality findings in trials of rofecoxib for Alzheimer disease or cognitive impairment: a case study based on documents from rofecoxib litigation. JAMA 299:1813–1817, 2008

Rennie D: Fair conduct and fair reporting of clinical trials. JAMA 282:1766–1768, 1999

Rosenthal R, Jacobson L: Pygmalion in the Classroom. New York, Holt, Rinehart & Winston, 1968

Rosenthal R, Rosnow RL: Essentials of Behavioral Research: Methods and Data Analysis, 2nd Edition. Boston, MA, McGraw-Hill, 1991

Ross JS, Hill KP, Egilman DS, et al: Guest authorship and ghostwriting in publications related to rofecoxib: a case study of industry documents from rofecoxib litigation. JAMA 299:1800–1812, 2008

Rothschild AJ, Locke CA: Reexposure to fluoxetine after serious suicide attempts by three patients: the role of akathisia. J Clin Psychiatry 52:491–493, 1991

Sackett DL, Haynes RB, Guyatt GH, et al: Clinical Epidemiology: A Basic Science for Clinical Medicine, 2nd Edition. Boston, MA, Little, Brown, 1991

Sackett DL, Straus SE, Richardson WS, et al: Evidence-Based Medicine: How to Practice and Teach EBM, 2nd Edition. New York, Churchill Livingstone, 2000

Safer DJ: Design and reporting modifications in industry-sponsored comparative psychopharmacology trials. J Nerv Ment Dis 190:583–592, 2002

Sarles RM: AACAP comment on pending pediatric antidepressants warning. September 28, 2004. Available at: http://www.aacap.org/cs/root/resources_for_families/psychiatric_medication/aacap_comment_on_pending_pediatric_antidepressants_warning. Accessed June 8, 2009

Schulz KF: Assessing allocation concealment and blinding in randomised controlled trials: why bother? Evid Based Ment Health 3:4–5, 2000

Sitthi-amorn C, Poshyachinda V: Bias. Lancet 342:286–288, 1993

Song F, Eastwood A, Gilbody S, et al: Publication and related biases, in The Advanced Handbook of Methods in Evidence Based Healthcare. Edited by Stevens A, Abrams K, Brazier J, et al. London, Sage, 2001, pp 371–390

Sterne JAC, Smith GD: Sifting the evidence: what's wrong with significance tests? BMJ 322:226–231, 2001

Straus SE, McAlister F: Applying the results of trials and systematic reviews to our individual patients. Evid Based Ment Health 4:6–7, 2001

Streiner D, Geddes J: Intention to treat analysis in clinical trials when there are missing data. Evid Based Ment Health 4:70–71, 2001

Szatmari P: Some useful concepts and terms used in articles about treatment. Evid Based Ment Health 1:39–40, 1998

Tandon R: Comparing antipsychotic efficacy. Am J Psychiatry 163:1645, 2006

Teicher MH, Gold C, Cole JO: Emergence of intense suicidal preoccupation during fluoxetine treatment. Am J Psychiatry 147:207–210, 1990

U.S. Food and Drug Administration: FDA statement regarding the anti-depressant Paxil for pediatric population (FDA Talk Paper). June 19, 2003. Available at: http://www.fda.gov/bbs/topics/ANSWERS/2003/ANS01230.html. Accessed June 8, 2009

U.S. Food and Drug Administration: Worsening depression and suicidality in patients being treated with antidepressant (FDA Public Health Advisory). March 22, 2004. Available at: http://www.fda.gov/Drugs/DrugSafety/PublicHealthAdvisories/ucm161696.htm. Accessed August 11, 2009

Walsh BT, Seidman SN, Sysko R, et al: Placebo response in studies of major depression: variable, substantial, and growing. JAMA 287:1840–1847, 2002

Woods SW, Stolar M, Sernyak MJ, et al: Consistency of atypical antipsychotic superiority to placebo in recent clinical trials. Biol Psychiatry 49:64–70, 2001

Working Group on Recommendations for Reporting of Clinical Trials in the Biomedical Literature: Call for comments on a proposal to improve reporting of clinical trials in the biomedical literature. Ann Intern Med 121:894–895, 1994

Yudkin PL, Stratton IM: How to deal with regression to the mean in intervention studies. Lancet 347:241–243, 1996

Zajecka J, Amsterdam JD, Quitkin FM, et al: Changes in adverse events reported by patients during 6 months of fluoxetine therapy. J Clin Psychiatry 60:389–394, 1999

Systematic Reviews and Meta-Analyses

Gregory E. Gray, M.D., Ph.D.

In Chapter 5, Taylor and I discussed individual studies of therapies. As we pointed out in that chapter, both false-positive and false-negative results can occur in clinical trials because of chance and bias. In particular, false-negative results are common because studies are often too small to detect important treatment effects. As a result, when attempting to answer a clinical question, it is best not to depend on the results of a single clinical trial. It is preferable instead to "average out" the results of all such clinical trials related to a specific clinical question because this will give a better estimate of the treatment effect than will the results of any single study. This is exactly what is done in a meta-analysis, and it is why systematic reviews rank at the top of the evidence hierarchy (Table 4–1, Chapter 4).

Narrative Reviews Versus Systematic Reviews

In the typical *journalistic* or *narrative* review article, the author attempts to present a coherent review of a topic, selectively citing the literature to support the statement made in the article. When studies of a treatment are not in agreement, the author of the review may tally the positive and negative results (sometimes called *vote counting*), indicating that controversy exists and that more research is needed to resolve the issue.

Although such reviews are common in medical journals (Rochon et al. 2002), they are often misleading, reflecting the author's biases in selectively reviewing the literature (D.J. Cook et al. 1998; Egger et al. 2001c; Greenhalgh 2001). Such reviews may contribute to delays in implementing changes in clinical practice that are based on important research findings (Egger et al. 2001c).

TABLE 6–1.   Steps in conducting a systematic review

1. **Formulate the question**

2. **Locate studies**

    Online databases (e.g., MEDLINE, EMBASE)

    Registers of clinical trials:

      ClinicalTrials.gov

      Cochrane Central Register of Controlled Trials

      *meta*Register of Controlled Trials

    Contact authors or manufacturers

    Check reference lists

    Perform manual searches

3. **Assess study quality**

    Rating scales

    Two or more reviewers

4. **Extract and summarize the data**

    Tables

    Forest plots

    Pooled effect size and confidence intervals

The systematic review is a better alternative to the traditional review (D.J. Cook et al. 1998; Egger et al. 2001c; Greenhalgh 2001). Such a review focuses on a specific clinical question, involves a comprehensive literature search, and often combines the study results mathematically through meta-analytic techniques (D.J. Cook et al. 1998).

Conducting a Systematic Review

The steps involved in conducting a systematic review are summarized in Table 6–1 and are described briefly in the following subsections. Readers who want more detail about the conduct of systematic reviews are referred to several textbooks (Clarke and Oxman 2002; Egger et al. 2001b; Glasziou et al. 2001). The National Health Service Centre for Reviews and Dissemination (2001) publishes a guide for systematic reviews that can be found at www.york.ac.uk/inst/crd/report4.htm.

Formulate the Question

The first step in the process is formulating the question. The process is similar to that of the evidence-based medicine (EBM) model (see Chapter 2) and involves a similar 4-part PICO question (patient/problem, intervention, comparison, and outcome; see Chapter 3).

Locate Studies

The second step in the process involves finding all of the relevant studies. Such a search involves using the online databases described in Chapter 4, but using filters for *sensitivity* (rather than for *specificity*) (Glasziou et al. 2001; Robinson and Dickersin 2002). Such a strategy will, however, miss many early (pre-1990) studies, non-English-language studies, and unpublished studies, so additional effort may be needed to identify such studies (Egger and Smith 1998; Egger et al. 2001a; Glasziou et al. 2001; Lefebvre and Clarke 2001). Methods that authors undertake to identify such studies include contacting authors of published studies or manufacturers of drugs, checking reference lists of published studies or prior reviews ("snowballing"), manually searching journals or proceedings abstracts that are not abstracted in MEDLINE or similar databases, and checking databases of clinical trials (Glasziou et al. 2001; Helmer et al. 2001; Lefebvre and Clarke 2001). The latter include the Cochrane Central Register of Controlled

Trials (available at www.mrw.interscience.wiley.com; also as part of Ovid's Evidence-Based Medicine Reviews database) and the *meta*Register of Controlled Trials (www.controlled-trials.com/mrct). If such measures are not taken, several sources of bias may influence the results of the review, including publication bias and language bias (Table 6–2).

Some meta-analyses rely on unpublished data or data requested from an investigator. Because negative studies may be more difficult to publish than positive studies (Dwan et al. 2008), a careful acquisition of unpublished data from well-conducted studies would allow for a more accurate appraisal of the effects of an intervention than simply using published studies. For instance, Turner et al. (2008) obtained reviews from the U.S. Food and Drug Administration (FDA) for studies of 12 antidepressant agents involving 12,564 patients. They then tried to identify matching publications in the medical literature. The effect size derived from the published reports was compared with the effect size derived from the entire FDA data set. About 74 FDA-registered studies (31%), accounting for 3,449 study participants, were not published. A total of 37 studies reviewed by the FDA as having positive results were published; only 1 study viewed as positive was not published. Studies viewed by the FDA as having negative or questionable results were, with three exceptions, either not published (22 studies) or published in a way that, in the opinion of Turner et al. (2008), conveyed a positive outcome. According to the published literature, it appeared that 94% of the trials conducted were positive. By contrast, the FDA analysis showed that 51% were positive. Separate meta-analyses of the FDA and journal data sets showed that the increase in effect size ranged from 11% to 69% for individual drugs and was 32% overall. One cannot assume that a review of published pharmaceutical studies represents the best estimate of the effect of the medication.

Publication bias, also known as the *file drawer problem*, refers to a tendency to preferentially publish "positive" results (Egger and Smith 1998; Egger et al. 2001a; Montori and Guyatt 2002; Montori et al. 2000; Rosenthal 1979; Sterne et al. 2001). Although it is clear that publication bias occurs, the reasons for it are a topic of some debate, but they include decisions by the investigators, journal editors and reviewers, and pharmaceutical company influences (Egger and Smith 1998; Egger et al. 2001a; Montori

TABLE 6–2.   Types of reporting bias in systematic reviews

Type of bias	Description
Publication bias	Results are more apt to be published if they are significant.
Time lag bias	Significant results are published sooner than nonsignificant results.
Language bias	Significant results are submitted to English-language journals, nonsignificant results to non-English-language journals.
Database bias	Studies with significant results are more likely to be published in a journal that is indexed in a database.
Citation bias	Likelihood of article being cited depends on results.
Duplicate publication bias	Results of study appear in more than one publication.
Outcome reporting bias	Selective reporting of some study results.

Source.   Adapted from Egger and Smith 1998; Egger et al. 2001a.

and Guyatt 2002; Montori et al. 2000; Olson et al. 2002; Song et al. 2001; Stern and Simes 1997; Thornton and Lee 2000).

Language bias can occur if English-language journals publish a greater proportion of positive studies than do non-English-language journals. Such a bias could occur if foreign investigators preferentially submit positive findings to English-language journals (Egger and Smith 1998; Egger et al. 2001a; Song et al. 2001). *Location bias*, a similar type of bias, refers to the tendency to publish lower-quality positive studies of complementary medicine in low-impact journals (Pittler et al. 2000). The extent to which language and location bias occurs seems to vary, depending on the medical specialty and the disease in question (Jüni et al. 2002; Moher et al. 2000b).

Assess Study Quality

Because the goal of the search strategy is to be as inclusive as possible to avoid missing relevant studies, a search typically will identify numerous studies, many of which are either irrelevant or of poor quality. Including such irrelevant or poor-quality studies in the review and subsequent meta-analysis yields misleading results. Statisticians refer to this as "garbage in, garbage out."

As was discussed in Chapter 5, evidence from less rigorously designed studies is more apt to be biased and misleading than is evidence from more rigorously designed studies (Greenhalgh 2001; Guyatt 2002; Lacchetti and Guyatt 2002; Schulz et al. 1995). It is therefore necessary to appraise the studies identified in the search and to limit further analysis to

those studies that meet certain quality criteria (Jüni et al. 2001). The method of doing so is similar to the approach used in Chapter 5 to appraise a randomized controlled trial (RCT). A standardized approach to appraisal, generally involving two reviewers, should be used to avoid biasing the review (Glasziou et al. 2001; Moher et al. 2001). A variety of instruments for rating the quality of studies have been developed for this purpose, but there is no single best instrument (Jüni et al. 2001; West et al. 2002).

Specific study quality aspects may have a greater effect on estimates of treatment effect than others, but this depends on the particular disease and treatment in question (Balk et al. 2002). Nonrandomized trials, trials with inadequate allocation concealment, and unblinded trials tend to overestimate the magnitude of a treatment's effectiveness, although this is not uniformly true for all diseases and their treatments (Altman and Schulz 2001; Ioannidis et al. 2001; Jüni et al. 2001; Kjaergard et al. 2001; Kunz and Oxman 1998; Lacchetti and Guyatt 2002; Schulz 2000). As a general rule, though, selecting higher-quality studies will lead to a less biased and generally less optimistic view of a treatment's effectiveness.

In the process of appraising study quality, an attempt also should be made to identify duplicate or overlapping publications. These can occur, for example, if preliminary data are first published, followed by a second (more complete) publication. It can also occur if different outcome measures are each presented in a separate publication. If such duplicate or overlapping publications are not identified, the same study may be overrepresented in any meta-analysis, a result known as *multiple publication bias* (Egger and Smith 1998; Tramer et al. 1997).

Extract and Summarize the Data

Once studies meeting the quality criteria are identified, data are abstracted. Such data include methodological details about the study population, intervention, and outcome measures, as well as study results. Such data are typically presented in tabular form in the review, with numerical results often displayed graphically and combined in a meta-analysis. A list of studies that were identified, appraised, and excluded from the review is generally included in the review, along with the reasons for exclusion.

Time and Effort Involved in Systematic Reviews

The process described earlier is conceptually simple; however, it is obviously quite time-consuming, especially if the literature search identifies many studies that then must be assessed for quality. Allen and Olkin (1999) found that systematic review requires 200–2,500 person-hours of effort (median=1,110 person-hours). About one-half of this effort is spent on the search and retrieval process.

A systematic review is generally a group effort because of the considerable effort involved in its production. Two international collaborative efforts that are involved in producing systematic reviews are the Cochrane Collaboration and the Campbell Collaboration (Antes and Oxman 2001; Cochrane Collaboration 1997; Davies and Boruch 2001).

Meta-Analysis

Meta-analysis refers to the statistical integration of the results of several independent studies (Egger and Smith 1997). In this section, I provide a short non-mathematical overview of meta-analysis. Readers who want an in-depth discussion are referred to several excellent texts (Egger et al. 2001b; Petitti 2000; Sutton et al. 2000).

Meta-analysis involves more than "vote tallying" or merely taking a simple average of the results of various studies. Instead, meta-analysis gives more weight to large studies than to small studies because the results of small studies are subject to more random variability (see Chapter 5). The specific methods by which this is accomplished depend on

whether the outcome variable is dichotomous or continuous.

Dichotomous Outcome Measures

As was discussed in Chapter 5, dichotomous outcome measures, such as dying, being readmitted to the hospital, achieving full remission, being rated as "improved" or "much improved," or having at least a 50% decrease in score on a rating scale, are often among the most clinically useful and readily understandable measures. Dichotomous measures are also favored in systematic reviews because of the ease of combining the data in meta-analyses.

Odds Ratio

The measure of treatment effect that is most commonly used in systematic reviews and meta-analyses is the odds ratio (OR). Calculation of the OR was described in Chapter 5. By convention, the outcome measures used in meta-analysis are adverse outcomes; therefore, effective treatments have ORs of 1.0 or less.

The reason that the OR is so frequently used in meta-analyses is that there are several straightforward methods of combining ORs from multiple studies (Deeks et al. 2001; Petitti 2000; Sutton et al. 2000). The two most common methods are the Mantel-Haenszel method (Mantel and Haenszel 1959) and the Peto method (Yusuf et al. 1985). Both methods involve producing a weighted average OR, with larger trials (which have narrower confidence intervals [CIs] for their ORs) being given greater weight than smaller trials (with wider CIs for their ORs), although they differ in the exact weighting used. Both methods assume a "fixed effects" model (see subsection "Fixed and Random Effects Models" later in this chapter). The DerSimonian and Laird (1986) method, used under the "random effects" model, gives somewhat more weight to smaller studies and produces a wider CI for the pooled OR estimate than do the other two methods.

The drawback of using the OR as a measure of treatment effectiveness is that it is not as easily interpretable as relative risk (RR) or number needed to treat (NNT) (Deeks and Altman 2001). Although the OR approximates RR when the frequency of rare outcomes is low (<10%), the two measures diverge as the outcome frequency increases, with the OR overestimating RR (Egger et al. 1997a). Under such circumstances, misinterpretation of an OR as RR will lead the reader to overestimate or underestimate the effects of a treatment (Deeks and Altman 2001).

Number Needed to Treat

Although NNT is believed by many to be the best expression of relative treatment effectiveness (R.J. Cook and Sackett 1995; Sackett et al. 1991, 2000), its mathematical properties are such that it cannot be directly used in a meta-analysis (Deeks and Altman 2001). NNT can, however, be calculated from the summary OR and the estimated control event rate (CER) with the formula in Appendix B. This approach assumes that the OR for a particular treatment comparison is independent of the CER. Empirically, this appears to be the case (Furukawa et al. 2002; McAlister 2002).

Continuous Outcome Measures

Continuous outcome measures, which include things such as body weight, intelligence quotient, or scores on a rating scale, are common in psychiatric research. In meta-analyses of continuous outcome measures, standardized mean differences, not the means of the outcome measures, are used as the measure of treatment effect (Deeks et al. 2001; Petitti 2000; Sutton et al. 2000). The results of each study are transformed into a standardized mean difference (represented by the letter *d*), using the following formula:

$$d = (\text{mean}_e - \text{mean}_c)/\text{SD}_p$$

where mean_e and mean_c are the means for the experimental and control groups, respectively, and SD_p is the pooled estimate of the standard deviation (SD) of the outcome measure. The results are then pooled by taking a weighted average of the *d*'s for each study, with the weight for a given study being the inverse of the variance of that study's effect size (Deeks et al. 2001; Petitti 2000; Sutton et al. 2000).

The standardized mean difference is a measure of the degree of overlap of the experimental and control group results, expressed in terms of SDs (Freemantle and Geddes 1998). If *d*=0, the means of the control and experimental groups are identical. If *d*=1, the mean of the experimental group is 1 SD above the mean of the control group. From a standard statistical table for a normal distribution, this is

equivalent to saying that 84% of the control group has scores below the mean of the experimental group. A table for interpreting the standardized mean difference is given in Appendix B–5.

Fixed and Random Effects Models

As noted earlier, there are both fixed effects and random effects models for combining the results of clinical trials. The choice of model is a topic of debate among statisticians, and readers are referred elsewhere for a more complete discussion (Egger et al. 2001b; Freemantle and Geddes 1998; Montori et al. 2002; Petitti 2000; Sutton et al. 2000). At the risk of oversimplifying a complex issue, it is probably sufficient to say that fixed effects models assume that there is no heterogeneity in study results, whereas random effects models assume that there is heterogeneity. As a result, the random effects model should be preferred when heterogeneity is present.

If there is no heterogeneity, both models will produce similar pooled estimates of the OR, but the CIs obtained with the random effects models are wider (less precise). As a result, the null hypothesis (i.e., that there is no difference between the two treatments) will be rejected less often if calculations are performed with the random effects model. This has led to the claim that the random effects model is overly conservative when minimal heterogeneity is present. In contrast, when there is heterogeneity, hypothesis testing, using the random effects model, gives the more appropriate results. (See Gray and Taylor, Chapter 5 in this volume, for further discussion of hypothesis testing.)

A second practical consideration is that the random effects model gives more equal weighting to large and small studies than does the fixed effects model, which gives more weight to large studies. If there is heterogeneity between the results of large and small studies as the result of either publication bias or differences in quality that vary by study size, the pooled estimate obtained with the random effects model will be more subject to such biases than the estimate obtained with the fixed effects model.

As a practical note, in most cases the two models give similar results. When the results differ, heterogeneity is generally present, and the causes for the heterogeneity need to be taken into account rather than relying on only the pooled estimate of treatment effect.

Forest Plots

Many systematic reviews present their results graphically, in the form of *forest plots* (Egger and Smith 2001; Egger et al. 1997a; Glasziou et al. 2001; Lewis and Clarke 2001; Sutton et al. 2000), also referred to as *blobbograms* (Freemantle and Geddes 1998). An example of a forest plot is given in Figure 6–1. In this example, the results of each individual study are given by a horizontal bar, with the width of the bar representing the 95% CI for the OR in that study. For each study, a black diamond is used to represent the OR; the size of the diamond is a measure of the size of the study (and hence the weight given to it). Unshaded diamonds are used to indicate the pooled OR, with the width of the diamond indicating the 95% CI for the pooled estimate.

Heterogeneity

Heterogeneity is present when the results from individual studies differ by more than what was expected by chance alone (Freemantle and Geddes 1998; Sutton et al. 2000). Heterogeneity can be assessed either informally (graphically) or through statistical techniques (Sutton et al. 2000).

The informal graphical approach uses forest plots. If there is considerable overlap between the CI bars for the various studies, no heterogeneity is present. Conversely, if the CI bars for some studies do not overlap those of other studies, heterogeneity is present. Figure 6–1 shows that four of the studies found no treatment effect, whereas two studies found the experimental treatment to be significantly better than the control treatment. It can also be seen that the CIs of the four *negative* studies overlap one another and that the CIs of the two *positive* studies also overlap each other. However, the bars for the positive studies do not overlap the Chandler-California study at all; in addition, they barely overlap the Lehman-Baltimore study. Thus, there is heterogeneity in the study results.

The formal statistical approach is to use a chi-square test for heterogeneity. This involves the calculation of a statistic, "Q," which has a chi-square distribution with 1 degree of freedom less than the number of studies. Details of the calculations are given elsewhere (Deeks et al. 2001; Petitti 2000; Sutton et al. 2000).

As noted earlier, when heterogeneity is detected, the random effects model gives a better estimate of pooled effect size than does the fixed effects model. However, the analysis should not stop there. Instead, an attempt should be made to assess the cause of the heterogeneity (Deeks et al. 2001; Glasziou et al. 2001; Petitti 2000; Sutton et al. 2000; Thompson

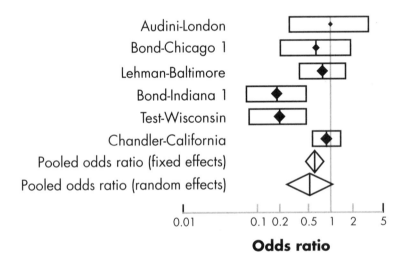

FIGURE 6–1. Example of a forest plot showing effects of assertive community treatment versus usual care on odds of hospitalization of patients with severe mental illness.

Source.   Reprinted from Freemantle N, Geddes J: "Understanding and Interpreting Systematic Reviews and Meta-Analyses, II: Meta-Analyses." *Evidence-Based Mental Health* 1:102–104, 1998. Copyright 1998 BMJ Publishing Group. Used with permission.

1994, 2001). Some of the causes of heterogeneity include differences between studies in patient population (e.g., disease severity or other prognostic factors), nature of the intervention (e.g., medication dose, frequency or number of psychotherapy sessions, or presence of co-interventions), compliance, outcome measures, study duration, study quality, and other sources of bias (Glasziou et al. 2001; Sutton et al. 2000).

If the source of the heterogeneity can be identified, it is sometimes useful to present the results by subgroup (Sutton et al. 2000). Unfortunately, differences in subgroups identified in this post hoc fashion may represent the effects of chance or bias rather than true differences in response to treatment (Smith and Egger 2001; Sutton et al. 2000). If, however, such subgroup differences are anticipated from the start of the meta-analysis process (i.e., prior to looking at the forest plot, combining the results, or testing for heterogeneity), then such subgroup analyses may be appropriate.

Funnel Plots and Publication Bias

As previously noted, publication bias is often a concern in systematic reviews. Furthermore, it can bias the results of a meta-analysis, especially if the random effects model is assumed.

Publication bias is usually assessed with a *funnel plot* (Egger et al. 1997b; Glasziou et al. 2001; Montori and Guyatt 2002; Montori et al. 2000; Sterne et al. 2001). In a funnel plot, the *x* axis is treatment effect, and the *y* axis is either study size or a measure of the study standard error, with standard error now considered the preferable measure (Sterne and Egger 2001).

Examples of funnel plots are given in Figure 6–2. Figure 6–2A shows a situation in which no publication bias exists. It can be seen that the plot is symmetrical. On average, the results of smaller studies are the same as those of larger studies; however, results from small studies are more variable. As a result, they deviate more from the mean, producing the funnel shape.

If there is publication bias, there will be a tendency to publish *positive* small study results, but not *negative* small study results. Such a tendency diminishes as the size of the study increases. In Figure 6–2A, the open circles represent the "negative" studies; these studies were not published. Removing these studies gives the asymmetrical funnel plot in Figure 6–2B.

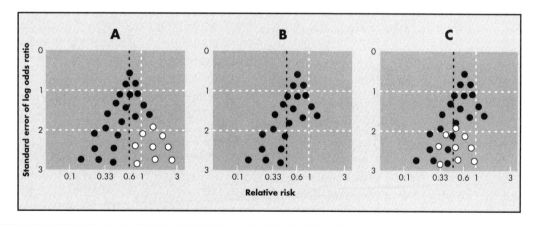

FIGURE 6–2. Examples of funnel plots.

(A) Symmetrical funnel plot demonstrating that results from all studies are centered around common relative risk but those from small studies vary more from the mean than do those from large studies.
(B) Publication bias occurs when small negative studies (shown as open circles in [A]) are not published. This results in the asymmetrical funnel plot shown in (B).
(C) Smaller studies are often of lower methodological quality, producing biased results (open circles). This can also produce an asymmetrical funnel plot.

Source.   Reprinted from Sterne JAC, Egger M, Smith GD: "Systematic Reviews in Health Care: Investigating and Dealing With Publication and Other Biases in Meta-Analysis." *BMJ* 323:101–105, 2001. Copyright 2001 BMJ Publishing Group. Used with permission.

Because small studies may be of lower methodological quality, they may be more likely to exaggerate the effects of a treatment (Kjaergard et al. 2001; Sterne et al. 2000, 2001). This situation, too, can produce an asymmetrical funnel plot, as demonstrated in Figure 6–2C.

Sensitivity Analysis

Questions often arise about whether a particular study or set of studies should be included in a meta-analysis because of differences in study design (e.g., patient population, treatment, co-intervention, outcome measure, duration, quality). In sensitivity analysis, the calculations are performed with and without a particular subset of studies to see whether this has any effect on the overall results (Egger and Smith 2001; Sutton et al. 2000).

A good example of the usefulness of sensitivity analysis comes from a systematic review of the effectiveness of antidepressants versus placebo in dysthymic disorder (Lima and Moncrieff 2002). Because the pre-1980 literature does not use the term *dysthymic disorder*, patients with this disorder were labeled as having *depressive neurosis, neurotic depression, depressive personality disorder*, and so forth. Lima and Moncrieff included studies of such patients but then used sensitivity analysis to show that the results were the same if the diagnosis were limited to *dysthymia* as they would be if these other studies were included.

Critical Appraisal Guide for Systematic Reviews

Even systematic reviews from respected sources can have methodological problems (Hopayian 2001; Olsen et al. 2001); therefore, all such reviews should be appraised by the reader. Several guides have been developed for the critical appraisal of systematic reviews (Badenoch and Heneghan 2002; Centre for Evidence-Based Medicine 2005; Freemantle and Geddes 1998; Geddes et al. 1998; Greenhalgh 2001; Oxman et al. 2002; Sackett et al. 2000; Seers 1999; Shea et al. 2001). One such guide appears in Table 6–3.

In 1996, a group of 30 clinical epidemiologists, clinicians, statisticians, editors, and researchers, concerned about the quality of meta-analyses, met to identify items they thought should be included in a checklist of standards. Whenever possible, checklist items were guided by research evidence suggest-

ing that failure to adhere to the item proposed could lead to biased results. The conference resulted in the QUOROM (Quality Of Reporting Of Meta-analyses) statement, a checklist, and a flow diagram (Moher et al. 2000a). The checklist describes the group's preferred way to present the abstract, introduction, methods, results, and discussion sections of a report of a meta-analysis. The QUOROM statement, checklist, and flow diagram can be obtained online at www.consort-statement.org/index.aspx?o=1065.

Did the Review Address a Clearly Defined Issue?

The first step in planning a systematic review is formulating the question. The authors of the review should indicate the 4-part PICO question (Chapter 3) that they are trying to address. Unless the question itself is clear, the subsequent literature search likely will be unfocused. As a result, if the clinical question is not clear, the clinician should probably try to find another review (Seers 1999). However, a review also may be either too broad or too narrow (Oxman et al. 2002). For example, a systematic review of psychotherapy for mental illness is such a broad topic that it is unlikely that the reviewers could do it justice within the confines of even a book-length review. Conversely, a systematic review of a topic that is too narrow may not generate appropriate studies, and such a review may be of limited generalizability.

Did the Authors Select the Right Sort of Studies?

As noted in Table 4–1 in Chapter 4, some study designs are better than others for answering particular types of clinical questions. For example, as was discussed in Chapter 5, the RCT is the preferred study design for answering therapy questions. The authors of a review should specify their inclusion criteria for which types of studies were selected, and these criteria should be appropriate to the clinical question being asked (Seers 1999).

Were All Relevant Studies Included?

Several questions can be asked with regard to the studies included. How comprehensive was the search strategy? Did the authors search only MEDLINE, or did they also search other online data-

TABLE 6–3.   Critical appraisal guide for systematic reviews

Did the review address a clearly defined issue?

Is the 4-part PICO question clearly identified?

Is the topic too broad or too narrow?

Did the authors select the right types of studies?

Are the inclusion criteria specified?

Do the authors specify the appropriate type of study to answer the question?

Were all relevant studies included?

How comprehensive was the search strategy?

Were appropriate electronic databases used?

Did the databases include non-English-language journals?

Did the authors go beyond electronic databases (e.g., personal contacts, manual searches)?

Was the quality of the studies addressed?

Were explicit criteria used?

Were two raters used, with a procedure for resolving differences?

Are the results similar from study to study? If not, was heterogeneity addressed?

Are the results clearly displayed (e.g., in a forest plot)?

Is there evidence of heterogeneity?

Are the reasons for the differences in study results discussed?

What are the overall results (with confidence intervals)?

What is the pooled effect measure, with confidence intervals?

Does it indicate that the two treatments are significantly different?

Can I apply the results to my patient?

Is my patient too different from those in the study?

What is the number needed to treat for my patient?

Is the treatment consistent with my patient's values and preferences?

Is the treatment feasible in my setting?

Note.   PICO=patient/problem, intervention, comparison, outcome.
Source.   Adapted from Centre for Evidence-Based Mental Health n.d.; Greenhalgh 2001; Oxman et al. 2002; Sackett et al. 2000; Seers 1999.

bases? Did the authors make other attempts to locate studies? For example, did they contact authors of published studies or manufacturers of drugs, check reference lists of published studies or prior reviews (i.e., snowballing), perform manual searches of journals or proceedings abstracts that are not abstracted in MEDLINE or similar databases, and check databases of clinical trials? If such measures are not taken, several sources of bias could influence the results, including publication bias and language bias (Table 6–2). Sampson et al. (2008) re-

cently reviewed the criteria used to perform various searches. They found no clear consensus regarding optimum reporting of systematic review search methods, and commonly recommended items were not optimally reported.

Was the Quality of the Studies Addressed?

As was discussed earlier and in Chapter 5, evidence from less rigorously designed studies is more apt to be biased and misleading than is evidence from more rigorously designed studies. The authors of the review should describe the criteria used for assessing quality, including the minimum quality needed for inclusion. For example, they may decide to include only RCTs with at least 80% follow-up and intention-to-treat analysis. Whatever the criteria, they should be explicit and decided in advance so that they are not influenced by study results (Silagy et al. 2002). In addition, the assessment of quality should generally involve two reviewers and a mechanism for resolving a difference between them (Glasziou et al. 2001; Oxman et al. 2002; Seers 1999). Reviews should list which studies were excluded from the analysis for quality reasons, and the reason for exclusion should be given.

Are the Results Similar From Study to Study?

Many systematic reviews present their results graphically in the form of forest plots. As previously discussed, forest plots can be used to assess whether the results are similar from study to study. The more formal statistical approach is to use a chi-square test for heterogeneity.

If heterogeneity is detected, an attempt should be made to assess the cause of the heterogeneity. Subgroup analysis may be appropriate if the rationale was identified beforehand. Sensitivity analysis also may indicate whether the inclusion of certain studies has a significant effect on the pooled measure of treatment effect.

What Are the Overall Results (With Confidence Intervals)?

The results of a meta-analysis generally will be presented as a forest diagram that includes a pooled effect measure and its CIs. For dichotomous outcome measures, this is an OR; for continuous measures, it is a standardized mean difference. If the CIs for the pooled OR include 1 or if the CIs for the standardized mean difference include 0, there is no statistically significant difference between the experimental and the control treatments.

Can the Clinician Apply the Results to His or Her Patient?

The final step in the appraisal process is to assess whether the clinician can apply the results to his or her patient. As with the discussion of a single therapy study in Chapter 5, several considerations enter into this assessment.

First, is the patient so different from those in the studies that the results do not apply? The question can be reframed in the following way: "Is the pathobiology of this patient so different from that of the study patients that the results cannot apply?" Typically, the answer to this question is "no," although there may be quantitative differences. To quantify the likelihood of a patient benefiting from a treatment, it is first necessary to convert the pooled estimate of the OR to NNT (McQuay and Moore 1998; Sackett et al. 2000) (see Appendix B).

Finally, the clinician must consider two additional questions before applying the treatment to his or her patient. First, is the treatment consistent with his or her patient's values and preferences? Second, is the treatment feasible in the clinician's setting? Assuming that the clinician has found a high-quality systematic review that has identified an effective treatment for the patient, the next steps in the EBM process (Table 2–1, Chapter 2) are to treat the patient and to evaluate the outcome.

References

Allen IE, Olkin I: Estimating time to conduct a meta-analysis from number of citations retrieved. JAMA 2892:634–635, 1999

Altman DG, Schulz KF: Statistics notes: concealing treatment allocation in randomised trials. BMJ 323:446–447, 2001

Antes G, Oxman AD: The Cochrane Collaboration in the 20th century, in Systematic Reviews in Health Care: Meta-Analysis in Context. Edited by Egger M, Smith GD, Altman DG. London, BMJ Books, 2001, pp 447–458

Badenoch D, Heneghan C: Evidence-Based Medicine Toolkit. London, BMJ Books, 2002

Balk EM, Bonis PAL, Moskowitz H, et al: Correlation of quality measures with estimates of treatment effect in meta-analyses of randomized controlled trials. JAMA 287:2973–2982, 2002

Centre for Evidence-Based Medicine: Critical Appraisal Worksheet for Systematic Review of Therapy [Centre for Evidence-Based Medicine Web site]. 2005. Available at: http://www.cebm.net/index.aspx?o=1157. Accessed June 28, 2009

Centre for Evidence-Based Mental Health: Critical appraisal form for an overview [Centre for Evidence-Based Mental Health Web site]. Available at: http://cebmh.warne .ox.ac.uk/cebmh/downloads/education_resources/ overview.pdf. Accessed June 28, 2009

Clarke M, Oxman AD (eds): Cochrane Reviewers' Handbook 4.1.6. [Cochrane Collaboration Web site]. April 2002. Available at: http://www.cochrane.org/cochrane/ hbook.htm. Accessed September 5, 2002

Cochrane Collaboration: The Cochrane Collaboration leaflet [Cochrane Collaboration Web site]. Available at: http://www.cochrane.org/resources/leaflet.htm. September 1997. Accessed June 18, 2002

Cook DJ, Mulrow CD, Haynes RB: Synthesis of best evidence for clinical decisions, in Systematic Reviews: Synthesis of Best Evidence for Health Care Decisions. Edited by Mulrow C, Cook D. Philadelphia, PA, American College of Physicians, 1998, pp 5–12

Cook RJ, Sackett DL: The number needed to treat: a clinically useful measure of treatment effect. BMJ 310:452–454, 1995

Davies P, Boruch R: The Campbell Collaboration does for public policy what Cochrane does for public health. BMJ 323:294–295, 2001

Deeks JJ, Altman DG: Effect measures for meta-analyses of trials with binary outcomes, in Systematic Reviews in Health Care: Meta-Analysis in Context. Edited by Egger M, Smith GD, Altman DG. London, BMJ Books, 2001, pp 313–335

Deeks JJ, Altman DG, Bradburn MJ: Statistical methods for examining heterogeneity and combining results from several studies in meta-analysis, in Systematic Reviews in Health Care: Meta-Analysis in Context. Edited by Egger M, Smith GD, Altman DG. London, BMJ Books, 2001, pp 285–312

DerSimonian R, Laird N: Meta-analysis in clinical trials. Control Clin Trials 7:177–188, 1986

Dwan K, Altman DG, Arnaiz JA, et al: Systematic review of the empirical evidence of study publication bias and outcome reporting bias. PLoS ONE 3(8):e3081, 2008

Egger M, Smith GD: Meta-analysis: potentials and promise. BMJ 315:1371–1374, 1997

Egger M, Smith GD: Bias in location and selection of studies. BMJ 316:61–66, 1998

Egger M, Smith GD: Principles and procedures for systematic reviews, in Systematic Reviews in Health Care: Meta-Analysis in Context. Edited by Egger M, Smith GD, Altman DG. London, BMJ Books, 2001, pp 23–42

Egger M, Smith GD, Phillips AN: Meta-analysis: principles and procedures. BMJ 315:1533–1537, 1997a

Egger M, Smith GD, Schneider M, et al: Bias in meta-analysis detected by a simple, graphical test. BMJ 315:629–634, 1997b

Egger M, Dickersin K, Smith GD: Problems and limitations in conducting systematic reviews, in Systematic Reviews in Health Care: Meta-Analysis in Context. Edited by Egger M, Smith GD, Altman DG. London, BMJ Books, 2001a, pp 43–68

Egger M, Smith GD, Altman DG (eds): Systematic Reviews in Health Care: Meta-Analysis in Context. London, BMJ Books, 2001b

Egger M, Smith GD, O'Rourke K: Rationale, potentials, and promise of systematic reviews, in Systematic Reviews in Health Care: Meta-Analysis in Context. Edited by Egger M, Smith GD, Altman DG. London, BMJ Books, 2001c, pp 3–19

Freemantle N, Geddes J: Understanding and interpreting systematic reviews and meta-analyses, II: meta-analyses. Evid Based Ment Health 1:102–104, 1998

Furukawa TA, Guyatt GH, Griffith LE: Can we individualize the "number needed to treat"? An empirical study of summary effect measures in meta-analysis. Int J Epidemiol 31:72–76, 2002

Geddes J, Freemantle N, Streiner D, et al: Understanding and interpreting reviews and meta-analyses, I: rationale, search strategy, and describing results. Evid Based Ment Health 1:68–69, 1998

Glasziou P, Irwig L, Bain C, et al: Systematic Reviews in Health Care: A Practical Guide. Cambridge, UK, Cambridge University Press, 2001

Greenhalgh T: How to Read a Paper: The Basics of Evidence Based Medicine, 2nd Edition. London, BMJ Books, 2001

Guyatt G: Therapy and harm: why study results mislead—bias and random error, in Users' Guides to the Medical Literature: A Manual for Evidence-Based Clinical Practice. Edited by Guyatt G, Rennie D. Chicago, IL, AMA Press, 2002, pp 223–231

Helmer D, Savoie I, Green C, et al: Evidence-based practice: extending the search to find material for the systematic review. Bull Med Libr Assoc 89:346–352, 2001

Hopayian K: The need for caution in interpreting high quality systematic reviews. BMJ 323:681–684, 2001

Ioannidis JPA, Haidich A-B, Pappa M, et al: Comparison of evidence of treatment effects in randomized and nonrandomized studies. JAMA 286:821–830, 2001

Jüni P, Altman DG, Egger M: Assessing the quality of randomised controlled trials, in Systematic Reviews in Health Care: Meta-Analysis in Context. Edited by Egger M, Smith GD, Altman DG. London, BMJ Books, 2001, pp 87–108

Jüni P, Holenstein F, Sterne J, et al: Direction and impact of language bias in meta-analyses of controlled trials: empirical study. Int J Epidemiol 31:115–123, 2002

Kjaergard LL, Villumsen J, Gluud C: Reported methodologic quality and discrepancies between large and small randomized trials in meta-analyses. Ann Intern Med 135:982–989, 2001

Kunz R, Oxman AD: The unpredictability paradox: review of hempirical comparisons of randomised and non-randomised clinical trials. BMJ 317:1185–1190, 1998

Lacchetti C, Guyatt G: Therapy and validity: surprising results of randomized controlled trials, in Users' Guides to the Medical Literature: A Manual for Evidence-Based Clinical Practice. Edited by Guyatt G, Rennie D. Chicago, IL, AMA Press, 2002, pp 247–265

Lefebvre C, Clarke MJ: Identifying randomised trials, in Systematic Reviews in Health Care: Meta-Analysis in Context. Edited by Egger M, Smith GD, Altman DG. London, BMJ Books, 2001, pp 69–86

Lewis S, Clarke M: Forest plots: trying to see the wood and the trees. BMJ 322:1479–1480, 2001

Lima MS, Moncrieff S: Drugs versus placebo for dysthymia, in The Cochrane Library, Issue 3. Oxford, UK, Update Software, 2002

Mantel N, Haenszel W: Statistical aspects of the analysis of data from retrospective studies of disease. J Natl Cancer Inst 22:719–748, 1959

McAlister FA: Commentary: relative treatment effects are consistent across the spectrum of underlying risks…usually. Int J Epidemiol 31:76–77, 2002

McQuay HJ, Moore RA: Using numerical results from systematic reviews in clinical practice, in Systematic Reviews: Synthesis of Best Evidence for Health Care Decisions. Edited by Mulrow C, Cook D. Philadelphia, PA, American College of Physicians, 1998, pp 23–36

Moher D, Cook DJ, Eastwood S, et al: Improving the quality of reports of meta-analyses of randomised controlled trials: the QUOROM statement. QUOROM Group. Br J Surg 87:1448–1454, 2000a

Moher D, Klassen TP, Schulz KF, et al: What contributions do languages other than English make on the results of meta-analyses? J Clin Epidemiol 5:964–972, 2000b

Moher D, Klassen TP, Jones AL, et al: Assessing the quality of reports of randomised trials included in meta-analyses: attitudes, practice, evidence and guides, in The Advanced Handbook of Methods in Evidence Based Healthcare. Edited by Stevens A, Abrams K, Brazier J, et al. London, Sage, 2001, pp 409–425

Montori V, Guyatt G: Summarizing the evidence: publication bias, in Users' Guides to the Medical Literature: A Manual for Evidence-Based Clinical Practice. Edited by Guyatt G, Rennie D. Chicago, IL, AMA Press, 2002, pp 529–538

Montori VM, Smieja M, Guyatt GH: Publication bias: a brief review for clinicians. Mayo Clin Proc 75:1284–1288, 2000

Montori V, Guyatt G, Oxman A, et al: Summarizing the evidence: fixed-effects and random-effects models, in Users' Guides to the Medical Literature: A Manual for Evidence-Based Clinical Practice. Edited by Guyatt G, Rennie D. Chicago, IL, AMA Press, 2002, pp 539–545

National Health Service Centre for Reviews and Dissemination [NHS CRD]: Undertaking systematic reviews of research on effectiveness: CRD's guidance for those carrying out commissioning reviews. CRD Report No 4, 2nd Edition [NHS CRD Web site]. March 2001. Available at: http://www.york.ac.uk/inst/crd/report4.htm. Accessed September 5, 2002

Olsen O, Middleton P, Ezzo J, et al: Quality of Cochrane reviews: assessment of sample from 1998. BMJ 323:829–832, 2001

Olson CM, Rennie D, Cook D, et al: Publication bias in editorial decision making. JAMA 287:2825–2828, 2002

Oxman A, Guyatt G, Cook D, et al: Summarizing the evidence, in Users' Guides to the Medical Literature: A Manual for Evidence-Based Clinical Practice. Edited by Guyatt G, Rennie D. Chicago, IL, AMA Press, 2002, pp 155–173

Petitti DB: Meta-Analysis, Decision Analysis, and Cost-Effectiveness Analysis: Methods for Quantitative Synthesis in Medicine, 2nd Edition. New York, Oxford University Press, 2000

Pittler MH, Abbot NC, Harkness EF, et al: Location bias in controlled clinical trials of complementary/alternative therapies. J Clin Epidemiol 53:485–489, 2000

Robinson KA, Dickersin K: Development of a highly sensitive search strategy for the retrieval of reports of controlled trials using PubMed. Int J Epidemiol 31:150–153, 2002

Rochon PA, Bero LA, Bay AM, et al: Comparison of review articles published in peer-reviewed and throwaway journals. JAMA 287:2853–2856, 2002

Rosenthal R: The "file drawer problem" and tolerance for null results. Psychol Bull 86:638–641, 1979

Sackett DL, Haynes RB, Guyatt GH, et al: Clinical Epidemiology: A Basic Science for Clinical Medicine, 2nd Edition. Boston, MA, Little, Brown, 1991

Sackett DL, Straus SE, Richardson WS, et al: Evidence-Based Medicine: How to Practice and Teach EBM, 2nd Edition. New York, Churchill Livingstone, 2000

Sampson M, McGowan J, Tetzlaff J, et al: No consensus exists on search reporting methods for systematic reviews. J Clin Epidemiol 61:748–754, 2008

Schulz KF: Assessing allocation concealment and blinding in randomised controlled trials: why bother? Evid Based Ment Health 3:4–5, 2000

Schulz KF, Chalmers I, Hayes RJ, et al: Empirical evidence of bias: dimensions of methodological quality associated with estimates of treatment effects in controlled trials. JAMA 273:408–412, 1995

Seers K: Systematic review, in Evidence-Based Medicine: A Primer for Health Care Professionals. Edited by Dawes M, Davies P, Gray A, et al. Edinburgh, Churchill Livingstone, 1999, pp 85–100

Shea B, Dube C, Moher D: Assessing the quality of reports of systematic reviews: the QUORUM statement compared to other tools, in Systematic Reviews in Health Care: Meta-Analysis in Context. Edited by Egger M, Smith GD, Altman DG. London, BMJ Books, 2001, pp 122–139

Silagy CA, Middleton P, Hopewell S: Publishing protocols of systematic reviews: comparing what was done to what was planned. JAMA 287:2831–2834, 2002

Smith GD, Egger M: Going beyond the grand mean: subgroup analysis in meta-analysis of randomised trials, in Systematic Reviews in Health Care: Meta-Analysis in Context. Edited by Egger M, Smith GD, Altman DG. London, BMJ Books, 2001, pp 143–156

Song F, Eastwood A, Gilbody S, et al: Publication and related biases, in The Advanced Handbook of Methods in Evidence Based Healthcare. Edited by Stevens A, Abrams K, Brazier J, et al. London, Sage, 2001, pp 371–390

Stern JM, Simes RJ: Publication bias: evidence of delayed publication in a cohort study of clinical research projects. BMJ 315:640–645, 1997

Sterne JAC, Egger M: Funnel plots for detecting bias in meta-analysis: guidelines on choice of axis. J Clin Epidemiol 54:1046–1055, 2001

Sterne JAC, Gavaghan D, Egger M: Publication and related bias in meta-analysis: power of statistical tests and prevalence in the literature. J Clin Epidemiol 53:1119–1129, 2000

Sterne JAC, Egger M, Smith GD: Systematic reviews in health care: investigating and dealing with publication and other biases in meta-analysis. BMJ 323:101–105, 2001

Sutton AJ, Abrams KR, Jones DR, et al: Methods for Meta-Analysis in Medical Research. New York, Wiley, 2000

Thompson SG: Why sources of heterogeneity in meta-analysis should be investigated. BMJ 309:1351–1355, 1994

Thompson SG: Why and how sources of heterogeneity should be investigated, in Systematic Reviews in Health Care: Meta-Analysis in Context. Edited by Egger M, Smith GD, Altman DG. London, BMJ Books, 2001, pp 157–175

Thornton A, Lee P: Publication bias in meta-analysis: its causes and consequences. J Clin Epidemiol 53:207–216, 2000

Tramer MR, Reynolds DJM, Moore RA, et al: Impact of covert duplicate publication on meta-analysis: a case study. BMJ 315:635–640, 1997

Turner EH, Matthews AM, Linardatos E, et al: Selective publication of antidepressant trials and its influence on apparent efficacy. N Engl J Med 358:252–260, 2008

West S, King V, Carey TS, et al: Systems to Rate the Strength of Scientific Evidence (Evidence Report/Technology Assessment, No 47). Rockville, MD, Agency for Healthcare Research and Quality, 2002

Yusuf S, Peto R, Lewis J, et al: Beta blockade during and after myocardial infarction: an overview of the randomized trials. Prog Cardiovasc Dis 27:335–371, 1985

Clinical Practice Guidelines

Gregory E. Gray, M.D., Ph.D.
C. Barr Taylor, M.D.

Clinical practice guidelines are generally defined as "systematically developed statements to assist practitioner decisions about appropriate health care for specific clinical circumstances" (Field and Lohr 1990, p. 1). Over the past two decades, there has been considerable interest and activity in developing these guidelines for a variety of clinical conditions, driven by concerns about variability in clinical practice, cost, quality, and legal liability (Birkmeyer 2001; Field and Lohr 1992; Greenhalgh 2001; Woolf et al. 1999b). We believe clinical practice guidelines are an invaluable source for improving patient care. Guidelines have many limitations, however, including the fact that most guidelines focus on a single disorder, that guidelines for treating one problem may conflict with aspects of guidelines for treating a comorbid problem in the same patient, and that many guidelines include recommendations that are not evidence based.

Role of Guidelines in Evidence-Based Practice

Most clinical practice guidelines represent an attempt to improve clinical care by focusing on effective evidence-based interventions. Although practice guidelines are sometimes equated with evidence-based medicine (EBM) (Grol 2001a), they should be viewed as distinct for several reasons (Gray 2002; Lipman 2000). First, as noted later in this chapter, not all practice guidelines are based on the best evidence, as derived from a systematic review of the medical literature (Browman 2001; Drake et al. 2001; Gray 2002; Greenhalgh 2001; Kahn et al. 1997; Woolf et al. 1999a, 1999b). All guidelines involve some degree of judgment and bias in their development (Browman 2001; Drake et al. 2001; Greenhalgh 2001; Greenhalgh and Peacock 2005), the extent of which is often unstated. In addition, clinical practice guidelines are often introduced as part of a "top-down" approach to changing clinician behavior, leading to clinician resistance (Haines and Jones 1994; Lipman 2000). Ideally, evidence-based psychiatric practice (EBPP) is a "bottom-up" approach in which clinicians make decisions on the basis of ability to search and appraise the medical literature.

From our standpoint, evidence-based clinical practice guidelines should play an important role in EBPP. Guidelines can serve as a very useful starting point for the practitioner to assess the major treatment principles that should be considered. Studies of practicing clinicians have found that clinicians often do not have the time to search and appraise the literature themselves but that they would welcome evidence-based guidelines when faced with clinical questions (McColl et al. 1998; Young and Ward 2001). In such cases, high-quality evidence-based guidelines can provide useful guidance (Feder et al. 1999; Grimshaw and Eccles 2001; Woolf et al. 1999b). In addition, such evidence-based guidelines generally either include or reference a systematic review of the relevant literature.

Sources of Guidelines

Clinical practice guidelines have been developed by a variety of organizations and are available for many DSM-IV-TR (American Psychiatric Association 2000) disorders. Some of the guidelines are evidence based; others are not. As described by Gray and Taylor in Chapter 4, a useful starting point in searching for evidence-based clinical practice guidelines is the National Guideline Clearinghouse (www.guideline .gov). A search function on the home page allows the user to find guidelines by disease, treatment, measures, and organization. Other resources include annotated bibliographies, expert commentaries, patient resources, syntheses, and comparison features. Other useful sources of guidelines are listed in Table 4–3.

American Psychiatric Association

The evidence-based guidelines most familiar to American psychiatrists are the ones developed by the American Psychiatric Association (APA) and represent a good starting point for the practitioner. These guidelines currently cover the major psychiatric disorders and are available both in print form (American Psychiatric Association 2006) and online (www .psychiatryonline.com). The APA guidelines are based on a systematic review of treatment options, with the use of expert opinion to synthesize the findings. One advantage of the APA guidelines is that they include a useful review of the relevant literature.

Expert Opinion

The APA, the Agency for Health Care Policy and Research (AHCPR), and the Agency for Healthcare Research and Quality (AHRQ) guidelines all involve expert opinion but with some quality assurance mechanisms, including standardized review of articles and databases, peer review and feedback, and public commentary. Also, several guidelines represent the opinion of experts. For instance, the *Expert Consensus Guidelines* (www.psychguides.com) provide a list of guidelines that can be purchased. In numerous instances, expert opinion on the treatment of medical conditions has been proved wrong by well-conducted research (Antman et al. 1992; Greenhalgh 2001; Mulrow 1994; Sackett et al. 1991); therefore, opinion does not necessarily provide the best guide to clinical practice. However, expert opinion can play a role in situations in which there is simply little or no evidence from well-conducted clinical trials. *Expert Review of Neurotherapeutics* (www.ingentaconnect.com/content/ftd/ern)provides expert reviews on the use of drugs and medicines in clinical neurology and neuropsychiatry. Coverage includes disease management, new medicines and drugs in neurology, therapeutic indications, diagnostics, medical treatment guidelines, and neurological diseases such as stroke, epilepsy, Alzheimer's disease, and Parkinson's disease. These are available by subscription. In Chapter 5, we noted the many potential biases in industry-sponsored trials. Expert opinion is also subject to many such biases.

Algorithms

Medication, and sometimes psychotherapy, algorithms are embedded in many guidelines. As mentioned in Chapter 4, several psychopharmacology algorithms are also available. Osser and Patterson have a Web site that lists many psychopharmacology algorithms (www.mhc.com/Algorithms). The project also lists the major guidelines and algorithm projects. The development and use of algorithms has been strongly influenced by the Texas Medication Algorithm Project (TMAP) started in 1996, which was designed to develop, implement, and evaluate a set of medication algorithms and an algorithm-driven treatment philosophy for major adult psychiatric disorders treated in the Texas public mental health sector. The ultimate goal of TMAP is to improve the quality of care and achieve the best possible patient outcomes for each dollar of resource expended. According to the developers, TMAP is a treatment philosophy for the medication management portion of care, consisting of 1) evidence-based, consensually agreed-on medication treatment algorithms; 2) clinical and technical support necessary to allow the clinician to implement the algorithm; 3) patient and family education programs that allow the patient to be an active partner in care; and 4) uniform documentation of care provided and resulting patient outcomes (Texas Medication Algorithm Project 2002). Currently, algorithms for schizophrenia, depression, and bipolar disorder are available (www.dshs.state.tx.us/mhprograms/ tima.shtm). As with the *Expert Consensus Guidelines* (2002), the TMAP algorithms include an evidence base but are strongly influenced by expert consensus (Gilbert et al. 1998).

The Sequenced Treatment Alternatives to Relieve Depression (STAR*D) trial has shown the benefit of using algorithms, particularly in the context of clearly defined and important clinical outcomes. The STAR*D trial is the largest study (N=4,041) ever conducted evaluating and comparing algorithmic treatment effectiveness in real-world patients experiencing a depressive episode as part of major depressive disorder (Trivedi et al. 2006). The STAR*D trial was supported by the National Institute of Mental Health (NIMH) and was implemented over a 5-year period. STAR*D was designed to assess effectiveness of treatments in generalizable samples and to ensure the delivery of adequate treatments, with the primary outcome measure being remission. The algorithm was designed to begin treatment with a selective serotonin reuptake inhibitor (SSRI). Citalopram was chosen as the initial drug (and SSRI) because of the absence of discontinuation symptoms, established safety in elderly and medically fragile patients, once-a-day dosing, few dose adjustment steps, and favorable drug-drug interaction profile (Trivedi et al. 2006). The protocol required that an adequate dose of citalopram be given for a sufficient time to ensure that an adequate treatment trial was conducted. A systematic but easily implemented approach to treatment, which the investigators referred to as *measurement-based care*, was developed.

Measurement-based care includes the routine measurement of symptoms and side effects at each treatment visit and the use of a treatment manual describing when and how to modify medication doses according to these measures. The details of how the algorithm can be implemented are provided by Trivedi and Kurian in Chapter 21, and the general algorithm has been described in many publications (Trivedi et al. 2006b). The study was designed to evaluate several issues, including identifying potential moderators of outcome. The overall results have been presented in many publications and should be familiar to most readers. The 8-week remission rates (28% for Hamilton Rating Scale for Depression; 33% for Quick Inventory of Depressive Symptomatology—Self-Report) were robust and similar to rates found in uncomplicated, nonchronic, symptomatic volunteers enrolled in placebo-controlled, randomized controlled trials with SSRIs (Agency for Health Care Policy and Research 1993b). These remission rates were better than those found in efficacy studies among patients with chronic depression

(22%) (Keller et al. 2000). This trial sets a new standard of care for the treatment of depression in clinical practice.

Differences Among Guidelines

As indicated in the previous section, not all guidelines are based on the best available evidence. Some guidelines are based on expert consensus and are not truly evidence based (Berg et al. 1997; Browman 2001). Guidelines also differ considerably in comprehensiveness, format, frequency of review, and ease of use. Milner and Valenstein (2002) have provided a useful comparison of several of the guidelines for the treatment of schizophrenia that details many of these differences. Those produced by the APA, AHRQ, and the other organizations listed in Table 4–3 in Chapter 4 are generally of high quality, but any guideline should be assessed before its use.

Developing Evidence-Based Practice Guidelines

The development of evidence-based clinical practice guidelines is generally viewed as a 6-step process (Eccles et al. 2001; Shekelle et al. 1999a, 1999b) (Table 7–1).

Identify the Topic

The first step in the guideline development process is to identify and refine the subject of the guideline. Given the large number of diagnoses and the time needed to develop guidelines, some prioritization must occur. Often this step is based on considerations such as the prevalence or economic effects of a disorder (Berg et al. 1997; Cook et al. 1998; Shekelle et al. 1999a, 1999b). Furthermore, decisions must be made on the scope of the guideline (e.g., whether it should be restricted to pharmacological treatment or whether it should include psychosocial interventions, patient education, etc.). Some authors suggest creating a "causal pathway" that diagrams the links between steps in a diagnostic or treatment process and the potential outcomes (benefits or harms) that could occur (Berg et al. 1997; Shekelle et al. 1999a, 1999b).

Convene a Group

The group convened to develop the guideline should include individuals with expertise in statistics and epidemiology, as well as clinical expertise related

TABLE 7–1.   Steps in developing evidence-based practice guidelines

1. **Identify and refine the topic of the guideline**

2. **Convene an appropriate group**

    Typically 6–20 members

    Requires both clinical and statistical expertise

    Should be multidisciplinary

3. **Gather and assess the evidence**

    Systematic review of literature

    Hierarchy of evidence

4. **Translate the evidence into recommendations**

    Some degree of clinical judgment always needed a) to weigh conflicting information and b) when there is little evidence

5. **Use outside reviewers to review the recommendations**

    Should include users, as well as experts

    Assess for validity and practicality

6. **Update the guideline periodically**

Source.   Adapted from Berg et al. 1997; Eccles et al. 2001; Shekelle et al. 1999a.

to the condition or treatment that will be the topic of the guideline (Berg et al. 1997; Shekelle et al. 1999a, 1999b). Such groups typically have 6–20 members, with one member serving as the group leader to moderate discussions, often supported by a project management team (Shekelle et al. 1999a, 1999b). It is best to convene a multidisciplinary group that includes representation from all of the stakeholders involved in implementing the guideline (Cook et al. 1998; Shekelle et al. 1999a, 1999b). Concerns have been raised regarding the extent to which pharmaceutical company relationships may influence decisions by members of guideline development groups (Choudhry et al. 2002; Greenhalgh 2001).

Gather and Assess the Evidence

The third step is to gather and assess the evidence regarding the subject of the guideline. Preexisting systematic reviews can be helpful in this step, provided that the systematic reviews themselves are valid (Browman 2001; Cook et al. 1998; Eccles et al. 2001; Shekelle et al. 1999a, 1999b). If they are not, then the guideline development group must develop

its own systematic review (see Gray, Chapter 6 in this volume).

In the process of assessing the evidence, different weight must be given to evidence from different study designs. As described in Chapter 4, hierarchies of evidence have been developed for this process (Badenoch and Heneghan 2002; Harbour and Miller 2001; Shekelle et al. 1999a, 1999b). For example, the National Institute for Health and Clinical Excellence (NICE) guidelines grade the level of evidence using the criteria provided in Table 7–2.

Translate the Evidence Into Recommendations

The fourth step is to translate the evidence into the recommendations that will make up the guideline. Clinical judgment is required in this step, both to weigh conflicting information and to make recommendations when little or no hard evidence exists (Harbour and Miller 2001; Shekelle et al. 1999a, 1999b). Various procedures have been developed to facilitate this process (Black et al. 2001; Kahn et al. 1997). Final recommendations should include an indication of the strength of evidence on which they are based (Harbour and Miller 2001; Pinsky and Deyo 2000; Shekelle et al. 1999a, 1999b). Again, the NICE guideline developers have developed a detailed procedure as to how to do this.

Forming and Grading the Statements and Recommendations

The standards and procedures developed by NICE are models for the field (National Institute for Health and Clinical Excellence 2007). As summarized from the guideline comparison search available through www.guideline.gov (and used in the comparison of guidelines discussed in the "Comparison of Guidelines" section later in this chapter), the NICE guidelines were developed as follows:

> The evidence tables and forest plots formed the basis for developing clinical statements and recommendations. For intervention studies, the statements were classified according to an accepted hierarchy of evidence. Recommendations were then graded A to C based on the level of associated evidence. In order to facilitate consistency in generating and drafting the clinical statements the guideline development group (GDG) utilised a statement decision tree. The flowchart was designed to assist with, but not re-

TABLE 7–2. Levels of evidence

I: Evidence obtained from a single randomized controlled trial or a meta-analysis of randomized controlled trials

IIa: Evidence obtained from at least one well-designed controlled study without randomization

IIb: Evidence obtained from at least one well-designed quasi-experimental study

III: Evidence obtained from well-designed nonexperimental descriptive studies, such as comparative studies, correlation studies, and case-control studies

IV: Evidence obtained from expert committee reports or opinions and/or clinical experience of respected authorities

Source. Adapted from National Institute for Health and Clinical Excellence 2007.

place, clinical judgment. Where a statistically significant summary statistic (effect size [ES]) was obtained (after controlling for heterogeneity), the GDG considered whether this finding was of clinical significance (i.e., likely to be of benefit to patients) taking into account the trial population, nature of the outcome, and size of the effect. On the basis of this consideration the ES was characterized as "clinically significant" or not. A further consideration was made about the strength of the evidence by examining the confidence interval (CI) surrounding the ES. For instance, for level I evidence, where the ES was judged to be clinically significant and had a CI entirely within a clinical relevant range, the result was characterised as "strong evidence" (S1).

The NICE guideline review process also includes the detailed methods used to answer a clinical question in the absence of appropriately designed high-quality research (National Institute for Health and Clinical Excellence 2007). The clinical recommendations are graded as follows:

- **Grade A**—At least one randomized controlled trial as part of a body of literature of overall good quality and consistency addressing the specific recommendation (evidence level I) without extrapolation
- **Grade B**—Well-conducted clinical studies but no randomized clinical trials on the topic of recommendation (evidence level II or III) or extrapolated from level I evidence
- **Grade C**—Expert committee reports or opinions and clinical experiences of respected authorities (evidence level IV) or extrapolated from level I or II evidence. This grading indicates that directly applicable clinical studies of good quality are absent or not readily available.

Obtain Outside Review

The fifth step in the guideline development process is external review to ensure that the guidelines are both valid and practical. This step should be done by potential users of the guidelines, as well as those with clinical and scientific expertise (Berg et al. 1997; Shekelle et al. 1999a, 1999b).

Update Guidelines Periodically

It is recognized that guidelines may become outdated as new diagnostic and treatment procedures are developed and as additional knowledge is acquired regarding the benefits and harms of existing procedures. On the basis of a review of published AHRQ guidelines, Shekelle et al. (2001) suggested that guidelines should be assessed for validity every 3 years, although the generalizability of this recommendation to other guidelines remains in doubt (Browman 2001). In any case, some strategy must exist for periodically evaluating new evidence and for updating guidelines as necessary (Browman 2001; Shekelle et al. 1999a, 1999b, 2001).

Critical Appraisal of Guidelines

Because of the variable nature of the guideline development process, with some guidelines linked more closely to the research evidence than others, it is necessary to critically appraise guidelines before following their recommendations (Feder et al. 1999). Several guidelines have been developed for the critical appraisal of clinical practice guidelines (Greenhalgh 2001; Grimshaw and Eccles 2001; Guyatt et al. 2002; Pinsky and Deyo 2000; Sackett et al. 2000; Snowball 1999). Table 7–3 presents one approach.

TABLE 7–3.   Critical appraisal guide for a clinical practice guideline

Is the guideline valid?

Did the developers carry out a systematic review of the literature?

Were all relevant treatment options and outcomes considered?

Did the developers specify and make explicit the values associated with various outcomes?

Did the developers indicate the level of evidence (and sources) upon which each recommendation was based?

Is the guideline applicable to my practice?

Is the burden of illness too low to warrant implementation?

Are the beliefs of my patients incompatible with the guidelines?

Are the costs and other barriers of implementation too high?

Source.   Adapted from Greenhalgh 2001; Guyatt et al. 2002; Sackett et al. 2000.

Is the Guideline Valid?

The first part of the appraisal concerns the validity of the clinical practice guidelines.

Did the Developers Carry Out a Systematic Review?

The development of a systematic review is what distinguishes evidence-based guidelines from opinion-based guidelines. The NICE methodology provides an excellent model for guideline development.

Were All Relevant Treatment Options and Outcomes Considered?

Several questions should be asked with regard to treatment options and outcome. For example, do the guidelines mention only pharmacotherapy, or do they include psychotherapy and other psychosocial interventions? Have the developers considered potential harms from the interventions, or have they considered only the benefits? It is more likely that these issues will be addressed if the group developing the guidelines is multidisciplinary rather than one limited by narrow expertise (Guyatt et al. 2002).

Did the Developers Specify Values Associated With Various Outcomes?

Reasonable people can make very different recommendations after considering the same evidence, depending on the value attached to different outcomes. In a review of atypical antipsychotics in the treatment of schizophrenia, Geddes et al. (2000) concluded that atypical and conventional antipsychotics were equal in effectiveness and tolerability. The authors then went on to recommend conventional antipsychotics as first-line drugs because of cost considerations. Kapur and Remington (2000) reached the opposite conclusion after reviewing the same data, giving more value to the differences in risk of extrapyramidal side effects and less value to other side effects and to economic considerations. In weighing benefits and risks, guideline developers should be clear as to how they arrive at a particular recommendation (Guyatt et al. 2002).

Did the Developers Indicate the Level of Evidence and Sources on Which Each Recommendation Was Based?

If guideline developers indicate the level of evidence and sources on which each recommendation is based, the user can determine which recommendations are based on strong evidence and which recommendations are based on opinion. Ideally, guidelines should be primarily based on research evidence rather than on opinion; however, guidelines typically have some recommendations based primarily on expert opinion, and these should be labeled as such.

Is the Guideline Applicable to My Practice?

Assuming that the guidelines are primarily evidence based (and that the recommendations that are opinion based are clearly indicated), the user still must decide whether to follow the recommendations.

Is the Burden of Illness Too Low to Warrant Implementation?

If a guideline involves screening for disease, is the risk high enough in your patient population to make this recommendation worthwhile? As discussed in

Chapter 9, screening low-risk populations produces far more false-positive than true-positive test results. Similarly, if the recommendation involves preventive measures, implementing them in a low-risk population may produce more harm than good (Sackett et al. 2000). Guidelines developed for use in tertiary care settings, where the severity of illness and degree of comorbidity are high, may not be applicable in primary care settings, where illness severity is lower (Greenhalgh 2001).

Are the Beliefs of My Patients Incompatible With the Guidelines?

If your patients prefer psychotherapy and the recommendation is for medications (or vice versa), the guideline will be difficult to implement.

Are the Costs and Other Barriers to Implementation Too High?

Perhaps the guideline recommends a type of therapy that is unavailable in your geographic area. Is it practical for someone to be trained in its application? Or perhaps the recommendation concerns a method of delivering services (e.g., assertive community treatment) that is not available in your setting. What are the costs and other barriers to implementation?

Comparison of Guidelines

Choosing one guideline over another can be a challenge. After reviewing and comparing guidelines, the clinician might decide to combine aspects of guidelines or even to include other recommendations. Presented with similar evidence, different guideline development groups might arrive at different conclusions. As an example, we compared the specific recommendations for the NICE and APA guidelines for the use of psychotherapies and medications in bulimia.

We began by using the comparison feature available on the National Guideline Clearinghouse Web site (www.guideline.gov) with the term *eating disorders*. To do this, we first searched the database to identify potentially useful guidelines and added two guidelines to our "collection": the National Collaborating Centre for Mental Health's *Eating Disorders: Core Interventions in the Treatment and Management of Anorexia Nervosa, Bulimia Nervosa and Related Eating Disorders* (NGC:003550) and the American Psychiatric Association's *Practice Guideline for the Treatment of*

Patients With Eating Disorders, American Psychiatric Association—Medical Specialty Society, 1993 (revised June 2006) (NGC:004987). We then went back to the home page to "Compare Checked Guidelines" and selected these two guidelines to compare. The program provided the basic characteristics of the two guidelines on several dimensions: guideline developers, sources of funding, composition of group that authored the guideline, conflicts of interest, guideline objectives, major outcomes considered, methods used to collect or select evidence, methods used to assess the quality and strength of the evidence, major recommendations, and so forth.

The NICE method seemed superior to the APA method, but both recommendations were worth considering. Unfortunately, the actual recommendations are difficult to compare. Both list more than 100 treatment recommendations (although many are specific to one disorder or another; e.g., anorexia or bulimia).

Another approach to comparing guidelines is to use the "Guideline Synthesis" function. For example, we used the "Guideline Synthesis" function to generate a list of available syntheses. We then selected "Management of Eating Disorders" from the list. The synthesis was conducted on three guidelines:

1. APA: *Practice Guideline for the Treatment of Patients With Eating Disorders*, 3rd Edition. Washington, DC, American Psychiatric Association
2. Finnish Medical Society Duodecim (FMSD): "Eating disorders among children and adolescents," in *EBM Guidelines: Evidence-Based Medicine* [Internet]. Helsinki, Finland, Wiley Interscience, John Wiley and Sons, 2007
3. National Collaborating Centre for Mental Health (NCCMH/NICE): *Eating Disorders: Core Interventions in the Treatment and Management of Anorexia Nervosa, Bulimia Nervosa and Related Eating Disorders*. Leicester, UK, British Psychological Society, 2004.

The first part of the synthesis provides much of the same information as does the comparison feature but goes further in providing a written guideline comparison. For instance, the content comparison notes, "While FMSD focuses on anorexia and bulimia nervosa, APA and NCCMH/NICE also address atypical eating disorders such as binge eating disorder and eating disorders not otherwise specified (EDNOS)." This implies that in searching for a guideline addressing atypical eating disorders, the FMSD would not be useful. More important, the synthesis examines areas of agreement and disagreement.

We then examined in more detail some specific recommendations related to the case of a young woman with bulimia presented in Chapter 18. The two guidelines would lead the clinician in somewhat different directions.

Table 7–4 lists the main psychotherapy recommendations for the two guidelines. The NICE guideline suggests starting with a self-help approach, which may not be feasible in private practice but might work well in a health maintenance organization. The NICE guideline also recommends cognitive-behavioral therapy (CBT) as the next choice. The APA notes that the evidence supports CBT as the most effective single intervention. However, the guidelines differ as to what to do if CBT fails or if the patient prefers another treatment. NICE states that interpersonal psychotherapy (IPT) should be considered as an alternative to CBT. The APA notes that IPT is effective in some cases but argues that CBT "is associated with more rapid remission of eating symptoms" and adds that "using psychodynamic interventions in conjunction with CBT and other psychotherapies may yield better global outcomes." A clinician curious about these different interpretations may want to go to the guideline to determine the database behind the recommendations, but this can be time-consuming. We searched PubMed with the terms *bulimia*, *psychotherapy* and with "limits of reviews," "summaries," and "meta-analyses." The most comprehensive review was by Wilson (2005), who stated:

> There is no evidence that an "integrated psychotherapy" is effective with BN [bulimia nervosa], let alone more effective than CBT alone. It has been suggested that complex cases characterized by comorbid personality disorders require a blend of CBT and psychodynamic psychotherapy....No evidence supports this speculation. Controlled studies of the effectiveness of psychodynamic therapies are still conspicuously lacking.

The guidelines also differ on the use of medications (see Table 7–5). NICE recommends SSRIs but grades the recommendation as a C. APA rates the use of fluoxetine as I. NICE does not recommend

other medications; APA notes that topiramate may be useful (III). We view these guidelines as sources of information.

Implementing Practice Guidelines and Algorithms

The reason that guidelines are usually developed is to attempt to improve the delivery of care within an organization, geographic area, or profession. The results of such attempts have been mixed (Bero et al. 1998; Davis and Taylor-Vaisey 1997; Greenhalgh 2001; Grimshaw and Russell 1993; Grol 2001b; Lipman 2000; National Health Service Centre for Reviews and Dissemination 1999; Owen et al. 2008; Oxman et al. 1995; Worrall et al. 1997). We mentioned in the beginning of the book that recent studies show that compared with treatment as usual, the use of algorithms and collaborative care approaches in the care of depressed patients enhances treatment outcomes by modifying practice procedures and treatment processes (Adli et al. 2006). Although implementation of STAR*D has not been compared with treatment without following STAR*D, the protocol is designed to achieve a clinically significant outcome. On the other hand, Owen et al. (2008) compared the effectiveness of a conceptually based, multicomponent "enhanced" strategy with a "basic" strategy for implementing antipsychotic management recommendations of Department of Veterans Affairs (VA) schizophrenia guidelines. Two VA medical centers in each of three Veterans Integrated Service Networks were randomly assigned to either a basic educational implementation strategy or the enhanced strategy, in which a trained nurse promoted provider guideline adherence and patient compliance. Patients with acute exacerbation of schizophrenia were enrolled and were assessed at baseline and 6 months, and their medical records were abstracted. The enhanced guideline implementation strategy increased addition of second-generation antipsychotic to first-generation antipsychotic therapy but did not significantly increase guideline-recommended switching from first-generation antipsychotic to second-generation antipsychotic monotherapy. Antipsychotic dosing was not significantly altered.

On the contrary, some organizations have found an improvement in quality of care and reduction of costs with the widespread implementation of guidelines (Mullaney 2005). Guidelines may be particu-

TABLE 7–4. A comparison of psychotherapy recommendations for treating bulimia for two guidelines

Area	NICE guideline	APA guideline
First step	**B**—As a possible first step, patients with bulimia nervosa should be encouraged to follow an evidence-based self-help program.	A variety of self-help and professionally guided self-help programs have been effective for some patients with bulimia nervosa **[I]**.
Cognitive-behavioral therapy (CBT)	**A**—CBT for bulimia nervosa (CBT-BN), a specifically adapted form of CBT, should be offered to adults with bulimia nervosa. The course of treatment should be for 16–20 sessions over 4–5 months.	For treating acute episodes of bulimia nervosa in adults, the evidence strongly supports the value of CBT as the most effective single intervention **[I]**.
If CBT does not work or patient prefers other treatments	**B**—When people with bulimia nervosa have not responded to or do not want CBT, other psychological treatments should be considered.	Some patients who do not respond initially to CBT may respond when switched to either interpersonal therapy (IPT) or fluoxetine **[II]** or other modes of treatment such as family and group psychotherapies **[III]**.
Interpersonal psychotherapy (IPT)	**B**—IPT should be considered as an alternative to CBT, but patients should be informed that it takes 8–12 months to achieve results comparable with those of CBT.	Controlled trials also have shown the utility of IPT in some cases **[II]**. In clinical practice, many practitioners combine elements of CBT, IPT, and other psychotherapeutic techniques. Compared with psychodynamic therapy or IPT, CBT is associated with more rapid remission of eating symptoms **[I]**, but using psychodynamic interventions in conjunction with CBT and other psychotherapies may yield better global outcomes **[II]**.

Note. APA=American Psychiatric Association; NICE=National Institute for Health and Clinical Excellence. **A**=At least one randomized controlled trial; **B**=Well-conducted clinical studies but no randomized clinical trials. **[I]**=Recommended with substantial clinical confidence; **[II]**=Recommended with moderate clinical confidence; **[III]**=May be recommended on the basis of individual circumstances.

Source. American Psychiatric Association: *Practice Guideline for the Treatment of Patients With Eating Disorders*, 3rd Edition. Washington, DC, American Psychiatric Association, 2006; National Collaborating Centre for Mental Health (NCCMH/NICE): *Eating Disorders: Core Interventions in the Treatment and Management of Anorexia Nervosa, Bulimia Nervosa and Related Eating Disorders*. Leicester, UK, British Psychological Society, 2004.

larly important when they recommend a treatment that is not widely used but might be associated with a better outcome. For instance, the algorithms for treating schizophrenia developed by TMAP, the International Psychopharmacology Algorithm Project, and the Psychopharmacology Algorithm Project at the Harvard South Shore Department of Psychiatry all recommend using clozapine after two adequate monotherapy trials of other antipsychotics in schizophrenia. The latest Clinical Antipsychotic Trials of Intervention Effectiveness data support this recommendation (McEvoy et al. 2006). Yet clinicians appear to prefer to try many additional monotherapy trials, various combinations of antipsychotics, and other polytherapy before starting clozapine. The reasons for not following this recommendation are not known but may be related to the fact that it is a more demanding treatment to implement for the physician and the patient. There may be concerns about adverse effects, additional time and effort to obtain consent, and the need for medical monitoring in addition to patient reluctance for some of the same reasons.

TABLE 7–5. Comparison of medication recommendations for treating bulimia for two guidelines

Area	NICE guideline	APA guideline
Initial medication	**C**—Selective serotonin reuptake inhibitors (SSRIs) (specifically fluoxetine) are the drugs of first choice for the treatment of bulimia nervosa.	To date, fluoxetine is the best studied of these SSRIs and is the only FDA-approved medication for bulimia nervosa. Sertraline is the only other SSRI that has been shown to be effective, as demonstrated in a small randomized controlled trial. In the absence of therapists qualified to treat bulimia nervosa with cognitive-behavioral therapy (CBT), fluoxetine is recommended as an initial treatment **[I]**.
Other drugs	None are recommended.	Small controlled trials have confirmed the efficacy of the anticonvulsant medication topiramate, but because adverse reactions to this medication are common, it should be used only when other medications have proved ineffective **[III]**.

Note. APA=American Psychiatric Association; FDA=U.S. Food and Drug Administration; NICE=National Institute for Health and Clinical Excellence.

C=Directly applicable clinical studies of good quality are absent or not readily available. **[I]**=Recommended with substantial clinical confidence; **[III]**=May be recommended on the basis of individual circumstances.

Source. Adapted from American Psychiatric Association: *Practice Guideline for the Treatment of Patients With Eating Disorders*, 3rd Edition. Washington, DC, American Psychiatric Association, 2006; National Collaborating Centre for Mental Health (NC-CMH/NICE): *Eating Disorders: Core Interventions in the Treatment and Management of Anorexia Nervosa, Bulimia Nervosa and Related Eating Disorders*. Leicester, UK, , British Psychological Society, 2004.

In general, the passive dissemination of guidelines has little effect on clinical practice (Bero et al. 1998; Davis and Taylor-Vaisey 1997; Oxman et al. 1995) or on patient outcome (Farmer et al. 2008). Guidelines are more apt to be adopted if they take account of local circumstances, are disseminated by active educational interventions, and are implemented using patient-specific reminders (Bero et al. 1998; Feder et al. 1999; Greenhalgh 2001; National Health Service Centre for Reviews and Dissemination 1999). Multifaceted interventions tend to be more effective, but they are also more expensive (Bero et al. 1998; Davis and Taylor-Vaisey 1997; Greenhalgh 2001; Grol 1997; National Health Service Centre for Reviews and Dissemination 1999; Oxman et al. 1995). In the cases presented in Chapters 17–34, we discuss ways to use guidelines more effectively.

Improving the Use of Guidelines

Reluctance and resistance to using guidelines come from many sources. Curiously, clinicians may agree with the recommendations when they are presented to them separately (Cabana et al. 1999). Many clinicians probably have a working set of guidelines in

their mind based on experience, training, and perhaps some updating of the literature.

With all these limitations, guidelines are still an important part of managing patients. As noted several times in this book, we review guidelines as a starting place. They are not a definitive source of patient care. However, clinicians should use guidelines as an important source of care options for their patients. The point is not to bring the patient to the guideline but to bring the guideline to the patient. The authors of some of the cases presented in this volume created checklists from the guidelines, and they used the checklists both to guide therapy and as a review to help them identify areas in which they could improve their practice.

Choosing Guidelines

Choosing which guideline or guidelines to follow for the complicated, comorbid cases we see in clinical practice is a challenge. Guidelines and medication algorithms are usually developed to treat most "single" disorders; few address comorbid problems. As illustrated in Chapter 18, a guideline for treating one disorder may be contradicted by a guideline for treating a comorbid disorder in the same patient. Many clinicians may prefer to follow only one guideline, presumably the one relevant to the primary problem. Other clinicians may wish to combine algorithms and guidelines drawn from various sources, as illustrated in Chapters 18, 20, and 34 among others. As therapy progresses, new problems, not covered by the initial guidelines and algorithms, may emerge and require consideration of other evidence bases and approaches.

The treatment setting and nature of the clinician's practice also affect which guidelines are selected. A guideline developed for a 20- to 30-minute patient visit might be very different from a guideline developed for a 50-minute visit. A guideline for a 50-minute session involving a nondirective psychodynamic approach will be quite different from a guideline for a 50-minute directive, structured session. Clinicians can find guidelines and algorithms appropriate for their practice setting and situation, and it is important for clinicians to continue to update them as a result of their experience and new information.

Another major problem in following guidelines is that they tend to focus on treatment planning rather than on implementation. The latter is much more challenging for most clinicians. In Chapters 17–34, experienced clinicians present examples of how they have used guidelines, algorithms, and other sources of EBPP to provide care for the individuals they discuss. We believe the cases in this volume provide wonderful examples of how EBPP can improve patient care!

References

Adli M, Bauer M, Rush AJ: Algorithms and collaborative-care systems for depression: are they effective and why? A systematic review. Biol Psychiatry 59:1029–1038, 2006

Agency for Health Care Policy and Research: Depression in primary care, Vol 2: Treatment of major depression. Clinical Practice Guideline No 5. Rockville, MD, U.S. Department of Health and Human Services, 1993b

American Psychiatric Association: Diagnostic and Statistical Manual of Mental Disorders, 4th Edition, Text Revision. Washington, DC, American Psychiatric Association, 2000

American Psychiatric Association: Practice Guidelines for the Treatment of Psychiatric Disorders, Compendium. Washington, DC, American Psychiatric Association, 2006

Antman EM, Lau J, Kupelnick B, et al: A comparison of results of meta-analyses of randomized control trials and recommendations of clinical experts: treatments for myocardial infarction. JAMA 268:240–248, 1992

Badenoch D, Heneghan C: Evidence-Based Medicine Toolkit. London, BMJ Books, 2002

Berg AO, Atkins D, Tierney W: Clinical practice guidelines in practice and education. J Gen Intern Med 12 (suppl 2):S25–S33, 1997

Bero LA, Grilli R, Grimshaw JM, et al: Closing the gap between research and practice: an overview of systematic reviews of interventions to promote the implementation of research findings. The Cochrane Effective Practice and Organization of Care Review Group. BMJ 317:465–468, 1998

Birkmeyer JD: Primer on geographic variation in health care. Eff Clin Pract 4:232–233, 2001

Black N, Murphy M, Lamping D, et al: Consensus development methods and their use in creating clinical guidelines, in The Advanced Handbook of Methods in Evidence Based Healthcare. Edited by Stevens A, Abrams K, Brazier J, et al. London, Sage, 2001, pp 426–448

Browman GP: Development and aftercare of clinical guidelines: the balance between rigor and pragmatism. JAMA 286:1509–1511, 2001

Cabana MD, Rand CS, Powe NR, et al: Why don't physicians follow clinical practice guidelines? A framework for improvement. JAMA 282:1458–1465, 1999

Choudhry NK, Stelfox HT, Detsky AS: Relationships between authors of clinical practice guidelines and the pharmaceutical industry. JAMA 287:612–617, 2002

Cook DJ, Greengold NL, Ellrodt AG, et al: The relation between systematic reviews and practice guidelines, in Systematic Reviews: Synthesis of Best Evidence for Health Care Decisions. Edited by Mulrow C, Cook D. Philadelphia, PA, American College of Physicians, 1998, pp 55–65

Davis DA, Taylor-Vaisey A: Translating guidelines into practice: a systematic review of theoretic concepts, practical experience and research evidence in the adoption of clinical practice guidelines. CMAJ 157:408–416, 1997

Drake RE, Goldman HH, Leff HS, et al: Implementing evidence-based practices in routine mental health settings. Psychiatr Serv 52:179–182, 2001

Eccles M, Freemantle N, Mason J: Using systematic reviews in clinical guideline development, in Systematic Reviews in Health Care: Meta-Analysis in Context. Edited by Egger M, Smith GD, Altman DG. London, BMJ Books, 2001, pp 400–409

Expert Consensus Guidelines: Psychiatric treatment guidelines for the most difficult questions facing clinicians [Expert Consensus Guidelines Web site]. April 3, 2002. Available at: http://www.psychguides.com. Accessed September 13, 2002

Farmer AP, Légaré F, Turcot L, et al: Printed educational materials: effects on professional practice and health care outcomes. Cochrane Database Syst Rev (3):CD004398, 2008

Feder G, Eccles M, Grol R, et al: Using clinical guidelines. BMJ 318:728–730, 1999

Field MJ, Lohr KN (eds): Clinical Practice Guidelines: Directions for a New Program. Washington, DC, National Academy Press, 1990

Field MJ, Lohr KN (eds): Clinical Practice Guidelines: From Development to Use. Washington, DC, National Academy Press, 1992

Geddes J, Freemantle N, Harrison P, et al: Atypical antipsychotics in the treatment of schizophrenia: systematic overview and meta-regression analysis. BMJ 321:1371–1376, 2000

Gilbert DA, Altshuler KZ, Rago WV, et al: Texas Medication Algorithm Project: definitions, rationale, and methods to develop medication algorithms. J Clin Psychiatry 59:345–351, 1998

Gray GE: Evidence-based medicine: an introduction for psychiatrists. J Psychiatr Pract 8:5–13, 2002

Greenhalgh T: How to Read a Paper: The Basics of Evidence-Based Medicine, 2nd Edition. London, BMJ Books, 2001

Greenhalgh T, Peacock R: Effectiveness and efficiency of search methods in systematic reviews of complex evidence: audit of primary sources. BMJ 331(7524):1064–1065, 2005

Grimshaw J, Eccles M: Identifying and using evidence-based guidelines in general practice, in Evidence-Based Practice in Primary Care, 2nd Edition. Edited by Silagy C, Haines A. London, BMJ Books, 2001, pp 120–134

Grimshaw JM, Russell IT: Effect of clinical guidelines on medical practice: a systematic review of rigorous evaluations. Lancet 342:1317–1322, 1993

Grol R: Personal paper: beliefs and evidence in changing clinical practice. BMJ 315:418–421, 1997

Grol R: Improving the quality of medical care: building bridges among professional pride, payer profit, and patient satisfaction. JAMA 286:2578–2585, 2001a

Grol R: Successes and failures in the implementation of evidence-based guidelines for clinical practice. Med Care 39 (suppl 2):II-46–II-54, 2001b

Guyatt G, Hayward R, Richardson WS, et al: Moving from evidence to action, in Users' Guides to the Medical Literature: A Manual for Evidence-Based Clinical Practice. Edited by Guyatt G, Rennie D. Chicago, IL, AMA Press, 2002, pp 175–199

Haines A, Jones R: Implementing findings of research. BMJ 308:1488–1492, 1994

Harbour R, Miller J: A new system for grading recommendations in evidence based guidelines. BMJ 323:334–336, 2001

Kahn DA, Docherty JP, Carpenter D, et al: Consensus methods in practice guideline development: a review and description of a new method. Psychopharmacol Bull 33:631–639, 1997

Kapur S, Remington G: Atypical antipsychotics. BMJ 321:1360–1361, 2000

Keller MB, McCullough JP, Klein DN, et al: A comparison of nefazodone, the cognitive behavioral-analysis system of psychotherapy, and their combination for the treatment of chronic depression. N Engl J Med 342:1462–1470, 2000

Lipman T: Evidence-based practice in general practice and primary care, in Evidence-Based Practice: A Critical Appraisal. Edited by Trinder L, Reynolds S. Oxford, UK, Blackwell Scientific, 2000, pp 35–65

McColl A, Smith H, White P, et al: General practitioners' perception of the route to evidence based medicine: a questionnaire survey. BMJ 316:361–365, 1998

McEvoy JP, Lieberman JA, Stroup TS, et al: Effectiveness of clozapine versus olanzapine, quetiapine, and risperidone in patients with chronic schizophrenia who did not respond to prior atypical antipsychotic treatment. Am J Psychiatry 163:600–610, 2006

Milner KK, Valenstein M: A comparison of guidelines for the treatment of schizophrenia. Psychiatr Serv 53:888–890, 2002

Mullaney TJ: Doctors wielding data. Business Week, November 21, 2005, pp 94, 98

Mulrow CD: Systematic reviews: rationale for systematic reviews. BMJ 309:597–599, 1994

National Health Service Centre for Reviews and Dissemination: Getting evidence into practice. Eff Health Care 5(1):1–16, 1999

National Institute for Health and Clinical Excellence: How NICE clinical guidelines are developed: an overview for stakeholders, the public and NHS. London, National Health Service, 2007

Owen RR, Hudson T, Thrush C, et al: The effectiveness of guideline implementation strategies on improving antipsychotic medication management for schizophrenia. Med Care 46:686–691, 2008

Oxman AD, Thomson MA, Davis DA, et al: No magic bullet: a systematic review of 102 trials of interventions to improve professional practice. CMAJ 153:1423–1431, 1995

Pinsky LE, Deyo RA: Clinical guidelines: a strategy for translating evidence into practice, in Evidence-Based Clinical Practice: Concepts and Approaches. Edited by Geyman JP, Deyo RA, Ramsey SD. Boston, MA, Butterworth-Heinemann, 2000, pp 119–123

Sackett DL, Haynes RB, Guyatt GH, et al: Clinical Epidemiology: A Basic Science for Clinical Medicine, 2nd Edition. Boston, MA, Little, Brown, 1991

Sackett DL, Straus SE, Richardson WS, et al: Evidence-Based Medicine: How to Practice and Teach EBM, 2nd Edition. New York, Churchill Livingstone, 2000

Shekelle PG, Woolf SH, Eccles M, et al: Developing clinical guidelines. West J Med 170:348–351, 1999a

Shekelle PG, Woolf SH, Eccles M, et al: Developing guidelines. BMJ 318:593–596, 1999b

Shekelle PG, Ortiz E, Rhodes S, et al: Validity of the Agency for Healthcare Research and Quality clinical practice guidelines: how quickly do guidelines become outdated? JAMA 286:1461–1467, 2001

Snowball R: Critical appraisal of clinical guidelines, in Evidence-Based Practice: A Primer for Health Care Professionals. Edited by Dawes M, Davies P, Gray A, et al. Edinburgh, Churchill Livingstone, 1999, pp 127–131

Texas Medication Algorithm Project: TMAP—a collaborative effort [Texas Medication Algorithm Project Web site]. April 3, 2002. Available at: http://www.dshs.state.tx.us/mhprograms/TIMA.shtm. Accessed July 1, 2009

Trivedi MH, Rush AJ, Wisniewski SR, et al: Evaluation of outcomes with citalopram for depression using measurement-based care in STAR*D: implications for clinical practice. Am J Psychiatry 163:28–40, 2006

Wilson GT: Psychological treatment of eating disorders. Annu Rev Clin Psychol 1:439–465, 2005

Woolf SH, Grol R, Hutchinson A, et al: Clinical guidelines: international overview [BMJ Web site]. February 20, 1999a. Available at: http://bmj.com/cgi/content/full/318/7182/527/DC1/1. Accessed September 24, 2002

Woolf SH, Grol R, Hutchinson A, et al: Potential benefits, limitations, and harms of clinical guidelines. BMJ 318:527–530, 1999b

Worrall G, Chaulk P, Freake D: The effects of clinical practice guidelines on patient outcomes in primary care: a systematic review. CMAJ 156:1705–1712, 1997

Young JM, Ward JE: Evidence-based medicine in general practice: beliefs and barriers among Australian GPs. J Eval Clin Pract 7:201–210, 2001

Measurement

C. Barr Taylor, M.D.

Measuring and monitoring patient progress are key to practicing evidence-based psychiatry. For many decades, researchers, policy makers, insurers, and some clinicians have noted the need to focus as much on outcomes as on process (Ellwood 1988; McGrath and Tempier 2003). Recently, the Sequenced Treatment Alternatives to Relieve Depression (STAR*D) investigators have argued that "measurement" should be the paradigm for psychiatric practice (Trivedi and Daly 2007; Trivedi et al. 2007). Yet few clinicians routinely monitor outcomes unless compelled to do so. Why? The main reason is probably that they have little incentive to do so and some good reasons not to. In a busy practice, the added paperwork could be seen as a needless addition to an already pressured schedule. Even simple assessment forms and instruments need to handed out, scored, stored, and interpreted, contributing to increased "charting burden." Some clinicians believe that paper assessment, at least beyond the initial sessions, can interfere with the therapeutic relationship—a piece of paper is substituted for a more meaningful interaction. The clinician might argue that if patients seem to be improving and seem satisfied with their care, then they should not make changes. Ultimately, the clinician must decide that the effort results in better patient care.

Fortunately, obtaining and using assessment instruments have become easier in recent years. First, numerous assessment instruments can be readily ob-tained or purchased online. Many instruments relevant to psychiatric practice are available on the CD-ROM that accompanies the American Psychiatric Publishing *Handbook of Psychiatric Measures*, 2nd Edition (Rush et al. 2008). Copyright protection and other issues may limit the use of some standardized assessment instruments, but alternative public domain instruments usually can be found to measure outcomes. Second, practice management software systems are now available that make assessment and record keeping easier, as discussed at the end of this chapter. Some of the cases illustrate how measurement can be incorporated into clinical practice. Third, many guidelines and algorithms use measurement to guide decision making, and adherence to such guidelines and algorithms may improve practice. Fourth, evidence-based medicine (EBM) and evidence-based psychiatric practice (EBPP) are based on measurement.

In this chapter, I discuss "what to measure," review how one can consider the reliability and validity of a measure, present examples of some "nonstandard" measures, and provide examples of how process and outcome measures have been implemented in several practice settings.

Which Outcomes to Measure

Several factors need to be considered in deciding what to measure.[1] The type of measures may be

---

[1] Instruments used to assess baseline function, psychological process, and other phenomena may be different from instruments used to assess outcome. In this section, we focus on outcome assessment instruments.

determined by the practice setting or by the insurer. For instance, the Department of Veterans Affairs (VA) is adopting outcome measures for a variety of problems. Some insurers ask providers to complete periodic assessments. Domains of outcome measurement to consider include symptomatology, patient functioning, quality of life, patient satisfaction, and even cost and cost-benefit ratio. We recommend a smorgasbord approach. If a clinician is using a guideline or algorithm that has a measure to guide treatment decisions, then that measure should be adopted. For instance, those who are following the STAR*D guidelines would want to use a version of the Quick Inventory of Depressive Symptomatology (QIDS), and those using the Beck model of cognitive-behavioral therapy (CBT) would want to use the Beck Depression Inventory–II (BDI-II) and also, perhaps, the QIDS because it has defined outcomes for remission and relapse.

If a clinician has decided to follow practice recommendations from the evidence base for a particular problem and the analyses have used an available instrument, that would be a logical choice as a measure. For example, the Hamilton Rating Scale for Depression (Ham-D) is a widely used measure for depression outcome studies and might serve as a good reference in helping clinicians determine how well their patients are doing against published standards.

The clinicians' values and interests should also guide what domains they assess. For instance, one might want to include a quality-of-life measure (see Chapter 30). Second, one should consider measuring behaviors, attitudes, and issues of relevance to individual patients but not necessarily covered in standard instruments. Table 16–1 in Chapter 16 lists the measures used by the therapists in the case presentations. Some of the measures are standardized outcomes, with extensive psychometric data (e.g., the Posttraumatic Stress Disorder [PTSD] Checklist, the QIDS–Self-Report, the Yale-Brown Obsessive Compulsive Scale). Others represent self-reports of behaviors (e.g., binge and purge frequency, alcohol use), relationships, symptoms (e.g., dizziness, panic attacks, trouble swallowing), or medical parameters (e.g., weight).

The *Handbook of Psychiatric Measures*, 2nd Edition (Rush et al. 2008), has provided an invaluable resource of standard measures for clinicians. Table 8–1 lists the categories of measures available in this pub-

lication. The text of the *Handbook* includes a description of each measure (e.g., number of items), the goals of the measure, practical issues (how long does it take to administer, where permission can be obtained), the psychometric properties of the instrument (reliability, validity), and the clinical utility (what useful information it provides).

Constructing a Measure

Given the importance of measures, it is worthwhile to consider how they are developed. Measures can be constructed in several ways. Many of the classic psychiatric measurement skills were developed by a researcher simply trying to identify the main features of a disorder and then finding a way to rate the frequency and intensity of these features. For instance, when Hamilton decided to develop a measure for depression in the 1950s, he presumably began by listing the main features: depressed mood, feelings of guilt, suicidality, insomnia, trouble with work and activities, psychomotor retardation, agitation, mental and somatic anxiety, gastrointestinal and other somatic symptoms, hypochondriasis, change in weight, change in insight, diurnal variation of mood, depersonalization and derealization, paranoia, and obessionality. He then developed a system to rate each of these items. Hamilton probably erred in mixing nominal and ordinal items and in assuming that each item was more or less equally as important as any other item (Babgy et al. 2004).

Beck developed his inventory (Beck et al. (1961; perhaps the most widely used self-report depression instrument in psychiatry) by first identifying symptoms and attitudes that were common in depressed patients but rare in nondepressed patients. These ideas were systematically consolidated into 21 symptoms and attitudes that could be rated from 0 to 3 in intensity. The items included mood, pessimism, sense of failure, lack of satisfaction, guilt, sense of punishment, sense of self-dislike, self-accusation, suicide wishes, crying, irritability, social withdrawal, fatigability, and loss of appetite. Seemingly, individuals who score higher are more depressed. Both the Ham-D and the BDI-II have undergone some revision, but the core measures remain much the same.

Both Hamilton and Beck used clinical observation to select items to measure. Some other approaches for scale construction are available. Another ap-

TABLE 8–1. Categories of measures available in *Handbook of Psychiatric Measures*

Measures are provided for:

    Diagnosis in adults

    General psychiatric symptoms

    Mental health status, functioning, and disabilities

    General health status, functioning, and disabilities

    Quality of life

    Adverse effects

    Patient perceptions of care

    Stress and life events

    Family risk factors

    Suicide risk

    Diagnosis and screening in children and adolescents

    Disorders usually first diagnosed in infancy, childhood, or adolescence

    Child and adolescent functional status

    Personality traits and defense mechanisms

    Delirium and behavioral symptoms of cognition

    Aggression

    Cognitive, substance use, psychotic, mood, anxiety, somatoform, factitious and malingering, dissociative, sexual dysfunction, eating, sleep, impulse-control, and personality disorders

Source. Rush AJ Jr, First MB, Blacker D (eds): *Handbook of Psychiatric Measures*, 2nd Edition. Washington, DC, American Psychiatric Publishing, 2008.

proach would be to develop a rating scale based on the standard items of some diagnostic system, such as DSM-IV-TR (American Psychiatric Association 2000). This was the approach used in developing the QIDS, which was used in the STAR*D project (Rush et al. 2003). Another approach is to ask many questions of a population of interest and then to use statistical methods to identify those items that best distinguish one population (such as depressed individuals) from another (nondepressed individuals). The items then can be used to form a scale. We used this approach several years ago when we wanted to develop a measure to identify students at risk for developing an eating disorder (Killen et al. 1993). We gave various standard eating disorder attitude and behavior scales to 967 sixth- and seventh-grade girls. A principal components analysis was conducted to reduce redundancy to find a set of independent variables. The result was a set of five items measuring worry about weight and body shape, weight gain, dieting, importance of weight, and feeling fat.

Once items are identified, the next issue in scale development is to determine how to rate them. Items can be rated in several ways. For instance, they can be rated in terms of frequency (never to very often) or intensity (not at all to very) across dimensions (see the Ham-D, item 5, for an example of this). Books and articles on scale development are available for the interested reader (e.g., DeVellis 2003). Before giving forms to a patient, it is a good idea for the clinician to fill out a copy to get a sense of exactly what is being asked.

Psychometric Properties of Scales

Scientific studies favor standard measures with known and acceptable reliability and validity.

Reliability

In statistics, *reliability* is the consistency of a set of measurements or a measuring instrument. Three types of reliability are reported, depending on the purpose of the measure and how it is administered. Clinical assessment instruments report the internal reliability (or consistency) of individual items, the test-retest reliability of the total score and/or items in the measurement instrument, and interrater reliability of the instrument. Reliability is inversely related to random error; that is, high reliability scores make one more confident that the scale is measuring what it is supposed to.

Internal consistency represents how well the items of a scale measure a single dimension of an underlying construct. Because individuals may use different words to describe some aspect of their functioning, a scale that assesses a dimension with several questions might allow for more people to be able to report more accurately. Some measurement instruments include several scales, each of which might have "good internal consistency." Good internal consistency of a scale may actually limit its usefulness for some purposes. For instance, an instrument to measure mania may assess both psychotic and neurovegetative symptoms. Because these symptoms are not strongly correlated in bipolar patients, the measure would have poor internal consistency, although it might accurately measure mania from a clinical standpoint.

Interrater reliability is a measure of agreement between two or more observers evaluating the same series of subjects and using the same information. Interrater reliability is best measured with the κ statistic, which is a measure of agreement corrected or changed (Fleiss 1981). For categorical measures, a κ value of 1 indicates perfect agreement; a κ of 0 indicates no agreement. In clinical trials, κ's of greater than 0.6–0.7 are considered adequate, and a κ greater than 0.8 is considered excellent (Landis and Koch 1977). The clinician should be wary of studies with a κ less than 0.5 because it suggests that two raters cannot agree on what they are judging. Reliability for continuous measures is more complicated. Suppose a rater is asked to determine whether a patient does not look at all sad, looks a little sad, looks somewhat sad, looks very sad, or looks very, very sad. It is harder for raters to agree on such levels, and statistical methods have been developed to account for this. Interrater reliability is extremely important for research studies.

Test-retest reliability measures whether the same observers or individuals completing a measure answer questions the same way from one time to the next, assuming there is no intervening change. Typically, the same test is repeated a few days or weeks apart. For retest reliability of scale items, a Pearson r greater than 0.70 is considered acceptable (Anastasia and Urbina 1997).

Validity

Reliability does not prove that a scale is valid. *Validity* refers to how well an instrument measures what it is supposed to. Types of validity of psychiatric rating scales include content, convergent, discriminant, factorial, predictive, and cultural validity.

Content validity is a nonstatistical type of validity. The basic issue is whether the content of the scale seems to cover a representative sample of the phenomenon to be measured. Content validity is assessed by examining scale items to determine correspondence with known features of a syndrome. Some of the very standard assessment instruments, such as the Ham-D, which was developed before the advent of the DSM-IV (American Psychiatric Association 1994) system, have been criticized for not including content relevant to the new diagnostic system, as discussed later in this chapter (Bagby et al.

2004) (see section "Reliability and Validity of the Hamilton Rating Scale for Depression"). The clinician also should determine whether the items measure areas that are expected to change with therapy.

Concurrent validity refers to the degree to which the measure correlates with other measures of the same construct measured at the same time. Concurrent validity is adequate when a scale shows Pearson r values of at least 0.50 in correlation with other measures of the same syndrome.

Other types of validity are important, depending on the purpose of the scale. *Discriminant validity* refers to how well the measure distinguishes groups differing in their diagnostic status. *Predictive validity* refers to how well the measure can predict the onset of symptom(s). *Cultural validity* refers to how well the measure works in various populations.

Sensitivity to Change

For outcome studies, measurements should be used that are likely to be able to detect change in the domain assessed. In general, sensitivity to change is reflected in the effect size (see Gray, Chapter 6 in this volume). Within a treatment group, effect size is often calculated as the difference between the mean score at time 1 and the mean score at time 2 for each subscale, divided by the standard deviation at time 1 or over time. Measures that have large standard deviations relative to the mean require either very strong interventions to show effects or very large sample sizes. An effect size of approximately 0.2 is generally somewhat arbitrarily considered to be small, one of 0.5 indicates moderate differences, and that of 0.8 or higher indicates large differences (Cohen 1988). Of course, an instrument may be very sensitive to change, but the change itself may be clinically meaningless. For this reason, some researchers argue that categorical measures (e.g., how many patients depressed at baseline are no longer depressed at posttreatment or follow-up on the basis of some criteria such as DSM-IV-TR) are more meaningful than ordinal measures.

A second approach is to define an outcome on a measure as indicated improvement; for instance, to expect at least a 50% reduction in a baseline measure or a score below a certain level on a scale such as the Ham-D. STAR*D provides guidelines for what constitutes remission or improvement (see Chapter 21). A third approach is to estimate how many patients fit into the "nondysfunctional" range of the outcome measure or measures. For example, in a study of panic attack interventions, Newman et al. (1997) and later Kenardy et al. (2003) used norms and test-retest reliability estimates from previous studies to determine the dysfunctional/functional range. A successful outcome would be that, following treatment, a participant was no longer in the dysfunctional range, and his or her change from pre- to posttest exceeded measurement error. In addition, Jacobson and Truax (1991) required subjects to meet both a reliable change index and a functional recovery criterion, which was defined as being panic attack free. A fourth approach is to determine what would be considered a minimal clinically important difference, defined as being the smallest difference in score in the domain of interest that patients perceive as beneficial and that would mandate, in the absence of troublesome side effects and excessive cost, a change in the patient's management (Jaeschke et al. 1989). This is a complicated issue, and some doubt exists that it is possible to arrive at a minimal clinically important difference (Beaton et al. 2002).

Reliability and Validity of the Hamilton Rating Scale for Depression

The Ham-D is the most frequently used measure for depression in psychopharmacology studies (Williams 2001), and changes in its score are used to judge the effectiveness of a medication. The Ham-D was developed in the late 1950s to assess the effectiveness of the first generation of antidepressants and was originally published in 1960 (Hamilton 1960). How reliable and valid is the Ham-D? To answer this question, Bagby et al. (2004) reviewed the psychometric properties of the 17-item Ham-D, perhaps the most widely used version. They used MEDLINE to identify all studies published during the period from January 1980 to May 2003 that addressed the psychometric properties of the Ham-D. Seventy articles met their selection criteria and were categorized into three groups on the basis of the major psychometric property examined—reliability, item response, or validity.

Reliability

The internal reliability of the Ham-D ranged from 0.46 to 0.97. However, 10 of 13 studies reported in-

ternal reliabilities greater than 0.70. All of the single items of the test also showed good reliability except for "loss of insight," which was quite variable. Overall, the Ham-D has good internal reliability, suggesting that the items measure one construct.

Interrater reliabilities were quite high: total Ham-D interrater reliabilities ranged from 0.82 to 0.98, and the intraclass r ranged from 0.46 to 0.99. However, a large range was seen on the individual items. This suggests that two individuals who were trained to administer the Ham-D and rated a depressed individual came up with similar scores, although they varied as to how negatively they rated one item to the next.

The overall retest reliability of the Ham-D was high, ranging from 0.81 to 0.98. However, the test-retest reliability of individual items ranged from 0.00 to 0.85. This suggests that over time with no intervening treatment, an individual is rated as having the same overall extent of depression from one time to the next. However, changes in particular items are much less reliable. Bagby et al. (2004) criticized how the scale was constructed, noting, for instance, that some items require ratings that may even cross dimensions. For example, the question of hypochondriasis is rated from self-absorption to delusions. Are hypochondriacal delusions on the same continuum as hypochondriacal symptoms?

Validity

Content Validity

Bagby et al. (2004) also questioned the content validity of the Ham-D, noting that the items were generated well before DSM-IV, and asked if the Ham-D accurately reflects depression as defined by DSM-IV. Important features of DSM-IV depression are buried within more complex items in the Ham-D and sometimes are not captured at all. The interested reader may want to examine the Depression Interview and Structured Hamilton (DISH), a structured interview developed for the National Heart, Lung, and Blood Institute's Enhancing Recovery in Coronary Heart Disease trial that combines the Ham-D and the clinical items of DSM-IV (Freedland et al. 2002).

Convergent Validity

The Ham-D has good *convergent validity* with many other scales given at the same time. In arguing, however, that the Ham-D does not reflect DSM-IV items, poor convergent validity between the Ham-D and the Structured Clinical Interview for DSM-IV was reported in a Turkish study. Language/translation issues might have been a factor in this result.

Discriminant Validity

The Ham-D, at cut-off points of greater than 1.0, had reasonable sensitivity (most studies reported sensitivities in the 0.7–0.8 range) and specificity (0.75–1.0).

Predictive Validity and Sensitivity to Change

Several very large meta-analyses involving thousands of patients and a variety of treatments have shown that the Ham-D is more sensitive to change than is the BDI, a widely used self-report instrument (Edwards et al. 1984; Lambert et al. 1986). Such studies also suggest that the instrument is sensitive to change.

Factorial Validity

Overall, the results from 15 studies suggested that the Ham-D is not unidimensional because separate sets of items seem to represent general depression and insomnia factors; however, the exact structure of its multidimensionality remains unclear.

Bagby et al. (2004) concluded that the Ham-D has adequate internal, interrater, and retest reliability and good convergent, discriminant, and predictive validity. They noted that the same is not true for individual items. For this reason, they recommended that the Ham-D should be replaced by other instruments and noted that the Inventory of Depressive Symptomatology (Rush et al. 1986) and the Montgomery-Åsberg Depression Rating Scale (Montgomery and Åsberg 1979), designed to address the limitations of the Ham-D, represent two potential replacement alternatives. The QIDS is obviously another one.

Critics of the Bagby et al. (2004) article noted that their analyses included studies in which the Ham-D was not used as intended, to measure change in depression, but to assess nondepressed populations (Corruble and Hardy 2005). A scale designed for one population may have excellent psychometric properties but do poorly in another population. For instance, in a "normal" population, in which very low scores on most items are expected, any small change may generate poor agreement. Carroll et al.

(2005), also critical of Bagby et al. (2004), argued that the Ham-D may not be perfect but that it captures the many different ways that depression presents and has proved sensitive to change, thus providing a useful outcome to determine the effectiveness of medications.

Changing a measure that has been the gold standard for evidence-based trials creates many problems. Whereas statistical approaches can "adjust" between measures, the same measure used in the same way for the same presenting problem allows for easy comparison. Although this is not a compelling reason to continue using the Ham-D, a PubMed search (July 20, 2008) identified hundreds of citations since Bagby et al. (2004) recommended that it be abandoned. It may not be perfect, but it endures. From a practical standpoint, a clinician could use the Ham-D total score to measure improvement but be less confident that changes in the individual items are meaningful. I favor use of the $QIDS-SR_{16}$ because it is tied into a measurement outcome–based protocol.

Practical Issues in Finding and Using Measures

An instrument with excellent psychometric properties may not be useful in clinical practice for several reasons. Some self-report measures include items that are reverse scored so that the clinician needs to have a scoring sheet or to have the form scored by a vendor or through software. The purpose of the reverse scoring is to help ensure that the person filling out the form reads each item and does not simply choose one end of the scale. Other assessments can be very lengthy and require a long time to complete. Many forms are also copyrighted. Simply because a form is available on the Internet does not mean that it is in the public domain and can be used for free or without permission. It is illegal and unethical to use a copyrighted test without buying it or receiving permission to use it from the owner of the copyright. American Psychiatric Publishing provides contact information for the use of the forms included on the CD-ROM accompanying the *Handbook of Psychiatric Measures* (Rush et al. 2008).

One may be surprised to learn that forms that have been used for some time are actually copyrighted. For instance, the Mini-Mental State Exam (MMSE) is now copyrighted and must be purchased. As an example of what forms cost, a package of 50

MMSE test forms costs $60. The American Psychiatric Publishing *Handbook of Psychiatric Measures*, 2nd Edition (Rush et al. 2008), includes a "Practical Issues" section for most measures that mentions how long it takes to complete the form, whether the form is copyrighted, and how it can be obtained.

Developing Your Own Assessment Measures

Some therapy goals can be measured without relying on standardized instruments. For instance, many behaviors, such as frequency of binge eating or drinking or the number of panic attacks experienced, can be assessed by self-report. The actual number of events can be counted, or the frequency can be described more generally. For instance, a patient may be experiencing nausea for psychological reasons. To get a sense of how the patient is doing, the clinician asks him to rate his nausea over the last week on the basis of how often he experienced it (Figure 8–1). The clinician also could ask the patient to rate it by severity (Figure 8–1). Table 16–1 in Chapter 16 of this volume lists cases in which the authors used a variety of nonstandardized measures to help guide their therapy.

A more complicated, and perhaps more interesting, issue is to determine how to "measure" complex phenomena specific to a particular patient. For instance, one might want to monitor the patient's "insight," satisfaction with relationships, confidence in conducting a job interview, or any number of the many phenomena that we address in therapy. Some-

times, I use a very simple satisfaction measure to assess progress. Figure 8–2 provides an example of a simple scale to measure confidence and satisfaction with dating in a patient with relationship issues (see also Chapter 18). The figure also uses a scale to rate the patient's confidence to use parenting skills. Such measures help remind me what the therapy is focused on and can be used to determine whether progress is occurring.

When I began to focus more on evidence-based practice, I decided to implement a very simple system that could work in most outpatient practice settings. I developed a weekly check-in form that evaluates mood (depression and anxiety) and includes measures specific to the patient. I also created a blank form that can be used to measure two target symptoms (per page) by frequency and severity, as appropriate. In the waiting room or at the beginning of the session, the patient is asked to complete the form, and if time permits and if relevant, we might plot the data together to see how the patient is progressing. These measures are meant to be guides. Single-item measures are subject to biases, but the form also helps ensure that my patients and I share similar goals. As one symptom or target behavior improves, or as events occur in the patient's life, we might add or refine our goals. I also include a general assessment of self-care activities that I consider to be important for most patients (exercise, stress management/relaxation/doing something fun, nutrition, social support, sleep hygiene) and treatment use (medication adherence, side effects, use of CBT or other strategies) and, as appropriate, use standard measures.

Target symptom 1: *Nausea*

In the last week, how often did you experience this? (circle an answer)			
never	almost never	a few times a week	a few times a day

In the last week, how severe was this symptom? (circle a number)									
not bad at all			moderate				severe		
1	2	3	4	5	6	7	8	9	10

FIGURE 8–1. **Example of a therapist-developed rating to assess therapy goals.**

Goal: *To improve my confidence and satisfaction when dating*

In the last week, how satisfied have you been with your relationships? (circle an answer)			
1 = not at all	2 = pretty unsatisfied	3 = pretty satisfied	4 = very satisfied

Goal: *To increase my confidence as a parent*

In the last week, how confident have you felt with your parenting skills? (circle an answer)			
1 = not at all	2 = somewhat	3 = pretty confident	4 = very confident

FIGURE 8–2. Two examples of simple, therapist-developed scales used to measure progress toward therapy goals.

Electronic Office Assessment Systems

In recent years, some software programs have been developed to facilitate measurement-based care and other electronic activities for psychiatric practice. For example, the Psychiatry Quality Measurement (PQM) is a computerized documentation and quality-measurement system (Joubert 2001). According to its developers, the PQM system was designed to document all aspects of a psychiatric patient's treatment, admission, and subsequent follow-up; reduce the time spent on administration; and increase the availability of data from a physician's practice. The system incorporates a program displaying descriptive statistics and can calculate a large range of quality measures, based either on the full population in the database or on preselected subgroups. Data can also be exported for more extensive statistical analysis (Joubert 2001).

One user noted, however, that entering data into the clinical charts is quite time-consuming.

Several other software packages are available for psychiatric practice. The following are examples of programs that have been advertised on the Internet (with no recommendation from me):

- *Valant Psychiatric EMR*—a powerful electronic medical record (EMR) software application that is specialty specific for psychiatrists but can accommodate psychologists as well.

- *A+ DELPHI Psychotherapy Billing Software*—a complete program designed specifically for mental health care professionals. It features extensive note taking for Psychotherapy and Progress Notes and Assessments and Intakes.
- *PatientTrac*—an EMR for psychiatrists and mental health facilities. Designed by board-certified psychiatrists, this EMR does not rely on templates but is a "living" system that can track differential data for subsequent visits.
- *MedEZ*—a medical office management and billing software that has modules designed for mental health centers, psychiatrists, and private practice facilities.
- *Q.D. Clinical EMR*—features hundreds of customizable templates, allowing mental health providers to alter the application to meet their needs.
- *OfficeEMR*—caters to small and mid-sized practices that want a fully integrated EMR and practice management system. OfficeEMR is Web based, Certification Commission for Healthcare Information Technology certified, and Health Insurance Portability and Accountability Act of 1996 compliant.
- *CollaborateMD*—a Web-enabled practice management and medical billing software system with free support and software updates. Requiring only an Internet connection, CollaborateMD manages all data backups and clearinghouse transmissions.

Examples of Electronic Data Systems to Facilitate Evidence-Based Psychiatric Practice

Example 1: A Measurement System to Facilitate Implementation of the STAR*D Guidelines

An example of a potentially useful office-based system is the one developed by Trivedi and Daly (2007) to help implement the STAR*D guidelines. In the STAR*D trial, poorer outcomes were most clearly associated with a failure to change medication after an extended (12–24 weeks) treatment trial that had not produced a meaningful benefit, as well as with a failure to increase the medication dose in a timely manner within the first 12 weeks, despite a lack of significant side effects (Trivedi and Daly 2007). The system developed by Trivedi and Daly (2007) incorporates the most current information about the treatment of depression and provides an easy-to-use interface allowing physicians to use this decision support tool within the context of a routine clinical visit. A computerized algorithm has been developed to facilitate the process of following the suggested dosing schedules and tactical recommendations by displaying the recommended dosages and pretreatment options at that point in time according to the decision. Additionally, all patient information, medication information, medication dosages, next appointments, and progress notes are accessible with a click of the computer mouse and recorded electronically. The program also provides a recommended time frame for the patient to return according to algorithm stage.

Example 2: An Electronic System to Help Monitor Symptom Severity, Plotted Against Clinical Activities

Sentiens has developed an e-health system to provide improved health care for the Western Australian population (see Chapter 30 for an example of how it was used in a clinical case). The system was designed to be used by practitioners to manage and monitor patients wherever they may be—whether close by in Perth, in less populated areas of Western Australia, or working overseas. The resultant HealthSteps system has been implemented in a few research trials, in both Australia (e.g., Barnes et al. 2007) and the United States (e.g., Harvey et al.

2007), to refine further its features and show its efficacy in the management of longer-term health conditions. The Sentiens system can be used to provide real-time data on symptom severity, plotted against clinical activities including medications.

Example 3: Clinical Research Information System at Duke University

Duke University has developed the Clinical Research Information System (CRIS), described as a comprehensive electronic behavioral health care management system (psychiatry.mc.duke.edu/CMRIS/CMRIndex.htm). CRIS was designed to integrate clinical care at all levels. CRIS also employs a clinical rules engine to help guide clinical practices and create a clinical outcomes data warehouse for retrospective decision support. Progress reports can also be generated in real time (http://psychiatry.mc.duke.edu/CMRIS/Image4Symptom.htm).

The cases presented in Parts II and III of this volume also provide examples of how measurement can be used in a variety of clinical settings.

References

American Psychiatric Association: Diagnostic and Statistical Manual of Mental Disorders, 4th Edition. Washington, DC, American Psychiatric Association, 1994

American Psychiatric Association: Diagnostic and Statistical Manual of Mental Disorders, 4th Edition, Text Revision. Washington, DC, American Psychiatric Association, 2000

Anastasia A, Urbina S: Psychological Testing, 7th Edition. New York, Macmillan, 1997

Bagby RM, Ryder AG, Schuller DR, et al: The Hamilton Depression Rating Scale: has the gold standard become a lead weight? Am J Psychiatry 161:2163–2177, 2004

Barnes C, Harvey R, Mitchell P, et al: Evaluation of an online relapse prevention program for bipolar disorder: an overview of the aims and methodology of a randomised controlled trial. Disease Management and Health Outcomes 15:215–224, 2007

Beaton DE, Boers M, Wells GA: Many faces of the minimal clinically important difference (MCID): a literature review and directions for future research. Curr Opin Rheumatol 14:109–114, 2002

Beck AT, Ward C, Mendelson M: An inventory for measuring depression. Arch Gen Psychiatry 4:561–571, 1961

Carroll BJ: Why the Hamilton Depression Rating Scale endures. Am J Psychiatry 162:2395–2396, 2005

Cohen J: Statistical Power for the Behavioral Sciences, 2nd Edition. Hillsdale, NJ, Erlbaum, 1988

Corruble E, Hardy P: Why the Hamilton Depression Rating Scale endures. Am J Psychiatry 162:2394, 2005

DeVellis RF: Scale Development: Theory and Applications, 2nd Edition. Thousand Oaks, CA, Sage, 2003

Edwards BC, Lambert MJ, Moran PW, et al: A meta-analytic comparison of the Beck Depression Inventory and the Hamilton Rating Scale for Depression as measures of treatment outcome. Br J Clin Psychol 23 (part 2):93–99, 1984

Ellwood PM: Shattuck lecture outcomes management: a technology of patient experience. N Engl J Med 318:1549–1556, 1988

Fleiss, JL. Statistical Methods for Rates and Proportions. Hoboken, NJ, Wiley Interscience, 1981

Freedland KE, Skala JA, Carney RM, et al: The Depression Interview and Structured Hamilton (DISH): rationale, development, characteristics, and clinical validity. Psychosom Med 64:897–905, 2002

Hamilton M: A rating scale for depression. J Neurol Neurosurg Psychiatry 23:56–62, 1960

Harvey R, Smith M, Abraham N, et al: The Hurricane Choir: remote mental health monitoring of participants in a community based intervention in the post Katrina period. J Health Care Poor Underserved 18:356–361, 2007

Jacobson NS, Truax P: Clinical significance: a statistical approach to defining meaningful change in psychotherapy research. J Consult Clin Psychol 59:12–19, 1991

Jaeschke R, Singer J, Guyatt GH: Measurement of health status: ascertaining the minimal clinically important difference. Control Clin Trials 10:407–415, 1989

Joubert AF: PQM—Psychiatry Quality Measurement. Int Clin Psychopharmacol 16 (suppl 3):S25–33, 2001

Kenardy JA, Dow MGT, Johnston DW, et al: A comparison of delivery methods of cognitive-behavioral therapy for panic disorder: an international multicenter trial. J Consult Clin Psychol 71:1068–1075, 2003

Killen JD, Taylor CB, Hammer LD, et al: An attempt to modify unhealthful eating attitudes and weight regulation practices of young adolescent girls. Int J Eat Disord 13:369–384, 1993

Lambert MJ, Hatch DR, Kingston MD, et al: Zung, Beck, and Hamilton Rating Scales as measures of treatment outcome: a meta-analytic comparison. J Consult Clin Psychol 54:54–59, 1986

Landis JR, Koch GG: The measurement of observer agreement for categorical data. Biometrics 33:159–174, 1977

McGrath BM, Tempier RP: Implementing quality management in psychiatry: from theory to practice—shifting focus from process to outcome. Can J Psychiatry 48:467–474, 2003

Montgomery SA, Åsberg M: A new depression scale designed to be sensitive to change. Br J Psychiatry 134:382–389, 1979

Newman MG, Kenardy J, Herman S, et al: Comparison of cognitive-behavioral treatment of panic disorder with computer assisted brief cognitive-behavioral treatment. J Consult Clin Psychol 65:173–178, 1997

Rush AJ, Giles DE, Schlesser MA, et al: The Inventory for Depressive Symptomatology (IDS): preliminary findings. Psychiatry Res 18:65–87, 1986

Rush AJ, Trivedi MH, Ibrahim HM, et al: The 16-Item Quick Inventory of Depressive Symptomatology (QIDS), clinician rating (QIDS-C), and self-report (QIDS-SR): a psychometric evaluation in patients with chronic major depression. Biol Psychiatry 54:573–583, 2003

Rush AJ Jr, First MB, Blacker D (eds): Handbook of Psychiatric Measures, 2nd Edition. Washington, DC, American Psychiatric Publishing, 2008

Trivedi MH, Daly EJ: Measurement-based care for refractory depression: a clinical decision support model for clinical research and practice. Drug Alcohol Depend 88 (suppl 2):S61–S71, 2007

Trivedi MH, Rush AJ, Gaynes BN, et al: Maximizing the adequacy of medication treatment in controlled trials and clinical practice: STAR(*)D measurement-based care. Neuropsychopharmacology 32:2479–2489, 2007

Williams JB: Standardizing the Hamilton Depression Rating Scale: past, present, and future. Eur Arch Psychiatry Clin Neurosci 251 (suppl 2):II6–II12, 2001

Diagnostic Tests

Gregory E. Gray, M.D., Ph.D.

Questions about diagnostic tests are most commonly related to the accuracy of the test, which is the focus of this chapter. For information on topics such as the clinical and economic impact of screening, clinical decision rules, and the differential diagnosis process, readers are referred to recent monographs (Hunink et al. 2001; Knottnerus 2002) and standard textbooks of clinical epidemiology (Fletcher et al. 1996; Sackett et al. 1991).

Evaluating Diagnostic Tests

The accuracy of a diagnostic test is generally assessed in a cross-sectional study, in which patients are evaluated with both the "gold standard" diagnostic procedure and the diagnostic test under evaluation (Knottnerus and Muris 2002; Knottnerus et al. 2002; Newman et al. 2001). Several important issues can affect the validity of such evaluations (Fletcher et al. 1996; Knottnerus and Muris 2002; Knottnerus et al. 2002; Newman et al. 2001; Sackett et al. 1991), but the two major issues are the choice of the gold standard and the choice of subjects.

Choice of Gold Standard

The first issue is related to the choice of the gold standard. In some branches of medicine, the gold standard might be a pathological diagnosis based on a biopsy or an autopsy; in psychiatry, we usually rely on the DSM-IV-TR criteria (American Psychiatric Association [APA] 2000).

Although the DSM-IV-TR diagnostic criteria are often used as the gold standard for evaluating diagnostic tests, they have limitations. First, there are unresolved issues concerning the validity of the criteria themselves (Goldstein and Simpson 2002; Kendell 1989; Kendler 1990).

The second issue relates to the method of eliciting symptoms from patients and of using this information to arrive at a diagnosis. In unstructured clinical interviews, clinicians may ignore or not inquire about certain symptoms and may choose not to follow the DSM criteria in arriving at a diagnosis (Robins 2002). As a result, unstructured interviews may not be reliable. For this reason, a variety of diagnostic instruments have been developed to standardize the process of psychiatric diagnosis, including structured clinical interviews (e.g., the Structured Clinical Interview for DSM-IV [SCID]) and structured interviews that may be administered by either a lay interviewer or a computer (e.g., the Composite International Diagnostic Interview [CIDI] and the Diagnostic Interview Schedule [DIS]) (Kobak et al. 2008). Although these standardized instruments increase the reliability of the diagnoses made, issues of validity remain (Murphy 2002; Narrow et al. 2002; Regier et al. 1998; Robins 2002).

For the assessment of particular symptoms or specific measures of cognitive function (e.g., memory or intelligence), well-established instruments are generally used as the gold standard. Descriptions of many of these are included in the *Handbook of Psychiatric Measures* (Rush et al. 2008)

Choice of Subjects

The other major issue relates to the choice of subjects. We administer diagnostic tests because we have uncertainty about a diagnosis. A cross-sectional study that includes a spectrum of patients who are similar to those to whom the test is expected to be administered in clinical practice is the most appropriate design. All too often, a test is evaluated in a population composed of a mix of very ill patients and a healthy control group. In such a population, the test performs much better in distinguishing the ill from the healthy than in actual practice. This is referred to as *spectrum bias* (Knottnerus et al. 2002; Newman et al. 2001).

Measures of Test Performance: Dichotomous Results

A variety of terms are used to describe the performance of a diagnostic test (Habbema et al. 2002). As an aid in discussing these terms, Table 9–1 displays the results of a hypothetical comparison of a new diagnostic test with an appropriate gold standard. In this section, we consider test results to be dichotomous (i.e., either positive or negative).

True Positive, True Negative, False Positive, and False Negative

If both the diagnostic test being evaluated and the gold standard yield positive results, the result of the diagnostic test is considered true positive (Table 9–1, cell A). Likewise, if both yield negative results, the result of the diagnostic test is considered true negative (Table 9–1, cell D). If the diagnostic test under evaluation gives a positive result, but the gold standard gives a negative result, the result of the diagnostic test is considered false positive (Table 9–1, cell B). Similarly, if the diagnostic test result is negative, but the gold standard result is positive, the result of the diagnostic test is considered false negative (Table 9–1, cell C).

Sensitivity and Specificity

Sensitivity refers to the proportion of patients with the disease (as assessed by the gold standard) who are detected by the diagnostic test. In Table 9–1, this is calculated as A/(A+C). A highly sensitive test is one that detects most cases of disease.

Specificity refers to the proportion of patients without the disease (as assessed by the gold standard) who are identified by the diagnostic test as *not* having the disease. In Table 9–1, this is calculated as

D/(B+D). A highly specific test is one that does not misidentify healthy individuals as having disease.

Although it may seem counterintuitive, highly sensitive diagnostic tests are most useful for ruling *out* diseases. This is because such tests seldom miss cases of disease. Sackett et al. (2000) have proposed the mnemonic SnNout (**Se**nsitive test, **N**egative result, rules **out** disease) as a teaching aid. Similarly, highly specific tests are most useful for ruling in diseases, because they seldom misidentify healthy individuals. The mnemonic for such tests is SpPin (**Sp**ecific test, **P**ositive test, rules **in** disease).

Confidence intervals (CIs) for specificity and sensitivity can be calculated using the tables given by Habbema et al. (2002).

Positive and Negative Predictive Values

The positive predictive value (PPV) is the proportion of positive test results that is true positives. Using Table 9–1, PPV is calculated as A/(A+B). The negative predictive value (NPV) is the proportion of negative test results that is true negatives. Using Table 9–1, NPV is calculated as D/(C+D).

PPV and NPV can also be looked at in terms of posttest probabilities of disease (Fletcher et al. 1996; Habbema et al. 2002). PPV represents the probability that an individual with a positive test result has the disease, whereas NPV represents the probability that an individual with a negative test result does not have the disease.

PPV and NPV are dependent on the prevalence of disease in the population being tested, which is also referred to as the *pretest probability of disease* (Fletcher et al. 1996). Mathematically, the relationship is as follows:

$$PPV = \frac{\text{sensitivity} \times \text{prevalence}}{(\text{sensitivity} \times \text{prevalence}) + [(1 - \text{specificity})(1 - \text{prevalence})]}$$

Because of this dependence on disease prevalence, screening for diseases in low-prevalence populations yields few true-positive test results, regardless of the sensitivity and specificity of the test (Fletcher et al. 1996). Baldessarini et al. (1983) have provided an excellent discussion of the effects of disease prevalence on PPV in psychiatric practice, using as their example the dexamethasone suppression test as a diagnostic test for depression.

TABLE 9–1. Possible results of a diagnostic test

	Disease present	Disease absent	Totals
Test results positive	**A** True positive	**B** False positive	**A+B**
Test results negative	**C** False negative	**D** True negative	**C+D**
Totals	**A+C**	**B+D**	

Sensitivity = A/(A+C)
Specificity = D/(B+D)
Positive predictive value = A/(A+B)
Negative predictive value = D/(C+D)

Likelihood ratio of positive test = [A/(A+C)]/[B/(B+D)]
Likelihood ratio of negative test = [C/(A+C)]/[D/(B+D)]
Error rate = (B+C)/(A+B+C+D)
Accuracy = (A+D)/(A+B+C+D)

Likelihood Ratios

Although PPV and NPV allow the clinician to estimate the probability of disease in a patient with a particular test result, they are both dependent on the prevalence of disease in the study population. Likelihood ratios (LRs), in contrast, are independent of disease prevalence.

The likelihood ratio of a positive test (LR+) is the ratio of the likelihood (probability) of a positive test result in the population with disease divided by the likelihood of a positive test result in the population without disease. This can be calculated as follows, using the data in Table 9–1:

$$\text{LR} + = \frac{A/(A+C)}{B/B+D} = \frac{\text{sensitivity}}{1 - \text{specificity}}$$

The likelihood ratio of a negative test result (LR–) is similarly the ratio of the likelihood of a negative test result in the population with disease divided by the likelihood of a negative test result in the population without disease. Once again, using the data in Table 9–1:

$$\text{LR} - = \frac{C/(A+C)}{D/(B+D)} = \frac{1 - \text{sensitivity}}{\text{specificity}}$$

Formulas for calculating CIs for LRs are given by Habbema et al. (2002).

One of the most useful features of LRs is that they can be used to estimate the probability that a given patient has an illness, given a particular test result. The following formula can be used for this estimate:

$$\text{posttest odds} = \text{pretest odds} \times \text{LR}$$

The odds of an event occurring is the ratio of the probability of an event occurring (P) divided by the probability of the event not occurring ($1-P$), or the odds = $P/(1-P)$.

The pretest probability of disease in a patient can be estimated from the prevalence of a disease in your own or similar patient populations, as derived from papers evaluating diagnostic tests, epidemiologic studies, or hospital statistics (Mant 1999; Sackett et al. 2000). For some medical conditions, clinical prediction rules may be used to better refine the estimated pretest probability (McGinn 2002). Sometimes published data are not available and a subjective estimate of pretest probability must be made, although this is subject to numerous biases (Elstein and Schwartz 2002; Hunink et al. 2001). When there is uncertainty about the pretest probability, it is best to estimate an upper and lower limit and to do the calculations with both values to see if it will change your management of the patient.

Once you have a pretest probability of disease, it is converted to the pretest odds, using the formula above. The pretest odds are then multiplied by the appropriate likelihood ratio (LR+ if the test is positive or LR– if the test is negative). The resulting posttest odds can then be converted to a posttest probability, using the following formula:

$$P = \frac{\text{odds}}{1+\text{odds}}$$

For those wishing to go directly from pretest probability to posttest probability, without having to go back and forth between probabilities and odds, nomograms and computer programs are available (Fagan 1975; Glasziou 2001).

Using diagnostic tests in this way to quantify the risk of disease in a patient and to then use these probabilities in clinical decision making has become an important field of study, but it is outside the scope this chapter. For further details, readers are referred to Hunink et al. (2001) and Sackett et al. (1991, 2000).

Error Rate and Accuracy

The error rate of a diagnostic test is the percentage of test results that is either false positives or false negatives (Habbema et al. 2002). Using the data in Table 9–1, error rate can be calculated as follows:

$$\frac{B+C}{A+B+C+D}$$

The term *accuracy* is sometimes used to describe the percentage of test results that is either true positives or true negatives (Fletcher et al. 1996; Greenhalgh 2001). Using the data in Table 9–1, accuracy is calculated as follows:

$$\frac{A+D}{A+B+C+D}$$

Accuracy can also be calculated as 1−error rate.

Diagnostic Odds Ratio

The diagnostic odds ratio (DOR) is sometimes used as a measure of overall test performance (Habbema et al. 2002). Using the data in Table 9–1, DOR is calculated as follows:

$$\frac{A \times D}{B \times C}$$

The DOR is sometimes used in systematic reviews and in meta-analyses because of its mathematical properties; however, it is not a statistic that is easy to interpret clinically (Deeks 2001).

Example of Calculations

Table 9–2 provides data from a study by Watkins et al. (2001) that evaluates the accuracy of a single question ("Do you often feel sad or depressed?") in screening for depression in stroke patients. In the study, answers to the question ("yes" or "no") were compared with the results of the Montgomery-Åsberg Rating Depression Rating Scale (MADRS), with a MADRS score >6 indicating depression. As can be seen from Table 9–2, the single question had a sensitivity of 86% and a specificity of 78%.

We can use LRs to see the impact of a positive or negative response to the question on the probability of a patient being depressed. Depression typically occurs in 25%–40% of patients with stroke and other neurologic conditions (APA 2000). Thus, the pretest odds for such a patient are between 25/75=0.33 and 40/60=0.67. If the patient answers "yes" to the question, the posttest odds are between 0.33×3.87=1.28 and 0.67×3.87=2.59, corresponding to posttest probabilities of 56%–72%. If the patient answers "no," the posttest odds are between 0.33×0.18=0.06 and 0.67×0.18=0.12, corresponding to posttest probabilities of 6%–11%.

Measures of Test Performance: Ordinal or Continuous Results

Although we often think of diagnostic test results as positive or negative, rating scales and many laboratory tests have more than just two values. Rating scales, for example, can have outcomes that are ordered categories (e.g., none, minimal, mild, moderate, or severe) or that yield a numerical score. Although a cutoff value is often chosen to convert such an outcome to a dichotomous measure, information is lost in the process.

Choosing a Cutoff Score

When a test result can take more than two values as described above, a decision must be made about a cutoff score if the results are to be viewed as either positive or negative. The choice of the cutoff value involves a trade-off between sensitivity and specificity (Fletcher et al. 1996).

Table 9–3 shows the results of a study of the CAGE questionnaire as a screening tool for diagnosing alcohol abuse in general medical patients (Buchsbaum et al. 1991). (CAGE is an acronym for certain key symptoms of alcohol abuse.) As can be seen, as the cutoff score is increased, the specificity increases, but the sensitivity decreases. At the usual cutoff score of 2 (Martino et al. 2008), the sensitivity is 74% and the specificity is 91%.

Receiver Operator Characteristic Curves

The data in Table 9–3 can also be displayed graphically, in the form of a receiver operator characteristic

TABLE 9–2. Accuracy of a single question ("Do you often feel sad or depressed?") in screening for depression in stroke patients

Answer to question	Depressed (MADRS>6)	Not depressed (MADRS ≤6)	Totals
Yes	37	8	45
No	6	28	34
Totals	43	36	79

Sensitivity=37/43=86%
Specificity=28/36=78%
Positive predictive value=37/45=82%
Negative predictive value=28/34=82%

Likelihood ratio of positive test=0.86/0.22=3.9
Likelihood ratio of negative test=0.14/0.78=0.18
Error rate=14/79=18%
Accuracy=65/79=82%

Note. MADRS=Montgomery-Åsberg Depression Rating Scale.
Source. Data from Watkins et al. 2001.

(ROC) curve (Figure 9–1). An ROC curve plots the sensitivity against (1–specificity) for each cutoff value (Fletcher et al. 1996; Sackett et al. 1991, 2000). The ROC curve can be used to identify a cutoff value, where a point near the upper left corner is the appropriate cutoff. ROC curves can also be used to compare two diagnostic tests; the better test is the one with its ROC curve closer to the upper left corner (Fletcher et al. 1996).

Likelihood Ratios

Intuitively, it would seem that converting numerical or ordered test results into just two categories would result in a loss of information. It would seem that a value greatly over the cutoff would be more indicative of disease than a value that is barely more than the cutoff. LRs allow these differences to be taken into account.

If a test result takes multiple values, LRs can be calculated for multiple scores, not just LR+ and LR–. This is illustrated in Table 9–4, using the same CAGE data found in Table 9–3 (Buchsbaum et al.

1991). It can be seen that as the CAGE score increases from 0 to 4, LRs increase from 0.14 to 100. Assuming a prevalence (pretest probability) of alcohol dependence of 5% (APA 2000), a CAGE score of 0 decreases the posttest probability to 1%. Using the same figures, a CAGE score of 2 increases the posttest probability to 19% and a CAGE score of 5 increases the posttest probability to 84%. Clearly, this provides more information than simply treating the results as *positive* (2+) or *negative* (0–1).

Systematic Reviews and Meta-Analyses of Diagnostic Tests

As with the evaluation of therapies, systematic reviews that are related to diagnostic tests may be conducted. However, there are several approaches to meta-analysis (Deeks 2001; Glasziou et al. 2001). One approach is to use one forest plot for sensitivities and their CIs and another for specificities and their CIs (see Chapter 6). Another approach is to plot the sensitivity against (1–specificity) on an

TABLE 9–3. Sensitivity and specificity of the CAGE questionnaire in screening for alcohol abuse in general medical patients

CAGE score cutoff	Sensitivity (%)	Specificity (%)
0 vs. 1+	89	81
<2 vs. 2+	74	91
<3 vs. 3+	44	98
<4 vs. 4+	25	100

Source. Data from Buchsbaum et al. 1991.

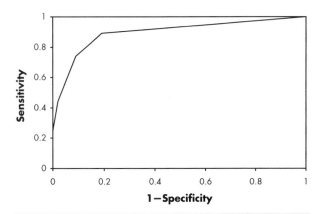

FIGURE 9–1. Receiver operator characteristic curve for CAGE questionnaire.

Source. Data from Buchsbaum et al. (1991).

TABLE 9–4. Likelihood ratios for specific CAGE scores in screening for alcohol abuse in general medical patients

CAGE score	Likelihood ratio
0	0.14
1	1.5
2	4.5
3	13
4	100

Source. Data from Buchsbaum et al. 1991.

ROC plot, with each study representing one point on the plot. Methods deriving pooled estimates of sensitivity, specificity, and LRs are also available. Finally, DORs can be pooled and this can be used to derive a summary ROC curve. Although such methods can demonstrate that a test is useful, if there is heterogeneity in results the summary statistics may not give a valid estimate of the probability associated with a specific test outcome (Deeks 2001).

Critical Appraisal Guide for Studies of Diagnostic Test Accuracy

Having discussed how diagnostic tests are evaluated and measures of their accuracy, we now turn to the critical appraisal of reports of such evaluations. A guide for critically appraising studies of diagnostic test accuracy is given in Table 9–5.

Is the Study Valid?

As discussed earlier in this chapter, the appropriate study design to assess the accuracy of a diagnostic test is a cross-sectional study in which patients are evaluated with both the gold standard diagnostic procedure and the diagnostic test under evaluation (Knottnerus and Muris 2002; Knottnerus et al. 2002; Newman et al. 2001). Both tests should be administered blindly to avoid observer bias (Fletcher et al. 1996), and the results of one test should not influence the decision to administer the other test. The gold standard itself should be appropriate, and

an appropriate spectrum of patients should be chosen to avoid spectrum bias (Knottnerus et al. 2002; Newman et al. 2001).

Are the Results Important?

Sensitivity and specificity are the usual measures of diagnostic test accuracy. Which of the two is more important will depend on the purpose of the test. Recall that highly sensitive diagnostic tests are most useful for ruling *out* diseases (SnNout: **Sen**sitive test, **N**egative result, rules **out** disease), whereas highly specific tests are most useful for ruling *in* diseases (SpPin: **Sp**ecific test, **P**ositive test, rules **in** disease) (Sackett et al. 2000).

PPV and NPV will provide estimates of the probabilities of disease in patients with positive or negative test results, respectively, in the study population. However, LR+ and LR– are more useful measures, because they can be generalized to other populations with different disease prevalences (Fletcher et al. 1996; Mant 1999).

Can I Apply the Results to My Patient?

The first question to ask is whether the test is feasible in your setting. Does it require specialized equipment or is it very expensive? Does it require expertise to administer or to interpret the test, and is such expertise available?

The next question is specific to your patient and relates to whether the results of the test will change your patient management. As described in more detail elsewhere (Hunink et al. 2001; Sackett et al. 1991, 2000), physicians make decisions about clinical management, based on their (often unstated) as-

TABLE 9–5. Critical appraisal guide for studies of diagnostic accuracy

Is the study valid?

Is it a cross-sectional study?

Was the test evaluated in an appropriate spectrum of patients?

Was there an independent blind comparison with a "gold standard"?

Were both tests administered, regardless of outcome?

Are the results important?

What is the sensitivity?

What is the specificity?

What is the positive predictive value?

What is the negative predictive value?

What is the likelihood ratio for a positive test result?

What is the likelihood ratio for a negative test result?

Can I apply the results to my patient?

Is the test available or feasible in my setting?

Do I have enough information to apply the test and to interpret the results?

Given reasonable pretest estimates of disease probability in my patient, what are the posttest probabilities if the test is positive? If it is negative?

Will these probabilities change my management of the patient?

Source. Based on Gilbert et al. 2001; Glasziou et al. 2001; Sackett et al. 2000.

sessments of the probability of disease in a given patient. If that probability is high, physicians treat the patient; if that probability is intermediate, physicians order more diagnostic tests; and if it is low, physicians do neither. The probability at or above which tests are ordered is termed the *test threshold*, and the probability at or above which treatment is begun is termed the *treatment threshold* (Hunink et al. 2001; Sackett et al. 2000).

If your patient's pretest probability is already above the treatment threshold, there is no point in ordering the diagnostic test. For example, if your diagnostic interview shows that your patient met the DSM-IV-TR criteria for major depression, there is no need to also use a rating scale developed to screen for depression. You have already established the diagnosis with enough certainty to begin treatment.

Conversely, if the posttest probability remains low even if the test result is positive, the test should probably not be performed because it is likely that any positive test result will be a false positive. Ordering the test under these circumstances would be both a waste of money and an unnecessary cause of anxiety for patients with false-positive results (Fletcher et al. 1996).

To do these sorts of calculations, you will need the LR+ and LR– from the article reporting the performance of the test in question and an estimate of your patient's pretest probability of disease. If your patient is similar to patients in the study population, the pretest probability can be derived from the study evaluating the diagnostic test. If not, the pretest probability can be estimated from epidemiologic data or from patient data from your hospital or health maintenance organization (Mant 1999; Sackett et al. 2000). If published data are not available, you may have to make a subjective estimate of the pretest. In this case, it is probably best to estimate an upper and lower limit and to do the calculations with both values.

If the test is valid and feasible and if the results will make a difference in patient management, you should use it.

References

American Psychiatric Association: Diagnostic and Statistical Manual of Mental Disorders, 4th Edition, Text Revision. Washington, DC, American Psychiatric Association, 2000

Baldessarini RJ, Finkelstein S, Arana GW: The predictive power of diagnostic tests and the effect of prevalence of illness. Arch Gen Psychiatry 40:569–573, 1983

Buchsbaum DG, Buchanan RG, Centor RM, et al: Screening for alcohol abuse using CAGE scores and likelihood ratios. Ann Intern Med 115:774–777, 1991

Deeks JJ: Systematic reviews of evaluation of diagnostic and screening tests. BMJ 323:157–162, 2001

Elstein AS, Schwartz A: Clinical problem solving and diagnostic decision making: a selective review of the cognitive research literature, in The Evidence Base of Clinical Diagnosis. Edited by Knottnerus JA. London, BMJ Books, 2002, pp 179–195

Fagan TJ: Nomogram for Bayes' theorem. N Engl J Med 293:257, 1975

Fletcher RH, Fletcher SW, Wagner EH: Clinical Epidemiology: The Essentials, 3rd Edition. Baltimore, MD, Williams & Wilkins, 1996

Gilbert R, Logan S, Moyer VA, et al: Assessing diagnostic and screening tests, II: how to use the research literature on diagnosis. West J Med 175:37–41, 2001

Glasziou P: Which methods for bedside Bayes? ACP J Club 135:A11–A12, 2001

Glasziou P, Irwig L, Bain C, et al: Systematic Reviews in Health Care: A Practical Guide. Cambridge, UK, Cambridge University Press, 2001

Goldstein JM, Simpson JC: Validity: definitions and applications to psychiatric research, in Textbook in Psychiatric Epidemiology, 2nd Edition. Edited by Tsuang MT, Tohen M. New York, Wiley-Liss, 2002, pp 149–163

Greenhalgh T: How to Read a Paper: The Basics of Evidence Based Medicine, 2nd Edition. London, BMJ Books, 2001

Habbema JDF, Eijkemans R, Krijnen P, et al: Analysis of data on the accuracy of diagnostic tests, in The Evidence Base of Clinical Diagnosis. Edited by Knottnerus JA. London, BMJ Books, 2002, pp 117–143

Hunink M, Glasziou P, Siegel J, et al: Decision Making in Health and Medicine: Integrating Evidence and Values. New York, Cambridge University Press, 2001

Kendell RE: Clinical validity. Psychol Med 19:45–55, 1989

Kendler KS: Toward a scientific psychiatric nosology: strengths and limitations. Arch Gen Psychiatry 47:969–973, 1990

Knottnerus JA (ed): The Evidence Base of Clinical Diagnosis. London, BMJ Books, 2002

Knottnerus JA, Muris JWM: Assessment of the accuracy of diagnostic tests: the cross-sectional study, in The Evidence Base of Clinical Diagnosis. Edited by Knottnerus JA. London, BMJ Books, 2002, pp 39–60

Knottnerus JA, van Weel C, Muris JWM: Evaluation of diagnostic procedures. BMJ 324:477–480, 2002

Kobak KA, Skodol AE, Bender DS: Diagnostic measures for adults, in Handbook of Psychiatric Measures, 2nd Edition. Edited by Rush AJ, First MB, Blacker D. Washington, DC, American Psychiatric Publishing, 2008, pp 35–60

Mant J: Is this test effective? In Evidence-Based Practice: A Primer for Health Professionals. Edited by Dawes M, Davies P, Gray A, et al. New York, Churchill Livingstone, 1999, pp 133–157

Martino S, Poling J, Rounsaville BJ: Substance use disorders measures, in Handbook of Psychiatric Measures, 2nd Edition. Edited by Rush AJ, First MB, Blacker D. Washington, DC, American Psychiatric Publishing, 2008, pp 437–470

McGinn T: Practice corner: using clinical prediction rules. ACP J Club 137:A10–A11, 2002

Murphy JM: Symptom scales and diagnostic schedules in adult psychiatry, in Textbook in Psychiatric Epidemiology, 2nd Edition. Edited by Tsuang MT, Tohen M. New York, Wiley-Liss, 2002, pp 273–332

Narrow WE, Rae DS, Robins LN, et al: Revised prevalence estimates of mental disorders in the United States: using a clinical significance criterion to reconcile 2 surveys' estimates. Arch Gen Psychiatry 59:115–123, 2002

Newman TB, Browner WS, Cummings SR: Designing studies of medical tests, in Designing Clinical Research: An Epidemiologic Approach, 2nd Edition. Edited by Hulley SB, Cummings SR, Browner WS, et al. Philadelphia, PA, Lippincott Williams & Wilkins, 2001, pp 175–191

Regier DA, Kaelber CT, Rae DS, et al: Limitations of diagnostic criteria and assessment instruments for mental disorders: implications for research and policy. Arch Gen Psychiatry 55:109–115, 1998

Robins LN: Birth and development of psychiatric interviews, in Textbook in Psychiatric Epidemiology, 2nd Edition. Edited by Tsuang MT, Tohen M. New York, Wiley-Liss, 2002, pp 257–271

Rush AJ, First MB, Blacker D (eds): Handbook of Psychiatric Measures, 2nd Edition. Washington, DC, American Psychiatric Publishing, 2008

Sackett DL, Haynes RB, Guyatt GH, et al: Clinical Epidemiology: A Basic Science for Clinical Medicine, 2nd Edition. Boston, MA, Little, Brown, 1991

Sackett DL, Straus SE, Richardson WS, et al: Evidence-Based Medicine: How to Practice and Teach EBM, 2nd Edition. New York, Churchill Livingstone, 2000

Watkins C, Daniels L, Jack C, et al: Accuracy of a single question in screening for depression in a cohort of patients after stroke: comparative study. BMJ 323:1159, 2001

Surveys of Disease Frequency

Gregory E. Gray, M.D., Ph.D.

Questions about disease frequency take various forms. A patient's family member or member of the public may wonder about the risk of developing a disease. An administrator may wonder about the number of patients who will need treatment. A clinician attempting to evaluate a patient's risk of disease, based on the results of a diagnostic test, will need information on the patient's pretest probability of disease (see Chapter 9).

All of these questions require quantitative information about the frequency of a particular illness in a defined population of interest, which is the subject of descriptive epidemiology. This chapter reviews the various measures of disease frequency and the methods of descriptive epidemiology, as background information for the critical appraisal of studies of disease frequency. For additional information, readers are referred to standard epidemiology texts (Fletcher et al. 1996; Gordis 2000; Hennekens et al. 1987; Lilienfeld and Stolley 1994) and reviews of psychiatric epidemiology (Regier and Burke 2000; Tsuang and Tohen 2002).

Measures of Disease Frequency

A number of terms, such as *incidence*, *prevalence*, and *lifetime prevalence*, are used—and often misused—to refer to the frequency of disease in a population.

Incidence

The *incidence* of disease is the number of new cases of disease in a defined population in a given period of time. It is measured by starting with a population (cohort) that is initially free of the disease in question and by then counting the cases that develop in a defined period of time. The incidence rate has "cases" as its numerator and "person-years at risk " as its denominator. The incidence rate is the measure of frequency of most interest to epidemiologists seeking to understand the cause of a disease, because it measures the actual risk of developing the disease.

Point Prevalence

When epidemiologists use the term *prevalence*, they are usually referring to the *point prevalence* (i.e., the number of cases of disease in a defined population at a given point in time). It is measured in a cross-sectional survey in which individuals are identified as either having or not having a disease at the time of the survey.

Point prevalence is of interest to health care planners, because it measures the burden of illness in a population. It is also of interest to clinicians, because it is a measure of a patient's pretest probability of disease (see Chapter 9).

Point prevalence is less helpful in understanding the causes of disease, because it reflects both the incidence (risk) of disease and the duration of the illness. In a *steady state* situation in which the incidence rate and average duration of illness are constant, the following relationship between incidence and point prevalence exists:

$$\text{point prevalence} = \text{incidence rate} \times \text{average duration of illness}$$

This relationship allows for the calculation of the third variable in the equation, if the other two variables are known.

Period Prevalence

Period prevalence is a measure of the proportion of individuals in a defined population who have an illness in a specified period of time. It is a hybrid measure that reflects both the proportion of patients who have the illness at the start of the time interval (prevalence), as well as the number of new cases that develop during the time period (incidence × time).

Although period prevalence is seldom used outside psychiatry (Hennekens et al. 1987), it is widely used in surveys of the frequency of psychiatric illnesses (Fleming and Hsieh 2002; Regier and Burke 2000). In the National Comorbidity Survey, for example, results were reported as 12-month prevalences, which indicates that an individual had the disorder in question at some time during the 12 months prior to the interview date (Kessler and Walters 2002).

The popularity of period prevalence in psychiatric epidemiology relates to the fact that many psychiatric illnesses have a recurring or episodic course; therefore, the period prevalence is believed to be a better reflection of disease burden in the population than is the proportion of patients who are symptomatic at a given point in time.

Lifetime Prevalence

Lifetime prevalence is a specific type of period prevalence used in psychiatric epidemiology. As used in the National Comorbidity Survey and in similar studies, *lifetime prevalence* is the proportion of the patients in population studies who have experienced an illness up to the point in their life that they are surveyed.

Defined in this way, lifetime prevalence has several limitations (Fleming and Hsieh 2002; Regier and Burke 2000). First, it is dependent on memory (recall bias). Second, it is highly dependent on the age structure of the population, with young people less likely to develop the disease than older people. Third, if the disease is associated with excess mortality from suicide or other causes, lifetime prevalence may decline with age.

Morbidity Risk

An alternative measure of lifetime risk, sometimes referred to as *lifetime expectancy*, is morbidity risk or morbid risk (Faraone et al. 2002; Slater and Cowie 1971). This measure corrects the denominator to reflect the fact that younger individuals have had less chance to develop the illness than older individuals and is a better estimate of the risk of developing the illness at some point during a normal lifespan.

Age- and Sex-Specific and Adjusted Rates

The incidence and prevalence of many psychiatric disorders vary with age and sex. The incidence of major depression, for example, is greater in women than in men (Horwath et al. 2002), and the incidence and prevalence of dementia increase with age, beginning at about age 65 years (Hybels and Blazer 2002). In determining the pretest probability of disease for an individual, using age- and sex-specific prevalences will be more accurate than using the prevalence figures for the population as a whole.

When comparing rates between geographic areas or over time, it is important to take demographic differences into account. For example, differences in the incidence of depression in two populations could reflect actual differences in risk for disease or they could simply reflect differences in age or sex distribution. To eliminate demographic differences as the explanation, rates can be standardized. In essence, this involves calculating a weighted average of the age- and sex-specific rates, using identical weights for both populations. Methods of standardization and details of the calculations can be found in standard epidemiology and biostatistics texts (Gordis 2000; Hennekens et al. 1987; Pagano and Gauvreau 2000).

Using Registries and Existing Records

There are several potential sources of existing or routinely collected information about the frequency of disease in a population. These resources include disease registries, reporting systems, and insurance or health plan statistics (Gordis 2000; Lilienfeld and Stolley 1994).

For some diseases (e.g., cancer and some infectious diseases), established disease reporting systems and case registries can provide considerable information about incidence or prevalence. In psychiatry, largely because of privacy concerns, such registers or reporting systems are largely nonexistent. Notable exceptions to this include case registers of psychiatric cases in Rochester, New York; in Denmark; and in Mannheim, Germany (Regier and Burke 2000). Information from such registers is largely limited to schizophrenia and to other serious mental illnesses that require hospitalization.

Records maintained by a health maintenance organization or a health plan can be used to provide useful information about the treated prevalence of mental illness in the health plan's members. Unfortunately, much illness goes untreated, so such records underestimate the actual frequency of mental illness in the health plan's members. As a result, surveys are required to better estimate the actual frequency of disease in a population.

Surveys of Disease Frequency

Two aspects of the design of surveys that are used to determine the incidence or prevalence of a disease in a population are of particular importance: who to survey and how to assess the presence of absence of disease.

Populations and Samples

The first decision involves deciding on the population of interest (Hulley et al. 2001). Although we often are interested in the frequency of disease in the general population, the prevalence of many psychiatric disorders is greater in specific settings (e.g., primary care settings or jails) and can vary with ethnicity (Burke 2002). Thus, there is a rationale for conducting surveys among subpopulations and in specific settings, as well as in the general population.

After deciding on the population of interest, the next step is to assemble a sample of individuals to actually study. A variety of techniques can be used for this purpose (Hulley et al. 2001). If the population is such that all members can be enumerated (e.g., members of a health plan), a simple random sample can be used. For community surveys, cluster sampling is often used. In cluster sampling, the investigators first randomly select census tracts or similar geographic areas, followed by a sample of addresses within the geographic area. Details of the various sampling methods, including methods of determining the sample size required for a certain precision in the estimate of the prevalence rate, can be found in standard texts on survey methods (Kalton 1983; Kelsey et al. 1996).

Assessment Instrument

The second decision relates to the method used to decide whether an individual has the disease of interest or not. Although we use the DSM-IV-TR diagnostic criteria (American Psychiatric Association [APA] 2000), we must also have a method of eliciting symptoms and for applying these criteria during a survey. The chosen method must be feasible, reliable, and valid (Regier and Burke 2000).

Reliability refers to the ability of an assessment instrument to yield a consistent result. In unstructured clinical interviews, clinicians may ignore or not inquire about certain symptoms and may choose not to follow DSM criteria in arriving at a diagnosis (Robins 2002). As a result, unstructured interviews may not be reliable. As noted in Chapter 9, a variety of diagnostic instruments have been developed to standardize and improve the reliability of the psychiatric diagnosis process, including structured interviews, administered either by a clinician (e.g., the Structured Clinical Interview for DSM-IV [SCID]) or by a lay interviewer (e.g., the Composite International Diagnostic Interview [CIDI] and the Diagnostic Interview Schedule [DIS]) (Kobak et al. 2008).

The other issue is *validity* (i.e., whether the instrument measures its intended parameters). Although the standardized instruments mentioned above have improved the reliability of the diagnoses made in surveys, issues of validity remain (Murphy 2002; Regier et al. 1998; Robins 2002). In particular, community surveys identify individuals who have less severe symptoms than those seen among individuals in treatment settings, and it is unclear if these represent milder cases of the same disorders or simply nonpathological transient responses to stressors (Narrow et al. 2002; Regier et al. 1998).

For the assessment of particular symptoms or specific measures of cognitive function (e.g., memory or intelligence), a variety of well-established instruments that are considered both reliable and valid are available. Descriptions of many of these are included in the *Handbook of Psychiatric Measures* (Rush et al. 2008).

Critical Appraisal of a Survey of Disease Frequency

Having discussed the various measures of disease frequency and how they are determined, we now turn to the critical appraisal of reports of disease frequency. A guide for critically appraising these studies is given in Table 10–1.

Is the Study Valid?

The first questions relate to the study design. For estimating prevalence, a cross-sectional survey, in which individuals are identified as either having or not having a disease either at the time of the survey or during some defined time period, is the appropriate design. Incidence rates are measured in cohort studies, in which a group of individuals who are initially free of the disease in question is followed over time, and cases of disease that develop in the cohort during the follow-up period are counted.

Regardless of study design, the individuals surveyed should be members of a defined population that is sampled in such a way as to give an unbiased estimate or incidence or prevalence rate. A convenience sample or the use of volunteers recruited from an advertisement cannot be considered representative of a defined population; it will give a biased estimate of disease frequency, which is referred to as *selection bias* (Daly and Bourke 2000).

Nonresponse bias is an additional concern, because individuals who refuse to participate in the survey may be systematically different from individuals who do participate (Aday 1996; Barker et al. 1998; Daly and Bourke 2000). For example, telephone follow-up of nonresponders in the National Comorbidity Survey found that they were more apt to have an anxiety disorder than were responders (Kessler and Walters 2002). In general, it is considered desirable to have as high a response rate as possible—generally, at least 75%–80% (Aday 1996; Barker et al. 1998; Kelsey et al. 1996).

It is essential to use standard criteria to decide whether an individual has a disorder or not, because prevalence will depend on the definition of what constitutes a case (Fletcher et al. 1996). In addition, as described above under "Surveys of Disease Frequency," the assessment instrument must have acceptable reliability and validity (Regier and Burke 2000).

Are the Results Important?

Which results are important will, of course, be related to your initial clinical question. At a minimum, you would expect to see an incidence or prevalence rate for each disorder surveyed, with confidence limits. If your goal is to apply the results to an individual pa-

---

TABLE 10–1.   Critical appraisal guide for surveys of disease frequency

Is the study valid?

Is the study design appropriate (cross-sectional survey for measuring prevalence or cohort study for measuring incidence)?

Was an appropriate sampling method used?

Was the response rate sufficiently high?

Was a standardized method used to determine the presence of disease?

Is the assessment instrument reliable and valid?

Are the results important?

What is the incidence or prevalence?

Are there important differences by age, sex, ethnicity, etc.?

How precise are the estimates?

Can I apply the results to my patient?

Does my patient come from a population similar to that surveyed?

Are there age- or sex-specific estimates (if appropriate) that apply to my patient?

Source.   Based in part on the criteria of Barker et al. 1998; Fletcher et al. 1996.

---

tient, rates specific to age, sex, and other demographic characteristics will be helpful. In contrast, if your interest lies in comparing the rates in two populations, standardized rates will be of more interest.

Can I Apply the Results to My Patient?

The first question to ask is whether the population is similar enough that the results can reasonably be generalized to your patient (Hulley et al. 2001). In addition, if your clinical question relates to a pretest probability of disease in your patient (see Chapter 9), the availability of age- and sex-specific prevalence rates will give you a more accurate estimate than will crude or standardized rates.

References

Aday LA: Designing and Conducting Health Surveys: A Comprehensive Guide, 2nd Edition. San Francisco, CA, Jossey-Bass, 1996

American Psychiatric Association: Diagnostic and Statistical Manual of Mental Disorders, 4th Edition, Text Revision. Washington, DC, American Psychiatric Association, 2000

Barker DJP, Cooper C, Rose G: Epidemiology in Medical Practice, 5th Edition. New York, Churchill Livingstone, 1998

Burke JD: Mental health services research, in Textbook in Psychiatric Epidemiology, 2nd Edition. Edited by Tsuang MT, Tohen M. New York, Wiley-Liss, 2002, pp 165–179

Daly LE, Bourke GJ: Interpretation and Uses of Medical Statistics, 5th Edition. Oxford, UK, Blackwell Scientific, 2000

Faraone SV, Tsuang D, Tsuang MT: Methods in psychiatric genetics, in Textbook in Psychiatric Epidemiology, 2nd Edition. Edited by Tsuang MT, Tohen M. New York, Wiley-Liss, 2002, pp 65–130

Fleming JA, Hsieh C-C: Introduction to epidemiologic research methods, in Textbook in Psychiatric Epidemiology, 2nd Edition. Edited by Tsuang MT, Tohen M. New York, Wiley-Liss, 2002, pp 3–33

Fletcher RH, Fletcher SW, Wagner EH: Clinical Epidemiology: The Essentials, 3rd Edition. Baltimore, MD, Williams & Wilkins, 1996

Gordis L: Epidemiology, 2nd Edition. Philadelphia, PA, WB Saunders, 2000

Hennekens CH, Buring JE, Mayrent SL: Epidemiology in Medicine. Boston, MA, Little, Brown, 1987

Horwath E, Cohen RS, Weissman MM: Epidemiology of depressive and anxiety disorders, in Textbook in Psychiatric Epidemiology, 2nd Edition. Edited by Tsuang MT, Tohen M. New York, Wiley-Liss, 2002, pp 389–426

Hulley SB, Newman TB, Cummings SR: Choosing the study subjects: specification, sampling, and recruitment, in Designing Clinical Research: An Epidemiologic Approach, 2nd Edition. Edited by Hulley SB, Cummings SR, Browner WS, et al. Philadelphia, PA, Lippincott Williams & Williams, 2001, pp 25–36

Hybels CF, Blazer DG: Epidemiology and geriatric psychiatry, in Textbook in Psychiatric Epidemiology, 2nd Edition. Edited by Tsuang MT, Tohen M. New York, Wiley-Liss, 2002, pp 603–628

Kalton G: Introduction to Survey Sampling. Newbury Park, CA, Sage, 1983

Kelsey JL, Whittemore AS, Evans AS, et al (eds): Methods in Observational Epidemiology, 2nd Edition. New York, Oxford University Press, 1996

Kessler RC, Walters E: The National Comorbidity Survey, in Textbook in Psychiatric Epidemiology, 2nd Edition. Edited by Tsuang MT, Tohen M. New York, Wiley-Liss, 2002, pp 343–362

Kobak KA, Skodol AE, Bender DS: Diagnostic measures for adults, in Handbook of Psychiatric Measures, 2nd Edition. Edited by Rush AJ, First MB, Blacker D. Washington, DC, American Psychiatric Publishing, 2008, pp 35–60

Lilienfeld DE, Stolley PD: Foundations of Epidemiology, 3rd Edition. New York, Oxford University Press, 1994

Murphy JM: Symptom scales and diagnostic schedules in adult psychiatry, in Textbook in Psychiatric Epidemiology, 2nd Edition. Edited by Tsuang MT, Tohen M. New York, Wiley-Liss, 2002, pp 273–332

Narrow WE, Rae DS, Robins LN, et al: Revised prevalence estimates of mental disorders in the United States: using a clinical significance criterion to reconcile 2 surveys' estimates. Arch Gen Psychiatry 59:115–123, 2002

Pagano M, Gauvreau K: Principles of Biostatistics, 2nd Edition. Pacific Grove, CA, Duxbury, 2000

Regier DA, Burke JD: Epidemiology, in Kaplan and Sadock's Comprehensive Textbook of Psychiatry, 7th Edition. Edited by Sadock BJ, Sadock VA. Philadelphia, PA, Lippincott Williams & Wilkins, 2000, pp 500–522

Regier DA, Kaelber CT, Rae DS, et al: Limitations of diagnostic criteria and assessment instruments for mental disorders: implications for research and policy. Arch Gen Psychiatry 55:109–115, 1998

Robins LN: Birth and development of psychiatric interviews, in Textbook in Psychiatric Epidemiology, 2nd Edition. Edited by Tsuang MT, Tohen M. New York, Wiley-Liss, 2002, pp 257–271

Rush AJ, First MB, Blacker D (eds): Handbook of Psychiatric Measures, 2nd Edition. Washington, DC, American Psychiatric Publishing, 2008

Slater E, Cowie V: The Genetics of Mental Disorder. New York, Oxford University Press, 1971

Tsuang MT, Tohen M (eds): Textbook in Psychiatric Epidemiology, 2nd Edition. New York, Wiley-Liss, 2002

Studies of Risk or Harm

Gregory E. Gray, M.D., Ph.D.

This chapter covers the appraisal of two types of studies: those that assess the *harm* associated with a therapy (e.g., medication side effects) and those that attempt to identify factors that increase the *risk* of developing a disease. A variety of study designs are presented, including case reports, randomized controlled trials (RCTs), cohort studies, and case-control studies (Levine et al. 2002; Turcotte et al. 2001) (Table 11–1).

Case Reports and Case Series

As noted in Chapter 5, case reports and case series are best viewed as sources of hypotheses for further testing (Fletcher et al. 1996; Hennekens et al. 1987). They have been used traditionally to describe rare clinical events and often provide the first warnings about rare—but clinically significant—adverse drug reactions (ADRs) (Brewer and Colditz 1999).

Unfortunately, case reports and case series may also include coincidental occurrences, and without a denominator it is impossible to determine the actual risk of an adverse event. For example, case reports have wrongly implicated beta-blockers as a cause of depression, which actually occurs no more frequently in patients on beta-blockers than in patients receiving placebos (Ko et al. 2002).

Randomized Controlled Trials

Although it would be unethical to conduct an RCT designed to cause harm to a subject, a considerable amount of information about common side effects of medications comes from Phase II and Phase III clinical trials (Jones 2001). Unfortunately, such reporting is often incomplete (Ioannidis and Lau 2001). Furthermore, premarketing trials are often of short duration, are limited to fewer than 2,000 patients, and simply do not have the statistical power to detect ADRs that occur in 1 of 10,000 drug exposures (for which 30,000 patients would have to be studied) (Brewer and Colditz 1999; Pirmohamed et al. 1998).

For common side effects, however, an RCT provides the best evidence that the side effect was caused by medication, not chance (Turcotte et al. 2001). A variety of statistical measures are used to assess the magnitude of the difference in adverse events between a control and experimental treatments. Most of these measures are discussed in Chapter 5; however, there are three measures that are unique to studies of harm: relative risk increase (RRI), absolute risk increase (ARI), and number needed to harm (NNH) (Sackett et al. 2000) (Table 11–2).

Relative Risk and Relative Risk Increase

If a therapy increases the risk of an adverse event, the experimental event rate (EER) is greater than the control event rate (CER), and relative risk (RR), calculated as EER/CER, is greater than 1. RRI is calculated using the following formula:

$$RRI = \frac{EER - CER}{CER} = RR - 1$$

Because RR and RRI are relative measures, they do not provide an estimate of the actual increase in frequency of an adverse event. For example, an EER

TABLE 11–1.   Study designs used to assess etiology or harm

	Case reports or case series	Randomized controlled trial (RCT)	Cohort study	Case-control study
Advantages	Used to describe rare or unusual events	Least biased study design Can demonstrate cause-effect relationship	Less apt to be biased than case-control study Better able to assess rare outcomes than RCT	Quicker, less expensive than cohort study Useful for rare diseases
Disadvantages	Cannot prove association or causality Often misleading	Cannot assess risk of rare side effects Unethical to conduct trial specifically to cause harm	Involves large numbers of subjects Loss to follow-up may limit validity	More prone to bias than RCT or cohort study Cannot measure absolute risks
Risk statistics	None	Relative risk increase Absolute risk increase Number needed to harm	Relative risk Risk difference Number needed to harm	Odds ratio

of 0.5% and a CER of 0.1% yield the same RR and RRI as an EER of 50% and an CER of 10%, yet the absolute magnitude of the increase in adverse events is greater in the latter case.

Absolute Risk Increase and Number Needed to Harm

ARI is calculated as EER–CER. Unlike RR and RRI, ARI provides a measure of the proportion of patients receiving treatment who will be harmed by it, which thus avoids some of the limitations of the relative measures of effect.

NNH is simply the reciprocal of ARI. It is analogous to NNT (see Chapter 5) as a measure of treatment effect; it indicates the number of patients who would need to be treated with the experimental treatment to produce one more adverse event than would have occurred with the control treatment.

Epidemiologic Studies

Because we do not ordinarily conduct experiments to prove that something is harmful to patients, much of our knowledge about the etiology of disease, as well as of less common medication side effects, comes from epidemiologic studies. In this section, the two most common study designs, cohort studies and case-control studies, are reviewed. The reader is referred to several excellent epidemiology texts for a

more complete discussion (Fletcher et al. 1996; Gordis 2000; Hennekens et al. 1987; Kelsey et al. 1996; Rothman 2002).

Cohort Studies

In a cohort study, a group of subjects (cohort) is followed over time, and the incidence of disease is determined (see Chapter 10). The members of the cohort can be classified as either *exposed* or *unexposed* to a medication or suspected risk factor for disease. Such characteristics are determined at the beginning of the study, before disease occurrence. If exposure increases the risk of disease, the incidence in the exposed group is greater than the incidence in the unexposed group.

TABLE 11–2.   Measures of risk: randomized controlled trial

	Experimental treatment	Control treatment
Harm	A	B
No harm	C	D
Total	A+C	B+D

Experimental event rate (EER) =A/(A+C)
Control event rate (CER) =B/(B+D)
Relative risk (RR) =EER/CER
Relative risk increase =(EER–CER)/CER=RR–1
Absolute risk increase (ARI) =EER–CER
Number needed to harm=1/ARI

Prospective Cohort Studies

Cohort studies can be either prospective or retrospective (Hennekens et al. 1987). In a prospective or concurrent cohort study, the cohort is assembled and the exposure status is determined; it is then followed over time to determine the incidence of disease. In a prospective cohort study, Takeshita et al. (2002) followed a cohort of more than 3,000 Japanese Americans for 6 years and found that those with depressive symptoms had an increased mortality rate, compared with those without depressive symptoms.

Retrospective Cohort Studies

In a retrospective cohort study, existing records are used to identify a historical cohort and to measure both exposures and outcomes of interest, all of which have occurred at the time the study is initiated. Doing so allows the study to be conducted more quickly and with less expense than if the cohort was actually followed for several years. Because retrospective cohort studies are dependent on existing records, issues of data quality often arise. An example of a retrospective cohort study is that of Gunnell et al. (2002), in which intellectual performance at age 18 was determined from military psychological records for a cohort of nearly 200,000 Swedish male conscripts examined several years earlier and was found to predict the subsequent development of schizophrenia and other psychoses over an average follow-up period of 5 years.

Bias and Confounding

Cohort studies are sometimes referred to as *natural experiments*, although they differ significantly in that the subjects are not randomly allocated in a cohort study (Gordis 2000; Rothman 2002). This is an important difference, in that bias and confounding become major considerations in interpreting the results. In an RCT, randomization minimizes the chance that differences in outcomes between the experimental and control groups are the result of preexisting differences in the subjects in the two groups. In a cohort study, preexisting differences between exposed and nonexposed subjects may influence the subsequent risk of disease.

Confounding is especially problematic in studies of medication side effects, where the prescription of particular medications may be influenced by the preexisting medical conditions of patients, which is called *confounding by indication* (Rothman 2002). For example, because olanzapine causes more weight gain than risperidone (Lawrie and McIntosh 2002), risperidone might be prescribed more frequently to patients predisposed to obesity or diabetes, thus confounding any observed relationship between medication and risk of diabetes. Confounding can be accounted for in the statistical analysis of the data, but only to the extent that the confounding factors have been identified and measured. Statistical methods to control for confounding in cohort studies include stratified analysis and Poisson regression, details of which can be found in more advanced texts (Kelsey et al. 1996; Rothman and Greenland 1998).

There are also several potential biases in cohort studies that could be problematic. These include differential misclassification as to disease and exposure status, losses to follow-up, and nonparticipation. Good discussions of biases and confounding in cohort studies can be found in most standard epidemiology texts (Gordis 2000; Hennekens et al. 1987; Rothman 2002).

Measures of Risk

In a cohort study, incidence rates are calculated for exposed and nonexposed groups. Several measures of risk can then be calculated, including absolute risk, RR, odds ratio (OR), and risk difference (RD) (Table 11–3). RD in a cohort study is analogous to ARI in an RCT, and NNH may be calculated as 1/RD. RR and OR are measures of the strength of association between an exposure and outcome, whereas RD and NNH are better measures of the potential for prevention (Gordis 2000; Sackett et al. 2000).

TABLE 11–3. Measures of risk: cohort study

	Exposed group	Nonexposed group
Harm	A	B
No harm	C	D
Total	A+C	B+D

Incidence in exposed group=A/(A+C)
Incidence in nonexposed group=B/(B+D)
Relative risk=incidence in exposed group/incidence in nonexposed group
Risk difference =incidence in exposed group–incidence in nonexposed group
Number needed to harm=1/RD

Case-Control Studies

The other major study design is the case-control study. In a case-control study, patients with a particular disease (cases) are compared with patients without the disease in question (i.e., controls) with regard to exposures and other characteristics. Case-control studies are especially useful in studying rare diseases, because cohort studies involve studying very large cohorts for extended periods of time for meaningful numbers of cases of rare diseases to occur.

By their nature, however, case-control studies are more susceptible to bias than are cohort studies and therefore rank lower on the hierarchy of evidence (Table 4–1, Chapter 4). Two of the major sources of bias relate to the choice of control subjects (selection bias) and the fact that information about exposure is gathered after the onset of disease (recall or information bias).

Choice of Controls

In a case-control study, control subjects must be chosen from the same source population as the cases, because control subjects are used to estimate the prevalence of exposure to a risk factor in the population from which the cases are drawn (Lewis and Pelosi 1990; Rothman 2002). In other words, if cases are identified from a particular clinic or hospital, control subjects must be individuals who similarly have obtained treatment from that same clinic or hospital if they have the disease in question. In many cases, there are multiple medical providers serving a geographic area; therefore, hypothetical source population is not defined by specific geographic boundaries, but rather by referral or care-seeking patterns.

Several potential sources of control subjects can be used, and each has its own advantages and limitations (Hennekens et al. 1987; Rothman 2002). Sources include general population controls, including those identified by random-digit dialing; hospital or clinic controls; and friends, relatives, or neighbors of the cases.

Although it is often convenient to draw control subjects from the same hospital or clinic as the cases, because they clearly come from the same source population, there are also some important limitations related to exposure status. In particular, hospitalized control subjects differ from individuals without disease in the frequency of exposures that are associated with the control subjects' own diseases. For example, if an investigator is interested in conducting a case-

control study to determine if alcohol use is a risk factor for deliberate self-harm, it might be tempting to identify both cases and controls from hospital emergency room patients. Because alcohol use is also a risk factor for accidental injuries, violence, and a number of other diseases, obtaining control subjects from an emergency room overestimates the use of alcohol in the population without disease and hence tends to obscure any association with self-harm.

The "nested" case-control study, which minimizes some of the issues in control selection, is a variant of the case-control study (Gordis 2000; Rothman 2002). In a nested case-control study, both cases and controls come from a previously assembled cohort; therefore, there is an enumerated source population from which to select the controls. An example of a nested case-control study is that of Koro et al. (2002), in which cases of patients with diabetes and control subjects were obtained from a cohort of over 19,000 patients with schizophrenia who were in a general practice research database. The authors then assessed prior use of antipsychotic medication by the patients with diabetes and the control subjects and were able to demonstrate that olanzapine use increased the risk of developing diabetes.

Recall Bias

The other serious concern in case-control studies is recall bias. Individuals with a disease often search their memories for possible causes and are therefore more likely to selectively recall exposures than are control subjects; this is sometimes called *rumination bias* or *effort after meaning* (Creed 1993; Gordis 2000). In psychiatric epidemiology, there is the added problem that the psychiatric illness may selectively influence memory (Lewis and Pelosi 1990). For example, patients with depression are more apt to remember negative life experiences than are nondepressed individuals (Creed 1993; Lloyd and Lishman 1976).

Reverse Causality

An additional problem with case-control studies is that of reverse causality (Creed 1993; Lewis and Pelosi 1990). In a case-control study, cases are asked about exposures prior to the onset of illness. For some psychiatric illnesses, it is difficult to determine the exact onset of illness. In addition, it may be difficult to determine retrospectively if an event, such as marital discord, truly preceded the onset of illness or if it was a consequence of the illness. This has been a particular problem with life events and depression research (Cooper and Paykel 1993; Creed 1993).

Odds Ratio

The odds ratio is the measure of risk in a case-control study (Table 11–4). For rare diseases, the OR approximates RR from a cohort study. Measures of absolute risk cannot be directly estimated from a case-control study. It is possible, however, to estimate NNH from the OR, if the incidence of disease in the unexposed population is known (Bjerre and LeLorier 2000). This method is described in Appendix B.

Causality in Epidemiologic Studies

There are several explanations for an association between an exposure and a disease in an epidemiologic study (Table 11–5), including bias, chance, confounding, and causality (Fletcher et al. 1996; Hennekens et al. 1987).

Bias

Bias refers to a systematic error that results in an incorrect estimate of the risk of disease associated with an exposure. Bias may occur as a result of the process of selecting subjects (selection bias) or from gathering information on exposures (information or recall bias). As noted earlier in this chapter, case-control studies are more susceptible to selection and information biases than are prospective cohort studies.

Chance

Chance is always a possible explanation for an observed association between an exposure and a disease. The likelihood that chance alone is responsible is assessed through tests of statistical significance (P values) and confidence intervals (see Chapter 5).

Confounding

Confounding involves the possibility that differences in subjects (other than the exposure under investigation) are responsible for the observed association between the exposure and the disease. For example, if women in a retirement community are, on average, older than men, an observed increased risk of Alzheimer's disease in women could be the result of an association with age rather than with female sex. In other words, age is a confounding factor. If there are potential confounding factors that have been measured in a study, the statistical analysis of the data can

TABLE 11–4. Measure of risk: case-control study

	Cases	Controls
Exposed	A	B
Nonexposed	C	D

Odds ratio = (A/C)/(B/D) = (AD)/(BC)

take them into account, either through stratified analysis or regression techniques (i.e., Poisson regression for a cohort study or logistic regression for a case-control study) (Kelsey et al. 1996; Rothman and Greenland 1998).

Causality

If bias, chance, and confounding are not the explanations for an association between exposure and disease, a causal relationship is likely. Bradford Hill (1965) described a variety of evidence that would support a causal relationship. Table 11–6 presents some of the criteria for causation suggested by Bradford Hill (1965) and others (Elwood 1998; Fletcher et al. 1996; Gordis 2000; Hennekens et al. 1987; Turcotte et al. 2001). Although Rothman (2002) has criticized such "checklists" as not reflecting more sophisticated notions of causality, many other epidemiologists continue to find them useful.

Critical Appraisal Guides for Studies of Etiology or Harm

Tables 11–7 through 11–9 are the critical appraisal guides for studies of etiology or harm. Separate guides are provided for RCT, cohort study, and case-control study, the three major study designs.

TABLE 11–5. Explanations for associations between exposure and disease in epidemiologic studies

Bias
Selection bias
Information bias

Chance

Confounding

Causality

TABLE 11–6.   Suggested criteria for causality in epidemiologic studies

Criterion	Description
Temporal relationship	Exposure precedes disease
Strength of association	Large relative risk or odds ratio
Dose–response relationship	Increasing exposure increases risk
Reversibility	Reducing exposure decreases risk
Consistency	Similar findings from other studies in different populations
Biological plausibility	Consistent with pharmacological or toxicological data
Analogy	Relationship established for similar cause and disease
Elimination of other explanations	Not the result of confounding or bias
Specificity	One cause, one effect

Source.   Adapted from Fletcher et al. 1996; Gordis 2000; Hennekens et al. 1987; Sackett et al. 2000.

Randomized Controlled Trial Reporting Harm

Is the Study Valid?

Before reviewing the results of the RCT, you should first ensure that the study is valid. The criteria for doing this are similar to those for appraising studies designed to evaluate the efficacy of a therapy (Table 5–6, Chapter 5). However, there are some additional considerations for a study of adverse effects.

First, were the adverse effects assessed in a systematic way (as opposed to self-reporting)? Some side effects (e.g., sexual side effects) may not be spontaneously reported because of embarrassment. Not asking about a specific side effect may lead to misleadingly low rates.

Second, was the size of the study sufficient to detect meaningful differences in rates of the side effects of interest? RCTs lack sufficient power to detect rare side effects; however, if a particular side effect (e.g., weight gain) is of interest, the study should have sufficient power to detect meaningful differences.

Are the Results Important?

In an RCT that reports adverse effects, NNH is the measure of interest. In addition, the severity of side effects, not only the frequency, is important.

Can I Apply the Results to My Patient?

As noted in Chapter 5, this question can be reframed as: "Is the pathobiology of my patient so different from that of the study patients that the results cannot apply?" Here the considerations regarding side effects become more complicated than with the assessment of beneficial effects. There are often significant differences in the risk of adverse effects, depending on patient characteristics. To take an obvious example, men and nonpregnant women are not at risk for the teratogenic side effects of a medication. Beyond this, however, there are a variety of physical illnesses that could be exacerbated by a medication or that could predispose a patient to a particular side effect. In addition, there are age-related changes in drug metabolism, and members of particular ethnic groups may be at increased risk of specific medication side effects, partly because of allelic variation in genes coding for drug-metabolizing enzymes (Cookson et al. 2002; Ruiz 2000). Thus, some judgment is required in deciding whether your patient is enough like those in the study that the results apply and whether your patient is at increased or decreased risk. In general, your patient will probably be similar enough to those studied that the results will apply, although the magnitude of the risk may differ.

In assessing the relative risks and benefits of treatment, the issue is one of comparing NNT as a measure of treatment effectiveness with NNH as a measure of treatment side effects. This can certainly be done informally by simply comparing NNT and NNH, together with a subjective assessment of the relative value the patient places on the benefit versus the risk. A more formal quantitative method of doing this has been described that involves calculating a statistic, the likelihood of being helped or harmed

TABLE 11–7. Critical appraisal guide for randomized controlled trials reporting harm

Is the study valid?

Is it a randomized controlled trial?

Was the randomization list concealed?

Were subjects and clinicians blinded to treatment being administered?

Were side effects assessed appropriately?

Was the trial of sufficient duration to detect the side effects of interest?

Were all subjects enrolled in the trial accounted for?

Were subjects analyzed in the groups to which they were assigned?

Despite randomization, were there clinically important differences between groups at the start of the trial?

Aside from the experimental treatment, were the groups treated equally?

Are the results important?

How large was the treatment effect (number needed to harm)?

How precise are the results (width of confidence intervals)?

Can I apply the results to my patient?

Is my patient too different from patients in the study?

How do the benefits and risks of treatment compare for my patient?

How does my patient value these benefits and risks?

Do the benefits outweigh the harms (likelihood of being helped or harmed)?

Source. Based in part on the criteria of Levine et al. 2002; Sackett et al. 2000.

(LHH) (Guyatt et al. 2002; Sackett et al. 2000). As a first approximation:

$$LHH = \frac{1/NNT}{1/NNH} = \frac{NNH}{NNT}$$

with values of LHH>1 indicating that the benefit outweighs the harm. This crude calculation weights benefits and side effects equally. A more sophisticated calculation, taking into account patients' relative preferences for side effects versus treatment

effects, (as well as patient-specific NNTs and NNHs) is given in Appendix B.

Cohort Studies of Etiology Or Harm

A critical appraisal guide for a cohort study of etiology or harm is given in Table 11–8.

Is the Study Valid?

Several questions should be asked to determine the validity of the study. First, how were the subjects selected? The cohort should consist of individuals who are initially free of the disease under investigation, but who are potentially at risk for developing the disease. In addition, the exposed and nonexposed groups should be selected in such a way as to avoid major differences other than exposure status.

Was the cohort large enough and was the follow-up period long enough? For rare outcomes, large numbers of individuals must often be studied for prolonged periods of time to detect statistically significant differences in risk.

How was exposure measured? If significant errors are made in classifying individuals as either "exposed" or not, the results will tend to be biased. Random misclassification will tend to bias the observed RR toward 1.0, whereas differential misclassification will result in either an overestimate or underestimate of the actual RR (Hennekens et al. 1987).

Were exposed and unexposed individuals assessed for outcomes with the same intensity and were outcomes assessed blindly (i.e., without knowledge of exposure status)? If not, any differences could be the result of measurement bias, not true differences (Fletcher et al. 1996).

Similarly, were there differences in dropout rates between the two groups? Because the outcomes of patients who drop out may differ from the outcomes of patients completing the study, differences in dropout rates between the two groups may lead to biased estimates of risk (Hennekens et al. 1987).

Were the exposed and nonexposed groups in fact similar, except for exposure? If not, then confounding may be responsible for any difference in risk that is observed. If there were differences in potential confounding factors, appropriate statistical techniques (stratification or multivariate techniques) should have been used in the data analysis.

TABLE 11–8.   Critical appraisal guide for cohort studies

Is the study valid?

Were the exposed and nonexposed groups similar (other than exposure) to the risk factor at the onset of the study?

If there were differences between groups at the start of the trial, did the statistical analysis take the differences into account?

Was the follow-up of the cohort sufficiently long for outcomes to develop?

Were outcomes measured in the same way in both groups?

Were there significant differences in losses to follow-up in the two groups?

Were any of the criteria for causality met (Table 11–6)?

Are the results important?

How strong is the association (relative risk)?

How large is the absolute increase in risk (risk difference)?

Can I apply the results to my patient?

Is my patient too different from patients in the study?

How do the benefits and risks of treatment compare for my patient?

How does my patient value these benefits and risks?

Do the benefits outweigh the harms (likelihood of being helped or harmed)?

Source.   Based in part on the criteria of Elwood 1998; Levine et al. 2002; Sackett et al. 2000.

Were any of the criteria for causality (Table 11–6) met? If so, the likelihood that the results were not the result of chance, bias, or confounding is increased.

Are the Results Important?

In a cohort study, RR measures the strength of association between the exposure and outcome, whereas NNH is a better measure of the potential harm to an individual patient (Sackett et al. 2000).

Can I Apply the Results to My Patient?

As with RCTs, this question can be reframed in the following way: "Is the biology of my patient so different from that of the study patients that the results cannot apply?"

If the clinical question is one that concerns the etiology of a disorder, the results will generally be applicable, assuming that your patient could be at risk for the outcome and bearing in mind that some outcomes are limited to patients who are of a particular age, sex, or childbearing status. With regard to etiology, the assumptions are that RR will apply to all individuals and that risks are generally multiplicative. In certain circumstances, however, interactions between risk factors that could either increase or decrease a particular patient's risk beyond what is expected by the RR associated with the individual risk factors are possible (Gordis 2000; Rothman 2002).

In assessing the absolute risk to an individual patient, however, NNH is used as the measure of risk. Unlike RR, this measure is sensitive to the individual's baseline risk and may need to be individualized.

As with an RCT, in assessing the relative risks and benefits of treatment, the issue is one of comparing NNT (usually derived from an RCT) with NNH from the cohort study, and the same considerations apply as discussed for LHH above.

Case-Control Study

A critical appraisal guide for a case-control study is given in Table 11–9.

Is the Study Valid?

The first question is how the cases were chosen. The cases should be representative of patients with the disease. In addition, they should be incident (newly diagnosed) cases, because a study of prevalent cases may reveal more about risk factors for chronicity than about the etiology of the disorder.

The next question is how the control subjects were chosen. In a case-control study, control subjects must be chosen from the same source population as the cases, because control subjects are used to estimate the prevalence of exposure to a risk factor in the population from which the cases are drawn (Lewis and Pelosi 1990; Rothman 2002). In other words, if the cases in a study were identified from a particular clinic or hospital, would the control subjects have obtained treatment from that same clinic or hospital if they had the disease in question? Control subjects can include general population controls; hospital or clinic controls; and friends, relatives, or neighbors of the cases. If more than one

TABLE 11–9. Critical appraisal guide for case-control studies

Is the study valid?

Did the method of selection of cases and control subjects introduce bias?

Were outcomes measured in the same way in both groups, independent of disease status?

Were confounding factors identified and dealt with in the analysis?

Were any of the criteria for causality met (Table 11–6)?

Are the results important?

How strong is the association (odds ratio)?

Can I apply the results to my patient?

Is my patient too different from patients in the study?

What is the number needed to harm for my patient?

How do the benefits and risks of treatment compare for my patient?

How does my patient value these benefits and risks?

Do the benefits outweigh the harms (likelihood of being helped or harmed)?

Source. Based in part on the criteria of Fletcher et al. 1996; Levine et al. 2002; Mant 1999; Sackett et al. 2000.

control group was used in a particular study, were the results similar? If so, it is less likely that the results were the result of selection bias.

The other serious concern in case-control studies is information or recall bias. Exposure history should be gathered without knowledge of whether the individual is a case or a control subject. In addition, using more than one information source may increase the validity of the information being collected, because individuals with a disease often search their memories for possible causes, and psychiatric illnesses may selectively influence memory.

Were the cases and the control subjects generally similar except for exposure? If not, confounding may be responsible for any difference in the amount of risk that is observed. If there were differences in potential confounding factors, appropriate statistical techniques (stratification or multivariate techniques) should have been used in the data analysis.

Were any of the criteria for causality (Table 11–6) met? If so, the likelihood that the results were not the result of chance, bias, or confounding is increased.

Are the Results Important?

In a case-control study, the OR measures the strength of association between the exposure and the outcome. Measures of absolute risk cannot be determined from a case-control study alone.

Can I Apply the Results to My Patient?

As in a cohort study, if the clinical question concerns the etiology of a disorder, the results will generally be applicable, assuming your patient could be at risk for the outcome. The assumptions are that the OR will apply to all individuals and that risks are multiplicative. There may be interactions between risk factors that may either increase or decrease a particular patient's risk beyond what would be expected from the OR associated with the individual risk factors (Gordis 2000; Rothman 2002).

Because measures of absolute risk cannot be directly estimated from a case-control study, the study itself will not yield NNH. It is possible, however, to estimate NNH from the OR if the probability of disease in the patient (usually estimated from the incidence of disease in the population) is known (Bjerre and LeLorier 2000). A method for calculating this estimation is given in Appendix B. As in an RCT or cohort study, the issue in assessing the relative risks and benefits of treatment becomes one of comparing NNT (usually derived from an RCT) with NNH (estimated from the OR and population incidence data).

References

Bjerre LM, LeLorier J: Expressing the magnitude of adverse effects in case-control studies: "the number of patients needed to be treated for one additional patient to be harmed." BMJ 320:503–506, 2000

Bradford Hill AB: The environment and disease: association and causation. Proc R Soc Med 58:295–300, 1965

Brewer T, Colditz GA: Postmarketing surveillance and adverse drug reactions: current perspectives and future needs. JAMA 281:824–829, 1999

Cookson J, Taylor D, Katona C: The Use of Drugs in Psychiatry: The Evidence from Psychopharmacology, 5th Edition. London, Gaskell, 2002

Cooper Z, Paykel ES: Social factors in the onset and maintenance of depression, in Principles of Social Psychiatry. Edited by Bhugra D, Leff J. London, Blackwell Scientific, 1993, pp 99–121

Creed F: Life events, in Principles of Social Psychiatry. Edited by Bhugra D, Leff J. London, Blackwell Scientific, 1993, pp 144–161

Elwood M: Critical Appraisal of Epidemiological Studies and Clinical Trials, 2nd Edition. Oxford, UK, Oxford University Press, 1998

Fletcher RH, Fletcher SW, Wagner EH: Clinical Epidemiology: The Essentials, 3rd Edition. Baltimore, MD, Williams & Wilkins, 1996

Gordis L: Epidemiology, 2nd Edition. Philadelphia, PA, WB Saunders, 2000

Gunnell D, Harrison G, Rasmussen F, et al: Associations between premorbid intellectual performance, early life exposures and early onset schizophrenia: cohort study. Br J Psychiatry 181:298–305, 2002

Guyatt G, Straus S, McAlister F, et al: Moving from evidence to action: incorporating patient values, in Users' Guides to the Medical Literature: A Manual for Evidence-Based Clinical Practice. Edited by Guyatt G, Rennie D. Chicago, IL, AMA Press, 2002, pp 567–582

Hennekens CH, Buring JE, Mayrent SL: Epidemiology in Medicine. Boston, MA, Little, Brown, 1987

Ioannidis JPA, Lau J: Completeness of safety reporting in randomized trials: an evaluation of 7 medical areas. JAMA 285:437–443, 2001

Jones TC: Call for a new approach to the process of clinical trials and drug registration. BMJ 322:920–923, 2001

Kelsey JL, Whittemore AS, Evans AS, et al (eds): Methods in Observational Epidemiology, 2nd Edition. New York, Oxford University Press, 1996

Ko DT, Hebert PR, Coffey CS, et al: Beta-blocker therapy and symptoms of depression, fatigue, and sexual dysfunction. JAMA 288:351–357, 2002

Koro CE, Fedder DO, L'Italien GJ, et al: Assessment of independent effect of olanzapine and risperidone on risk of diabetes among patients with schizophrenia: population based nested case-control study. BMJ 325:243–245, 2002

Lawrie S, McIntosh A: Schizophrenia. Clin Evid 7:920–944, 2002

Levine M, Haslam D, Walter S, et al: Harm, in Users' Guides to the Medical Literature: A Manual for Evidence-Based Clinical Practice. Edited by Guyatt G, Rennie D. Chicago, IL, AMA Press, 2002, pp 81–100

Lewis G, Pelosi AJ: The case-control study in psychiatry. Br J Psychiatry 157:197–207, 1990

Lloyd G, Lishman A: The effect of depression on speed of recall of pleasant and unpleasant experiences. Psychol Med 5:173–190, 1976

Mant J: Case-control studies, in Evidence-Based Practice: A Primer for Health Care Professionals. Edited by Dawes M, Davies P, Gray A, et al. Edinburgh, Churchill Livingstone, 1999, pp 73–84

Pirmohamed M, Breckenridge AM, Kitteringham NR, et al: Adverse drug reactions. BMJ 316:1295–1298, 1998

Rothman KJ: Epidemiology: An Introduction. New York, Oxford University Press, 2002

Rothman KJ, Greenland S (eds): Modern Epidemiology, 2nd Edition. Philadelphia, PA, Lippincott-Raven, 1998

Ruiz P (ed): Ethnicity and Psychopharmacology (Review of Psychiatry Series, Vol 19, No 4). Washington, DC, American Psychiatric Press, 2000

Sackett DL, Straus SE, Richardson WS, et al: Evidence-Based Medicine: How to Practice and Teach EBM, 2nd Edition. New York, Churchill Livingstone, 2000

Takeshita J, Masaki K, Ahmed I, et al: Are depressive symptoms a risk factor for mortality in elderly Japanese American men? The Honolulu-Asia Aging Study. Am J Psychiatry 159:1127–1132, 2002

Turcotte K, Raina P, Moyer VA: Above all, do no harm. West J Med 174: 325–329, 2001

Studies of Prognosis

Gregory E. Gray, M.D., Ph.D.

Questions about prognosis are frequently raised by patients and by their families. Such questions take many forms. When will I get better? Will I be completely well? What are the chances of the disease recurring? Such questions are studied by following groups of patients over time (i.e., in a cohort study). Some such studies are purely descriptive, whereas other studies attempt to find prognostic factors that predict a good or bad outcome. The latter types are similar to the cohort studies of risk described in Chapter 11 and are subject to the same design and analysis issues. This chapter focuses on descriptive studies of prognosis and briefly reviews some of the issues in their design and analysis before discussing their critical appraisal.

Selecting Patients

The selection of patients in a cohort study of prognosis is of considerable importance. The two key issues are the populations from which the subjects are obtained and whether they are newly diagnosed cases or patients currently in treatment.

Source of Patients

One can think of several populations of patients with the same illness: patients in the general population who are in treatment with non–mental health practitioners, those in outpatient treatment with mental health professionals, those in specialized mental health clinics (e.g., an academic mood disorders clinic), and those who are hospitalized for their conditions. In general, patients seen at academic medi-

cal centers have more severe disease, more comorbid conditions, and are more likely to be treatment resistant or chronically ill than are those in community settings (Cohen and Cohen 1984; Hulley et al. 2001; Randolph et al. 2002). We know far less about the prognosis of individuals in the community who do not seek treatment (Regier et al. 1998), but it is believed that they have a better prognosis and more social supports (Cohen and Cohen 1984).

An example of such a difference in prognosis comes from a study of the duration of major depressive episodes in the general population conducted by Spijker et al. (2002). In this study, cases were identified as part of a prospective epidemiological study in a community, so the authors were able to identify cases that did not seek treatment, as well as those that did. Median durations of the depressive episode were 3.0 months for patients who had no professional care, 4.5 months for patients treated in primary care settings, and 6.0 months for patients who entered the mental health system.

There is no "right" population to study, but the population studied affects the generalizability of the results (Gordis 2000; Randolph et al. 2002). Results obtained from a study of patients in an academic medical center may not apply to individuals in the community.

Incident Versus Prevalent Cases

The other major issue concerns whether to select new (incident) cases or existing (prevalent) cases. There is a temptation to begin with a cohort of patients already in treatment (a survival cohort), but such a sample would contain an overrepresentation of chronic patients and hence lead to a biased estimate of prognosis (Cohen and Cohen 1984; Fletcher et al. 1996). Instead, an inception cohort (a group of people assembled near the onset of disease) should be studied (Fletcher et al. 1996).

A related issue is that of the starting point or *zero time* (Fletcher et al. 1996; Gordis 2000). This could either be at the onset of symptoms, when treatment was first begun, or when a diagnosis was made. Regardless of what is chosen as the zero time, it should be used consistently as the starting point (Fletcher et al. 1996).

Follow-up and Attrition

One of the major sources of bias in cohort studies of prognosis concerns patients lost to follow-up. If patients lost to follow-up differ in outcomes from patients who remain in the study, estimates of prognosis will be biased. This is called *migration bias* (Fletcher et al. 1996).

One way of dealing with losses to follow-up in the analysis is to perform a *best case/worst case* analysis, a form of sensitivity analysis in which outcome statistics are first calculated assuming all of those lost to follow-up did well, then recalculated assuming all of those lost to follow-up had a bad outcome (Fletcher et al. 1996; Sackett et al. 2000). Ideally, researchers should attempt to minimize losses to follow-up through periodic contact and other means (Cummings et al. 2001).

Outcomes and Data Analysis

There are two commonly used approaches for describing the prognosis of a cohort: reporting on outcomes at specified follow-up times and measuring time to an event.

Outcomes at Specific Follow-Up Times

Investigators will sometimes recontact a cohort at specified times and collect data for a variety of outcome measures. Such an approach was taken by Wiersma et al. (2000) when they used several measures of social disability to assess a cohort of patients with schizophrenia at 1, 2, and 15 years after diagnosis. The advantage of this approach is that considerable information can be collected at each follow-up interview. The disadvantage is that no information is

gathered between the set follow-up intervals, and the losses that follow lead to data that are based on smaller and smaller numbers of subjects at each subsequent interview.

Time-to-Event Outcomes: Survival Analysis

The use of time-to-event as an outcome measure in studies of prognosis is more common than the use of specified follow-up times. The event may be a negative one (e.g., death, relapse, rehospitalization, or dropping out of treatment) or a positive one (e.g., recovery). Such data are analyzed using statistical techniques called *survival analysis* or *failure time analysis*.

Survival analysis acknowledges that patients may be lost to follow-up; however, the analysis does include these patients until such time as they are lost. A basic statistical assumption, however, is that the prognosis of patients lost to follow-up (i.e., censored) will be the same as for patients who continue in the study (Bland and Altman 1998; Gordis 2000). Survival curves, such as the one in Figure 12–1, are calculated using the Kaplan-Meier method, the details of which are given in standard biostatistics texts (e.g., Altman 1991; Pagano and Gauvreau 2000). The log-rank test can be used to test for differences in survival times between subgroups (Altman 1991; Peto et al. 1977).

Critical Appraisal Guide for Studies of Prognosis

Guidelines for appraising cohort studies of prognosis are given in Table 12–1. As with other types of studies, validity should be assessed before considering the results.

Is the Study Valid?

The study should be based on an inception (incidence) cohort. If it is based on a survival cohort of patients at various stages of illness, it is simply not a valid study of prognosis.

The next question concerns follow-up losses. Sackett et al. (2000) have suggested using the "5 and 20" guideline, where <5% of patients lost to follow-up is probably not significant, whereas >20% lost to follow-up seriously threatens the validity of the study.

Finally, it is important that study outcomes be assessed in a uniform way.

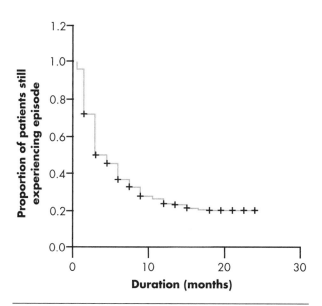

FIGURE 12–1. Survival curve of a cohort with newly originated major depression in the community.

Source. Reprinted from Spijker J, DeGraaf R, Bijl RV, et al: "Duration of Major Depressive Episodes in the General Population: Results From The Netherlands Mental Health Survey and Incidence Study (NEMESIS)." *British Journal of Psychiatry* 181:208–213, 2002. Copyright 2002 Royal College of Psychiatrists. Used with permission.

What Are the Results?

If measures other than time-to-event data are used, results should be presented with confidence intervals. Time-to-event data are generally presented in the form of a survival curve, often omitting confidence intervals for the curve itself but providing some information in the text on precision of the estimates.

Can I Apply the Results to My Patient?

As noted above, the prognosis of a community sample may differ significantly from that obtained from various treatment settings. Whenever possible, an attempt should be made to find a study reporting on a population from a setting similar to that of your patient. If this is not possible, the results may still be usable, keeping in mind the general rule that cohorts assembled from an academic medical center or specialty mental health program will often contain a greater number of poor-prognosis patients than will cohorts assembled from primary care or community settings.

TABLE 12–1. Critical appraisal guide for studies of prognosis

Is the study valid?

Is it a cohort study based on an inception cohort?

Was the follow-up relatively complete (>80% and preferably >95%)?

Were outcomes assessed in a uniform, unbiased manner?

What are the results?

What are the outcome data at various points in time?

Is there a survival curve?

How precise are the estimates?

Can I apply the results to my patient?

Were the patients similar to my patients in diagnosis and comorbidity?

Were the patients derived from a similar treatment setting?

Was the management similar to that in my practice?

Source. Based in part on data from Randolph et al. 2002; Sackett et al. 2000.

A secondary consideration has to do with comorbidity and other patient attributes that may affect prognosis. Again, there are no hard and fast rules, but patients with comorbid conditions frequently have a worse prognosis than do patients without comorbid conditions. Once again, although this does not invalidate a study, some mental adjustment of the results must be made in applying them to your patient.

References

Altman DG: Practical Statistics for Medical Research. Boca Raton, FL, Chapman & Hall, 1991

Bland JM, Altman DG: Survival probabilities (the Kaplan-Meier method). BMJ 317:1572, 1998

Cohen P, Cohen J: The clinician's illusion. Arch Gen Psychiatry 41:1178–1182, 1984

Cummings SR, Newman TB, Hulley SB: Designing an observational study: cohort studies, in Designing Clinical Research: An Epidemiologic Approach, 2nd Edition. Edited by Hulley SB, Cummings SR. Philadelphia, PA, Lippincott Williams & Wilkins, 2001, pp 95–105

Fletcher RH, Fletcher SW, Wagner EH: Clinical Epidemiology: The Essentials, 3rd Edition. Baltimore, MD, Williams & Wilkins, 1996

Gordis L: Epidemiology, 2nd Edition. Philadelphia, PA, WB Saunders, 2000

Hulley SB, Newman TB, Cummings SR: Choosing the study subjects: specification, sampling, and recruitment, in Designing Clinical Research: An Epidemiologic Approach, 2nd Edition. Edited by Hulley SB, Cummings SR. Philadelphia, PA, Lippincott Williams & Wilkins, 2001, pp 25–35

Pagano M, Gauvreau K: Principles of Biostatistics, 2nd Edition. Pacific Grove, CA, Duxbury, 2000

Peto R, Pike MC, Armitage P, et al: Design and analysis of randomized clinical trials requiring prolonged observation of each patient, II: analysis and examples. Br J Cancer 35:1–39, 1977

Randolph A, Bucher H, Richardson WS, et al: Prognosis, in Users' Guides to the Medical Literature: A Manual for Evidence-Based Clinical Practice. Edited by Guyatt G, Rennie D. Chicago, IL, AMA Press, 2002, pp 141–154

Regier DA, Kaelber CT, Rae DS, et al: Limitations of diagnostic criteria and assessment instruments for mental disorders: implications for research and policy. Arch Gen Psychiatry 55:109–115, 1998

Sackett DL, Straus SE, Richardson WS, et al: Evidence-Based Medicine: How to Practice and Teach EBM, 2nd Edition. New York, Churchill Livingstone, 2000

Spijker J, DeGraaf R, Bijl RV, et al: Duration of major depressive episodes in the general population: results from The Netherlands Mental Health Survey and Incidence Study (NEMESIS). Br J Psychiatry 181:208–213, 2002

Wiersma D, Wanderling J, Dragomirecka E, et al: Social disability in schizophrenia: its development and prediction over 15 years in incidence cohorts in six European cities. Psychol Med 30:1155–1167, 2000

Evaluating Your Performance of Evidence-Based Medicine

Gregory E. Gray, M.D., Ph.D.

Psychiatry residents are expected to acquire positive attitudes toward lifelong learning, and more specifically, according to the Accreditation Council for Graduate Medical Education (ACGME): "The physician shall recognize limitations in his or her own knowledge base and clinical skills, and understand and address the need for lifelong learning." In this chapter, the focus is on evaluating evidence-based medicine (EBM) skills. In the next chapter, we focus on the broader issues of evaluating one's practice.

In the 5-step EBM model (see Gray, Chapter 2 in this volume), the final step is assessing the outcome. In ordinary clinical practice, we assess whether a particular treatment worked or whether a diagnostic test provided helpful information. In the EBM model, assessment has the added component of evaluating the clinician's performance in the EBM process.

The model for such an evaluation, as suggested by Sackett et al. (2000) and Wolf (2000), focuses on skills in performing each of the five steps in the EBM process (Table 13–1). A more in-depth discussion of the evaluation of clinical skills in general—and of EBM skills in particular—can be found in the works of Sackett et al. (1991, 2000).

Formulating Clinical Questions

The first necessary skill is formulating the 4-part clinical questions (see Gray, Chapter 3 in this volume). Such a skill is important because it leads to a more efficient search strategy (Cabell et al. 2001),

yet it is still one with which physicians may have difficulty (Ely et al. 2002).

The first question to ask is whether the clinician understands the concept of the 4-part PICO clinical question (i.e., patient/problem, intervention, comparison, and outcome, as described in Chapter 3) and whether he or she was able to formulate such questions before beginning the most recent search for information. The next question to ask is whether the clinician routinely formulates such questions in his or her clinical practice.

Clinical questions arise every day in clinical practice, but we often do not have the ability to answer them on the spot (Del Mar and Glasziou 2001). To incorporate EBM into daily practice requires that we have a way of keeping track of the most important questions so that they can be answered at a later time.

Searching for Answers

The next step in the process is searching for an answer to the clinical question. In evaluating a particular search, barriers to finding the information should be identified. Common barriers include lack of time and information resources, as well as the search strategy itself (Cabell et al. 2001; Craig et al. 2001; Ely et al. 2002; McColl et al. 1998). Furthermore, many practitioners either lack awareness of the Cochrane Database of Systematic Reviews and other resources or do not use them, even if available (Kerse et al. 2001; McColl et al. 1998).

TABLE 13–1. Self-evaluation of evidence-based medicine skills

Formulating clinical questions

Do I understand what a 4-part PICO clinical question is?

Was I able to formulate a 4-part PICO question this time?

Do I routinely keep track of clinical questions that arise in my practice and attempt to find answers to them?

Searching for answers

Do I know the common databases and how to search them?

Did this particular search go well or could I have been more efficient?

Do I routinely attempt to answer clinical questions through searches or do I still rely primarily on textbooks?

Appraising the evidence

Do I understand how to critically appraise research articles and other evidence?

Was I able to apply the critical appraisal guide in this case, including considering my patient's individual risks, needs, and preferences?

Are my critical appraisal skills improving over time?

Applying the evidence

Do I incorporate the evidence that I have appraised (and have found to be valid) into my clinical practice?

What proportion of my clinical decisions is based on current best evidence?

Evaluating the results

Do I routinely evaluate my evidence-based medicine skills?

Are there particular aspects of the evidence-based medicine process that I need to review?

Note. PICO=Patient/Problem, Intervention, Comparison, and Outcome.

In evaluating one's own performance, the first question to ask is whether you have an understanding of the basic search process (as outlined by Gray and Taylor in Chapter 4 in this volume), including the roles of the various databases that are available. The second question relates to the ability to perform the particular search and whether another search

strategy would have proved more efficient. The final question to ask is whether you are routinely searching for answers in appropriate databases in your clinical practice rather than relying on textbooks.

Appraising the Evidence

Critical appraisal skills are the most commonly taught aspect of EBM (Green 1999), yet clinicians often remain unfamiliar with many of the basic concepts (LeClair et al. 1999; McColl et al. 1998; Young et al. 2002). Such skills, however, are associated with the ability and willingness to apply the results of systematic reviews in clinical practice (Doust and Silagy 2000).

In evaluating yourself, the first question to ask is whether you have an understanding of the methods of critical appraisal, including the use of critical appraisal worksheets. (To review this information, see Chapters 5–11.) The next question to ask is whether you had any difficulties in appraising the evidence from this particular search. This also involves considering whether the evidence was applicable to your patient, being able to individualize the results for your patient, and assessing whether it was consistent with patient needs and preferences. Finally, you should ask whether your appraisal skills are improving over time as a result of practice.

Applying the Evidence

The fourth step involves applying the evidence to a particular patient. This is when clinicians often falter (Wolf 2000). The most important question to ask here is whether one's practice is becoming more evidence based. This can be done informally; for example, as the clinician sees patients, he or she should ask whether the treatment provided, diagnostic test ordered, and so forth were supported by good evidence. This may encourage clinicians to conduct searches for some common treatments that are being used, and the results may surprise them. It can also be done in a more formal way, as part of a quality improvement project (Baker and Grol 2001).

Evaluating the Results

Finally, clinicians should reflect on their own performance of EBM. In Chapter 14, Taylor addresses the issue of evaluating one's practice in more detail, and in Chapter 15, Gray and Taylor provide resources to be used in teaching and learning EBM. Remember that skill in EBM is like any other skill: it gets easier with practice.

Learning Evidence-Based Medicine

Clinicians who need more training in EBM have several options to increase their knowledge and skills.

Books and Journals

This book covers the basics of EBM (and evidence-based psychiatric practice) as applied to psychiatric practice. Other excellent EBM texts, each with a slightly different orientation, provide additional information about various aspects of the EBM process. These include books by Dawes et al. (1999), Greenhalgh (2001), Guyatt and Rennie (2002a, 2002b), and Sackett et al. (2000). The texts by Dawes et al. (1999), Greenhalgh (2001), and Guyatt and Rennie (2002a) are similar in scope to the current volume, whereas the texts of Guyatt and Rennie (2002b), Sackett et al. (2000), and Straus et al. (2005) provide a more in-depth coverage of topics. Although the texts are more oriented toward internists or family practitioners, they can profitably be read by anyone who wants to apply EBM to psychiatric practice.

In addition to books specifically about EBM, books about the basic sciences behind EBM (i.e., clinical epidemiology and biostatistics) may be helpful. The best starting point for learning more about clinical epidemiology is the brief clinically oriented text by Fletcher et al. (1996); Gordis (2000) has written a useful text that is slightly more detailed. Among the many biostatistics texts, the monograph by Daly and Bourke (2000) stands out for its clarity and clinical relevance. Several journals also regularly include useful overviews of EBM concepts, including the *ACP Journal Club*, *Evidence-Based Mental Health*, and the general medical journals *BMJ* and *JAMA*.

Internet Resources

In addition to print resources, several online resources may be useful in learning more about various aspects of EBM. Some general resources are listed in Table 15–2 in Chapter 15 of this volume. A search of the Internet identifies numerous Internet-based courses as well.

Courses

Most medical libraries regularly offer courses about MEDLINE and other databases. In addition, medical librarians can be quite helpful in teaching you how to improve your search techniques.

Also, several regularly offered courses on EBM use active small-group teaching strategies. Many of these can be found by searching the Web sites listed in Table 4–2 in Chapter 4 of this volume. The American Psychiatric Association has also offered 1-day workshops at its annual meetings.

References

Baker R, Grol R: How to assess the effectiveness of applying the evidence, in Evidence-Based Practice in Primary Care, 2nd Edition. Edited by Silagy C, Haines A. London, BMJ Books, 2001, pp 83–97

Cabell CH, Schardt C, Sanders L, et al: Resident utilization of information technology: a randomized trial of clinical question formation. J Gen Intern Med 16:838–844, 2001

Craig JC, Irwig LM, Stockler MR: Evidence-based medicine: useful tools for decision making. Med J Aust 174:248–253, 2001

Daly L, Bourke GF: Interpretation and Uses of Medical Statistics, 5th Edition. Hoboken, NJ, Wiley-Blackwell, 2000

Dawes M, Davies P, Gray A, et al (eds): Evidence-Based Practice: A Primer for Health Care Professionals. New York, Churchill Livingstone, 1999

Del Mar CB, Glasziou PP: Ways of using evidence-based medicine in general practice. Med J Aust 174:347–350, 2001

Doust JA, Silagy CA: Applying the results of a systematic review in general practice. Med J Aust 172:153–156, 2000

Ely JW, Osheroff JA, Ebell MH, et al: Obstacles to answering doctors' questions about patient care with evidence: qualitative study. BMJ 324:710–713, 2002

Fletcher RH, Fletcher SW, Wagner EH: Clinical Epidemiology: The Essentials, 3rd Edition. Baltimore, MD, Williams & Wilkins, 1996

Gordis L: Epidemiology, 2nd Edition. Philadelphia, PA, WB Saunders, 2000

Green ML: Graduate medical education training in clinical epidemiology, critical appraisal, and evidence-based medicine: a critical review of the curricula. Acad Med 74:686–694, 1999

Greenhalgh T: How to Read a Paper: The Basics of Evidence Based Medicine, 2nd Edition. London, BMJ Books, 2001

Guyatt G, Rennie D (eds): Users' Guides to the Medical Literature: Essentials of Evidence-Based Clinical Practice. Chicago, IL, AMA Press, 2002a

Guyatt G, Rennie D (eds): Users' Guides to the Medical Literature: A Manual for Evidence-Based Clinical Practice. Chicago, IL, AMA Press, 2002b

Kerse N, Arroll B, Lloyd T, et al: Evidence databases, the Internet, and general practitioners: the New Zealand story. N Z Med J 114:89–91, 2001

LeClair BM, Wagner PJ, Miller MD: A tool to evaluate self-efficacy in evidence-based medicine. Acad Med 74:597, 1999

McColl A, Smith H, White P, et al: General practitioners' perceptions of the route to evidence based medicine: a questionnaire survey. BMJ 316:361–365, 1998

Sackett DL, Haynes RB, Guyatt GH, et al: Clinical Epidemiology: A Basic Science for Clinical Medicine, 2nd Edition. Boston, MA, Little, Brown, 1991

Sackett DL, Straus SE, Richardson WS, et al: Evidence-Based Medicine: How to Practice and Teach EBM, 2nd Edition. New York, Churchill Livingstone, 2000

Straus SE, Richardson WS, Glasziou P, et al: Evidence-Based Medicine: How to Practice and Teach EBM, 3rd Edition. Edinburgh, Churchill Livingstone, 2005

Wolf FM: Lessons to be learned from evidence-based medicine: practice and promise of evidence-based medicine and evidence-based education. Med Teach 22:251–259, 2000

Young JM, Glasziou P, Ward JE: General practitioners' self ratings of skills in evidence based medicine: validation study. BMJ 324:950–951, 2002

Evidence-Based Psychiatric Practice

C. Barr Taylor, M.D.

The goals of evidence-based psychiatric practice are to improve patient care and to help ensure that patients receive the most effective treatments available. In a broader sense, the goal for the clinician also should be to frequently assess and improve his or her clinical skills and acumen. The Accreditation Council for Graduate Medical Education now requires residents to learn how to use practice guidelines as part of the systems-based competency (Andrews and Burruss 2004). In recent decades, the knowledge base in all aspects of psychiatry has increased dramatically, with new findings of relevance to patient care reported frequently in the scientific literature. Modern clinicians need to enhance their psychotherapy skills and techniques and to be conversant with new developments in medicine, psychotherapy, and psychopharmacology that may affect their patients' care. Keeping up to date on this knowledge requires the ability both to find information relevant to a particular patient and to monitor information that may be relevant to one's overall practice. In this chapter, I consider how clinicians can focus on the quality of care of their practice.

Evaluating one's practice is more complicated than finding an answer to a particular therapeutic question. In this case, the clinician would want to know not only about the choice of therapies but also how well the quality of his or her work measures up to standards in the field or literature and the clinician's own personal standards. Learning how to evaluate and improve their practice as needed is one of the core competencies psychiatry residents are now expected to acquire in the course of training. Evaluating one's practice is also a core feature of lifelong learning. In this chapter, I discuss several approaches to doing so.

Evaluating One's Practice

Sir William Osler, one of the founders of modern medicine, encouraged clinicians to classify cases as "clear cases, doubtful cases and mistakes." He argued that "It is only by getting your cases grouped in this way that you can make any real progress in your post-collegiate education; only in this way you gain wisdom with experience" (Cushing 1940, p. 328). He also said that "It is a common error to think the more a physician sees the greater his experience and more he knows," the implication being that experience is not sufficient for lifelong learning. Yet from an evidence-based standpoint, what constitutes a "clear case, doubtful case, and mistake"? A clinician may prescribe a medication that is immediately followed by a significant improvement in the patient's symptoms, but the time course of improvement may be too soon for the medication to have had an effect. A major life event also may have led to a significant improvement in the symptom. The patient discussed in Taylor, Chapter 19 of this volume, had multiple problems and showed substantial improvement over the course of therapy, but it was not clear that the therapy led to the improvement. The same can be said about a doubtful case in which the outcome is not as expected. Here again, several interceding factors can affect the patient in ways that may reduce an otherwise effective approach. Both "clear" and "doubtful" outcomes must be considered as only one source of information about one's practice, but they can serve to help the clinician consider what he or she may be doing well or where he or she might be able to improve.

Peer Review

One approach to evaluating one's performance is to discuss cases with peers routinely during case conferences, during private consultations, or in other settings. The evidential quality of the feedback will be determined by the expertise of the group and the type of information that is presented. Such clinical feedback groups usually focus on particular therapeutic issues or problems rather than on outcomes. Some practice groups may hire individuals with particular expertise, such as an academic psychopharmacologist with a focus on bipolar disorder, to discuss treatment approaches. Such expert advice may be useful, particularly if the expertise is supported by evidence.

Measurement-Based Practice

A more demanding approach is to consider how well a patient is doing relative to some evidence-based standard. Such an evaluation could focus on implementation or outcome. With an implementation-based focus, clinicians would evaluate how well they are adhering to the guidelines and algorithms they favor. With an outcome-based focus, clinicians would focus on how well they are achieving their designated outcomes. An outcome focus has the advantage of helping to ensure that the patients are being provided optimal care, assuming of course that the outcomes are relevant to the patient's needs and that the therapies leading to these outcomes have been shown to be consistent. Outcome-based approaches, with frequent assessments linked to algorithms and other stepped care approaches that delineate and/or suggest practices and decisions, may lead to improved care. This approach has been called *measurement-based care* (Trivedi and Daly 2007; Trivedi et al. 2007). The advantages of measurement-based care are illustrated by Trivedi and Kurian in Chapter 21. This case, written by one of the lead investigators of Sequenced Treatment Al-

ternatives to Relieve Depression (STAR*D) and one of his colleagues, illustrates how a patient's progress is used to determine treatment decisions. Critics of STAR*D might argue that it does not adequately address or incorporate psychosocial issues or interventions, does not deal with comorbidities, and has an important but limited outcome. Even so, patients deserve to achieve *at least* the rate of depression remission and symptom reduction suggested by STAR*D while also achieving gains in other areas. Other cases also indicate that patients' progress can be considered in relation to measures, outcomes, guidelines, and algorithms.

In the cases presented in Parts II and III of this book, we asked the authors to discuss their choice of guidelines and algorithms and reflect on what they learned from the case presented that might affect how, if at all, they could do a better job next time.

Guideline- and Algorithm-Based Psychiatry Practice

With guideline-based psychiatric practice, clinicians would begin by choosing the guidelines or combination of guidelines most relevant to the patient being treated. Clinicians might then "check off" their practices against these guidelines and perhaps at the end of treatment, as illustrated in Chapters 16–19 and 34 of this volume.

For example, suppose a clinician wants to evaluate her care of a patient presenting with both depression and substance abuse. The clinician would identify the appropriate guidelines and outcomes and determine how and when these outcomes would be assessed. In Chapter 8, I discussed how the clinician can identify measures appropriate to his or her practice and patients. For this case, the clinician would focus on depression outcomes and substance use. For instance, the clinician might choose to follow the general American Psychiatric Association depression guidelines but to modify the pharmacology to follow the STAR*D algorithm (see Chapter 21). In accordance with STAR*D, the clinician decides that the patient should experience a 50% reduction in his depressive symptoms by 12 weeks and should be in remission by 6 months, as measured by the Quick Inventory of Depressive Symptomatology self-report version (QIDS-SR) (see Chapter 21 for definitions of remission). The pharmacological intervention would begin with citalopram, with an increase in dose and use of alternative medications and/or cognitive-behavioral therapy (CBT) as per the STAR*D algorithm (see Chapter 21).

For substance abuse, the clinician decides to generally follow the American Psychiatric Association substance use guidelines but to add a time frame for achieving the predetermined outcomes. Because the guidelines are not very specific, the clinician uses her own standards and experience to define the goals and time frame. For instance, as seen in Table 14–1, for the goal of "motivate the patient to change," the clinician arbitrarily sets a personal standard of achieving this by 3 weeks. The clinician also believes in abstinence and feels that this should be achieved by 2 months into treatment. The clinician agrees that it is important for the patient to "repair disrupted relationships and enhance familial and interpersonal relationships that will support an abstinent lifestyle" and would hope to have the patient do so by 6 months and to help the patient develop social and vocational skills, also by 6 months. For the next goal, "help the patient learn, practice, and internalize changes in attitudes and behaviors conducive to relapse prevention," the clinician wants to accomplish this once the patient has become abstinent before termination. She plans to use a relapse prevention approach.

At week 3, the clinician evaluates how much progress has been made on motivating the patient to take steps toward abstinence. If the patient has not made progress, she reviews how the problem is being approached. The clinician may decide that a different approach is needed (e.g., to put more emphasis on motivational interviewing or establish a new time frame to achieve this goal).

After 8 weeks of therapy, after having generally followed the STAR*D guidelines, she gives the patient another QIDS-SR to assess his depressive symptoms. The QIDS-SR score has declined by more than 50% to a 5, and the depression is in remission. If the patient had not improved, the clinician would continue "down" the STAR*D algorithm with dose escalation, augmentation, and use of CBT, as appropriate and desired by the patient. With this approach, STAR*D achieved an overall remission rate of 67% (Rush et al. 2006).

Following STAR*D makes evaluation of overall practice relatively easy because each case is considered relative to some standards. But many clinicians, for a variety of reasons, might prefer not to use STAR*D or all aspects of STAR*D. Should clinicians using non-STAR*D approaches to treating major depressive disorder be expected to achieve results similar to those with STAR*D (i.e., an overall 67% remission)? In some settings, depending on the patients being treated, this is an unrealistic target. STAR*D indicated that some patients will not benefit even from this very aggressive approach. For instance, the remission rates were 37%, 31%, 14%,

TABLE 14–1. Problem, goals, time frame, and measures

Goal	Time frame[b]	Intervention/activity	Process measure
Motivate the patient to change: patients are in action phase of change, taking steps or abstinent.[a]	By week 3	Motivation interview	Self-report
Achieve abstinence.	At 2 months	Motivation interview/ Cognitive-behavioral therapy	Self-report
Repair disrupted relationships and enhance familial and interpersonal relationships that will support an abstinent lifestyle.[a]	Improvement by 6 months	Family, couples therapy if appropriate	Self-report
Develop social and vocational skills.[a]	Improvement by 6 months	Vocational training	Self-report
Help the patient learn, practice, and internalize changes in attitudes and behavior conducive to relapse prevention.[a]	Before termination	Relapse prevention	Self-report

[a]American Psychiatric Association substance use guidelines.
[b]Time frame added by author.

and 13% for the first, second, third, and fourth acute treatment steps, respectively (Rush et al. 2006). The clinician might take a moment to ask him- or herself: What are my treatment goals for depression, and am I achieving them?

Evaluating one's psychotherapeutic competency is an even more complicated process than evaluating pharmacological practice and outcomes. Suppose a clinician decides that the use of CBT would reduce relapse rates in depressed patients and wants to add this to his or her therapeutic approach. CBT researchers have defined a set of skills appropriate for providing effective CBT and a criterion, representing the sum of these scores, that is arbitrarily considered to reflect competency (Trepka et al. 2004). The instrument is meant to be scored by an experienced rater, but for the practicing clinician, it could be self-scored. Clinicians might consider assessing themselves on how adequately they are applying the basic therapeutic strategies: setting an agenda, providing feedback, being understanding, being interpersonally effective and collaborative, pacing the sessions, and using the time efficiently. Clinicians also might consider how they are teaching skills they wish patients to acquire. For instance, Strachowski et al. (2008) provide an example of how they monitored their patients' use of CBT or engagement in behaviorally activating actions. Assessing practice competence of the more structured interventions, such as CBT, is much simpler than evaluating one's psychotherapeutic competence of less well-defined strategies.

For alcohol abuse, the clinician's first goal (Table 14–1) was to motivate the patient to consider abstinence by week 3. Even though the clinician thought that she did a good job of providing motivational interview techniques, the patient is still drinking and not convinced that he should abstain or even that he has alcoholism. When patients are not progressing as expected, it is reasonable to review diagnosis, assessment, and treatment but also to examine the therapeutic relationship. In this case, the clinician evaluates her treatment according to the Working Alliance Inventory (Horvath and Greenberg 2008). This scale measures client's views of the therapy goals and tasks and of the bond between him or her and the clinician. The clinician finds a large discrepancy between her goals for one aspect of therapy— abstinence from alcohol—and those of the patient— to cut down. She finds that the patient perceives her as caring and understanding. The clinician wonders,

however, if she has not been direct enough in confronting the patient's denial about what she perceives as his alcohol dependence.

Overall Practice Performance

If the clinician collected data on a few patients with similar problems and presentations, she could use these types of data to evaluate her overall practice, looking for relevant standards in the scientific literature. However, this can be time-consuming, and such standards may be hard to come by. Although standards for practice seem to be a worthy goal, figuring out how to find and use them is a problem. In the following section, I discuss some approaches, realizing that I am simplifying a very complicated issue and using some relatively easy examples. Yet even these examples illustrate the difficulties of doing evidence-based practice evaluation.

For depression, the clinician might want to assess how the patient is doing compared with STAR*D remission and relapse rates. As noted earlier, an overall target might be 67%. She decides that at least 10 sessions of CBT are necessary to achieve a positive outcome and establishes this as a goal. If fewer than half of her patients are seen for the targeted number of 10 sessions, she might want to examine this aspect of her practice. The clinician has established an abstinence goal at 16 weeks for patients who present with alcohol abuse or dependence and who are drinking. However, she has difficulty finding studies that have used abstinence as a major outcome because many recent alcohol trials report measures such as percentage of days abstinent or days of heavy drinking (Anton et al. 2006). She decides also to use the COMBINE study improvement criteria, which enrolled more than 1,300 patients for a study that compared nine different alcohol abuse treatments (Anton et al. 2006), as one source of information to judge how she is doing. In this study, the main outcomes were percentage of days abstinent over the 8 weeks of the study and time to first heavy drinking day (five standard drinks per day for men; four for women). The mean percentage of days abstinent was about 65%, or 2 days out of 3. The clinician thought that this was a minimal standard, which she defined as the number of patients in her practice with a diagnosis of alcohol abuse or dependence who were sober more than 65% of the time, in the last 2 months of this treatment. She then looked at 10 patients she had treated in the past year and found that 3 were abstinent for the last 2 months of treatment, and the rest were sober about 50% of the time. On average, the patients were sober more than 65% of the time, meeting the criteria, and had reduced number of heavy drinking episodes. It was difficult for her to know, however, if these results meant that she was doing well or how she could improve her practice.

Checking one's practice against guidelines or algorithms and outcomes is one of many approaches to evidence-based psychiatric practice. The American Psychiatric Association provides a set of tools to make this easier, including a resource for measures (Rush et al. 2008), and the guidelines themselves are designed to improve practice. For illustrative purposes, I translated some of the guidelines into checklists and measured my performance against these guidelines for Chapters 16, 17, and 19.

Performance Measures

Many clinical settings have adopted standards of care and performance measures. These are usually used to determine how well an overall practice of clinicians is doing. For instance, The Joint Commission and the National Association of Psychiatric Health Systems (NAPHS), the National Association of State Mental Health Program Directors (NASMHPD), and the NASMHPD Research Institute, Inc. (NRI), have developed a set of core performance measures for hospital-based inpatient psychiatric services (www.jointcommission.org) that affect all the providers within that system. For instance, inpatient psychiatric health systems need to prove that they screen patients for violence risk, substance use, psychological trauma history, and patient strengths and show that a postdischarge continuing care plan was created and transmitted to the next level of care provider on discharge, among other activities.

Such measures tend to focus on process rather than outcome, although they are presumably developed to ensure better outcomes in the domains assessed. However, they are not necessarily evidence based.

The Department of Veterans Affairs routinely assesses clinician performance on several measures with the goal of 100% compliance to the measure. For instance, through chart review, clinicians may be evaluated on the number of people they screen for alcohol use who were due to be screened or whether they provided a timely suicide assessment and behavior evaluation for patients whose screening results were positive.

The American Psychiatric Association Web site lists several mental health performance measures, as listed in Table 14–2. Links to the source documents and databases are provided at this site.

Standards of care are often related to performance measures. Clinicians also may want to examine how they are doing relative to standards. For instance, the American Diabetes Association, American Psychiatric Association, American Association of Clinical Endocrinologists, and North American Association for the Study of Obesity have created a consensus statement of monitoring weight, blood pressure, glucose, and lipids for patients who are taking second-generation antipsychotics (American Diabetes Association 2004). Many such standards exist relative to mental health practice.

Mistakes and Improvement

Osler urged us to learn from our mistakes, but both identifying mistakes and admitting to them are difficult. Medical errors with serious consequences are common. In 2000, the Institute of Medicine (IOM) reported that 44,000–98,000 people die in hospitals each year as the result of medical errors (Kohn et al. 2000). About 7,000 people per year are estimated to die from medication errors alone—about 16% more deaths than the number attributable to work-related injuries. Unfortunately, very few data exist on the extent of the problem outside of hospitals or in mental health practice settings. The IOM report indicated, however, that many errors are likely to occur outside the hospital. For example, in a recent investigation of pharmacists, the Massachusetts Board of Registration in Pharmacy estimated that 2.4 million prescriptions are filled improperly each year in the state. The IOM emphasized that most of the medical errors are systems related and not attributable to individual negligence or misconduct and that the key to reducing medical errors is to focus on improving the systems of delivering care and not to blame individuals. Many performance measures are designed to reduce errors.

In March 2001, the IOM released a second report on its research into the safety of health care in the United States (Kohn et al. 2001). This report focuses on 13 specific recommendations designed to

TABLE 14–2.　Mental health performance measures

Resource	Comments
Quality Measure Inventory. From: Center for Quality Assessment and Improvement in Mental Health (CQAIMH)	Searchable database of more than 300 mental health performance measures
Experience of Care and Health Outcomes Survey (ECHO)	Mental health patient experience-of-care survey instrument
MDD Measures. From: Foundation for Accountability	Legacy documents maintained by the Markle Foundation
Healthcare Effectiveness Data and Information Set (HEDIS) 2008. From: National Committee for Quality Assurance (NCQA)	Health plan–level measures, including several mental health measures
Hospital-Based Inpatient Psychiatric Services (HBIPS) Core Measure Set. From: The Joint Commission	
Health Disparities Collaboratives (HDC) Depression Measures. From: Health Resources and Services Administration (HRSA)	
Behavioral Health Guidelines. From: Institute for Clinical Systems Improvement (ICSI)	MDD and ADHD guidelines, including performance measures
National Quality Measures Clearinghouse (NQMC). From: Agency for Healthcare Research and Quality (AHRQ)	Searchable compendium of performance measures from many domains of health care, including mental health
Physician Consortium for Performance Improvement MDD Measures. From: American Medical Association	
Quality Measures for Schizophrenia. Compiled by New York State Office of Mental Health	
Standards for Bipolar Excellence (STABLE) Project. Maintained by CQAIMH	
VA/DoD Clinical Practice Guidelines. From: U.S. Department of Veterans Affairs	Includes guidelines and measures for MDD, psychoses, and substance use disorder
Washington Circle Substance Use Disorder Measures	Core set of performance measures for alcohol and other drug services for public- and private-sector health plans

Note.　ADHD=attention-deficit/hyperactivity disorder; MDD=major depressive disorder.

Source.　Adapted from http://www.psych.org/MainMenu/PsychiatricPractice/QualityImprovement/PerformanceMeasures/MentalHealthPerformanceMeasures.aspx.

provide a guide for organizations to use in their efforts to improve patient safety. (An online course is available at www.criticalconceptsusa.com/online_coursesPME/PME_UPDATE.html).

Before clinicians can change practice procedures, they need to be able to identify that an error has been made and admit that one has made or contributed to an error. In this highly litigious practice environment, it is frightening to admit errors, particularly if they had adverse consequences, and to take steps to improve one's practice, which could be seen as an "admission of guilt." Among the barriers to being able to admit errors are resistance to change, fear of discipline, fear of licensure sanction, hindsight bias, need to blame, need to rationalize a negative event, legal system that focuses on fault-finding, and exposure to liability. The issues involved in discussing and disclosing errors with patients, colleagues, and others are beyond the scope of this chapter. The reader is referred to the

IOM report (Kohn et al. 2001) to consider how the IOM recommendations might be used to improve one's practice. The best approach is to prevent errors and for the clinician to monitor practice parameters before having a bad outcome.

However, some minor "mistakes" that clinicians make in practice have no major consequences. In addition to ensuring that they establish practice procedures to avoid serious errors, clinicians also should realize that they could probably do things a little better with almost every patient. The notion that clinicians also should be trying to improve their practice and outcomes is at the heart of evidence-based psychiatric practice. At the end of each case, I asked the authors to reflect on what they might have learned from that case and how they might provide better care to the next patient on the basis of their review. When I compared my actual practice with those suggested by the guidelines I had chosen, I was sometimes surprised to see how many "little" things I had omitted that might have made a difference in the outcome.

References

American Diabetes Association, American Psychiatric Association, American Association of Clinical Endocrinologists, North American Association for the Study of Obesity: Consensus development conference on antipsychotic drugs and obesity and diabetes. Diabetes Care 27:596–601, 2004

Andrews LB, Burruss JW: Core Competencies for Psychiatric Education: Defining, Teaching, and Assessing Resident Competence. Washington, DC, American Psychiatric Publishing, 2004

Anton RF, O'Malley SS, Ciraulo DA, et al: Combined pharmacotherapies and behavioral interventions for alcohol dependence: the COMBINE Study—a randomized controlled trial. JAMA 295:2003–2017, 2006

Cushing H: The Life of William Osler. New York, Oxford University Press, 1940

Horvath AO, Greenberg LS: Working Alliance Inventory (WAI), in Handbook of Psychiatric Measures, 2nd Edition. Edited by Rush AJ Jr, First MB, Blacker D. Washington, DC, American Psychiatric Publishing, 2008, pp 187–191

Kohn LT, Corrigan JM, Donaldson MS (eds): To Err Is Human: Building a Safer Health System. Washington, DC, Institute of Medicine, Committee on Quality of Health Care in America, National Academy Press, 2000

Kohn LT, Corrigan JM, Donaldson MS (eds): Crossing the Quality Chasm: A New System for the 21st Century. Washington, DC, Institute of Medicine, Committee on Quality of Health Care in America, National Academy Press, 2001

Rush AJ, Trivedi MH, Wisniewski SR, et al: Acute and longer-term outcomes in depressed outpatients requiring one or several treatment steps: a STAR*D report. Am J Psychiatry 163:1905–1917, 2006

Rush AJ Jr, First MB, Blacker D (eds): Handbook of Psychiatric Measures, 2nd Edition. Washington, DC, American Psychiatric Publishing, 2008

Strachowski D, Khaylis A, Conrad A, et al: The effects of directed cognitive behavior therapy on depression in older patients with cardiovascular risk. Depress Anxiety 25:E1–10, 2008

Trepka C, Rees A, Shapiro DA, et al: Clinician competence and outcome of cognitive therapy for depression. Cognit Ther Res 28:143–157, 2004

Trivedi MH, Daly EJ: Measurement-based care for refractory depression: a clinical decision support model for clinical research and practice. Drug Alcohol Depend 88 (suppl 2):S61–S71, 2007

Trivedi MH, Rush AJ, Gaynes BN, et al: Maximizing the adequacy of medication treatment in controlled trials and clinical practice: STAR(*)D measurement-based care. Neuropsychopharmacology 32:2479–2489, 2007

Teaching Evidence-Based Medicine and Evidence-Based Psychiatric Practice to Psychiatry Residents

Gregory E. Gray, M.D., Ph.D.
C. Barr Taylor, M.D.

This chapter is intended as a brief overview for residency directors and faculty who are responsible for teaching evidence-based medicine (EBM) to their residents. Other useful sources of information about teaching EBM include the works of Davies (1999), Gray (2001), Green (2000), and Sackett et al. (2000). The Evidence-Based Medicine Resource Center (www.ebmny.org/teach.html) sponsors a Web site that provides access to the Centre for Evidence-Based Medicine teaching materials and presentations, a list of EBM courses on the Web, and other materials. The Accreditation Council for Graduate Medical Education (ACGME) Outcome Project provides a variety of resources related to teaching and assessing EBM and related competencies. The ACGME (2005) also has developed a booklet to promote education in practice-based learning and improvement. The booklet includes a list of resources and examples for teaching and assessing this competency. The American Psychiatric Association also publishes a book providing overviews of the core competencies and how to teach them (Andrews and Burruss 2004).

Why Teach Evidence-Based Medicine and Evidence-Based Psychiatric Practice?

For more than a decade, teaching medical students and residents the fundamentals of clinical epidemiology and EBM has been viewed as a way of enabling them to keep up with the medical literature and of improving clinical care (Evidence-Based Medicine Working Group 1992; Sackett et al. 1991). More recently, however, it has become a required part of residency education in the United States. The ACGME introduced general competencies for residents that are to be included in the requirements for all specialties (Scheiber et al. 2003). The six general areas of core competencies are 1) patient care, 2) medical knowledge, 3) interpersonal and communications skills, 4) practice-based learning and improvement, 5) professionalism, and 6) systems-based practice. As seen in Table 15–1, the core competencies for practice-based learning and improvement for psychiatry are directly related to EBM and evidence-based psychiatric practice (EBPP). For instance, competency 4 states that "the physician shall demonstrate an ability to critically evaluate relevant medical literature," and competency 5 states that the physician shall demonstrate the ability to learn from

TABLE 15–1.   Psychiatry core competencies related to evidence-based medicine and evidence-based psychiatric practice

1. The physician shall recognize limitations in his or her own knowledge base and clinical skills and understand and address the need for lifelong learning.

2. The physician shall demonstrate appropriate skills for obtaining and evaluating up-to-date information from scientific and practice literature and other sources to assist in the quality care of patients. This shall include, but not be limited to, the following:

    Use of medical libraries

    Use of information technology, including Internet-based searches and literature databases (e.g., MEDLINE)

    Use of drug information databases

    Active participation, as appropriate, in educational courses, conferences, and other organized educational activities at both the local and the national levels

3. The physician shall evaluate caseload and practice experience in a systematic manner. This may include the following:

    Case-based learning

    Use of best practices through practice guidelines or clinical pathways

    Review of patient records and outcomes

    Obtaining evaluations from patients (e.g., outcomes and patient satisfaction)

    Obtaining appropriate supervision and consultation

    Maintaining a system for examining errors in practice and initiating improvements to eliminate or reduce errors

4. The physician shall demonstrate an ability to critically evaluate relevant medical literature. This ability may include the following:

    Use of knowledge of common methodologies employed in psychiatric and neurological research

    Researching and summarizing a particular problem that derives from the physician's caseload

5. The physician shall demonstrate the ability to do the following:

    Review and critically assess scientific literature to determine how quality of care can be improved in relation to practice (e.g., reliable and valid assessment techniques, treatment approaches with established effectiveness, practice parameter adherence). Within this aim, the physician shall be able to assess the generalizability or applicability of research findings to patients in relation to their sociodemographic and clinical characteristics.

    Develop and pursue effective remediation strategies that are based on critical review of scientific literature

    Learn from one's own and other specialties

Source.   Adapted from Scheiber et al. 2003.

one's practice, the subject of the previous chapter. In addition, one of the systems-based practice requirements is to be able to use practice guidelines.

What to Teach

The ACGME general competencies require that psychiatry residents become competent in using the EBM process to answer questions about therapies

and diagnostic tests. At a minimum, therefore, residents should be taught how to formulate a clinical question (Chapter 3); perform a literature search (Chapter 4); appraise clinical trials, systematic reviews, guidelines, and diagnostic tests (Chapters 5–7 and 9); and apply the results to their patients. A more complete course would include appraisal of articles on disease frequency (Chapter 10), etiology or harm (Chapter 11), and prognosis (Chapter 12) and learning how to apply these results to their practice (Chapter 13 and as illustrated in the cases in the remainder of this volume).

In providing this instruction, it is important to realize that most residents are not interested in clinical epidemiology or in learning some of the more advanced EBM skills (Guyatt et al. 2000). The goal instead should be to ensure that residents are able to find answers efficiently by using the preappraised information sources we described in Chapter 4 (Evans 2001; Guyatt et al. 2000) and to understand how to use measures, algorithms, guidelines, and similar resources in practice. However, at times, preappraised sources will not yield an answer, or it may be necessary to discuss the evidence in more detail with a colleague or patient. Under these circumstances, it is necessary to have the kind of deeper knowledge that is covered in an advanced course (Woodcock et al. 2002). Furthermore, a deeper understanding of EBM allows clinicians to better appraise the quality of guidelines developed by others and to better understand and incorporate the results from systematic reviews into clinical practice (Doust and Silagy 2000; Laupacis 2001).

One of the more important aspects of teaching EBM to psychiatry residents is teaching the philosophy of EBM and EBPP, not just the methodology. Residents often have some misconceptions about EBM (Bilsker and Goldner 1999; Padrino 2002). In addition to providing an overview of what EBM is and what it is not (see Taylor and Gray, Chapter 1 in this volume) and discussing some of the misconceptions about EBM (Straus and McAlister 2000), it may be helpful to distribute the humorous article by Isaacs and Fitzgerald (1999), in which they describe alternatives to EBM, such as *eminence-based medicine* ("experience is worth any amount of evidence"), *vehemence-based medicine* ("substitution of volume for evidence"), and *eloquence-based medicine*. This article is also helpful to residents in coping with situations in which the opinions of their supervisors are at odds with the evidence in the literature.

Methods of Teaching Evidence-Based Medicine and Evidence-Based Psychiatric Practice

The ACGME Outcome Project has a Web site that showcases examples of activities that may be used to

teach and assess the general competencies (www .acgme.org/outcome/implement/rsvp.asp). The descriptions are provided directly by the program or institution. The user is advised to communicate directly with the contact person listed for each project for further information. Most of the examples are not related to practice-based learning and do not directly address psychiatry or psychiatric competencies.

Seminars and Small-Group Sessions

Some material can best be introduced in seminars or in small-group sessions. In the University of Southern California program, the topics (e.g., critical appraisal of clinical trials) were presented to a small group in the form of a brief presentation and discussion. This was then followed by the critical appraisal of an article related to the topic under discussion (e.g., an article reporting the results of a randomized controlled trial). To do the appraisal, the residents were given a copy of the article along with a worksheet that incorporates the appropriate critical appraisal guidelines. After the residents had completed the worksheet, individual items on it were discussed. Although such sessions are useful for introducing a topic or method, they do not provide sufficient practice for the residents to become proficient; for this, other approaches are more useful.

Computer Laboratory and Library Sessions

The best way to become familiar with the various databases and how to use them is through hands-on practice, not by reading about them or through a lecture. Most medical schools have computer laboratories or library classrooms equipped with computers that can be used for demonstrations and hands-on practice in a group setting. Most medical libraries offer classes on searching MEDLINE and other databases, and librarians will often customize courses for the needs of particular users.

Evidence-Based Journal Clubs

Journal clubs, a staple of residency education programs, are the most common sites for teaching critical appraisal skills (Green 1999, 2000). Sackett et al. (2000) have described a novel approach to journal clubs—the evidence-based journal club—as a method for teaching the EBM process.

In an evidence-based journal club, the starting point is a clinical question suggested by one of the residents, preferably one that is based on an actual patient care issue. The group agrees on the 4-part PICO question (a question that uses the mnemonic aid "patient/problem, intervention, comparison, and outcome"), and a resident is assigned to conduct a literature search to find the best evidence to answer the question. The resident assigned to the task tries to find the evidence that is highest in the hierarchy (Table 4–1, Chapter 4). At the next journal club meeting, the resident distributes the article that was found, and the group as a whole uses a critical appraisal worksheet to evaluate the article. The question, search process, results, and applicability are then discussed.

The evidence-based journal club format has become popular in psychiatry training programs in the United Kingdom (Dhar 2001; Walker 2001; Warner and King 1997).

Rounds and Supervision

It is generally recommended that EBM not be taught in isolation but instead be incorporated in other clinical teaching activities (Dobbie et al. 2000; Green 1999, 2000; Sackett et al. 2000). In some institutions, this can be done through real-time literature searches during rounds or supervision, but on-line database access is still the exception in most hospital settings (Green 2000). Sackett et al. (2000) and the Evidence-Based Medicine Working Group (1992), for example, describe settings in which on-line searches can be conducted during rounds. Chapter 33 in this volume provides an example of EBM on a consultation-liaison service.

The Department of Psychiatry at Duke University has a model for providing the weekly Chairman's Rounds in an evidence-based format (http://psychiatry.mc.duke.edu/Residents/Quest.html).

The issues for teaching EBPP are more complicated than are those for teaching EBM, and few curricula exist on how to do this. Dr. Tan, who was supervised by the author, provides an example of how a resident-in-training can incorporate aspects of EBPP to develop a treatment plan, determine treatment strategies, and evaluate outcome (see Chapter 34).

Online Teaching Resources

A variety of Web sites provide useful information (such as curriculum guides and online syllabi) for the teaching of EBM (Table 15–2).

An Example of Teaching Evidence-Based Medicine on an Inpatient Service

Mascola (2008) described a curriculum integrated into an inpatient teaching service. The trainees are e-mailed a syllabus before the rotation that specifies the EBM objectives to be learned, practiced, and assessed during the 1-month rotation. The syllabus includes six brief discussion modules designed to teach residents how to apply the key elements of the EBM model in a busy clinical setting. EBM knowledge and skills are assessed before and after the rotation. In a pilot study, Mascola (2008) reported that the knowledge and skills increased significantly relative to baseline in a sample of 24 consecutive trainees who underwent the program. Chapter 33 illustrates how Mascola used EBM on a consultation-liaison service.

A Model Curriculum

The Duke University Department of Psychiatry identifies the teaching of EBM as one of its three primary missions. According to the Web site (www.psychres.duke.edu/residency/general.html):

> Interns begin with an EBM Start-Up course in July of their PGY-1 year, followed by intensive practice writing CATs or Critically Appraised Topics for presentation in our weekly Chairman's Rounds. Our chief residents receive training in how to teach EBM and meet with the presenting residents to guide him/her through the process of selecting a relevant clinical problem from their patient experience, forming a researchable question, searching the literature for the best evidence and appraising that evidence for its validity. Residents practice generating the most relevant summary statistic for the study's results and evaluating the applicability of the study to their patient. Residents receive additional practice writing CATs for other seminars and conferences throughout their training. And an EBM Review course for all residents runs year-round during our Academic Half-day....[R]esidents are challenged to practice these skills on the wards and in the clinic. EBM-trained attendings and supervisors apply an evidence-based approach to resident supervision, whether the topic is a medication or a psychosocial therapy question.

Aspects of this program are described in March et al. (2007). The grand rounds are presented as evidence-based summaries and reviews and posted online as noted earlier.

TABLE 15–2. Useful sites for teachers of evidence-based medicine

Organization	Address
Centre for Evidence-Based Medicine (Oxford)	http://www.cebm.net/index.asp
Centre for Evidence-Based Medicine (Toronto)	http://www.cebm.utoronto.ca/teach
Centre for Evidence-Based Mental Health	http://www.cebmh.com
Evidence-Based Medicine Resource Center	http://www.ebmny.org

Evaluating Evidence-Based Medicine Skills

Most evaluations of EBM have focused on critical appraisal skills of knowledge of EBM terminology and concepts, generally using multiple-choice examinations (Green 1999, 2000; Hatala and Guyatt 2002). Such approaches are subject to many criticisms, including the lack of validation of instruments and failure to assess the entire EBM process.

One promising approach for appraising a broader range of EBM skills is that of Smith et al. (2000), who developed a written test that focuses on four different skills: formulation of questions, literature searches, quantitative understanding, and appraisal of study quality and clinical relevance. Other authors have suggested the use of objective structured clinical examination–type stations to assess specific skills (Dobbie et al. 2000).

Evaluating whether residents are applying EBM skills in their day-to-day practices is as yet an unmet need. Such assessments generally have relied on self-reports, which may not be accurate (Green 1999, 2000). For example, Cabell et al. (2001) found that resident self-reports overestimated the actual use of online databases.

The ACGME Outcome Project (Accreditation Council for Graduate Medical Education 2001) provides several approaches to assessing practice-based learning and improvement competency. Included are self-administered diaries, portfolios, and instruments to assess opinions about EBM and information technology; and knowledge of EBM concepts and critical appraisal skills.

Evaluating Evidence-Based Medicine Teaching Programs

The Centre for Evidence-Based Medicine has a freely accessible Web site (www.cebm.utoronto.ca)

developed by the Department of Medicine at Toronto General Hospital. The goal of the Web site is "to help develop, disseminate, and evaluate resources that can be used to practise and teach EBM for undergraduate, postgraduate and continuing education for health care professionals from a variety of clinical disciplines." A self-evaluation toolkit that can be used by the teachers of EBM is available on the Web site. It suggests that EBM educators ask themselves questions such as the following:

- When did I last issue an educational prescription?
- Am I helping my trainees learn how to ask answerable questions?
- Am I teaching and modeling searching skills?
- Am I teaching and modeling critical appraisal skills?
- Am I teaching and modeling the generation of critically appraised topics?
- Am I teaching and modeling the integration of best evidence with my clinical expertise and my patients' preferences?
- Am I developing new ways of evaluating the effectiveness of my teaching?
- Am I developing new EBM educational material?
- Am I a member of an EBM-style journal club?
- Have I participated in or tutored at one of the workshops on how to practice or teach EBM?
- Have I joined the evidence-based health e-mail discussion group?
- Have I established links with other practitioners or teachers of EBM?

The ACGME Web site offers examples of assessment tools, as noted earlier.

Resident Views of Evidence-Based Medicine

Psychiatry residents often have some exposure to EBM as medical students, although this is not necessarily true for international medical graduates. Residents often have some ambivalence toward EBM, wondering if it ignores the humanistic side of psychiatric practice (Bilsker and Goldner 1999). However, as they develop a better understanding of EBM and the roles of clinical judgment and patient preference, coming to realize that EBM and patient-centered care are complementary, such concerns generally lessen (Bilsker and Goldner 1999; Hope 2002).

Some residents are intimidated by the quantitative emphasis of EBM (Bilsker and Goldner 1999). This generally can be overcome by setting realistic goals and by remembering that the focus should be on preparing users of evidence, not researchers (Guyatt et al. 2000; Sackett et al. 2000).

A barrier to teaching EBM and EBPP may be the negative opinions of some faculty members (Ball 1999; Evidence-Based Medicine Working Group 1992). Faculty development efforts may be needed to address the negative opinions (Bilsker and Goldner 1999; Evidence-Based Medicine Working Group 1992; Neale et al. 1999), although some residents are able to educate their supervisors about the concepts (Ball 1999).

Finally, it is important to emphasize that many residents find the practice of EBM to be empowering (Ball 1999; Padrino 2002). As Padrino (2002) said, "I feel more confident in my medical decisions when I can say 'the data show this' or 'the data show that.' Even when I have to say 'there are no data for this,' I feel my decision is more valid" (p. 13). Being able to incorporate the best evidence from the research literature into patient care decisions is what EBM is all about, and residents are quite capable of learning how to use evidence to improve their clinical decision making.

References

Accreditation Council for Graduate Medical Education: Practice-based learning and improvement: assessment approaches [ACGME Outcome Project Web site]. 2001. Available at: http://www.acgme.org/outcome/assess/PBLI_Index.asp. Accessed October 29, 2002

Accreditation Council for Graduate Medical Education: Advancing Education in Practice-Based Learning & Improvement: An Educational Resource From the ACGME Outcome Project. 2005. Available at: http://www.acgme.org/outcome/implement/complete_PBLI Booklet.pdf. Accessed June 28, 2009

Andrews LB, Burruss JW: Core Competencies for Psychiatric Education: Defining, Teaching, and Assessing Resident Competence. Washington, DC, American Psychiatric Publishing, 2004

Ball C: Evidence-based medicine on the wards: report from an evidence-based minion. Evid Based Med 3:101–103, 1999

Bilsker D, Goldner EM: Teaching evidence-based practice in mental health. Evid Based Ment Health 2:68–69, 1999

Cabell CH, Schardt C, Sanders L, et al: Resident utilization of information technology: a randomized trial of clinical question formation. J Gen Intern Med 16:838–844, 2001

Davies P: Teaching evidence-based health care, in Evidence-Based Practice: A Primer for Health Care Professionals. Edited by Dawes M, Davies P, Gray A, et al. New York, Churchill Livingstone, 1999, pp 223–242

Dhar R: Evidence-based journal clubs and the critical review paper: candidate's perspective. Psychiatr Bull 25:67–68, 2001

Dobbie AE, Schneider ED, Anderson AD, et al: What evidence supports teaching evidence-based medicine? Acad Med 75:1184–1185, 2000

Doust JA, Silagy CA: Applying the results of a systematic review in general practice. Med J Aust 172:153–156, 2000

Evans M: Creating knowledge management skills in primary care residents: a description of a new pathway to evidence-based practice. ACP J Club 135:A11–A12, 2001

Evidence-Based Medicine Working Group: Evidence-based medicine: a new approach to teaching the practice of medicine. JAMA 268:2420–2425, 1992

Gray JAM: Evidence-Based Healthcare: How to Make Health Policy and Management Decisions, 2nd Edition. New York, Churchill Livingstone, 2001

Green ML: Graduate medical education training in clinical epidemiology, critical appraisal, and evidence-based medicine: a critical review of curricula. Acad Med 74:686–694, 1999

Green ML: Evidence-based medicine training in graduate medical education: past, present, and future. J Eval Clin Pract 6:121–138, 2000

Guyatt GH, Meade MO, Jaeschke RZ, et al: Practitioners of evidence-based care. BMJ 320:954–955, 2000

Hatala R, Guyatt G: Evaluating the teaching of evidence-based medicine. JAMA 288:1110–1112, 2002

Hope T: Evidence-based patient choice and psychiatry. Evid Based Ment Health 5:100–101, 2002

Isaacs D, Fitzgerald D: Seven alternatives to evidence based medicine. BMJ 319:1618, 1999

Laupacis A: The future of evidence-based medicine. Can J Clin Pharmacol 8 (suppl A):6A–9A, 2001

March JS, Chrisman A, Breland-Noble A, et al: Using and teaching evidence-based medicine: the Duke University child and adolescent psychiatry model. Child Adolesc Psychiatr Clin N Am 14:273–296, viii–ix, 2005

March JS, Szatmari P, Bukstein O, et al: AACAP 2005 Research Forum: speeding the adoption of evidence-based practice in pediatric psychiatry. J Am Acad Child Adolesc Psychiatry 46:1098–1110, 2007

Mascola AJ: Guided mentorship in evidence-based medicine for psychiatry: a pilot cohort study supporting a promising method of real-time clinical instruction. Acad Psychiatry 32:475–483, 2008

Neale V, Roth LM, Schwartz KL: Faculty development using evidence-based medicine as an organizing curricular theme. Acad Med 74:611, 1999

Padrino S: Evidence-based psychiatry: fad or fundamental? Psychiatr News 37(16):13, 2002

Sackett DL, Haynes RB, Guyatt GH, et al: Clinical Epidemiology: A Basic Science for Clinical Medicine, 2nd Edition. Boston, MA, Little, Brown, 1991

Sackett DL, Straus SE, Richardson WS, et al: Evidence-Based Medicine: How to Practice and Teach EBM, 2nd Edition. New York, Churchill Livingstone, 2000

Scheiber JC, Kramer TAM, Adamowski SE: The implications of core competencies for psychiatric education and practice in the US. Can J Psychiatry 48:215–221, 2003

Smith CA, Ganschow PS, Reilly BM: Teaching residents evidence-based medicine skills: a controlled trial of effectiveness and assessment of durability. J Gen Intern Med 15:710–715, 2000

Straus SE, McAlister FA: Evidence-based medicine: a commentary on common criticisms. CMAJ 163:837–841, 2000

Walker N: Evidence-based journal clubs and the critical review paper. Psychiatr Bull 25:237, 2001

Warner JP, King M: Evidence-based medicine and the journal club: a cross-sectional survey of participants' views. Psychiatr Bull 21:532–534, 1997

Woodcock JD, Greenley S, Barton S: Doctors' knowledge about evidence-based medicine terminology. BMJ 324:929–930, 2002

II

Case Studies:
Evidence-Based Medicine
Applied to Major DSM-IV Disorders

Introduction to the Cases

C. Barr Taylor, M.D.

The cases presented in the remainder of this volume are designed to illustrate the principles and practices of evidence-based psychiatric practice (EBPP). As discussed in Chapter 1, EBPP is based on the following:

1. Accurate evaluation and treatment planning
2. Consideration of treatment algorithms, guidelines, and best practices when planning and providing treatment
3. Use of measures to determine progress of an individual patient
4. Review of a patient's progress against personal and published standards
5. Consideration of "evidence and experts" in clinical decisions
6. Expertise in providing a range of therapies or in making them available through other resources or providers

In addition to improving patient care, EBPP is a method of achieving practice-based learning and improvement, one of the core competencies now expected of all graduating residents. Having directed a residency training program for over a decade, I have found that this is one of the more difficult competencies for faculty to teach and practitioners to enact. I began this project in part to find better ways to teach residents how to learn from patients and improve their care and found that it helped improve my own practice. These cases are presented to illustrate how I and others have used EBPP in our practice.

I asked each of the authors to follow a general outline as follows:

Setting. Provide a brief description of your practice setting, patient population/focus, and treatment orientation/philosophy.

Illustration. List several applications of expert/evidence-based psychiatry that will be illustrated.

Chief complaint. Use present tense for statement of the chief complaint.

Present illness. The case should be "real" but, for ethical reasons, the identity of the individuals should be changed so that they cannot be identified by others (e.g., change age, sex, occupation, personal details). While real data are ideal, it may be necessary to combine data from patients. Keep it brief.

Other significant findings from assessment. Present only relevant findings (including negative ones if they are pertinent). Keep it brief.

Differential diagnosis (if appropriate).

DSM-IV-TR assessment.

Treatment plan considerations. Identify the main and secondary problems and issues. As appropriate for your practice and the patient, describe the guidelines, algorithms, measures, or other sources of EBPP you used.

Treatment goals, measures, and methods. Include a time frame for measurement/improvement, preferably as a table.

Course. Provide a brief discussion of the course. An important aspect of these cases is to let the reader into how you were thinking about the problem over the course of therapy. If you deviated from expert practices, why? How did you use the manual, self-help materials, brochures, and other sources, if at all? How did you consider problems that emerged and were not covered by guidelines and algorithms? How did you coordinate care if you referred to other practitioners (e.g., for marital therapy or substance abuse treatment)? Were there issues you researched using EBM [evidence-based medicine] methods?

Figure/graph/table of improvement (if appropriate and available).

Summary (including use of guidelines/algorithms, other issues).

Ways to improve practice. What did you learn from this case (if anything) that might help you improve your practice?

One challenge of writing about real clinical cases, as mentioned earlier, is the need to protect the privacy of the individuals being discussed. For this reason, I have asked the authors to change the age, sex, job, revealing personal details, and, even when it was not essential, the history of the patient and the course of treatment.

Another challenge is to make the case "come alive." In my practice I usually cover the core of the American Psychiatric Association (2002) practice guidelines baseline assessment and obtain a detailed history and mental status. However, in my cases, I present only information relevant to the case or illustrative of the issues addressed. I asked the other authors to do the same. I also do not discuss general therapy issues and techniques, the focus of much of

my work with patients, and I didn't expect the other authors to. To do so would make the cases very long and cover material familiar to most clinicians.

When I first began working on this book, my initial idea was to write up a dozen or so illustrative cases taken from my own practice. In the end, I decided to restrict the cases I present to anxiety, eating, and affective disorders and comorbidities, the most common problems presenting in my clinic, and to invite specialists in other areas to prepare evidence-based case reports around problems they routinely address so that examples of evidence-based treatment would be available for many of the major DSM-IV-TR (American Psychiatric Association 2000) disorders where guidelines are available. I also felt it was important to provide examples of EBPP in a variety of different treatment settings.

The cases address a number of ways to undertake EBPP. Table 16–1 presents an overview of the case diagnoses, the guidelines/algorithms followed, and the outcome measures. I encouraged the authors to present real cases, including those where the outcome was not as expected. In such cases, I also asked the authors to consider what they might have done differently, if anything. The cases are meant to be illustrative of how to treat the cases presented. I suspect the readers will have their own views as to how they might have approached the cases in different and perhaps better ways.

References

American Psychiatric Association: Diagnostic and Statistical Manual of Mental Disorders, 4th Edition, Text Revision. Washington, DC, American Psychiatric Association, 2000

American Psychiatric Association: Practice Guidelines for the Treatment of Psychiatric Disorders, Compendium. Washington, DC, American Psychiatric Association, 2006

TABLE 16–1. Case authors, disorders, guidelines/algorithms, and outcome measures

Chapter	Authors	Disorder(s)/Issues	Guidelines/Algorithms	Outcome measures
17	Taylor	Panic disorder	NICE—anxiety disorders	QIDS-SR$_{16}$ Self-report: panic attack frequency, dizziness, depression (severity)
18	Taylor	MDD Bulimia Relationship issues	APA—depression, STAR*D NICE—eating disorders	QIDS-SR$_{16}$ Self-report: bulimic episodes, relationship issues (satisfaction), depression
19	Taylor	MDE Weight loss/ food refusal Relationship issues	APA—depression	QIDS-SR$_{16}$ Weight Self-report: difficulty swallowing, depression
20	Taylor	Anorexia OCD Depression Psychosis NOS	APA—anorexia APA—OCD	QIDS-SR$_{16}$, Weight Obsessions (frequency/severity) BPRS Depression
21	Trivedi & Kurian	MDD	STAR*D	QIDS-C$_{16}$ FIBSER
22	Rothschild	MDD	APA—MDD	BPRS DAS Ham-D Stress, self-report
23	Wang & Ketter	Bipolar II	TIMA	Bipolarity Index, self-report: mood and elation
24	Das & Koran	OCD MDD	APA—OCD	Y-BOCS Ham-D
25	Rait & Glick	Schizophrenia	APA—schizophrenia (section on family therapy)	Global functioning Global relationship functioning
26	Lembke & Humphreys	Substance abuse	VHA-DoD—substance use disorders	Abstinence
27	Reich	Personality disorders	APA—borderline personality disorder APA—OCD WFSBP—personality disorders	Self-report: personality disorder symptoms
28	Marino & Mitchell	Bulimia	APA—bulimia	Binge/purge frequency

TABLE 16–1. Case authors, disorders, guidelines/algorithms, and outcome measures

Chapter	Authors	Disorder(s)/Issues	Guidelines/Algorithms	Outcome measures
29	Lindner & Lindley	PTSD Substance abuse	VHA-DoD—PTSD	PTSD Checklist Alcohol abstinence Hours of sleep Housed Employed
30	Tannenbaum & Spiranovic	Depression Panic disorder	APA—depression APA—panic disorder RANZCP—depression NICE—depression	Depression Severity Questionnaire Quality of Life Side Effects Scale
31	May & Reynolds-May	Postpartum depression	ACOG Various others	Relationship satisfaction
32	Shanteau	Bipolar I	TMAP	PHQ-9 Self-report
33	Mascola	Dementia, delirium, or depression	Various evidence-based practices on a C-L service	Structured clinical interview
34	Tan	Alcohol abuse, depression	APA—substance use disorders	Alcohol use, alcohol craving, depression

Note. ACOG=American College of Obstetricians and Gynecologists; APA=American Psychiatric Association; BPRS=Brief Psychiatric Rating Scale; C-L=consultation-liaison; DAS=Delusional Assessment Scale; FIBSER=Frequency, Intensity, and Burden of Side Effects Rating; Ham-D=Hamilton Rating Scale for Depression; MDD=major depressive disorder; MDE=major depressive episode; NICE=National Institute for Health and Clinical Excellence; NOS=not otherwise specified; OCD=obsessive-compulsive disorder; PHQ-9=Patient Health Questionnaire (nine questions); PTSD=posttraumatic stress disorder; QIDS-C$_{16}$=Quick Inventory of Depressive Symptomatology–Clinician Rating; QIDS-SR$_{16}$=Quick Inventory of Depressive Symptomatology–Self-Report; RANZCP=Royal Australian and New Zealand College of Psychiatrists; STAR*D=Sequenced Treatment Alternatives to Relieve Depression; TIMA=Texas Implementation of Medication Algorithms; VHA-DoD=Veterans Health Administration, Department of Defense; WFSBP=World Federation of Societies of Biological Psychiatry; Y-BOCS=Yale-Brown Obsessive Compulsive Scale.

Panic Disorder

C. Barr Taylor, M.D.

Introduction

General Therapeutic Approach

I am an "eclectic psychiatrist," expert in a number of types of therapy but with a bias toward more empirically derived approaches. In general, I prefer to consider a set of techniques that may be helpful for a particular patient rather than to rigidly follow any specific school or approach. I usually provide both psychotherapy and psychopharmacology.

I generally see patients for 50 minutes. I begin my session with a review of how the patient has being doing since the last visit, noting any important events and issues. If the patient has completed the presession assessment in the waiting room, I quickly go over it; otherwise, I review salient aspects (such as depression and/or anxiety and target symptoms or behaviors), medication (side effects, adherence, change in other medications), and homework (if assigned). I then set an agenda, beginning with therapeutic issues related to the most pressing issues raised by the patient, but ensure that I also have time for teaching and practicing new therapeutic strategies, establishing goals and assignments, and setting up a new appointment. I look for indications that the therapeutic alliance is strong. At times the patient may be in crisis, and I drop this agenda to spend as much time as needed to deal with urgent issues or other therapeutic issues that may arise.

Charting Patient Progress

In preparing cases for this book, I decided to keep graphs or charts of the patient's progress and to combine three types of measurements:

1. *Simple scales of depression and anxiety.* As appropriate, I ask the patient, if he or she has not completed the form in the waiting room: "In the past week, what was your average level of depression, where 0=none/no symptoms to 10=severe?" I use the same question adapted for anxiety. (If you use this system it is important to "anchor" the points by asking the patient what his or her point of reference is in rating anxiety or depression as moderate or severe.) I also ask the patient what his or her maximum anxiety or depression was in the past week if appropriate, but I don't graph the data.

2. *Standard measures.* If the patient's problems are appropriate for the Sequenced Treatment Alternatives to Relieve Depression (STAR*D) algorithm, I have the patient complete, or I complete with the patient, the Quick Inventory of Depressive Symptomatology–Self-Report (QIDS-SR$_{16}$) every 6 weeks or so. I may add another standard measure to assess a problem, such as the Yale-Brown Obsessive Compulsive Scale for obsessive-compulsive disorder.

3. *Measures of target symptoms/problems.* I use one or two other measures targeted specifically to the patient's problems. I may monitor the frequency of a symptom, asking the patient, "In the last week, how often did you experience this?" and have the patient rate it as "never," "almost never," "a few times a week," or "a few times a day." I may also plot actual frequencies of behaviors or symptoms, such as panic attacks or binges. Or I may monitor the severity of a symptom by asking, "On average, how severe (bothersome) was the symptom over the past week?"

I have the patient rate it from 0=not bad at all to 10=severe. Working with the patient, I may develop some other simple measure to reflect the patient's progress toward his or her goals. For instance, if I am dealing with a patient with social phobia who wants to date more, I may decide to use a general measure of how comfortable he feels in dating. I may also use a measure that focuses on satisfaction, for instance, "How satisfied are you with your relationships with women you date?" The data will give me, and the patient, an idea of how he is doing and help determine if I need to change treatment strategies, for example, if the patient is not adequately improving relative to his or my expectation of what progress would be appropriate at that point in therapy. I provide examples of all these types of measures collected over time in the following cases.

There are many challenges in collecting such data, and I believe we should use the data we collect. One challenge is to relate the patient's visit number to the week he or she has been in therapy. To make it easier, I attach a simple chart to the front of the case that looks like this:

Visit	Date	Week
1	09/07/06	0 (baseline)
2	09/13/06	1
3	10/05/06	6
4	10/18/06	13
(etc.)		

The chart allows me to plot the data, by visit, in real time. I usually share the information on the chart with the patient. Doing so allows me to review the patient's goals and keeps me focused on helping the patient achieve progress.

In truth, keeping up even this simple data system is a bit of a nuisance. Patients may resent filling out the forms or find them repetitive or unnecessary, a session may run over, or I may have limited time between sessions or other more urgent issues to attend to. My first priority in charting is to complete the clinical note; the graph is optional. However, it is rarely necessary to keep data at each patient session.

Guidelines

Having been trying to focus on evidence-based psychiatric practice for the past several years, I thought I was familiar with the guidelines. However, in formally reviewing my cases against guidelines, I find that I sometimes deviate more than I should. I felt

the reader would benefit from my discussion about these deviations. I decided to turn the guidelines into checklists and then to examine my practice against the guideline as a standard. I used this review as one source for evaluating how I could do a better job with a similar patient in the future.

When patients are not improving as I would expect them to based on my experience or some other source of information, I ask myself: Is my diagnosis/assessment correct? Are my therapeutic choices appropriate and/or being applied (e.g., are there adherence or implementation problems)? Are there problems in the therapeutic relationship? Searches applying methods of evidence-based medicine can be useful to help me determine if I have missed some useful information or approach that might aid the patient.

Setting

I practice in a general outpatient clinic in a private university medical center department of psychiatry. The clinic serves mostly insurance patients. I have set up my office so that my computer is to my left and my patients sit to my right in a chair at the corner of my desk.

Illustration

This study illustrates:

- Application of guidelines to a single disorder
- Use of manualized treatments/self-help
- Monitoring of symptoms
- Dealing with relapse

Chief Complaint

Mr. C.W. is a 32-year-old male engineer who presents with a chief complaint of panic attacks.

Present Illness

Mr. C.W. said that his problems had begun about 3 months prior to presentation when he was driving to work and crossing over a bridge. He experienced a sudden, intense feeling of panic that was accompanied by a sharp pain in the back of his head and a rapid heart rate. He drove himself to an emergency room (ER) where he received medical tests and "no abnormalities" were found. A week later he had another attack when he was again driving to work.

He returned to the ER and received a CT scan, chest X ray, ECG, and other tests, which all yielded "normal" results. He began to find it impossible to cross over the bridge on the way to work without being accompanied by a friend, and he started to avoid work altogether, even though he had not had another panic attack. He also began to experience severe dizziness nearly constantly. He went to his internist, who told him he had anxiety and prescribed citalopram, starting at 10 mg/day, and clonazepam 0.5 mg prn. On the day after the patient took the citalopram he became "severely" depressed, felt like crying, and had suicidal thoughts. He stopped the citalopram on his own but stayed on the clonazepam. He continued to be driven to work by a friend and had a number of episodes when he felt his heart was beating fast on his way to work even when not on a bridge. He then self-referred to the psychiatry outpatient clinic, where I first saw him.

The patient had been keeping detailed notes since the first event. For instance, his notes from one day were as follows:

- 6:45 A.M. heart beating fast
- 7:30 A.M. anxiety, dizzy
- 8:00 A.M. at work, dizzy
- 12:00 P.M. weak and faint
- 1:00 P.M. weak and faint
- 7:00 P.M. feel better, dizzy

When asked what he thought was causing the problem, he suggested, "Work stress, maybe chemicals at work, or maybe I have a brain tumor."

Other Significant Findings From Assessment

The patient exercised one to two times per week (jogging for about 40 minutes on Saturday and Sunday). He was happy with his diet and weight. He reported being isolated, although he socialized with people at work on Friday nights and sometimes on the weekend. He considered himself to be an agnostic. He denied smoking, drinking, or taking any over-the-counter or herbal or other nonprescribed products or medicines. He avoided any foods or drinks with caffeine. There were no medical problems contributing to onset of panic attacks. He reported moderate and increasing stress at work, with long hours. His STAR*D QID-SR$_{16}$ score=8 (low to

moderate depression; see Chapter 21). On his baseline form, he rated his average level of depression over the past week as being about a 3 (moderate, on a scale of 0=no symptoms and 10=severe symptoms) and his maximum depression about the same. He rated his average anxiety as being 5/10 with his maximum as 8/10. He said he experienced panic a few times a week. He rated his dizziness as a 6/10.

DSM-IV-TR Diagnosis

Axis I   Panic disorder with agoraphobia
Axis II   None
Axis III   None (cause of dizziness was not clear)
Axis IV   Work stress; social isolation
Axis V   Global Assessment of Functioning (GAF) score: 50

Treatment Plan Considerations

Panic Attacks/Avoidance

On first assessment Mr. C.W. seemed to present a fairly straightforward case of panic disorder with agoraphobia and secondary depression. He was having about two to three "panic episodes" every week although these were rarely full-blown panic attacks, perhaps because of his avoidance and use of benzodiazepines.

Selecting a Guideline

Having reviewed both the American Psychiatric Association (APA) and National Institute for Health and Clinical Excellence (NICE) guidelines (and others) for an article for *BMJ* (Taylor 2006), I ended up preferring the NICE guideline, which was most consistent with my own practice and publications. I provide the guideline at the end of the case and review where I adhered to or deviated from the guideline (www.nice.org.uk/Guidance/CG22).

Given that the guideline lists cognitive-behavioral therapy (CBT) as the therapy of first choice, the first major therapeutic decision for the patient was to determine if medications were appropriate for this case and, if so, which medications to use. CBT would certainly be appropriate in the long run, but would it be sufficient to deal with the patient's distress? The patient was quite impaired (GAF=50), requiring a friend to drive him to work and feeling miserable most of the day. He also had a number of depressive symptoms (feelings of sadness, fatigue, being slowed down, and thoughts that life is empty or not worth living). I felt he would benefit from an adequate trial of antidepressant both for the panic and for the depressive symptoms. The patient also was reluctant to use only CBT, and his job required some flexibility as to when I could schedule sessions. The guideline does not suggest that CBT be used in lieu of medication but suggests that CBT should be used first.

Having decided to use a medication, should I choose a selective serotonin reuptake inhibitor (SSRI) other than citalopram or start on another type of antidepressant? The patient had become very depressed on the citalopram when he first tried it. (I made a mental note to see what I could find out about using another SSRI when a patient had a "depressive reaction.") The patient would not try citalopram again, even at half the dose, so I decided to start him on sertraline at a very low dose (a quarter of a 25 mg tablet for 3 days followed by half a tablet for 3 days). The patient was told to stop the medication if he felt worse.

From the NICE guideline perspective, the use of the clonazepam was problematic. The guideline states that benzodiazepines are not to be used, on the basis that "outcome studies argue that patients given benzodiazepines do worse over time." The guideline would imply that I should stop the clonazepam that the patient was already on. I *assumed* that a combination of antidepressant medication and CBT would reduce panic, depression, and avoidance and that the benzodiazepines would be stopped. However, the patient said that the clonazepam had been helpful. The patient might feel worse if it was stopped, and stopping it might be associated with some rebound or withdrawal effects. I decided to continue it for another week. I told the patient that I would consider stopping it or cutting down at the next visit.

Dizziness

Dizziness is a common symptom of patients with panic, which may represent some underlying disturbance in the vestibular system (Tecer et al. 2004) and can be related to hyperventilation or occur from other, unknown reasons. Dizziness can also represent a number of medical problems. The patient's medical evaluation had focused on his cardiovascular but not ear, nose, and throat (ENT) system. His interpretation of the symptom was that he might have a brain tumor, and if not that, some other seri-

ous medical problem. Should I recommend further medical evaluation? The patient felt that his worst symptom was the one that seemed to interfere the most with his work and that it served as a major cue for his feeling like something was seriously wrong. I weighed the advantages and need of further medical workup against the effect that such a workup could have on reinforcing his sense that he had a "medical problem." An important aspect of care, and implied in the guideline, is the need to help patients understand how their symptoms might have a psychological rather than medical origin. I also assumed that treatment of the panic would result in reduction in dizziness. The dizziness would be used as part of in vitro exposure therapy and in helping the patient learn new breathing techniques. I decided not to make a referral at this time but to follow up if the dizziness did not diminish as expected.

Onset/Stressors

As is often the case, the reason for the onset of the panic was not clear. Stress at work appeared to be a contributing factor, although the patient had had many times at work when he felt under intense stress without feeling panicky. There were no other obvious lifestyle habits (such as caffeine use, cessation of smoking, drug use) or medical precipitants. I wondered if stress management might be useful at some point, but the patient was not interested. The guideline does not recommend stress management for treating panic, but there appeared to be another reason to offer it, that is, for reducing stress and improving coping.

Avoidance

The patient had developed significant avoidance that could eventually cost him his job. I was confident that exposure therapy would reduce his avoidance. I considered this to be my number one goal (the patient was more concerned about his dizziness.) As suggested in the guideline, "massed" exposure, that is, intensive exposure over a short time, can be used and appears as effective as more prolonged exposure. (The focus would be on driving and crossing bridges.) My schedule does not permit providing massed exposure and it is not available in the community, so I decided against using this potentially rapid treatment of his avoidance. I also felt it was important to first develop a relationship with the patient, to help reduce the dizziness, at which point he might be open to more demanding interventions such as exposure therapy.

Interpersonal Isolation

The patient reported that he had a lot of friends but no close relationships. He said that he had thought about getting married and at one point was engaged, but his then-girlfriend had moved from the area and he didn't pursue the relationship. He spent weekends running in the mountains with a group of other runners. He would sometimes go to a bar with his coworkers but otherwise spent most of his time at home. I felt that his social isolation was an important aspect of his life that should be addressed; however, he was not interested in addressing it, at least initially.

With these considerations, I discussed an initial treatment plan and approach with the patient. I mentioned that I would periodically monitor how he was doing, but I didn't give him the same time frame of improvement reflected in Table 17–1; I only mentioned that he should be feeling better in a few weeks. He agreed to my initial treatment plan as follows: I prescribed 1) sertraline one-quarter tablet for 3 days, then half a tablet, explaining the side effects and telling him to call me if his mood got worse and to stop the medications; and 2) use of a relaxation tape three times a week. I scheduled a visit in 1 week.

Course

Visit 2 (Week 2)

The patient said that he was feeling less anxious and had not had a full-blown panic attack although he had a few episodes of feeling panicky. His mood had improved slightly. He kept records of how he was feeling and brought them in for review. He practiced relaxation as prescribed. He was still avoiding going to work. I asked him to decrease his clonazepam, I increased his sertraline to 25 mg, and I asked him to continue use of his relaxation tape. Much of the session was spent in discussing the nature of panic, as per CBT (Barlow and Craske 2006). I printed out and gave him the National Institute of Mental Health information handout on panic disorder. I considered using a structured treatment program (e.g., Barlow and Craske 2006, which we keep on hand and sell to patients at cost), but I didn't feel it was necessary because the patient was already self-

monitoring and I could provide the treatment. I also did in vivo exposure for dizziness and taught him breathing exercises (per Craske and Barlow 2006).

Visit 3 (Week 3)

The patient reported depression, dizziness, and panic similar to the previous week. I continued to provide CBT/psychoeducation and increased sertraline to 50 mg. I continued in vivo exposure and prescribed relaxation training and breathing practice. The in vivo exposure followed Craske and Barlow (2006) and included spinning in his chair while monitoring symptoms, feelings, and cognitions. I also began graduated in vitro exposure focusing on driving and crossing bridges.

Visit 4 (Week 5)

The patient felt depressed on increased sertraline. The patient called the on-duty resident, who recommended that he decrease sertraline to 25 mg and restart clonazepam, which he did. The patient was feeling better and maintained sertraline at 25 mg and clonazepam 0.25 mg prn. I decided to begin bupropion (25 mg) because I felt the patient continued to have depressive symptoms and I was reluctant to go up on the sertraline. If I followed the NICE guidelines, I should have considered imipramine or clomipramine as the next choice and even stopped sertraline. Why did I deviate? I was worried about anticholinergic side effects from tricyclics in a patient with very high somatic concerns. I was also concerned about risk of an overdose and I wanted to use a drug with different pharmacological action. However, there is only anecdotal evidence of the use of bupropion and panic, and it would be an off-label use (Simon et al. 2003).

Visit 5 (Week 7)

The patient said that he felt close to normal. No panic or anxiety, and he was now driving to work on his own. We set a goal of his flying back East to visit his family.

Visit 6 (Week 10)

The patient said he continued to feel some anxiety in the morning (mainly muscle tension). He felt a little more panicky when driving over the bridge but had no panic attacks, and he was not feeling depressed. We reviewed his "exposure work" (assignments to

TABLE 17–1.   Initial treatment goals, measures, and methods

Treatment goal	Measure	Method
Reduce panic attack frequency to 0 within 2 months	Self-report of weekly panic attacks	Pharmacotherapy Psychoeducation/cognitive-behavioral therapy
Reduce dizziness from 10 to 3 within 3 months	Self-report: 10=as bad as it gets, 0=no dizziness	Pharmacotherapy Cognitive-behavioral therapy with emphasis on in vitro exposure, breathing training, and relaxation
Reduce depression by 50% or more, by 8 weeks	QIDS-SR$_{16}$	Pharmacotherapy
Reduce avoidance, return to driving to work within 2 months	Self-report	Exposure therapy would be a key part of the cognitive-behavioral therapy
Reduce stress at work	Self-report	Deferred, per patient preference

Note.   QIDS-SR$_{16}$=Quick Inventory of Depressive Symptomatology–Self-Report.

drive to work, cross bridges, etc.) in terms of feelings/symptoms, behaviors, and cognitions.

Visit 7 (Week 15)

The patient continued to do well with no depression, minimal anxiety, and no avoidance. He continued to drive to work. He had bought a ticket to go back East but was worried about having a panic attack on the plane. I gave him instructions on breathing and suggested he could use clonazepam if he was experiencing significant anxiety before the flight. I asked if he wanted to address the issue of dating, and he agreed but seemed ambivalent and did not want to set any goals related to dating at this time.

Visit 8 (Week 18)

The patient continued to do well with minimal anxiety, depression, and no panic. He decided he did not want to work on dating or on stress issues at work. We discussed moving into maintenance/relapse prevention after the next session.

Visit 9 (Week 22)

The patient continued to do well. We discussed relapse prevention techniques and scheduled a follow-up visit to review medication use.

Visit 10 (Week 38)

This was the maintenance visit. The patient continued to do well with no panic, depression, or anxiety. He wanted to stop medications. I explained that the guideline recommends that he continue medication

for 6 months after he has been symptom free and explained the rationale. He was willing to continue for another 3 months. He was informed of how to stop the medications and alerted to discontinuation effects.

Relapse

About 9 months after the last visit, the patient called to say that he had had another panic attack out of the blue. He said that about 3 months after his last visit he stopped the bupropion, and because he continued to feel very good, he also stopped the sertraline. About 1 week prior to his call, he had another panic attack and decided to restart the sertraline and clonazepam on his own. One day after restarting the medication he became depressed and frightened. He was worried that he would fall right back into his old patterns. I scheduled a visit within the next week, suggested he continue the sertraline but at a lower dose, and invited him to call me if he felt worse. I reminded him of the importance of his breathing exercises, which he had stopped. At our session a week later, he reported having had no panic attacks and his mood was much improved (3/10; maximum dysphoria 4/10). Surprisingly, he had no dizziness. He was not doing his breathing or relaxation but was not avoiding. I suggested he continue the sertraline but decrease the clonazepam. In this instance, the onset seemed to be related to a significant increase in his workload and the feeling that he was falling behind and not doing a good job. However, he did not want to discuss these issues in detail. Based on his relapse, longer-term use of the medication (at least another year) seemed advisable. For the panic,

How often did you experience panic attacks/episodes in the past week?
(1=none, 2=once, 3=a few times a week, 4=a few times a day)

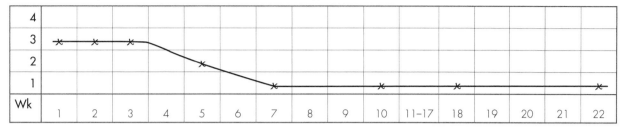

FIGURE 17–1. Panic attacks/episodes.

In the past week, what was your average level of depression or dizziness? (0=none/no symptoms to 10=severe)

FIGURE 17–2. Depression (X–X) and dizziness (O–O) trends.

stress reduction/coping skills might have reduced his stress at work.

Figures 17–1 and 17–2 show the patient's progress over the first 22 weeks of therapy.

Summary of Guideline Use

Table 17–2 summarizes the guidelines applied to this patient and whether or not the guideline was followed. Although an SSRI was used as the first medication of choice, the actual practice was more complicated because the patient had had an adverse reaction to the first drug prescribed in that class and a second SSRI was started at a unusually small dose.

Benzodiazepines were prescribed by the patient's internist and were continued for several weeks, which would seem to go against the spirit of the guideline. The guideline stresses that "CBT should be delivered only by suitably trained and supervised people who can demonstrate that they adhere closely to empirically grounded treatment protocols." Treatment protocols are available for panic disorder (and many other problems), for instance, through the Treatments That Work series (www.oup.com/us/catalog/general/series/TreatmentsThatWork/?view=usa).[1] Since I have extensive experience in treating panic, it didn't seem necessary to strictly follow such a protocol. The guideline also expects CBT to be com-

---

[1] The author is an unpaid member of the Treatments That Work Scientific Advisory Board.

TABLE 17–2.   NICE guideline recommendations for panic disorder

Area	Recommendation	Followed
Shared decision making	Include review and benefit of therapies, alternative therapies	√
Patient education	Provide information on nature, course, and treatment, including medication use and side effects	√
	Use everyday, jargon-free language	√
Medication	*Step 1:* SSRIs are medications of first choice	√
	Step 2: If an SSRI is not suitable or there is no improvement after a 12-week course and if a further medication is appropriate, imipramine or clomipramine	No, we preferred bupropion
	Benzodiazepines are not to be used	No, patient was already on benzodiazepines
	Sedating antihistamines or antipsychotics should not be used	NA
	Consider medication in terms of age, previous treatment response, risk, likelihood of overdose/self-harm, tolerability, patient preference, cost (where equal effectiveness is demonstrated)	√
	Doses at the upper end of the indicated dose range may be necessary and should be offered if needed	NA
	Long-term treatment may be necessary for some people and should be offered if needed	NA
	If the patient is showing improvement on treatment with an antidepressant, the medication should be continued for at least 6 months after optimal dose, then the dose can be tapered	√
	Patient should be advised to take medication as prescribed, discontinuation/withdrawal symptoms should be discussed	√
Psychotherapy	CBT is therapy of first choice	√
	Adherence to CBT treatment guidelines	No, adapted to patient needs
	7–14 hours over 12–16 weeks or brief CBT (6–8 hours) with self-help	9 hours over 22 weeks without self-help
	Intensive "massed exposure"	Not available
	Relapse prevention	√
Self-help	Bibliotherapy based on CBT should be offered	√, NIMH sheet given
Support groups	Information on support groups should be offered	Not needed
Exercise	The benefits of exercise should be discussed	Already exercising
Monitoring	Short self-report questionnaires can be used	I used Likert-like scales
	Use psychometrically sound measures as appropriate	
	Baseline assessment	√
	Process assessments	√
	12-week review	Done at 10 weeks

Note. CBT=cognitive-behavioral therapy; NA=not applicable to patient; NICE=National Institute for Health and Clinical Excellence; NIMH=National Institute of Mental Health; SSRI=selective serotonin reuptake inhibitor.
Source.   Adapted from www.nice.org.uk/Guidance/CG22 for panic disorder.

pleted in 4 months, although this was not possible with the patient's schedule.

I find that keeping track of the patient's progress is the most useful aspect of the guideline. Medication algorithms are designed so that failure to improve by a certain period leads to other medication choices. This is not the case with psychotherapy, where failure to improve leads to another set of recommendations. I would expect a patient with uncomplicated panic to have significantly improved by six sessions (Kenardy et al. 2003; Taylor 2006). If the patient had not improved, I would ask myself, as noted in the introduction: 1) Is this the right therapy? 2) Is the therapy being followed (e.g., am I doing the CBT properly, is the patient taking the medication?) or 3) Am I missing something? (e.g., wrong diagnosis, a medical problem, secondary gain, the patient's dissatisfaction with me or the therapy). In this case, the patient had improved as expected.

Ways to Improve Practice

In reviewing the guideline and my practice, I identified some areas where I could improve and some questions where I would like more information. I could improve by ensuring that self-help manuals are available when needed (e.g., order a supply in advance, sign up for a supplementary program). Although I am confident in my ability to provide CBT, a manual helps to ensure that the patient is provided the core information. I might have focused more attention on how the patient might cope or avoid relapse.

References

Barlow DH, Craske HG: Mastery of Your Anxiety and Panic: Workbook (Treatments That Work). New York, Oxford University Press, 2006

Craske HG, Barlow DH: Mastery of Your Anxiety and Panic: Therapist Guide (Treatments That Work). New York, Oxford University Press, 2006

Kenardy JA, Dow MGT, Johnston DW, et al: A comparison of delivery methods of cognitive-behavioral therapy for panic disorder: an international multicentre trial. J Consult Clin Psychol 71:1068–1075, 2003

Simon NM, Emmanuel N, Ballenger J, et al: Bupropion sustained release for panic disorder. Psychopharmacol Bull 37(4):66–72, 2003

Taylor CB: Panic disorder. BMJ 332:951–955, 2006

Tecer A, Tükel R, Erdamar B, et al: Audiovestibular functioning in patients with panic disorder. J Psychosom Res 57:177–182, 2004

Major Depressive Disorder and Bulimia Nervosa

C. Barr Taylor, M.D.

Introduction and Setting

See Chapter 17.

Illustration

This study illustrates:

- Use of American Psychiatric Association (APA) major depressive disorder guidelines
- Use of Sequenced Treatment Alternatives to Relieve Depression (STAR*D) guidelines
- Reconciliation of National Institute for Health and Clinical Excellence (NICE) guidelines for bulimia nervosa with APA guidelines for major depressive disorder
- Use of self-help materials
- Stepped care for bulimia; marginal outcome

Chief Complaint

Ms. S.W. is a 24-year-old female Hispanic law student who presents with a chief complaint of depression and frequent vomiting.

Present Illness

Ms. S.W. said that she had been very depressed for the last 3 months following a breakup with her boyfriend. She said that her relationship with her boyfriend had been on and off again for a number of years but after their last breakup he began dating another woman. For the past 2 months she had felt sad

nearly every day and had a loss of interest in her usual activities, fatigue, feelings of worthlessness, and trouble concentrating but no change in weight or sleep. She denied thoughts of suicide. Her symptoms had begun to interfere with her being able to concentrate on her class work. She denied any previous episodes of depression. She had seen a therapist about 3 years ago, when she was in college, around issues of her breaking up with another boyfriend.

She reported bingeing two or three times a day with at least one episode followed by vomiting. She said this habit had been going on for about 4 years and that it was her way of controlling her weight. (Her weight, body mass index = 21, was well within the normal range and had not changed since she was an adolescent.) Typically she would overeat or binge at lunch or dinner and then vomit an hour or so after the meal. She would occasionally binge and purge at night as well. When she wasn't able to vomit, for instance, because she was at an after-dinner party in a friend's apartment, she became very anxious, almost frantic.

Other Significant Findings From Assessment

The patient denied tobacco or caffeine use. She exercised every day. She said she sometimes would drink two to three glasses of wine on a weekend. She reported no drug use or other pharmaceuticals (such as over-the-counter diet pills). She saw her general practitioner 1 month prior to her initial visit. Physical exam and electrolyte levels were normal. She did not have dental erosion or enlarged parotid glands. Her STAR*D Quick Inventory of Depressive Symptomatology—Self-Report (QIDS-SR$_{16}$) score was 13 (moderate depression). On her baseline assessment, she rated her average level of depression over the past week as being about a 6 or 7 (on a scale of 0=no depression, 10=moderate to severe depression) and her maximum depression about the same. She rated her average anxiety as being a 6 or 7 and maximum at 8. (She did not consider anxiety to be a major problem.)

DSM-IV-TR Diagnosis

Axis I   Major depressive episode
            Bulimia nervosa
Axis II   None
Axis III   None
Axis IV   Breakup with boyfriend
Axis V   GAF score: 75

Treatment Plan Considerations

Depression and Bulimia

The patient's main problems were depression and bulimia. She was much more concerned about her depression than her bulimia but felt that she wanted to address both issues. She felt the depression was entirely due to her breakup with her boyfriend.

Selecting a Guideline

I considered four guidelines and algorithms: 1) the APA guideline for major depressive disorder (www.psychiatryonline.com/pracGuide/pracGuide-home.aspx), 2) the STAR*D guideline (Rush et al. 2003), 3) the APA guideline for eating disorders (www.psychiatryonline.com/pracGuide/pracGuide-home.aspx), and 4) the NICE guideline for treating bulimia (www.nice.org.uk/CG009niceguideline).

The APA general depression guidelines provide an excellent overview and general principles of treatment (see Table 18–1). I added a row to the guideline to indicate the need to assess and address exercise. Clinicians should consider evaluating the evidence for practices they consider useful and adding them to their personalized guidelines. For example, I used the five-step approach discussed in Chapter 2 of this volume to address the question,

"Does exercise help treat depression?" The results are summarized in Table 18–2. I felt there was enough evidence to include exercise in this patient's regimen and to add it to my guideline.

An important consideration for Ms. S.W. was whether to use psychotherapy and/or medications. The patient preferred psychotherapy (including cognitive-behavioral therapy [CBT]) but was willing to consider medications. I was confident the patient would improve on either or both. However, I felt that a CBT approach would be necessary for her bulimia nervosa where medication was less likely to be useful. By using both medication and CBT, I felt that I would be able to provide treatment for her depression (with pharmacotherapy) and to spend the psychotherapy focusing on the eating disorder and relationship issues.

The medication algorithm embedded in the APA guidelines for depression is excellent, but given the extensive use of the STAR*D algorithms and the definitions of response and phases, I think the latter is preferable, in part because of its real-world approach (see Chapter 21 for a detailed presentation of STAR*D) (Gaynes et al. 2008). A critical issue in all the guidelines is to define what represents response and what represents remission. STAR*D defines *response* as a significant improvement in depressive symptoms, although residual symptoms may be present. It is generally defined as a 50% improvement or greater reduction from baseline score on a standard measure such as the Hamilton Rating Scale for Depression, Beck Depression Inventory, or QIDS-SR$_{16}$. Remission is considered full restoration of a patient's normal capacity for psychosocial and occupational function with no residual symptoms, as defined by a score of ≤7 on the 17-item Hamilton Rating Scale for Depression or <5 on the QIDS-SR$_{16}$. *Relapse* is defined as recurrence of symptoms and impairment following response. *Treatment-resistant depression* is defined as failure to respond to at least two or three antidepressants given at therapeutic doses for more than 4 weeks (see Chapter 21 and Trivedi et al. 2007 for more details on the STAR*D algorithm).

I debated between the APA eating disorder guideline and the NICE guideline. The NICE guideline is more specific than the APA guideline and is closer to my therapeutic approach. Furthermore, members of our clinic have written a patient treatment guide with an accompanying manual (Agras and Apple

TABLE 18–1. Modified American Psychiatric Association general recommendation for major depressive disorder through remission

Recommendation		Followed
Psychiatric management	Basic clinical requirements	
	Diagnostic evaluation (including safety, functional impairment, etc.)	√
	Establish and maintain a therapeutic alliance	√
	Monitor transference/countertransference	√
	Monitor status and safety	√
	Provide education to patient	√
	Provide education to families	No, per patient
	Enhance medication treatment adherence by emphasizing:	
	When and how often to take	√
	Typical 2- to 4- week lag to benefit	√
	Continue medication even when feeling better	√
	Consult with medical doctor if problems arise	√
	Review side effects	√
	What to do if problems arise	√
	Address early signs of relapse	√
Acute treatment	Select initial treatment modality	
	Antidepressant medication or	
	Psychotherapy or	
	Psychotherapy plus antidepressant medication and	√
	Consider ECT	NA
	CBT and interpersonal therapy have best-documented efficacy	
	Must be integrated with psychiatric management and other treatments	NA
	Response to therapy should be carefully monitored	√
	Care needs to be coordinated	NA
	Patients should be treated until a complete response occurs. If moderate improvement or less is not achieved in 4–8 weeks, treatment needs to be reviewed.	√, used STAR*D criteria
	No or partial response (change medications; add or change psychotherapy; consider ECT)	√
	Reassess in 4–8 weeks	√
	The benefits of exercise should be discussed and program initiated if appropriate[a]	*Already exercising*
Continuation phase (16–20 weeks following remission)	Patients should continue on medications, generally at the dose used in the acute phase	√
	Psychotherapy effective for relapse prevention should be used (frequency of visits is not clear)	NA

Note. CBT=cognitive-behavioral therapy; ECT=electroconvulsive therapy; NA=not applicable to patient; STAR*D=Sequenced Treatment Alternatives to Relieve Depression.

[a] Author's addition.

Source. http://www.psychiatryonline.com/pracGuide/pracGuidehome.aspx.

TABLE 18–2.   Using the 5-step evidence-based medicine process to evaluate the effects of exercise on depression

Process	Evaluation
Step 1. Formulate the question	Does exercise help treat depression? (If yes, other important issues would need to be considered, such as type, intensity, frequency, and setting.)
Step 2. Search for answers	Several reviews suggested that regular aerobic exercise is effective in reducing depressive symptoms (e.g. Barbour et al. 2007) but that it is not recommended as a primary treatment, at least in older adults (Steinman et al. 2007). An older meta-analysis (Lawlor and Hopker 2001) concluded, "The effectiveness of exercise in reducing symptoms of depression cannot be determined because of a lack of good quality research on clinical populations with adequate follow up."
Step 3. Appraise the evidence	The advantage of searching for reviews and meta-analyses is that others have appraised the evidence. The results and conclusions are not always consistent, however, as suggested in the two reviews above, and I am left to draw my own conclusions. I don't find convincing evidence that exercise should be the primary treatment for depression. Having been involved in a number of exercise intervention studies, I am also aware of the time and resources required, the potential medical risks (falls, sprains, cardiovascular events), and the generally poor adherence. I conclude, as reflected in Table 18–1 (which comes not only from this review, but my own work in the field) that the benefits of exercise should be discussed and a program initiated if appropriate.
Step 4. Apply the results	Ms. S.W. was already exercising. (My general approach to provide exercise programs for patients is presented in Miller and Taylor 1995).
Step 5. Assess the outcome	The APA guideline includes periodic assessment of depression, and I use frequent single-item assessments. However, it is often difficult to attribute change to any one practice when patients are being provided a number of activities. I think it is important to assess adherence to exercise, and I routinely ask patients to report how many times a week they exercise as a global assessment.

2008a, 2008b) that can be used to provide the CBT approach recommended by NICE.

The NICE guideline for the pharmacological treatment of bulimia nervosa is not consistent with the STAR*D and APA guidelines for major depressive disorder. The NICE guideline (Table 18–3) states that fluoxetine is the medication of first choice; STAR*D recommends citalopram (although probably any selective serotonin reuptake inhibitor could be substituted). NICE states that the patient should be told to expect rapid improvement with pharmacology (based on a limited number of studies); APA emphasizes the need to inform patients of more gradual improvement. NICE recommends reassessment at 4–5 months (based on expected time course for bulimia treatment); the STAR*D guidelines suggest reassessment at 8 weeks.

Another consideration was what assessment instruments to use for bulimia nervosa. Although a number of standardized instruments are available to assess eating disorder attitudes and behaviors, I decided to focus only on purging episodes as the main outcome measure.

Relationship Issues

The patient's depression was related to the breakup of a relationship, and this would be a focus of therapy. I am not aware of guidelines for treating relationships, although therapeutic practices of relevant interventions such as interpersonal therapy (IPT) have been clearly defined. I planned to use IPT techniques to deal with the relationship issue and CBT techniques to deal with the bulimia and depression. Many of the core ideas of these therapies cross pa-

TABLE 18–3. Modified NICE guidelines for bulimia nervosa

Recommendation		Followed
Psychological interventions	As a first step, encourage use of evidence-based self-help program	No, given manual
	If self-help is declined, offer CBT	
	16–20 sessions over 4–5 months	√
	Reassess at 4–5 months	√
	If CBT is declined or no response (per guideline), offer other psychological treatments. IPT should be considered as an alternative to CBT but patient should be told it may take 8–12 months.	±
Pharmacological interventions	As an alternative or additional first step, offer antidepressant	√
	Fluoxetine is first choice. Dose for bulimia nervosa is higher than for depression.	Used STAR*D
	Inform patients that long-term effects are not known; beneficial effects will be rapidly apparent	
Medical management	If patient is vomiting frequently or taking many laxatives, assess fluid and electrolyte balance	No
	If electrolyte disturbance is detected, focus on behavior change or oral supplementation	NA

Note. CBT=cognitive-behavioral therapy; IPT=interpersonal therapy; NICE=National Institute for Health and Clinical Excellence; NA=not applicable to patient; STAR*D=Sequenced Treatment Alternatives to Relieve Depression.

Source. http://www.nice.org.uk/CG009niceguideline.

tient issues. For instance, negative thoughts related to body image are likely to cause both depression and excessive focus on weight and shape concerns. The NICE guideline for eating disorders states that if IPT is used, the patient should be cautioned that it might take up to a year. But with any recommendations derived from trials that restrict therapy to one approach, the recommendation does not fit the real world where we use several synergistic approaches.

Another issue was how to measure progress in the patient's relationships. Relating involves a number of factors, including confidence, skills, interest, and behavior. I decided to use a very simple metric by asking the patient every few sessions how satisfied she was with her relationships, from 1=not at all to 4=very satisfied, with the idea that I could explore the components as it seemed appropriate. I assumed she would need to overcome her sense of loss and impaired self-esteem from the breakup with her boyfriend before she would want to explore and develop new relationships. Routine use of even this simple question would remind me to keep relation-

ship issues as part of the agenda, because this was the patient's main concern, and also allow me to determine if she was making progress. From my clinical experience I would expect her relationships to improve to a score of 3 or 4 after 6 months of therapy.

With these considerations, I discussed an initial treatment plan and approach with the patient. I mentioned that I would periodically monitor how she was doing. She agreed to my initial treatment plan, listed in Table 18–4.

I prescribed citalopram 10 mg, increasing to 20 mg as tolerated. I explained the side effects and told her to stop the medication if she got worse. I scheduled a visit in 1 week.

Course

Visit 2 (Week 2)

The patient had no side effects from the citalopram and had increased it to 20 mg per day. About half the session was spent reviewing her relationship with her ex-boyfriend. It appeared that he had pushed

TABLE 18–4.   Initial treatment goals, measures, and methods

Treatment goal	Measure	Method
Reduce depressive symptoms by 50% by 8 weeks	QIDS-SR$_{16}$	Pharmacotherapy Supportive therapy
Reduce bulimic episodes by 50% by 8 weeks	Self-report (episodes/week)	Cognitive-behavioral therapy Pharmacotherapy?
Deal with relationship issues	Self-report (qualitative)	IPT embedded in cognitive-behavioral therapy Supportive psychotherapy

Note.   IPT = interpersonal therapy; QIDS-SR$_{16}$=Quick Inventory of Depressive Symptomatology–Self-Report.

her away as she was trying to achieve a closer relationship. She interpreted this as "I am not worthy or attractive" and "Nobody will ever want me"—thoughts appropriate for CBT intervention. The second part of the session was spent providing an overview of CBT treatment for bulimia nervosa. She was provided a self-help patient treatment manual, *Overcoming Eating Disorders* (Agras and Apple 2008a). According to the therapist guide (Agras and Apple 2008b), following evaluation, for the first session I should have undertaken the steps listed in Table 18–5. I followed most of these activities although I knew I would need to have some flexibility in scheduling.

Visit 3 (Week 3)

The patient was feeling less depressed and had no side effects from the medication. She had not completed her daily food records or read the first chapter of the workbook. We spent about 30 minutes on relationship issues, which was what she wanted to talk about. We then returned to discuss the importance of keeping the food records and reading the first several chapters of the manual. In reviewing the therapist guide (Agras and Apple 2008b), I found there was little said about very noncompliant patients, although much has been written about this in the CBT literature. I reemphasized the importance of keeping the records and examined her thoughts about doing so. The patient said that she didn't have time and felt too conspicuous carrying them around. We problem-solved ways for her to keep the records (such as writing the items down before she went to sleep) and even focused on accurate record keeping for a few days but not the entire week. I had the impression the patient was not motivated to change her bingeing/purging. I decided to wait another week or

so to confront, giving me more time to build a therapeutic relationship.

Visits 4–8 (Weeks 4–12)

The patient's mood had improved. She no longer met criteria for depression by week 8 and would be considered in remission. She was feeling much better about herself in general except for her bingeing/purging. It was evident to her that her bingeing/purging was a factor in her break-up with her boyfriend and would be a factor in future relationships, but she was not motivated to stop. She firmly believed that her bingeing/purging was controlling her weight. Overall adherence to the CBT practices was less than 50%. She was not "able" to follow a prescribed diet plan. Although her binge frequency, by her report, had dropped by 25%–50% and she had days when she was binge/purge free, I felt it was important for me to review why the patient was not doing better. I didn't feel her diagnosis or assessment was wrong, but she had very little motivation to change her behavior or to question her core beliefs and attitudes about bingeing/purging. We reviewed treatment options, including whether she might want to see someone else or change or increase her antidepressant, all of which she declined.

Weeks 13–36

The patient remained in remission from her depression for the next 4 months and wanted to stop her medication. She was feeling much better about herself and her relationships and had started dating. However, she continued to binge/purge at a high rate. I did a literature search to see if there were some new approaches that might prove beneficial, following the five-step approach discussed in Chapter 2 of this volume (see Table 18–6). The search

TABLE 18–5. First session of cognitive-behavioral therapy for bulimia nervosa, therapist activities

Activity	Followed	Comment
Provide rationale for therapy	√	
Emphasize importance of regularizing eating patterns	√	
Explain the three phases of treatment (behavior change, binge triggers, relapse prevention)	√	
Outline the session structure	No	I planned to focus on several issues, including medication and relationships
Provide evidence base of outcome	√	
Provide rationale for self-monitoring and introduce the daily food records	√	
Introduce the patient workbook	√	
Assign homework	√	Read first chapter in workbook, and complete daily food records

Source. Agras and Apple 2008b.

identified topiramate as a possible adjunct, but I felt the evidence for the use of topiramate was marginal. I discussed the risk/benefit with the patient, and she wanted to try it. After several weeks, and at a dose of 150 mg, the patient had seen no benefit and asked to stop the medication.

We stopped therapy after 36 weeks. The patient had accepted a job as an intern at a law firm in New York for the summer, and we decided this was a good time for her to take a break from therapy with the notion we would reevaluate treatment options in the fall when she returned, if she wanted to.

TABLE 18–6. Using the 5-step evidence-based medicine (EBM) process to evaluate pharmacological approaches to reducing bingeing/purging

Process	Evaluation
Step 1. Formulate the question.	Are there medications that can be used to reduce bingeing/purging (aside from those discussed in guidelines)?
Step 2. Search for answers.	After a more general search, I found some reports of the potential benefits of topiramate (Kotwal et al. 2003; Nickel et al. 2005). I could not find the Kotwal article online through my medical library (limited access to many journal articles is a major problem for EBM in clinical practice). Nickel et al. 2005 found that about 30% of the topiramate group had reduced binge frequency by 50% or more, compared with 3% in the control group. The medication was started at 25 mg and increased to 250 mg over 6 weeks. No side effects were noted. I also reviewed the basic pharmacology of topiramate.
Step 3. Appraise the evidence.	The evidence for the use of topiramate was marginal. I discussed the risk/benefit with the patient, however, and she wanted to try it.
Step 4. Apply the results.	Ms. S.W. was started on topiramate at 25 mg, with the goal of increasing the dose to 250 mg over 6 weeks.
Step 5. Assess the outcome.	After 4 weeks, and at a dose of 150 mg, the patient had seen no benefit and asked to stop the medication.

In the past week, what was your average level of depression? (0=none/no symptoms to 10=severe)

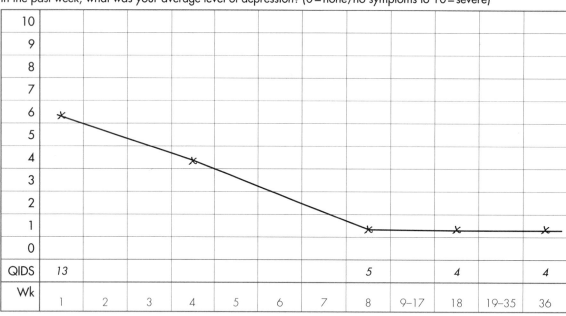

FIGURE 18–1.   Depression trends (X–X).

QIDS=Quick Inventory of Depressive Symptomatology–Self-Report (QIDS-SR$_{16}$).

Figures 18–1 through 18–3 show the patient's progress in mood and depression, purging, and relationships over the first 36 weeks of therapy. Her depression and her relationships improved; there was little change in her purging.

Summary of Guideline Use

At the end of 36 weeks I reviewed my use of the guidelines. I followed the APA guidelines for depression fairly well (see Table 18–1). The guidelines suggest that the therapist review transference/countertransference issues. While I hope I do this routinely, I

think I became more invested in the patient not being bulimic than she was. I was frustrated that she had not responded as anticipated to the manualized CBT approach. The patient responded to the first step of the STAR*D guideline. However she did not want to continue her medication for a full 12 months.

The NICE guideline recommends self-help as the first step and I provided the patient with a manual, but since she was in therapy it seemed appropriate to provide additional therapeutic guidance. I was not very successful at implementing a course of CBT for bulimia via a manualized treatment. However, I was able to have the patient use the basic skills

How often did you experience purging episodes in the past week? (1=none, 2=once a week, 3=a few times a week, 4=a few times a day)

FIGURE 18–2.   Purging episodes.

How satisfied are you with your relationships?
(1 = not at all; 2 = pretty unsatisfied; 3 = pretty satisfied; 4 = very satisfied)

FIGURE 18–3.   Relationship satisfaction.

(food monitoring, meal planning, identifying binge triggers) by tailoring the approach to her preferences. The NICE guideline suggests that I might have moved from CBT to IPT, if CBT was unsuccessful. However, a focus of IPT would have been on her relationships, which had improved substantially. The NICE guideline also suggests that IPT needs to be provided for a year, but I didn't think this was justified. The NICE guideline says that no medications other than fluoxetine should be used. As mentioned, I decided to use citalopram following STAR*D and was not convinced that fluoxetine was required. A PubMed search identified topiramate as a possible adjunct. Alternatively, I could have increased the dose of citalopram. The NICE guideline recommends review of electrolytes, which I failed to do. The patient's physical exam and electrolyte levels were normal at baseline; a reassessment would have been appropriate and would also have provided an indication of my concern about the potential medical consequences of her behavior. I believed I had generally followed the guidelines and a stepped-care approach with benefit for her depression, self-image, and relationship issues but with little impact on her bingeing.

Ways to Improve Practice

I identified several aspects of my practice that might have benefited this patient. First, I might have been more conscientious in how I delivered the manualized treatment. I might have put greater emphasis on the need for her to use it and examined her resistance more effectively. Second, I might have presented this case to the clinical case conference where other experts could present ideas relevant to the pa-

tient's care. This would also have given me an opportunity to examine the therapeutic relationship. Finally, I should have monitored her electrolytes periodically to help emphasize the potential negative effects of her persistent purging.

References

Agras WS, Apple R: Overcoming Eating Disorders: A Cognitive-Behavioral Treatment for Bulimia Nervosa and Binge-Eating: Patient Manual (Treatments That Work). Oxford, UK, Oxford University Press, 2008a

Agras WS, Apple R: Overcoming Eating Disorders: A Cognitive-Behavioral Treatment for Bulimia Nervosa and Binge-Eating—Therapist Guide (Treatments That Work). Oxford, UK, Oxford University Press, 2008b

Barbour KA, Edenfield TM, Blumenthal JA: Exercise as a treatment for depression and other psychiatric disorders: a review. J Cardiopulm Rehabil Prev 27:359–367, 2007

Gaynes BN, Rush AJ, Trivedi MH, et al: The STAR*D study: treating depression in the real world. Cleve Clin J Med 75:57–66, 2008

Kotwal R, McElroy SL, Malhotra S: What treatment data support topiramate in bulimia nervosa and binge eating disorder? What is the drug's safety profile? How is it used in these conditions? Eat Disord 11:71–75, 2003

Lawlor DA, Hopker SW: The effectiveness of exercise as an intervention in the management of depression: systematic review and meta-regression analysis of randomised controlled trials. BMJ 322:763–767, 2001

Miller NH, Taylor CB: Lifestyle Management for Patients With Coronary Heart Disease. Champaign, IL, Human Kinetics, 1995

Nickel C, Tritt K, Muehlbacher M, et al: Topiramate treatment in bulimia nervosa patients: a randomized, double-blind, placebo-controlled trial. Int J Eat Disord 38:295–300, 2005

Rush AJ, Trivedi M, Fava M: Depression, IV: STAR*D treatment trial for depression. Am J Psychiatry 160:237, 2003

Steinman LE, Frederick JT, Prohaska T, et al: Late life depression Special Interest Project (SIP) panelists: recommendations for treating depression in community-based
older adults. Am J Prev Med 33:175–181, 2007

Trivedi MH, Rush AJ, Gaynes BN, et al: Maximizing the adequacy of medication treatment in controlled trials and
clinical practice: STAR(*)D measurement-based care.
Neuropsychopharmacology 32:2479–2489, 2007

Depression, Refusal to Eat, and Nasopharyngeal Carcinoma

C. Barr Taylor, M.D.

Introduction and Setting

See Chapter 17.

Illustration

This study illustrates:

- Application of guidelines to psychiatric and medical comorbid problems
- Monitoring of symptoms
- Emergence of new problems
- A threat to the therapeutic relationship

Chief Complaint

Ms. P.A. is a 60-year-old woman who presents with a chief complaint of depression and being unable to eat.

Present Illness

The patient said she was fine until 3 months prior to admission, when she was diagnosed with nasopharyngeal carcinoma. She began radiation therapy followed by chemotherapy that needed to be stopped after two rounds because of side effects. About 6 weeks prior to admission she began to feel very depressed and was started on citalopram 20 mg but felt that the medication only had a mild benefit and caused her mouth to be drier. She said that food has no taste and that eating foods was very painful. She reported feeling sad most of the day, had no appetite or motivation to eat, had trouble concentrating, used sleep to escape, had no interest in sex, and had fatigue and no energy. She denied any suicidal intent. She reported attending a group for cancer survivors, seeing an acupuncturist for pain control, and using several compounds prescribed by a Chinese herbalist. She would sometimes use the dietary supplement Ensure to increase her caloric intake.

Past Psychiatric History

Ms. P.A. said she was a recovering alcoholic and had been abstinent for over 5 years. She attended Alcoholics Anonymous (AA) for 2 years after she quit drinking but had not been to AA since.

Medical History

The patient underwent radiation and chemotherapy for nasopharyngeal carcinoma. No nodes were found, and neck dissection was not recommended. Her weight dropped from 140–150 lb prior to cancer treatment to her current weight of 114 lb. She was told that she would need to have a feeding tube if she did not start to gain weight.

Social History

The patient was married for 30 years and had two adult children (both women). She worked at home as a part-time accountant. The patient felt that her cancer treatment had had a very negative impact on her family and marriage. She had lost interest in sexual activity and worried that her husband was very frustrated (she had asked him about this and he didn't complain) and that she had let down her daughters by not being stronger in simply eating "at any cost."

Other Significant Findings From Assessment

The patient used to play tennis two to three times a week and play golf but now reported walking three to four times a week for 30 minutes. She denied tobacco or caffeine use. On the mental status examination, she was tearful. There was no evidence of cognitive impairment. She scored 17 (moderate to severe depression) on the Quick Inventory of Depressive Symptomatology–Self-Report (QIDS-SR$_{16}$); 4/10 on the self-report of depression; and 1/10 on anxiety. Her Mini-Mental State Examination score was 29.

DSM-IV-TR Diagnosis

Axis I	Major depressive episode
	History of ethanol abuse
Axis II	None
Axis III	Radiation and chemotherapy for nasopharyngeal carcinoma with secondary pain upon swallowing, loss of taste
Axis IV	Stress/trauma related to cancer, possible marital discord
Axis V	GAF score: 60

Treatment Plan Considerations

Depression

The patient presented with major symptoms of depression probably related to the effects of being diagnosed and treated for cancer, with loss of taste and pain on swallowing, resulting in reluctance to eat and weight loss. She felt that she had let her family down because she was not eating. She was desperate to begin eating because she was terrified of having a feeding tube placed. The use of unidentified compounds from the Chinese herbalist presented a problem of potential adverse interactions among their use and psychopharmacology. (I made a mental note to do a quick search on the use of antidepressants and herbs and Chinese medicines when I had time and told the patient to try to find the names of the compounds she was using.)

Selecting a Guideline

As in the case presented in Chapter 18, the American Psychiatric Association (APA) major depressive disorder guideline would be appropriate for general management and the Sequenced Treatment Alternatives to Relieve Depression (STAR*D) guideline would be appropriate for medication (see Chapter 21 for a detailed presentation of STAR*D). The STAR*D guideline would call for 8 weeks of citalopram at an adequate dose; the patient had been at an adequate dose for 6 weeks. She also felt that her mouth was drier on citalopram than it had been before she started the medication, but ensuing rounds of radiation and chemotherapy are likely to have reduced her salivation. STAR*D suggests sertraline, venlafaxine extended release, or bupropion sustained release as an alternative if citalopram is not effective or is unacceptable. I was concerned that sertraline might cause more drowsiness without improving salivation; I decided to use fluoxetine based on my clinical impression that it can be more activating and has little effect on salivation (evidence: soft and clinical). (The use of monoamine oxidase inhibitors, or MAOIs, to be considered if the patient did not respond to the first three steps, would be contraindicated by her use of meperidine before eating to reduce the pain of swallowing.) As noted in the APA guideline, coordination of care with her other treatment providers would be important.

The APA guideline for depression would suggest that cognitive-behavioral therapy (CBT) and interpersonal therapy would be appropriate. I felt that a very structured, behavioral approach would be needed to help her with eating. I also felt that supportive therapy would be most appropriate following the general principles discussed in Winston et al. (2004).

Weight Loss/Food Refusal

The patient's main goal was to resume eating. Her problems in eating were probably related to her depression (loss of appetite) but also to her loss of taste and pain on swallowing. It hurt to eat. There are no guidelines for food refusal that I could find. We decided to establish two measurement parameters: weight gain and difficulty swallowing. I assumed, based on my experience with cancer patients who had gone through this type of treatment, that swallowing would improve, but gradually and subtly. I felt that the patient would benefit by seeing progress on a graph, even if slow. If progress didn't occur, it would help to consider other treatment approaches. A note in her medical chart indicated that she had been prescribed 45 mg of zinc sulfate tablets three times per day with food "in order to potentially provide some benefit to her taste function as previously described in the literature."

Stressors/Trauma of Cancer

A number of clinical approaches to treating cancer trauma have been described (Spiegel and Classen 2000). I have had positive experiences with online groups as one method of providing this service (Winzelberg et al. 2003). Encouraging the patient to use Internet resources, such as searching for ways to help treat her pain and improve her swallowing, would also seem appropriate.

Relationships Issues

The patient felt that her medical problems and depression had adversely affected her relationships. I decided to provide supportive therapy as noted above to help her with these problems and to consider referral to couples therapy (see Table 19–1).

I prescribed fluoxetine 20 mg one tablet in the morning and the use of a relaxation tape three times a week. I also gave her an individualized food record and asked her to write down everything she ate and, for at least one meal a day, what her thoughts were around eating (e.g., "I want my food to taste better,"

"I will never get better"). I also encouraged her to explore foods that might be easier to swallow and relatively more satisfying. I scheduled an appointment in a week.

Course

Visit 2 (Week 2)

The patient reported progress in being able to eat and found the logs useful. She was proud of herself when she could eat and hard on herself when she was not able to. She found that her mood varied throughout the week and at times she "felt normal" and other times felt frustrated and down. Evening meals were much harder for her. She was not preparing meals for her family, in part because she resented the fact that she couldn't eat what she prepared. She decided it would be important for her self-esteem if she began to prepare meals even if she wasn't able to eat them. The patient's depression scores, average level of eating/swallowing difficulty, and weight can be seen in Figures 19–1 and 19–2.

Visit 3 (Week 3)

The patient had lost another pound and was feeling discouraged. She realized that she would never be able to gain weight or even maintain her weight unless she increased her supplementation. She set a goal of using enough daily nutrition supplements to ensure weight maintenance. When discussing the use of supplements she said, "I don't want to spend

TABLE 19–1. Initial treatment goals, measures, and methods

Treatment goal	Measure	Method
Reduce depressive symptoms by 50% by 8 weeks	QIDS-SR$_{16}$	Pharmacotherapy Supportive therapy
Weight gain	Weekly weights	Supportive and behavioral therapy Pharmacotherapy Medical therapy
Reduce difficulty eating	Self-report	Supportive and behavioral therapy Pharmacotherapy Medical therapy
Reduce cancer trauma/stress	None	Supportive therapy Pharmacotherapy
Address relationship issues	Self-report, global	Supportive therapy, monitoring Couples therapy?

Note. QIDS-SR$_{16}$=Quick Inventory of Depressive Symptomatology–Self-Report.

In the past week, what was your average level of depression? (0=none/no symptoms to 10=severe)

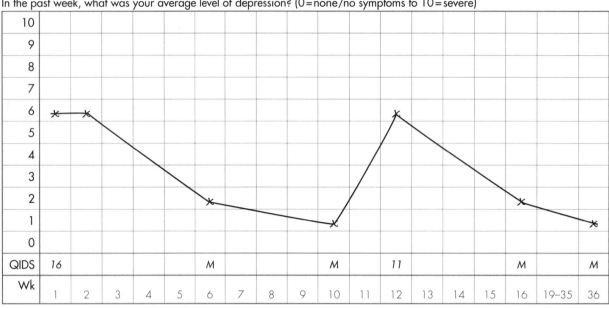

FIGURE 19–1. Depression trends (X—X).

M=missing; QIDS=Quick Inventory of Depressive Symptomatology–Self-Report (QIDS-SR$_{16}$).

the rest of my life drinking this crap." We discussed alternative thoughts (e.g., "If I gain weight I will feel better," "I only have to do this for another few months," "If I can hold my weight steady I won't need a tube"). The patient was going to be out of town the following week, so the next visit was scheduled for 2 weeks.

Visit 4 (Week 5)

The patient's mood had improved and intake was up until 2 days before the visit when a magnetic resonance imaging scan found an "abnormality" in her colon. She was scheduled for a colonoscopy (and would need to be NPO [nothing by mouth]) and was terrified that her cancer had metastasized or that she might have some other medical problem. We discussed this new event as being a major trauma. From her food records, she had found it useful to think of her eating as, "This is what it's going to be like. If I have the odd good moment, yippee." We scheduled a visit after her colonoscopy.

Visit 5 (Week 6)

The colonoscopy was negative and the patient's mood was demonstrably improved. However, she continued to lose weight. We reviewed her food records, looking for strategies to improve eating and

examining negative and catastrophic cognitions ("I hate this food. I will always hate this food"), as well as identifying activities that might give her some pleasure or fun or even relatively more pleasure or fun.

Visits 6–10 (Weeks 7–11)

(Not all visits were graphed.) The patient's mood continued to improve, and she was able to maintain her weight at 109–110 lb.

Visit 11 (Week 12)

The patient developed an infection at the back of her tongue which made eating almost impossible. Her weight dropped by another 2 lb. She also said that her husband told her that their relationship was unsatisfactory. Her mood worsened. She scored an 11 on the QIDS-SR$_{16}$. It would have been appropriate to consider other antidepressants, but her worse mood seemed related to her infection and her issues with her husband. When I started to focus on the food records and her weight, she became annoyed and insisted, "I need to talk about my marriage." I dropped my agenda and listened. She was very tearful in talking about how frightened she was that her marriage might not last or that her husband was frustrated with her progress. I asked if she wanted him to come to a session or if marital therapy might

In the past week, what was your average level of difficulty eating and swallowing? (0=not at all to 10=severe)

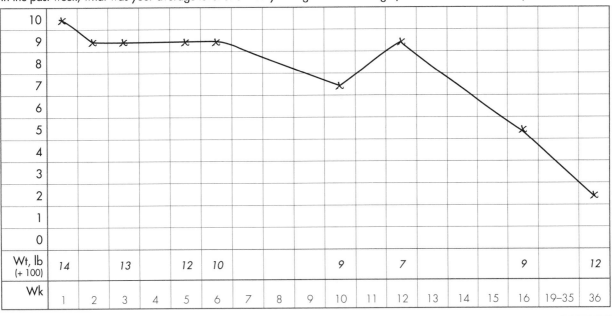

FIGURE 19–2. Eating/swallowing severity.

be appropriate. She said that she felt that their relationship was strong and had weathered other problems. A friend had invited them to spend some time with them in the desert. "If things aren't better when we get back, maybe we could see someone then." I *gently* encouraged her to continue her food records and weight monitoring while she was gone and thanked her for being very assertive about what she needed to talk about.

Visit 12 (Week 16)

The patient returned from the desert in a much better mood. Her QIDS-SR$_{16}$ was now at 8, and her weekly average mood was a 2/10. She said that she had long talks with her husband and it seemed to help that he could "vent." They committed to continuing to work on their relationship. Her weight was 109 lb, which she felt was acceptable given all that had happened.

Final Visits

The patient continued to improve over the next several months. Her swallowing improved dramatically and she was able to eat regular, although soft, foods and to consume less Ensure. Taste remained a problem but she was optimistic; from what she had heard from online discussions and her support group, that

would improve. Mood was normal. We scheduled a follow-up session in 3 months.

Summary of Guideline Use

I followed the general APA recommendations for major depressive disorder. I did not follow a strict CBT approach (use of thought records, etc.) but instead focused on the patient's need to maintain weight in the face of extreme discomfort.

I deviated from the STAR*D guideline as discussed above in minor ways for initial choice of medication. The patient had also "relapsed" by week 12 and, strictly on the basis of QIDS-SR, other interventions should have been considered. However, given the patient's exacerbated medical condition and relationship problems, it did not seem advisable to make a change until I had a sense of what would happen to her mood, assuming these problems would improve.

Sometimes, I follow the guidelines and manualized procedures too closely. If the patient had not interrupted me at week 12 to demand that we talk about what was really on her mind, I might not have been able to help her, could have overlooked an important contributing factor to her progress, and could have seriously impaired our therapeutic relationship. It can be challenging to listen carefully to patients' concerns while trying to adhere strictly to structured interventions.

Ways to Improve Practice

In reviewing my notes and the guidelines (not reflected in the brief case discussion above), I realized that I was not carefully monitoring some aspects of the patient's care, especially in monitoring the use of Chinese herbs and alternative treatments. I also was adhering too rigidly to my treatment program at the expense of being insensitive to the patient.

References

Spiegel D, Classen C: Group Therapy for Cancer Patients: A Research-Based Handbook of Psychosocial Care. New York, Basic Books, 2000

Winston A, Rosenthal RN, Pinsker H: Introduction to Supportive Psychotherapy. (Core Competencies in Psychotherapy Series; Gabbard GO, series ed.). Washington, DC, American Psychiatric Publishing, 2004

Winzelberg AJ, Classen C, Alpers GW, et al: Evaluation of an Internet support group for women with primary breast cancer. Cancer 7:1164–1173, 2003

Anorexia, Obsessive-Compulsive Disorder, and Depression

C. Barr Taylor, M.D.

Introduction and Setting

See Chapter 17.

Illustration

This study illustrates:

- Use of obsessive-compulsive disorder (OCD) and anorexia guidelines
- Adaptation of guidelines and practices for a patient with limited financial resources
- Consideration of a new guideline as a new problem emerges

Chief Complaint

Ms. C.J. is a 35-year-old married woman who is self-referred for treatment of obsessive thoughts and anorexia.

Present Illness

Ms. C.J. said that about 4 months prior to admission (PTA), she began to have sexual fantasies about someone she worked with and also imagined that he had fallen in love with her. She was terrified that she was having these thoughts and wrote an e-mail to the man, indicating that she was not interested. Her husband was looking at her e-mail and discovered the note. He became very upset and threatened to divorce her. She told her husband that there was "nothing going on" and she would quit her job,

which she did, to avoid further contact. However, she continued to obsess about her coworker. "I just can't get him out of my mind." She also began to feel that there were "germs" in her food. The thoughts seem to be getting worse and made her feel hopeless and depressed.

On the Yale-Brown Obsessive Compulsive Scale (Goodman et al. 1989a, 1989b), she reported current contamination, sexual, and somatic obsessions and fears, and hand-washing compulsions—she reported washing her hands about 20 times/day.

In addition, she reported a long history of food restriction and one episode of being hospitalized for anorexia about 5 years ago. About 2 months prior to assessment she began to reduce her food intake, but she said it was because of loss of appetite and not because of fear of germs. Over the previous 2 months, her weight had dropped from about 115 to 100 lb. She denied laxative use, purging, or driven exercise and said she wanted to weigh more.

One week prior to assessment her internist started her on sertraline 50 mg for her depression and she said that it helped but made her very "sluggish."

Other Significant Findings From Assessment

The patient reported no medical problems. She denied any alcohol or drug use. She reported multiple family members with depression. Her sister took fluoxetine with "good benefit." The patient was married for 12 years, with 2 children ages 3 and 11.

She was a high school dropout. On the mental status examination, her affect was very guarded and somewhat flat. There was no evidence of a thought disorder, and she denied hallucinations or delusions. Her baseline Quick Inventory of Depressive Symptomatology–Self-Report (QIDS-SR$_{16}$) was 5, in the normal range. This rating seemed inconsistent with her affect, which seemed sad. She reported a baseline level of 7/10 for depression, 6/10 for anxiety, intrusive thoughts a few times per week, with the thoughts being 7/10 in terms of severity (on a 0- to 10-point rating scale, with 0=no symptoms, 10=severe symptoms). Her weight was 100 lb.

Differential Diagnosis

The patient met DSM-IV-TR (American Psychiatric Association 2000) criteria for OCD. She did not meet criteria for a current depressive episode, but her answers were inconsistent as she reported significant depression on a one-item scale but few symptoms on the QIDS-SR$_{16}$ and attributed her 15-lb recent weight loss to a loss of appetite. She had a history of anorexia but denied current symptoms. However, she was very guarded on the initial interview and seemed to minimize symptoms. She was very uncomfortable in talking about her obsessive thoughts.

DSM-IV-TR Diagnosis

Axis I	OCD
	Probable current anorexia nervosa
	Major depressive episode?
Axis II	None
Axis III	None
Axis IV	Deferred
Axis V	GAF score: 50

Treatment Plan Considerations

The patient's main concerns related to her obsessive thoughts. She felt that her depressive symptoms were secondary to these thoughts and that she "desperately" wanted them to stop. The family's limited financial resources would be a factor in determining treatment. The patient lost her insurance coverage when she quit her job. Her husband's insurance had limited psychiatric benefits, and the family's income was just above the poverty line. A major focus of the initial sessions would be to build a sense of trust. I

had the impression that she was afraid of revealing "too much."

Selecting a Guideline and Outcomes

The American Psychiatric Association (APA) OCD guideline (www.psychiatryonline.com/pracGuide/pracGuidehome.aspx) seemed to be an appropriate guideline to follow, at least initially. The selection of the guideline was complicated by the possibility of the patient having an eating disorder. The OCD treatment guideline states that treatment outcome targets include <1 hour/day spent obsessing and performing compulsive behaviors, no more than mild OCD-related anxiety, an ability to live with OCD-associated uncertainty, and little or no interference of OCD with the tasks of daily living. I decided to focus on a simple measure of frequency ("In the past week, how often did you experience upsetting thoughts?" rated from "never" to "a few times a day," and "In the last week, how severe was this symptom?" rated from "not bad at all" to "severe").

Anorexia

The APA eating disorders guideline would be reasonable to consider. Initially I decide to focus on weight gain and monitor how she was doing and to get a better sense of her attitudes and behaviors related to eating.

Depression and Anxiety Symptoms

The patient did not meet criteria for a depressive disorder but I was struck by her weight loss, which might have been due to depressive symptoms or anorectic food refusal (she denied the latter). Her score on the QIDS-SR$_{16}$ was in the normal range, but I worried that she was minimizing symptoms. I decided to monitor depression and anxiety weekly and to entertain a focus on either depending on her course. Medication for her OCD would likely help her depression as well.

Treatment Plan and Initial Treatment

The OCD guideline states that the first-line treatments for OCD are cognitive-behavioral therapy (CBT) and serotonin reuptake inhibitors (SRIs). The guideline recommends that CBT focus on exposure and response prevention but notes the patient must be agreeable to and able to use the techniques. Having provided CBT to a number of

OCD patients, I was concerned that the patient would not have time to learn the techniques and that we would also need our limited number of sessions to deal with her eating and other problems. The anorexia guideline recommends fluoxetine (at a higher than usual dose). Because the patient was having unpleasant side effects on the sertraline, I decided to switch to fluoxetine. Other considerations in choosing fluoxetine were that her sister had done well on it and it is less expensive in case she needed to purchase the medication herself.

The OCD guideline recommends a course of CBT. However, the patient had a high school education and limited reading and writing skills, and her insurance coverage was limited to 10 sessions/year. The focus on therapy would need to be on medication and supportive therapy. I also mentioned that I would be weighing her before each session. I decided I would include CBT techniques as appropriate and as I had time (see Table 20–1).

Course

Visits 2–3 (Weeks 2 and 3)

The patient reported doing a little better in terms of improved mood, but her OCD thoughts remained unchanged. I printed out the National Institute of Mental Health handout on OCD to give her some background on the illness. The sessions focused on obtaining more information but also on providing some encouragement to eat. The patient felt that her continued obsessive thoughts about her former coworker were driving a wedge between her and her husband, and she wanted to find ways to spend more time with her husband. I also gave her a relaxation tape to help reduce her anxiety and increased the fluoxetine from 20 mg to 40 mg. Figures 20–1 and 20–2 show the course of her depressive and OCD symptoms and her weight.

Visit 4 (Week 6)

The patient reported that her mood had improved. She also felt some decrease in the frequency of her obsessive thoughts (not graphed in Figure 20–2) but no change in intensity of symptoms. She also reported significant problems eating; she was not able to increase her intake as requested—in fact, she wanted to further restrict. She did, however, report an improvement in her appetite. Her wish to restrict, history of anorexia, and thin-body ideal suggested that her weight loss was related to anorexia. We discussed the advantages of finding a support group for eating disorders. She continued to have difficulties with her husband. We discussed seeking a counselor, perhaps through her church.

The OCD guideline notes that it may take 8–12 weeks, including 4–6 weeks at a maximally tolerable dose, for the pharmacotherapy to be effective. The patient might have been able to tolerate a higher dose of fluoxetine, and using a higher dose would be consistent with the anorexia treatment guideline. However, as she had shown improvement, I decided not to increase the medication at this time. Adding CBT would be ideal but was not feasible for reasons mentioned above. I decided to start her on a low dose of risperidone (0.25 mg) to see if this might help her anxiety and help her gain weight. I gave the patient a self-monitoring food log to use at home. She was asked to simply note for each meal whether or not she ate "too little" or "enough."

TABLE 20–1. Initial treatment goals, measures, and methods

Treatment goal	Measure	Method
Reduce obsessive-compulsive disorder symptoms	Self-report frequency and severity: 50% reduction in frequency and severity in 6 months	Pharmacotherapy Supportive therapy Cognitive-behavioral therapy?
Weight gain	Weekly weights: target weight 110 lb in 6 months	Supportive and behavioral therapy
Reduce depressive symptoms	Self-report: 50% improvement by 8 weeks	Pharmacotherapy Supportive and behavioral therapy

In the past week, what was your average level of depression? (0=none/no symptoms to 10=severe)

FIGURE 20–1.   Depression trends (X—X).

QIDS=Quick Inventory of Depressive Symptomatology–Self-Report (QIDS-SR$_{16}$).

Visit 5 (Week 8)

Ms. C.J. reported that her mood was much better and her anxiety much less. She had gained 2 lb. She discussed wanting to go back to work.

Visit 6 (Week 10)

The patient reported that her obsessive thoughts had gotten much worse. On careful questioning she reported that she had been "hearing voices." She felt that her former coworker had actually been talking to her. "I can hear his voice in my head." She said this had happened to her before she first came to see me, but she was afraid to tell me for fear of being "locked up." I reviewed my diagnosis and treatment plan. She reported a slight increase in her depression but did not meet criteria for major depressive episode with psychotic features. She did, however, meet the criteria for psychotic disorder not otherwise specified.

I reviewed the schizophrenia treatment guidelines. The APA practice guideline recommends the Brief Psychiatric Rating Scale (BPRS; Overall and Gorham 1962) and the Positive and Negative Syndrome Scale (PANSS; Kay et al. 1987) for monitoring psychopathology. The PANSS needs to be purchased and requires 30–40 minutes to administer and score (Kay et al. 1987), making it impractical in

a clinical setting. On the BPRS, the patient had symptoms of anxiety, emotional withdrawal, guilt, hallucinatory behavior, and blunted affect for a total score of 19. A score of less than 18 is considered improved. I added the BPRS to her monitoring form (see Figure 20–2).

Although she had received some initial benefit from the risperidone, the dosage was below the therapeutic range used, for instance, in the Clinical Antipsychotic Trials of Intervention Effectiveness (CATIE) (Lieberman et al. 2005) or for augmenting treatment of OCD (Maina et al. 2008). Cost was a major factor. I discussed the cost/benefit of using perphenazine or haloperidol. She wanted to continue with the risperidone. I increased the risperidone to 0.5 mg/day and encouraged her to increase it over the next week to 2.0 mg/day.

Visit 7 (Week 15)

The patient reported a decrease in the voices, that her mood was slightly better, and that her OCD symptoms had returned to their level of a month or so ago. She said, however, that she had not increased the risperidone because she was not able to afford it. She had also gained 3 lb, which she was able to tolerate. Because of cost, she wanted to return in 3 months.

In the past week, what was your average level of severity of obsessive-compulsive thoughts?
(0=none/no symptoms to 10=severe)

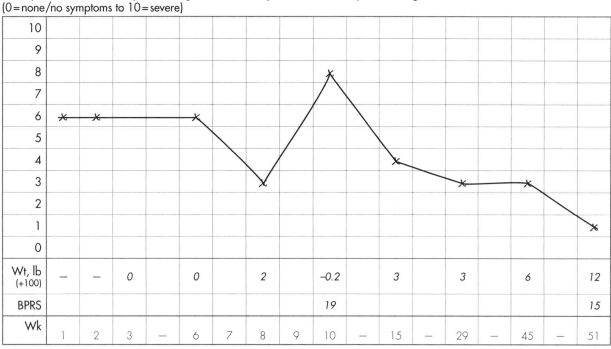

FIGURE 20–2. Severity of obsessive-compulsive thoughts (X—X).

BPRS=Brief Psychiatric Rating Scale.

Visit 8 (Week 29)

The patient reported that she had been doing OK. Her OCD symptoms were much less bothersome. She said she only heard occasional voices. She had maintained her 3-lb weight gain. I focused on issues related to her eating and weight and the need for her to continue taking her medication.

Visit 9 (Week 45)

A week after visit 8 the patient called to say that she stopped the risperidone because she had run out and couldn't afford it. After she had stopped the medication she still heard voices but she said they were less bothersome. She said that her "obsessive thoughts" (which she distinguished from the voices) were less. I prescribed a low dose of perphenazine. She had not attended a support group for eating disorders because she said that she had no one to leave her children with. We problem-solved ways for her to find support for her attending such a group.

Visit 10 (Week 51)

The patient never filled the perphenazine prescription. However, she continued to feel less depressed

and anxious. She still had mild obsessive thoughts and heard occasional voices, but they continued to be less troublesome. She was also able to gain another 6 lb. The patient planned to move from the area. We discussed options for her continued care, including going to a community mental health center when she had settled into another area.

Summary of Guideline Use

This patient presented a number of challenges, including the need to address a number of complex issues in a limited number of sessions with a patient with limited financial resources and little support from her husband. Four different guidelines provided useful guidance for her treatment. I began by following the APA OCD guideline. As seen in Table 20–2, I followed the General Psychiatric Management principles (A1–8). For the initial treatment, CBT was recommended, but the patient was not able to afford the required number of sessions and didn't seem to be a good candidate for self-help. (I have not included my checklist for the rest of the guidelines.) At week 6, I decided to augment with an atypical antipsychotic because she was still having

TABLE 20–2. American Psychiatric Association general recommendations for obsessive-compulsive disorder

	F	C
A. Psychiatric management		
1. Establish and maintain a therapeutic alliance		
Tailor communication style to the patient's needs and abilities	√	
Allow patients with excessive worry or doubting time to consider treatment decisions; repeat explanations if necessary	NA	
Attend to transference and countertransference, which may disrupt the alliance and adherence	√	
Consider how the patient's expectations are affected by his or her cultural and religious background, beliefs about the illness, and experience with past treatments	√	
2. Assess the patient's symptoms		
Use DSM-IV-TR criteria for diagnosis	√	
Consider using screening questions to detect commonly unrecognized symptoms	√	
Differentiate OCD obsessions, compulsions, and rituals from similar symptoms found in other disorders	√	
3. Consider rating the patient's symptom severity and level of function. The following instruments are useful:		
For symptoms: Yale-Brown Obsessive Compulsive Scale	√	
For self-rated depression: Patient Health Questionnaire (PHQ-9), Beck Depression Inventory–II, Zung Depression Scale, and the patient versions of the Inventory of Depressive Symptoms (IDS) or Quick Inventory of Depressive Symptomatology (QIDS)	√	
For disability: Sheehan Disability Scale	No	
For quality of life: Quality of Life Enjoyment and Satisfaction Questionnaire or the more detailed World Health Organization Quality of Life Survey	No	
4. Enhance the safety of the patient and others		
Assess for risk of suicide, self-injurious behavior, and harm to others	√	
Consider obtaining collateral information from family members and others		√
Take into consideration factors associated with increased risk of suicide, including specific psychiatric symptoms and disorders and previous suicide attempts		√
Evaluate the patient's potential for harming others, either directly or indirectly (e.g., when OCD symptoms interfere with parenting)		√
5. Complete the psychiatric assessment		
See APA's (1995) *Practice Guideline for the Psychiatric Evaluation of Adults*	√	
Assess for common co-occurring disorders, including mood disorders, other anxiety disorders, eating disorders, substance use disorders, and personality disorders	√	
6. Establish goals for treatment; goals of treatment include decreasing symptom frequency and severity, improving the patient's functioning, and helping the patient to improve his or her quality of life	√	
Reasonable treatment outcome targets include < 1 hour/day spent obsessing and performing compulsive behaviors, no more than mild OCD-related anxiety, an ability to live with OCD-associated uncertainty, and little or no interference of OCD with the tasks of daily living; despite best efforts, some patients will be unable to reach targets	√	

TABLE 20–2. American Psychiatric Association general recommendations for obsessive-compulsive disorder *(continued)*

		F	C
7.	Establish the appropriate setting for treatment		√
	Generally choose least restrictive setting that is safe to allow for effective treatment		√
	Is hospitalization indicated?		√
	Is home-based treatment needed?		√
8.	Enhance treatment adherence		
	Recognize that the patient's fears, doubting, and need for certainty can influence his or her willingness and ability to cooperate with treatment and can challenge the clinician's patience	√	
	Provide education about the illness and its treatment, including expected outcomes and time and effort required	±	
	Inform the patient about likely side effects (SEs), inquire about SEs the patient may be unwilling to report (e.g., sexual SEs), respond quickly to concerns about SEs, and schedule follow-up appointments soon after starting or changing medications	√	
	Address breakdowns in the therapeutic alliance	NA	
	Consider the role of the patient's family and social support system		√
	When possible, help the patient to address practical issues such as treatment cost, insurance coverage, and transportation	√	

Note. The APA guidelines contain both recommended actions and areas for consideration. As in the author's example above, you may use the columns to the right to indicate that a recommendation was followed (F) or considered (C), as appropriate. You may also indicate NA for "not applicable."
APA=American Psychiatric Association; OCD=obsessive-compulsive disorder.

Source. Adapted from http://www.psychiatryonline.com/pracGuide/pracGuidehome.aspx.

disabling symptoms and extensive anxiety. Following the OCD guidelines, I might have increased the fluoxetine and waited several more weeks before trying an atypical antipsychotic.

I also considered the APA general eating disorder guidelines and those specific to anorexia (see Table 20–3 for those related to anorexia). The general guideline encourages the therapist to address a number of "underlying themes and correct core maladaptive thoughts and attitudes" (B.6). I did not have time to address many of these issues. Unfortunately, there is no strong evidence to guide treatment of adult anorexia patients (Keel and Haedt 2008). I might have done a better job in providing some simple psychoeducational materials. Overall, I don't think I provided enough homework activity; more might have served as a bridge between sessions.

The APA schizophrenia guideline was also relevant. This was not a major focus of therapy as the patient's "auditory hallucinations" seems to respond to a low dose of risperidone, and in fact they remained

improved even when she no longer took the medication. The APA depression guideline also provided useful and different information on how to manage this patient. Because the use of this guideline is presented in Chapter 18, I don't go over it here. Overall, I ended up selecting pieces of the guidelines, perhaps at the expense of not providing some important therapeutic procedures. Would I have done better, for instance, to focus on only one type of CBT practice, such as thought-stopping? Would this even have clarified the relationship between her thoughts and her "hallucinations"?

Ways to Improve Practice

The patient did much better than I expected. As presented, the use of the fluoxetine would seem to have been a major factor in her improvement, but I suspect other nonspecific elements may have been important, such as providing a supportive and trusting relationship, which allowed her to discuss a number

TABLE 20–3. **Specific recommendations for anorexia adapted from American Psychiatric Association eating disorders guideline**

	F
a. Nutritional rehabilitation	
Establish goals for seriously underweight patients	√
Restore weight	±
Normalize eating patterns	√
Achieve normal perceptions of hunger and satiety	No
Correct biological and psychological sequelae of malnutrition	NA
Help the patient to resume eating and gain weight (see guidelines for details)	√
Help the patient to maintain weight	NA
b. Psychosocial treatments	
Establish goals, including to help the patient	√
Understand and cooperate with nutritional and physical rehabilitation	√
Understand and change the behaviors and dysfunctional attitudes related to the eating disorder	√
Improve interpersonal and social functioning	√
Address comorbid psychopathology and psychological conflicts that reinforce or maintain eating disorder behaviors	±
Establish and maintain a psychotherapeutically informed relationship with the patient	√
Provide formal psychotherapy once weight gain has started.	No
c. Medications	
Use psychotropic medications in conjunction with psychosocial interventions, not as a sole or primary treatment for patients with anorexia nervosa	√
Whenever possible, defer making decisions about medications until after weight has been restored	NA
Be aware of and manage general side effects	√
Consider antidepressants to treat persistent depression or anxiety following weight restoration	√
Consider approaches to restore lost bone mineral density	No

Note.   F=followed; NA=not applicable.

Source.   http://www.psychiatryonline.com/pracGuide/pracGuidehome.aspx.

of distressing issues. In reviewing the case and my use of guidelines, here are two ways in which I could improve my practice: 1) use higher doses for longer periods of the initial SRI in treating patients with OCD, and 2) find low-literacy, simple psychoeducational materials to supplement therapy. Given the unusual picture and complexity of this patient's -psychopathology, a consult with a peer would have been warranted.

References

American Psychiatric Association: Practice guideline for the psychiatric evaluation of adults, 2nd edition, in Practice Guidelines for the Treatment of Psychiatric Disorders, Compendium. Washington, DC, American Psychiatric Publishing, 2006, pp 1–60

Goodman WK, Price LH, Rasmussen SA, et al: The Yale-Brown Obsessive Compulsive Scale, I: development, use, and reliability. Arch Gen Psychiatry 46:1006–1011, 1989a

Goodman WK, Price LH, Rasmussen SA, et al: The Yale-Brown Obsessive Compulsive Scale, II: validity. Arch Gen Psychiatry 46:1012–1016, 1989b

Kay SR, Fiszbein A, Opler LA: The Positive and Negative Syndrome Scale (PANSS) for schizophrenia. Schizophr Bull 13:261–276, 1987

Keel PK, Haedt A: Evidence-based psychosocial treatments for eating problems and eating disorders. J Clin Child Adolesc Psychol 37:39–61, 2008

Lieberman JA, Stroup TS, McEvoy JP, et al: Clinical Antipsychotic Trials of Intervention Effectiveness (CATIE) investigators: effectiveness of antipsychotic drugs in patients with chronic schizophrenia. N Engl J Med 353:1209–1223, 2005

Maina G, Pessina E, Albert U, et al: 8-week, single-blind, randomized trial comparing risperidone versus olanzapine augmentation of serotonin reuptake inhibitors in treatment-resistant obsessive-compulsive disorder. Eur Neuropsychopharmacol 18:364–372, 2008

Overall JE, Gorham DR. The Brief Psychiatric Rating Scale. Psychol Rep 10:799–812, 1962

Major Depressive Disorder

A Measurement-Based Care Approach

Madhukar H. Trivedi, M.D.
Ben Kurian, M.D., M.P.H.

Setting

The following case is based on a patient who participated in the Sequenced Treatment Alternatives to Relieve Depression (STAR*D), a research trial using measurement-based care (MBC) to treat major depressive disorder (MDD) in real-world outpatients with depression.

Illustration

This study illustrates:

- Use of a nonpsychotic major depressive episode sequential treatment algorithm
- Use of STAR*D MBC guidelines
- Personalized treatment of MDD and disease self-management

Chief Complaint

Ms. S.W. is a 40-year-old married white female who works as a truck driver and presents with symptoms of depression.

Present Illness

Ms. S.W. stated that she had been depressed for the last 6 months, following the death of her mother,

and the depression had gotten particularly worse in the past 2 months. The patient stated that her mother had a history of high blood pressure and high cholesterol and had died suddenly from a heart attack 6 months prior to the patient's initial clinic presentation. For the past 2 months the patient felt sad nearly every day and had decreased sleep (initial insomnia), decreased interest in her usual activities, increasing fatigue, and feelings of worthlessness and guilt. In addition, the patient reported increasing difficulties with concentration but denied change in appetite or weight. She also denied any thoughts of suicide or preoccupation with death. Her symptoms had worsened to the point at which they interfered with her ability to concentrate while at work, with the patient stating that in the past 2 months she had gotten lost while driving (which was very unusual for her). Ms. S.W. had remarried recently (about 3 months ago), although she denied any significant stress associated with this event.

Past Psychiatric History

The patient reported one prior major depressive episode, approximately 10 years ago while undergoing a divorce from her first husband. At that time, the patient noted her primary care physician started her on sertraline and titrated her dose up to 100 mg/day, which she took for 1 year with good results. She stopped the sertraline on her own because she felt she "no longer needed it." In addition to sertraline, the patient stated her primary care physician also prescribed Ambien (zolpidem) to assist with initial insomnia.

Medical History

- Hypertension (stable)—taking hydrochlorothiazide 25 mg
- Gastroesophageal reflux disease (stable)—taking pantoprazole 40 mg
- Tension headaches (stable)—taking ibuprofen as needed
- Hysterectomy 16 years ago—not taking hormone replacement

Social History

The patient denied tobacco use. She drank approximately two to three cups of coffee daily. She reported no routine exercise. She stated that she rarely had alcohol (approximately one glass of wine per month). She denied use of drugs or other pharmaceuticals (i.e., herbal medications). The patient lived with her husband and his teenage son. She had been living with her current husband for some time before they got married. She has one prior marriage with two now-adult children. The patient graduated from high school but reported no further schooling.

There was no significant family history of depression or mental illness. The patient's mental status examination was significant for a depressed affect with limited range of emotion. Her thought process and content were intact, and her Mini-Mental State Examination score=30; however, the patient subjectively reported distress with short-term memory and concentration. Her physical exam and vital signs were within normal limits. Her baseline Quick Inventory of Depressive Symptomatology–Clinician Rated (QIDS-C$_{16}$) score was 19, in the severe range (see below for interpretation of scores):

QIDS-C$_{16}$ scoring criteria:
Normal	≤5
Mild	6–10
Moderate	11–15
Severe	16–20
Very severe	21–27

DSM-IV-TR Diagnosis

Axis I	Major depressive disorder, recurrent, current episode severe, without psychotic features
Axis II	None
Axis III	Hypertension, gastroesophageal reflux disease, tension headaches
Axis IV	Recent loss of mother
Axis V	GAF score: 55

Treatment Plan Considerations

Major Depressive Disorder and Uncomplicated Bereavement

The patient's main problem was her depression. She was concerned that if it continued, it would affect her new marriage. She stated that the grief surrounding her mother's sudden death had improved a few months previously but that she was still depressed. The patient felt guilty that she remained depressed despite recently getting remarried. She had not had any counseling/psychotherapy regarding her recent loss and wished to first try pharmacological treatment for MDD.

MDD Treatment Guideline Selection

A number of treatment algorithms and guidelines are available to clinicians considering the treatment of MDD: 1) the STAR*D guideline (Rush et al. 2004), 2) the American Psychiatric Association (2000) guidelines for MDD, and 3) the TMAP guideline for nonpsychotic MDD (Crismon et al. 1999).

The goal of treatment for all patients with MDD, as outlined in Rush et al. (2006b), is to achieve remission of depressive symptoms (i.e., the patient is symptom free). The TMAP guideline for MDD introduced the concept of using critical decision points (CDPs) at defined intervals to objectively assess symptom and side-effect burden and to adjust treatment accordingly (Crismon et al. 1999). STAR*D further refined the objective assessments of symptoms and side effects with the introduction of measurement-based care (Trivedi and Daly 2007; Trivedi et al. 2006b, 2007b).

MBC promotes the use of rating scales or questionnaires to measure symptoms, side effects, and adherence at every visit as well as to guide tactics to modify dosage and treatment duration. In addition, MBC integrates these objective measurements and targets for full symptom remission. Most clinicians do not routinely use specific measures of depressive symptoms at patient visits; rather, they tend to use global measures (Biggs et al. 2000). Results from level 1 of STAR*D reveal that the use of MBC may lead to greater remission rates than those seen in efficacy studies for patients with chronic depression (Trivedi et al. 2006b).

STAR*D used the QIDS, a 16-item questionnaire based on DSM-IV-TR criteria for MDD, developed as a measure of depressive symptom severity (www.ids-qids.org). The QIDS is quick and easy to use, with good reliability and validity. Both clinician and self-rated versions are available free of charge and have been validated and translated into other languages (Rush et al. 2003, 2006a; Trivedi et al. 2004). To comply with the STAR*D MBC guidelines, we present the QIDS in this case presentation, but we recognize that alternative symptom ratings such as the Patient Health Questionnaire–9 (PHQ-9; Kroenke et al. 2001), Beck Depression Inventory–II (Steer et al. 1999), and others can be used. With regard to systematically measuring side effects, MBC guidelines recommend using the Frequency, Intensity, and Burden of Side Effects Rating (FIBSER; Wisniewski et al. 2006).

Table 21–1 reflects MBC for the acute treatment phase of MDD. Clinical status (e.g., remission, partial response) and side-effect tolerability at each CDP determine the treatment plan for that visit. Remission was defined by QIDS-$C_{16} \leq 5$, partial response was defined as QIDS-$C_{16} = 6-8$, and nonresponse essentially was defined as QIDS-$C_{16} \geq 9$. Clinic visits in STAR*D were generally recommended at weeks 0, 2, 4, 6, 9, and 12 at each treatment stage (level) or until an adequate remission or response was obtained, with CDPs occurring at each of these visits (except week 2).

TABLE 21–1. Critical decision points (CDPs) and tactics for acute phase treatment of major depression

Critical decision point	Clinical status	Plan
Week 0 (CDP #1)	Symptomatic	Initiate medication; adjust dose to lower end of therapeutic dose range or serum level
Week 4 (CDP #2)	Remission (QIDS-$C_{16} \leq 5$)	Continue current dose
	Partial response (QIDS-$C_{16} = 6-8$)	Continue current dose Consider increasing dose
	Nonresponse (QIDS-$C_{16} \geq 9$)	Increase dose
Week 6 (CDP #3)	Remission (QIDS-$C_{16} \leq 5$)	Continue current dose
	Partial response (QIDS-$C_{16} = 6-8$)	Increase/maximize dose
	Nonresponse (QIDS-$C_{16} \geq 9$)	
Week 9 (CDP #4)	Remission (QIDS-$C_{16} \leq 5$)	Continue current dose
	Partial response (QIDS-$C_{16} = 6-8$)	Increase dose Go to the next level
	Nonresponse (QIDS-$C_{16} \geq 9$)	Discontinue and go to the next level
Week 12 (CDP #5)	Remission (QIDS-$C_{16} \leq 5$)	Go to follow-up phase
	Partial response (QIDS-$C_{16} = 6-8$)	Go to the next level Increase dose and reevaluate in 2 weeks

Note. QIDS-C_{16}=Quick Inventory of Depressive Symptomatology–Clinician Rated.

Course

Level 1 Treatment Course (Citalopram)

CDP 1 (Week 0)

Prior to entering a patient into any treatment algorithm, one should conduct a thorough diagnostic evaluation to confirm a primary diagnosis of MDD and to uncover any other potential comorbid medical and psychiatric conditions. Antidepressant selection should be based on individual patient characteristics (e.g., history of prior treatment response) and patient preference. Additional consideration for side-effect profiles, potential drug interactions, and comorbid medical and psychiatric conditions may favor the choice of one particular medication over another.

In this case example, the patient, diagnosed with MDD without psychotic features (QIDS-C_{16}=19), was started on citalopram 20 mg. However, at this treatment stage, it is acceptable to prescribe any of the U.S. Food and Drug Administration (FDA)–approved selective serotonin reuptake inhibitors (SSRIs; e.g., fluoxetine, paroxetine, sertraline, citalopram, and escitalopram); serotonin and norepinephrine reuptake inhibitors (SNRIs; e.g., venlafaxine XR and duloxetine), or bupropion SR or XL. While head-to-head comparisons are not available for all antidepressants, data from the FDA and comparison trials suggest that all these antidepressants are similar in efficacy in treatment-naïve patients (level A data; Hansen et al. 2005).

The patient was counseled on potential medication side effects and the potential increased risk of suicidal thinking and behavior (i.e., suicidality), in accordance with FDA guidelines (U.S. Food and Drug Administration, Center for Drug Evaluation and Research 2004). Additionally, prior to starting a patient on an antidepressant, both the patient and the patient's family should be educated regarding the need to monitor for suicidality and associated symptoms, including anxiety, agitation, insomnia, irritability, hostility, aggressiveness, impulsivity, akathisia (psychomotor restlessness), hypomania, mania, or any other unusual changes in behavior. These symptoms, if present, are likely to emerge early in the course of treatment, and therefore a return visit was scheduled for this patient in 2 weeks. Furthermore, a telephone follow-up was scheduled with the patient 1 week after initiating citalopram to assess tolerability and suicidality.

The following figures reflect the practical application of the STAR*D level 1 algorithm for the present case, at each of the critical decision points, beginning with Figure 21–1, CDP week 0.

Week 1

A phone screen was conducted between the patient and a research assistant 1 week after initiating citalopram 20 mg to assess tolerability and adherence, and specifically to assess for any increase in suicidal thoughts and/or behavior. The patient reported mild gastrointestinal side effects (i.e., cramps, diarrhea); however, overall she tolerated citalopram 20 mg and reported no missed doses. Additionally, the patient denied any suicidal thoughts or associated symptoms and was reminded of her follow-up appointment in 1 week.

Week 2

At week 2 visit, once again side effects, tolerability, and adherence were measured. The patient reported resolution of gastrointestinal side effects and once again denied suicidal ideation. She did report two missed medication doses, when she forgot to take her medication with her while staying with her mother. The next visit, week 4, included a CDP to determine a treatment decision based on measurement of symptoms, side effects, and tolerability.

CDP 2 (Week 4)

According to the STAR*D MBC algorithm, the second CDP took place at week 4 (Figure 21–2). At this visit the patient had three domains of treatment measured: symptom severity (measured by the QIDS-C_{16}), side effects (measured by the FIBSER), and medication adherence. After 4 weeks of treatment with citalopram 20 mg, the patient's QIDS-C_{16} was measured at a 13. The patient noted slight improvements in mood and concentration; however, insomnia and anhedonia still persisted. The patient reported no side effects related to medication treat-

CDP, Week 0	STAR*D Level 1
	Start patient on citalopram 20 mg/day
Return to clinic:	Return in 2 weeks

FIGURE 21–1. Critical decision point (CDP) 1 (level 1).

CDP, Week 4	STAR★D Level 1
Symptom Improvement (SEs tolerable)	
QIDS-C$_{16}$ ≥ 9	Increase dose to 40 mg/day
QIDS-C$_{16}$ = 6–8	Continue current dose, *or* Increase dose to 40 mg/day
QIDS-C$_{16}$ ≤ 5	Continue current dose
Improved, but SEs are intolerable	Continue current dose and address SEs, *or* Go to the next level
Not improved and SEs are intolerable	Go to the next level
Return to clinic:	Return in 2 weeks

FIGURE 21–2.   Critical decision point 2 (level 1).

QIDS-C$_{16}$=Quick Inventory of Depressive Symptomatology; SEs=side effects.

ment. This was reflected by the FIBSER, which measured the frequency, intensity, and burden of side effects (the patient reported "no side effects" to all). Furthermore, the patient reported no additional missed doses of medication since the last visit. Specifically, because the patient's QIDS score remained≥9 and the side-effect profile was tolerable, the MBC algorithm dictated that the dose of citalopram be increased to 40 mg/day. Had the patient's side-effect profile for citalopram been intolerable, the algorithm does allow the clinician to go to the next level of treatment (i.e., switch to another antidepressant) at week 4 and beyond. Lastly, as was done at every visit, suicidal behavior and associated symptoms were assessed (patient reported none), and the patient was scheduled for follow-up visit in 2 weeks.

CDP 3 (Week 6)

At week 6 the patient scored a 14 on her QIDS-C$_{16}$ and reported no significant improvement in depressive symptom severity. She also reported a new side effect she believed was induced by citalopram: daytime sleepiness (the patient had been taking citalopram daily in the morning), most notably present at work. According to the FIBSER, the patient reported daytime somnolence as present 25% of the time with mild intensity and impairment, but still tolerable. It was suggested to the patient to try and switch the time of citalopram dosing to evening to see if this improved side effect. Once again, accord-

ing to the MBC algorithm (Figure 21–3), the daily dose of citalopram was increased to 60 mg, given acceptable side effects and persistence of depressive symptoms. Follow-up was scheduled in 3 weeks.

CDP 4 (Week 9)

The patient returned at week 9, after having taken citalopram 60 mg for 3 weeks. This visit was the first CDP that allowed for the clinician to move to the next treatment level due to an inadequate treatment response, despite tolerable side effects (Figure 21–4). At this visit the patient's depressive symptoms were virtually unchanged from the previous visit, QIDS-C$_{16}$=13, and only mildly improved from baseline. The side effect of daytime somnolence resolved, and the patient was uncertain whether this was secondary to switching the medication dosing time to evening or whether the increase to 60 mg daily played a role. Regardless, the patient reported no presence of side effects, with no intensity and no functional impairment on the FIBSER, and once again the patient also had not missed any medication doses in the past 3 weeks. However, with a QIDS≥9 after 9 weeks of treatment with citalopram, the clinician and patient elected at this CDP to move to the next level of treatment. According to the STAR*D algorithm, treatment options at level 2 are divided into switch and augmentation (Rush et al. 2004). The decision to switch or augment is determined by treatment response and medication tolerability. For example, if a patient has had no treatment response or has intol-

CDP, Week 6	STAR ⋆ D Level 1
Symptom Improvement (SEs tolerable):	
QIDS-C$_{16}$ ≥ 9	Increase dose to 60 mg/day
QIDS-C$_{16}$ = 6–8	Increase dose to 60 mg/day, *or* Continue current dose
QIDS-C$_{16}$ ≤ 5	Continue current dose
Improved, but SEs are intolerable	Continue current dose and address SEs, *or* Decrease dose and continue for 2 additional weeks, *or* Go to the next level
Not improved and SEs are intolerable	Go to the next level
Return to clinic:	Return in 3 weeks

FIGURE 21–3.   Critical decision point 3 (level 1).

erable side effects, a switch to another medication is recommended. According to STAR*D, switch options for level 2 include any of the following: sertraline, bupropion, venlafaxine, or cognitive therapy. However, if a patient has a tolerable side-effect profile and a partial treatment response, as is the case in this example, then a treatment augmentation is recommended. Level 2 treatment options for augmentation per the STAR*D algorithm include one of the following: buspirone, bupropion, or cognitive therapy (Rush et al. 2004). Figure 21–5 shows the patient's STAR*D level 2 treatment.

At the week 9 CDP visit, augmentation treatment options were discussed with the patient, and the only treatment she was unwilling to accept was cognitive therapy. According to STAR*D level 2 results, buspirone and bupropion are both efficacious as augmentation agents; however, bupropion is associated with better tolerability and greater reduction in self-reported depressive symptoms (Trivedi et al. 2006a). Therefore, bupropion XL (bupropion SR is also acceptable) was chosen as the level 2 augmentation agent, and the MBC algorithm for bupropion XL augmentation was initiated.

CDP, Week 9	STAR ⋆ D Level 1
Symptom Improvement (SEs tolerable):	
QIDS-C$_{16}$ ≥ 9	Go to the next level
QIDS-C$_{16}$ = 6–8	Increase dose to 60 mg/day, if not done before, *or* Go to the next level
QIDS-C$_{16}$ ≤ 5	Continue current dose
SEs are intolerable	Go to the next level
Return to clinic:	Return in 3 weeks

FIGURE 21–4.   Critical decision point 4 (level 1).

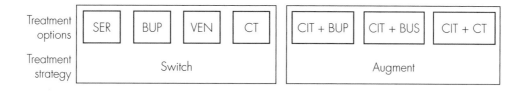

FIGURE 21–5. STAR*D level 2 treatment.

BUP=bupropion; BUS=buspirone; CIT=citalopram; CT=cognitive therapy; SER=sertraline; VEN=venlafaxine.

Source.   Adapted from Rush AJ, Fava M, Wisniewski SR, et al: Sequenced Treatment Alternatives to Relieve Depression (STAR*D): rationale and design. *Controlled Clinical Trials* 25:119–142, 2004.

Level 2 Treatment Course (Citalopram + Bupropion XL)

CDP 1 (Week 0)

Prior to initiating any second treatment options, switch or augmentation, the clinician should reassess the diagnosis of MDD, with specific care to rule out a bipolar diathesis. For this case, after confirmation of diagnosis, the patient was continued on citalopram 60 mg, and bupropion XL 150 mg daily was initiated (Figure 21–6). In fact, during level 2 treatment, assuming tolerability it was recommended that the patient continue citalopram at the last acceptable dosage from level 1 (in this case 60 mg). Side-effect profile of bupropion XL and precautions to watch for increase in suicidal thoughts/behavior and associated symptoms were once again discussed with the patient. Follow-up was scheduled in 2 weeks.

Week 2

The patient returned for week 2 visit and underwent a routine clinic visit. She noted a mild headache the first week after bupropion was initiated with resolution of side effect in the days leading up to week 2 visit. She noted feeling better and denied any missed doses of either medication. Follow-up visit was scheduled in 2 weeks.

CDP 2 (Week 4)

Systematic measurement of symptoms, side effects, and adherence once again guided the level 2 CDP. At this visit, the patient noted significant improvement in depressive symptoms, with a QIDS-C$_{16}$=6, and specific improvements in mood, energy, concentration, and guilt. In fact, the only depressive symptom that the patient continued to complain of was anhedonia. The patient denied any continuing side effects (i.e., headache), and according to the FIBSER, side effects were determined to be tolerable. Additionally, the patient denied any suicidal thoughts/behavior or associated symptoms. At this stage, MBC provides the clinician with the choice of continuing on the current dose of the augmentation medication or increasing the dose if acceptable to the patient (Figure 21–7). The clinician and the patient jointly decided to increase the bupropion to 300 mg with a goal of targeting full symptom remission (QIDS-C$_{16}$≤5), and the patient was scheduled for follow-up in 2 weeks.

An emphasis has been placed on remission in recent years, and the American College of Neuropsychopharmacology Task Force advocates remission as the goal of treatment for patients with MDD (Rush et al. 2006b). This is largely due to the conse-

CDP, Week 0	STAR ☀ D Level 2: Citalopram + Bupropion XL
	Start patient on bupropion 150 mg/day in addition to current dose of citalopram
Return to clinic:	Return in 2 weeks

FIGURE 21–6.   Critical decision point 1 (level 2).

CDP, Week 4	STAR✶D Level 2: Citalopram + Bupropion XL
Symptom Improvement (SEs tolerable)	
$QIDS\text{-}C_{16} \geq 9$	Increase dose to 300 mg/day
$QIDS\text{-}C_{16} = 6\text{-}8$	Continue current dose, or Increase dose to 300 mg/day
$QIDS\text{-}C_{16} \leq 5$	Continue current dose
Improved, but SEs are intolerable	Continue current dose and address SEs, or Go to the next level
Not improved and SEs are intolerable	Go to the next level
Return to clinic:	Return in 2 weeks

FIGURE 21–7.   Critical decision point 2 (level 2).

quence of not achieving remission. Paykel and colleagues found that patients with residual depressive symptoms have an increased risk for and a shorter time to relapse of MDD (Paykel et al. 1995).

CDP 3 (Week 6)

The patient returned for her week 6 visit in high spirits. She noted feeling "so much better," and this was confirmed with a $QIDS\text{-}C_{16}=3$. Improvements were noted in all domains, and the patient officially achieved remission status. She was able to tolerate the 300 mg dose of bupropion XL without side effects, and the

FIBSER again revealed no side-effect frequency, intensity, or burden. Furthermore, the patient was compliant with prescribed medications and reported no missed doses. Thus, the patient was continued on citalopram 60 mg and bupropion XL 300 mg (Figure 21–8), with a follow-up visit scheduled in 3 weeks.

CDP 4 (Week 9)

Results from week 9 visit mirrored the findings from week 6, in that the patient continued to remit and showed acceptable tolerability. Once again, the patient denied any suicidal thoughts/behavior or asso-

CDP, Week 6	STAR✶D Level 2: Citalopram + Bupropion XL
Symptom Improvement (SEs tolerable)	
$QIDS\text{-}C_{16} \geq 9$	Increase dose to 450 mg/day.
$QIDS\text{-}C_{16} = 6\text{-}8$	Increase dose to 450 mg/day, or Continue current dose.
$QIDS\text{-}C_{16} \leq 5$	Continue current dose.
Improved, but SEs are intolerable	Continue current dose and address SEs, or Decrease dose and continue for 2 additional weeks, or Go to the next level.
Not improved and SEs are intolerable	Go to the next level.
Return to clinic:	Return in 3 weeks.

FIGURE 21–8.   Critical decision point 3 (level 2).

CDP, Week 9	STAR⋆D Level 2: Citalopram + Bupropion XL
Symptom Improvement (SEs tolerable)	
QIDS-C$_{16}$ ≥ 9	Go to the next level
QIDS-C$_{16}$ = 6–8	Increase dose to 450 mg/day if not previously done, *or* Go to the next level
QIDS-C$_{16}$ ≤ 5	Continue current dose
SEs are intolerable	Go to the next level
Return to clinic:	Return in 3 weeks

FIGURE 21–9. Critical decision point 4 (level 2).

ciated symptoms. Given that the patient's QIDS-C$_{16}$=2 and the FIBSER remained acceptable, she was continued on prior medication dosages (Figure 21–9) and rescheduled for follow-up CDP visit in 3 weeks.

CDP 5 (Week 12)

The patient returned for her week 12 visit on time (Figure 21–10). The QIDS-C$_{16}$ was scored as a 2, the FIBSER revealed no side effects, and the patient reported 100% medication adherence. Continued remission into week 12 represents the end of acute phase treatment and signifies moving the patient into the continuation phase of treatment.

Continuation Phase

The continuation phase is the next stage in the pharmacological treatment of MDD. Classification in the continuation phase dictates that the patient achieve full remission of depressive symptoms. The current recommendation for the duration in which psychopharmacological medications are continued in this phase of treatment is a minimum of 6 to 9 months (Keller 2002). In addition to pharmacological treatments, increasing evidence supports the use of evidence-based psychotherapies in the continuation phase of treatment to reduce the risk of relapse (Hollon et al. 2005; Jarrett et al. 2001). Additionally, Fava and colleagues (2004) showed that cognitive-behavioral therapy that sequentially follows a successful course of pharmacotherapy reduces the rates of MDD relapse. With specific regard to this case, after the patient completed participation in the research study, she was referred back to her primary care physician for continued medication management, and follow-up with a cognitive therapist was arranged to help reduce the risk of relapse.

CDP, Week 12	STAR⋆D Level 2: Citalopram + Bupropion XL
Symptom Improvement (SEs tolerable)	
QIDS-C$_{16}$ ≥ 9	Go to the next level
QIDS-C$_{16}$ = 6–8	Continue current dose and go to follow-up,[1] *or* Go to the next level
QIDS-C$_{16}$ ≤ 5	Continue current dose and go to follow-up
SEs are intolerable	Go to the next level
Return to clinic:	If remitted, return in 3 months or as needed If starting new level, return in 2 weeks

FIGURE 21–10. Critical decision point 5 (level 2).

[1]Because of the severity level of some patients, clinicians may choose to keep patient on current dose and move to follow-up if at week 12 the patient has maintained a score of 6–8 on the QIDS-C$_{16}$ or if the patient does not want to change medications and/or the patient is satisfied with the level of improvement.

Personalized Treatment and Disease Self-Management

Another important component of clinical care with significant promise in the continuing treatment of MDD is counseling patients on disease self-management (Trivedi et al. 2007a). In the case described above, the patient was given a copy of the self-report QIDS-SR$_{16}$ (www.ids-qids.org) with instructions to routinely check for return or worsening of depressive symptoms and contact information for follow-up. Providing patients with the components of MBC are in line with the National Institute of Mental Health's (NIMH) new strategic initiative to target and personalize the treatment of individuals with mental illness. In the plan, Strategy 3.2 aims to "expand and deepen the focus to personalize intervention research." As a part of this strategy, it is suggested that traditional outcome measures used in clinical efficacy studies be expanded to include functional measures and "other indicators of recovery," which must include targeted symptoms and specific symptom profiles. It is hoped that this more personalized treatment will provide patients with depression and other mental illnesses with more thorough recovery.

In conclusion, MBC converges with the NIMH's initiative to personalize treatment and provides patients with education regarding their depressive illness, thereby promoting disease self-management.

Summary

Results from STAR*D indicate the majority of patients will not achieve full remission of depressive symptoms by the end of their first treatment (Trivedi et al. 2006b). On the basis of our clinical experience, determining what subsequent treatments to initiate should be done systematically while paying close attention to objective measures of symptom severity and side-effect burden. These domains constitute the treatment construct known as measurement-based care (Trivedi and Daly 2007; Trivedi et al. 2006b, 2007b). In research settings, measuring these domains is accomplished with the aid of a research assistant; however, in routine clinical practice the same can be done with a nurse or an administrative staff member. The FIBSER is a self-rated measure of side effects, and the QIDS has both a clinician

version and a self-rated version that the patient can fill out in the waiting room, with the results easily conveyed to the clinician. The primary goal of MBC is to individualize antidepressant treatment and dosing in an effort to minimize side-effect burden and maintain safety, while enhancing the therapeutic efficacy for each patient. Utilizing a treatment strategy such as MBC in clinical practice provides objective evidence to address key antidepressant treatment questions, such as: At what dose, for what duration, and when do I switch or augment? In addition, MBC can provide ongoing monitoring of symptomatic improvement and side-effect burden in the continuation and maintenance phases of treatment.

References

American Psychiatric Association: Practice guideline for the treatment of patients with major depressive disorder (revision). Am J Psychiatry 157 (suppl 4):1–45, 2000. Available at: http://www.psychiatryonline.com/pracGuide/pracGuideTopic_7.aspx. Accessed June 20, 2009

Biggs MM, Shores-Wilson K, Rush AJ, et al: A comparison of alternative assessments of depressive symptom severity: a pilot study. Psychiatry Res 96:269–279, 2000

Crismon ML, Trivedi M, Pigott TA, et al: The Texas Medication Algorithm Project: report of the Texas Consensus Conference Panel on Medication Treatment of Major Depressive Disorder. J Clin Psychiatry 60:142–156, 1999

Fava GA, Ruini C, Rafanelli C, et al: Six-year outcome of cognitive behavior therapy for prevention of recurrent depression. Am J Psychiatry 161:1872–1876, 2004

Hansen RA, Gartlehner G, Lohr KN, et al: Efficacy and safety of second-generation antidepressants in the treatment of major depressive disorder. Ann Intern Med 143:415–426, 2005

Hollon SD, DeRubeis RJ, Shelton RC, et al: Prevention of relapse following cognitive therapy vs medications in moderate to severe depression. Arch Gen Psychiatry 62:417–422, 2005

Jarrett RB, Kraft D, Doyle J, et al: Preventing recurrent depression using cognitive therapy with and without a continuation phase: a randomized clinical trial. Arch Gen Psychiatry 58:381–388, 2001

Keller MB: Long-term treatment strategies in affective disorders. Psychopharmacol Bull 36 (suppl 2):36–48, 2002

Kroenke K, Spitzer RL, Williams JB: The PHQ-9: validity of a brief depression severity measure. J Gen Intern Med 16:606–613, 2001

Paykel ES, Ramana R, Cooper Z, et al.: Residual symptoms after partial remission: an important outcome in depression. Psychol Med 25:1171–1180, 1995

Rush AJ, Trivedi MH, Ibrahim HM, et al: The 16-Item Quick Inventory of Depressive Symptomatology (QIDS), clinician rating (QIDS-C), and self-report (QIDS-SR): a psychometric evaluation in patients with chronic major depression. Biol Psychiatry 54:573–583, 2003

Rush AJ, Fava M, Wisniewski SR, et al: Sequenced Treatment Alternatives to Relieve Depression (STAR*D): rationale and design. Control Clin Trials 25:119–142, 2004

Rush AJ, Carmody TJ, Ibrahim HM, et al: Comparison of self-report and clinician ratings on two inventories of depressive symptomatology. Psychiatr Serv 57:829–837, 2006a

Rush AJ, Kraemer HC, Sackeim HA, et al: Report by the ACNP Task Force on response and remission in major depressive disorder. Neuropsychopharmacology 31:1841–1853, 2006b

Steer RA, Ball R, Ranieri WF, et al: Dimensions of the Beck Depression Inventory–II in clinically depressed outpatients. J Clin Psychol 55:117–128, 1999

Trivedi MH, Daly EJ: Measurement-based care for refractory depression: a clinical decision support model for clinical research and practice. Drug Alcohol Depend 88 (suppl 2):S61–S71, 2007

Trivedi MH, Rush AJ, Ibrahim HM, et al: The Inventory of Depressive Symptomatology, Clinician Rating (IDS-C) and Self-Report (IDS-SR), and the Quick Inventory of Depressive Symptomatology, Clinician Rating (QIDS-C) and Self-Report (QIDS-SR) in public sector patients with mood disorders: a psychometric evaluation. Psychol Med 34:73–82, 2004

Trivedi MH, Fava M, Wisniewski SR, et al: Medication augmentation after the failure of SSRIs for depression. N Engl J Med 354:1243–1252, 2006a

Trivedi MH, Rush AJ, Wisniewski SR, et al: Evaluation of outcomes with citalopram for depression using measurement-based care in STAR*D: implications for clinical practice. Am J Psychiatry 163:28–40, 2006b

Trivedi MH, Lin EH, Katon WJ: Consensus recommendations for improving adherence, self-management, and outcomes in patients with depression. CNS Spectr 12:1–27, 2007a

Trivedi MH, Rush AJ, Gaynes BN, et al: Maximizing the adequacy of medication treatment in controlled trials and clinical practice: STAR(*)D measurement-based care. Neuropsychopharmacology 32:2479–2489, 2007b

U.S. Food and Drug Administration, Center for Drug Evaluation and Research: Antidepressant use in children, adolescents and adults. March 22, 2004. Available at: http://www.fda.gov/cder/drug/antidepressants/default.htm. Accessed May 2, 2007.

Wisniewski SR, Rush AJ, Balasubramani GK, et al: Self-rated global measure of the frequency, intensity, and burden of side effects. J Psychiatr Pract 12:71–79, 2006

Major Depressive Disorder, Severe With Psychotic Features

Anthony J. Rothschild, M.D.

Setting

I practice in a psychiatry outpatient clinic at a university medical center. The majority of the patients in my practice have major depression. Although like most psychiatrists my role in the care of patients is the prescription of pharmacotherapy, I am a trained psychotherapist, and I do formal psychotherapy with some patients. Even for patients whom I see for "psychopharmacology visits," I provide some psychotherapy during our sessions (i.e., I am not just handing the patients an envelope with information and instructions as to how to take their pills).

Illustration

This study illustrates:

- Difficulty diagnosing psychotic symptoms in major depression
- Decision process involved for electroconvulsive therapy (ECT) versus medications
- Issues in continuation and maintenance therapy: risk of relapse versus medication side effects

Chief Complaint

Mr. P.W. is a 49-year-old male engineer who presents with a chief complaint of "I am very depressed." He was referred by his primary care doctor.

Present Illness

Mr. P.W. stated that about 4–5 months ago he began to feel depressed and "lost interest in life." He thought that the onset of his depression had coincided with a new supervisor at work with whom he had been having trouble getting along. He reported that he feels depressed every day for most of the day. He has lost 9 lb over the past 2 months (current weight, 161 lb), without dieting, because he did not feel like eating. He reported that he has trouble falling asleep almost every night and wakes up at 3:30 A.M. 3–4 nights a week (he normally gets up at 6:30 A.M.). He said he has had no energy for the past 2 months and that it is a struggle to get himself out of bed and to work each day. Once at work, he has trouble completing tasks and concentrating and will frequently sit at his desk and stare out the window for hours at a time. This, he believes, is part of the reason he recently received a poor quarterly performance review at work. He denied suicidal ideation presently but acknowledged that he occasionally feels like "the world would be better off if he died in his sleep." He denied ever having thought of ways to harm himself.

Other Significant Findings From Assessment

Mr. P.W. denied any previous psychiatric history. He has one brother with depression who he thinks responded to sertraline, but he does not know at what dosage. He denied any history of hypomania or mania. He has a glass of wine with dinner and has another glass of wine before he goes to bed. He has been married for 20 years, and he and his wife have two children, ages 18 and 16. He has been employed for 10 years with his current company, where he is involved with the design and production of weapons systems for the United States military. He denied drug use. He said he does not exercise. Physical examinations and the results of laboratory testing including complete blood count, electrolytes, blood urea nitrogen, creatinine, calcium, glucose, thyroid function tests, folate, and vitamin B_{12} were within normal limits. Mr. P.W.'s primary care doctor had ordered a head magnetic resonance imaging scan because Mr. P.W. had thought he had a brain tumor and insisted that a scan be done. The scan was normal. On mental status examination, Mr. P.W. was cooperative and psychomotorically retarded. He answered most questions with short answers, often simply saying "yes" or "no." He denied symptoms of paranoia or hallucinations. He reported no unusual thoughts or delusions. He was worried that his inability to concentrate and the poor performance review he received might result in his losing his job. He reported that he is still going to work.

Differential Diagnosis

Mr. P.W. meets DSM-IV-TR (American Psychiatric Association 2000a) criteria for major depressive disorder. He exhibits five (or more) symptoms of major depression (depressed mood, loss of interest or pleasure, insomnia, weight loss, trouble concentrating, loss of energy, psychomotor retardation, and thoughts of death), which have been present during the same 2-week period and represent a change from previous functioning. The symptoms are not due to a general medical condition. There is nothing in Mr. P.W.'s history to suggest he has bipolar disorder.

DSM-IV-TR Diagnosis

Axis I   Major depressive disorder, single episode, severe, without psychotic features (296.23)
Axis II   None
Axis III   None
Axis IV   Work stress
Axis V   GAF score: 55

Treatment Plan Considerations

Major Depression, Single Episode

On first assessment Mr. P.W. appears to have a fairly straightforward case of major depressive disorder. He has many symptoms, which indicates that this is a severe episode. His depressive symptoms appear to have affected his ability to function particularly at work. However, he is still going to work. He does not have suicidal ideation at initial assessment and has no active plans for suicide.

Because he is not actively suicidal, homicidal, or psychotic and is still going to work, hospitalization is not indicated, and I decide to treat him as an outpatient. According to the American Psychiatric Association's current practice guideline for the treatment of patients with major depressive disorder (American Psychiatric Association 2000b), in the acute phase the psychiatrist may choose between several initial treatment modalities, including pharmacotherapy, psychotherapy, the combination of medications plus psychotherapy, or ECT. Given that this is Mr. P.W.'s first episode of depression and that he is not actively suicidal or psychotic, I do not believe that ECT is indicated. According to the guideline, because he meets criteria for a severe episode of major depressive disorder Mr. P.W. should be prescribed medication unless he is receiving ECT. I discuss with him the options of medication, psychotherapy, or the combination, and he declines psychotherapy because he feels he does not have enough time or interest to pursue it. He would like to be treated with an antidepressant.

Normally I would review with the patient the previous antidepressant trials received, whether the patient had responded, and whether he or she experienced any side effects. In the case of Mr. P.W., he has never been treated with an antidepressant, so in theory one could prescribe any number of possible antidepressants. However, because he reported that his brother had responded to sertraline, I suggest that he should try sertraline as well. Although there is no firm evidence that if a first-degree relative has responded to a particular antidepressant, it is more likely that the patient will respond as well, in my experience it does seem to increase the likelihood of a response, perhaps just for psychological reasons. Therefore, after reviewing the possible side effects of sertraline with Mr. P.W. and discussing with him how to take the medication, I prescribe sertraline

50 mg/day to be taken in the morning. I advise him to give me a phone call in 3–4 days to report how he is tolerating the medication and have him schedule an appointment to see me again in 10 days.

Treatment Goals, Measures, and Methods

The initial goal for Mr. P.W. is to be able to tolerate the antidepressant medication so he can stay on it long enough to have an antidepressant response. That is the first goal, and it is an important one given that noncompliance with antidepressant medication is a big problem (Melfi et al. 1998). That is one of the reasons I ask patients to call me a few days after starting the medication. Another reason is to make sure that the patient's illness is not getting worse. I will also be monitoring Mr. P.W.'s depressive symptoms with the Hamilton Rating Scale for Depression (Ham-D; Hamilton 1960). In some situations I may formally administer the scale; in others, I ask the same questions that are on the scale during my clinical interview. For Mr. P.W., I will use the Ham-D.

Course

Phone Call (Day 4)

Mr. P.W. calls to report that he has had no side effects from the medication. He also reports that he called in sick to work today because he did not have the energy to get out of bed but plans to go to work tomorrow.

Visit 2 (10 Days)

Mr. P.W. returns for his second visit accompanied by his wife. She asks if she can speak to me. With Mr. P.W.'s permission, she joins the beginning of the appointment. Mr. P.W. reports that he is unchanged and still feels depressed. He again denies symptoms of hallucinations, suicidal ideation, or unusual thoughts, and no delusions are noted. At this point, his wife urges him to "Tell Dr. Rothschild about the car across the street," whereupon the patient described a parked car that he believed contained FBI agents on a stakeout who were following him everywhere he went. The patient then explained a rather detailed delusional system that he was being targeted as part of an investigation of a foreign country's attempt to purchase military secrets. Although this was seemingly plausible given his line of work, his wife reported that neither her husband nor her

husband's company worked on classified information requiring a security clearance and, in any case, the cars he was worried about belonged to neighbors. Mr. P.W. had answered in the negative to questions regarding paranoia and unusual thoughts, because to him, the delusional system was "real" and was not an example of unusual thoughts or a reflection of paranoia.

Revised DSM-IV-TR Assessment

After the second visit with the patient and his wife, it became clear that Mr. P.W. had major depressive disorder, single episode, severe with psychotic features (296.24). When I presented my reassessment to Mr. P.W., he was adamant that I was mistaken. In part, this was because the word "psychotic" was frightening to him, and I think it had pejorative connotations for him. Thus I have found using the term "irrational worries" instead of "psychosis" more acceptable to patients and have found its use to result in a greater likelihood of patients telling me what is on their mind (Rothschild 2009). Mr. P.W. felt better with this description of his illness. He, himself, began to refer to his illness as major depressive disorder with "irrational worries."

Axis I	Major depressive disorder, single episode, severe with psychotic features (296.24)
Axis II	None
Axis III	None
Axis IV	Work stress
Axis V	GAF score: 55

Additional Treatment Plan Considerations

Mr. P.W.'s main problem is major depression with psychotic features (psychotic depression), a serious illness during which a person has the dangerous combination of depressed mood and psychosis, with the psychosis commonly manifesting itself as nihilistic delusions that "bad things are about to happen." The American Psychiatric Association's practice guideline for the treatment of patients with major depressive disorder (American Psychiatric Association 2000b) recommends, with substantial clinical confidence, the use of either ECT or the combination of an antipsychotic and an antidepressant for the treatment of psychotic depression. Several algorithms have recently been proposed, incorporating the current evidence base, to help guide the clinician in the use of somatic treatments for psychotic depression (Hamoda and Osser 2008; Rothschild 2009). Mr. P.W. and his wife were concerned about possible side effects of confusion and memory disruption from ECT and stated that they preferred medication treatment. Because Mr. P.W. was not suicidal, and his current clinical situation was not life threatening, I agreed with their preference for a trial of medication (for further discussion of the decision-making process when deciding between ECT and medications for psychotic depression, see Rothschild 2009).

Of the two recently published algorithms, I followed my own (it is never a good thing not to follow your own published guidelines!), which is based on the evidence base of randomized controlled clinical trials. In the algorithm I point out that there are four combinations of antidepressant plus antipsychotic medications that have been studied and shown to be effective in randomized controlled clinical trials in patients with psychotic depression. These include sertraline plus olanzapine (Meyers et al. 2009; 259 subjects), fluoxetine plus olanzapine (Rothschild et al. 2004; 249 subjects), venlafaxine plus quetiapine (Wijkstra et al. 2008; 122 subjects), and amitriptyline plus perphenazine (Spiker et al. 1985; 51 subjects). Other combinations of antidepressants and antipsychotics have not been studied in randomized controlled clinical trials. After discussion with Mr. P.W. (and, with his permission, his wife), we decided to treat him with a trial of sertraline plus olanzapine. We also decided to dose the medication aggressively, as was done in the National Institute of Mental Health Study of the Pharmacotherapy of Psychotic Depression (STOP-PD; Meyers et al. 2009). The daily dosages of medications in the STOP-PD study (Meyers et al. 2009) were as follows:

1. Initial dosages of 50 mg sertraline/placebo and 5 mg of olanzapine as tolerated
2. Increase the dosage of sertraline/placebo by 50 mg/day and of olanzapine by 5 mg/day every 3 days as tolerated
3. Attempt to achieve minimum dosages of 100 mg/day of sertraline/placebo and 10 mg/day of olanzapine by the end of week 1

4. Increase dosages to 150 mg/day of sertraline/placebo and 15 mg/day of olanzapine during week 2
5. Allow dosages of 200 mg/day of sertraline/placebo and 20 mg/day of olanzapine for residual symptoms beginning in week 3

Because Mr. P.W. is already taking 50 mg/day of sertraline, I advise him to increase the dosage of sertraline to 100 mg/day for 3 days and then to take 150 mg/day. I also start him on olanzapine 5 mg at bedtime (after reviewing possible side effects) and advise him to increase the dosage to 10 mg at bedtime after 3 days. I plan to see him back in 7 days but instruct him to contact me before the appointment if he has trouble tolerating the medications or if his symptoms worsen.

In addition to the pharmacotherapy, I plan to use psychoeducational/cognitive therapy. I use a modified version of cognitive-behavioral therapy based in large part on the work of Gaudiano et al. (2007).

I also advise Mr. P.W. to take a leave of absence from work. This is in part due to the fact that his delusional system involves work. In addition, Mr. P.W. himself admits that he is having trouble functioning and concentrating at work and agrees that a leave of absence is a good idea. He will use accumulated sick time.

Treatment Goals, Measures, and Methods

Table 22–1 outlines my initial treatment goals, measures, and methods.

The initial goal for Mr. P.W. is for him to be able to tolerate the antidepressant and antipsychotic medication combination. In my experience, the psychotic symptoms in psychotically depressed patients can improve quickly, whereas the depressive symptoms may take considerably longer to improve. In the psychotically depressed patient, one can monitor the psychotic symptoms with the Brief Psychiatric Rating Scale (BPRS; Overall and Gorham 1962) and the Delusional Assessment Scale (DAS; Meyers et al. 2006); I will continue to monitor the depressive symptoms with the Ham-D. As mentioned earlier, in some situations I may formally administer the scales, whereas in other situations I ask the same questions that are on the scales during my clinical interview. For Mr. P.W., I will use the Ham-D and the BPRS.

Although the person with an episode of psychotic depression can expect to make a full recovery and re-

TABLE 22–1.   Initial treatment goals, measures, and methods

Treatment goal	Measure	Method
Eliminate psychotic symptoms within 10 days	Brief Psychiatric Rating Scale, self-report, probing questions	Pharmacotherapy
Reduce depressive symptoms by 50% or more by 8 weeks	Hamilton Rating Scale for Depression, self-report	Pharmacotherapy Cognitive-behavioral therapy/ psychoeducation
Reduce stress at work	Self-report	Pharmacotherapy (delusional re: work) Use sick time until no longer delusional Return part-time at first Return full-time

turn to full occupational and social functioning in the community, how soon that will happen is highly variable. Some patients will respond quickly to treatment, with fast resolution of depressive and psychotic symptoms, whereas others may have only partial improvement in symptoms, with a significant period of time elapsing until full recovery (Rothschild 2009). In my experience, the patient who is likely to return to full social and occupational functioning quickly is someone who meets the following criteria: first episode, a good response to the somatic treatment prescribed (whether pharmacotherapy or ECT), age between 30 and 65 years, and good premorbid functioning (Rothschild 2009). Mr. P.W. meets several of the criteria for someone likely to have a full recovery quickly.

His Ham-D score is 30, and his BPRS score is 55.

Course (Continued)

Visit 3 (17 Days)

Mr. P.W. reports that he is feeling better. He reports no side effects from the medication. He says he is "no longer concerned about the men in the cars." He states that they are still present across the street, but they are "no longer that interested" in him. I consider this improvement. Although he is still delusional, the "delusions," according to Mr. P.W., are losing interest in him. He reports no change in his depressive symptoms. His Ham-D score is 28, and his BPRS score is 40. I advise him to keep the sertraline at 150 mg/day in the morning and increase the olanzapine to 15 mg at bedtime.

I was torn between holding the olanzapine at 10 mg/day and making the increase to 15 mg/day. An argument for staying at 10 mg/day is that he is

improving, whereas arguments for advancing to 15 mg/day include the following:

1. He is still psychotic.
2. The STOP-PD study used 15 mg/day of olanzapine as a target (Meyers et al. 2009).
3. Other studies of psychotic depression that used olanzapine in combination with an antidepressant had a mean dosage of olanzapine between 12.4 and 13.9 mg/day (Rothschild et al. 2004).
4. The serious morbidity and mortality of psychotic depression requires more aggressive treatment.

Visit 4 (24 Days)

Mr. P.W. reports that he has continued to improve. He reports no side effects from the medication except he experienced some morning drowsiness for a few days after the olanzapine was increased to 15 mg/day. He reports no change in appetite or weight. He reports that the "men in the cars" still occasionally drive by his house, but they appear to be doing so less frequently, and he believes they are "losing interest" in him. He still reports a number of depressive symptoms and still feels sad. He is sleeping well. He still has no appetite. His Ham-D score is 16, and his BPRS score is 32. He worries that his poor performance at work and his current leave of absence may cost him his job. He would like to return to work. I advise him that it is still premature to return to work and that it could be counterproductive for him to return to work before he is well. I reassure him that he will get better and that his improvement to date is a good prognostic sign. I advise him to continue his medications at sertraline 150 mg in the morning and olanzapine 15 mg at bedtime.

Visit 5 (31 Days)

For the first time since I have been seeing him, I notice that Mr. P.W. smiles appropriately. He is not aware of this (in my experience, seeing a depressed person smile for the first time when they had not done so before is frequently a harbinger of future improvement). He feels only mildly depressed. No delusional thinking is noted on examination. He says that the people watching him are "gone." His Ham-D score is 11 and his BPRS score is 25. He complains that he has gained 2 lb since he last weighed himself (2 weeks ago) and says that he is eating more. He is concerned that the weight gain is related to his medication. I point out to him that although it is possible that his increased appetite and weight gain are related to the medication, he did lose 9 lb in the 2 months prior to coming to see me and that the increased appetite and weight gain may be related to the improvement in his depression. We will continue to monitor his weight. He again asks about returning to work. I advise that I would prefer to see him have at least another week (2 weeks in total) of no serious depressive symptoms and no "irrational worries." I suggested to him that he contact his supervisor as to whether he could return part-time in about 9–10 days from today (after our next appointment). I also advise continuation of his current medication regimen of sertraline 150 mg/day in the morning and olanzapine 15 mg/day at bedtime.

Phone Call (40 Days)

I receive a phone call from Mr. P.W.'s wife to let me know that he appears to be back to "his old self."

Visit 6 (41 Days)

Improvement has continued. Mr. P.W. denies depression. When I ask about the men in the cars across the street he looks at me with a surprised look and says, "I now know that I had those thoughts because I was ill. I cannot believe I thought that." We then discuss the delusional thoughts, "the irrational worries," he had experienced. It becomes very clear that Mr. P.W. is having a very hard time reconciling that he has had these thoughts. This is a very good sign. When a patient with psychotic depression has insight that the unusual thoughts were part of the illness and almost has a cognitive dissonance that they had once believed them, I am confident that they are in the process of making a full recovery. His Ham-D

score is 9, and his BPRS score is 21. Mr. P.W. reports that his supervisor said he could return to work with a note from me. I write a note stating that he can return to work at 50% time for 1 week and full-time after that. (My plan was to see Mr. P.W. again after he had been back at work part-time for 1 week before deciding whether he was ready to return full-time.) I advise continuation of his current medication regimen of sertraline 150 mg/day in the morning and olanzapine 15 mg/day at bedtime.

Visit 7 (Week 9)

Mr. P.W. reports that his week back at work went well and that his supervisor would like him to return to work full-time. He denies any symptoms of depression. His Ham-D score is 7. No delusions are noted on examination. His BPRS score is 20. He complains again about increased appetite and weight gain. Now up to 170 lb, Mr. P.W. has gained 9 lb since I began treating him and is back to his starting weight before he was depressed. I reassure him that we will continue to monitor his weight. I write him a note to return to work full-time. He is to continue on sertraline 150 mg/day in the morning and olanzapine 15 mg/day at bedtime.

Visit 8 (Week 13)

Mr. P.W. is doing well. Work is also going well. He has had no depressive or psychotic symptoms. His Ham-D score is 7, and his BPRS score is 20. His weight is 172 lb.

Visit 9 (Week 17)

He is still doing well. Work is also still going well. No depressive or psychotic symptoms. His Ham-D score is 7, and his BPRS score is 20. His weight is 173 lb.

Visit 10 (Week 21)

He is still doing well. Work is also still going well. No depressive or psychotic symptoms. His Ham-D score is 7, and his BPRS score is 20. His weight is 174 lb.

Visit 11 (Week 25)

He is still doing well. Work is also still going well. No depressive or psychotic symptoms. His Ham-D score is 7, and his BPRS score is 20. His weight is 174 lb.

Visit 12 (Week 29)

He is still doing well. Work is also still going well. No depressive or psychotic symptoms. His Ham-D score is 7, and his BPRS score is 20. His weight is 176 lb. At this point, Mr. P.W. has gained 6 lb above his premorbid weight of 170 lb and has been stable psychiatrically for at least 4 months. Based on studies of the continuation and maintenance treatment of psychotic depression (Rothschild 2009), it has been my practice to leave a patient on the combination of the antidepressant/antipsychotic to which he or she responded to for 4 months. After 4 months, if the patient has continued to remain in remission, I begin a gradual taper of the antipsychotic medication, leaving the patient on the antidepressant. If the patient is having significant side effects (e.g., signs of tardive dyskinesia with an older antipsychotic medication or metabolic syndrome symptoms with a newer antipsychotic agent), I may start the taper earlier than 4 months. On the other hand, if the patient is not having any side effects, and/or is still symptomatic, I may delay the taper of the antipsychotic medication beyond 4 months. I usually will leave the patient on the antidepressant indefinitely, given the high rate of relapse in psychotic depression and the significant morbidity and mortality associated with relapses. Given Mr. P.W.'s current stability for at least 4 months and gradual weight gain, I begin a gradual taper of the olanzapine by 5 mg every 4 weeks. He is to remain on sertraline at 150 mg/day.

Visit 13 (Week 33)

He is still doing well. Work is also still going well. No depressive or psychotic symptoms. He is taking olanzapine 10 mg/day and sertraline 150 mg/day. His Ham-D score is 7, and his BPRS score is 20. His weight is 175 lb.

Visit 14 (Week 37)

He is still doing well. Work is also still going well. No depressive or psychotic symptoms. He is taking olanzapine 5 mg/day and sertraline 150 mg/day. His Ham-D score is 7, and his BPRS score is 20. His weight is 174 lb.

Visit 15 (Week 41)

Mr. P.W. is now taking just sertraline 150 mg/day. He is doing well, and work is going well. No depressive or psychotic symptoms. His Ham-D score is 7, and his BPRS score is 20. His weight is 173 lb.

Visit 16 (Week 46)

Mr. P.W. continues on sertraline 150 mg/day. He is doing well, and work is going well. No depressive or psychotic symptoms. His Ham-D score is 7, and his BPRS score is 20. His weight is 172 lb.

Summary of Guideline Use

I followed the practice guidelines for treatment of the patient with psychotic depression, which recommend either the combination of an antidepressant and an antipsychotic or ECT (American Psychiatric Association 2000b; Hamoda and Osser 2008; Rothschild 2009). A delay in the implementation of these guidelines occurred when the diagnosis of psychotic depression was initially missed because PW's delusional thinking was not readily apparent. This, unfortunately, is a not an infrequent occurrence (Rothschild et al. 2008), even among experts.

Ways to Improve Practice

In reviewing my practice, I could have improved the care of Mr. P.W. by detecting his psychotic features earlier. Had I asked more probing questions or involved his wife earlier, I might have learned earlier about his paranoid delusional thoughts.

I now refer to delusional thinking with my depressed patients as "irrational worries" and find that my patients have an easier time accepting this concept than "psychotic thinking." This then results in their feeling more comfortable about telling me what is worrying them and what is on their mind.

References

American Psychiatric Association: Diagnostic and Statistical Manual of Mental Disorders, 4th Edition, Text Revision. Washington, DC, American Psychiatric Association, 2000a

American Psychiatric Association: Practice guideline for the treatment of patients with major depressive disorder, 2nd edition, in Practice Guidelines for the Treatment of Psychiatric Disorders, Compendium. Washington, DC, American Psychiatric Association, 2006, pp 763–840

Gaudiano BA, Miller IW, Hebert JD: The treatment of psychotic major depression: is there a role for adjunctive psychotherapy? Psychother Psychosom 76:271–277, 2007

Hamilton M: A rating scale for depression. J Neurol Neurosurg Psychiatry 23:56–62, 1960

Hamoda HM, Osser DN: The psychopharmacology algorithm project at the Harvard South Shore Program: an update on psychotic depression. Harv Rev Psychiatry 16:235–247, 2008

Melfi CA, Chawla AJ, Croghan TW, et al: The effects of adherence to antidepressant treatment: guidelines on relapse and recurrence of depression. Arch Gen Psychiatry 55:1128–1132, 1998

Meyers B, English J, Gabriele M, et al: A delusion assessment scale for psychotic major depression: reliability, validity and utility. Biol Psychiatry 60:1336–1342, 2006

Meyers BS, Flint AJ, Rothschild AJ, et al: A double-blind randomized controlled trial of olanzapine plus sertraline vs olanzapine plus placebo for psychotic depression: the Study of Pharmacotherapy of Psychotic Depression (STOP-PD). Arch Gen Psychiatry 66:838–847, 2009

Overall JE, Gorham DE: The Brief Psychiatric Rating Scale. Psychol Rep 10:799–812, 1962

Rothschild AJ (ed): Clinical Manual for the Diagnosis and Treatment of Psychotic Depression. Washington, DC, American Psychiatric Publishing, 2009

Rothschild AJ, Williamson DJ, Tohen MF, et al: A double-blind, randomized study of olanzapine and olanzapine/fluoxetine combination for major depression with psychotic features. J Clin Psychopharmacol 24:365–373, 2004

Rothschild AJ, Winer J, Fratoni S, et al: Missed diagnosis of psychotic depression at 4 academic medical centers. J Clin Psychiatry 69:1293–1296, 2008

Spiker DG, Weiss JC, Dealy RS, et al: The pharmacological treatment of delusional depression. Am J Psychiatry 142:430–436, 1985

Wijkstra JJ, Burger, D, van den Broek WW, et al: Pharmacological treatment of psychotic depression: a randomized, double-blind study comparing imipramine, venlafaxine and venlafaxine plus quetiapine. Presented at the annual meeting of the American Psychiatric Association, Washington, DC, May 2008

Patient and Family Resources

Families for Depression Awareness (www.familyaware .org)

Rothschild AJ (ed): Clinical Manual for the Diagnosis and Treatment of Psychotic Depression. Washington, DC, American Psychiatric Publishing, 2009

23

Acute Bipolar Depression

Po W. Wang, M.D.
Terence A. Ketter, M.D.

Setting

The patient was seen in an academic outpatient practice setting. The surrounding population is of high educational attainment and upper socio-economic status and ethnically diverse. The patient population is sophisticated in their approach to accessing Internet-based information. The treatment strategy used was evidence-based pharmacotherapy with a combination of psychoeducation and cognitive-behavioral therapy (CBT).

Illustration

This study illustrates:

- Importance of differentiating bipolar from unipolar depression
- Use of standardized clinical monitoring forms
- Use of medication tracking forms
- Use of standardized adverse effects monitoring and tracking
- Use of standardized mood severity ratings
- Application of guideline-based treatment for bipolar depression
- Integrating manualized psychoeducation
- Application of manualized CBT

Chief Complaint

Ms. M.S. is a 28-year-old married Caucasian woman who reports a long history of "mood swings" since adolescence and presents with treatment-resistant

depression. She arrives for the evaluation with her husband.

Present Illness

The patient reported depressive episodes manifested by depressed mood and anhedonia with social isolation. Despite sleeping 10–14 hours per night, she has low energy and psychomotor retardation during the day. Each of these symptoms meets DSM-IV-TR (American Psychiatric Association 2000) criteria for being pervasively present nearly all day and nearly every day over at least the past 2 weeks prior to her presentation to the clinic. Appetite has increased, but without significant weight gain. She has had thoughts of suicide at times during the week but not any plans or intentions to end her life. She has ruminated on her poor performance in school, past failed relationships, and current financial difficulties. In addition, she has had anxiety with palpitations and mild tremors sporadically, but no shortness of breath, diaphoresis, or nausea. The current episode is 3 weeks in duration. A completed Clinical Monitoring Form is shown in Figure 23–1A.

These episodes began in elementary school, as far as Ms. M.S. could recall. In the past, these episodes ranged in duration from 2 to 4 weeks, followed by 2 to 4 weeks during which her mood returned to a baseline level of poor self-esteem and sleeping 9–10 hours per night, but with good function in school, relationships, and work. Her mood would continuously alternate between these two states of low self-

Clinical Monitoring: Treatment and Symptoms

Date **A** / __ / __

Name: **M.S.** _____ ID# __ __ - __ __ - __ __ __ __ Others: _____ Physician: **PW** CPT code ____ Visit Type: ____

Over the past 10 days, how many days have you been/had . . .

	days	Severity (0-4)	DSM Criteria	DSM Criteria Satisfied		
				No	Probable	Definite
... depressed **most of day**:	**100**%	**3**	Depressed most of the day nearly every day for ≥2wk			**X**
... less interest in **most** activities or found you **couldn't enjoy even pleasurable activities** through **most of the day**:	**100**%	**3**	Decreased interest or diminished pleasure in most activities most of the day nearly every day for ≥2wks			**X**
... **any period of** abnormal mood elevation	**0**%	**0**	Mood Elevation (high, euphoric, expansive) to a significant degree over a 4 - 7 day period	**X**		
... **any period of** abnormal irritability	**30**%	**3**	Irritability to a significant degree over a 4 -7 day period	**X**		
... **any** abnormal anxiety	**100**%	**2**				

Rate Associated Symptoms for PAST WEEK

Much more **+2** —— **0** —— **-2** Much less
0= usual/none

MDE
requires ≥ 5
(including depressed mood and/or interest)

Depression	Sleep	Interest	Guilt / SE	Energy	Conc / Distr	Appetite	PMR / PMA	SI
+1	**+1**	**-1**	**+1** or **-1**	**-1**	**-1** or **+1/2**	**+1/2**	**+1** or **+1/2**	**+1/2**

Sleeps **10-14** hours **+** EBT **+** DFA **▪** MCA **▪** EMA **+** DGOOB **▪** Naps **+** anhedonia **+** LNWL **▪** Passive **▪** Active

Elevation
Mania/hypomania requires ≥ 3 unless only irritable, then ≥ 4 moderate sxs are required (do not count elevation or irritability) toward dx of hypomania or mania

Increased Self Esteem	Decreased Need for sleep	Talking	FOI/Racing thoughts	Distractible	Goal directed activity /PMA	High Risk Behavior
0	**0**	**0**	**0**	**+1/2**	**0** or **+1/2**	**0**

Y **(N)** New major stressor, if yes _____

Y **(N)** Substance abuse ____ d-use/wk   **4** c/d caffeine   **0** ppd nicotine   Onset of menses **03** / **04** / ____ early late **(NA)**

Y **(N)** Alcohol abuse ____ d/wk   **(Y)** N Headache   **(Y)** N Binge/Purge   Y **(N)** Additional Psych tx: OP ER Hosp

    (Y) N Migraine   Y **(N)** Panic attacks   Y **(N)** Additional Gen Med tx: OP ER Hosp

Y **(N)** Significant Medical illness , if yes _____   Actual / Reported **Weight**: __**160**____

Current Treatments

	Dose Mg 24 total	Mg Missed Past 7 days		Dose Mg 24 total	Mg Missed Past 7 days
Bimodal Agents					
Anxiolytics/Hypnotics					
Antidepressants					
Dopamine Blockers					
			Imitrex	PRN **1 tab** x **3**	
				PRN x	

Adverse Effects

	Severity 0-4
Tremor	**0**
Dry Mouth	**1**
Sedation	**0**
Constipation	**0**
Diarrhea	**0**
Headache	**2**
Poor Memory	**2**
Sexual Dysfunction	**0**
Increased Appetite	**0**
Rash	**0**
Nausea	**1**

Selected Mental Status	Severity 0-4	
PI **0**	IOR **0**	OC **0**
Hallucinations **0**	Delusions **0**	

Last Labs	Date / /
Li = __	VPA= __ TSH= __
Creat= __	

Current Clinical Status (check one)
X Depression ___ Continued Sx
___ Hypomania ___ Recovering
___ Mania ___ Recovered
___ Mixed* ___ Roughening

If new episode, estimate onset date: / /
Other Dx: _____

CGI **5** GAF **45** GAF **45**
(1-7) week (0-90) month (0-90)

Psychosocial Interventions **0** /mo ECT ___ /mo Other ___ /mo   EPS ____ **0**
Yes No Significant Noncompliance, if yes

Comments: **28 yo MWF with BD-II, currently in MDE, with rapid cycling course of illness.
Discussed history, diagnosis, and treatment options (LTG, QTP) with pt.
Discussed dermatology precautions with pt.
Discussed mood charting, psychotherapy, collaborative care model.**

Plan: **LTG starter pack.
Referral to CBT therapist.**

RTC **2 weeks**

Signature _____

FIGURE 23–1. Clinical monitoring form–representative time points (A).

A, Initial intake. B, Four weeks after starting lamotrigine. C, Regular follow-up visit during 2½ years of euthymic mood.
D, Subsyndromal mood elevation during euthymic mood period.

Clinical Monitoring: Treatment and Symptoms

Date **B**/ __ / __

Name: __**M.S.**__   ID# __ __ __ - __ - __ __ __ __ __   Others: _____   Physician: __**PW**__ CPT code ____   Visit Type: _____

Over the past 10 days, how many days have you been/had . . .

	% days	Severity (0-4)	DSM Criteria	No	Probable	Definite
				DSM Criteria Satisfied		
... depressed **most of day**:	**100**%	**3**	Depressed most of the day nearly every day for ≥2wk	__	__	**X**
... less interest in **most** activities or found you **couldn't enjoy even pleasurable activities** through **most of the day**:	**100**%	**2**	Decreased interest or diminished pleasure in most activities most of the day nearly every day for ≥2wks	__	__	**X**
... **any period of** abnormal mood elevation	**0**%	**0**	Mood Elevation (high, euphoric, expansive) to a significant degree over a 4 - 7 day period	**X**	__	__
... **any period of** abnormal irritability	**10** %	**2**	Irritability to a significant degree over a 4 -7 day period	**X**	__	__
... **any** abnormal anxiety	**80**%	**2**				

Rate Associated Symptoms for PAST WEEK

Much more +2 —— **0** —— -2 Much less
0= usual/none

MDE
requires ≥ 5
(including depressed mood and/or interest)

Depression	Sleep	Interest	Guilt / SE	Energy	Conc / Distr	Appetite	PMR / PMA	SI
+1	**0**	**-1**	**0** or **-1/2**	**-1/2**	**-1/2** or **0**	**0**	**+1/2** or **0**	**0**

Sleeps **8** - **9** hours ▪EBT ▪DFA ▪MCA ▪EMA ▪DGOOB ▪Naps **+** anhedonia ▪ LNWL ▪ Passive ▪ Active

Elevation

Mania/hypomania requires ≥ 3 unless only irritable, then ≥ 4 moderate sxs are required (do not count elevation or irritability) toward dx of hypomania or mania

Increased Self Esteem	Decreased Need for sleep	Talking	FOI/Racing thoughts	Distractible	Goal directed activity /PMA	High Risk Behavior
0	**0**	**0**	**0**	**0**	**0** or **0**	**0**

Y (N) New major stressor, if yes _____

Y (N) Substance abuse ____ d-use/wk   **2** c/d **caffeine**   **0** ppd **nicotine**   Onset of menses **04** / **02** / ____ early late (NA)

Y (N) Alcohol abuse ____ d/wk   (Y) N Headache   Y (N) Binge/Purge   (Y) N Additional Psych tx: (OP) ER Hosp

(Y) N Migraine   Y (N) Panic attacks   Y (N) Additional Gen Med tx: OP ER Hosp

Y (N) Significant Medical illness , if yes   Actual / Reported **Weight:** __**160**__

Current Treatments / Adverse Effects

Bimodal Agents	Dose Mg 24 total	Mg Missed Past 7 days		Dose Mg 24 total	Mg Missed Past 7 days	**Adverse Effects** Severity 0-4	
Lamictal	**200**	**0**				Tremor	**0**
Anxiolytics/Hypnotics						Dry Mouth	**1**
						Sedation	**0**
Antidepressants						Constipation	**0**
						Diarrhea	**0**
Dopamine Blockers						Headache	**2**
				Imitrex	PRN **1 tab** x 1	Poor Memory	**0**
					PRN ___ x	Sexual Dysfunction	**0**
						Increased Appetite	**0**
						Rash	**0**
						Nausea	**0**
						Hair loss	**1**

Selected Mental Status Severity 0-4
PI **0**   IOR **0**   OC **0**
Hallucinations **0**   Delusions **0**

Last Labs   Date / /
Li = ____   VPA= ____   TSH= ____
Creat= ____

Current Clinical Status (check one)
__ Depression   __ Continued Sx
__ Hypomania   **X** Recovering
__ Mania   __ Recovered
__ Mixed*   __ Roughening
If new episode, estimate onset date: / /
Other Dx: _____

Psychosocial Interventions **4**/mo ECT ___/mo Other _____/mo
Yes (No) Significant Noncompliance, if yes

EPS ____ **0**

CGI **3** GAF **65** GAF **55**
(1-7) week (0-90) month (0-90)

Comments: 28 yo MWF with BD-II - MDE, with rapid cycling course of illness. Improvement noted by family and therapist; pt endorses on prompting. Tolerated LTG titration.

Started weekly CBT therapy.

Plan: Meds status quo.

RTC 4 weeks

© Gary Sachs, MD 2005   _____ Signature

FIGURE 23–1.   Clinical monitoring form–representative time points (B).

A, Initial intake. **B,** Four weeks after starting lamotrigine. C, Regular follow-up visit during 2½ years of euthymic mood. D, Subsyndromal mood elevation during euthymic mood period.

Clinical Monitoring: Treatment and Symptoms

Date **C** / __ / __

Name: **M.S.** _____ ID# __ __ - __ __ - __ __ __ __ Others: _____ Physician: **PW** CPT code ____ Visit Type: _____

Over the past 10 days, how many days have you been/had . . .

	% days	Severity (0-4)	DSM Criteria	DSM Criteria Satisfied		
				No	Probable	Definite
… depressed **most of day:**	**0**%	**0**	Depressed most of the day nearly every day for $\geq$2wk	**X**	__	__
… less interest in **most** activities or found you **couldn't enjoy even pleasurable activities** through most of the day:	**0**%	**0**	Decreased interest or diminished pleasure in most activities most of the day nearly every day for $\geq$2wks	**X**	__	__
… **any period of** abnormal mood elevation	**0**%	**0**	Mood Elevation (high, euphoric, expansive) to a significant degree over a 4 - 7 day period	**X**	__	__
… **any period of** abnormal irritability	**0**%	**0**	Irritability to a significant degree over a 4 -7 day period	**X**	__	__
… **any** abnormal anxiety	**20**%	**2**				

Rate Associated Symptoms for PAST WEEK   Much more **+2** ——— **0** ——— **-2** Much less
                                                              0= usual/none

MDE	Depression	Sleep	Interest	Guilt / SE	Energy	Conc / Distr	Appetite	PMR / PMA	SI
requires $\geq$ 5 (including depressed mood and/or interest)	**0**	**0**	**0**	**0** or **0**	**-1/2**	**-1/2** or **0**	**0**	**0** or **0**	**0**

Sleeps **8 - 9** hours   ▪ EBT _ DFA ▪MCA ▪ EMA   **+** DGOOB ▪ Naps   ▪ anhedonia   ▪ LNWL ▪ Passive ▪ Active

Elevation
Mania/hypomania requires $\geq$ 3 unless only irritable, then $\geq$ 4 moderate sxs are required (do not count elevation or irritability) toward dx of hypomania or mania

Increased Self Esteem	Decreased Need for sleep	Talking	FOI/Racing thoughts	Distractible	Goal directed activity /PMA	High Risk Behavior
0	**0**	**0**	**0**	**0**	**0** or **0**	**0**

Y Ⓝ New major stressor, if yes _____

Y Ⓝ Substance abuse ____ d-use/wk   **2** c/d caffeine   **0** ppd nicotine   Onset of menses **07**/ **24**/ ____ early late ⓃⒶ

Y Ⓝ Alcohol abuse ____ d/wk   Ⓨ N Headache   Y Ⓝ Binge/Purge   Ⓨ N Additional Psych tx: ⓄⓅ ER Hosp

                                          Y Ⓝ Migraine   Y Ⓝ Panic attacks   Ⓨ N Additional Gen Med tx: OP ⒺⓇ Hosp
Ⓨ N Significant Medical illness , if yes ___**UTI**_____   Actual / Reported **Weight: 160**

Current Treatments / Adverse Effects

Bimodal Agents	Dose Mg 24 total	Mg Missed Past 7 days		Dose Mg 24 total	Mg Missed Past 7 days	Adverse Effects Severity 0-4	
Lamictal	**200**	**0**	**Cipro**	**1000**	**500**	Tremor	**0**
Anxiolytics/Hypnotics						Dry Mouth	**1**
						Sedation	**0**
						Constipation	**0**
Antidepressants						Diarrhea	**0**
						Headache	**2**
						Poor Memory	**0**
Dopamine Blockers						Sexual Dysfunction	**0**
						Increased Appetite	**0**
			Imitrex	PRN **1 tab** x **0**		Rash	**0**
				PRN x		Nausea	**0**

Selected Mental Status Severity 0-4
PI **0**   IOR **0**   OC **0**
Hallucinations **0**   Delusions **0**

Last Labs   Date / /
Li = ___   VPA= ___   TSH= ___
Creat= ___

Current Clinical Status (check one)
__ Depression   __ Continued Sx
__ Hypomania   __ Recovering
__ Mania   **X** Recovered
__ Mixed*   __ Roughening

— If new episode, estimate onset date: / /
— Other Dx: _____

Psychosocial Interventions **4**/mo ECT ___/mo Other _____ ___/mo
Yes Ⓝⓞ Significant Noncompliance, if yes _____

EPS_____ **0**

CGI **2** GAF **75** GAF **75**
(1-7)   week (0-90) month (0-90)

Comments: **28 yo MWF with BD-II – recovered since May.**

Plan: **Meds status quo. Use CBT for residual anxiety.**

RTC **2-3 months**

Signature _____

FIGURE 23–1.   Clinical monitoring form–representative time points (C).

A, Initial intake. B, Four weeks after starting lamotrigine. **C,** Regular follow-up visit during 2½ years of euthymic mood. D, Subsyndromal mood elevation during euthymic mood period.

Clinical Monitoring: Treatment and Symptoms

Date **D** / **09**/ **12**

Name: **M.S.** ID#_ _ _ - _ _ - _ _ _ _ _ Others:_____ Physician: **PW** CPT code _____ Visit Type:_____

Over the past 10 days, how many days have you been/had . . .

DSM Criteria Satisfied

	% days	Severity (0-4)	DSM Criteria	No	Probable	Definite
... depressed **most of day:**	**30**%	**1**	Depressed most of the day nearly every day for ≥2wk	**X**	__	__
... less interest in **most** activities or found you **couldn't enjoy even pleasurable activities** through **most of the day:**	**0**%	**0**	Decreased interest or diminished pleasure in most activities most of the day nearly every day for ≥2wks	**X**	__	__
... **any period of** abnormal mood elevation	**0**%	**0**	Mood Elevation (high, euphoric, expansive) to a significant degree over a 4 - 7 day period	**X**	__	__
... **any period of** abnormal irritability	**40**%	**2**	Irritability to a significant degree over a 4 -7 day period	__	__	**X**
... **any** abnormal anxiety	**50**%	**3**				

Rate Associated Symptoms for PAST WEEK

Much more **+2**——— **0** ——— **-2** Much less
0= usual/none

MDE
requires ≥ 5
(including depressed mood and/or interest)

	Depression	Sleep	Interest	Guilt / SE	Energy	Conc / Distr	Appetite	PMR / PMA	SI
	+1/2	**-1**	**0**	**0** or **0**	**0**	**0** or **+1/2**	**0**	**0** or **+1**	**0**

Sleeps **6** - **8** hours   ▪ EBT **+**DFA ▪ MCA ▪ EMA   ▪ DGOOB ▪ Naps   ▪ anhedonia   ▪ LNWL ▪ Passive ▪ Active

Elevation
Mania/hypomania requires ≥ 3 unless only irritable, then ≥ 4 moderate sxs are required (do not count elevation or irritability) toward dx of hypomania or mania

Increased Self Esteem	Decreased Need for sleep	Talking	FOI/Racing thoughts	Distractible	Goal directed activity /PMA	High Risk Behavior
0	**-1**	**+1/2**	**+1/2**	**+1/2**	**0** or **+1**	**0**

Y (N) New major stressor, if yes _____

Y (N) Substance abuse _____ d-use/wk   **2** c/d **caffeine**   **0** ppd **nicotine**   Onset of menses **09** / **1** / ____ early late (NA)

Y (N) Alcohol abuse _____ d/wk   Y (N) Headache   Y (N) Binge/Purge   Y N Additional Psych tx: (OP) ER Hosp

Y (N) Migraine   Y (N) Panic attacks   Y (N) Additional Gen Med tx: OP ER Hosp

Y (N) Significant Medical illness, if yes _____   Actual / Reported **Weight: 155**

Current Treatments

Bimodal Agents	Dose Mg 24 total	Mg Missed Past 7 days		Dose Mg 24 total	Mg Missed Past 7 days
Lamictal	**200**	**400**	**OCP**	**1 tab**	**1 tab**

Anxiolytics/Hypnotics

Antidepressants

Dopamine Blockers

		PRN	
Imitrex	**1 tab**	x **0**	
Ambien	PRN **10**	x **2**	

Adverse Effects

	Severity 0-4
Tremor	**2**
Dry Mouth	**2**
Sedation	**0**
Constipation	**0**
Diarrhea	**0**
Headache	**0**
Poor Memory	**0**
Sexual Dysfunction	**0**
Increased Appetite	**0**
Rash	**0**
Nausea	**0**
_____	__
_____	__
EPS_____	**0**

Selected Mental Status **Severity 0-4**

PI **0**   IOR **0**   OC **0**

Hallucinations **0**   Delusions **0**

Last Labs Date / /
Li = __   VPA= ___   TSH= ___

Creat= __

Current Clinical Status (check one)
__ Depression   __ Continued Sx
__ Hypomania   __ Recovering
__ Mania   __ Recovered
__ Mixed*   **X** Roughening

__ If new episode, estimate onset date: / /

__ Other Dx: _____

CGI **4**   GAF **55**   GAF **55**
(1-7)   week (0-90)   month (0-90)

Psychosocial Interventions **2**/mo   ECT ___/mo   Other _____ /mo

Yes (No) Significant Noncompliance, if yes

Comments: **28 yo MWF with BD-II – subsyndromal hypomania.**

Discussed increase LTG versus CBT and better sleep hygiene.

Plan: **Use CBT. Reassess LTG dose next visit.**

RTC **2 weeks**

_____
Signature

FIGURE 23–1.   Clinical monitoring form–representative time points (D).

A, Initial intake. B, Four weeks after starting lamotrigine. C, Regular follow-up visit during 2½ years of euthymic mood. **D**, Subsyndromal mood elevation during euthymic mood period.

esteem to more prominent and functionally disabling depressive episodes.

Approximately 6 years after the onset of these episodes, Ms. M.S. first sought psychiatric care, and she was diagnosed with "double depression" (major depressive disorder plus dysthymic disorder). Citalopram was used for 2 months without significant change in mood but with intolerable nausea and agitation. Sertraline remained ineffective after a 2-month trial and was associated with nausea and irritability. Duloxetine was effective within days of use, and the patient began to feel as if her whole life had been abnormally depressed until therapy with duloxetine. She began to see that there were many new opportunities for her life, and colors appeared brighter. After 2 months of treatment with duloxetine, however, her depression symptoms returned. The patient lost confidence in treatment and did not see a psychiatrist for another 2 years. On returning to psychiatric care, the patient was started on bupropion, which caused intolerable irritability and agitation. Due to the inefficacy of prior antidepressant medication trials, a consultation was sought.

Other Significant Findings From Assessment

During the consultation, in addition to the chronic depression overlaid with periods of more pervasive symptoms, other episodes with 2-week periods of time during which the patient was described by others as "weird" were elicited. Ms. M.S. remembered that between her more pronounced depressive episodes, she would have periods of improved mood in which she would try to catch up on her lost productivity, actually feeling that she could do anything and engaging in enough projects to more than make up for the periods of decreased productivity. During these periods, she would be more jovial. She slept 8 hours, in contrast to requiring the usual 9–10 hours, and she felt energetic during the day. Her thoughts would flow quickly, and her physical activity was increased to the level that peers commented that she was acting "weird." She would spend more and have increased libido but did not act outside her current relationships on these drives. She did not recall that these episodes were problematic at the time, until her husband reminded her of the associated irritability and that she would occasionally get into arguments with her boss and husband during these times.

These hypomanic episodes were present beginning in her mid-20s but have decreased in intensity over the years.

She has described more recent periods of increased irritability with difficulty sitting still for very long and thoughts jumping between different goals she felt she needed to pursue. During these times, she sleeps a "normal" amount of 7–8 hours. These periods intersperse the long periods of depression and last only 2 to 3 days.

Ms. M.S. has no significant medical problems. She used marijuana between the ages of 15 and 18 but has not used any other illicit drugs or alcohol.

Ms. M.S. does report a family history of depression in a brother, her mother is on divalproex and paroxetine for bipolar disorder, and her maternal grandmother received electroconvulsive therapy after a postpartum depression.

Ms. M.S. had a Bipolarity Index score of 60: Episode Characteristics=10 points, Age of Onset= 15 points, Course of Illness=5 points, Response to Treatment=10 points, Family History=20 points (Figure 23–2).

DSM-IV-TR Diagnosis

Axis I   Bipolar disorder, type II, current major depressive episode with rapid cycling course of illness
Axis II   None
Axis III None
Axis IV   Moderate stressors (school, relationships, finances)
Axis V   GAF score: 50

Treatment Plan Considerations

Bipolar Depression

Based on the obtained history, supported by the Bipolarity Index score of 60, the probable diagnosis of bipolar depression was made. In addition, the rapid cycling course of illness would also direct treatment decisions.

Major depressive episodes are commonly seen in the context of a major depressive disorder, but importantly, at least one in four cases may be related to an underlying bipolar disorder (Hasin et al. 2005). Prognostic and treatment differences between a major depressive episode occurring in the context of either bipolar disorder or major depressive disorder

BIPOLARITY INDEX

For each of the items below, circle the score next to the characteristic that best describes the patient.
Characteristics' scores range from 0 (no evidence of bipolar disorder) to 20 (most convincing characteristic of bipolar disorder).

I. Episode Characteristics

20	• Documented acute mania or mixed episode with prominent euphoria, grandiosity, or expansiveness and no significant general medical or known secondary etiology.
15	• Clear-cut acute mixed episode or dysphoric or irritable mania with no significant general medical or known secondary etiology.
(10)	• Clear-cut hypomania with no significant general medical or known secondary etiology. • Clear-cut cyclothymia with no significant general medical or known secondary etiology. • Clear-cut mania secondary to antidepressant use.
5	• Clear-cut hypomania secondary to antidepressant use. • Episodes with characteristic sxs of hypomania, but sxs, duration, or intensity are subthreshold for hypomania or cyclothymia. • A single MDE with psychotic or atypical features (Atypical is 2 of the following sxs: hypersomnia, hyperphagia, leaden paralysis of limbs) • Any postpartum depression.
2	• Any recurrent typical unipolar major depressive disorder. • History of any kind of psychotic disorder (i.e., presence of delusions, hallucinations, ideas of reference, magical thinking).
0	• No history of significant mood elevation, recurrent depression, or psychosis.

II. Age of Onset (1st affective episode/syndrome)

20	• 15 to 19 years
(15)	• before age 15 or between 20 and 30
10	• 30 to 45 years
5	• after age 45
0	• No history of affective illness (no episodes, cyclothymia, dysthymia, or BP NOS).

III. Course of Illness / Associated Features

20	• Recurrent, distinct manic episodes separated by periods of full recovery.
15	• Recurrent, distinct manic episodes with incomplete inter-episode recovery. • Recurrent, distinct hypomanic episodes with full inter-episode recovery.
10	• Comorbid substance abuse. • Psychotic features only during acute mood episodes. • Incarceration or repeated legal offenses related to manic behavior (e.g., shoplifting, reckless driving, bankruptcy).
(5)	• Recurrent unipolar MDD with 3 or more major depressive episodes. • Recurrent, distinct hypomanic episodes without full inter-episode recovery. • Recurrent medication non-compliance. • Comorbid borderline personality disorder, anxiety disorders, or eating disorders, or history of ADHD. • Engagement in risky behaviors that pose a problem for patient, family, or friends. • Behavioral evidence of perimenstrual exacerbation of mood symptoms.
2	• Baseline hyperthymic personality (when not manic or depressed). • Marriage 3 or more times (including remarriage to the same individual. • In two or more years,, has started a new job and changed jobs after less than a year. • Has more than two advanced degrees.
0	• None of the above.

IV. Response to Treatment

20	• Full recovery within 4 weeks of therapeutic treatment with mood stabilizing medication.
15	• Full recovery within 12 weeks of therapeutic treatment with mood stabilizing medication or relapse within 12 weeks of discontinuing tx. • Affective switch to mania (pure or mixed) within 12 weeks of starting a new antidepressant or increasing dose.
(10)	• Worsening dysphoria or mixed symptoms during antidepressant treatment subthreshold for mania. • Partial response to one or two mood stabilizers within 12 weeks of therapeutic treatment. • Antidepressant-induced new or worsening rapid-cycling course.
5	• Treatment resistance: lack of response to complete trials of 3 or more antidepressants. • Affective switch to mania or hypomania with antidepressant withdrawal.
2	• Immediate near complete response to antidepressant withdrawal.
0	• None of the above, or no treatment.

V. Family History

(20)	• At least one first degree relative with documented bipolar illness.
15	• At least one second degree relative with documented bipolar illness. • At least one first degree relative with documented, recurrent unipolar MDD and behavioral evidence suggesting bipolar illness.
10	• First degree relative with documented, recurrent unipolar MDD or schizoaffective disorder. • Any relative with documented bipolar illness or recurrent unipolar MDD and behavioral evidence suggesting bipolar illness.
5	• First degree relative with documented substance abuse. • And relative with possible bipolar illness.
2	• First degree relative with possible recurrent unipolar MDD. • First degree relative with diagnosed related illness: anxiety disorders, eating disorders, ADD/ADHD.
0	• None of the above, or no family psychiatric illness.

60 ← Total score (0 – 100)

FIGURE 23–2. Bipolarity Index.

need to be considered carefully, because treatment priorities differ between these diagnoses. Guidelines on the treatment of bipolar depression integrate both efficacy data and adverse effects considerations laying out an evidence-based hierarchy of treatment options.

The correct diagnosis of bipolar disorder often is delayed by up to 10 years (Hirschfeld et al. 2003). Bipolar depression has the same diagnostic criteria as major depressive disorder, and this may partially account for the delay in accurate diagnosis of bipolar disorder. However, some clinical factors may be discriminating (Table 23–1). Historically defined "atypical depressions" are often more typical for bipolar depression presentations (Akiskal 2005). Symptoms of bipolar depression are often the reverse of symptoms during mania. Thus, decreased need for sleep, decreased appetite, and psychomotor agitation in mania may switch to increased sleep, increased appetite and weight gain, and psychomotor retardation during the depressive phase. An earlier age of onset is more typical of bipolar disorder. In fact, nearly half of childhood (Geller et al. 2001) and nearly 50% of young adult or adolescent (Goldberg et al. 2001) severe depressions eventually develop into bipolar disorder instead of major depressive disorder. That clinical factor alone doubles the risk of bipolar outcome from one out of four to one out of every two patients with major depressive episodes. A family history of bipolar disorder in a first-degree relative is associated with at least a 20% chance of bipolar disorder in any given individual, which is considerably higher than the general population rate of 3% (Hasin et al. 2005).

Collaborative Care Model

Including family members or other sources of collateral information is particularly important in identifying hypomanic episodes. Oftentimes, patients do not recognize the association between mood symptoms and overperformance or underperformance. Family members are often the best source of objective historical information. In addition, family members are often the best subsequent support system for patients. Manualized family-focused therapy for bipolar disorder, in combination with pharmacotherapy, has been shown to be more effective at minimizing mood symptoms recurrence and maximizing medication compliance than usual pharma-

TABLE 23–1. Discriminating between bipolar and unipolar depression

Bipolar more likely	Unipolar more likely
Symptoms	
Oversleeping	Insomnia
Overeating	Decreased appetite
Sluggishness	Restlessness
Delusions or hallucinations	Physical complaints
Mood swings or elevations	
Onset and course	
Onset age < 25	Onset age > 25
≥5 depressions total	Current depression > 6 months
Family history	
Bipolar disorder	No bipolar disorder

Source. Adapted from Mitchell et al. 2008.

cotherapy with crisis management (Miklowitz et al. 2003). Although brief family psychoeducation is included as part of the standard initial clinical evaluation, for this case we chose manualized CBT for bipolar disorder as the psychotherapeutic adjunctive treatment. The choice of type of adjunctive psychotherapy is further discussed later.

Guideline Selection

The most recent guideline available at the time the patient was seen was the Texas Implementation of Medication Algorithm (TIMA), which integrates benefits and risks based on the most currently available clinical trials, with particular focus on double-blind, placebo-controlled trials. The last American Psychiatric Association guideline for treatment of bipolar disorders available at the time we saw this patient was published in 2002, although a contemporary revision has been published.

Currently, TIMA suggests a tiered approach to treatment of bipolar depression (Table 23–2; Suppes et al. 2005). At the first stage of treatment, lamotrigine monotherapy or lamotrigine plus an antimanic agent is suggested, based on a post hoc analysis of lamotrigine monotherapy in bipolar I depression

TABLE 23–2.   Texas Implementation of Medication Algorithm for bipolar I depression

Therapy

Stage 1	Lamotrigine + antimanic agent *or* Lamotrigine monotherapy (optimize lithium if already on lithium)
Stage 2	Quetiapine *or* olanzapine-fluoxetine combination (OFC)
Stage 3	Combination from lithium, lamotrigine, quetiapine, *or* OFC
Stage 4	Any of the following: lithium, lamotrigine, quetiapine, OFC, valproate, carbamazepine combined with any of the following: selective serotonin reuptake inhibitor, bupropion, venlafaxine *or* Electroconvulsive therapy
Stage 5	Monoamine oxidase inhibitor, tricyclic antidepressant, pramipexole, atypical antipsychotic, oxcarbazepine, inositol, stimulants, thyroid augmentation

Source.   Adapted from Suppes et al. 2005.

(Calabrese et al. 1999). The combination therapy is recommended for patients with history of severe manic episodes, because lamotrigine is only modestly preventive of manic episodes (Goodwin et al. 2004) and has no acute antimanic efficacy (Bowden et al. 2000). For patients already receiving lithium therapy, optimizing the lithium dose to target a blood level of 0.8 mEq/L is also a first-line recommendation (Nemeroff et al. 2001).

At the next stage of treatment, two U.S. Food and Drug Administration–approved treatments are suggested, including olanzapine plus fluoxetine and quetiapine monotherapy, based on robust placebo-controlled trials (Calabrese et al. 2005; Thase et al. 2006; Tohen et al. 2003). Despite the faster onset of action and more robust studies, both of these medications have greater adverse effects burden and so are recommended at the second stage of treatment. A more clinically understandable and useful way to understand this balance between efficacy and risk data is to use number-needed-to-treat (NNT) and number-needed-to-harm (NNH) calculations (Ketter 2010). Thus, although olanzapine and quetiapine had NNTs for acute bipolar depression response, compared with placebo, of 4 and 6, respectively, they had NNHs for at least 7% weight gain (olanzapine) and sedation (quetiapine), compared with placebo, of 6 and 5, respectively—meaning that side effects were about as likely as was response, making these agents lower-priority treatment options (Ketter 2010).

The third stage of treatment combines therapies from the first and second stages of treatment. It is not until the fourth stage of treatment that antidepressant medications are suggested.

Use of Antidepressant Medications in Bipolar Disorder

Whereas first-line treatment of major depressive disorder is antidepressant medication, bipolar disorder treatment guidelines suggest mood stabilizer medications such as lithium, lamotrigine, and quetiapine (Suppes et al. 2005). Despite the available literature demonstrating efficacy of such mood stabilizers for bipolar depression, the community standard is still antidepressant medications. In fact, about one-half of patients with bipolar disorder are initially prescribed an antidepressant medication, whereas in stark contrast less than one-quarter were prescribed mood stabilizers (anticonvulsants 17% and lithium 8%) (Baldessarini et al. 2007). Adjunctive antidepressant medications have not been adequately studied in bipolar depression, and some studies do not suggest efficacy beyond mood stabilizer treatment alone (Nemeroff et al. 2001; Sachs et al. 2007). Antidepressant medications also have been implicated in inducing mania or accelerating mood cycle recurrences in patients with bipolar disorder. Up to two-thirds of mood episodes in patients with bipolar disorder may be antidepressant-associated mood episodes (Altshuler et al. 1995). Some studies suggest that among the classes of antidepressant medications, the dual-acting (serotonin-norepinephrine reuptake inhibitors, e.g., venlafaxine) may be worse at inducing mood cycling than either selective serotonin reuptake inhibitors or bupropion (Post et al.

2006). Coupled with these potential risks, antidepressant medication use for bipolar depression in the community may be excessive.

Cognitive-Behavioral Therapy for Bipolar Disorder

Intensive psychotherapy (CBT, Family-Focused Therapy [FFT], or Interpersonal and Social Rhythm Therapy) has been shown to be superior to a short course of psychoeducation in augmenting pharmacotherapy to stabilize bipolar disorder symptoms (Miklowitz et al. 2007). CBT with psychopharmacology has been shown to be specifically superior to medication management alone for maintaining bipolar disorder stability (Lam et al. 2003). For this case, CBT was selected for psychotherapy due to the availability of therapists trained in manualized CBT compared with the other therapies.

An important tool used in CBT for bipolar disorder is mood charting (see Figure 23–3 for example) (Denicoff et al. 1997). The mood chart is a focal point for collaboration between the patient, the psychiatrist, and the therapist. Mood is tracked prospectively so that pharmacological treatment decisions are not based on state-dependent memory. Therapists can use the mood changes and noted psychosocial stressors to more accurately recall cognition–mood–behavior interactions. Patients, as more active participants in their own care, may have greater treatment compliance.

Rapid Cycling Course of Illness

Approximately one-third of patients with bipolar disorder have a rapid cycling course of illness (Schneck et al. 2008). Documenting at least four full DSM-IV-TR mood episodes per year (at least 4 days of pervasive hypomanic symptoms and at least 2 weeks of depressive symptoms) can be challenging. Using a semistructured interview for the initial intake and subsequent clinical follow-up improves the documentation of such episodes. Oftentimes, patients can only recall "mood cycling" as a constellation of depressive and hypomanic symptoms without consideration of daily pervasiveness or meeting full duration criteria. In these situations, patients are often treated for depression as the prevailing presentation, whereas subsyndromal (by time and symptom count criteria) mixed episodes may be the relevant clinical syndrome. Antidepressant medica-

tion may worsen such clinical states, whereas mood-stabilizing medications have had more consistent evidence suggesting treatment efficacy. Mood charting may more accurately capture rapid cycling than patient recall alone.

Anxiety Symptoms

Approximately one-third of patients with bipolar disorder also have comorbid anxiety. Antidepressant medications, the mainstay of treatment for anxiety disorders, may be counterproductive for treatment of bipolar disorder; therefore, anxiety symptoms are frequently treated only if remaining after adequate mood stabilization and first targeting mood cycling and depression. CBT, on the other hand, may be used without the liability of antidepressant medications. Thus, the high comorbidity of anxiety symptoms with bipolar disorder may be another reason to preferentially use CBT as the intensive psychotherapy of choice for bipolar disorder.

Course

Ms. M.S. was started on lamotrigine, following the recommended slow titration. The risk of rash was discussed. At 200 mg/day of lamotrigine, she began to feel improvement in her mood. Mood improvement was tracked with the Clinical Monitoring Form, noting a generally steady improvement in overall symptoms even though depressed mood did not improve until approximately 4–5 weeks after starting lamotrigine. It was useful to have a standardized list of symptoms to monitor at each visit to show the patient that her mood is more than the single symptom of depressed mood or anhedonia. CBT was concurrently started and continued on a weekly basis initially. Mood charting was introduced during the initial consultation with the psychiatrist and was reinforced and discussed in depth at each CBT sessions. The psychiatrist and the therapist used the patient-generated mood chart as the focus of collaboration. Anxiety symptoms remained, but at a lower level of severity. Medication or CBT were offered as treatment options, and the patient chose CBT based on the risk-benefit discussion.

The patient remained in euthymic mood for approximately 2½ years. During that time, her visits to the psychiatrist decreased to approximately every 3 months. Her visits with her therapist continued at

Mood Chart: _____ M.S. _____ Month: _____ Sept 2007

		01	02	03	04	05	06	07	08	09	10	11	12	13	14	15	16	17	18	19	20	21	22	23	24	25	26	27	28	29	30	31
Elevation	Severe																															
	Moderate High																															
	Moderate Low																															
	Mild																															
Depression	Mild																															
	Moderate Low																															
	Moderate High																															
	Severe																															

	01	02	03	04	05	06	07	08	09	10	11	12	13	14	15	16	17	18	19	20	21	22	23	24	25	26	27	28	29	30	31
Sleep	9	9	9	8	7	6	7	8	7	6	7	8	7	6	7	7	8	7	7	6	7	8	9	8	9	8	9	10	10	9	
Lamictal 200 mg	0	1	1	1	0	1	1	1	1	0	0	1	1	1	1	1	0	1	0	1	1	1	1	1	1	1	1	1	1	1	
Ambien 10 mg											1	1							1	1											
OCP	1	1	1	1	1	1	1	1	1	1	0	1	1	1	1	1	1	1	1	1	1	1	1	1	1	1	1	1	1	1	
Imitrex																												2	1		

Medications

Life Events: Neg comment from boss; Overwhelmed at work; Hiking with family; Appt with psychiatrist; Appt with psychiatrist; Migraine headache; Migraine headache

FIGURE 23–3. Mood charting—corresponds approximately to Clinical Monitoring Form, time point D.

HA=headache; OCP=oral contraceptive pill.

twice per month, then decreased to once per month. During the first year of euthymic mood, the patient had a slight, subsyndromal mood elevation around Labor Day, which was noticed only as the minor decreased sleep noted on the mood charting (Figure 23–3). The therapist asked the patient to call the psychiatrist to discuss a medication reevaluation. Reinitiating weekly CBT sessions was chosen instead of increasing the lamotrigine. Symptoms never reached DSM-IV-TR syndromal level and resolved within 3 weeks. The patient then returned to her quarterly psychiatric and monthly therapist visits.

The patient then became interested in becoming pregnant. She had tried to decrease lamotrigine dosage for the planned pregnancy, but she returned to 200 mg/day when some irritability returned. When she did become pregnant, the pregnancy was otherwise unremarkable. She returned to twice-monthly therapy and monthly psychiatric visits. Within 1 month postpartum she had a major depressive episode, despite arranging weekly therapist and twice-monthly psychiatric visits. Mood stabilized after lamotrigine was increased to 225 mg/day, and she remained stable for another 15 months until the birth of her second child. She had another major depressive episode within 1 month of delivery, but she has since been stable for 3 years after lamotrigine was increased to 300 mg/day.

Summary of Guideline Use

For this patient with bipolar depression, we used the TIMA guidelines suggesting an initial trial with either lamotrigine or lithium. Given the better tolerability profile of lamotrigine compared with lithium, we started this patient on a trial of lamotrigine, which led to improvement at the target dosage of 200 mg/day given as a single daytime dose. Although quetiapine is listed as a second-stage treatment option due to greater adverse effects burden, it may be considered as an initial treatment based on a faster onset of action. Lamotrigine is slower to onset of improvement but better tolerated, whereas quetiapine may show benefit by the first week of treatment but generally has more tolerability challenges. It should also be considered that quetiapine has benefits for anxiety symptoms, which were present in this patient. This patient was not overburdened by a severely functionally disabling illness, so lamotrigine was chosen for its greater tolerability.

Even prior to using a specific treatment guideline, for bipolar disorder it is even more imperative to make an accurate diagnosis. Bipolar disorder is an important consideration in a patient who presents with a major depressive episode, due to differences in evidence-based treatment preferences. Utilizing collateral sources of information serves dual purposes of providing more objective clinical history and establishing a collaborative care model.

Clinical monitoring of patient with bipolar disorder requires a collaborative approach involving family and peer supports, and therapists as well. TIMA advocates combined pharmacotherapy and psychotherapy but does not indicate a preference for any specific psychotherapy, owing to a lack of direct comparisons between psychotherapies. CBT is usually chosen in our setting due to the availability of therapists in our community with specialized training in CBT.

Mood charting played a pivotal role in identifying the subsyndromal mood elevation during a period in this patient's follow-up when symptoms had remitted for many months and the frequency of clinical visits with psychiatrist and therapist were decreasing. Collaboration with the therapist clearly closed the information loop for having the patient inform the psychiatrist about the mood elevation symptoms. Tracking specific symptoms at each visit with the Clinical Monitoring Form improved sensitivity for noting clinical improvement early in treatment and some mood destabilization later in ongoing clinical management.

Based on treatment guidelines, we could have either increased lamotrigine or added lithium or an atypical antipsychotic medication for this noted subsyndromal mood elevation. Instead, to control this mood recurrence, we offered these medication options or increasing psychotherapy frequency to improve sleep hygiene and medication compliance and decreasing external stimulus. Based on the collaborative care model, patient input is equally important, so the decision was made to increase psychotherapy sessions. In addition, we scheduled a follow-up visit within 2 weeks to ensure that pharmacological interventions were always available.

Ways to Improve Practice

Patients and families often would like to investigate their illness on their own. The Internet is a vast but sometimes too unregulated resource. We have offered various consumer-oriented books on bipolar disorder, but a resource list compiled by consumers may be more effective.

CBT is an effective adjunctive treatment for patients with bipolar disorder, and it is broadly applicable to many patients. However, the main reason that FFT and Interpersonal and Social Rhythm Therapy were not used was the lack of reliable referral options. A better understanding is needed of the availability of community resources for these evidence-supported therapies.

Patients frequently benefit from peer-support groups as a further adjunct to treatment. However, most clinicians only have a basic understanding of the workings of local peer-support groups. We have started to serve as medical advisors to several local groups in order to extend the concept of collaborative care further.

Family involvement is greatest at the initiation of care due to the acuity of illness. However, over time, with longer periods of euthymic mood and prolonged normality, family involvement diminishes. We cannot help but wonder whether continuing to actively involve family and/or peer supports would have caught the subsyndromal mood elevation earlier. Involving family and peer supports throughout the acute and stable periods may somewhat destigmatize coming to the psychiatrist's office. We will consider regularly inviting family and/or peer supports to attend office visits.

References

Akiskal HS: The dark side of bipolarity: detecting bipolar depression in its pleomorphic expressions. J Affect Disord 84:107–115, 2005

Altshuler LL, Post RM, Leverich GS, et al: Antidepressant-induced mania and cycle acceleration: a controversy revisited. Am J Psychiatry 152:1130–1138, 1995

American Psychiatric Association: Diagnostic and Statistical Manual of Mental Disorders, 4th Edition, Text Revision. Washington, DC, American Psychiatric Association, 2000

American Psychiatric Association: Practice guideline for the treatment of patients with bipolar disorder. Am J Psychiatry 151 (12 suppl)1–36, 2002. Available at: http://www.psychiatryonline.com/pracGuide/pracGuideTopic_8.aspx.

Baldessarini RJ, Leahy L, Arcona S, et al: Patterns of psychotropic drug prescription for U.S. patients with diagnoses of bipolar disorders. Psychiatr Serv 58:85–91, 2007

Bowden C, Calabrese J, Ascher J, et al: Spectrum of efficacy of lamotrigine in bipolar disorder: overview of double-blind placebo-controlled studies. Paper presented at the 39th annual meeting of the American College of Neuropsychopharmacology, San Juan, Puerto Rico, December 2000

Calabrese JR, Bowden CL, Sachs GS, et al: A double-blind placebo-controlled study of lamotrigine monotherapy in outpatients with bipolar I depression. Lamictal 602 Study Group. J Clin Psychiatry 60:79–88, 1999

Calabrese JR, Keck PE Jr, Macfadden W, et al: A randomized, double-blind, placebo-controlled trial of quetiapine in the treatment of bipolar I or II depression. Am J Psychiatry 162:1351–1360, 2005

Denicoff KD, Smith-Jackson EE, Disney ER, et al: Preliminary evidence of the reliability and validity of the prospective life-chart methodology (LCM-p). J Psychiatr Res 31:593–603, 1997

Derry S, Moore RA: Atypical antipsychotics in bipolar disorder: systematic review of randomised trials. BMC Psychiatry 7:40, 2007

Geller B, Zimerman B, Williams M, et al: Bipolar disorder at prospective follow-up of adults who had prepubertal major depressive disorder. Am J Psychiatry 158:125–127, 2001

Goldberg JF, Harrow M, Whiteside JE: Risk for bipolar illness in patients initially hospitalized for unipolar depression. Am J Psychiatry 158:1265–1270, 2001

Goodwin GM, Bowden CL, Calabrese JR, et al: A pooled analysis of 2 placebo-controlled 18-month trials of lamotrigine and lithium maintenance in bipolar I disorder. J Clin Psychiatry 65:432–441, 2004

Hasin DS, Goodwin RD, Stinson FS, et al: Epidemiology of major depressive disorder: results from the National Epidemiologic Survey on Alcoholism and Related Conditions. Arch Gen Psychiatry 62:1097–1106, 2005

Hirschfeld RM, Calabrese JR, Weissman MM, et al: Screening for bipolar disorder in the community. J Clin Psychiatry 64:53–59, 2003

Ketter TA (ed): Handbook of Diagnosis and Treatment of Bipolar Disorders. Washington, DC, American Psychiatric Publishing, 2010

Lam DH, Watkins ER, Hayward P, et al: A randomized controlled study of cognitive therapy for relapse prevention for bipolar affective disorder: outcome of the first year. Arch Gen Psychiatry 60:145–152, 2003

Miklowitz DJ, George EL, Richards JA, et al: A randomized study of family focused psychoeducation and pharmacotherapy in the outpatient management of bipolar disorder. Arch Gen Psychiatry 60:904–912, 2003

Miklowitz DJ, Otto MW, Frank E, et al: Psychosocial treatments for bipolar depression: a 1-year randomized trial from the Systematic Treatment Enhancement Program. Arch Gen Psychiatry 64:419–426, 2007

Mitchell PB, Goodwin GM, Johnson GF, et al: Diagnostic guidelines for bipolar depression: a probabilistic approach. Bipolar Disord 10:144–152, 2008

Nemeroff CB, Evans DL, Gyulai L, et al: Double-blind, placebo-controlled comparison of imipramine and paroxetine in the treatment of bipolar depression. Am J Psychiatry 158:906–912, 2001

Post RM, Altshuler LL, Leverich GS, et al: Mood switch in bipolar depression: comparison of adjunctive venlafaxine, bupropion and sertraline. Br J Psychiatry 189:124–131, 2006

Sachs GS, Nierenberg AA, Calabrese JR, et al: Effectiveness of adjunctive antidepressant treatment for bipolar depression. N Engl J Med 356:1711–1722, 2007

Schneck CD, Miklowitz DJ, Miyahara S, et al: The prospective course of rapid-cycling bipolar disorder: findings from the STEP-BD. Am J Psychiatry 165:370–377; quiz 410, 2008

Suppes T, Dennehy EB, Hirschfeld RM, et al: The Texas implementation of medication algorithms: update to the algorithms for treatment of bipolar I disorder. J Clin Psychiatry 66:870–886, 2005

Thase ME, Macfadden W, Weisler RH, et al: Efficacy of quetiapine monotherapy in bipolar I and II depression: a double-blind, placebo-controlled study (the BOLDER II study). J Clin Psychopharmacol 26:600–609, 2006

Tohen M, Vieta E, Calabrese J, et al: Efficacy of olanzapine and olanzapine-fluoxetine combination in the treatment of bipolar I depression. Arch Gen Psychiatry 60:1079–1088, 2003

Obsessive-Compulsive Disorder

Bibi Das, M.D.
Lorrin M. Koran, M.D.

Setting

The patient was seen in a private practice setting. The population in the surrounding area is of high educational attainment and upper socioeconomic status and is ethnically diverse. The patient population is also quite sophisticated in accessing information on the Web.

The treatment strategy utilized is evidence-based pharmacotherapy combined with cognitive-behavioral therapy (CBT).

Illustration

This study illustrates:

- Combining medications (selective serotonin reuptake inhibitors [SSRIs]) and psychotherapy (CBT) in the treatment of obsessive-compulsive disorder (OCD)
- The importance of family involvement in the treatment to eliminate family accommodation to the symptoms
- Cognitive restructuring in an attempt to increase motivation for exposure and response prevention (ERP)
- Repeated Yale-Brown Obsessive Compulsive Scale (Y-BOCS; Goodman et al. 1989) assessments of the severity of the disorder
- The steps taken to improve adherence
- The utility of assessing common co-occurring disorders

Chief Complaint

Ms. D.B., a 19-year-old single Caucasian female, presents with a long history of "taking hours to get anything done."

Present Illness

Ms. D.B. reported that she has been "stuck in life." She is unable to get anything done "because everything I do takes forever." She has intrusive thoughts of hurting her family that make her feel "sick to the stomach." She relieves her anxiety by washing her hands or saying a prayer under her breath. Over the years, she has developed elaborate rituals that dictate how she showers, eats, drives, studies, and carries out many other activities. She spends 7–8 hours a day doing her rituals.

Ms. D.B. is afraid that she is getting "stupid and crazy because I do things that make no sense." She feels helpless in the face of her thoughts because she cannot stop herself from carrying out her rituals.

Ms. D.B. reported that she has had rituals "ever since I was playing with dolls." In the previous 5 months, however, her symptoms had worsened, so that she stopped going to school and was unable to drive or leave the house. She believes that the acute stressor was her having been accepted to a college far from home.

She also acknowledged that in the past month she had struggled with pervasive sad mood and low energy and has had difficulty enjoying herself. She

TABLE 24–1. Past medication trials

Medication	Daily dosage	Duration	Side effects	Efficacy
Fluoxetine	20 mg	4 months	Agitation	Mild
Citalopram	20 mg	3 months	Sexual	None
Olanzapine	10 mg	1 month	Weight gain	None
Clonazepam	0.5 mg, prn	with citalopram	None	Most helpful

feels "either guilty or stupid all the time" and has had feelings of worthlessness. She denies any hopelessness, suicidal ideation, and symptoms of mood elevation. Appetite and memory are normal. She has had problems falling asleep but denies any mid-cycle awakening, nightmares, early morning awakening, or daytime sedation. She also complained of problems with focus and distractibility. Ms. D.B. has had free-floating anxiety but denied any panic attacks. She has had no impulse-control problems.

Past Psychiatric History

Ms. D.B. has no history of substance abuse.

Her compulsions began in childhood, when her little brother was born. She went to the store and bought three candies even though they were four siblings. She remembers feeling "like a monster because I wanted one of them to die." As a child she could not talk about this to anyone and controlled her anxiety by creating rituals "that would neutralize the bad thoughts."

She denies any history of depression before the current episode. At age 17, she sought treatment from her pediatrician. She had tried several medications (Table 24-1) prescribed by her pediatrician with "little help." I verified her medication history by asking her pharmacy to fax me records. All medications had been refilled on time, indicating that Ms D.B. adhered to treatment. She had not had a trial of psychotherapy.

Medical History

- Euthyroid (checked in the previous year during her annual physical)
- No history of head injury, seizures, loss of consciousness, sexually transmitted disease, or any risk factor for HIV
- No known drug allergies

Family History

- Motor tics in a maternal cousin
- A maternal aunt with major depressive disorder and anxiety disorder (the specific type was unknown to the patient), who responded well to escitalopram
- A brother with generalized anxiety disorder who had been treated successfully with escitalopram 10 mg/day

DSM-IV-TR Diagnosis

Axis I   Obsessive-compulsive disorder
          Major depressive disorder, currently moderate severity

Treatment Plan Considerations

1. Compulsions—Y-BOCS score 16
2. Obsessions—Y-BOCS score 16
3. Depression—Hamilton Rating Scale for Depression (Ham-D; Hamilton 1960) score 24

A "gold standard" OCD severity measure is the Y-BOCS. A score of 32 (16+16) falls in the "severe" range (Goodman et al. 1989).

Secondary Points in the Plan

Psychoeducation will emphasize understanding that the cause of the disorder is unknown and that it represents a chemical problem in the brain and is not a weakness of character and cannot be willed away, has a waxing and waning course that seems influenced by stress, is treatable and responds to both medications and to CBT, and usually does not go away completely. We will emphasize the need for adherence to treatment in order to reap the benefits, and we will set a realistic expectation of recovery in terms of symptom relief and the time needed to reach this goal.

Treatment Goals

- Compulsions: Less than 30 minutes a day and not interfering with functioning
- Obsessions: Less than 30 minutes a day and not interfering with functioning.
- Depression: Remission

Treatment Goal Measures

- Y-BOCS: Score less than 8 (Simpson et al. 2006)
- Ham-D: Score less than 7

Course

Week 1

The options of using medications alone, CBT with ERP alone, or a combination of these two treatments were discussed (Simpson and Liebowitz 2005).

I (Dr. B.D.) prefer to meet my patients once a week if I am providing medication management together with CBT. The literature and expert opinions suggest that CBT sessions should be scheduled at least once weekly (March et al. 1997; Whittal et al. 2005). The number of treatment sessions, their length, and the duration of an adequate trial have not been established, but expert consensus recommends 13–20 weekly sessions "for most patients" (March et al. 1997). I share these data with my patients so that they can have a realistic expectation of when they can expect to start feeling better. Also, this helps them decide whether they are willing to make the time and the emotional and financial commitment required to fully participate in the therapy process.

Ms. D.B. was started on escitalopram 5 mg/day. She had tried two other SSRIs that had not brought significant symptom control and had caused some side effects. Although clinical trials indicate that all SSRIs are equally efficacious in treating both depression and OCD (Koran et al. 2007), I decided to start her on escitalopram because her brother had responded to this drug. The common side effects were discussed. In some patients, drug-drug interactions, particular unwanted side effects, and insurance coverage are important additional factors to consider, but in Ms. D.B.'s case these factors were not relevant.

I also asked Ms. D.B. to take 1,000 mg/day of eicosapentaenoic acid (EPA), an omega-3 fatty acid (available in fish oil capsules), in view of studies suggesting that at this dosage it may be a beneficial augmentation strategy in depressive disorders (Freeman et al. 2006), and encouraged her to add 800 μg/day of folic acid to help treat her depression, again based on studies suggesting possible benefit (Alpert et al. 2002; Coppen and Bailey 2000).

I provided Ms. D.B. with a reading list and asked her to procure *The OCD Workbook* (Hyman and Pedrick 2005) and *Brain Lock* (Schwartz 1996). Her assignment for the first week was to make an Anxiety/Exposure List and to grade the severity of anxiety aroused in different fear-provoking situations using the Subjective Units of Distress Scale (SUDS), with each item rated from 1 to 100 points.

Before initiating CBT, I explained the nature of the treatment, including its here-and-now focus, the rationale of underlying treatment procedures, and what she would be required to do.

At the start of therapy, I used the Y-BOCS symptom checklist (Goodman et al. 1989) to help her create a list of target symptoms, including obsessions, compulsions, and items or situations that are avoided because of OCD concerns. The patient ranked the listed items from least to most anxiety provoking.

In CBT consisting of ERP, patients are taught to confront feared situations and objects (i.e., exposure) and to refrain from performing rituals (i.e., response prevention). Exposures may include in vivo confrontations (e.g., setting the dials of the thermostat to the wrong number, wearing unlucky clothes) and imagining feared consequences. Exposures that provoke moderate anxiety are prescribed first, followed as quickly as tolerable by exposures of increasing difficulty. Patients must face their fears for a prolonged period without ritualizing, allowing the anxiety or discomfort to dissipate on its own ("habituation"). The goal is to weaken the connections between feared stimuli and distress and between ritualizing and relief from distress.

She was also encouraged to visit the Obsessive Compulsive Foundation Web site, www.ocfoundation.org, to learn more about OCD and to look for a local OCD support group sponsored by the foundation. Unfortunately, she was unable to join a group because of time constraints.

Week 2

Ms. D.B. came back after having taken escitalopram 5 mg/day for a week. She had tolerated the medication with no side effects but reported no symptom improvement. I increased the dosage by 5 mg to 10 mg/

TABLE 24–2. Obsessions/compulsions and subjective distress levels

Obsession or compulsion	SUDS level (0–100)
Thinking about, talking about, or seeing pirates	35
Locking the front door once, checking twice, and walking away	45
Leaving the bed in the morning without doing ritual	65
Not adjusting the car temperature or radio station to the correct number while driving	70
Not checking all kitchen appliances before going to bed	75
Not saying a prayer when parents leave the house	85
Not doing elaborate bath ritual	100

Note. SUDS=Subjective Units of Distress Scale.

day, because 5 mg/day was far lower than the dosage (20 mg/day) demonstrated quite effective in a controlled clinical trial (Stein et al. 2007). In contrast to improvement in depression, OCD improvement takes longer and often requires higher SSRI dosages (often above U.S. Food and Drug Administration–approved maximum dosages) (Koran et al. 2007). Many articles suggest waiting 8–12 weeks before increasing the SSRI dosage or considering a switch. However, I tend to increase the dosage faster for two reasons:

1. Delay in initial response often leads to noncompliance. Also, because it appears that higher dosages are more effective than lower dosages in treating OCD (Koran et al. 2007), slow titration wastes precious time before the patient can experience relief of symptoms.
2. SSRI side effects tend not to be strongly dose dependent, so once we reach remission with favorable tolerability, I slowly back off on the dosage over several months while being vigilant for returning symptoms. The goal is to obtain maximum symptom control with minimum medication.

Ms. D.B. had prepared an inventory of some of her OCD symptoms, as shown in Table 24–2. She reported that her obsessions revolved around fears that if she did not do her rituals, a member of her family would get into an accident and die or some natural calamity would befall that person. She reported that even though she knew that this made "no logical sense, I am a prisoner to my thoughts."

While I am working on ERP, I like to also work on the cognitive distortions that underlie OCD and try to teach the patient formal cognitive techniques aimed at changing these dysfunctional beliefs. Even though data comparing ERP alone to CBT alone remain inconclusive (Koran et al. 2007), many experts suggest that a combined approach is most fruitful. Dysfunctional beliefs that are common in OCD include magical thinking (e.g., a bathing ritual will keep my family safe), an inflated sense of responsibility for unwanted events, overestimation of the probability of feared events, the assumption that thoughts are morally equivalent to actions or inevitably lead to action ("thought-action fusion"), perfectionism, the belief that anxiety/discomfort will persist forever, and the need for control.

We decided that we would start with the OCD symptom that caused least anxiety and then move up the anxiety ladder. Thus we started with the patient's anxiety about "pirates."

Table 24–3 shows Ms. D.B.'s mini-list for her pirate anxiety. Because a SUDS level of 20 was not distressing enough, we started with writing the word "pirate." We worked on trying to spell the word, which Ms. D.B. did with little anxiety. Then, we wrote the word in the air, and finally, on paper. We

TABLE 24–3. Pirate anxiety and subjective distress levels

Activity	SUDS level
Thinking about pirates	10
Hearing someone talk about pirates	20
Writing the word *pirate*	25
Seeing a picture of a pirate	30
Seeing a movie with pirates	35

Note. SUDS=Subjective Units of Distress Scale.

TABLE 24–4. Response to intrusive thoughts

Intrusive thought	Response (talking back to your brain)
If I have bad thoughts, it means I am a bad person.	"It's only my overactive brain chemicals."
Maybe I will act on my bad thoughts.	"It's not me, it's my OCD."
Maybe this is not OCD.	This is more evidence that this is OCD.

obtained several pictures of pirates from the Internet, and I asked Ms. D.B. to look at them. The feared consequence of ritual prevention that cropped up was "my family will get hurt by bad guys."

We decided that Ms. D.B. would try to do the writing/looking at the picture exercise when with her family.

Week 3

Ms. D.B. was now taking 10 mg/day of escitalopram. She reported a 40% decrease in her sad mood and overall anxiety. She also reported that she was getting better-quality sleep and waking up feeling more refreshed. She had some constipation, however, for which she was taking Metamucil.

Her Ham-D score reflected the improvement in her depressive symptoms, having decreased from 23 to 12. Her Y-BOCS score remained almost the same (15 obsessions + 16 compulsions). As expected, her depressive symptoms responded earlier than her OCD symptoms.

Ms. D.B. reported that she was able to do her ERP exercise in spite of increased anxiety. She was so excited by her success that she rented *Pirates of the Caribbean* and was able to watch 30 minutes of it.

We looked at "self-talk strategies" that she could use in order to plow through the exposure. We reviewed the concept of being an "impartial observer" as outlined in *Brain Lock* (Schwartz 1996). The idea is to pay attention to one's inner dialogue and talk back to the intrusive thoughts with logical and directive statements rather than giving in to them (Table 24–4).

We decided to target the next OCD symptom, locking the front door and checking it. We made a mini-list, breaking down the locking and checking behavior (Table 24–5).

The mini-list was used to do the ERP in the following steps:

1. Choose the item that produces at least moderate anxiety by bringing it on and confronting it with an adequate level of anxiety.
2. Allow the discomfort to rise and tolerate it rather than trying to neutralize it.
3. Practice ritual prevention while doing the exposure (i.e., do not pray under your breath).
4. Repeat the task again and again till the SUDS decreases to 20 or less.

We also increased Ms. D.B.'s escitalopram dosage to 20 mg/day, the dosage demonstrated more effective in OCD (Stein et al. 2007), because she had tolerated 10 mg/day quite well.

Week 4

Ms. D.B. came back the following week reporting that she was able to cut down her checking behavior to three times that week. However, the anxiety had been

TABLE 24–5. Locking and checking behaviors and subjective distress levels

Behavior	SUDS level
Locking the front door once, checking twice, and walking away	45
Locking the front door once, checking once, and walking away	65
Locking the front door once, checking once, and walking away and staying away for 1 hour	85
Locking the front door once, checking once, and walking away and staying away for 4 hours	95
Locking the front door once, checking once, and walking away and staying away overnight	100

Note. SUDS=Subjective Units of Distress Scale.

so intense that she had had her mother check the door for her and reassure her that the door was safely locked. I learned that her family had often "helped her out" when she was unable to get started or move on.

I explained to her that this "help" would be counterproductive to her improvement. We decided to have her family come in for the next session (Renshaw et al. 2005).

Week 5

During the family meeting I explained how family/caregivers could inadvertently act in ways that are counterproductive to the patient's recovery. Participating or "enabling" is a family's way to protect the loved one in the face of suffering, thus offering immediate relief from OCD distress. I elaborated some typical ways that the family was vicariously participating in OCD behavior:

- Assisting with checking rituals
- Reassuring the patient that things are "safe"
- Trying to reason the OCD away by recounting endless reasons and facts that show how unreasonable the OCD fears are. (In the process, the family may be counterproductively neutralizing the obsessive thought, giving it credence and perpetuating the cycle.)

I asked the family to come up with examples of how they had fallen into any of these traps. We then did some role-playing regarding how the family members could be helpful by being coaches and cheerleaders for Ms. D.B. The following guidelines were established:

1. Anticipate that Ms. D.B. will notice an increase in anxiety before it finally subsides
2. Decrease participation gradually to reach complete disengagement at an agreed-upon time, which is non-negotiable
3. Expect resistance and possibly anger
4. When demands are made for reassurance, the family member should calmly remind Ms. D.B. that, "because I love you, I cannot participate in harmful OCD behavior."

Weeks 6–13

From week 6 to week 13 Ms. D.B. moved down the OCD symptom target list carrying out ERP. She continued to keep her ERP log, and her Y-BOCS scores dropped from 30 to 20. However, when we reached her bathing ritual, we hit a roadblock. At this point she was unable/unwilling to do any of the exposure. She reported severe anxiety and terrible feelings of guilt. She thought that "if the rituals are for my family's safety, I cannot let them go. I feel I am a bad daughter/sister if I challenge the rituals." We tried to use the strategy of "relabeling" as outlined in *Brain Lock* (Schwartz 1996). When relabeling, she would try to identify these thoughts as OCD thoughts and say to herself, "It's not me, it's my OCD." This would allow her to not regard the thoughts as part of her normal thinking and to get perspective on how absurd they are.

From week 11 to week 13 Ms. D.B. appeared to reach an impasse in confronting her remaining OCD symptoms (Figure 24–1). We tried to augment the effect of escitalopram by adding clonazepam 0.5 mg as needed (not to exceed 1 mg/day) for anxiety. She had a history of experiencing anxiety relief with clonazepam, so I tried it first. We could have tried other augmentation strategies, for example, atypical antipsychotics, clomipramine, or buspirone (Koran et al. 2007), but it seemed to me that she just needed a little help in doing her exposure, via relief from heightened anxiety.

Week 14

Ms. D.B. returned with worsening depressive symptoms (Figure 24–2). She reported that her inability to do the ERP was making her "feel like a failure," yet trying to do the exposure "just makes me way too guilty." She wanted a "guarantee that nothing will happen to my family if I try." She also said that, "deep down I must really want them dead if I have this OCD."

We tried to address the cognitive distortions that were getting in the way of her recovery. Prominent among them were the following:

- *Magical thinking/thought-action fusion:* If I think of a pirate, bad things will happen to my family.
- *All-or-nothing thinking:* If I do not shower properly, I am totally dirty.
- *Perfectionism:* It is intolerable until I do it perfectly.
- *Overresponsibility:* I must at all times be on alert so that I do not harm any innocent person.
- *What-if thinking:* What if I make a mistake? …it is not OCD? …Dr. Das is wrong?

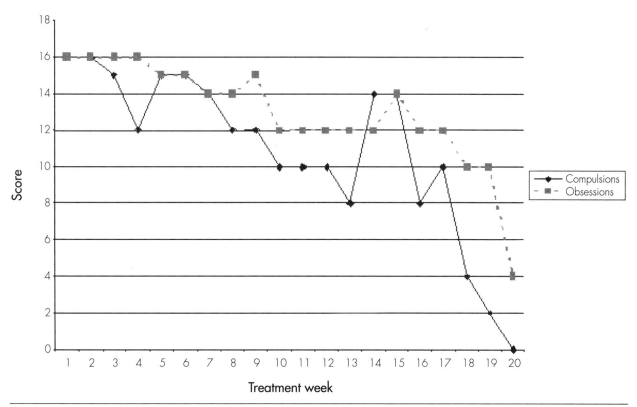

FIGURE 24–1. Patient's Yale-Brown Obsessive Compulsive Scale scores by week.

- *The exclusivity error:* All bad things will happen to my loved ones.

Ms. D.B. was to try to keep a "thought log" and to try to recognize any of these cognitive distortions if they occurred. We also decided that it would be a good idea to have a second family meeting.

Week 15

At the family meeting I had two agenda items: First, I wished to address Ms. D.B.'s guilt. I told her that maybe her OCD revolved around her family's safety because that was the dearest thing to her heart rather than the other way around. There were no data to suggest that this was a fact, but I pointed out that one can only feel intense anxiety when it involves something dear. Second, I asked all the family members if they would give Ms. D.B. permission to do her exposure. They unanimously agreed. We also agreed that if a harmful event did happen in the next few weeks, the family (and, it is hoped, Ms. D.B.) would regard it as having occurred independent of her exposure therapy.

Weeks 16–20

Ms. D.B. was able to go forward with her ERP with renewed vigor. Her Y-BOCS total score came down to 4. She continued escitalopram 20 mg/day. By week 19, she had stopped using clonazepam. We discussed the importance of medication adherence.

Ms. D.B. was to start college. I encouraged her to find a clinician to work with when she moved and gave her names of psychiatrists in the new city. I also had her sign a release of information so that I could transfer records and facilitate continuity of care.

Ways to Improve Practice

Obtain Previous Records

Obtaining records from the previous treating clinician is a good idea. In this case, Ms. D.B. knew what medications she had taken, including how long she took each one and whether it was effective. Her mother had kept records of when she had started each medication, the dosage, and how long Ms. D.B. had taken it. However, patients often do not remember such details, and time may be lost trying something that has already proved ineffective.

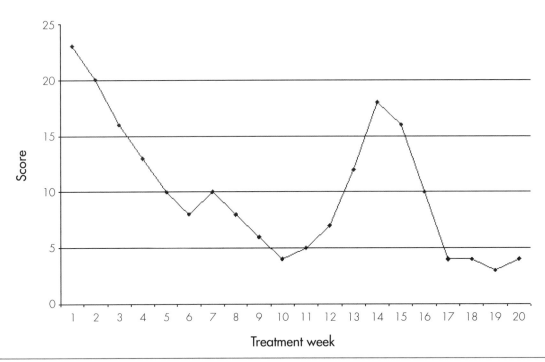

FIGURE 24–2.   Patient's Hamilton Rating Scale for Depression scores by week.

Recognize Resistance

In hindsight, when I looked at Ms. D.B.'s Ham-D graph, it was obvious that she had gotten more depressed as she faced some of the challenges with ERP. The spike seen from week 6 to week 13 was due to an increase in the way she rated her "guilt." If I had paid more careful attention to the ratings and to the symptom subgroups, I could have helped her conquer her fears about doing the exposures.

References

Alpert JE, Mischoulon D, Rubenstein GE, et al: Folic acid (Leucovorin) as an adjunctive treatment for SSRI-refractory depression. Ann Clin Psychiatry 14:33–38, 2002

Coppen A, Bailey J: Enhancement of the antidepressant action of fluoxetine by folic acid: a randomized, placebo controlled trial. J Affect Disord 60:121–130, 2000

Freeman MP, Hibbeln JR, Wisner KL, et al: Omega-3 fatty acids: evidence basis for treatment and future research in psychiatry. J Clin Psychiatry 67:1954–1967, 2006

Goodman WK, Price L, Rasmussen S, et al: The Yale-Brown Obsessive Compulsive Scale (Y-BOCS), part I: development, use, and reliability. Arch Gen Psychiatry 46:1006–1011, 1989

Hamilton M: A rating scale for depression. J Neurol Neurosurg Psychiatry 23:56–62, 1960

Hyman BM, Pedrick C: The OCD Workbook: Your Guide to Breaking Free From Obsessive Compulsive Disorder, 2nd Edition. Oakland, CA, New Harbinger Publications, 2005

Koran LM, Hanna GL, Hollander E, et al: Practice guideline for the treatment of patients with obsessive-compulsive disorder. Am J Psychiatry 164(suppl):1–53, 2007. Available at: http://www.psychiatryonline.com/pracGuide/pracGuideTopic_10.aspx. Accessed June 18, 2009

March JS, Frances A, Carpenter D, et al: The Expert Consensus Guideline Series: treatment of obsessive-compulsive disorder. J Clin Psychiatry 58(suppl):3–72, 1997

Renshaw KD, Steketee G, Chambless DL: Involving family members in the treatment of OCD. Cogn Behav Ther 34:164–175, 2005

Schwartz JM: Brain Lock: Free Yourself From Obsessive-Compulsive Behavior. New York, HarperCollins, 1996

Simpson HB, Liebowitz MR: Combining pharmacotherapy and cognitive-behavioral therapy in the treatment of OCD, in Concepts and Controversies in Obsessive-Compulsive Disorder. Edited by Abramowitz J, Houts A. New York, Springer, 2005, pp 359–376

Simpson HB, Huppert JD, Petkova E, et al: Response versus remission in obsessive-compulsive disorder. J Clin Psychiatry 67:269–276, 2006

Stein DJ, Andersen EW, Tonnoir B, et al: Escitalopram in obsessive-compulsive disorder: a randomized, placebo-controlled, paroxetine-referenced, fixed-dose, 24-week study. Curr Med Res Opin 23:701–711, 2007

Whittal ML, Thordarson DS, McLean PD: Treatment of obsessive-compulsive disorder: cognitive behavior therapy vs. exposure and response prevention. Behav Res Ther 43:1559–1576, 2005

Schizophrenia

A Family Psychoeducational Approach

Douglas S. Rait, Ph.D.

Ira D. Glick, M.D.

The current American Psychiatric Association (APA) practice guidelines for the treatment of schizophrenia (Lehman et al. 2004) offer a striking example of how family interventions have returned to the mainstream in contemporary psychiatric practice. Indeed, as Heru (2008) has pointed out, APA practice guidelines already recommend early couple and family involvement as well as family-based interventions for Axis I disorders, including, but not limited to, schizophrenia, bipolar disorder, major depression, panic disorder, and eating disorders. The family's role in the treatment of schizophrenia has certainly come full circle in that the very roots of the family therapy field can be found in the schizophrenia research conducted more than half a century ago by the field's founders.

These early efforts hypothesized unidirectional parent–child causal effects that, at the time, were thought to possibly explain the etiology of schizophrenia. However, the focus of family researchers in schizophrenia gradually shifted to looking at family processes that maintain the disorder (Kaplan and Rait 1993; Lehman et al. 2004; McFarlane et al. 2003). They identified a host of family factors—such as expressed emotion, stigma, isolation, and caregiver burden—implicated in the ongoing maintenance of serious psychiatric illness (Butzlaff and Hooley 1998; Kavanaugh 1992). These findings

gave rise to family-centered interventions that, in tandem with psychopharmacology advances, reduce patient relapse rates and psychiatric symptoms, enhance medication compliance, and contribute to improved patient and family coping and quality of life (Cohen et al. 2008; Kaplan and Rait 1993; McFarlane et al. 2003; Pitschel-Walz et al. 2004).

Expressed emotion, perhaps the most well-known of these dimensions, is characterized by high levels of criticism, hostility, and overinvolvement on the part of family members. Research has shown that high expressed emotion is a robust predictor of relapse not only in schizophrenia but also in many psychiatric illnesses (that create caregiver burden), such as depressive disorders, bipolar disorder, and alcoholism (Hooley and Teasdale 1989; Miklowitz et al. 1988; O'Farrell et al. 1998; Rait and Glick 2008). At the same time, caregiver research has identified the high emotional and practical burdens of caring for relatives with psychiatric illnesses (Chakrabarti et al. 1992; Drapalski et al. 2008; Ferro et al. 2000).

Family psychoeducation, multiple family therapy psychoeducational groups, behavioral interventions, psychosocial rehabilitation, and self-help advocacy groups (e.g., the National Alliance on Mental Illness [NAMI]) specifically address areas of family functioning that can accelerate illness progression or, alternately, mitigate distress and enhance coping not only for patients but also for families (Cohen et al. 2008; Dixon et al. 2009; McFarlane et al. 2003). As a result, current standards of treatment for the seriously mentally ill recognize the importance of family members' roles in the promotion of long-term recovery. Through empathic engagement, education about the illness, the expansion of social support, accessing appropriate clinical resources during periods of crisis, and the development of communication and problem-solving skills, family psychoeducation in particular has repeatedly been shown to improve both patient recovery and family well-being (Baucom et al. 1997; Glick et al. 2000; Glynn et al. 2008; McFarlane et al. 2003; Pinsof and Wynne 1995; Pitschel-Walz et al. 2004).

On the consumer front, Rolland and Walsh (2005) have also noted that both patients and family members have increasingly advocated for health care that attends to the physical and psychosocial challenges of major health conditions for all family members (not just the sickest person). Heru (2008) has suggested that "improving the family environment has important health implications equivalent to the reduction of risk factors for chronic illness" (p. 966). With this context in mind, we now look at a case example that will serve as a paradigm for the evidence-based practice in the treatment of schizophrenia. Rather than describing a single empirically validated treatment approach, *evidence-based practice* is defined as "the conscientious, explicit, and judicious use of the best evidence in making decisions about the care of individual patients" (Sackett 1999, p. 120). The assessment of and treatment decisions in this case were informed by the clinical data emerging from recent work in the area of schizophrenia, family process, and family psychoeducational interventions.

Setting

Treatment occurred in an academic medical center–based practice of psychiatry involving both brief inpatient hospitalization and long-term outpatient treatment. A flexible family systems orientation was used that combined medication management, individual and family therapy and psychoeducation, and close alliance with a consumer support network involving NAMI. The clinic's patient population covers all socioeconomic groups.

Illustration

This study illustrates the application of a flexible, evidence-based treatment of schizophrenic disorder based on APA practice guidelines. The APA practice guideline for schizophrenia emphasizes the importance of psychopharmacology combined with family intervention, during both the acute phase and the stable phase of the illness (Lehman et al. 2004):

> The acute phase is…the best time for the psychiatrist to initiate a relationship with family members, who tend to be particularly concerned about the patient's disorder, disability, and prognosis during the acute phase and during hospitalization [I]. Educational meetings, "survival workshops" that teach the family how to cope with schizophrenia, and referrals to local chapters of patient and family organizations such as NAMI may be helpful and are recommended [III]. Family members may be under considerable stress, particularly if the patient has been exhibiting dangerous or unstable behavior…. [During the stable phase:] Provide patient and family education and therapies. Work with patients to recognize early symptoms of relapse in order to prevent full-blown illness exacerbations. Educate the family about the nature of the illness and coping strategies to diminish relapses and improve quality of life for patients.

This combined treatment includes individual supportive psychotherapy, medication management, family psychoeducation, and building a network of social support for both patient and family (McFarlane et al. 2003).

Chief Complaint

The patient, Nick, is a 23-year-old single white male with a history of schizophrenia, paranoid type, and substance abuse. He was initially seen a year earlier for psychiatric follow-up (medication maintenance) several weeks after his second hospitalization. The family, also involved in his care, is middle-class and consists of Rob, the father, age 55, a sales representative; Meghan, the mother, age 52, a teacher; a son, Nick (the patient), age 23, who did not complete community college, is a part-time sales clerk, developed paranoid schizophrenia at the age of 19, and smokes marijuana; a daughter, Pam, age 20, a part-time college student who holds a full-time job; and a son, Dave, age 17, a senior in high school. All three children still live at home. They were referred for follow-up after Nick's second hospitalization for the exacerbation of paranoid schizophrenia. Nick is currently being treated with 15 mg/day of olanzapine—a second-generation rather than a first-generation agent—although his compliance with the medication is inconsistent. He complains of side effects, primarily weight gain and sedation.

Present Illness

What Is the Current Family Problem?

Nick has both positive psychotic symptoms, characterized by auditory hallucinations, paranoid thinking, and worries about being attacked by strangers, and negative symptoms that include apathy, flat affect, and inability to seek or hold a job. He also has moderate cognitive impairment. Following his second brief inpatient stay, he was restarted on olanzapine 15 mg/day and referred back to his psychiatrist for follow-up. At the same time, family therapy was also recommended due to intensified family conflict, and the family met with a psychologist/family therapist. Stressors at home prior to that hospitalization included increased conflict around Nick's failure to show up at work, sibling conflicts, and parental conflict about whether to "force him to go to work" or allow him to stay at home and reorganize himself. Given his spotty academic and employment history, his father strongly advocated Nick's going to work "even if he didn't always like it." His mother believed this approach was counterproductive, and she urged her husband and son to "ease up on Nick" because he could not deal with the heightened stress. As a result, heated conflict between the mother and father, with increasing criticism leveled at Nick, ensued.

Why Does the Family Come for Treatment at This Time?

Following the second hospitalization, Meghan felt it was time to intensify treatment in order to develop a strategy that would address the chronic and mounting family conflict surrounding Nick's condition, the stresses undermining Nick's recovery, and the question of whether he should move out on his own. The family had already been referred by the inpatient team to NAMI's family-to-family support program, and they had received individual and family psychoeducation on the unit through lectures and group meetings.

The family reported that about the time Nick announced that he was going to move out, days after he was discharged from the hospital, the parents' long-standing quarreling intensified. The mother went to her family doctor seeking medication for her own anxiety, and she considered finding her own individual therapist because her husband "simply would not listen" to her. Upon discharge, Meghan had also tried to convene a family meeting to develop a plan.

She was unable to find a time when all family members would agree to meet ("How will talking help? He just needs to do something!"), and she requested additional family sessions with the family therapist to formulate next steps. She was joined in these sentiments by her daughter and, eventually, her younger son. However, she felt that nobody would help her and that she could not get any cooperation from the family members in supporting Nick, not to mention in doing regular household chores.

What Is the Background of the Family Problem?

Nick began to develop paranoid symptoms during high school. Rob has worked in high-tech sales for different companies over an extended period of time. Although he had been steadily employed, there were extended periods where he lost jobs, engaged in a job search, and found new work opportunities. Although this boom/bust cycle has been a common fact of life in their area, his wife felt increasingly worried about finances and the "poor role model my husband is offering to the children." Throughout this time, Meghan worked as a middle-school English teacher and managed most of the household duties. The children were all good students, although Nick was thought to have a learning disability for reading (diagnosed in middle school) that had served as an explanation for his increased apathy in class.

Family support had become more of an issue because the parents of both Rob and Meghan had had serious health problems while the children were still in the local public school. Following the death of Meghan's father due to a stroke, Meghan's mother developed dementia. The mother lived nearby and was residing in a nursing facility. Although there is no documented history of schizophrenia in the family, an uncle on Meghan's mother's side and two cousins on Meghan's father's side were similarly described as "odd, eccentric, and difficult to spend time with." Both of Rob's parents were in poor health and lived in the Midwest near his brother and sister.

Current Interactional Patterns

The situation at home had progressively worsened during the 2 months prior to Nick's rehospitalization. Nick began to skip days at work, stay up all night, and show increased irritability. His parents engaged in intensifying conflict, with Rob accusing Nick of being the "cause for all the family's misery" while Meghan defended Nick, claiming that he was "sick," that Rob was insensitive and out of control, and that he (Rob) was the reason her level of stress was unmanageable. As the young adult children entered the conflict, Pam first joined Rob in criticizing Nick, whereas Dave loyally allied with his mother. This pattern of alliances, with Rob and Pam in coalition against Nick, Meghan, and Dave, had been pointed out to the family many times in their family sessions in the hospital. As Rob's complaints about Nick and the "indulgent" attitude shown by Meghan increased, however, Pam eventually joined Meghan in her defense, saying that although she agreed with her father's point about Nick's laziness, pot smoking, and unwillingness to take responsibility, it "isn't fair to attack Mom."

Differential Diagnosis

The patient met the criteria for schizophrenic disorder, paranoid type. In addition, his marijuana use met the criteria for substance abuse, rule out substance dependence. Finally, due to family conflict, parent–child problem was also diagnosed.

DSM-IV-TR Diagnosis

Axis I   Schizophrenic disorder, paranoid type. Substance abuse. Parent–child problem.
Axis II   None
Axis III   None
Axis IV   Deferred
Axis V   GAF score: 30.
            Family's score on the Global Assessment of Relational Functioning Scale: 45.

Treatment Plan Considerations

Although Nick had been treated individually for nearly 2 years without much organized family in-

volvement (one of his parents occasionally accompanied him to monthly appointments), it was determined during his recent inpatient admission that a more consistent family intervention might be helpful in preventing relapse and future inpatient hospitalizations. The family had already been referred to NAMI, but they had never attended a meeting, nor had they attended any outpatient family support meetings offered through the clinic. Although Nick and his family accepted that schizophrenia is a brain disorder, his functional and behavioral dysfunction created ample opportunities for family members to continue to debate whether Nick was "lazy" or "sick."

Given the fact that this family had not previously participated in any organized family intervention program, developing an alliance and shared set of goals was crucial. Family members reported feeling "alone" with the problems they were experiencing, frustrated with Nick's unwillingness to take positive steps on his own behalf, and tired of the arguments and family strife. Because each family member had a busy life, with the exception of the patient, scheduling appointments where everyone could meet invariably presented a challenge. This practical challenge was addressed by setting up a loose schedule, after the initial set of intensive sessions, where meetings were scheduled monthly well in advance, with the option of meeting more frequently during periods of particular stress.

Treatment Goals, Measures, and Methods

The principal components of family psychoeducation outlined by Kaplan and Rait (1993) and McFarlane et al. (2003) include 1) coordinating all elements of treatment and rehabilitation so that everyone is working toward the same goals in a collaborative fashion; 2) paying attention to the social as well as the clinical needs of the patient; 3) providing optimal medication management; 4) assessing and supporting family strengths while acknowledging family limitations in dealing with the patient; 5) improving communication and resolving family conflict; 6) addressing feelings of grief and loss; 7) providing relevant information for family members at appropriate times; 8) developing an explicit crisis plan and response; 9) encouraging family members to expand their social systems of support to combat stigma, caregiver burnout, and social isolation; and 10) in-

TABLE 25–1. Self-reported progress and global functioning scores, by stage

Goal	Early stage	Mid-stage	Late stage
Decrease positive symptoms of disorder	x	x	x
Increase individual coping skills in work, social, and family contexts		x	x
Increase patient and family knowledge about schizophrenia	x	x	x
Reduce expressed emotion and family conflict		x	x
Normalize feelings and reduce emotional burnout	x	x	x
Reduce social isolation and increase individual and family support	x	x	x
Increase problem-solving skills and communication		x	x
Enhance patient's medication compliance	x		x
Decrease patient's marijuana abuse	x		
Global Assessment of Functioning score	30	40	50
Global Assessment of Relational Functioning score	45	55	62

creasing agency and competence and instilling hope in the face of extreme psychosocial challenges.

Specific treatment goals for Nick and his family were to increase knowledge about schizophrenia; reduce expressed emotion and family conflict; normalize family members' feelings and reduce emotional burnout; reduce social isolation and increase family support; increase family problem-solving skills and communication; encourage the patient's functioning in work, social, and family contexts; and support the patient's medication compliance.

Medication goals included decreasing positive symptoms of schizophrenia, over the long run, and improving the negative symptoms and cognition. Here, a second-generation antipsychotic, olanzapine, was used because it has somewhat better efficacy over time and causes fewer extrapyramidal effects. Olanzapine can produce weight gain, so metabolic parameters would have to be constantly monitored. In addition, given Nick's marijuana use, an additional treatment goal was to refer Nick to a substance abuse program, because comorbid substance abuse drastically lowers prognosis (Dickey et al. 2002).

In this particular case, no formal measures were used to track the problem areas or treatment goals. General progress was assessed with treatment notes in the desired areas for improvement, and estimates of progress are provided in Table 25–1 in order to show how treatment progress could be charted.

In a case in which the clinicians are using formal assessment measures to track progress, a range of rating scales and self-report instruments are available. Looking at potential measurable outcomes of family psychoeducation interventions, Cohen et al. (2008) proposed the following: greater rates of ongoing contact between family and patient's treatment team; increased empowerment for family members; increased knowledge about psychiatric illness, treatment, and resources for family members; an improved subjective recovery trajectory (such as perceived control and well-being) of the patient participating in family-based services; enhanced perceptions of family support by patients participating in family services; and improved coping and reduced stress and conflict among all involved family members. Consistent with their emphasis on evidence-based care, they also identified specific instruments to assess each of these dimensions (Cohen et al. 2008).

Course

Early Stage

In the initial family meetings, family members were introduced to the family psychoeducational approach (Heru 2008; Lehman et al. 2004). Information was shared about the etiology and various presentations of the illness, the importance of medication compliance, including the pros and cons of different medications, and the range of services and extrafamilial social supports that were available to them. Initial goals also included recognizing and normalizing family members' emotional reactions of anger, shame, guilt, stigma, and isolation. Finally, family members learned about the structure of the family psychoeducational meetings that would serve as a format for subsequent sessions.

These psychoeducational meetings for the family followed a predictable series of steps. After a brief period of socialization and reconnecting at the session's outset, family members were asked to identify what they would like to gain from the session. Following this "go-round," a particular problem would be selected for the family to address. Then, the therapist would guide the family through a process of problem solving in which the problem would be defined and elaborated, solutions would be entertained and discussed, and a plan would then be adopted.

This process, repeated from meeting to meeting, became a reliable format that family members could use. Problems they identified included focusing on the family's pattern of alliances or "teams," the level of criticism and anger directed toward Nick, a debate over whether to return to the hospital, how to handle problems and disappointments at work, the question of whether Nick should find his own apartment, how to get Nick into a substance abuse program, ways to handle the stress of the grandmother's dementia, strategies for reducing burnout and demoralization, the issue of whether the mother should continue to teach, and how to ensure that Nick was taking his psychiatric medications. Skills for problem solving and communication were also addressed and modeled in every meeting, and the family's continuing involvement with self-help advocacy and support groups was reinforced. In collaboration with his psychiatrist, Nick complied with medication changes and had regular follow-up visits at increasingly spaced intervals. He followed a diet and exercised two to three times a week.

Individual supportive psychotherapy and medication management were started on a weekly basis during the acute phases and gradually increased to monthly sessions as Nick stabilized and his positive symptoms decreased. Family sessions were initially conducted every other week (with more frequent meetings during periods of particular crisis). After Nick's hospitalization, the family convened to discuss whether Nick should move out of the family home. Rob's disappointment and irritation because Nick had stopped going to work regularly was identified as the first problem to solve, and family

members thoughtfully reexamined their roles and alliances with one another. During the session, Nick admitted that he felt he should leave because his father no longer wanted him at home. Rob reassured his son, yet he disclosed how hopeless and frustrated he was that Nick was not taking more responsibility. After all, this had been "an enormous strain for everyone." Nick's mother and siblings were able to understand Rob's feelings, and they shared their concern that Nick would deteriorate more if he lived alone and that he might smoke marijuana to excess, avoid working, and avoid taking care of himself.

Mid-Stage

Over time, Nick's positive symptoms decreased, and communication within the family improved. The family was able to find common ground when Nick agreed that he would stay at home, return to his job, and attend support groups focusing on his marijuana abuse. This concrete plan was ratified, and the family agreed to continue meeting to evaluate progress in each of the areas and to consider the longer-term question of whether Nick might find his own living situation. Feelings on the part of both siblings were addressed, and the parents reported feeling relieved that they had an "agreement that was comfortable for everyone." During periods of extreme stress and increased positive symptoms, both individual and family appointments were more frequent (as was the collaboration between the clinicians in the case). Both patient and family were engaged in treatment consisting of family psychoeducation, individual supportive psychotherapy and medication management with the psychiatrist, and social support though the family-to-family groups at the local chapter of NAMI.

Late Stage

Family meetings continued on an intermittent basis, and regular follow-up was maintained with the psychiatrist. Nick continued to refuse to deal directly with his marijuana use, and neither the family sessions nor the psychiatrist's urging resulted in his locating a treatment program that he would commit to attending. Nick's problem-solving and social skills improved. At the same time, his attendance and performance at his job improved, as he switched (because of his cognitive impairment) to a more suitable position in the stockroom instead of on the sales floor.

As Table 25–1 shows, family members reported a decrease in overall conflict, increased understanding and acceptance of Nick's illness and its consequences, and fewer feelings of frustration, anger, and demoralization. In general, the family's ability to respond to changes in Nick's behavior and affect showed greater flexibility. Family members also highlighted their ability to communicate more clearly, solve problems more effectively, and appropriately identify community and medical resources. Their final Global Assessment of Relational Functioning Scale score was 62.

Ways to Improve Practice

Although no formal measures of treatment progress were used in this case, using formal rating scales or questionnaires could provide data to both the clinicians and family members about their progress together (Cohen et al. 2008). Additionally, this flexible treatment approach combining supportive psychotherapy, medication management, family psychoeducation, and new sources of social support can be replicated in many settings, from a hospital-based practice to the private practice setting to a community mental health context. We do not recommend family therapy alone (i.e., without medication) for treatment of schizophrenia in either acute or chronic phases (Glick 2004; Kaplan and Rait 1993).

Understanding that both the biological and psychosocial aspects of the disorder and the patient's care must be recognized and respected, medical and nonmedical clinicians can work in a collaborative fashion, as is described in the case of Nick and his family, or the psychiatrist can handle both aspects of the care. In some settings that have a more developed family support program for schizophrenia and other serious mental illnesses, families can join family psychoeducational groups that serve many of the same functions as the individual family meetings described here. These groups, however, add the important dimension of social learning and additional social support that emerge when family members from different families facing similar challenges take an interest in, and literally "cross-parent" one another, while encouraging validation, problem solving, and emotional support.

Conclusions

For clinicians helping patients and families deal with the overwhelming experiences associated with schizophrenia, the proposed model of practice provides a helpful framework for an evidence-based practice that builds on considerable clinical research and satisfies current APA practice guidelines (Alexander et al. 2002; Cohen et al. 2008; Lehman et al. 2004; Patterson et al. 2004). The trajectory of schizophrenia over the patient's and family's lifetime requires a flexible treatment approach. We have described a model that combines individual and family support, psychopharmacology, education about the disorder and its consequences, skill building in the areas of family communication and problem solving, the alleviation of conflict and emotional burnout, and a recognition that appropriate involvement of both medical and extrafamilial social supports is essential.

The early work by pioneers in the field of family therapy has been updated and improved by contemporary researchers and clinicians working with patients with schizophrenia. At the same time, there is strong research support for the continued integration of family psychoeducation and other family-centered treatments with prudent psychopharmacological intervention and community support (Cohen et al. 2008; McFarlane et al. 2003). As a result of these developments, current evidence-based practices and principles of family psychoeducation, which can be administered in any clinical setting, can assist every clinician in providing optimal care to every patient and family struggling with this crippling disorder. Psychiatric training and practice would do well to emphasize the identification and application of new ways to enlist the critical involvement of family members in the care of people with schizophrenia.

References

Alexander JF, Sexton TL, Robbins MS: The developmental status of family therapy in family psychology intervention sciences, in Family Psychology: Science-Based Interventions. Edited by Liddle HA, Santisteban DA, Levant RF, et al. Washington, DC, American Psychiatric Association, 2002, pp 17–40

Baucom D, Shoham V, Muester K, et al: Empirically supported couples and family interventions for marital distress and adult mental health problems. J Consult Clin Psychol 66:53–88, 1998

Butzlaff R, Hooley J: Expressed emotion and psychiatric relapse. Arch Gen Psychiatry 55:547–552, 1998

Chakrabarti S, Kulhara P, Verma S: Extent and determinants of burden among families of patients with affective disorders. Acta Psychiatr Scand 86:247–252, 1992

Cohen AM, Glynn SM, Murray-Swank AB, et al: The family forum: directions for the implementation of family psychoeducation for severe mental illness. Psychiatr Serv 59:40–48, 2009

Dickey B, Normand SL, Weiss R, et al: Medical morbidity, mental illness, and substance use disorders. Psychiatr Serv 53:861–867, 2002

Dixon L, Goldberg R, Iannone I, et al: Use of a critical time intervention to promote continuity of care after psychiatric inpatient hospitalization. Psychiatr Serv 60:451–458, 2009

Drapalksi A, Marshall T, Seybolt D, et al: Unmet needs of families of adults with mental illness and preferences regarding family services. Psychiatr Serv 59:655–662, 2008

Ferro T, Verdeli H, Pierre F, et al: Screening for depression in mothers bringing their offspring for evaluation or treatment of depression. Am J Psychiatry 157:375–379, 2000

Glick ID: Adding psychotherapy to pharmacotherapy: data, benefits, and guidelines for integration. Am J Psychother 58:186–208, 2004

Glick I, Berman E, Clarkin J, et al: Marital and Family Therapy, 4th Edition, Washington, DC, American Psychiatric Press, 2000, pp 647–648

Glynn SM, Dixon LB, Cohen AM, et al: The family member provider outreach program. Psychiatr Serv 59:934, 2008

Heru A: Family psychiatry: from research to practice. Am J Psychiatry 163:962–968, 2008

Hooley J, Teasdale J: Predictors of relapse in unipolar depressives: expressed emotion, marital distress and perceived criticism. J Abnorm Psychol 3:229–235, 1989

Kaplan F, Rait D: Partnerships for schizophrenia: reconciling professional models. Workshop presented at the 51st annual conference of the American Association of Marriage and Family Therapy, Anaheim, CA, October 1993

Kavanaugh D: Recent developments in expressed emotion and schizophrenia. Br J Psychiatry 160:601–620, 1992

Lehman AF, Lieberman JA, Dixon LB, et al: American Psychiatric Association Steering Committee on Practice Guidelines: practice guideline for the treatment of patients with schizophrenia, 2nd ed. Am J Psychiatry 161(suppl):1–56, 2004

McFarlane W, Dixon L, Lukens E, et al: Family psychoeducation and schizophrenia: a review of the literature. J Marital Fam Ther 29:223–246, 2003

Miklowitz D, Goldstein M, Nuechterlein K, et al: Family factors and the course of bipolar affective disorder. Arch Gen Psychiatry 45:225–231, 1988

O'Farrell T, Hooley J, Fals-Stewart W, et al: Expressed emotion and relapse in alcoholic patients. J Consult Clin Psychol 66:744–752, 1998

Patterson JE, Miller RB, Carnes S, et al: Evidence based practice for marriage and family therapists. J Marital Fam Ther 30:183–195, 2004

Pinsof W, Wynne L: The efficacy of marital and family therapy: an empirical overview, conclusions, and recommendations. J Marital Fam Ther 21:585–613, 1995

Pitschel-Walz G, Leucht S, Bäuml J, et al: The effect of family interventions on relapse and rehospitalization in schizophrenia: a meta-analysis. Focus 2:78–94, 2004

Rait D, Glick I: Reintegrating family therapy training in psychiatric residency programs: making the case. Acad Psychiatry 32:76–80, 2008

Rolland J, Walsh F: Systemic training for healthcare professionals: The Chicago Center for Family Health approach. Fam Process 44:283–301, 2005

Sackett DL: How evidence-based medicine will change the way you practice. Med Econ 76:120–128, 1999

Substance Use Disorder Presenting as a Mood Disorder

Anna Lembke, M.D.
Keith Humphreys, Ph.D.

Setting

We practice at a university medical center with no specialty treatment program for substance use disorders. Our patients with addictive disorders are typically seeking treatment for psychiatric and/or medical issues rather than openly presenting complaints related to substance abuse.

General Treatment Approach

Our treatment approach is targeted at helping patients with addictive disorders understand that substance use is a problem and likely a contributor to their psychiatric symptoms. The challenge is to invite the patient into an honest discussion of substance use while maintaining a therapeutic alliance and addressing the chief complaint.

Illustration

This study illustrates:

- Screening for substance use disorders, specifically focusing on how to use the Timeline Followback (TLFB) method
- Differentiating primary from secondary (i.e., substance-induced) psychiatric symptoms
- Treating substance use disorders using the Veterans Health Administration/Department of Defense (VHA/DoD) *Clinical Practice Guidelines for the Management of Substance Use Disorders*

Chief Complaint

Ms. R.D., a 19-year-old female freshman undergraduate, has been referred to our outpatient psychiatric treatment clinic from the campus health center for assessment and treatment of "mood swings, insomnia, and anxiety" lasting for at least 2 months.

Present Illness

Ms. R.D. reports feeling "very sad" for 3 weeks prior to her initial presentation in our clinic, with bouts of crying, difficulty completing her schoolwork, and thoughts of suicide but no specific plan to take her life. She also reports excessive sleep, often not getting out of bed until midday, and episodes of severe anxiety, during which she begins to hyperventilate and "feel overwhelmed." She also describes a pattern of mood fluctuation, in which for up to 5 days at a time she feels happy, even euphoric, with high energy, extreme garrulousness, and decreased need for sleep—i.e., not feeling tired even if she only sleeps 3 hours the night before. She also describes some high-risk behaviors at these times: excessive spending and unprotected sex with multiple partners. She

Keith Humphreys was supported by grants from the Veterans Affairs Health Services Research and Development Service and the Robert Wood Johnson Foundation.

has not experienced an elevated mood in the past 3 weeks.

Based on her self-report narrative, Ms. R.D. appears to meet full criteria for bipolar disorder, characterized by periods of depression alternating with periods of mania/hypomania. Her mood at the time of presentation is depressed for 3 weeks, with thoughts of suicide but no specific intent or plan. Her recent behavior has put her at risk for sexually transmitted diseases.

Ms. R.D. does not mention substances in her chief complaint or opening narrative. This is not atypical, even when substances are a prominent problem in the patient's life. The reasons for this omission are manifold, having to do with but not limited to clinical inattention, stigma, and unwillingness to surrender the rewarding aspects of substance use. Therefore it falls upon the treatment provider to screen for substance use, a task that is all too frequently neglected by psychiatrists (Danielsson et al. 1999; Himelhoch and Daumit 2003).

Other Significant Findings From Assessment

Screening for Substance Use Disorders

With all of our patients, we introduce substance use screening early in the evaluation process and document our findings in a separate section just after the "History of Present Illness." We usually label it "Substance Use Patterns and History." We prioritize substance use screening for several reasons. Epidemiological studies, corroborated by our clinical experiences, tell us that 30%–40% of individuals with a lifetime mood disorder will meet criteria for a substance use disorder (Kessler et al. 1996). Likewise, many individuals dependent on nicotine, alcohol, or illegal drugs will also have a depressive disorder (Kessler et al. 2003). If substance use is detected as a problem early on, this discovery informs the rest of the interview process. It becomes necessary to delineate what relationship the presenting psychiatric symptoms have with the substance use. Substance use can mimic many psychiatric symptoms and disorders.

Many individuals, addicted or not, are poor at recalling substance use accurately, even if they are comfortable disclosing it candidly to the clinician. Therefore, asking about specific amounts and spe-

cific days using the Timeline Followback method is, in our opinion, a very effective way to begin assessment. The TLFB method charts the amounts and patterns of substance use in the preceding 1–2 weeks, independent of consequences or compulsivity of use (Sobell and Sobell 1995). This method often results in a more valid assessment of actual substance use than if the interviewer simply asks: "How much do you drink in a given week?" By keeping to specifics and a timeline, there is a markedly decreased chance of the patient minimizing consumption, mixing up drinking occasions, or mentally averaging drinking over the period of interest.

We ask the patient to begin with the day prior to our encounter and move backward, remembering how much alcohol he or she consumed on each day in the preceding 1–2 weeks. Where appropriate, we offer concrete events to stimulate memory, for example, "Let's start with Monday, that was the first day of the week before midterm exams." When asking about alcohol, it is vital to ask about the type of alcoholic beverage consumed and the size of the drink (see Table 26–1 for definitions). By knowing the type and exact amounts, we can calculate the number of standard drinks consumed in a week. Hazardous drinking for men is 14 or more standard drinks in a week or 5 or more standard drinks in a sitting. Hazardous drinking for women is 7 or more standard drinks in a week or 4 or more in a sitting (see Table 26–1). The TLFB method was developed and validated primarily for alcohol, but we also find it a useful means for other substances. It is important to remember when screening for other substances that there are no unequivocal quantity or frequency risk thresholds for hazardous use, and nearly all daily nicotine users are nicotine dependent (Veterans Health Administration/Department of Defense 2001).

Using the TLFB method with Ms. R.D., we assess amounts and patterns of alcohol use:

Interviewer: Do you drink alcohol?
R.D.: Yes.
Interviewer: Today is Wednesday. How much, if anything, did you drink last night?
R.D.: Nothing.
Interviewer: How about Monday night?
R.D.: Nothing.
Interviewer: And Sunday night—that was when the Oscars were on.
R.D.: Yes, I always watch. I didn't drink anything.

TABLE 26–1. Hazardous alcohol use screening

Definition	Comments	Male	Female
Typical drinks *per week* (U.S. Preventive Services Task Force 1996)	Standard drinks: 0.5 fluid ounces of absolute alcohol 12 ounces of beer 5 ounces of wine 1.5 ounces of 80-proof spirits	≥14	≥7
Maximum drinks *per occasion* (SAMHSA 2008)	May vary depending on age, ethnicity, medical and psychiatric comorbidity, pregnancy, and other risk factors	≥5	≥4

Interviewer: O.K., How about Saturday night? That was the night after the presidential debate.

R.D.: Well, my sorority gave a party, so of course I drank a lot.

Interviewer: How much?

R.D.: Oh, I don't know. Maybe four or five drinks.

Interviewer: What kinds of drinks did you have?

R.D.: Well, I started with a couple glasses of wine, and then I had some tequila shots. And then some vodka shots.

Interviewer: About how many ounces do you think were in each glass of wine?

R.D.: An average size glass.

Interviewer: About 5 ounces in each glass? *(gesturing with hand to mark size)*

R.D.: That looks about right.

Interviewer: And how many ounces in the tequila and vodka shots?

R.D.: I guess about an ounce.

Interviewer: And how many shots total?

R.D.: Well...maybe five...or six.

By using this method, we discover that Ms. R.D. drank eight standard drinks on the preceding Saturday night, as opposed to the "four or five" she originally quoted. By continuing the TLFB method for the remainder of the week, we discover that Ms. R.D. had consumed 18 standard drinks in the week preceding the interview. Even she is surprised by the actual amounts once it is all added up. Clearly her level of consumption is in the hazardous range (see Table 26–1) and alerts us (based on amounts and pattern of use alone) to the probability of a substance use disorder. With that information we put more time and emphasis on eliciting a detailed substance use history, now focused on DSM-IV-TR (American Psychiatric Association 2000) criteria for abuse and dependence, which primarily have to do with consequences of substance use and the compulsive drive to use.

Substance Use Patterns and History

Ms. R.D. first began using substances at age 15, when she started smoking marijuana two or three times per month. At age 17 she began to drink alcohol heavily and at age 18 began snorting cocaine. For the past 4 or 5 months, she reports drinking much more than usual for her, drinking on average three times a week, typically consuming between five and seven drinks in a single sitting. As the TLFB method revealed, she had consumed 18 standard drinks in the week preceding the interview. She reports drinking even more if there are parties in the dormitories.

She has tried to cut back on her own in the preceding couple of months but has been unable to do so. She also reports that once she begins drinking, even if she only intends to have one or two, she finds she is not able to stop drinking. She admits she plans her entire day, and even her week, around going out to drink and that it is the only thing she looks forward to all day long. She states that she lives in a sorority and that her entire social life revolves around going out and "partying" with her friends.

When asked about other drugs currently used, she endorses habitual cocaine use for 3 months, up until 3 weeks ago, when she "stopped cold turkey." Prior to 3 weeks ago, she "snorted one to two lines" during the week, and up to four or five lines per night on the weekends. She smokes approximately five cigarettes a day but can smoke up to a pack in a single sitting if she has been drinking heavily: "Then I smoke until my throat hurts."

Differentiating Primary From Secondary Psychiatric Symptoms

After gathering a detailed substance use history, we obtain a detailed mood history with the intention of sorting out the relationship, if any, between the psychiatric symptoms and the substance use. This method creates a more objective view of the relationship between substance use and psychiatric symptoms than if we asked the patient "Which came first, the depression or the drinking?" In our experience, a question asked in that way will more likely than not get a response that attributes substance use to the psychiatric illness (the "self-medication hypothesis"), even when the actual pattern is not consistent with this explanation. This is not always because patients are intentionally duplicitous, but rather because the human brain is seeking to ascribe a rational cause to an irrational behavior (i.e., substance abuse) and because framing substance use as a side effect of illness may alleviate shame in the patient's mind.

In obtaining this history, we are particularly interested in periods of sustained sobriety when we might analyze the patient's mood patterns free of the cycle of intoxication and withdrawal. We also focus on time of onset, although both mood disorders and substance use disorders tend to progress insidiously, making differentiation between primary and secondary mood disorders difficult (Mueser et al. 1998). Due to retrospective bias, clarification of primary versus secondary psychiatric symptoms is best done with prospective charting of mood during a period of confirmed abstinence.

Ms. R.D. reports that her mood swings started in high school, fluctuating wildly up and down, but that she never sought or received professional treatment for this problem and that it never impaired her functioning. She states that her mood problems predated her substance use problems and that she began drinking to "self-medicate" her depression, although this information is at odds with the substance use history she gave earlier in the interview, in which she stated that alcohol and marijuana use began at age 15, around the same time her mood problems began. When asked to clarify, she reports that she would go for a month at a time without drinking or using marijuana in high school and still had mood problems, although she has had no period of abstinence longer than a month since matriculating high school.

Focusing on more recent events, Ms. R.D. describes extreme euphoric moods alternating with depression, her primary reason for presenting to our clinic. Her high moods generally coincide with cocaine intoxication, and the low moods with cocaine withdrawal. She has been persistently depressed in the 3 weeks prior to presenting in our clinic, after her abrupt discontinuation of cocaine. Before beginning heavier cocaine use 3–4 months ago, her mood would fluctuate, but not to such an extreme.

With this information, we are now ready to make a preliminary diagnosis.

DSM-IV-TR Diagnosis

Axis I   Substance-induced mood disorder; rule out primary mood disorder (major depressive disorder vs. bipolar disorder); alcohol dependence, binge type; nicotine dependence; cocaine dependence; marijuana abuse; cocaine withdrawal

Axis II   Deferred

Axis III   At risk for sexually transmitted diseases

Axis IV   Compromised role functioning, trouble with schoolwork

Axis V   GAF scale score: 50, moderate to severe, with role impairment and passive suicidal ideation

Differential Diagnosis

We do not make a diagnosis of mood disorder at this time, because we feel based on her history and presenting symptoms that all of Ms. R.D.'s problems may be substance induced. Her euphoric moods may be entirely explained by cocaine intoxication, and her recent persistent depression by cocaine withdrawal. Her more remote history of mood fluctuations is so intertwined with substance use, without any clear antecedent or sustained period of sobriety (greater than 1 month), that we are unable to differentiate substance-induced mood fluctuations from mood disorder. Ms. R.D.'s recent anxiety and insomnia are certainly also attributable to her ongoing hazardous alcohol use and daily cigarette smoking. Nonetheless, we are not ruling out the possibility that she has an independent mood disorder, and we will use prospective analysis during a period of sobriety to make a more definitive conclusion.

Treatment Plan Considerations

Developing a specific treatment guideline for substance use disorders is difficult, because although addiction can broadly be conceptualized as one disorder, treatment interventions vary greatly depending on the types of substances being abused, the severity of the substance use disorder, an individual's readiness for change, the treatment setting, and the presence of co-occurring medical and psychiatric disorders. Of necessity then, guidelines for substance use disorders tend to be vague. Nonetheless, they are useful in promoting evidence-based strategies, particularly if they delineate not only the substance being abused but also the other parameters described earlier that influence patient care, such as readiness for change.

The American Psychiatric Association guidelines contain many useful lessons but are written at a general level, which does not substantially inform the care process step by step. In contrast, the VHA/DoD *Clinical Practice Guideline for the Management of Substance Use Disorders in the Primary Care Setting* (Veterans Health Administration/Department of Defense 2001) was most useful. [This guideline has since been replaced; see Veterans Health Administration/Department of Defense 2009.] This VHA/DoD treatment guideline is organized as an algorithm with five modules, and recommendations vary depending on treatment setting, severity of substance use, and readiness for change. The guideline focuses on assessment and management in a primary care setting. At first it may seem odd to use a primary care guideline in a psychiatry setting, but our practice is similar to primary medical practice in that our patients present for help with self-identified problems that typically have nothing to do with addiction, and those with substance abuse tend to have somewhat less severe problems than would typical be encountered in a specialty setting, for example, a substance abuse inpatient or residential program. We have outlined the VHA/DoD treatment guideline recommendations in Table 26–2, following the algorithm as it applies to our patient, Ms. R.D. In the following sections, we provide a brief review of the treatment course of Ms. R.D., comparing and contrasting our intervention with those recommended by the VHA/DoD guideline. Missing in most guidelines is the "how" to achieve these goals, and so we present in a detailed manner the exact language we use in communicating with our patients and the specific strategies we apply to achieving each clinical intervention.

Recommendation #1

- Give feedback about screening results, relating the risks of negative health effects to the patient's presenting health concerns.

In giving feedback to Ms. R.D. about her substance use, we make a conscious effort not to replicate the nagging insistence of exhausted, worried, and overwhelmed spouses/parents/friends. Instead, we take a matter-of-fact approach, emphasizing that we are partners in this endeavor of getting her well and that she is an autonomous adult who will have to make her own decisions based on the information that we provide.

Our first step is to talk about the results of the TLFB method regarding her alcohol consumption and ask what she thinks about the amount of alcohol she consumes in a week. Not surprisingly, Ms. R.D. says that she drinks no more than her friends. It is helpful to introduce the scientific finding that individuals who drink heavily tend to select in to social networks where heavy drinking is common. Thus, although she may consume the same amount as her friends, this makes it neither healthy nor by any means "normal." In fact, most young adults her age are not using substances at the same frequency and amount she does. Ms. R.D. is genuinely surprised to learn that, for example, the average 19-year-old consumes a mere fraction of the amount of alcohol she is consuming. Based on the National Survey on Drug Use and Health, 45% of women in the age range of 18–25 do not drink any alcohol in a typical week, and only 2% of 18- to 25-year-old women drink 15 or more drinks in a typical week (see Figure 26–1; Substance Abuse and Mental Health Services Administration 2008). With this information, Ms. R.D. can see that her alcohol consumption is well outside the "normal" range for women her age.

After discussing the results of the TLFB method and discussing "normal" alcohol use for a woman her age, we read aloud the diagnostic criteria for substance abuse and dependence from DSM-IV-TR. We ask Ms. R.D. if she thinks any of the criteria apply to her. She is able to endorse the compulsivity

TABLE 26–2.   VHA/DoD clinical practice guideline for the management of substance use disorders for patient R.D.

Area	Recommendation	Followed
Initial assessment	Obtain history, physical examination, laboratory tests, mental status examination, and medication.	√
	Is patient medically or psychiatrically unstable or acutely intoxicated?	√ Passive suicidality present but no plan or intent: Assessed with CIWAR and not at risk for dangerous alcohol withdrawal
	Does patient exhibit hazardous substance use or abuse or dependence or risk of relapse? If yes, then...	√ Yes
Provide brief intervention	Give feedback about screening results, relating the risks of negative health effects to the patient's presenting health concerns.	√
	Inform the patient about safe consumption limits and offer advice about change.	√
	Offer to involve family members in this process to educate them and solicit their input (consent is required).	No, but took an ecological approach
	Assess patient's degree of readiness for change (e.g., "How willing are you to consider reducing your use at this time?").	√
	Negotiate goals and strategies for change.	√
	If indicated, treat with pharmacotherapy for addiction.	No, and perhaps should have considered this
	Schedule an initial follow-up appointment in 2–4 weeks.	Scheduled a follow-up in 1 week after first visit, given suicidal ideation at first presentation
	Monitor changes at follow-up visits by asking patient about use, health effects, and barriers to change.	√
	Is patient nicotine dependent? If yes, then treat.	√
	Treat concurrent psychiatric disorders, including concurrent pharmacotherapy.	√
Monitoring	Establish a specific system for monitoring substance use.	Not done, an error on our part

Note.   CIWAR=Clinical Institute Withdrawal Assessment of Alcohol; VHA/DoD=Veterans Health Administration/Department of Defense.

Source.   Veterans Health Administration/Department of Defense 2009.

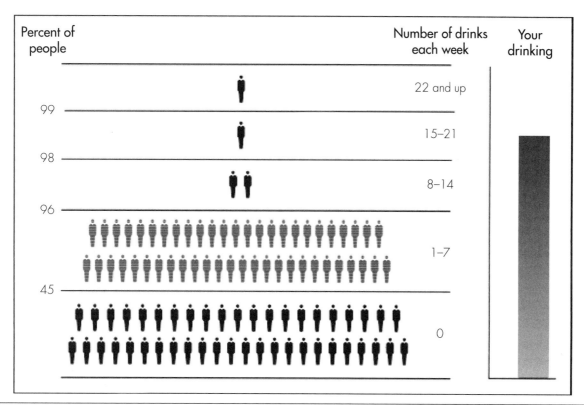

FIGURE 26–1. Rates of alcohol consumption, based on standard drinks, for women in the United States ages 18–25 years and for patient R.D.

Source. Kenneth R. Weingardt, Center for Health Care Evaluation, VA Palo Alto Health Care System and Stanford University School of Medicine; National Survey on Drug Use and Health (SAMHSA 2008).

and out-of-control nature of her use but is not able to clearly state any negative consequences. We help her identify some of the negative consequences, including exposing herself to sexually transmitted diseases; doing poorly at school; and possibly causing depression, anxiety, and insomnia, in the short-term and liver and lung damage in the long term. We talk about the cognitive and emotional problems that can result as a direct response to substance use. When the patient reports that substances "feel good" in the short term, no effort is made to argue. Following the precepts of the evidence-based treatment known as motivational interviewing, we do not try to argue patients out of what they perceive as the positives of their behavior. Rather, we attempt to balance these immediate rewards with information about longer-term costs. Ms. R.D. is able to tolerate hearing this information, but she responds with "I really don't think I am an alcoholic. If I really wanted to, I could stop drinking." Here is our opportunity then, to ask her to do just that (see Recommendation #2). Again following motivational interviewing

principles, in suggesting an abstinence trial we do not label her as "alcoholic." Rather, we ask her to conduct an experiment, so to speak, to help her and us understand how serious her drinking is.

We revisit Ms. R.D.'s specific chief complaint: "mood swings, insomnia, and anxiety" and feeling "very sad" in the 3 weeks prior to her appointment. We reiterate that dysphoria, insomnia, and anxiety are the most common and pervasive symptoms of withdrawal from any addictive substance, no matter the type, and although substances may help with these symptoms in the short term, they will create these symptoms once the individual is in the cycle of intoxication and withdrawal. Many patients presenting to our clinic insist that their depression, insomnia, anxiety, and so on cause them to use substances and that if we would only "cure" their psychiatric problems, their substance use would disappear. We know based on evidence in the literature and our own clinical experience that treating the mood or anxiety disorders seldom if ever resolves the substance use disorder and that psychiatric symptoms are in general very resistant to treatment in the context of a co-occurring substance use disorder. Numerous studies treating mood problems prospectively in patients with co-occurring substance use problems demonstrate that substance use problems do not generally resolve when mood issues are treated (Nunes and Levin 2004). Addiction appears to have an illness course independent of mood outcomes and needs its own treatment strategy. For an excellent review addressing the question of which came first, the substance use or the mood problems, please see "Dual Diagnosis: A Review of Etiological Theories," by Mueser et al. (1998). It is our very important job to educate patients that even if relief from negative emotions is what causes them to initiate substance use, the pattern of abuse and dependence is a disorder distinctly its own and needs and deserves to be treated as well.

Recommendation #2

- Inform the patient about safe consumption limits and offer advice about change.

We inform Ms. R.D. that hazardous alcohol use for an adult woman is more than seven drinks in a single week, and more than four drinks in a single sitting, and that all-cause morbidity and mortality is lowest for women who consume fewer than two standard drinks per week (Swift 1999). However, in the context of out-of-control and compulsive use, abstinence from all substances may be the best alternative, primarily because individuals with alcohol dependence have great difficulty limiting their use. Abstinence is also a recommended course of action when psychiatric symptoms are prominent, in order to help clarify what fraction of the patient's symptoms is substance induced and what fraction represents another Axis I disorder, such as major depression or panic disorder. We tell Ms. R.D. that smoking even a single cigarette a day adversely impacts her lifetime morbidity and mortality and possibly contributes to her symptoms of depression and anxiety.

After challenging Ms. R.D.'s misperception about normal substance use, discussing the criteria for a substance use disorder, educating her about the adverse consequences of substance abuse, and offering information about safe consumption, we make our first suggestions for change. For outpatients like Ms.

R.D. who do not self-identify as having a substance use disorder and who present for treatment of psychiatric problems other than substance use, we typically begin by suggesting an agreed-upon period of abstinence as a test of the patient's control over substances and as a means by which to better evaluate their presenting psychiatric problems. We also let them know that even if they are unable to adhere to the contract, they may want to consider the possibility that they do not have the control they thought they had, in which case we might need a more specific and extended intervention for a substance use disorder, such as Alcoholics Anonymous. Practice guidelines recommend referral of all serious cases of drinking problems to Alcoholics Anonymous or other self-help groups, and both research literature and our clinical experience support this suggestion (Humphreys 2004).

Less commonly appreciated in cases like that of Ms. R.D., self-help groups can actually benefit patients who never attend them, because for the average person, needing to go to Alcoholics Anonymous meetings is a common-sense sign that their alcohol problem is indeed quite serious. This may be quite motivating during a trial of abstinence (e.g., "I would rather quit on my own than have to admit that I need Alcoholics Anonymous").

We also ask our patients to consider stopping smoking. Psychiatrists tend to defer smoking cessation treatment to a time when the patient is not in acute crisis. However, there is mounting evidence that depressed smokers are both willing and able to quit smoking at rates similar to nondepressed smokers and that the risk of depression in the wake of smoking cessation is much less than previously believed. Furthermore, stopping smoking may improve psychiatric symptoms over the life course. Our approach to this issue is discussed in detail later in this chapter.

Recommendation #3

- Offer to involve family members in this process to educate them and solicit their input (consent is required).

We typically ask patients to involve family members, as long as the specific family member is clearly a positive influence and understands the process of recovery from addiction. In Ms. R.D.'s case, her father is an active alcoholic and her mother a chronic bulimic, not to mention that they are both living on the other side of the country from our patient. In cases like these, we do not involve family members but instead embark on a discussion of the environmental factors contributing toward a patient's substance use. An ecological approach to addiction treatment underscores the importance of context and social relations in the cycle of addiction.

Ms. R.D. lives in a sorority with a reputation for partying and has a circle of friends, including a boyfriend, with whom she habitually drinks to get drunk. In other words, the network of people at the center of her life use substances. It is essential to explore with substance use–disordered patients how the relationships in their lives will be affected if they stop using substances. Not uncommonly, removing the major shared activity—and one that at least part of the time is quite rewarding—can threaten the foundation of the relationship. We try to acknowledge that stopping substances may have a destabilizing effect on the patient's social milieu. Likewise, we ask patients to identify who in their lives might help them stop using substances and encourage them to seek out settings in which substances are not used, which may range from religious organizations to cultural/civic clubs to athletic teams or study groups. Depending on the arrangements available on the campus, another possibility when necessary is to shift living arrangements to a dry floor in a dormitory.

Recommendation #4

- Assess patient's degree of readiness for change (e.g., "How willing are you to consider reducing your use at this time?").

Ms. R.D. is willing to make changes and agrees to a 4-week trial of abstinence from all substances. She is motivated by the prospect that her insomnia and mood swings might improve and by her own acknowledgment that her substance use is not where she would like it to be.

Recommendation #5

- Negotiate goals and strategies for change.

As mentioned earlier, we recommend that Ms. R.D. identify individuals and activities that might help her avoid substance use. We discuss triggers for substance use, such as sorority parties, and talk about whether she could avoid the parties altogether or, if not, develop strategies to abstain from substance use while attending the parties. We recommend getting rid of all substances and substance paraphernalia, including running water over her remaining cigarettes before disposing of them in her garbage can, and so on. Importantly, we emphasize to Ms. R.D. that whether or not she is successful in this 4-week trial of abstinence, we want to see her, we want to hear from her, we are here to care for her. We give her our contact information and carte blanche to call us with any questions or concerns. We warn her again that initially her symptoms of low mood, anxiety, and insomnia may get worse before they get better, due to early withdrawal, but that if she is able to remain abstinent or even substantially reduce her use, we believe she will begin to feel better in 2–4 weeks. If at that time, with abstinence, she continues to have psychiatric symptoms, we assure her that we will proceed with treatment for a mood disorder. We warn her about more serious withdrawal symptoms, such as delirium tremens and seizure, although we do not feel she is at risk for these. Although withdrawal risk is not extremely high in Ms. R.D.'s case, it is worth mentioning that in many cases, particularly those that are more severe, we often refer to the Clinical Institute Withdrawal Assessment for Alcohol (Sellers et al. 2008). This instrument screens medical and surgical patients for the risk of developing alcohol withdrawal syndrome and is published in the *Handbook of Psychiatric Measures* by Rush et al. (2008). It can also be found on the Internet.

Recommendation #6

- Treat with pharmacotherapy for addiction, if indicated.

We do not recommend or even discuss pharmacotherapy specifically for addiction with Ms. R.D. According to the VHA/DoD guideline, Ms. R.D. is a good candidate for naltrexone or disulfiram, particularly given her combined alcohol and cocaine dependence (see Table 26–3). Given that her alcohol

TABLE 26–3. Indications for using naltrexone and disulfiram for alcohol dependence, according to VHA/DoD guidelines

Naltrexone	Disulfiram[a]
Alcohol dependence with:	**Alcohol dependence with:**
Ability to achieve at least 3–5 days of abstinence to rule out the need for detoxification	Abstinence >24 hours and blood alcohol level=0
Drinking within the past 30 days and/or reports of craving	Combined cocaine and alcohol dependence
Most effective when the patient is engaged in addiction-focused counseling	Failure of or contraindication to naltrexone
	Previous response to disulfiram
	Patient preference
	Capacity to appreciate risks and benefits and to consent to treatment

Note. VHA/DoD=Veterans Health Administration/Department of Defense.
[a]Most effective with monitored administration (e.g., in clinic or with spouse or probation officer).

Source. Veterans Health Administration/Department of Defense 2004.

dependence is not extremely advanced, her readiness for change, and the lack of any recent prior quit attempts, we decide to bypass addiction pharmacotherapy, at least initially. However, we do offer low-dose trazodone, an antidepressant which is an effective, nonaddictive sleep aid. She declines.

Recommendation #7

- Schedule an initial follow-up appointment in 2–4 weeks.

Given the severity of Ms. R.D.'s substance use, including a severe binge drinking pattern and the use of illicit drugs as well as her passive suicidal ideation, we feel it is important to see her back within a week and to establish a safety contract for her to call us if she gets much worse in the interim. Ms. R.D. agrees to this plan, yet she does not appear for her next appointment.

We frequently experience this phenomenon: A patient expresses willingness to a trial of reduced substance use or abstinence and then does not appear at the follow-up appointment. It represents an important juncture in the treatment of addicted patients. It is essential that we call the patient at this time and emphasize to them that we want to see them, that we care about them, and that this is true even if they were not able to adhere to the contract

of reduced or abstinent substance use. If the patient is not able to reduce or abstain from substances, their shame often leads them to consciously or unconsciously forget their appointment with us. Therefore it becomes essential for us to initiate contact and reemphasize our involvement in their treatment, no matter their current substance use. In our experience, a phone call like this usually brings the patient in. If the clinician does not call the patient, the patient will likely not return to treatment.

We call Ms. R.D., and she states that she had forgotten the appointment but says she is doing better, has drastically reduced her alcohol consumption, and is not using any other substances except for "occasional" nicotine. She is unable to be specific as to the precise amounts of substances consumed, although we believe her report of substantial reduction. We emphasize how important it is for her to come in and see us, and indeed the next week she comes to her appointment. Her mood seems upbeat, and she reports that she is sleeping better than she has in years, and her mood is much steadier. She has decided to tell everyone in her sorority, and her boyfriend, that she has had to stop drinking and using drugs, and to her great surprise, they are very supportive. Her boyfriend apparently comments that he likes her "better off drugs" because she "isn't so loopy." Life is looking up, and we continue the same treatment plan, encouraging her to try to further reduce her alcohol consumption down to nothing and to even try to abstain from cigarettes, which she is now smoking at the rate of three or four per week. We schedule an appointment for 2 weeks from now.

Recommendation #8

- Offer and recommend smoking cessation treatment to every patient who is dependent on nicotine. Use the VHA/DoD *Clinical Practice Guideline for the Management of Tobacco Use* (Veterans Health Administration/Department of Defense 2004).

Nicotine dependence is a diagnosis that is too often ignored and minimized by mental health care providers (Himelhoch and Daumit 2003). We feel strongly that nicotine dependence should be included in the diagnoses and aggressively treated, and this viewpoint is supported by the VHA/DoD guideline as well as most other guidelines. Although most clinicians would have stronger concern about alcohol and cocaine use in cases like that of Ms. R.D., the epidemiologic reality is that, on average, nicotine is far more likely to result in death over the lifespan of such individuals. Nicotine addiction is the highest contributor toward morbidity and mortality in this country, taking up to 350,000 lives every year. It is important for mental health care providers to identify nicotine dependence as a health care issue and to discuss treatment options, lest they covertly communicate that smoking is not a problem (Lembke et al. 2007).

Ms. R.D. is initially able to reduce her daily cigarette consumption but not cut cigarettes out altogether. We take time at her third visit to address nicotine again and to encourage her to stop smoking completely. We offer a U.S. Food and Drug Administration–approved smoking cessation remedy, namely bupropion (Wellbutrin or Zyban) and nicotine replacement therapy, and encourage her to set a specific quit date, both interventions that have been associated with the best outcomes. Ms. R.D. accepts a smoking cessation trial intervention with bupropion; however, 3 days into treatment with bupropion, prior to quitting smoking, she calls to report she is feeling very jittery and "amped" and is unable to sleep. Her mood is euthymic with brief period of feeling down, lasting less than half a day. She has maintained a lower level of alcohol consumption

and continues to be abstinent from cocaine and marijuana. We immediately call her back and suggest she stop the bupropion until further discussion at her next visit, scheduled for the next week.

Recommendation #9

- Monitor changes at follow-up visits by asking patient about use, health effects, and barriers to change.

When Ms. R.D. presents for her fourth appointment, 5 weeks from her initial presentation, she reports that her sleep has continued to be poor, even after stopping the bupropion, although still not as bad as before she initially presented. She also reports that her mood is consistently low nearly all day, 2–3 days a week. She is not suicidal, she has continued to abstain from marijuana and cocaine, and her alcohol consumption has gone down to zero for the past week, in the hope that complete abstinence would buoy her mood. Despite these efforts, she finds herself getting progressively more depressed. She is still smoking, and even increased her cigarette use to five or six per week, or approximately one per day. Although we are of course concerned about Ms. R.D.'s downturn in mood, we are very encouraged that she called us about it and that she continues to refrain from hazardous substance use, because it suggests we have been successful in making a strong therapeutic alliance, despite a somewhat rocky start.

Recommendation #10

- Treat concurrent psychiatric disorders, including concurrent pharmacotherapy.

There is no evidence base by which to judge how long a patient needs to abstain from substances before one can determine whether psychiatric symptoms are substance induced or represent a *forme fruste* mental illness other than a substance use disorder. DSM-IV-TR recommends a minimum of 4 weeks, and in working in our clinic, we like to see a minimum of 4 weeks of abstinence (or at worst, minimal use) before we make the diagnosis. Every case is different, however, and there is no hard-and-fast rule that can eliminate the need for clinical judgment when one is making these difficult determinations. In the case of Ms. R.D., we feel that her downturn in mood after 4–5 weeks of significant substance reduction and abstinence from many substances she had previously been abusing, along with her long history of mood instability, is enough to convince us that she probably has a mood disorder as well. Given her predominantly depressed mood with prominent anxiety and insomnia, and her poor reaction to bupropion, we decide to start her on the selective serotonin reuptake inhibitor citalopram.

She responds well, with improvements in sleep, mood, and anxiety. She remains largely abstinent from substances, and when she does use alcohol and/ or nicotine she does so in moderation. She continues to struggle with affect regulation and self-esteem, and for these issues we refer her to psychotherapy and a skills training group, which emphasizes distress tolerance and mindfulness meditation. She does well for 8 months and then completely disappears from treatment after the summer break from school. We have not seen her in several years.

Summary

The patient presents with a chief complaint of mood instability marked most recently by depression with fleeting suicidal ideation, but no imminent threat to herself or others. A careful screening for alcohol consumption, focusing initially on amounts and frequency in the past week using the TLFB, reveals a level of alcohol consumption far above what is considered safe and well within the hazardous range. This discovery prompts an in-depth substance use screening and history, which in turn reveals nicotine dependence, cocaine dependence, marijuana abuse, and probably cocaine withdrawal. Keeping the patient's chief complaint in mind, we give feedback about the substance use screening results, educate her about safe levels of drinking, challenge normalization of her substance use, and negotiate strategies for change, using her chief complaint as incentive to target substance use. Four to five weeks after the patient commits to change and markedly reduces her substance use, she still experiences symptoms of depression, at which point we begin treatment with an antidepressant medication, even as we continue to assess and intervene in the substance use problems. We also offer a psychotropic agent for smoking cessation treatment, but the patient does not tolerate the medication and discontinues it. Four to five

months into treatment, the patient's mood and functioning is significantly improved, and she has largely eliminated all substance use, except for the occasional alcoholic beverage and cigarette. She continues to do well for the entirety of the academic year but is lost to treatment after the summer break.

Ways to Improve Practice

We made a significant error in this case by not working out a system for the patient to track her consumption during treatment. We were thus left to accept her account of "substantial reduction" in alcohol consumption and "occasional" use of nicotine without knowing the exact meaning of these terms. Careful monitoring is desirable in several respects (Kanfer and Scheft 1988). First, monitoring reduces the behavior through reactance. Second, it allows both the patient and provider to see change over time, which can be motivating and informative for care planning. Patients like Ms. R.D. who drink in social situations are often averse to monitoring, and in such cases it is useful to develop a covert strategy, for example, moving a coin from the right pocket to the left for each drink that is taken.

References

American Psychiatric Association: Diagnostic and Statistical Manual of Mental Disorders, 4th Edition, Text Revision. Washington, DC, American Psychiatric Association, 2000

Danielsson PE, Rivara FP, Gentilello LM, et al: Reasons why trauma surgeons fail to screen for alcohol problems. Arch Surg 134:564–568, 1999

Himelhoch S, Daumit G: To whom do psychiatrists offer smoking-cessation counseling? Am J Psychiatry 160:2228–2230, 2003

Humphreys K: Circles of Recovery: Self-Help Organizations for Addictions. Cambridge, UK, Cambridge University Press, 2004

Kanfer FH, Scheft BK: Guiding the Process of Therapeutic Change. Champaign, IL, Research Press, 1988

Kessler RC, Nelson CB, McGonagle KA, et al: The epidemiology of co-occurring addictive and mental disorders: implications for prevention and service utilization. Am J Orthopsychiatry 66:17–31, 1996

Kessler RC, Berglund P, Demler O, et al: The epidemiology of major depressive disorder: results from the National Comorbidity Survey Replication (NCS-R). JAMA 289:3095–3105, 2003

Lembke A, Johnson K, DeBattista C: Depression and smoking cessation: does the evidence support psychiatric practice? Neuropsychiatr Dis Treat 3:1–7, 2007

Mueser KT, Drake RE, Wallach MA: Dual diagnosis: a review of etiological theories. Addict Behav 23:717–734, 1998

Nunes EV, Levin FR: Treatment of depression in patients with alcohol or other drug dependence: a meta-analysis. JAMA 291:1887–1896, 2004

Rush AJ, First MB, Blacker D (eds): Handbook of Psychiatric Measures, 2nd Edition. Washington, DC, American Psychiatric Publishing, 2008

Sellers EM, Sullivan JT, Somer G, et al: Clinical Institute Withdrawal Assessment for Alcohol (CIWA-AD), in Handbook of Psychiatric Measures, 2nd Edition. Edited by Rush AJ, First MB, and Blacker D. Washington, DC, American Psychiatric Publishing, 2008, pp 460–461

Sobell LC, Sobell MB: Alcohol Timeline Followback Users' Manual. Toronto, ON, Canada, Addiction Research Foundation, 1995

Substance Abuse and Mental Health Services Administration [SAMHSA]: Results from the 2007 National Survey on Drug Use and Health: national findings (NSDUH Series H-34, DHHS Publ No SMA 08–4343). Rockville, MD, Substance Abuse and Mental Health Services Administration, Office of Applied Studies, 2008

Swift RM: Drug therapy for alcohol dependence. N Engl J Med 340:1482–1490, 1999

U.S. Preventive Services Task Force: Guide to Clinical Preventive Services, 2nd Edition. Washington, DC, Office of Disease Prevention and Health Promotion, 1996

Veterans Health Administration/Department of Defense: Clinical Practice Guideline for the Management of Substance Use Disorders. VA Office of Quality and Performance. Washington, DC, Department of Veterans Affairs/Department of Defense, 2001

Veterans Health Administration/Department of Defense: Clinical Practice Guideline for the Management of Tobacco Use. Management of Tobacco Use Working Group. Washington, DC, Department of Veterans Affairs, 2002. Available at: http://www.healthquality.va.gov/tuc/tuc_fulltext.pdf

Veterans Health Administration/Department of Defense: Clinical Practice Guideline for the Management of Substance Use Disorders: Guideline Summary, v.2.0. Management of SUD Working Group. Washington, DC, Department of Veterans Affairs, 2009. Available at: http://www.healthquality.va.gov/sud/sud_sum_v2_0.pdf

A Complex Personality Disorder Case

James Reich, M.D.

Setting

I work as a solo practitioner doing outpatient psychiatry. My specialty is difficult-to-treat anxiety disorders, which are often comorbid with personality disorders.

Illustration

This study illustrates:

- Management of a complex case of two personality disorders as well as a comorbid Axis I disorder, obsessive-compulsive disorder (OCD)
- Use of expert guidelines for borderline personality disorder (American Psychiatric Association 2001) and OCD (American Psychiatric Association 2007)
- Psychopharmacology of personality disorders (Herpertz et al. 2007)

Chief Complaint

The patient, Mr. X, presents as a 30-year-old single male with significant social avoidance, obsessive thoughts, and impulsive behavior. He wishes to stabilize his symptoms so he can pursue work.

Present Illness

Mr. X was a 30-year-old single lawyer. His obsessions began in his teenage years but did not interfere with his ability to finish high school or, ultimately,

college and law school. However, he had had unstable relationships with sudden shifts between feeling very positive toward someone and feeling that the same person had no redeeming qualities. This caused difficulty at work, although he tried to be professional. He had some identity disturbance in which he questioned who he was, including having doubts about his sexuality. He had had impulsive behavior with regard to alcohol and sex. At times he would feel intense anger. At one point he faced the possibility of serious legal repercussions for assault, but fortunately this did not happen. He had intense dysphoric anxious episodes with extreme self-doubt, which would go away only to recur. He also had chronic feelings of emptiness.

Mr. X had an intense fear of rejection. It was hard for him to follow up on job leads; often he would call back when he doubted there would be someone to answer. He was intensely afraid of being criticized at job interviews, leading him to postpone or cancel them. His social insecurity affected his ability to date, and he was not dating despite opportunities to do so.

He had some strengths as well. In addition to completing his schooling, Mr. X had worked at a law firm for several years and gotten some good experience. He was capable of forming friendships, though this was difficult for him, and seemed to be liked by his friends. He had a good relationship with his family.

Mr. X had worked with a number of psychiatrists and psychologists intermittently. Medication classes he had been on included antidepressants, antipsychotics, antianxiety agents, and mood stabilizers. In general, the medications had been given during periods of significant exacerbation of symptoms at relatively high dosages and then tapered off. At the time he presented to me he was on a very low dose of a selective serotonin reuptake inhibitor (SSRI) and a medication for sleep as needed.

Other Significant Findings From Assessment

Mr. X had had periods of depression that were treated with antidepressants, raising the possibility of major depressive disorder.

His binge drinking, although not frequent, could involve as many as 10 drinks in an evening and result in risky behavior.

His lack of structure and his anxiety had resulted in a somewhat reversed sleep-wake cycle.

Differential Diagnosis

Most of the diagnostic issues were fairly straightforward. The only real question was whether some of the personality symptoms were due to state effects that would be reduced by treatment of the comorbid Axis I disorder(s) (Reich 2007).

DSM-IV-TR Diagnosis

Axis I	OCD
	Alcohol abuse
	Rule out major depression
Axis II	Borderline personality disorder
	Avoidant personality disorder
Axis III	No significant medical problems
Axis IV	Unemployment, lack of structure
Axis V	GAF score: 52

Treatment Plan Considerations

Primary Problems and Guideline Selection

Personality pathology was clearly a major problem for this patient. There are no algorithms for the treatment of personality disorder in general, but the American Psychiatric Association does have guidelines for the treatment of borderline personality disorder (Oldham et al. 2001). In addition, the World Federation of Societies of Biological Psychiatry has guidelines for the biological treatment of personality disorders (Herpertz et al. 2007)

The obsessive symptoms were also clearly a major problem. Here we follow the American Psychiatric Association guidelines for treatment (Koran et al. 2007).

Secondary Problems and Issues

Of concern is Mr. X's episodic binge drinking. Although not frequent, it could have significant life consequences. Another secondary issue is his depression, which although not current would represent a potential future problem.

Treatment Goals, Measures, and Methods

Table 27–1 shows the treatment goals, measures, and methods for Mr. X's case.

Course

The guidelines for borderline personality disorder and OCD, cited earlier, emphasize the formation of a good therapeutic relationship with the patient, stressing psychotherapy. Mr. X and I set up weekly meetings and decided on a cognitive-behavioral approach, which fit both the treatment guidelines for borderline personality disorder and OCD and the patient's own preferences. Initially we made no changes to his medications, but we spent time understanding Mr. X's symptoms and establishing a relationship.

It became clear that Mr. X had such overwhelming anxiety that we would need to proceed with some medication relief to allow him to be calm enough to make progress. He had had sexual side effects on increased SSRI dosage in the past and was reluctant to try another antipsychotic, which he also had tried in the past. Benzodiazepines were contraindicated by the borderline personality disorder treatment guidelines because they could exacerbate impulsive behavior and might not be helpful for binge drinking. The World Federation of Societies of Biological Psychiatry guidelines (www.wfsbp.org/treatment-guidelines.html) indicated that avoidant personality disorder might be treated similarly to generalized social phobia, which would respond to benzodiazepines (Reich 2009). Ultimately we tried a combination of clonazepam 0.5 mg in the morning and alcohol education, alcohol counseling, and very careful alcohol and drug intake monitoring.

TABLE 27–1.   Treatment goals, measures and methods

Treatment goal	Measure	Method
Establish a treatment relationship to work together in psychotherapy (ability to communicate difficulties and collaboratively work out plans to approach them)	Attendance and treatment compliance	Weekly cognitive and behavioral psychotherapy
Reduce personality symptoms characterized by avoidance	Ability to follow through in feared situations such as job interviews[a]	Medication and cognitive and behavioral therapy
Reduce personality symptoms characterized by impulsivity and anger	Episodes of socially inappropriate anger or impulsive behavior	Medication and developing alternate strategies to deal with uncomfortable feelings
Reduce obsessive symptoms	Level of obsessive thoughts[a]	Medication and cognitive and behavioral therapy
Reduce frequency of episodic binge drinking	Episodes of binge drinking	Alcohol education and counseling

[a]Measured on a nonstandardized 0–10 scale.

The use of a benzodiazepine in a patient with impulse-control problems and binge drinking was clearly a difficult risk management decision. I chose a longer-acting benzodiazepine to reduce addictive potential and used this medication in small regular doses. There were to be no "as needed" doses, and Mr. X understood that any escalation in dosage or change in drinking patterns would result in stopping the clonazepam. To ensure compliance, prescription amounts and dates were closely monitored. Also, at least at first, each session would involve discussion of alcohol and/or use and relevant education.

Mr. X's anxiety was reduced enough to focus on some of the OCD symptoms. Following medication treatment consistent with both borderline and OCD guidelines we increased his SSRI incrementally to 100 mg (where side effects precluded going higher) and ultimately added the antipsychotic quetiapine 50 mg at night. The quetiapine helped both his OCD symptoms and his reversed day/night cycle and was consistent with borderline personality disorder guidelines. The medication was combined with behavioral and cognitive techniques, which he was able to apply reasonably well. We used these same techniques to work on his social avoidance. I felt this was an area in which progress could be made and that would give Mr. X more self-confidence.

The alcohol treatment started with Mr. X coming to the conclusion he would want to stop drinking at some point (not then). He tried limiting his drinking in social situations but was not very successful. He made an attempt at abstinence that failed. Later, he made a second attempt at abstinence that went better and that he thought helped his overall mental health.

His functional status improved somewhat, and he signed up for education classes to bolster his areas of expertise, but progress was not as fast as we hoped. Very far into the therapy Mr. X brought up a sexual trauma that he had experienced as a teenager, which seemed to have a connection with his impulsivity and anger. The therapy then focused on this area, which is ongoing.

The goals to establish a relationship with a significant other and return to the workplace are works in progress.

Tables of Improvement

Tables 27–2 through 27–6 describe the patient's improvement during the course of treatment.

Ways to Improve Practice

There are real challenges to using guidelines when a patient has multiple significant problems. These challenges include lack of guidelines (i.e., treatment of avoidant personality disorder or a mixture of personality disorders); the possibility of conflicting advice as to the use of a particular technique (e.g., use

TABLE 27–2.   Establishment of treatment relationship

Weeks 0–10	Weeks 11–20	Week 21 onward
Occasional missed appointments without agreed prior notice	Some changes in medication use without consultation (mainly discontinuation due to side effects)	Reasonably good attendance and discussion of medication and therapeutic issues

TABLE 27–3.   Reduction of personality symptoms characterized by avoidance

Weeks 2–10	Weeks 11–20	Weeks 21–40	Week 41 onward
Trials and discussion of trials of different medications (many of which did not work or could not be tolerated) Score=9	Some successful adjustment of current medications (selective serotonin reuptake inhibitor) and addition of new medications (benzodiazepine and atypical antipsychotic) Score=6.5	Largely therapy to encourage use of cognitive-behavioral techniques Score=5	Use of earlier techniques plus discussion and self exposure of feelings of defectiveness related to teenage sexual trauma Score=4

TABLE 27–4.   Reduction of personality symptoms characterized by impulsivity and anger

Weeks 0–10	Weeks 11–40	Week 41 onward
Review of prior anger and impulsive actions with discussion on their effects on client's life Client always recognized the destructive aspects of these incidents Score=6	Discussed and examined anger and impulse issues as they came up; seemed to be improvement with reduction of other symptoms and especially with gradual control of alcohol use Score=3	Added to earlier treatment was discussion of how early sexual trauma created feelings of defectiveness and how this related to anger and impulsive actions Score=2

TABLE 27–5.   Reduction of obsessive symptoms

Weeks 0–10	Weeks 11–20	Weeks 21–30	Weeks 31–40	Week 41 onward
Trials and discussion of different medications (many of which did not work or could not be tolerated) Score=9	Some successful adjustment of current medications (selective serotonin reuptake inhibitor) and addition of new medications (atypical antipsychotic) Score=6	Cognitive and behavioral techniques with much emphasis on exposure and response prevention Score=4	Continued use of all of the earlier techniques Score=3	Specific discussions of sexual obsessions Score=2

TABLE 27–6. Reduction of frequency of episodic binge drinking

Weeks 0–5	Weeks 6–15	Weeks 16–20	Week 21 onward
Assessment of problem and education Client believed he might someday wish to stop drinking but at present wished to try to become a "social drinker"	Continued assessment of motivation to change and education Social drinking not successful; several significant binges	Client decided to try abstinence but rejected formal programs such as Alcoholics Anonymous At week 20 attended wedding with old college drinking friends—binge drinking	Therapy for fears related to not drinking (will have no social life, etc.) and specific behaviors to avoid the beginning of a binge Client still rejects formal programs Abstinent so far

of benzodiazepines for avoidant personality disorder vs. borderline personality disorder); and prioritizing which steps to take first.

Nonetheless I found the guidelines quite helpful. When all the guidelines agreed on certain interventions, these obviously rose to the top. In this case all of the guidelines emphasized the importance of forming a therapeutic relationship and the use of at least two categories of medication (SSRIs and atypical antipsychotics). Even when the guidelines conflicted to some extent, they helped in the formation of a risk-benefit decision.

The guidelines can also help us reflect on our own practice patterns. For myself, this case showed me how hard it is not to use benzodiazepines in cases with considerable anxiety even when there are contraindications.

Although the guidelines do not anticipate every contingency and do not replace clinical judgment (the emergence of sexual trauma as an issue in this case came as a surprise to me and was not really anticipated by the various guidelines), they do provide a solid base of advice and a measure to examine your own treatment approaches.

References

American Psychiatric Association: Practice guidelines for the treatment of patients with borderline personality disorder. Am J Psychiatry 158:1–52, 2001

American Psychiatric Association: Practice Guideline for the Treatment of Patients With Obsessive-Compulsive Disorder. Washington, DC, American Psychiatric Association, 2007. Available at: http://www.psychiatry-online.com/pracGuide/pracGuideChapToc_10.aspx. Accessed September 18, 2009

Herpertz SC, Zanarini M, Schultz CS, et al: World Federation of Societies of Biological Psychiatry (WFSBP) guidelines for biological treatment of personality disorders. World J Biol Psychiatry 8:212–244, 2007

Koran LM, Hanna GL, Hollander E, et al: Practice guideline for the treatment of patients with obsessive-compulsive disorder. Am J Psychiatry 164(suppl):1–53, 2007. Available at: http://www.psychiatryonline.com/pracGuide/pracGuideTopic_10.aspx. Accessed June 18, 2009

Reich J: State and trait in personality disorders. Ann Clin Psychiatry 19:37–44, 2007

Reich J: Avoidant personality disorder and its relationship to social phobia. Curr Psychiatry Rep 11:89–93, 2009

Bulimia Nervosa

Joanna M. Marino, M.A.
James E. Mitchell, M.D.

Setting

Patients with bulimia nervosa, most of whom present for treatment in their late teens or 20s, generally can be treated successfully in outpatient settings. Exceptions include patients who are medically unstable; patients for whom comorbid conditions, such as severe depression and suicidality, dictate the need for inpatient treatment; and patients with severe comorbid personality problems who may benefit from a structured partial hospitalization program. However, for the average patient, outpatient treatment either in an individual or group format is both adequate and preferable. Our treatment setting includes a team approach composed of psychologists, dietitians, a physician, and advanced practice nurses, because this approach targets the psychological, behavioral, nutritional, and medical needs of eating disorder patients.

Illustration

The following case provides an example for discussion of the application of the American Psychiatric Association (2006) *Practice Guideline for the Treatment of Patients With Eating Disorders*. Initial assessment of eating disorder symptoms should include height, weight, and body mass index (BMI) measurements. The assessment should review the patient's history of eating behaviors, compensatory behaviors, and beliefs about weight, shape, and food. Gathering a general psychosocial history in order to identify stressors and assess comorbid psycho-

pathology provides helpful information for the course and outcomes of treatment.

Chief Complaint

Allison is a 22-year-old female who presents with complaints of depressed mood, anxiety, and binge eating and purging episodes.

Present Illness

Allison reported her binge eating and vomiting developed at age 16 and seemed to help her "relax," especially in the evenings when her binge/purge episodes typically occurred. She reported binge eating and vomiting up to four times each evening. She hoped to avoid these episodes but was afraid of gaining weight. Her current weight was 120 lb and her height was 5'4" (BMI=20.6).

Past Psychiatric History

The patient reported a history of depressed mood and anxiety since age 15. She denied a specific event that precipitated her mood symptoms. She had had suicidal ideation at age 15, although she reported no current plan or intent. At age 15, she often felt as if she was "not good enough or pretty enough," especially when compared with other girls at school. She experienced bouts of unprovoked crying, anhedonia, concentration difficulties, and worry about the future, which caused her to have difficulty falling asleep. She reported that these symptoms have continued since age 15 but "aren't as intense" as they were when they first occurred. She denied past psychological treatment for any mental health concerns.

At age 15, Allison began to gain weight. Her highest weight was 140 lb. She then began to diet, reducing her intake to 1,200 calories per day. She reported that this dieting lasted about a month and that she lost approximately 8 lb. On a Saturday when her parents were away, she experienced a binge eating episode. She then developed a pattern of binge eating every weekend and then restarting her dieting pattern every Monday. After about 2 months in this pattern, Allison experienced a binge eating episode that was larger than her prior episodes. She felt the urge to vomit in order to "feel just a little less stuffed." Vomiting came easily to Allison and she thought she could be successful at losing more weight if she vomited after each dinner. Allison's binge/purge cycle then became more frequent and was occurring at least once per day by the time she was 17.

History of Substance Abuse

The patient reported drinking one or two alcoholic drinks once monthly. She smoked marijuana on three occasions in tenth grade and related this to "peer pressure." She denied use of any other substances.

Exercise, Diet, and Stress Management

Allison exercised five times weekly for 1.5 hours during each episode. Her exercise routine included running for 60 minutes and a weight-lifting routine lasting 30 minutes. She reported exercising even though on most days she felt fatigued. She had had some dizziness when running. Her meal plan was also quite stringent, including a diet of 1,500 calories per day and limited fat intake. However, on most days she reported being unable to follow her diet and feeling "ravenous" when arriving home from work at 6 P.M. She did not experience the urge to binge eat during the day; however, when leaving work she became anxious about her performance during the day. She reported intrusive thoughts of binge eating on her drive home from work and feeling compelled to stop at the grocery store for a few items to prepare for dinner. Her binge eating episodes always involved high-fat food items such as pizza, cookies, chocolate milk, and chips.

Allison reported eating quickly and feeling as if she "blacked out" when she had a binge eating episode. She stated, "I know what I'm doing, bingeing on all that food, I just can't stop." She became overwhelmed with a sense of guilt after her eating episodes and then vomited several times. The vomiting decreased her anxiety and "clears my head... I don't have to worry when I'm binge eating and I can then just get rid of the food." Allison related her depressed mood to her inability to control her food intake and "feeling fat." She desired to weigh 110 lb (BMI=18.9).

Social History

Allison reported three or four close friends throughout her schooling and several acquaintances. She had been involved in soccer and tennis during eighth grade; however, she quit both teams to pursue her interest in playing piano, drawing, and painting. At the time of her evaluation she had very few friends. She denied involvement in a romantic relationship.

Educational and Occupational History

The patient completed the twelfth grade and attained her associate's degree in graphic design at a local community college. She worked at a fast food restaurant during high school and then began working at a well-known local graphic design studio after meeting the owner through an acquaintance.

Family History

Allison was raised by her biological mother and father. She had one older brother who was studying medicine. She reported that her upbringing was "good...just typical, I guess." Her father was employed as an executive at a local grocery store, and her mother was an administrative assistant. She reported a "good" relationship with her brother and parents but suggested her mother was sometimes critical of her, accepting only "A" grades as "good." Allison was on the "B honor roll," and this was often a point of contention with her mother. Her mother was often concerned about what other members of her church thought about the family and was focused on appearing "worry-free...or perfect."

Other Significant Findings From Assessment

Review of Systems

- Unremarkable except for occasional headaches, primarily frontal and usually relieved by aspirin
- Occasional palpitations and tachycardia post vomiting
- Problems with intermittent constipation and diarrhea; occasional upper abdominal pain associated with binge eating
- Had two episodes in which she found trace amounts of blood in her vomitus

Physical Examination

Patient was a well-developed, well-nourished female in no acute distress. Her blood pressure was 110 over 62, right arm sitting; her pulse was 64 and regular; and her respiratory rate was 12. Physical examination was essentially negative except for some evidence of scar formation on the dorsum of her right hand where she had traumatized the skin while self-inducing vomiting. This is known as Russell's sign.

Diagnostic Tests

Allison's diagnostic tests were within normal limits. Of particular importance in this testing is obtaining a serum electrolyte determination, because this is the blood chemistry most commonly affected by bulimia nervosa. Of particular concern is the risk of severe hypochloremia, metabolic alkalosis, and hypocholemia.

Psychological Tests

Allison completed the Beck Depression Inventory–II and attained a raw score of 21, suggesting moderate depressive symptoms. She also completed the Beck Anxiety Inventory with a score of 30, suggesting moderate symptoms of anxiety. The results of Allison's Eating Disorder Inventory–3 revealed clinical elevations (i.e., T/Composite Score≥50) on Drive for Thinness (T=52), Bulimia (T=56), Interpersonal Alienation (T=61), Personal Alienation (T=60), Perfectionism (T=58), and Affective Problems (T=58). The elevations appeared to align with Allison's reported dieting and binge/purge behavior as well as her lack of social support, perfectionistic tendencies, and mood problems.

DSM-IV-TR Diagnosis

Axis I	Bulimia nervosa
	Major depressive disorder, single episode, moderate
	Anxiety disorder not otherwise specified
Axis II	No diagnosis on Axis II
Axis III	Patient reports headaches; see medical record
Axis IV	Occupational stressors, limited social support
Axis V	GAF score: 60

Treatment Plan Considerations

In general, treatments for bulimia nervosa have focused on pharmacological and psychotherapeutic approaches. Antidepressants were first used for the treatment of this condition because of the observation that many patients with bulimia were comorbidly depressed, and it was assumed that if their depression improved their eating disorder would improve as well. However, research has shown that the presence of depression does not predict response to antidepressant treatment in these patients. A variety of antidepressants have been studied, including monoamine oxidase inhibitors, tricyclic antidepressants, and most recently serotonin reuptake inhibitors. Currently the only drug approved by the U.S. Food and Drug Administration for the treatment of bulimia nervosa is fluoxetine. It is notable that the drug seems to work best in high dosages, at approximately 60 mg/day. Many patients will tolerate this as the initial dosage. By analogy, most practitioners prescribe fairly high dosages of other antidepressants if alternative medications are being used. The controlled treatment literature suggests that most of these drugs work reasonably well. However, fluvoxamine may be ineffective, and bupropion should be avoided because it seems to have a high propensity for causing seizures in this patient population.

Relative to psychotherapeutic interventions, a variety of psychotherapies have been described in the literature, but much of the work has focused on the use of cognitive-behavioral techniques in either group or individual formats. It is safe to conclude that currently cognitive-behavioral therapy (CBT) is the treatment of choice for bulimia nervosa. This treatment is usually delivered in a twice-weekly format for the first month or so, and this seems to be an important variable in determining treatment outcome. There is also literature to suggest that interpersonal therapy may be effective, although the data are more limited and the treatment response seems to be somewhat delayed. In addition, there is some indication that dialectical behavior therapy can be helpful for some patients.

The question often arises as to whether antidepressant therapy and CBT should routinely be used in combination in the initial treatment of patients. Studies that have examined this question have found some modest benefit for the addition of antidepressants to CBT, but it is not clear that this outweighs the added costs and risks involved. Many practitioners recommend beginning with CBT and adding antidepressant treatment if there is no evidence of a fairly prompt response, demonstrated by reductions in the frequency of targeted behaviors, early in treatment.

As mentioned, individual and group psychotherapeutic interventions have been helpful in treating patients with bulimia nervosa. Dietary consultation is also beneficial in combination with psychotherapy. Family-based interventions are especially useful for adolescents because interpersonal issues can be discussed in the context of eating-disordered behavior. Self-help and support groups are also being studied for their effectiveness.

The American Psychiatric Association guideline's suggested aims for the treatment of individuals with bulimia nervosa are incorporated into Table 28–1. Note that the treatment interventions utilized target pharmacological, medical, and psychological interventions. A team approach to treating patients with bulimia is valuable, especially when considering the need for continued medication management and psychological interventions. Additionally, patients with medical or psychology comorbidities will need continued assessment to determine the appropriate level of care, especially if the patient fails to respond to outpatient treatment. The treatment guideline provides detailed information regarding the appropriate level of care for eating disorder patients based on several factors, including age, control over eating disorder behaviors, medical status, and location.

The outpatient clinic where Allison received her psychological treatment was composed of psychologists and psychiatrists. After the initial assessment, the importance of a treatment team was discussed with Allison. She was given referrals to a dietitian

and a primary physician. The team of providers had worked together for several patients and had a strong history of good communication about patient needs and progress. This open communication was an essential component, especially when she became resistant to normalizing her eating out of fear of gaining weight. The dietitian communicated with the therapist through a hospital-wide computer system about progress and topics to address in therapy. Allison was referred to a dentist outside of the hospital system to address dental erosion secondary to her purging behavior.

Allison's initial assessment revealed comorbid anxiety and depression, which is common in eating disorder patients. Medication use can be implemented at the beginning of treatment or as treatment progresses, depending on the severity of the comorbid psychological condition. It is important to consider that mood and anxiety symptoms, especially depression, can remit as binge/purge episodes subside, providing one reason for delaying the use of pharmacological agents.

In addition to her psychological assessment, Allison was seen by a primary practice physician. Results of her medical assessment were largely within normal limits. Given her medical stability, Allison was a good candidate for outpatient treatment. She was followed monthly by the primary physician to ensure medical stability.

Treatment Goals, Measures, and Methods

The goals, measures, and methods for this treatment are outlined in Table 28–1.

Course

Allison met with the therapist twice weekly for the first 4 weeks of therapy, as is often indicated in CBT for bulimia nervosa. The beginning of psychotherapy was marked by a focus on developing a therapeutic alliance. The therapist validated the role the eating disorder behaviors served for Allison and provided a supportive and open environment to discuss concerns about the treatment course. This allowed for an environment in which Allison would feel comfortable disclosing her eating and weight concerns. The therapist provided Allison with psychoeducation regarding the hypothesized model that

TABLE 28–1. Treatment goals, measures, and methods for a patient with bulimia nervosa

Treatment goal	Measure	Method
Reduce binge/purge episodes to zero times per week	Self-report of weekly binge/purge episodes and review of self-monitoring logs	Psychoeducation CBT Add SSRI if lack of early response
Reduce body image concerns within six sessions	Self-report, EDI-3	CBT
Reduce depression and anxiety by 50% or more by week 8	BDI-II, BAI	Consider pharmacotherapy CBT
Provide psychoeducation regarding healthy nutrition and eating patterns	Self-report	Psychoeducation Consultation with dietitian
Diminish food restriction behaviors and thoughts (e.g., "safe foods" or "dieting")	Food monitoring logs	CBT Consultation with dietitian
Increase motivation to fulfill treatment requirements	Attend all therapy sessions. Complete Motivational Enhancement Decisional Balance Sheet	Psychoeducation Treatment contract Therapeutic alliance
Treat all physical complications	Laboratory reports	Consultation with general medical provider
Discuss relapse prevention	Create a relapse prevention plan	CBT
Utilize social support by enlisting one family member or friend to support treatment	Discuss family therapy options, if applicable. Participation by family or friends during therapy sessions	Psychoeducation CBT IPT

Note. BAI=Beck Anxiety Inventory; BDI-II=Beck Depression Inventory–II; CBT=cognitive-behavioral therapy; EDI-3=Eating Disorder Inventory-3; IPT=interpersonal therapy; SSRI=selective serotonin reuptake inhibitor.
Source. Goals adapted from American Psychiatric Association 2006.

diagrammed the development and continuation of her eating disorder as a means of helping Allison understand the impact emotions, cognitions, social settings, and behaviors can have on her eating disorder. The therapist also worked with Allison to create a treatment plan, which was a way to help her feel in control of her treatment and think of herself as a member of a collaborative relationship. The practitioner also suggested to Allison that use of a self-help guide could be a valuable aid understanding eating disorders. Notably, the American Psychiatric Association treatment guideline provides a recommended list of readings that are beneficial to specific patient groups and for families of those with eating disorders. A practitioner may also consult the treatment guideline for a list of recommended reading about the CBT treatment manuals and guides.

Allison was provided with monitoring logs to detail her eating episodes throughout the day (see Figure 28–1). These monitoring logs provided valuable information about the pattern of eating Allison experienced during the day. In addition to the monitoring logs, psychoeducation regarding the importance of normalized eating was incorporated throughout the sessions. Allison was quite resistant to accepting the idea that eating throughout the day would not lead her to become "fat," and she continued to have episodes of morning restricting throughout the first half of treatment. Targeted behavioral interventions such as preplanning and packing meals was somewhat helpful in addressing her restricting behavior, although her beliefs that feeling full meant she was "fat" likely hindered her ability to change her eating patterns. Figure 28–2 depicts the reduction in Allison's binge/purge episodes. As shown, her binge/purge episodes decreased steadily, but she continued to have periodic episodes. We began discussing alternative behaviors and coping skills that Allison was able to implement when she had urges to binge eat and purge. Allison, unlike

Date: ___/___/___

Time	Intake (food/fluid)	Setting	Binge eat Y/N	Vomit Y/N	Laxative Y/N	Comments

FIGURE 28–1.   Food log.

Source.   Adapted from Fairburn 2008.

some patients, enjoyed monitoring her eating behavior. Some patients feel that monitoring eating behaviors makes them focus too much on their consumption habits. This tends to resolve in many patients when they begin to see the benefit of analyzing their eating behavior during the session.

In the case of Allison, her binge/purge episodes persisted and her mood remained depressed during the first 4 weeks of therapy. A selective serotonin reuptake inhibitor (SSRI) was then added at week 4, and a steady decrease in symptoms resulted. Various pharmacological interventions have been effective in treating bulimia symptoms, and an SSRI was chosen because of its general tolerability by many patients. Allison reported decreases in her depression and overall level of anxiety; however, she continued to experience anxiety related to her strenuous work

environment. Relaxation techniques and coping skills were used to target these anxiety symptoms.

Allison was referred to a dietitian to address her concerns regarding "safe" foods and to gain additional information about nutrition. Allison continued to have "bad" or "unsafe" foods in her diet, which at times would trigger a binge episode. She was comfortable avoiding these foods during therapy. As the eating patterns began to stabilize over the second half of the treatment course, Allison was able to expose herself to these feared foods and then utilize her distraction behavior until the foods became more tolerable.

The final steps of Allison's treatment involved discussing a relapse prevention plan. Allison and the therapist worked on identifying triggers to a lapse in eating-disordered behavior and the use of problem-

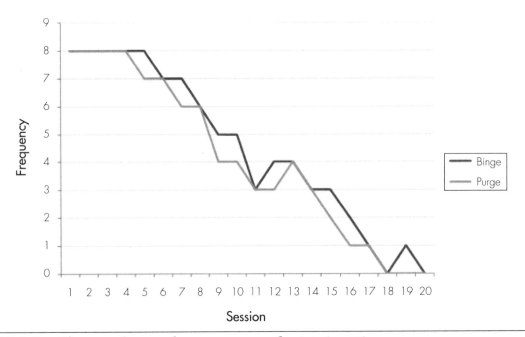

FIGURE 28–2.   Binge and purge frequency over the treatment.

Sessions were biweekly during the first 4 weeks of therapy.

solving skills to avoid a full relapse. Allison became aware that minor setbacks were likely. Figure 28–2 displays the continued trouble Allison had in fully stopping her binge eating episodes. The therapeutic relationship and collaboration that was established in the beginning of treatment remained helpful in motivating Allison to continue to journey toward remission of binge/purge episodes.

In treating adolescents with eating disorders, family therapy is an important component because of the continuous interaction with parents and food in the home. In adults, involving relationship partners in adjunct therapy sessions can be beneficial, especially to aid in the monitoring of behavior or supporting behavioral changes. Treatment manuals are available for family-based therapy, and recommended readings are listed in the treatment guideline.

Allison was uninterested in involving her parents in the therapy process, even with continued discussion about the benefits of additional family therapy. Allison was very hesitant about disclosing her behavior to her family. Her situation did, however, present an ideal opportunity for the involvement of parents, especially because Allison has limited social support. She recognized that some of her anxiety and beliefs about weight were likely related to her mother's distorted beliefs about appearance and perfection. If Allison had been willing to involve her family in therapy, supplemental sessions would have occurred to address the role of families in eating disorder etiology and treatment.

Summary/Conclusion

The challenges in treating eating disorder patients are the necessities of a multidisciplinary team approach, continued assessment of medical symptomatology, and the risk of chronicity of the disorders. The treatment guideline provides valuable, explicit information regarding treatment settings and level of care (i.e., inpatient versus outpatient), medical assessments, and targets of psychotherapy. Unfortunately, not all patients are motivated for treatment, and attrition in therapy can be high. Additionally, the preponderance of eating disorder cases seem to fall into the Eating Disorder Not Otherwise Specified category, highlighting the importance of developing a treatment plan tailored to the needs of the patient.

Ways to Improve Practice

In the case described, two improvements to treatment could be considered. Allison's frequency of binge eating and purging decreased more slowly when compared with most reports in the literature regarding response patterns of bulimia nervosa patients being treated with CBT. The use of antidepressants was indicated here and was implemented in Allison's case. The addition of a third therapy session per week could also have been very helpful in reducing the frequency in these behaviors. A relapse prevention plan that included follow-up visits would also have been beneficial. Literature has suggested that patients with bulimia may not necessarily pursue follow-up treatment if they experience relapses after a successful CBT intervention (Mitchell et al. 2004). Developing a schedule of monthly follow-up sessions could be helpful in preventing full-blown relapse.

References

American Psychiatric Association: Practice Guideline for the Treatment of Patients With Eating Disorders, 3rd Edition. Washington, DC, American Psychiatric Association, 2006. Available at: http://www.psychiatryonline.com/pracGuide/pracGuideTopic_12.aspx. Accessed June 18, 2009

Beck AT, Steer RA, Brown GK: Beck Depression Inventory-II Manual. San Antonio, TX, Psychological Corporation, 1996

Fairburn CG: Cognitive Behavior Therapy and Eating Disorders. New York, Guilford, 2008

Garner DM: Eating Disorder Inventory-3 (EDI-3) Professional Manual. Lutz, FL, Psychological Assessment Resources, 2004

Mitchell JE, Agras WS, Wilson GT, et al: A trial of a relapse prevention strategy in women with bulimia nervosa who respond to cognitive-behavior therapy. Int J Eat Disord 35:549–555, 2004

Suggested Readings

Fairburn CG: Overcoming Binge Eating. New York, Guilford, 1995

Mitchell JE, Wonderlich S, Agras S: The treatment of bulimia nervosa: where are we and where are we going? Int J Eat Disord 40:94–101, 2007

Mitchell JE, Peterson CB: Assessment of Eating Disorders. New York, Guilford, 2007

National Institute for Clinical Excellence: Eating Disorders: Core Interventions in the Treatment and Management of Anorexia Nervosa, Bulimia Nervosa and Related Eating Disorders: Clinical Guideline 9. London, National Institute for Clinical Excellence, 2004

III

Case Studies:
Evidence-Based Psychiatric Practice
in Different Settings

Dual Diagnosis (PTSD/SUD) Treated in a Veterans Affairs Health Care Facility

Gretchen Lindner, Ph.D.
Steven E. Lindley, M.D., Ph.D.

Setting

Treatment was performed in a specialized outpatient posttraumatic stress disorder (PTSD) program at a Veterans Affairs (VA) health care facility. The PTSD program utilizes a multidisciplinary model wherein psychiatrists, psychologists, social workers, and nurses are all represented on the team. Veterans are typically referred to the program by other outpatient mental health programs in the hospital, psychiatric inpatient units, or primary care. The start of treatment typically involves a period of thorough assessment and treatment planning, followed by the provision of an appropriate PTSD-specific treatment. Treatment options include short-term individual therapy, short-term and long-term group therapy, couples/family therapy, medication management, and case management. The primary author was a psychology fellow in this setting and, as such, had the opportunity to work with this veteran for up to a year, functioning as the primary individual and group psychotherapist. The second author was not a treating provider but reviewed the treatment plan and outcome.

Illustration

This study illustrates:

- Application of guidelines to PTSD

- Adjustment of guidelines for comorbid PTSD and substance abuse
- Use of manualized treatments (e.g., stress management, exposure therapy, Seeking Safety)
- Concurrent use of individual therapy, group therapy, and medication management
- Coordination of care

Chief Complaint

Mr. B.H. is a 49-year-old divorced Caucasian male Army veteran who was referred to the PTSD program after he screened positive for both military sexual trauma (MST) and PTSD during a routine mental health screening in primary care. He presents to mental health with a 25-year history of intrusive memories, nightmares, insomnia, feelings of shame, and excessive alcohol use after being sexually assaulted while in the military. At the time of the rape, the veteran was 24 years old, in the U.S. Army, and stationed in Italy. While walking alone through a public park one evening, Mr. B.H. was sexually assaulted and severely beaten by five civilian men who then left him alone "to die" in the park. In addition to this sexual assault as an adult, the patient has a history of being sexually molested, between the ages of 8 and 10, by an uncle. He never discussed either the childhood molestation or military sexual assault with anyone.

Mr. B.H. states that after being assaulted in the military, he began to drink heavily in order to cope with his intense psychological reaction to the trauma. The veteran is living in a residential treatment program for homeless veterans with substance abuse problems. Although he has been clean and sober for 6 months, he continues to struggle with PTSD symptoms. He has PTSD reexperiencing symptoms that include nightmares about his assault, daily intrusive thoughts and images about the rape and his earlier molestation, and significant physical and emotional reactions in response to trauma-related cues (e.g., psychotherapy groups with other men in the program, news stories about rape, having to share a room with a man). He also has avoidance/numbing symptoms including significant avoidance of trauma-related activities (e.g., talking about his rape, touch/sex, close relationships with men), as well as numerous obsessive "safety" behaviors (e.g., showering five times a day, cleaning sheets multiple times a week). He also describes emotional numbing and severe social isolation from both friends and family. In the hyperarousal domain of PTSD symptoms, Mr. B.H. reports that he struggles with significant sleep difficulties (e.g., sleeping 2–3 hours per night), hypervigilance, irritability, and an exaggerated startle response. His score on the PTSD Checklist—Civilian Version (PCL-C) is 70.

Substance Abuse History

Mr. B.H. states that he began drinking alcohol at the age of 15, but heavy and problematic drinking began the night of his MST. He has drunk alcohol consistently for the last 25 years. Although he has had periods of productive employment (e.g., worked as a dental assistant, received numerous accolades as a program manager), the alcohol abuse progressively worsened and negatively affected his consistency at work and in relationships. He has had multiple failed marriages, long periods of unemployment, chronic homelessness, and multiple DUIs. Over the last 10 years, Mr. B.H. has enrolled in three different substance abuse programs, none of which led to substantial periods of sobriety (longest prior sobriety was 4 months). He has been participating in a homeless veterans' residential treatment program for the last 4 months and has been clean and sober for the last 6 months. The residential treatment program provides him with numerous weekly recovery-oriented group psychotherapies and weekly contact with a case manager but provides no PTSD-specific treatment.

Other Relevant Findings

Mr. B.H. reports two suicidal gestures in his life. He once played Russian roulette with a loaded gun and once lay in a bathtub with a broken bottle while strongly considering cutting his wrists.

Mr. B.H. is the youngest of four children, with two brothers and one sister. For the last 20 years he has been disconnected from his family until he recently reconnected with his sister and her children. He denies having any friends or a support system with which he feels connected, finding it difficult to trust people. He has no significant medical problems, and his medical exams have all been normal.

DSM-IV-TR Diagnosis

Axis I	Posttraumatic stress disorder
	Alcohol dependence, early full remission
Axis II	None
Axis III	None
Axis IV	Social isolation, unemployment, recent homelessness
Axis V	GAF score: 40

Treatment Plan Considerations

Main Problem

Mr. B.H.'s presenting problem was PTSD. Although present throughout his adult life, his symptoms appeared to have worsened significantly over his 6-month period of sobriety. He described current problems with all three clusters of PTSD symptoms (reexperiencing, avoidance/numbing, and hyperarousal).

Secondary Problem

Although the veteran was not currently using alcohol or other drugs, his long-standing history of severe dependence and his brief period of sobriety complicated treatment planning. He described a cycle of drinking in response to worsening PTSD symptoms as well as worsening PTSD symptoms during periods of sobriety. As such, there appeared to be a reciprocal relationship between his experiencing PTSD symptoms and alcohol consumption.

It was important to consider how to help the veteran develop additional coping skills to decrease his reliance on alcohol as the primary means of coping with PTSD symptoms. In addition, it was essential to consider how to provide relapse prevention work while also addressing his PTSD symptoms. Lastly, considerations of how to adjust traditional PTSD treatments to increase the likelihood of sustained sobriety were critical.

Selecting a Guideline

I (G.L.) began by reviewing the available guidelines for the treatment of PTSD, including the American Psychiatric Association (2004) practice guidelines for the treatment of patients with acute stress disorder and posttraumatic stress disorder, the Expert Consensus Guideline for treatment of posttraumatic stress disorder (Foa et al. 1999), *Effective Treatments for PTSD: Practice Guidelines From the International Society for Traumatic Stress Studies* (Foa et al. 2000), and the VA/DoD *Clinical Practice Guideline for the Management of Post-Traumatic Stress* (VA/DoD Management of Post-Traumatic Stress Working Group 2004). My predominant impression from reviewing these multiple sources was that the majority of the recommendations are similar across treatment guidelines and relied on the same body of literature. I decided to use the VA/DoD guideline in my treatment of this veteran because this guideline seemed the most appropriate given that I was working in a VA setting. This guideline also encapsulated many of the treatment recommendations highlighted in the other guideline. (See Table 29–1 for a summary of the VA/DoD guidelines and the ways in which I adhered to or made changes in the recommendations.)

The VA/DoD guideline strongly recommends several psychotherapy treatments that have been shown to have significant benefit for PTSD symptoms, including cognitive therapy, exposure therapy, stress inoculation training, and eye movement desensitization and reprocessing (EMDR). In addition, the guideline recommends using medication management as a first-line treatment for PTSD, strongly recommending the use of a selective serotonin reuptake inhibitor (SSRI), which has been shown to be effective for reducing symptom severity for all three PTSD symptom clusters, although less so in VA populations. The guideline also encourages practitioners to consider incorporating patient edu-

cation and group therapy into interventions. Given these recommendations, I decided immediately to refer Mr. B.H. for medication management with one of the psychiatrists on the PTSD team. In addition, I decided on a plan for stress inoculation, exposure therapy, and cognitive therapy with this veteran. I decided against providing EMDR because the research suggests that exposure therapy and EMDR have similar outcomes, and dismantling studies suggest that the active ingredient in EMDR is the exposure (Davidson and Parker 2001). Furthermore, I have had extensive training in exposure therapy, and my clinical experience is that this is an extremely effective treatment for PTSD.

Although these seemed like appropriate treatment considerations for someone with PTSD, I also had questions about how to ensure that I was addressing treatment of his substance abuse in my plan. The VA/DoD guideline does not provide recommendations about what additional treatments, if any, should be provided when treating a veteran with comorbid substance abuse problems. As such, I went back to the research literature to identify any studies specifically addressing how to treat individuals with comorbid PTSD and substance abuse. Although traditionally the model for treatment of this population has been to first treat the substance abuse problems and then treat the PTSD problems (Brady et al. 2004), researchers have shown the effectiveness of a new manualized group-based treatment called *Seeking Safety* (Najavits 2002) that addresses both substance abuse and PTSD issues simultaneously. This 25-session group-based protocol is present centered and builds additional coping skills through cognitive, behavioral, and interpersonal modules. It is explicitly designed as a first-phase treatment of PTSD and substance dependence with a goal of increasing stabilization and safety. Given the research support for this treatment, I thought it would be appropriate to add this to my treatment plan.

Another issue during treatment planning was whether the PTSD interventions needed to be adjusted in order to treat safely those with comorbid substance abuse problems and minimize the chances of relapse. Although it is clear that exposure therapy is one of the most efficacious treatments for PTSD (Institute of Medicine 2007), the guideline gives no advice about the possible risks for those with substance abuse problems. When I was talking with treatment team members about providing exposure

TABLE 29–1.   Summary of VA/DoD clinical practice guideline for the management of posttraumatic stress disorder (PTSD)

Area	Description	Followed
Interventions with significant benefit		
Medication management[a]	Medications with significant or some benefit include SSRIs, TCAs, MAOIs, sympatholytics, and novel antidepressants.	√ Referred to team psychiatrist to address medication needs
Cognitive therapy	Structured, short-term, present-centered therapy focusing on thoughts. Include thought records, thought patterns, challenging thoughts, identifying/challenging trauma-related thoughts, and distorted core beliefs.	√
Exposure therapy	Typically 8- to 12-session therapy in which patients face trauma-related feared thoughts, images, and situations through graded, repeated exposure. Can use imaginal or in-vivo exposure techniques.	√ Adjusted approach to address substance dependence history
Stress inoculation training	Teaching patients a set of skills or "toolbox" for managing anxiety and stress. The education and training of coping skills.	√
Eye movement desensitization and reprocessing	Exposure to traumatic images while shifting eyes in back-and-forth motion while also thinking of positive self-referring cognition.	Not necessary given positive response to exposure
Interventions with some benefit		
Imagery rehearsal therapy	Changes content of the patients' nightmares through imagery control.	Addressed through medications and exposure
Psychodynamic therapy	Explores psychological meaning of posttraumatic response by shifting and sorting through fantasies, fears, and defenses stirred up by traumatic event. Typically long term.	Not appropriate given VA's more short-term orientation to treatment
Other interventions to consider		
Patient education	Educate patients about the symptoms of PTSD and the multiple treatment options.	√
Group therapy	Group therapy that addresses PTSD symptoms. No clear differences/recommendations between supportive, psychodynamic, or cognitive-behavioral groups.	√

Note.   MAOIs=monoamine oxidase inhibitors; TCAs=tricyclic antidepressants; SSRIs=selective serotonin reuptake inhibitors; VA/DoD=Veterans Affairs/Department of Defense.

[a]There are additional explicit guidelines for medication management, not summarized here because the primary author referred to the team psychiatrist to manage psychiatric medication.

therapy with this veteran, many people voiced concerns about the high probability of relapse upon engagement in imaginal exposure. I again turned to the literature to see what the research suggests about whether the risks for relapse are too high with exposure therapy. There generally was a paucity of research in this area; however, four non–randomized controlled trial studies showed support for the benefit of exposure therapy for PTSD patients with substance dependence (Brady et al. 2001; Donovan et al. 2001; Najavits et al. 2005; Triffleman et al. 1999). A clinical observation article by Najavits and colleagues (2005) summarizes the positive results of combining Seeking Safety and exposure therapy with dual diagnosis patients. In this article they provide explicit recommendations for how to adjust exposure therapy techniques when working with someone who has a history of substance abuse. The authors suggest creating an explicit, extensive, written set of safety parameters, as well as allowing patients to process more fluidly multiple events. They also suggest encouraging patients to process both trauma and substance use memories. Lastly, the authors indicate that it is important to conduct the exposure more flexibility and to decide collaboratively on pacing and quantity of exposure. The summary of clinical experiences and research articles encouraged me to employ exposure therapy with this veteran, but with significant modifications as delineated previously.

The last major issue that arose around treatment planning was identifying the order in which the multiple treatments should be delivered. Again, the VA/DoD guidelines do not provide explicit instructions. Thus, I used my clinical intuition and experience to help me answer this question. Because Mr. B.H. was early in sobriety, I decided that it would be most appropriate to start with treatments that were present centered and skill based. In addition, the veteran indicated a preference for starting with skill building and then transitioning to trauma-focused work if the first-line interventions were not effective. Therefore we began with individual therapy that addressed both his PTSD and substance abuse issues, utilizing cognitive therapy, stress inoculation/skill building, and relapse prevention interventions. In addition, I referred him to a 12-week stress management for PTSD group that I was co-leading based on stress inoculation and cognitive-behavioral models. I would have preferred to send him directly to a Seeking Safety group for skill building, but there were no available group openings at the time of treatment planning. We therefore planned to enroll him in Seeking Safety as soon as there was an opening. Depending on his response to these interventions, I also considered exposure therapy as a follow-up treatment if his symptoms persisted despite skill building and cognitive interventions.

Treatment Goals, Measures, and Methods

Table 29–2 summarizes our treatment goals, measures, and methods for this patient.

Course

The course of our therapy is best described as having occurred in two phases. The first phase of treatment consisted of Mr. B.H. seeing me for individual therapy focused on skill building, relapse prevention, and cognitive therapy. The veteran also concurrently participated in a 12-week stress management group co-led by me and a psychology trainee. In this phase of treatment I also referred the veteran for medication management with a PTSD team psychiatrist and coordinated care with him throughout treatment. In the second phase of treatment, when the veteran's PTSD symptoms remained elevated, the veteran participated in individual exposure therapy with me as well as a Seeking Safety group co-led by myself and another psychology fellow.

Phase 1: Individual Psychotherapy and Stress Management Group

Individual Skill-Based Psychotherapy

The first step in treatment was beginning an individual, skill-based, weekly psychotherapy. Mr. B.H. and I met together 22 times before we decided to begin exposure therapy. The first two sessions consisted of PTSD assessment and treatment planning. After our second session, I also spoke to the veteran's case manager from the residential treatment program to ensure coordination of care. She indicated that she was providing him unstructured, supportive meetings, and as such his participation in a structured, PTSD-specific treatment with me would not represent a conflict or overlapping treatment.

During the subsequent 19 sessions, I utilized cognitive-behavioral interventions to help the veteran build additional relapse prevention skills (e.g., identifying triggers, developing coping plans, encour-

TABLE 29–2.   Summary of treatment goals, measures, and methods

Treatment goals	Measure	Method
Increase quality of sleep by increasing number of hours of sleep per night (>5 per night) within 3 months	Self-report	Coordinating care with psychiatrist
		Psychoeducation
		Individual and group stress inoculation
Decrease PTSD symptoms, as measured by the PTSD Checklist—Civilian Version (PCL-C <50) within 12 months	Self-report PCL-C	Coordinating care with psychiatrist
		Individual and group stress inoculation
		Cognitive therapy
		Exposure therapy
		Seeking Safety
Maintain sobriety from alcohol for duration of treatment	Self-report	Coordinating care with residential treatment program
		Self-help groups/AA
		Relapse prevention
		Stress inoculation
		Seeking Safety
Increase social network (e.g., increase identified safe/helpful friendships, reconnect with family, access support groups)	Self-report	Multiple group therapies
		Self-help groups/AA
		Exposure therapy to decrease shame
Increase psychosocial functioning, as indicated by securing employment and housing	Self-report	Coordinating care with residential treatment program
		Stress inoculation
		Seeking Safety
		Exposure therapy

Note.   AA=Alcoholics Anonymous; PTSD=posttraumatic stress disorder.

aging attendance at Alcoholics Anonymous [AA] meetings); engaged in stress inoculation training, helping the veteran to enhance his coping resources (e.g., grounding, affect regulation); and employed cognitive interventions to help Mr. B.H. identify his automatic thoughts and thinking patterns and challenge his cognitive distortions. I also utilized basic interpersonal therapy interventions to build a strong therapeutic alliance and encourage engagement with the veteran. This became especially important during times of increased stress that occurred near the beginning of therapy. For example, during the fourth session the veteran reported that a good friend of his was murdered in a dangerous area after

relapsing to alcohol. I used a more process-oriented, nondirective approach in helping the veteran process his feelings of grief, fear, and anger around this incident.

Psychopharmacology

Mr. B.H. was referred to the PTSD team psychiatrist after the second session. The primary complaint of the patient was frequent and intense nightmares related to the trauma in the military. He reported that the nightmares occurred almost every night and were frightening, awakened him from sleep, and were increasing over the last 2 months. He had also been feeling more depressed, although he did not meet the criteria for major depression. Because he was reluctant to try medication, it was decided to take a focused approach to treating his nightmares with the off-label use of prazosin (listed in the guideline as a secondary treatment option with some limited evidence-base support). Mr. B.H. was taking hydrochlorothiazide for his hypertension and was warned about possible orthostatic hypotension. He was started on prazosin 1 mg qhs for 3 days, then 2 mg qhs for 5 days, then 4 mg qhs. He returned to his psychiatrist 2 weeks later stating his sleep was better, "a solid 3 hours." He was taking only 3 mg qhs and was instructed to increase to 4 mg qhs and then 6 mg qhs. Upon returning another 2 weeks later, he stated that he had felt nauseous and uncomfortable on 6 mg and reduced the dose back to 4 mg. The veteran had noticed a decrease in nightmares and more restful sleep. He did not return for further psychopharmacology appointments but remained at the same dose of prazosin for the remainder of this treatment period.

Stress Management Group

Mr. B.H. began to participate in the stress management for PTSD group after our ninth session of individual therapy and participated in all twelve 75-minute classes. We used an unpublished manualized treatment that is utilized in multiple VA PTSD programs. The group consisted of Mr. B.H. and seven other veterans, all of whom had PTSD symptoms and many of whom also struggled with substance abuse issues. The group always began with a brief check-in, followed by 45 minutes of psychoeducation about stress and stress management techniques. It ended with a 15- to 20-minute experiential stress reduction technique (e.g., diaphragmatic breathing, progressive muscle relaxation, guided imagery, meditation). Veterans were asked to practice these relaxation techniques between sessions and report on their experience in the check-in process. Throughout the course of therapy the veteran participated actively in group and practiced the stress-reduction techniques between sessions. He was able to identify two particular relaxation techniques, diaphragmatic breathing and guided imagery, that worked best for decreasing his anxiety. However, he did not report feeling connected to other group members and overall did not feel that participating in the group reduced his PTSD symptoms.

Evaluation After Phase 1

After Mr. B.H. had participated in 22 individual sessions and 12 stress management group sessions, we decided to reevaluate his symptoms and discuss additional treatment considerations. The veteran indicated that he was sleeping significantly better, averaging 5–6 hours of unbroken sleep per night. In addition, the veteran reported that he felt stronger in his sobriety, now having maintained sobriety from alcohol for 11 months. He described having significantly more coping resources that he utilized to cope with both urges to drink and PTSD symptoms. He was practicing his breathing exercises daily and finding these very helpful in decreasing his overall level of anxiety. However, he stated that he continued to experience significant PTSD symptoms, especially intrusive thoughts/images, social isolation, numbing, hypervigilance, and irritability. He also described continuing to feel socially isolated from others in the treatment program, friends, and family. His PCL-C score at this point in therapy was 62, indicating a decrease from his baseline score of 70 but still a clinically significant level of PTSD symptoms.

I proposed exposure therapy as a next step, and the veteran stated that he felt ready to engage in this treatment. I again contacted both his psychiatrist and his case manager to let them know about the change in the treatment plan and the potential short-term increase in his anxiety when first starting exposure therapy. I also encouraged the veteran to let others in his life know that he might need additional support for the next few months (e.g., roommate at program, sister, AA sponsor). Additionally, a new Seeking Safety group was starting at the same time, and so the veteran decided to participate in this group co-led by myself and another psychology fellow. The veteran reported feeling excited to have a place to continue to discuss and build coping skills.

Phase 2: Exposure Therapy and Seeking Safety

Individual Exposure Therapy

Mr. B.H.'s exposure therapy consisted of 30 individual sessions over a 5-month period, typically meeting twice weekly. Of the individual sessions, 16 were 90-minute sessions in which the veteran participated in imaginal exposure. The other 14 were shorter sessions (typically 60 minutes) where the veteran processed the feelings that arose for him while retelling the story of his trauma or listening to his trauma tapes. In each of the 16 imaginal exposure sessions the veteran audio taped his trauma retelling and then listened to it once or twice during the following week. As such, the veteran listened to his trauma tapes 30 times during the course of therapy.

The first session was spent providing psychoeducation about exposure therapy and creating a thorough safety plan for potential increases in anxiety and alcohol cravings. I spent time explaining the structure of the therapy and the rationale for exposure. We identified 10 ways of coping with anxiety and urges that might arise during the course of exposure and wrote them down on a "coping card" that he carried with him at all times. We also discussed that he could call me during VA hours if he needed to check in or listen to my voice mail after hours in order to become grounded. Lastly, we identified the primary trauma that would be the focus of exposure therapy. Because most of his nightmares and intrusions were related to his MST, as opposed to his childhood molestation, we decided to focus on this as the primary event for the trauma retelling. Between the first and second sessions the veteran decided to begin the process of exposure by creating a written account of the trauma and its impact on him. The following is an excerpt from his writing, which highlights the strong link between his PTSD and substance use:

> I was so afraid of being asked what was going on with me that I cut all my friends off and became a loner. I would go off alone and drink. I don't know what people thought and I did not care. Nobody was going to find out the truth. Nobody. You don't tell the army you were raped. Not if you're a man.... I could not go home.... I kept stuffing what happened to me by drinking...the more I drank the more I could be who I wanted to be, 'cause I did not want to be me.... I felt at fault for everything bad that happened then and now.... I deserved it 'cause I did not fight back enough.... I drank to forget and to be anyone but me. I had so much shame and guilt that I just could not let anyone know me, because they might find out my secret. I need to know who I am because I have not known since that night.

During the second session of exposure therapy, the veteran spent 55 minutes telling the story of his rape for the first time while being audio taped. Mr. B.H. connected to his affect readily during session and was extremely tearful throughout the entire re-

counting of the trauma. During much of the retelling he was clenching his body, and he made absolutely no eye contact. In addition, at the most difficult part of the story the veteran became extremely anxious and vomited. During the processing time after the trauma account the veteran described feeling significant sadness, anxiety, fear, and anger. He felt shame about what had happened and for having shared it with me and continued to have difficulty making eye contact. Given his reactions in this first session, it became clear that part of the goal of exposure would be to help the veteran relax his body while recounting the trauma and to move toward more eye contact after the retelling. In addition, we decided to monitor his vomiting and the number of daily showers to ensure that these decreased over time.

During the third through sixth sessions the veteran recounted the trauma two more times and also spent time discussing the strong emotional reactions he was having both in and out of session. He shared that he was experiencing a significant increase in anxiety as well as urges to use alcohol. It therefore became extremely important for me to adjust the exposure therapy protocol and allow additional time for processing his feelings of anxiety, sadness, anger, and shame, and every week to discuss coping strategies for dealing with his urges to use. At the end of the sixth session the veteran completed the PCL-C and his score was 60, indicating that his PTSD symptoms had not yet improved.

In the seventh session (the fourth in-session recounting of the trauma), the veteran remembered and shared an additional piece of information about the trauma that was particularly difficult for him to say aloud. Although he had been able to recount having been raped with objects, this was the first time that he was able to share the whole rape story, which included having been raped by another man. This felt like the first "whole" recounting and the veteran was extremely sad and angry throughout the retelling. We spent additional time at the end of the session ensuring that his anxiety decreased by 50% prior to ending the session and ensuring that we developed an explicit safety plan for him that day.

In sessions 8 through 30 the veteran continued to recount his trauma and to listen to the tapes between sessions. Each week his trauma recounting became easier, and he described progressively less anxiety. Although decreasing the tensing of his body was very hard for him at first, because he reported that he felt as if clenching was the only "protection" he still had, by the final retelling his whole body was relaxed when recounting the trauma. In addition, after the sixth recounting of the trauma the veteran no longer experienced vomiting and his showering stabilized at three times per day, as opposed to the previous rate of five times per day. In addition, in the final recounting the veteran was able to tell the whole story while also looking at me, representing a significant decrease in his feelings of shame. In the "processing" sessions in which the veteran explored his affective and cognitive reactions to the trauma, Mr. B.H. discussed further the ways that retelling his trauma story also affected his feelings and thoughts toward his childhood molestation. Thus, the processing often occurred for both traumas, even though the recounting only occurred around the MST.

After every in-session and between-session imaginal exposure the veteran filled out a form asking him about his thoughts and feelings. In the processing sessions we would discuss the information on these sheets at length. The following quotes exemplify the progression of his responses during the course of treatment, representing a significant and meaningful shift in his relationship to the trauma:

Question: What are your feelings and thoughts right now?

I feel sorry and sad for that guy on the tape. What those fucking bastards did to him changed his life forever. I feel anger and rage and sick to my stomach. I have to go throw up.

I feel pretty helpless right now. I don't believe that anyone could do that to me. I want them to pay for this.

My feelings are confused. I still have some anger, but not as much. Mostly sadness. I feel alone.

I am not feeling as bad as I have. I know what's coming and know that I have to deal with it.

I must be getting better 'cause my thoughts are pretty clear. What happened, happened. As much as I want to change it, that doesn't change. So, I'm in therapy getting healthy and dealing with it.

I've had a positive week, so right now I feel sadness and empathy, not just for myself but kind of for the assholes that did that to me. How sick they must be.

Question: What did you do that you should be able to feel good about? Can you allow yourself to feel that?

The only thing I feel good about is that I crawled out of there and survived. No!!!

I do feel relief that I'm not running away right now.

I came here and took risks to trust others with this. It's too heavy for me to carry alone.

I feel good that I can listen to the tapes and relive the evil without walking out and killing someone.

I lived and made it back to the U.S. I feel good about where I am at right now in my life. Maybe by going through all that, that's how I got here!!

In addition to these significant shifts in his affective and cognitive reactions to the trauma, Mr. B.H. also experienced a significant decrease in his PTSD symptoms. His PCL-C score at the end of the exposure therapy was 42, representing a significant decrease in PTSD symptoms and falling below the 50-point recommended cutoff for PTSD in veterans. In addition, during the course of exposure therapy the veteran obtained a job, moved into his own apartment, and began reconnecting with family members. He also developed a friendship with a man at the residential treatment community and at the end of treatment decided to share the story of his rape with this male friend. The veteran maintained his sobriety throughout the course of the exposure therapy.

Seeking Safety Group

During the same time that Mr. B.H. participated in the exposure therapy, he also participated in a Seeking Safety group that consisted of the patient and three other veterans. He participated in all 25 sessions of this 60-minute group over a 6-month period. Seeking Safety is a manualized, group-based treatment for individuals with comorbid PTSD and substance abuse/dependence. Each of the groups began with a check-in process and the review of a topic-relevant quote. Veterans then spent 30–45 minutes reviewing psychoeducation/skill-building handouts that are provided and discussing how the topic is relevant to their own experience with PTSD and substance abuse. The group then ends with a checkout in which veterans identify a committed action that they will take before the next group. Mr. B.H. participated actively in this group and reported that he found the topics extremely beneficial. The most notable difference between his participation in this group and the stress management group is that here, the veteran connected very well with other group members. They would often meet up before group or stay after group to continue the social process. In addition, midway through group, group members shared their telephone numbers with each other and often had out-of-group contact with one another.

Evaluation After Phase 2

After Mr. B.H. completed exposure therapy and while he finished the Seeking Safety group, we met for a final eight sessions to evaluate progress, discuss the course of treatment, identify lessons learned, and process termination. My fellowship was ending, and thus the veteran was going to be transferred to another treatment provider. We discussed at length his multiple areas of progress over the course of the year, including maintaining his sobriety, decreasing his PTSD symptoms, improving his sleep, enhancing his social network, and increasing his psychosocial functioning (e.g., obtaining employment and independent living). We also spent significant time discussing his feelings about the end of the therapeutic relationship, because he felt very connected to me given the emotional intensity of the work that we did together. It represented growth that the veteran was able to process and discuss his feeling of grief about saying goodbye. Lastly, we discussed next steps in therapy, including engaging in in vivo exposure to address a few continued avoidance behaviors and continuing to challenge trauma-related cognitive distortions.

Summary of Guideline Use

Table 29–1 summarizes the guideline recommendations that applied to this patient and whether the recommendations were followed or adjusted. The major complication in applying the VA/DoD treatment guideline to this case was the lack of guidance in treatment options and adjustments for veterans with a long history of alcohol dependence. A particular concern was whether exposure therapy could be employed without increasing the odds of relapse to alcohol. This was addressed by turning to the literature for an evidence-supported treatment (Seeking

Safety) as well as noncontrolled clinical observations. Based on these reports from outside the guideline, a treatment plan was established that included the addition of a set of safety parameters while conducting exposure therapy and the concurrent application of Seeking Safety group therapy. These additional interventions allowed for the safe and successful application of exposure therapy.

Although the VA/DoD guideline strongly recommended initiating pharmacological treatment with an SSRI, Mr. B.H. was resistant to trying medications, despite having agreed to a consult. The veteran agreed on a targeted approach with prazosin for nightmares. Thus, patient preference resulted in a deviation from the guideline. The dosing of prazosin was below that in the guideline (which recommends 6–12 mg) because of side effects experienced at doses above 6 mg. Verbal communication with researchers involved in investigating prazosin suggested that lower dosages can be efficacious. Because the targeted symptom of nightmares improved and the veteran was engaged in exposure therapy, no further pharmacological treatments were attempted.

The focal treatment intervention in this case, exposure therapy, also deviated somewhat from that described in the literature because of the veteran's significant history of substance dependence. The number of sessions was able to be titrated in part because of the primary author's more flexible schedule as a trainee. This flexibility is not available in many treatment settings but may have improved the chances of successful treatment response with this veteran.

Ways to Improve Practice

Although this veteran was treated as part of an integrated treatment team, it was still difficult to integrate fully the psychotherapy and pharmacotherapy interventions into a uniform treatment plan. This was in part because of Mr. B.H.'s reluctance to take medications. In an ideal setting, an evidence-based pharmacological intervention would be given that either would work synergistically with the psychotherapy or even pharmacologically enhance the exposure therapy, as has been proposed by some researchers.

As stated, because this case occurred while the primary author was a trainee, there was the ability to provide more sessions than is described generally in the literature. It is possible the same level of effectiveness could have been accomplished with a decreased number of sessions, but because the number of sessions was not a significant limitation in this case, the greater number of sessions increased the probability the interventions could be applied safely.

The primary outcome measure used was the PCL-C. This is a cumbersome measure to apply in a normal clinic setting in which time is a limiting factor. The lack of validated briefer measures of PTSD is a significant limitation in monitoring treatment responses while administering evidence-based treatments. This case could have benefited from more measures aimed at monitoring improvements in social functioning, sense of well-being, and interpersonal interactions.

References

American Psychiatric Association: Practice Guideline for the Treatment of Patients With Acute Stress Disorder and Posttraumatic Stress Disorder. 2004. Available at: http://www.psychiatryonline.com/pracGuide/pracGuideTopic_11.aspx. Accessed March 4, 2009

Brady KT, Dansky BS, Back SE, et al: Exposure therapy in the treatment of PTSD among cocaine-dependent individuals: preliminary findings. J Subst Abuse Treat 21:47–54, 2001

Brady KT, Back SE, Coffey SF: Substance abuse and posttraumatic stress disorder. Curr Dir Psychol Sci 13:206–209, 2004

Davidson PR, Parker KC: Eye movement desensitization and reprocessing (EMDR): a meta-analysis. J Consult Clin Psychol 69:305–316, 2001

Donovan, B, Padin-Rivera E, Kowaliw S: "Transcend": initial outcomes from a posttraumatic stress disorder/substance abuse treatment program. J Trauma Stress 14:757–772, 2001

Foa EB, Davidson JRT, Frances A: The expert consensus guideline series: treatment of posttraumatic stress disorder. J Clin Psychiatry 60 (suppl 16), 1999

Foa EB, Keane TM, Friedman MJ (eds): Effective Treatments for PTSD: Practice Guidelines From the International Society for Traumatic Stress Studies. New York, Guilford, 2000

Institute of Medicine: Treatment of Posttraumatic Stress Disorder: An Assessment of the Evidence. Washington, DC, National Academies Press, 2007

Najavits LM: Seeking Safety: A Treatment Manual for PTSD and Substance Abuse. New York, Guilford, 2002

Najavits LM, Schmitz M, Gotthardt S, et al: Seeking Safety plus exposure therapy: an outcome study on dual diagnosis men. J Psychoactive Drugs 37:425–435, 2005

Triffleman E, Carroll K, Kellogg S: Substance dependence posttraumatic stress disorder therapy: an integrated cognitive-behavioral approach. J Subst Abuse Treat 17:3–14, 1999

VA/DOD Management of Post-Traumatic Stress Working Group: VA/DoD clinical practice guideline for the management of post-traumatic stress. Washington, DC, Veterans Health Administration/Department of Defense, 2004. Available at: http://www.healthquality.va.gov/ptsd/ptsd_full.pdf. Accessed July 18, 2009

Severe, Recurrent Depression Managed in a Remote Setting Via the Internet

An Example of Remote Care Using the HealthSteps System

Dennis Tannenbaum, M.B.Ch.B., FRANZCP

Caroline Spiranovic, Ph.D.

As practitioners, we are aware that despite implementing evidence-based treatment plans with our patients, many will not adhere to treatment and will cease treatment prematurely as a result of intolerable side effects (Nemeroff 2003). Furthermore, large-scale clinical trials of antidepressant medications indicate that remission may be difficult to achieve even in medication-compliant depressed patients (Rush et al. 2006). Also, relapse rates are relatively high (i.e., 67%) in the long term for patients with severe depression even when they are compliant with medications and achieve remission in the acute stage of treatment (Kennedy et al. 2003). To ensure that the maximum number of patients achieve remission and maintain this state in the long term, there need to be systems in place that supplement the work we can physically do as practitioners.

These systems would need to allow for regular monitoring of patient compliance and side-effect burden as well as measurement of treatment response.

The case study we present here outlines the use of the HealthSteps (www.healthsteps.net.au) Internet-based system, developed by Sentiens, to deliver care and monitor remotely a depressed patient from a rural and isolated town in Australia. The patient was seen by the first author (D.T., hereafter referred to in the first person) in his private practice in early 2002. The patient agreed to be managed remotely using an emergent version of the e-health system developed by Sentiens. This example is somewhat of a departure from typical practice, in which the patient would be seen via face-to-face consultation, or occasionally via telepsychiatry, and the HealthSteps system would be employed as an adjunct to regular treatment.

To the best of our knowledge, elements of the HealthSteps system developed by Sentiens are already existent in commercial disease management systems in the United States, but the outcome data for these systems is rarely available for public scrutiny.

Setting

Sentiens is a private specialist mental health clinic that operates a busy outpatient clinic and a day hospital with a 52-patient capacity. Sentiens is based in Perth, Western Australia.

Western Australia is Australia's largest state in area, comprising one-third of Australia's total coastline. Despite this, the population size of Western Australia is approximately 2.1 million and therefore accounts only for 10% of Australia's total population. Over 70% of Western Australian's population resides in Perth, the capital city (Australian Bureau of Statistics 2008). Providing medical services for this vast state is difficult, particularly given that a substantial minority of the population is employed in mining in the remote Goldfields region and hence works on a fly in, fly out (FIFO) basis (Australian Bureau of Statistics 2003).

To provide improved health care for the Western Australian population, Sentiens has pioneered an e-health system that can be used by practitioners to manage and monitor patients wherever they may be: close by in Perth, in rural Australia, or working overseas. The resultant HealthSteps system has been implemented in a number of research trials, both in Australia (e.g., Barnes et al. 2007) and the United States (e.g., Harvey et al. 2007), to further refine its features and demonstrate its efficacy in the management of longer-term health conditions.

Illustration

This study illustrates:

- Monitoring and maintenance of progress
- Patient self-empowerment
- Maintaining adherence

Chief Complaint

Mr. P.J. is a 50-year-old man who requests that I manage a recurrence of his depression that has been progressively worsening. The patient completed Sentiens's online assessment battery, which confirmed the telephone history of severe major depression with diurnal mood variation, early morning wakening, daily depression, agitation, and anxiety with two to three low-grade panic attacks occurring weekly. He was finding it hard to motivate himself and was finding each day interminable. He has fleet-ing suicidal thoughts but no plan or intention to commit suicide.

His general practitioner (GP) had started him on 20 mg/day of paroxetine 3 weeks prior to our consultation, and this had resulted in a small reduction in panic attack intensity. I wrote to his GP to undertake a number of blood tests and perform a physical examination. The test results from the patient's GP confirmed that Mr. P.J. is in good physical health.

Patient History

Mr. P.J. was well known to me because previously I had treated him intermittently for depression over a 10-year period beginning in the early 1990s. Mr. P.J. initially came to see me for assistance in managing what appeared to be a mild episode of depression and to develop strategies to cope with the difficulties he was experiencing in his marriage. His wife, who was in poor health, was becoming progressively more anxious and depressed and was acting in an aggressive manner toward him and the children.

With regard to the patient's history, Mr. P.J. had performed well academically at university, was socially well adjusted, and was the CEO of a successful company. He had a family history of depression, and his mother had been admitted to a psychiatric hospital on several occasions in the past for severe depression that was treated with electroconvulsive therapy (ECT). Just prior to our first consultation, Mr. P.J. had had a very comprehensive recent medical evaluation from his company, and he was deemed to be in very good physical health.

I initially saw Mr. P.J. for three to four sessions of cognitive-behavioral therapy (CBT) before he decided to cease therapy because of an improvement in his situation. However, he returned to see me within 1 month of ceasing therapy because his depressive symptoms had worsened considerably. He indicated he would prefer to persist with CBT because he was resistant to the idea of taking medications. He felt that "taking medication would prove [he] had the family illness" and he wanted to "sort [himself] out without it."

After a further 2 weeks of CBT, it was clear that his condition was worsening and he agreed to try an antidepressant medication. (He initially was started on fluoxetine because this selective serotonin reuptake inhibitor [SSRI] had been recently made available in 1990 and was the first of the SSRIs on the Australian market.) Fluoxetine was not successful. Mr. P.J.'s condition deteriorated rapidly, and he required inpatient admission.

In the hospital, he was started on dothiepin, a tricyclic antidepressant (TCA) that was still commonly prescribed in Australia during the early 1990s. The patient made a rapid recovery on dothiepin at 150 mg/day and returned to work after 4 weeks.

After 4 months, he ceased the medication without discussing it with me, claiming he was well.

I thereafter saw Mr. P.J. on an intermittent basis for approximately 10 years. During this time he frequently ceased taking his medication without prior consultation and would subsequently relapse.

Other Significant Findings From Assessment

The online assessment battery completed by Mr. P.J. indicated that he was struggling to cope with his day-to-day activities.

DSM-IV-TR Diagnosis

Axis I	Major depression with comorbid panic disorder
Axis II	None
Axis III	None
Axis IV	Work stress
Axis V	GAF score: 50

Treatment Plan Considerations

My current assessment of this patient indicated that the primary problem was major depression with comorbid anxiety associated with low-intensity and low-frequency panic attacks. Although the patient's anxiety and panic symptoms had been relieved somewhat by the paroxetine prescribed 3 weeks earlier by his GP, he was still experiencing severe levels of depression and this was affecting his day-to-day functioning. He had a poor level of functioning (GAF=50) that was affecting his ability to work, socialize, and even self-care.

The patient had recently moved to a small town some distance from Perth and was managing a small business. His poor level of functioning was placing his developing business at risk, and hence the patient recognized he needed treatment. However, he was limited in his ability to leave his workplace for the time

needed to visit me in Perth without sustaining significant financial loss because he had no cover for himself in his newly developing business. He was also caring for his now ex-wife, who was chronically ill and unable to care for herself. He requested I manage him by telephone and advise his local GP on treatment.

The primary aim of treatment was to achieve a remission in the patient's symptoms and maintain this progress so that the patient could function well and make a success of his life. The patient previously had a satisfactory response to a TCA, namely dothiepin, but this antidepressant gave rise to side effects that he complained about and was prepared to tolerate only because he was unable to achieve success on another medication. His treatment adherence had not been persuasive, as he had lowered and ceased his medication only to subsequently relapse on a number of occasions. In order to achieve and maintain a remission of symptoms in this patient, it was essential that he be treated with an antidepressant that was associated with a lower side-effect burden. The American Psychiatric Association (APA) released their revised guideline on the treatment of major depression in 2000. This guideline provided ample information regarding the side-effect profiles of newer antidepressants, and there were many newer-generation antidepressants available in Australia that had a lower side-effect profile than TCAs (see Mant et al. 2004).

However, given the patient's prior history of severe and recurrent depressive episodes, he would be considered at high risk for relapse. The patient was going to require regular monitoring as well as early intervention in not only the acute phase of treatment but also in the long term, particularly with regard to managing side-effect burden. Although the APA (2000) practice guideline did not specify a minimum length of time required for continuation and maintenance therapy with patients who had recurrent and severe episodes of depression, there was evidence available at the time to suggest that this patient would benefit from maintenance therapy using pharmacotherapy for at least a 2-year period (Ellis and Smith 2002).

Treatment Goals, Measures, and Methods

The primary aim of treatment was to improve the patient's mood and function with an antidepressant that has a tolerable side-effect burden and provide therapy to help him return to and maintain an optimal level of function. I discussed the medication options with Mr. P.J., and he agreed to remain on the paroxetine prescribed by his GP in the interim. Paroxetine was an accepted SSRI in the treatment of both major depression and comorbid anxiety and panic disorder (American Psychiatric Association 2000). Moreover, SSRIs are typically associated with a lower side-effect profile than older-generation antidepressants (American Psychiatric Association 2000), and the patient reported in the interim that he was tolerating the side effects. Medications were to be prescribed and monitored by his local GP, who was happy to monitor the patient weekly. I discussed this with the patient's GP via telephone, and she agreed to take primary responsibility for the patient's care.

I discussed the option of using the HealthSteps online program for depression with Mr. P.J., and he agreed to enroll in this program. I wanted my patient to use this program because it would allow me to monitor remotely his progress, provide him with relevant psychoeducational material, and communicate with him via a secure e-consultation facility. The program allows both the patient and practitioner to access and print out a progress report that provides a graph of the patient's progress on the key measures over time and details the patient's medication chart and self-reported medication compliance. This HealthSteps program would measure the patient's progress on three measures developed by Sentiens: the Depression Severity Scale (DSS), the Quality of Life (QOL) measure, and the Side Effects Scale (SES). As opposed to using validated measures that were freely available in the public domain, we chose to construct our own measures for use in HealthSteps to avoid the possibility of future royalty claims or liabilities.

The DSS is a 20-item measure developed by Sentiens to assess severity of depressive symptoms. Respondents rate the frequency with which they have experienced each listed symptom on a 4-point Likert scale (never, sometimes, often, most of the time). From this measure, three subscale scores (general depression symptoms, self-harm, mood symptoms) and a total score may be derived, with higher scores indicative of greater depressive symptoms.

The psychometric properties of the DSS were demonstrated in an unpublished report by Ree in 2002. The DSS was administered to a sample of 169 psychiatric patients of Sentiens clinic, the majority of whom were male (57.4%), with a mean age of 42.17

years (SD = 12.35). The DSS demonstrated a high degree of internal consistency, with a Cronbach's alpha for the total scale of 0.94 ($n=141$). Factor analysis using generalized least squares with oblique rotation supported a three-factor solution: general depression symptoms, self-harm, and mood symptoms. The convergent validity for the DSS was demonstrated using the 42-item version of the Depression Anxiety Stress Scales (DASS; Lovibond and Lovibond 1995) as a benchmark measure of depression, wherein the DSS total score ($r=0.86$) and DSS mood symptoms scale ($r=0.80$) had good convergent validity with the DASS depression scale ($P<0.01$). The DSS self-harm subscale demonstrated low convergence with the DASS depression scale ($r=0.54$, $P<0.01$), which was to be expected given that the DASS depression scale does not assess self-harm/suicidal ideation. The discriminant validity of the DSS was not well supported, as moderate correlations were obtained between the DSS total score and the DSS mood symptoms subscale and the DASS anxiety and stress scales ($P<0.01$). However, there were also moderate to high correlations between the DASS depression scale and the anxiety and stress scales ($P<0.01$), thus demonstrating the commonality of underlying causes and characteristics of these constructs.

The QOL was designed by Sentiens as a brief screening scale comprising 8 items that measure the degree to which the patient's symptoms are having a negative impact on quality of life. The QOL is used simply to detect changes in impairment associated with symptoms and was not intended as a tool for determining clinically defined levels of functioning. Although the psychometric properties of the QOL have not been established, this measure was designed to be representative of the constructs commonly measured in such scales. Respondents rate the extent to which their symptoms have affected various aspects of their lives on a 4-point Likert scale (not at all, a little, very much so, severely). This measure yields a total score as well as four subscale scores (relationships, risk behaviors, social, work and money) with high scores indicating that symptoms are having a greater negative effect on quality of life.

Finally, Sentiens developed the Side Effects Scale to measure the level of medication side effects experienced by patients completing pharmacotherapy. This scale was designed specifically for descriptive purposes to gauge the level and type of side effects reported, and thus its psychometric properties have not been evaluated. Respondents rate the extent to which they have been experiencing 30 items relating to medication side-effects on a 4-point Likert scale (not at all, a little, very much so, severely). From the SES, a total score may be derived as well as six subscale scores (akathisia, attention and mood, involuntary movements, parkinsonism, physical difficulties, and sexual problems). Higher scores are indicative of a greater side-effect burden.

With regard to the treatment schedule, the patient was willing to complete monitoring questionnaires on a once-weekly basis for 6 weeks or until a satisfactory response was achieved. The patient also agreed to communicate with me regularly via e-consultation and telephone as necessary. It was agreed that after a satisfactory improvement, the frequency of monitoring questionnaires and e-consultations could be reduced gradually provided the patient remained compliant and continued to improve. The primary aim was to continue treatment with antidepressants until the patient's depressive symptoms were reduced to a normal range and were consequently having minimal impact on his quality of life. I would then maintain the patient with pharmacotherapy for at least 12 months. A secondary aim was to greatly reduce the side-effect burden of the medications he was taking because this would in turn greatly enhance the patient's likelihood of adherence and remission in the long term.

Course

I monitored the patient's progress closely on the DSS, QOL, and SES for a period of 46 weeks. After this time, I primarily monitored and communicated with the patient via e-consultation and telephone for an additional 12 months. The progress graphs for the DSS, QOL, and SES are presented in Figures 30–1, 30–2, and 30–3, respectively. Plotted against the scale scores in each of these three figures is the patient's medication chart, as well as events of interest that arose during our e-consultations. It should be noted that the patient had been taking paroxetine for 3 weeks prior to commencement of this 46-week period of monitoring.

Initially, paroxetine at 40 mg/day did not result in any noticeable change in symptoms (see Figure 30–1). The patient's quality of life was worsening (Figure 30–2), and the SES (Figure 30–3) indicated he was experiencing substantial side effects. An increase

in paroxetine dosage to 60 mg resulted in minimal improvement in depressive symptoms (Figure 30–1) and quality of life (Figure 30–2), and he was still scoring in the severe range for depression. During this time, there was a noticeable improvement on the SES (Figure 30–3) that indicated the medication side effects were dissipating.

However, the patient subsequently and abruptly ceased taking the paroxetine without consultation. He reported he was experiencing significant sleep disturbances, which included episodes of nocturnal sleepwalking. When the patient ceased taking the paroxetine there was a noticeable worsening in his quality of life, as demonstrated in Figure 30–2. By this time point, the patient had been taking paroxetine for a total of 8 weeks, having commenced this medication 3 weeks prior to our consultation, and I had now been monitoring him for 5 weeks. The APA (2000) guideline recommends that it is appropriate to undertake a review of the treatment plan and medications if a moderate improvement in symptoms is not observed after 6–8 weeks of pharmacotherapy.

Thus, approximately 8 weeks into pharmacotherapy, the patient was recommenced on paroxetine at 40 mg/day. I decided to continue the patient on this lower dose of paroxetine rather than switch to another antidepressant, because of the effectiveness of this SSRI in treating symptoms of both depression and anxiety. The difficulty was that paroxetine at 40 mg as a monotherapy would not produce a sufficient response for this patient and the patient was experiencing significant sleep disturbances. I was aware that in this instance, where a partial response was obtained, the APA practice guideline would recommend the addition of an augmenting agent such as lithium, thyroid hormone (namely triiodothyronine: T_3), or buspirone (a 5-HT_{1A} receptor antagonist) in addition to the SSRI. However, these augmentation strategies were unlikely to alleviate the insomnia experienced by the patient.

Hence, mirtazapine, a norepinephrine-serotonin modulator, at 45 mg/day, was added for its additive antidepressant effect and to alleviate the patient's problems with sleep. In support of this choice, the current Texas Medication Algorithm for major depression supports the switch to a sedating antidepressant medication such as mirtazapine to address insomnia as a side effect (Suehs et al. 2008). Furthermore, there was also evidence available at the time to

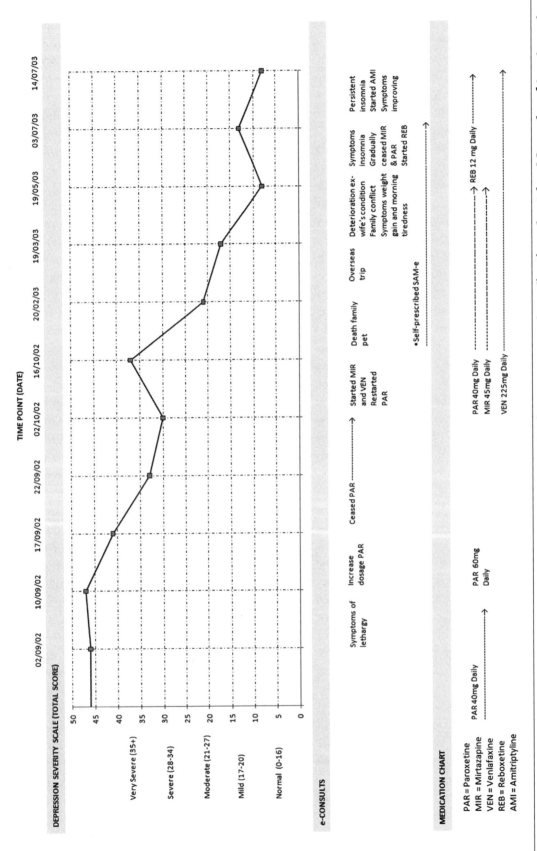

FIGURE 30–1. Total Depression Severity Scale scores, e-consultation events, and medication chart for 46 weeks of treatment.

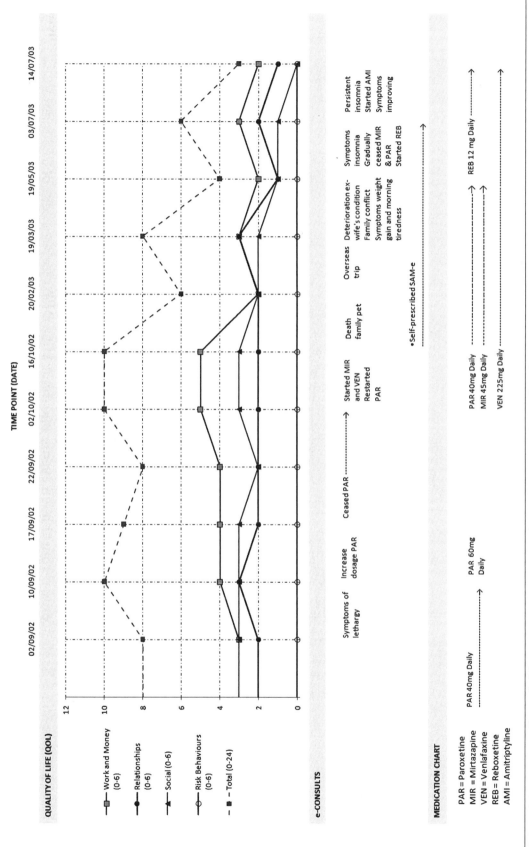

FIGURE 30–2.   Quality of Life scores, e-consultation events, and medication chart for 46 weeks of treatment.

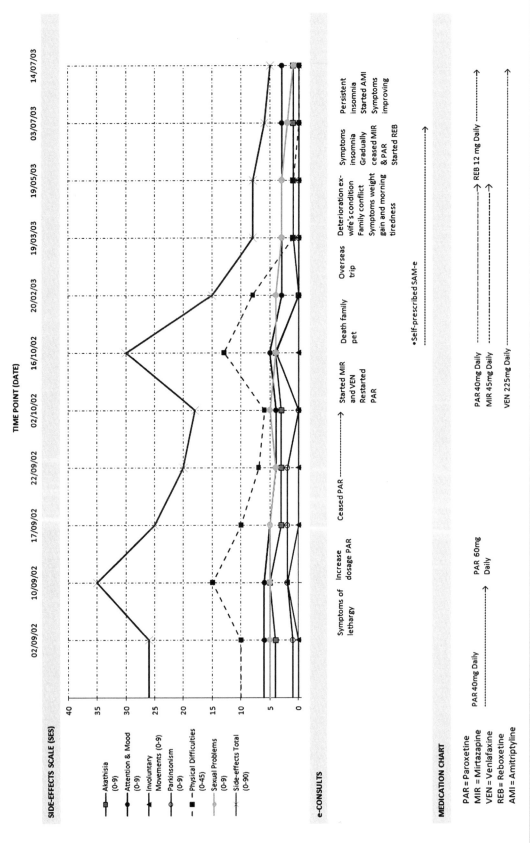

FIGURE 30–3.   Side Effects Scale scores, e-consultation events, and medication charts for 46 weeks of treatment.

suggest that the addition of mirtazapine might be particularly helpful given its dual serotonergic and noradrenergic action (Fava et al. 2003).

In addition, venlafaxine, a serotonin-norepinephrine reuptake inhibitor (SNRI), at 225 mg/day, was added because of its strong antidepressant action and suitability as a relatively safe adjunct medication to SSRIs. I was aware that the combination of mirtazapine and venlafaxine was the final step of treatment in the STAR*D trials for those patients who had demonstrated relatively high levels of treatment-resistant depression (Fava et al. 2003). Furthermore, this combination was associated with a lower side-effect profile and higher adherence rates than alternatives for treatment-resistant depression such as tranylcypromine, which is a monoamine oxidase inhibitor (McGrath et al. 2006). I was also aware that mirtazapine and venlafaxine had superior safety indices when compared with MAOIs (Kent 2000). It was therefore reasonable to assume that this powerful combination of antidepressants would be tolerated by the patient and would result in a rapid improvement in symptoms and functioning.

Upon commencing the combination of mirtazapine, venlafaxine, and paroxetine, the patient initially experienced an increase in depressive symptoms (see Figure 30–1), which could largely be attributed to a sudden increase in medication side effects (see Figure 30–3). However, this initial increase in symptoms and side effects was to be expected with this powerful combination of medications. The patient thereafter progressively improved, although progress was slower than anticipated. Within 18 weeks of commencing these new medications, the patient's depressive symptoms (see Figure 30–1) had decreased from the very severe range to within the moderate range. This was a marked improvement, indicating that the trial was in part a success. However, the ultimate aim was to achieve a full remission in symptoms, as indicated by a score on the DSS within the normal range. Coinciding with this reduction in depressive symptoms over the 18 weeks was a marked improvement in the patient's quality of life (see Figure 30–2), particularly with regard to work and money, and the medication side effects had lessened considerably (see Figure 30–3).

Further improvement in symptoms, quality of life, and side effects were gained over the next 3 months, to the point where the patient's depressive symptoms were scored in the normal range. It was interesting to observe that these improvements in the patient's depressive symptoms (see Figure 30–1) occurred at a somewhat tumultuous time during which the patient was experiencing significant psychosocial stressors, such as the death of a family pet, as well as a further deterioration in his ex-wife's condition that was resulting in substantial family conflict. These significant stressors also, surprisingly, had little bearing on the patient's quality of life (see Figure 30–2), as he was able to maintain an acceptable level of functioning during this time. These improvements despite adversity indicated to me that the medications were having the desired effect.

During this time of substantial progress, it is noteworthy that the patient, without consultation, commenced a self-prescribed dosage of *S*-adenosyl-L-methionine (SAMe). At the time of my consultations with this patient, there were no guidelines concerning the use of SAMe as an alternative treatment for major depression. There was relatively sparse and inconclusive evidence regarding the efficacy of this naturally occurring psychotropic substance, and studies were typically limited by methodological issues such as small sample size. However, there was some evidence to suggest that this substance exhibited antidepressant effects and that its use was associated with acceptable levels of safety and tolerability in patients (Agency for Healthcare Research and Quality 2002; Pancheri et al. 2002). Given that the patient believed in the efficacy of this substance and I could see no harm in its use as an adjunctive treatment, I was happy for the patient to remain on SAMe. In fact, although I could not rule out the possibility of a placebo effect, given the inclusive evidence regarding use of SAMe, the patient's recent improvements did appear to coincide with the commencement of SAMe.

It is noteworthy that the patient was willing to continue treatment despite adverse effects until a substantial improvement had been obtained. Once these gains in symptoms and functioning had been achieved, the patient was no longer willing to tolerate the medication side effects. About 30 weeks after commencing the combination of mirtazapine, venlafaxine, and paroxetine, the patient reported he was experiencing substantial difficulties with weight gain and morning tiredness, and hence requested a change in medications.

At that point in time, newer generation antidepressants associated with lower side-effect profiles than their predecessors had become available in Australia. I instructed the patient to start on reboxetine, a norepinephrine reuptake inhibitor. At the time, reboxetine was a relatively new antidepressant, but I was aware of clinical trials that indicated reboxetine was well tolerated and had similar levels of clinical efficacy to many SSRIs (Kent 2000). However, I was also aware that clinical trials indicated reboxetine was associated with impotence in some male patients (Kent 2000), and my own experiences in treating patients through private practice confirmed this. I discussed the side-effect profile of reboxetine with my patient, who had also read widely on this subject, and he indicated he would prefer to try reboxetine because he was unwilling to tolerate the weight gain associated with mirtazapine.

The reboxetine failed to result in an initial improvement, and the dosage was increased to 12 mg/day. This dose had the desired effect of maintaining remission while also lowering side-effect burden. However, the patient's tolerance lessened somewhat and he experienced worsening symptoms of insomnia. In response, venlafaxine was ceased and amitriptyline, a tricyclic antidepressant, was added for its known sedative properties (Phillips et al. 2000) approximately 46 weeks into treatment. Although the APA (2000) guideline would recommend trazodone in this instance, this antidepressant was not available in Australia. Furthermore, benzodiazepine-related compounds were not an adjunctive option because the patient was previously unable to tolerate such compounds. I largely chose to use amitriptyline over other sedative antidepressants because the patient had previously tolerated tricyclics and did not experience the weight gain often associated with such medications (APA 2000).

Clinically, this case brought to light the importance of tailoring treatments to suit individual patients' needs and, in particular, managing intolerances. The combination of reboxetine and amitriptyline appeared to produce sufficiently strong antidepressant effects and also side effects that were below threshold levels of tolerance. This combination was successful in the long term, as the patient continued on reboxetine at 12 mg/day and amitriptyline at 50 mg/day for 12 months before ceasing pharmacotherapy. Furthermore, the patient has maintained contact with me since this cessation and has not relapsed, to the best of my knowledge, in over 5 years.

Summary of Guideline Use

Utilizing this online monitoring system, it is apparent that the patient's progress was markedly slower than the APA guideline would suggest (American Psychiatric Association 2000). At approximately 9 months into treatment, the patient achieved remission. Remission was maintained over the following months, and changes in medications appeared to have the desired effect of further lowering side-effect burden. Although progress was slower than expected, research would suggest that remission is more difficult to achieve in patients with severe and recurrent depression (Kennedy et al. 2003).

Current guidelines recommend longer periods of continuation and maintenance therapy for patients with severe and/or recurrent depression because such patients are at an increased risk for relapse (American Psychiatric Association 2000; National Institute for Health and Clinical Excellence 2007; Royal Australian and New Zealand College of Psychiatrists Clinical Practice Guidelines Team for Depression 2004). In accordance with these guidelines, I maintained the patient on reboxetine and amitriptyline for an additional 12 months to preserve remission.

Although I was aware of the APA (2000) guideline for treatment of depression, I also knew that the side-effect burden was going to be an important issue to resolve with this patient. It is all too often the case that patients with high levels of side-effect burden cease taking their medications, despite improvements in symptoms, and consequently relapse (Nemeroff 2003). Hence, an essential goal of the treatment plan was to achieve a minimal level of side-effect burden. The present patient, as with many patients, initially improved upon commencement of psychotherapy with SSRIs. Despite the benefits of these medications, it was difficult to maintain an acceptable balance between efficacy and side effects. In the present case, augmentation of antidepressant medications to below side-effect threshold levels proved to be a worthwhile strategy because remission was achieved and maintained for 12 months while also obtaining an acceptably low side-effect burden.

In order to achieve these long-term gains, I was required at times to diverge from what would be considered an ideal approach. For instance, in my experience as a practitioner, the majority of male patients are unable to tolerate reboxetine. However, this patient was a very intelligent and educated man who had read widely on the available antidepressants. He believed that the side effects of reboxetine would be better tolerated than the weight gain associated with the current medications he was taking. Although I discussed the issue of efficacy versus side effects of this medication, the patient was willing and motivated to tolerate these effects. As was predicted given available guidelines (American Psychiatric Association 2000), the reboxetine resulted in complaints of insomnia, but these were ameliorated with the amitriptyline. This combination was clearly successful in the long term because the patient was able to tolerate the side effects and maintained a remission in symptoms.

This case clearly illustrates the importance of compromise because for many patients the side effects can outweigh the efficacy of many antidepressant medications, and many patients are only willing to maintain pharmacotherapy if a low level of side-effect burden can be achieved. It would be beneficial for future guidelines to outline the processes a practitioner may follow to minimize side-effect burden and dropout while also improving quality of life and, hence, achieving the best results for a given population.

This case study also highlights the importance of the capacity to monitor patient progress, as outlined in the guidelines developed for treating depression (American Psychiatric Association 2000; National Institute for Health and Clinical Excellence 2007; Royal Australian and New Zealand College of Psychiatrists Clinical Practice Guidelines Team for Depression 2004). Despite these guidelines, practitioners typically find it practically difficult to monitor patients frequently and in great detail. Through the use of the HealthSteps online system, I was able to respond to my patient's concerns regarding side effects in a timely manner and quickly detect any changes in symptoms or quality of life. I believe this capacity to monitor and intervene early was the key to success with this patient because previous to this my patient often ceased medications without consultation and experienced multiple episodes of relapse. Also, and equally important, the HealthSteps system enabled me to develop rapport and establish a working relationship with my patient in the absence of face-to-face contact. The system enabled us regularly to discuss and review such issues as medication efficacy versus side effects, and together we decided on the best course of action.

Ways to Improve Practice

This case study has demonstrated the utility of online disease management systems in monitoring patients with longer-term health conditions. The HealthSteps system developed by Sentiens was designed as an adjunct tool to monitor and manage large numbers of patients over long periods of time. The system facilitates the evaluation of different strategies to maintain patients in treatment through monitoring of symptoms, quality of life, and side-effect burden. As this case study illustrates, patients typically require frequent monitoring to ensure medication compliance. However, it is often the case that practitioners experience barriers, such as heavy caseloads, that preclude frequent and detailed monitoring of patients. Although the system developed by Sentiens can address many of these barriers, it is evident that practitioners may require additional support to effectively monitor and manage large numbers of patients. To address this issue, recently we have begun to explore the possibilities for utilizing the time and expertise of allied health professionals. Allied health professionals may take on the role of case manager and can facilitate practitioners by regularly monitoring patients using the online system and may contact patients who are not progressing well.

In conclusion, developments in information and communication technologies, as evidenced by the emergent HealthSteps system, offer infrastructures that may be used by practitioners to improve their management of patients. These infrastructures enable us to better monitor and maintain patients so that we may break the iterant cycle of relapse and achieve our long-term goal of remission.

References

Agency for Healthcare Research and Quality: S-Adenosyl-L-methionine for treatment of depression, osteoarthritis, and liver disease (Evidence Report/Technology Assessment, No 64). August 2002. Available at: http://www.ahrq.gov/clinic/epcsums/samesum.htm. Accessed March 5, 2009

American Psychiatric Association: Practice guideline for the treatment of patients with major depressive disorder (revision). Am J Psychiatry 157 (suppl 4):1–45, 2000

Australian Bureau of Statistics: Western Australian Statistical Indicators (cat no 1367.5). June 2003. Available at: http://www.abs.gov.au/ausstats. Accessed March 7, 2009

Australian Bureau of Statistics: Western Australia at a Glance (cat no 1306.5). 2008. Available at: http://www.abs.gov.au/ausstats. Accessed March 7, 2009

Barnes C, Harvey R, Mitchell P, et al: Evaluation of an online relapse prevention program for bipolar disorder: an overview of the aims and methodology of a randomised controlled trial. Disease Management and Health Outcomes 15:215–224, 2007

Ellis PM, Smith DA: Treating depression: the beyondblue guidelines for treating depression in primary care. Med J Aust 176:S77–S83, 2002

Fava M, Rush AJ, Trivedi MH, et al: Background and rationale for the Sequenced Treatment Alternatives to Relieve Depression (STAR*D) study. Psychiatr Clin N Am 26:457–494, 2003

Harvey R, Smith M, Abraham N, et al: The Hurricane Choir: remote mental health monitoring of participants in a community based intervention in the post Katrina period. J Health Care Poor Underserved 18:356–361, 2007

Kennedy N, Abbott R, Paykel ES: Remission and recurrence of depression in the maintenance era: long-term outcome in a Cambridge cohort. Psychol Med 33:827–838, 2003

Kent JM: SNaRIs, NaSSAs, and NaRIs: new agents for the treatment of depression. Lancet 355:911–918, 2000

Lovibond SH, Lovibond PF: Manual for the Depression Anxiety Stress Scales, 2nd Edition. Sydney, Psychology Foundation, 1995

Mant A, Rendle VA, Hall WD, et al: Making new choices about antidepressants in Australia: the long view 1975–2002. Med J Aust 181:S21–S24, 2004

McGrath PJ, Stewart JW, Fava M, et al: Tranylcypromine versus venlafaxine plus mirtazapine following three failed antidepressant medication trials for depression: a STAR*D report. Am J Psychiatry 163:1531–1541, 2006

National Institute for Health and Clinical Excellence: Depression (amended): management of depression in primary and secondary care (clinical guideline 23). April 2007. Available at: http://www.nice.org.uk/guidance/CG23. Accessed March 7, 2009

Nemeroff CB: Improving antidepressant adherence. J Clin Psychiatry 64:S25–S30, 2003

Pancheri P, Scapicchio P, Delle Chiaie R: A double-blind, randomized parallel-group, efficacy and safety study of intramuscular S-adenosyl-L-methionine 1,4-butanedisulphonate (SAMe) versus imipramine in patients with major depressive disorder. Int J Neuropsychopharmacol 5:287–294, 2002

Phillips MA, Bitsios P, Szabadi E, et al: Comparison of the antidepressants reboxetine, fluvoxamine and amitriptyline upon spontaneous papillary fluctuations in healthy human volunteers. Psychopharmacology 149:72–76, 2000

Royal Australian and New Zealand College of Psychiatrists Clinical Practice Guidelines Team for Depression: Australian and New Zealand clinical practice guidelines for the treatment of depression. Am J Psychiatry 38:389–407, 2004

Rush AJ, Trivedi MH, Wisniewski SR, et al: Acute and longer-term outcomes in depressed outpatients requiring one or several treatment steps: a STAR*D report. Am J Psychiatry 163:1905–1917, 2006

Suehs B, Argo TR, Bendele SD, et al: Texas Medication Algorithm Project Procedural Manual: major depressive disorder algorithms. Austin, Texas Department of State Health Services, 2008. Available at: http://www.dshs.state.tx.us/mhprograms/pdf/TIMA_MDD_MDD AlgoOnly_080608.pdf. Accessed November 3, 2008

Postpartum Depression Treated in Private Practice

Matthew H. May, M.D.
Margaret F. Reynolds-May, B.A.

Setting

Dr. Matthew May operates a private practice in Menlo Park, California, that consists mainly of self-paying or insured individuals presenting with depression, anxiety, interpersonal, and/or transitional life issues. He combines psychopharmacology and psychotherapy based on the TEAM (Testing, Empathy, Agenda Setting, Methods) framework created by Dr. David Burns. TEAM is a structured treatment methodology incorporating many novel techniques that can be combined creatively to address a variety of mood and relationship problems, addictions, and unwanted habits. Emphasis is placed on testing and information gathering, building and sustaining rapport, collaboration at the motivational level, as well as classic cognitive and behavioral strategies. All techniques and excerpts from publications by Dr. Burns are used with permission.

Illustration

This study illustrates:

- Multimodal treatment of severe postpartum depression using cognitive-behavioral therapy (CBT), electroconvulsive therapy (ECT), and medication management
- Guidelines for assessment and treatment of postpartum depression
- Symptom assessment and monitoring
- Agenda setting in CBT
- Relapse prevention

Chief Complaint

Jane is a well-educated, married, professionally successful 26-year-old Caucasian woman with recurrent major depressive episodes.

Three weeks following the birth of her first child, the patient experienced dysphoria, reduced energy, and crying spells. She interpreted her symptoms as "baby blues" and intended to discuss the problem with her obstetrician. Unfortunately, she became distracted by her child's crying during the office visit and did not report her symptoms. Aside from weight gain, her physiologic recovery from the delivery was normal, including resumption of her menses and lactation (reducing the concern for Sheehan's syndrome). During the next 4 months postpartum, she developed progressively worsening depression, including intense feelings of hopelessness and worthlessness, anhedonia, difficulty making decisions, prolonged daily crying spells, severe anxiety, reduced energy and libido, and suicidal ideation. This late presentation is not atypical and underscores the importance of screening and early treatment by primary care physicians and mental health professionals (Cho et al. 2008; Cox et al. 1987; Dennis and Hodnett 2007; Peindl et al. 2004; Rychnovsky and Brady 2008).

Present Illness

The patient attempted suicide by suffocation on three separate occasions, all within 1 year of the birth of her child. There were elements of impulsivity and desperation in her attempts. She was hospitalized on each occasion and treated with antidepressants, including high doses of sertraline, escitalopram, bupropion, and duloxetine both alone and in combination. She reported little improvement in her symptoms with these medications.

During her third hospital stay, while being treated with bupropion, escitalopram, and duloxetine, she was observed to have some increased mood lability and impulsivity. The question of bipolarity was raised, and she was tapered off of antidepressants and treated with olanzapine for mood stabilization and clonazepam for anxiety. She responded well to this regimen for several days, although she struggled with somnolence. Modafinil was added to alleviate this problem. She also had difficulty with weight gain and glucose metabolism while on olanzapine and was transitioned to aripiprazole. Her mood continued to decline. Having failed standard antidepressant treatment modalities, the patient was offered ECT. After a total of seven ECT treatments, the patient had significant improvements in mood (Montgomery-Åsberg Depression Rating Scale [MADRS] score fell from 45 to 9 during this 6-week hospitalization). Once stabilized, she was discharged to my outpatient practice with maintenance ECT.

DSM-IV-TR Diagnosis

Axis I	Major depressive disorder, recurrent, severe, with postpartum onset; consider bipolar affective disorder
Axis II	None
Axis III	None
Axis IV	Problems with social environment (child care), problems with primary support group, occupational problem
Axis V	GAF scores: 35–40

Treatment Plan Considerations

Suicide and Infanticide Risk

The patient was clearly at high risk for completing suicide (Appleby et al. 1998) and at some increased risk for infanticide (Taguchi 2007). Reliable early screening for suicide risk, infanticide risk, and psychosis was paramount for the success of this case.

Treatment of Postpartum Depression

There is limited evidence for a variety of modalities in the treatment of postpartum depression, both biological and nonbiological (Dennis 2004; Dennis and Stewart 2004). In light of the limited data, we are forced to rely on expert consensus guidelines (Altshuler et al. 2001). The consensus for initial treatment of nonpsychotic, severe postpartum depression is to combine psychosocial interventions with pharmacotherapy (antidepressants). Preferred antidepressants include sertraline followed by paroxetine (safety during pregnancy and lactation is frequently a concern, as discussed later in this section). In terms of psychotherapy, experts preferred CBT and interpersonal therapy (IPT). In the case of failure to respond to medication or in the presence of psychotic features, ECT was agreed upon as an acceptable treatment modality, although no randomized controlled trials exist (Forray and Ostroff 2007; Rabheru 2001). Most experts agreed that providing support in the home for the mother was appropriate and encouraged including the spouse in the psychotherapy.

In the case presented here, trials of antidepressants had either failed or appeared to pose the threat of a "switch" to mania (Altshuler et al. 1995), hence the choice of ECT and atypical antipsychotics for their mood-stabilizing effects. I decided to use a CBT model developed by Dr. David Burns (TEAM), as it is a flexible model with many interpersonal components. In addition, it incorporates meaningful scales to measure the efficacy of each therapy session and progress over the long-term course of therapy. The inpatient team had arranged for support in the home (a full-time professional nanny), and the patient was to attend a partial hospitalization program.

The specific treatment goals for this patient are outlined in Table 31–1.

Treatment of Depression in Bipolar Disorder

There is good evidence for the use of mood stabilizers, especially lithium, in the treatment of bipolar depression (Baldessarini et al. 2003). Although there is evidence that tricyclic antidepressants may increase the risk of causing mania or hypomania, several studies suggest that treating bipolar depression acutely

TABLE 31–1. Initial treatment goals, measures, and methods

Treatment goal	Measure	Method
Reduction in depressive symptoms and suicidal ideation/suicide attempts	Brief Mood Survey and self-report	TEAM–CBT ECT Psychopharmacology
Reduction in anxiety symptoms	Brief Mood Survey	Exposure (increased time in mothering role) Response prevention (decreasing assistance from child care services) Cognitive restructuring
Increased independence and improved functioning	Self-report, observation	TEAM–CBT
Improvement in relationship	Brief Mood Survey	Patient declined treatment initially

Note.   CBT=cognitive-behavioral therapy; ECT=electroconvulsive therapy; TEAM=Testing, Empathy, Agenda Setting, Methods.

(6–12 months) with antidepressants, especially selective serotonin reuptake inhibitors (SSRIs), is less likely to result in a "switch" to mania or hypomania than previously was thought (Gijsman et al. 2004; Leverich et al. 2006; Sachs et al. 2007). Meanwhile, longer-term treatment with antidepressants does seem to promote mood destabilization, especially if there are manic symptoms present (Ghaemi et al. 2008; Goldberg et al. 2007). Whether antidepressants are actually effective in reducing the symptoms of bipolar depression is debatable, especially when manic symptoms are also present (in which case there appears to be an increased risk of mania but no reduction in depressive symptoms) (Gijsman et al. 2004; Goldberg et al. 2007; Sachs et al. 2007).

There are data showing an increased chance of recovering from depressive symptoms and earlier recovery when patients are taking part in intensive psychotherapy (as compared with patients who are not participating in therapy) (Miklowitz and Otto 2007). Therapy focusing on interpersonal problems and sleep patterns has empirical evidence of its effectiveness (Ellen Frank's Interpersonal and Social Rhythm Therapy [Frank 2005]). There are other special considerations in treating bipolar illness, including recognizing prodromal phases, the importance of psychoeducation (especially of the genetic nature of the illness and the chronic course of the illness), and measuring compliance with medication (Leahy 2007).

Treatment of Anxiety

The patient experienced nearly paralyzing anxiety. Anxiety is known to exacerbate depressive symptoms and is a risk factor for suicide (Bolton et al. 2008). I felt it was necessary to measure anxiety regularly throughout the therapy and to address this symptom using a combination of cognitive and behavioral exercises. Many potential sources of anxiety exist for first-time mothers:

- Fears of inadequacy as a mother and worries about making parenting errors
- Financial worries as the household takes on additional expenses and may be losing income (depending on the employment arrangements of the mother)
- Fears of losing friends and social support; feeling pressured to maintain friendships despite exhaustion; feeling self-conscious
- Stressors stemming from problems in the partnership and frustrations in the sexual relationship
- Difficulties acknowledging and expressing (productively) feelings of anger or resentment toward family, friends, and the partner

Because of the etiological complexity of anxiety and other mood problems, one of the most important initial steps was to narrow the focus of the psychotherapy, custom tailoring it to the needs of the patient.

TABLE 31–2. Psychotropic medications in pregnancy and lactation

Medication type	FDA pregnancy risk category	Lactation risk category
Benzodiazepines (e.g., clonazepam, diazepam, lorazepam)	D	L3 (diazepam=L4 if used chronically)
Benzodiazepines for insomnia (e.g., estazolam, flurazepam, temazepam)	X	L2/L3
Nonbenzodiazepine anxiolytics and hypnotics		
Buspirone and zolpidem	B	L2/L3
Eszopiclone and zaleplon	C	
Tricyclic and heterocyclic antidepressants (e.g., amitriptyline, clomipramine, desipramine)	C (maprotiline=B)	L2/L3 (doxepin=L5)
Selective serotonin reuptake inhibitors (e.g., citalopram, fluoxetine, sertraline)	C (paroxetine=D)	L2/L3
Other antidepressants (e.g., bupropion, venlafaxine, mirtazapine, nefazodone)	C (bupropion=B)	L3 (nefazodone=L4)
Atypical antipsychotics (e.g., olanzapine, risperidone, quetiapine)	C (clozapine=B)	L2: olanzapine L3: aripiprazole, clozapine, risperidone L4: quetiapine, ziprasidone

Note. U.S. Food and Drug Administration (FDA) pregnancy risk categories: A=controlled studies show no risk; B=no evidence of risk in humans; C=risk cannot be ruled out; D=positive evidence of risk; X=contraindicated in pregnancy. Lactation risk categories: L1=safest; L2=safer; L3=moderately safe; L4=possibly hazardous; L5=contraindicated.

Source. Adapted from ACOG Practice Bulletin Number 92, April 2008; see original publication for greater detail.

Breastfeeding and Psychotropic Medication

The American College of Obstetricians and Gynecologists (ACOG) regularly updates its safety guidelines for the use of psychotropic medications during pregnancy and lactation. For women with bipolar illness who are pregnant or in the puerperium, the risks and benefits of psychopharmacological treatment must be balanced for the individual and the specific agent (Dodd and Berk 2006). All psychotropic medications enter breast milk, and none have been proved conclusively to be safe to the child. Some of these medications are more safe than others, and there are several options among antidepressants in the "L2" category (with L1 being safest and L5 contraindicated; see Table 31–2) (ACOG Committee on Practice Bulletins—Obstetrics 2008).

Although mothers with depression frequently would prefer not to expose their child to any risk, most physicians concur that depression itself poses a threat to the child (ACOG Committee on Practice Bulletins—Obstetrics 2008; Murray et al. 1996; O'Hara et al. 2000). Mothers with severe depression who are tempted to forego treatment should know that untreated depression is associated with its own risks. In the April 2008 Practice Bulletin, ACOG summarizes this concern concisely:

> Maternal Psychiatric Illness, if inadequately treated or untreated, may result in poor compliance with prenatal care, inadequate nutrition, exposure to additional medication or herbal remedies, increased alcohol and tobacco use, deficits in mother-infant bonding and disruptions within the family environment.

Hence the decision is complicated by the necessity to weigh several options simultaneously: the pros and cons of breastfeeding with or without medication and bottle-feeding with or without medication. This is complicated further by emerging evidence that breastfeeding may be quite beneficial to the child's health (Ip et al. 2007). In this case, the patient decided against breastfeeding, which afforded a wider array of options pharmacologically. Foregoing breastfeeding may be interpreted as a sign of inadequacy in women with depression.

Risk of Future Episodes and Family Planning

Women who have had an episode of postpartum depression appear to be at higher risk of subsequent episodes of postpartum depression (Harlow et al. 2007). Women who are depressed during pregnancy are more likely to have children with lower birth weights, growth retardation, and increased postnatal complications (ACOG Committee on Practice Bulletins 2008; Murray et al. 1996). There is some limited evidence that psychotherapy and psychopharmacology can be employed to reduce this risk, but this must be weighed against the findings that most commonly used antidepressants—SSRIs—have been associated with reduced birth weight for gestational age and increased risk for respiratory distress and cesarean section (Newham et al. 2008; Oberlander et al. 2008; Ramos et al. 2008).

Course

Visit 1

The early visits were 2 hours in duration, twice per week. The patient was enrolled in a partial hospitalization, was undergoing maintenance ECT every other week, and had in-home child support. She had been familiarized with a "gradual exposure" model, in which she would slowly, over the course of several weeks, return to the home and acquire increasing responsibilities as a mother. Presession and postsession scores for depression, anxiety, anger, and relationship satisfaction over the course of therapy, assessed by using using the Brief Mood Survey (Burns 2007), are presented in Figures 31–1 through 31–4.

Testing/Information Gathering

I took a detailed history in the initial visit, facilitated by conversations with her inpatient providers. We paid particular attention to the events surrounding previous depressive episodes and her cognitions at those times as well as her recent depression and suicide attempts.

Initial Conceptualization

When depressed, the patient saw herself as fundamentally inadequate, defective, and flawed. She "compensated" for these perceived deficiencies by being meticulous and cautious and setting very high goals for herself. This behavior had given her certain advantages both academically and professionally, including an impressive attention to detail as well as a tendency to consider and prepare for nearly every potential negative outcome. So long as her performance was acceptable to her, she had a good deal of confidence and self-esteem. However, she felt overwhelmed by the new and unfamiliar responsibilities of motherhood. Whenever she did not live up to her own high standards, she would criticize herself ruthlessly. She would worry excessively about even minor decisions and became convinced that she was a bad mother. Suicidal ideation occurred when she believed this thought so completely that she became convinced that her family would be better off without her. She also felt some pull toward believing she was inadequate and defective because this offered her, both in fantasy and reality, an escape from the responsibilities of motherhood.

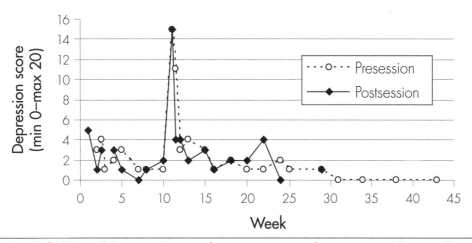

FIGURE 31–1. Brief Mood Survey depression scores over time pre– and post–therapy session.

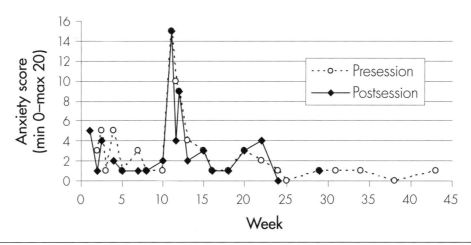

FIGURE 31–2.   Brief Mood Survey anxiety scores over time pre– and post–therapy session.

FIGURE 31–3.   Brief Mood Survey anger scores over time pre– and post–therapy session.

FIGURE 31–4.   Brief Mood Survey relationship satisfaction scores over time pre– and post–therapy session.

Empathy

One thing I like about the TEAM model is that if I forget what I am supposed to be doing or get stuck somewhere, I can often simply repeat the acronym and discover where I went wrong. Usually it is somewhere in the middle, either empathy or agenda setting. One of those instances, when I felt like a deer in the headlights, was when my patient said, "I'm a bad mother. My family would be better off without me." This was no cocktail conversation. It will seem easy if you just read along at this point, so in some ways it is better if you imagine what you might say to a patient in that situation or write down what you would say after they say "I'm a bad mother. My family would be better off without me." Of course there would be no right or wrong answer; much is dependent on the relationship with the patient and the setting. I tried to resist the urge to offer advice or reassurance, which is almost never effective and often sounds patronizing. Instead I tried to express my understanding and my own feelings in a curious and respectful manner:

> My heart goes out to you, Jane. You believe you are a bad mother and that your family would be better off without you. I can imagine that you're feeling inadequate and defective as well as discouraged and frustrated. I admire you for telling me that and for how much you care about your family. Do I understand the situation correctly?

Meanwhile, I noted to myself (for later use in agenda setting) that one possible piece of resistance to overcoming depression is that she may believe that her depression is necessary to prevent harm from befalling her family and that recovery would mean greater exposure to the child and hence greater damage to the child. I am not saying this is objectively true, just that it might be true from the patient's perspective.

Safety

I have to admit that this patient made me a little nervous, considering the number of recent suicide attempts she had made. However, she convinced me that she would not attempt suicide again and that she would be accountable for her own safety, including going to the hospital if necessary. She had never had thoughts of harming her child but agreed to share any such thoughts if they were to occur rather than acting on these thoughts.

Visit 2

We discussed her medication regimen, and she expressed an interest in discontinuing aripiprazole because she was noticing increased appetite on this medication and, despite regular exercise, was struggling to lose the weight from her pregnancy. I was concerned about taking her off of a mood-stabilizing agent and suggested adding a different mood stabilizer before discontinuing aripiprazole, to which she agreed. Lithium was perhaps the best choice for mood stabilization, especially in the presence of suicidal ideation. However, with ongoing ECT treatments, this was not an option in the short term (Baldessarini et al. 2006b). I considered lamotrigine to be a reasonable alternative based on evidence that this drug prevented relapse (Calabrese et al. 2003). After discussing risks/benefits and alternatives, she was started on 25 mg/day.

We worked briefly on communication strategies to improve her relationship with her husband and family. This later became a focus of our work, although it will not be described further in this chapter. A gradual improvement in her relationship satisfaction scores can be seen throughout the therapy.

Visit 3

We used a daily mood log to begin to identify her negative cognitions. The situation we identified was a time at home when she, her nanny, and her child were together. She felt 100% inferior and inadequate, 100% hopeless, 100% ashamed, 100% sad, 90% upset and disappointed with herself, and 75% resentful. She had the following thoughts:

- I'm a bad mom.
- I'll always be a bad mom.
- I'm a failure.
- My friends will be disappointed in me.
- I will lose my friends.
- I should never have had a child.
- If I hadn't had a child, I'd still be happy.
- I shouldn't think that.
- I deserve to suffer.

She chose to work on the thought "I should never have had a child" because this resulted in extreme amounts of shame and self-directed anger and resentment.

Decision Point

The patient had identified a disturbing negative thought with which she would like help. CBT is rife with methods to defeat negative cognitions, and I wanted to help the patient. I decided to apply a technique called "identify the distortions." We searched for logical errors in the structure of the negative thought. For example, her thought "I should never have had a child" is using harsh language or "should" statements that are inflicting unnecessary suffering; she is "fortune telling" because only in hindsight could she possibly know that having a child would cause her such suffering; she is applying meaningless labels to herself such as "bad mom"; she is blaming herself for factors outside her control; she is reasoning emotionally by telling herself that because she *feels* bad she *is* bad, and so on. In fact, when we looked closely, we found elements of every cognitive distortion in this thought and its supporting thoughts. Upon identifying the distortions, I switched to an "externalization of voices" model in which I played the role of the patient's negative thoughts, attacking her with these thoughts, and giving her the opportunity to defeat or revise them—with which she did fairly well. I was about to pat myself on the back for being a brilliant therapist when I discovered that she was not feeling any better and was even a little upset with the way the session was going…then I realized I had made a huge agenda-setting error!

To better understand agenda setting, by way of analogy, imagine coming across a friend who is flogging his or her own back with a whip. You might be tempted to point out how illogical this is or try to take the whip away, apply some soothing ointment to the wounds, and so on. This would be the equivalent of applying one of the many different *M*ethods in the TE*A*M model without having the appropriate framework in place. The problem is that intervening without permission can result in resistance. The individual who is self-flagellating must have, in his or her mind, at least one "good reason" to be inflicting such punishment. To avoid forcing the patient to dig in his or her heels when we try to help, we use *A*genda setting (TE*A*M). That means asking whether the patient wants help or just need us to understand what they are feeling. If he or she wants help, rather than chasing our tail talking about every moment the patient had that problem, we narrow the scope to one specific time they were having

problems, who was there, what happened, and so on. Agenda setting is also about understanding the type of problem being faced so we can avoid resistance by anticipating and paradoxically aligning ourselves with it. In essence, we become the voice of their resistance. The patient can then choose to argue against his or her own resistance or he or she can agree with us and accept him- or herself proudly.

This is a win-win situation for the therapist. It can sometimes be difficult to imagine the advantages of believing a negative thought, however. Often I simply ask my patient whether he or she can think of any reason to maintain his or her negative thought and make a list with them of advantages to *believing* in the negative thought. Can you imagine any advantages to believing "I should never have had a child"? Here are a few that the patient came up with:

Advantages to Believing "I Should Never Have Had a Child"

- It allows me to recall and fantasize about the "good old days," prior to having a child.
- This will remind me to be more careful in the future so I can avoid such errors. It motivates and facilitates self-improvement.
- It feels morally correct to use such punishing language on myself, since I made an error.
- I can insist on being better, rather than having to accept being an "average mom" or one who makes mistakes.
- It prevents me from being angry with my child or my husband, focuses the blame on me, sparing them.
- If I blame myself and punish myself, other people can't. They will have to take pity on me and help me.
- I can avoid the stress of being a mother and continue to feel the safety of being taken care of by my family.
- If I accept defeat early, then I don't have to try and I can't fail.

Examples of Agenda Setting: How to Discuss Resistance With a Patient

"Jane, I think you're right that this thought is causing some of your shame and hopelessness, and I think we could defeat this thought and lift your spirits today. I'm a little hesitant to do that, however, because I've noticed that this thought reflects positively on you as a person. You've chosen to blame yourself rather than be upset with your husband or your child for all that has happened to you. This thought is an example of your love and willingness to self-sacrifice. Why change this?"

"If we were to defeat this thought and your depression went away entirely, would you be concerned about what others might expect of you? Wouldn't you be even more stressed than you are now with the responsibilities and demands of motherhood?"

"Are you certain that you would be willing to feel good about yourself considering the fact that you sometimes regret having had a child? Isn't it appropriate for you to feel ashamed of thoughts like that? What would be the moral basis of our eliminating your shame?"

Visit 4

I realized my error in the latter part of visit 3 and dropped back to empathy and agenda setting. After a few agenda-setting questions, the patient was ready to apply techniques and motivated to overcome her self-defeating thoughts, which we did in that session and the following sessions.

Methods

The reason we have over 50 techniques in CBT is that we often need to fail at 5 or 10 or 15 before coming upon the technique that is effective. In this case we used many different techniques in rapid succession, each with the understanding that they were unlikely to be effective and we were eliminating options until we could find the right tool for her. For example, we tried identifying the distortions with a straightforward technique, a downward arrow technique, a cost-benefit analysis technique, and so on.

The most helpful technique ended up being a role-play called the "double standard," which allowed her to be a "good mother" to herself. In this exercise, I pretended to be a clone of her, someone who was exactly the same in every way and had experienced everything she had, made all the same decisions, and felt and thought the same as well. I told my story, how I'd been through a painful and difficult pregnancy, how I'd developed a deep depression that required hospitalizations, and how I was sure I had made a mistake by having a child. The patient readily spoke to me (her clone) in an incredibly supportive way. She would say, "No, you're a fantastic mom, you've just been through a lot and you can't

expect to be perfect." I would challenge this, saying, "I'm feeling a bit better, but are you just telling me what I want to hear?" This was our first breakthrough in therapy, and her mood improved significantly over the course of those two sessions. I stored away this technique, reminding myself that what works once will probably work again.

Visit 5

Focus shifted away from her mood, which was increasingly less of an issue for her, and onto her relationship, especially tension between herself and her husband. She seemed to expect that her husband should be doing more in the relationship to be kind to and respectful of her, that he should be less critical of her and be more respectful toward her family. She was disappointed and angry with him but reluctant to express these emotions because of a conflict phobia (fear that expressing her feelings would make the problem worse and there would be no solution). She was unwilling to work individually on this problem because she felt he should be doing more of the changing. She agreed to have her husband come in to the next visit.

Visit 6

As planned, her husband came to this visit. He spoke with me individually, giving his perspective on Jane's illness. He had noticed her perfectionism and negative self-talk when goals were not met. He wanted Jane to express more caring and compassion for him. He felt betrayed and thought that Jane had favored her family over him.

Visit 7

Between sessions the patient experienced a complication with ECT, possibly due to insufficient paralysis. She described unilateral myalgias that were so intense that she could not walk normally. The patient's pain had not responded entirely to nonsteroidal anti-inflammatory drugs. I called in a prescription for four tablets of Vicodin and four tablets of clonazepam. The patient responded well and was feeling better by the time I saw her. We discussed ECT during this visit and she said she disliked going back to the hospital because it was a painful reminder of where she had been and the severity of her illness. She was afraid to discuss her discontent with the physician providing ECT, however.

Visit 8

Jane was essentially euthymic at this point. She was very happy to be home full-time after completing day treatment, although she was still disappointed with her husband. We decided that we could not work on that problem because she felt it was mostly his fault. She had selected a new nanny and had some negative thoughts that she brought in to work on, especially the thought that, because she had to have a nanny, this meant she was defective and inadequate. We did some brief agenda setting and then tried a few techniques. Not surprisingly, it was the double standard technique that was able to beat the thought. Her mood improved immediately in session.

Visit 9

Jane was doing well, but one day after increasing her dosage of lamictal to 100 mg/day, she developed a rash on her arms. There was no mucosal involvement and no lymphadenopathy, myalgia, fever, chills, or lethargy. She was aware of what to look for in terms of Stevens-Johnson rash, and we decided to continue with lamictal at the 100 mg dose and see if her body would adjust to the drug. She was motivated by the fact that she was still having trouble losing weight (and therefore did not want to revert to aripiprazole, which she felt had increased her appetite). We again worked on her negative thoughts; as she engaged more and more in the role of mother, she developed new concerns and new negative thoughts. After we wrote those thoughts down, we again applied the double standard technique:

Example of Double Standard Technique

Negative thought (expressed by the therapist):
"I should have been around and not so fearful. Then my child would be running to me."
"I'm her mom. My child should be just as bonded if not more to me because I carried her inside me for so long and I breastfed her, and above all else she should be bonded to me the most."

Positive thought (expressed by the patient):
"You were sick for so long that your child needs some time to be more bonded with you. It just takes more time; it doesn't happen overnight."

Aside from the patient's rash, I was feeling quite confident that this therapy was going to be a success.

Visit 10

Relapse! The patient was clearly deeply depressed again. She was convinced that she was a "horrible mother" and had an assortment of other negative thoughts. Her affect was constricted, and there was psychomotor retardation. She continued to have a rash on her arms that was itchy. There still was no mucosal involvement, but we decided to have her discontinue the drug for the time being. She cried during the session, which she found cathartic, but we did not have time to do any cognitive exercises, and she left feeling horrible. We scheduled another visit in 2 days, the day after her ECT.

Visit 11

The patient was feeling a bit better after receiving ECT the day before. Her depression score had fallen from 15 to 11 on the Brief Mood Survey. We worked hard in this session and added several techniques, including "be specific," "examine the evidence," and "acceptance paradox," to our favorite "double standard." We worked systematically, using a double column with negative thoughts on one side being replaced with positive thoughts on the other (Table 31–3). After this session, her depression score fell to a 4 on the Brief Mood Survey.

Subsequent Visits

It turned out that the patient's depression, when in full force, required several different techniques working in tandem. She used the four techniques described in visit 11 several times on her own and together in session with me to overcome relapses that came up in the next 30 weeks. She became increasingly self-sufficient. She convinced me that she was able to discontinue her medication and did so without event. I monitored her for some time, but her depression continued to improve. She lost the weight and her relationship improved as well. She created an emergency worksheet that she kept in a safe place that contained the list of techniques and how to use them in case of relapse. We did relapse prevention. She decided there wasn't much need for her to visit me anymore, and I told her I would be available in the future if she wanted to meet with me. We terminated and I have not heard from her since.

TABLE 31–3. Negative thought/positive thought and associated methods

Negative thought		Positive thought (methods)
You're a bad mother.	→	Some of the time or all of the time? (be specific technique)
All of the time.	→	That would be impossible. Even if I tried to be a bad mother all the time I'd accidentally be a good mother occasionally. (self-defense technique)
Some of the time, then, you're a bad mother.	→	That's undoubtedly true. When was a time that I was a bad mother? (acceptance paradox and be specific techniques)
You were a bad mother yesterday.	→	Probably. I forget: What happened? (acceptance paradox and be specific techniques)
You didn't love your child enough.	→	There's probably some truth in that. One can probably always improve when it comes to expressing one's love, and I'd be grateful for any pointers you have. Perhaps we could see if we could think of three things I did to express my love for my child and three ways in which I could improve. (acceptance paradox, be specific, and examine the evidence techniques)

Summary of Guideline Use

In the absence of a strong body of evidence-based algorithms on best practices in postpartum depression, we are forced to rely on expert consensus guidelines. The most recent consist of a 2005 report, commissioned by the Agency for Healthcare Research and Quality, which systematically reviewed evidence-based practices related to perinatal depression, and a 2001 study by Altshuler et al. reviewing depression in women (Altshuler et al. 2001; Gaynes et al. 2005). In addition, a 2008 publication by a group of nurse practitioners in Ontario formulated 10 evidence-based recommendations for nurses related to screening, treatment, and prevention of postpartum depression (Gaynes et al. 2005; McQueen et al. 2008). Biological and nonbiological treatment modalities for postpartum depression have been systematically reviewed as recently as 2008 (Dennis and Hodrett 2007; Dennis and Stewart 2004). Recommendations from these sources have been pooled and presented in Table 31–4.

One of the key questions is how to identify postpartum depression. Postpartum depression is generally understood as a modifier ("postpartum onset") of a major depressive episode as outlined in DSM-IV-TR (American Psychiatric Association 2000), indicating the episode commenced within 12 weeks of delivery, although some claim this period can last up to 12 months (Forray and Ostroff 2007; Gaynes

et al. 2005). Screening is one important method to identify women experiencing postpartum depression but may not be as necessary in a psychiatric setting in which patients are often already referred for a psychiatric concern (versus a primary care, OB/GYN, or pediatric setting). However, measures to evaluate and track progress of symptoms during treatment are still necessary and useful. One screening/tracking measure that has been used extensively in Europe is the Edinburgh Postnatal Depression Scale, consisting of 10 questions regarding mood and symptoms, and using a 4-point Likert scale (none of which are specific to the postpartum period). A number of trials have shown a score greater than 12 on this scale during the postpartum period provided reasonable specificity for postpartum depression (Gaynes et al. 2005). The Postpartum Depression Screening Scale, available at a cost, and the Beck Depression Inventory have also been used in the literature. There exist concerns about the low sensitivity of these screening methods.

Although it remains unclear whether postpartum depression has a specific unique etiology, evaluation of symptoms continues to mirror that of major depression. In my own practice, I have found Dr. Burns's TEAM approach to be very valuable in identifying, measuring, and treating mood and anxiety disorders. In addition to a comprehensive initial screening and evaluation form, the Brief Mood Survey and Therapy Evaluation form is used at the

TABLE 31–4.   General recommendations for postpartum depression

Area	Recommendation
Screening and evaluation	
Screening and diagnostic tools	Depending on setting, specific screening tools (Edinburgh Postnatal Depression Scale, Postpartum Depression Screening Scale) or standard depression instrument (e.g., Beck Depression Inventory, Brief Mood Survey) may be useful.
Exclude medical causes	Exclude medical causes for mood disturbance such as thyroid dysfunction, anemia, and Sheehan's syndrome. Initial evaluation should include a thorough history, physical examination, and routine laboratory tests.
Information gathering	If necessary, seek additional information from other providers of patient (e.g., primary care, obstetrics, pediatrics).
Evaluate risk for bipolarity and psychosis	It is important to assess the risk of bipolarity (current and previous symptoms, past manic or hypomanic episodes, family history), and postpartum psychosis to devise treatment plan and avoid "switch" to mania with use of antidepressants.
Evaluate suicidality	Treatment strategy (modalities and setting) will depend in part on risk of suicidality.
Treatment	
Shared decision making	Includes review of both pharmacological and nonpharmacological therapies and discussion that inadequate treatment increases the risk of morbidity in both mother and infant. Preferably occurs before pregnancy commences.
Patient education	Provide information on nature, course, and treatment, including medication use and side effects as well as nonpharmacological treatment options. Use clear, appropriate language.
Devise treatment plan	Work together with patient to devise a clear and acceptable treatment plan (see Treatment Plan Considerations section in text) based on the severity of the symptoms, including setting (e.g., inpatient versus outpatient).
Nonpharmacological treatment options	
Psychotherapy	Individual therapy: CBT and IPT are therapies of choice. Group therapy may also be useful, depending on case. Couples therapy: involvement of spouse may be helpful.
Psychoeducational or support groups	May be especially attractive to patients who feel alone and/or would like to join a community.

TABLE 31–4. General recommendations for postpartum depression *(continued)*

Area	Recommendation
Nonpharmacological treatment options *(continued)*	
Other at-home support measures	If feasible, at-home interventions such as social work visits or household/child care help (either from paid employees or temporary family help) may be appropriate.
Other self-help measures (e.g., bibliotherapy)	Bibliotherapy based on CBT (e.g., David Burns's book *Feeling Good*) should be offered.
ECT	ECT should be considered in cases of severe postpartum depression, especially those with active suicidal ideation. ECT is considered rapid and safe and can be effective.
Light therapy	Two case studies suggest that incorporating a 100,000-lux box for 60 minutes daily beginning with 10 minutes of awakening for at least 3–5 weeks may be helpful.
Medication options	Use standard antidepressant dosages. Typically symptoms diminish in 2–4 weeks.
Step 1: SSRIs are medications of first choice	Consider medications in terms of previous treatment response, risk to patient, lactation concerns, weight gain, likelihood of overdose/self-harm, tolerability, patient preference, and cost.
	Limited RCT evidence is available to show benefit of SSRIs; prophylactic sertraline and fluoxetine treatment after onset have shown some efficacy.
Step 2: If an SSRI is not suitable, there is no improvement after a 12-week course, or if symptoms remain or side effects become intolerable, further medication substitutions or additions may be appropriate.	SNRIs such as venlafaxine, duloxetine, and bupropion may be effective. If patient is breastfeeding, nefazodone should be avoided.
	Tricyclic antidepressants such as nortriptyline may be useful for women with sleep disturbances; however, evidence does not indicate robust efficacy. If breastfeeding, avoid doxepin.
	Anxiolytic agents such as lorazepam and clonazepam may be useful as adjunctive treatment in patients with anxiety and/or sleep disturbances. Avoid diazepam in breastfeeding women.
	Small observational trials indicate that transdermal and/or oral estrogen (200 μg 17beta-estradiol plus 10 mg cyclical dydrogesterone) may boost mood, especially with concomitant antidepressant use.

Notes for medication options:

6–12 months of treatment is recommended. For women with recurrent major depression, long-term maintenance treatment with an antidepressant is indicated.

If there is a risk of bipolarity, atypical antidepressants may be more appropriate for mood stabilization; weight gain should be monitored. If patient is breastfeeding, quetiapine and ziprasidone should be avoided.

Women should be informed that all psychotropic medications are secreted into breast milk; concentrations can vary widely. Infant serum blood levels are not typically monitored except for lithium use, which is typically not advised because of case reports of neonatal lithium toxicity.

TABLE 31–4.   General recommendations for postpartum depression *(continued)*

Area	Recommendation
Monitoring	
Use of monitoring tools	Self-report questionnaires (e.g., Brief Mood Survey) can be used before and after each therapy session.
	Baseline assessment
	Session assessments
	12-week review
	Record response to and satisfaction with therapist/therapy
Response to evaluation	Therapist should respond to evaluations of performance and therapy direction/goals.
Prevention	
Relapse prevention	Therapy work should address potential methods of relapse prevention and identification.
Early screening and identification	Women at risk for postpartum illness should be identified prior to delivery; use of screening tools (listed previously) may aid identification.
Prophylactic treatment	There is limited and divided evidence both for and against prophylactic pharmacological treatment in postpartum depression; sertraline may be efficacious at preventing relapse during subsequent postpartum periods. Antidepressants may be started during pregnancy (see Table 31–2).

Note.   CBT=cognitive-behavioral therapy; ECT=electroconvulsive therapy; IPT=interpersonal therapy; RCT=randomized controlled trial; SNRI=serotonin-norepinephrine reuptake inhibitor; SSRI=selective serotonin reuptake inhibitor.

beginning and end of each therapy session to track efficacy of therapy modalities—both in the immediate sense and also over the long-term course of the therapy. These forms have been used in a number of studies and have undergone both reliability and validity testing where applicable (Burns and Eidelson 1998; Burns and Nolen-Hoeksema 1992; Burns et al. 1994).

As described in this patient's treatment considerations, a combination of medication and psychotherapy modalities, as well as an at-home intervention (full-time nanny) was used. These and other recommendations for postpartum depression are presented in Table 31–4. In general, recommendations emphasize combining pharmacological and psychotherapy treatments to achieve the best results. However, because of the lack of randomized placebo-controlled trials of medications in this specific subpopulation, expert consensus guidelines and practices are limited in the scope of their evidence. For example, only three placebo-controlled trials of antidepressants for postpartum depression have been published. The first showed that prophylactic treatment of postpartum depression with nortriptyline in women at risk did *not* prevent recurrence any greater than placebo (Wisner et al. 2001). Using the same study design, the second trial did show a significant benefit of sertraline in preventing recurrence (Wisner et al. 2004). In yet another controlled trial in which fluoxetine with CBT was compared to placebo with CBT in women diagnosed with postpartum depression, the authors found no difference between fluoxetine with one CBT session and placebo with six CBT sessions. This finding suggests that CBT may be as effective as an SSRI intervention (Appleby et al. 1997). Despite the lack of strong evidence for treatment with antidepressant medications, many physicians still consider this approach a standard of care.

Other treatment modalities are based purely on small observational trials or case studies, such as the use of estrogen therapy alone or in conjunction with antidepressants (Ahokas et al. 1999, 2001; Dennis 2004; Gregoire et al. 1996). Similarly, bright light therapy has been endorsed in two case studies but remains to be examined in a randomized controlled trial (Corral et al. 2000; Dennis 2004; Oren et al. 2002). These should be considered experimental treatment modalities, but because they pose minimal risk to appropriate patients they may prove helpful adjunct options.

Ways to Improve Practice

Considering the history of suicide attempts and the possibility of bipolarity, I was even more interested than usual in the topic of safety (Baldessarini et al. 2006a). Despite this concern, I believe I relied too heavily on information provided by the inpatient team during my initial risk assessment. Not surprisingly to veterans of our profession, it is a sad truth that some patients who are depressed often speak less of suicide and experience a brightening of their affect as the date of discharge approaches, knowing that soon they will be free to kill themselves without interruption. Sadly, I covered only a fraction of the information in a structured suicide risk interview, relying instead on "signs." For example, she seemed to have an interest in the future and in scheduling appointments, and she denied suicidal urges at the time of our meeting. To my credit, I did ask, and she agreed to meet with me before acting on any suicidal urges that might develop in the future.

In retrospect, I would have preferred to have used a detailed, structured suicide risk assessment instrument such as that created by Dr. David Burns (Burns 2007). Topics to cover in assessing patients' suicide risk include, but are not limited to, the following:

- History of prior attempts, including whether the attempt(s) were planned or impulsive, whether a note was left and what it said, whether a will was created, how long the individual had been feeling suicidal before the attempt, the situation surrounding the attempt (where they were, who was with them, who said what, what they were drinking), what means were used and some crude sense of how lethal this method might be and how lethal it seemed from their own perspective at the time, any conscious or potential unconscious motive or intent, the reason the attempt did not succeed, and the effects on them physically and psychologically (e.g., did they quit work or file for disability)
- General attitudes toward death and suicide in particular, including a listing of all possible reasons they may want to end their life as well as reasons not to end their life, what they expect the

process to feel like and the moment of death to be like, and their sense of what might come after

- Identification of specific situations in which they would be tempted to end their life
- Current, recent, and lifetime history of depressive symptoms, especially the intensity of hopelessness, anger, and anxiety and patterns of substance use
- Current desire to end their life and what plans they have and whether they intend to act on those plans
- Their attitudes toward being hospitalized, whether they would be willing to go to the hospital if they became suicidal or if this would not be acceptable
- Their attitudes toward communicating suicidality to the provider, including how trustworthy they seem to be, whether they would agree to call if they felt suicidal, whether they would prefer to retain the right to end their life
- Other factors that might place them at higher or lower risk (e.g., primary diagnosis, reports of pain or debilitation, troubles with insomnia, family history of suicide, religious beliefs, significant relationships, future events they look forward to, their support network)
- Would they be willing to make an absolute guarantee of their safety in the future, regardless of how hopeless or desperate they feel?

Along these same lines, my initial intake could have been strengthened by inquiring more about the patient's expectations and motivations. Many patients have unrealistic expectations at the outset of therapy that lurk like hidden icebergs in the North Atlantic. Having experienced my fair share of disappointments in therapy, I now use psychoeducational memos and surveys to assess motivation and the risk of premature termination. The best source that I have found for surveys that provide information about motivation for, resistance to, and attitudes toward therapy that are likely to result in early termination and failure if not addressed early are found in *Therapist's Toolkit*, available from David Burns online at www.feelinggood.com.

An example of a common misconception among patients is the notion that all progress will be confined to the time spent with the therapist, and little change or effort will be required on their part. Meanwhile, there is substantial evidence that indi-

viduals who participate in psychotherapy homework are more likely to improve than those who simply talk about their problems (Cowan et al. 2008; Legeron 1991). Unfortunately, there are many good reasons why someone might not want to do psychotherapy homework. Some patients might say "I didn't feel like it," others, "I just knew it wouldn't work," and so on. Before reading the next paragraph, imagine what you would say to a patient who made such a statement.

Most of us would try to convince the patient to do homework. We might try logic and reason, threats of never getting better, begging, and groveling. Most of this will either not work or backfire and result in even greater resistance because the patient will feel that he or she is not accepted as is. Another approach is to agree with them that they have a right *not* to do homework and respect their decision, observing that this might not be a problem they want to work on right now and is there something else they want help with? The Buddhists had it right all along: true power comes from letting go. When we do this, the patient will lead the way.

This has been one of the hardest lessons for me to learn as a therapist, especially a psychiatrist trained in the medical model. I have a strong desire to help those who are suffering and I am sometimes tempted to believe that I can "fix" people without their cooperation or make lasting changes in only an hour per week of talking. It has been humbling to discover otherwise.

One major problem in this patient's therapy had to do with medication management. As I mentioned, I chose lamotrigine because of the evidence available to me that this medication increased the interval between depressive episodes. One flaw with the referenced study on lamotrigine, however, was selection bias. The research, funded by the manufacturer, had included in the treatment group only individuals who had already tolerated and responded to lamotrigine. It was later revealed that they had not published results of five negative studies of lamotrigine for depression (Calabrese et al. 2008).

As I developed more experience with the patient's depression, I came to realize that it might not be primarily chemically mediated. For example, the patient responded much more robustly, when at the height of her depressive episode, to a single 2-hour psychotherapy session than to a session of ECT she received a few days before. In my practice, I have found that acute improvements in mood are not unusual when I am using the TEAM model of psychotherapy. I have also found that when proper relapse prevention is incorporated future relapses can be avoided or their duration limited to the time necessary for the patient to employ, on their own, the techniques that were helpful initially.

Conclusions

The case presented illustrates the complexity involved in treating one individual who is suffering from severe depression arising in the postpartum period. There is much debate about the etiology of this illness, yet there is little in the way of encouraging data on the efficacy of any one particular treatment or preventative strategy. This is not for a lack of treatment options: medications, electric shock, acupuncture, hormone replacement, light therapy, fish oils, and so on, have all been investigated. An ideal treatment would be safe, rapid, and effective for the patient and in the context of breastfeeding. Psychotherapy would meet many of these criteria, though this option is used less frequently than before among psychiatrists, perhaps because of increased medication options or payment schedules that favor prescribing (Mojtabai and Olfson 2008). Then there are questions of efficacy. Seldom does psychotherapy outperform medication in randomized trials. Meanwhile, the efficacy of medication in the treatment of depression is being called into question (Turner et al. 2008). Clearly we need more effective treatment options for patients with depression, one of the leading causes of morbidity and mortality in the developed world (McKenna et al. 2005). TEAM, a structured treatment framework for psychotherapy, was developed by Dr. David Burns and incorporates a wide array of models and techniques for testing and information gathering; building and sustaining rapport; altering motivation; and facilitating change in mood, relationships, and habits/addictions (Burns 2007). The TEAM approach has frequently surprised the author, especially regarding the rapid rate of improvement in single sessions and the reproducibility of results from one session to the next. Whether it will stand the test of more rigorous testing and comparison remains to be seen.

References

ACOG Committee on Practice Bulletins—Obstetrics: ACOG Practice Bulletin: clinical management guidelines for obstetrician-gynecologists number 92, April 2008 (replaces practice bulletin number 87, November 2007). Use of psychiatric medications during pregnancy and lactation. Obstet Gynecol 111:1001–1020, 2008

Ahokas A, Kaukoranta J, Aito M: Effect of oestradiol on postpartum depression. Psychopharmacology (Berl) 146:108–110, 1999

Ahokas A, Kaukoranta J, Wahlbeck K, et al: Estrogen deficiency in severe postpartum depression: successful treatment with sublingual physiologic 17beta-estradiol: a preliminary study. J Clin Psychiatry 62:332–336, 2001

Altshuler LL, Post RM, Leverich GS, et al: Antidepressant-induced mania and cycle acceleration: a controversy revisited. Am J Psychiatry 152:1130–1138, 1995

Altshuler LL, Cohen LS, Moline ML, et al: The Expert Consensus Guideline Series. Treatment of depression in women. Postgrad Med (March):1–107, 2001

American Psychiatric Association: Diagnostic and Statistical Manual of Mental Disorders, 4th Edition, Text Revision. Washington, DC, American Psychiatric Association, 2000

Appleby L, Warner R, Whitton A, et al: A controlled study of fluoxetine and cognitive-behavioural counselling in the treatment of postnatal depression. BMJ 314:932–936, 1997

Appleby L, Mortensen PB, Faragher EB: Suicide and other causes of mortality after post-partum psychiatric admission. Br J Psychiatry 173:209–211, 1998

Baldessarini RJ, Tondo L, Hennen J: Lithium treatment and suicide risk in major affective disorders: update and new findings. J Clin Psychiatry 64 (suppl 5):44–52, 2003

Baldessarini RJ, Pompili M, Tondo L: Suicide in bipolar disorder: risks and management. CNS Spectr 11:465–471, 2006a

Baldessarini RJ, Tondo L, Davis P, et al: Decreased risk of suicides and attempts during long-term lithium treatment: a meta-analytic review. Bipolar Disord 8:625–639, 2006b

Bolton JM, Cox BJ, Afifi TO, et al: Anxiety disorders and risk for suicide attempts: findings from the Baltimore Epidemiologic Catchment area follow-up study. Depress Anxiety 25:477–481, 2008

Burns DD: Therapist's Toolkit: Comprehensive Assessment and Treatment Tools for the Mental Health Professional. Philadelphia, PA, D.D. Burns, 2007

Burns DD, Eidelson RJ: Why are depression and anxiety correlated? A test of the tripartite model. J Consult Clin Psychol 66:461–473, 1998

Burns DD, Nolen-Hoeksema S: Therapeutic empathy and recovery from depression in cognitive-behavioral therapy: a structural equation model. J Consult Clin Psychol 60:441–449, 1992

Burns DD, Sayers SL, Moras K: Intimate relationships and depression: is there a causal connection? J Consult Clin Psychol 62:1033–1043, 1994

Calabrese JR, Bowden CL, Sachs G, et al: A placebo-controlled 18-month trial of lamotrigine and lithium maintenance treatment in recently depressed patients with bipolar I disorder. J Clin Psychiatry 64:1013–1024, 2003

Calabrese JR, Huffman RF, White RL, et al: Lamotrigine in the acute treatment of bipolar depression: results of five double-blind, placebo-controlled clinical trials. Bipolar Disord 10:323–333, 2008

Cho HJ, Kwon JH, Lee JJ: Antenatal cognitive-behavioral therapy for prevention of postpartum depression: a pilot study. Yonsei Med J 49:553–562, 2008

Corral M, Kuan A, Kostaras D: Bright light therapy's effect on postpartum depression. Am J Psychiatry 157:303–304, 2000

Cowan MJ, Freedland KE, Burg MM, et al: Predictors of treatment response for depression and inadequate social support—the ENRICHD randomized clinical trial. Psychother Psychosom 77:27–37, 2008

Cox JL, Holden JM, Sagovsky R: Detection of postnatal depression. Development of the 10-item Edinburgh Postnatal Depression Scale. Br J Psychiatry 150:782–786, 1987

Dennis CL: Treatment of postpartum depression, part 2: a critical review of nonbiological interventions. J Clin Psychiatry 65:1252–1265, 2004

Dennis CL, Hodnett E: Psychosocial and psychological interventions for treating postpartum depression. Cochrane Database Syst Rev (4):CD006116, 2007

Dennis CL, Stewart DE: Treatment of postpartum depression, part 1: a critical review of biological interventions. J Clin Psychiatry 65:1242–1251, 2004

Dodd S, Berk M: The safety of medications for the treatment of bipolar disorder during pregnancy and the puerperium. Curr Drug Saf 1:25–33, 2006

Forray A, Ostroff RB: The use of electroconvulsive therapy in postpartum affective disorders. J ECT 23:188–193, 2007

Frank E: Treating Bipolar Disorder: A Clinician's Guide to Interpersonal and Social Rhythm Therapy. New York, Guilford, 2005

Gaynes BN, Gavin N, Meltzer-Brody S, et al: Perinatal depression: prevalence, screening accuracy and screening outcomes, AHRQ Evidence Report No 119 (AHRQ Publ No 05-E006-2). Rockville, MD, Agency for Healthcare Research and Quality, 2005

Ghaemi SN, Wingo AP, Filkowski MA, et al: Long-term antidepressant treatment in bipolar disorder: meta-analyses of benefits and risks. Acta Psychiatr Scand 118:347–356, 2008

Gijsman HJ, Geddes JR, Rendell JM, et al: Antidepressants for bipolar depression: a systematic review of randomized, controlled trials. Am J Psychiatry 161:1537–1547, 2004

Goldberg JF, Perlis RH, Ghaemi SN, et al: Adjunctive antidepressant use and symptomatic recovery among bipolar depressed patients with concomitant manic symptoms: findings from the STEP-BD. Am J Psychiatry 164:1348–1355, 2007

Gregoire AJ, Kumar R, Everitt B, et al: Transdermal oestrogen for treatment of severe postnatal depression. Lancet 347:930–933, 1996

Harlow BL, Vitonis AF, Sparen P, et al: Incidence of hospitalization for postpartum psychotic and bipolar episodes in women with and without prior pregnancy or prenatal psychiatric hospitalizations. Arch Gen Psychiatry 64:42–48, 2007

Ip S, Chung M, Raman G, et al: Breastfeeding and maternal and infant health outcomes in developed countries. Evid Rep Technol Assess (Full Rep):1–186, 2007

Leahy RL: Bipolar disorder: causes, contexts, and treatments. J Clin Psychol 63:417–424, 2007

Legeron P: [Predictive factors of a good response to cognitive therapies in depression]. Encephale 17:405–409, 1991

Leverich GS, Altshuler LL, Frye MA, et al: Risk of switch in mood polarity to hypomania or mania in patients with bipolar depression during acute and continuation trials of venlafaxine, sertraline, and bupropion as adjuncts to mood stabilizers. Am J Psychiatry 163:232–239, 2006

McKenna MT, Michaud CM, Murray CJ, et al: Assessing the burden of disease in the United States using disability-adjusted life years. Am J Prev Med 28:415–423, 2005

McQueen K, Montgomery P, Lappan-Gracon S, et al: Evidence-based recommendations for depressive symptoms in postpartum women. J Obstet Gynecol Neonatal Nurs 37:127–136, 2008

Miklowitz DJ, Otto MW: Psychosocial interventions for bipolar disorder: a review of literature and introduction of the systematic treatment enhancement program. Psychopharmacol Bull 40:116–131, 2007

Mojtabai R, Olfson M: National trends in psychotherapy by office-based psychiatrists. Arch Gen Psychiatry 65:962–970, 2008

Murray L, Fiori-Cowley A, Hooper R, et al: The impact of postnatal depression and associated adversity on early mother-infant interactions and later infant outcome. Child Dev 67:2512–2526, 1996

Newham JJ, Thomas SH, MacRitchie K, et al: Birth weight of infants after maternal exposure to typical and atypical antipsychotics: prospective comparison study. Br J Psychiatry 192:333–337, 2008

Oberlander TF, Warburton W, Misri S, et al: Effects of timing and duration of gestational exposure to serotonin reuptake inhibitor antidepressants: population-based study. Br J Psychiatry 192:338–343, 2008

O'Hara MW, Stuart S, Gorman LL, et al: Efficacy of interpersonal psychotherapy for postpartum depression. Arch Gen Psychiatry 57:1039–1045, 2000

Oren DA, Wisner KL, Spinelli M, et al: An open trial of morning light therapy for treatment of antepartum depression. Am J Psychiatry 159:666–669, 2002

Peindl KS, Wisner KL, Hanusa BH: Identifying depression in the first postpartum year: guidelines for office-based screening and referral. J Affect Disord 80:37–44, 2004

Rabheru K: The use of electroconvulsive therapy in special patient populations. Can J Psychiatry 46:710–719, 2001

Ramos E, St-Andre M, Rey E, et al: Duration of antidepressant use during pregnancy and risk of major congenital malformations. Br J Psychiatry 192:344–350, 2008

Rychnovsky JD, Brady MA: Choosing a postpartum depression screening instrument for your pediatric practice. J Pediatr Health Care 22:64–67, 2008

Sachs GS, Nierenberg AA, Calabrese JR, et al: Effectiveness of adjunctive antidepressant treatment for bipolar depression. N Engl J Med 356:1711–1722, 2007

Taguchi H: [Maternal filicide in Japan: analyses of 96 cases and future directions for prevention] (in Japanese). Seishin Shinkeigaku Zasshi 109:110–127, 2007

Turner EH, Matthews AM, Linardatos E, et al: Selective publication of antidepressant trials and its influence on apparent efficacy. N Engl J Med 358:252–260, 2008

Wisner KL, Perel JM, Peindl KS, et al: Prevention of recurrent postpartum depression: a randomized clinical trial. J Clin Psychiatry 62:82–86, 2001

Wisner KL, Perel JM, Peindl KS, et al: Prevention of postpartum depression: a pilot randomized clinical trial. Am J Psychiatry 161:1290–1292, 2004

Bipolar Disorder Treated in the Kaiser Permanente Health Care System

Richard E. Shanteau, M.D.

Setting

The patient was seen in an outpatient clinic located in the South San Francisco Kaiser Permanente Medical Center. Kaiser Permanente is an integrated managed care organization. Hospital stays were in local contracted psychiatric units. The outpatient clinic offers crisis intervention, short-term individual therapy, and ongoing medication management. Numerous types of group therapies are offered, including day treatment group programs.

Illustration

- Application of guidelines to bipolar disorder
- Monitoring of symptoms
- Use of multidisciplinary team in HMO setting
- Dealing with relapse

Chief Complaint

Mr. E.S. is a 45-year-old tour boat owner/operator who presents with the chief complaint of bipolar manic episode.

Present Illness

This gentleman first came to my office shortly after he had been discharged from a local psychiatric unit where he had spent 2 weeks for treatment of a severe manic episode. He had been on a cruise ship from San Diego to San Francisco when his wife had become alarmed at his agitation and delusional ideas. He was convinced that the ship was full of CIA and Homeland Security agents who were spying on him and whom he was also helping to train. He sent 20 letters to the captain of the ship in 2 days. He had racing thoughts, slept very little for 7 days, was irritable, and was concocting grandiose schemes to get the country straightened out. Three months prior to his admission he had begun to show increasing manic symptoms. He talked of many new inventions that seemed brilliant to him. He gave $10,000 to his daughter for no clear reason and without discussing it with his wife. He bought his wife a new car that she did not want and planned to give his $800,000 warehouse to his boating community. He sold a $30,000 boat for $1. When he revealed his delusional ideas to his wife during the cruise, his family called Kaiser, brought him to the emergency department, and he was placed in the hospital on a Section 5150 legal involuntary psychiatric hold for grave disability.

Other Significant Findings From Assessment

The patient's premorbid personality had been hard-driving and highly productive, with some irritability. An adult son told the outpatient psychiatrist that his father had been showing manic symptoms for 2 years, with decreased sleep, euphoria, irritability, impulsiveness, anger, and anxiety. He did not use alcohol or drugs, and had never received any psychiatric treatments. His father and paternal grandfather had both committed suicide. His mother had a diagnosis of bipolar disorder and had been on lithium for many years. He had a stable marriage with three children. Medically he only had mild hypertension, treated with hydrochlorothiazide. He was active in a Protestant church and did not use tobacco or caffeine. He was by all measures a successful businessman and citizen.

At the time of admission to the outpatient service he completed the Patient Health Questionnaire–9 (PHQ-9) and scored 8 of a possible 27, placing him in the mildly distressed range. He did not claim any anhedonia or depression, only indicating some sleep, energy, and concentration problems. He denied any suicidality.

DSM-IV-TR Diagnosis

Axis I   Bipolar I disorder, most recent episode manic with psychotic features
Axis II   None
Axis III   Hypertension, mild
Axis IV   Conflicts with wife
Axis V   GAF score (at time of discharge from hospital): 55

Treatment Plan Considerations

Selecting a Guideline

Kaiser Permanente of Northern California promotes the use of the Texas Medication Algorithm Project (TMAP) guideline (Suppes et al. 2005) for medication treatment of bipolar disorder. The more comprehensive American Psychiatric Association (APA) practice guideline (2006) uses nearly identical algorithms for medications for the manic, mixed, and depressed phases of this illness. In the discussion to follow in this chapter, I compare and contrast any differences between the two sets of guidelines as applied to this case.

Manic Episode

Mr. E.S. did not present any diagnostic challenges, coming in with a straightforward history of premorbid hypomanic traits, no drug or alcohol use, a clear-cut family history of bipolar and perhaps other affective disorders, and a full-blown manic episode of psychotic proportion for his first entry into the psychiatric care system. One wonders why the family did not pressure him to come for consultation before the mania reached psychotic levels.

He arrived at my office with the first decisions having already been made by the treating psychiatrist at the hospital. Because he presented with psychotic features, the use of olanzapine and lithium was correct by both guidelines, although the TMAP suggests olanzapine as an alternate stage 1 choice because of safety concerns (stage 1 agents listed by TMAP are lithium, depakote, aripiprazole, quetiapine, risperidone, and ziprasidone; stage 1b choices are olanzapine and carbamazepine, with metabolic and hematologic concerns). The treating psychiatrist noted that his family history included successful treatment with lithium. Lithium levels were monitored several times during his 2-week stay, reaching a maximum of 1.5 mm/L, which prompted a reduction of dose to 900 mg/day. He was started on olanzapine 20 mg/day, which was raised to 40 mg/day after 1 week. Zolpidem 10 mg was given to improve his sleep pattern. The APA guideline mentions short-term use of a benzodiazepine as sometimes useful, and TMAP suggests use of hypnotics for insomnia. His manic and delusional behaviors gradually quieted.

Mr. E.S. had been treated in the past with hydrochlorothiazide for hypertension; this was discontinued because of the interaction of the diuretic with lithium excretion, and he was placed on clonidine, which effectively managed this issue. TMAP suggests clonidine as adjunctive treatment for agitation or aggression as well. He also had some constipation, which was treated with docusate sodium.

Although he remained hyperverbal and not entirely convinced that his beliefs were delusional, he improved enough to be discharged to home and outpatient follow-up.

Posthospital Management in the Kaiser System

Mr. E.S. was now entering the more difficult part of his recovery, that of adapting to new realities and regaining function, hopefully at a level equal to or better than his premorbid functioning. The APA guideline stresses the need to establish a therapeutic alliance, educate the patient and family about the illness, monitor symptoms, ensure safety, promote awareness of stressors and regular patterns of activity and sleep, and manage functional impairments. In the Kaiser system of psychiatric care, nearly all patients who are discharged from inpatient stays are enrolled in a short course of day treatment, labeled intensive outpatient (IOP). At the South San Francisco Clinic where this gentleman was enrolled, the day treatment meets for 3 hours every Monday, Wednesday, and Friday mornings, in a group room. The format is interactive group didactic lectures and videos, with training given in relaxation techniques, stress and anger management, cognitive-behavioral therapy (CBT), dialectical behavior therapy (DBT), substance abuse issues and recovery, and psychotropic medications. Social workers, psychologists, a registered nurse, and a physician meet with the 8 to 20 patients in various combinations. Each patient is assigned to a staff member who meets with him or her individually at least once a week. The normal course is 2–4 weeks of attendance, sometimes more. During their IOP course the patients meet with the psychiatrist on their case one or more times per week of attendance. This format of care allows for meeting all the recommendations published in the APA's sensible guideline.

Treatment Goals, Measures, and Methods

1. Achieve euthymia within 2 months, as reported by patient and family, scored on the PHQ-9, and observed by treatment staff, using pharmacotherapy, psychoeducation, CBT, and group and family support. The PHQ-9 (Spitzer et al. 1999) is a nine-item instrument used in the Kaiser system for a quick assessment of depression.
2. Return to full functioning in his work within 2 months, measured by self-report of satisfactory performance, using pharmacotherapy and supportive therapy for patient and his wife.

Course

Mr. E.S. presented to IOP and his initial outpatient evaluations as disheveled, fidgety, with loud voice and pressured rambling speech, though he was generally logical. He seemed to understand that he had been delusional but would occasionally offer rationalizations, which hinted that he was unsure. He was cooperative with the treatments outlined, but somewhat reluctant. He attended dutifully, however. He was

taking olanzapine 40 mg/day, lithium 900 mg/day, zolpidem 10 mg at bed, and clonidine for his hypertension. Weight was 182 lb (body mass index=28), slightly below his normal weight of 190 lb. My assessment of him was that he was probably always hypomanic, but never truly manic until this episode. I believed he was responding fairly well to the lithium and olanzapine, but likely would need to switch to another neuroleptic soon, because of metabolic issues of weight gain and altered glucose metabolism. His fasting blood sugar was mildly elevated on repeated checks.

He attended IOP every Monday, Wednesday, and Friday mornings as requested, participating actively. I saw him for 10 to 20 minutes individually during most of these mornings, with his wife often present for the interviews with me. He seemed to be clearing up steadily at first, becoming more normal in appearance and speech. He began to complain of feeling weak, which he blamed on the olanzapine. I elected to lower the olanzapine dosage to 30 mg/ day to address this complaint. Serum lithium level was 0.6 mEq/L.

By 2 weeks after discharge from the hospital he reported feeling ready to return to work but continued to complain of side effects, this time complaining of erectile dysfunction. He and his wife met with me to report that they had unilaterally decided to stop the olanzapine 2 days earlier. At that time he looked improved, with no return of manic symptoms, so I reluctantly agreed with their decision, in order to maintain our developing therapeutic alliance. I scheduled a follow-up appointment in 2 weeks.

Unfortunately he deteriorated rapidly, developing suicidal ideation 8 days after stopping the olanzapine. He had also by this time stopped taking the lithium, a medication that he feared. He rarely took any medications, even aspirin. His father had committed suicide after being recommended to take lithium. His wife brought him in for an urgent appointment, and they resumed lithium 900 mg/day at my prompting.

A week later he returned looking very sad, talking of guilt and failure in his career, complaining of not sleeping, feeling hopeless, acting withdrawn, sitting motionless. He denied ongoing suicidality at this visit. I diagnosed a switch into the depressed phase of the illness, and resumed his olanzapine at 20 mg/day. TMAP calls for raising the lithium level to 0.8 mEq/ L or above, continuing the second antimanic agent, and adding lamotrigine. I delayed starting the lamotrigine because of the earlier good response to lithium and olanzapine, hoping he would respond to resumption of those medications. I planned to see him two or three times a week, so I could change treatments rapidly as indicated.

Second Hospitalization

Two days later he came to the emergency department of the hospital, where the on-call psychiatrist diagnosed a severe depression, near catatonic level. He presented as disheveled, with poor hygiene, psychomotor retardation, blunted depressed affect, and tangential thoughts; he was preoccupied with poor business decisions made while manic and with his current inability to work. The doctor placed him in a psychiatric unit again, on a legal hold for grave disability, potential suicide risk, and treatment noncompliance.

The hospital psychiatrist found an elevated random glucose level of 156. That, combined with his complaints of fatigue and weakness on olanzapine, prompted the doctor to change his olanzapine to ziprasidone 40 mg bid. The doctor also started lamotrigine 25 mg bid for the depression, and continued his lithium. Within 5 days he was noticeably better and was discharged to home.

Return to Outpatient Setting

Week 8

Mr. E.S.'s wife called to report he was very depressed, with little interest in doing anything. She asked for help with ideas on how to lift him out of his depression. She was reminded to bring him in for his appointments the next day. She was noncommittal about family support group sessions. He came in for IOP and psychiatric visits, looking quite depressed, saying "my thoughts are locked up, like my mind has erased itself."

At this point he had been on the lamotrigine for 2 weeks. He had come out of the hospital on ziprasidone 40 mg bid, but it had been lowered to once daily by the on-call psychiatrist when he called in and complained of feeling too tired. He was taking zolpidem at the 20 mg level and was free of suicidal ideation and delusions. When he came to my office I let the lower ziprasidone level remain and increased his lamotrigine to 75 mg/day for 2 weeks. Again I felt constrained against loading up this man with

standard dosages of medications, given the vocal opposition to medications both the patient and his wife expressed.

Week 9

Over the weekend the patient had done poorly, being observed to stand in one place and stare. His wife thought he was responding to internal stimuli. In the Monday morning group he looked worse, apparently slipping back into catatonic behaviors. He expressed extreme guilt feelings, worrying about exhausting his wife and letting his employees down. He was very pessimistic about getting better. In my office he was moving somewhat stiffly and showed a fine tremor of his hands and tongue, but had no cogwheeling or dyskinetic movements. I had him increase his ziprasidone to 40 mg bid again and added clonazepam 0.5 mg to 1 mg bid-tid for anxiety and sleep. TMAP supports use of benzodiazepines targeted to anxiety and hypnotics for sleep. I also added bupropion 100 mg/day for 2 days, then to increase to 200 mg/day. This is listed as a stage 4 maneuver by TMAP. For stages 2 and 3, TMAP suggests using lithium and lamotrigine plus quetiapine or olanzapine/fluoxetine combination, which I was avoiding because of the metabolic issues here. By Friday, 4 days after making these medication changes, he was beginning to look somewhat better, with better color in his face and describing being more able to take care of some chores at home. He had a determined attitude by then, relaying the impression that he would soldier ahead through his ordeal.

Discussion

This sequence of events shows the importance of not lowering medications too soon because of bothersome side effects. Perhaps we could not have persuaded this couple to continue the dosages he was on when he came out of the hospital, but he probably would have had a smoother course of recovery from his psychotic episode if the olanzapine and lithium had not been lowered and stopped. He might have slipped into depression anyway, but one suspects that the second hospital stay could have been avoided. And when he did end up hospitalized again, the ziprasidone was lowered almost immediately after discharge, and he suffered an apparent worsening of his depression after that. He responded within 5 days of returning it to 80 mg (40 mg bid), plus having bupropion and clonazepam added.

Week 10

On Monday he still looked and acted fairly depressed. He complained of memory problems and had amnesia for calling a helper to meet him at 6 A.M. He had set his alarm clock for 6 P.M. His serum lithium level was 0.5 mEq/L on 900 mg, so it was raised to 1,200 mg for 3 days and then to 1,500 mg, seeking a level of 0.8–1.0 mEq/L. He was showing signs of improving in that he was speaking up more in groups. I encouraged him to try to return to a reduced schedule of work. I also had him lower his zolpidem dosage from 20 mg to 10 mg/day.

Two days later he returned to report that he had successfully run his boat tours the day before and was feeling better because of this. His wife reported that he was slowly returning to normal, watching TV, sleeping more normally. He still had a mildly depressed affect but was improving rapidly. I raised his lamotrigine to 50 mg bid and had him switch his zolpidem and clonazepam to prn only. I reduced his clonidine to 0.1 mg bid from tid because his blood pressure readings were normal and we wanted to reduce his overall medication load.

He was able to graduate from IOP that Friday, with obvious progress having been made in 1 week. He even expressed optimism about his future and gratitude toward the staff. He registered for a depression class and agreed to have some individual therapy as well as his psychiatric visits.

Discussion

When Mr. E.S. came out of the hospital the second time, his wife was much more accepting of guidance about the medications. I spent a lot of time in our joint sessions explaining the illness to them and coaching them that we needed to make changes more carefully and slowly over time. I reassured them that it was in my interest as well that he be taking only the necessary number and quantity of medications, to minimize side-effect burden on him and to reduce costs.

Week 14

Mr. E.S. and his wife reported he was doing well, especially when working, which he was doing every other day. No tardive dyskinesia or other side effects were mentioned. He showed no evidence of mania or depression and no further amnestic episodes. He was sleeping 8 hours without zolpidem. He was taking lithium 1,200 mg, ziprasidone 80 mg, bupropion 200 mg, lamotrigine 100 mg, and clonazepam 1.5 mg daily, as well as clonidine 0.1 mg bid.

Week 19

Mr. E.S. continued to do well. His only side effect was minor tremor of the hands. He had gained weight and reached 193 lb, slightly above his usual weight. He did not wish to change any medications at this visit. I recommended he modify his diet to lose weight slowly and see his primary care physician for a checkup.

Week 23

The patient continued to do well. His wife reported he was better tempered now than he was premorbidly, when he was more irritable and angry. He was working 2 days per week for himself, being careful not to overdo things. He would help out a colleague on some other days. He and his wife planned another cruise soon. His internist switched him from clonidine to a lisinopril/hydrochlorothiazide combination. He was taking lithium 1,200 mg, ziprasidone 80 mg, bupropion 300 mg, and lamotrigine 100 mg daily, as well as clonazepam prn.

Week 29

The patient and his wife went on a Caribbean cruise and did well except that he was uncomfortable for a few hours, remembering his manic episode during his previous cruise. He had a mildly elevated fasting blood sugar level, and his lithium level was 0.8 mEq/L. He remained euthymic but complained of erectile dysfunction. In response, I lowered his ziprasidone to 40 mg/day for 4 weeks and then discontinued it. My assumption was that any of the medications could be causing the sexual dysfunction, and the guidelines call for removing the atypical neuroleptics when the patient is stable. Again, I encouraged exercise and weight loss as aids to his overall health and potency.

Week 38

He had been off ziprasidone for 3 weeks and continued to function adequately, but he and his wife both commented that he was not as happy-acting as he had been. He was still having erectile dysfunction and low libido. His sleep was fine, and he was using a treadmill daily. He had lost weight and was now at 180 lb. I had him lower his lithium to 900 mg/day and stop the clonazepam to lower his overall medication burden. I also added trazodone in hopes of assisting with the sexual issues, using it instead of prn clonazepam for sleep. I e-mailed his internist to ask for clearance to use sildenafil as an aid.

Week 47

PHQ-9=1 (no depression). Again the patient and his wife reported he was doing well, continuing to walk and lose weight, sleeping well, able to socialize comfortably even in large groups. He continued to have erectile dysfunction, with incomplete erections and infrequent intercourse. Serum lithium level was 0.8 mEq/L on 900 mg, weight was down to 172 lb. His affect had improved to be quite relaxed and natural, no longer with a flattened quality. I had him take all his lamotrigine at bedtime and reduced the trazodone to prn use only. He took a sildenafil prescription with him, pending approval by his internist.

Week 55

PHQ-9=2 (no depression). He continued to do well. They had gone on another cruise and reported that the sexual issues had resolved with the use of sildenafil. He discussed some guilt at things that had transpired between himself and his son during his initial hospitalization. His weight and lab values remained stable, within normal limits except for a mildly elevated fasting blood sugar level of 94.

Tables 31–1 and 31–2 list the TMAP algorithms for bipolar disorder, manic and depressed phases, and summarizes how closely they were followed in this case.

Ways to Improve Practice

This case illustrates the danger of lowering therapeutic medications too early and too rapidly in the bipolar individual. In retrospect, I would have spent more time with this patient and his wife in trying to slow down their attempts at withdrawing the medications. Since sexual performance problems proved to be a major concern later, perhaps they were causing some of the early resistance to the medications, and discussing sexual issues earlier would have been helpful.

Also, I will more quickly return to the same levels of medicines that were working before, and not be as hesitant to perhaps cause a few extra side effects. I already move quite slowly and deliberately when withdrawing such people from medications, if they permit me to guide them thusly.

I will also be much more likely to consistently use measurement tools such as the PHQ-9. The Young Mania Rating Scale also would have been useful after his first hospital stay, as he was recovering from the manic episode. The act of completing the scale could serve as an important educational moment for the patient and his wife.

Perhaps most importantly, the work of writing up this case has illustrated to me the value of referencing the published treatment guidelines from time to time in order to reduce uncertainty for the clinician and speed recovery for the patient.

References

American Psychiatric Association: Practice Guidelines for the Treatment of Psychiatric Disorders, Compendium. Washington, DC, American Psychiatric Publishing, 2006

Spitzer RI, Kroenke K, Williams JBW: Validation and utility of a self-report version of PRIME-MD: the PHQ primary care study—Primary Care Evaluation of Mental Disorders, Patient Health Questionnaire. JAMA 282:1737–1744, 1999

Suppes T, Dennehy EB, Hirschfeld M, et al: The Texas Implementation of Medication Algorithms: update to the algorithms for treatment of bipolar disorder. J Clin Psychiatry 66:870–886, 2005

TABLE 32–1. TMAP recommendations for bipolar disorder, currently hypomanic/manic

	Recommendation	Followed
Stage 1	Monotherapy with lithium, valproate, aripiprazole, quetiapine, risperidone, ziprasidone, or Stage 1b, olanzapine or carbamazepine, plus targeted adjunctive treatments	Inpatient physician put him on stage 2 treatment immediately
Stage 2	Two-drug combination of lithium, valproate, or atypical antipsychotic, plus targeted adjunctive treatments such as benzodiazepines, hypnotics	Yes. Lithium plus olanzapine and zolpidem
Stage 3	Try another two-drug combination of lithium, valproate, atypical antipsychotics, carbamazepine, oxcarbazepine, typical antipsychotics, plus targeted adjunctive treatments	Not needed
Stage 4	Electroconvulsive therapy or add clozapine or lithium+valproate or carbamazepine or oxcarbazepine+atypical antipsychotic	Not needed

TABLE 32–2. TMAP algorithm for the treatment of bipolar disorder, currently depressed

	Recommendation	Followed
Stage 1	Antimanic + lamotrigine. If lithium, increase dose to ≥0.8	Patient was on lithium and olanzapine for mania before switching to depressed phase.
Stage 2	Antimanic + lamotrigine + quetiapine *or* olanzapine/fluoxetine combination (OFC)	Lamotrigine was started at the second hospital stay (for depression).
Stage 3	Combination from lithium, lamotrigine, quetiapine, *or* OFC	Ziprasidone replaced olanzapine because of metabolic and other side effects.
Stage 4	Lithium, lamotrigine, quetiapine, OFC, valproate, *or* carbamazepine+SSRI, bupropion, or venlafaxine; *or* ECT	Bupropion was added.
Stage 5	MAOIs, tricyclics, pramipexole, other atypical antipsychotics, oxcarbazepine, other	Clonazepam, zolpidem, and trazodone were used.

Note. ECT=electroconvulsive therapy; MAOIs=monoamine oxidase inhibitors; SSRI=selective serotonin reuptake inhibitor.

Consultation-Liaison Psychiatry

Anthony J. Mascola, M.D.

Setting

The psychiatric consultation-liaison service provides psychiatric care and support to patients admitted to the medical and surgical services of the medical center. It is a unique practice environment that provides many opportunities to apply the tenets of the evidence-based medicine (EBM) model. Disturbances of mood and behavior in the setting of serious medical illness might reasonably be considered psychological reactions to the extreme stressors present in such an environment. They could represent exacerbations of a preexisting psychiatric illness. There exists also the possibility of a much broader differential diagnosis of potential causative factors given the high pretest probability of medical, pharmacological, and surgical conditions associated with psychiatric symptoms in these settings. Teasing these factors apart and assigning a diagnosis that might optimally assist the clinician in easing the suffering of the patient can be challenging. The focus of this case is on using an evidence-based approach to diagnosis.

Recommended Prior Knowledge

If you are unfamiliar with the evidence-based diagnostic process, it is highly recommended that you read the introductory chapters in part I of Steven McGee's excellent text on evidence-based physical diagnosis (McGee 2007) or the introductory article by Sackett (1992) before proceeding.

Illustration

This study illustrates:

- Common biases affecting our diagnostic methods
- Importance of the first step in the EBM cycle—assessment:
  - Importance of, and methods for generating, a reasonable differential diagnosis for the patient's symptoms
  - Importance of carefully considering the pretest probabilities of the conditions in the differential diagnosis
  - Making use of the operating characteristics of tests, including those describing diagnostic accuracy (likelihood ratios) and reliability (kappa)
  - Combining pretest probability estimates with likelihood ratios to estimate the posttest probability of a given diagnosis in the differential
- Asking focused, answerable clinical questions to search the medical literature
- Acquiring information
- Appraising information on diagnostic tests for validity and relevance
- Applying information using a shared decision-making model that incorporates published evidence, clinical judgment, and patient and family preferences
- Assessing both patient outcomes and the process of decision making used

315

Chief Complaint/Reason for Consultation

Mr. C.K. is a 79-year-old married man of Polish American descent admitted to the hospital for surgical removal of a recurrent squamous cell carcinoma of his vocal cord. His surgery occurred 4 days prior to our being consulted to "evaluate and treat the anxiety and depression affecting his postoperative course."

Present Illness and History

From the information available in the chart and the verbal information shared from the consulting physician, Mr. C.K. had a long history of cigarette use, smoking about one pack per day for 45 years. He quit smoking 17 years prior to admission when he was diagnosed with coronary artery disease and had a two-vessel coronary artery bypass graft performed. He was diagnosed as having an in situ squamous cell carcinoma of the right vocal cord 2 years prior to admission and received radiation treatment. He was thought to be in remission until he began noticing increasing hoarseness of his voice. He was evaluated and found to have a recurrent moderately differentiated squamous cell carcinoma of the right vocal cord staged T3 N0 M0. He was readmitted to the hospital for a modified radical neck dissection, supracricoid laryngectomy with cricohyoidopexy, and tracheostomy.

In addition to his coronary artery disease, Mr. C.K. had intermittent atrial fibrillation. He was not taking warfarin. He also suffered from hypertension, hypercholesterolemia, gastroesophageal reflux disease (GERD), and benign prostatic hypertrophy (BPH) and was status post transurethral prostatectomy. Little was known about Mr. C.K.'s past psychiatric, substance use, developmental history, or social history. He was noted at times in the presurgical consultation notes to appear "anxious" when discussing his treatment options; he was known to be married but his current living situation was not specified. There was no mention of his previous education level, employment history, or any past psychiatric diagnoses or treatment. As an outpatient, he was prescribed tamsulosin hydrochloride for BPH, omeprazole for GERD, amlodipine/benazepril for hypertension, atorvastatin for hyperlipidemia, and aspirin for coronary artery disease.

Mr. C.K. was felt to be an appropriate candidate for surgery for his laryngeal tumor despite the multiple other comorbid medical problems that made him a high-risk surgical candidate, because without intervention the tumor would likely continue to expand and cause increasing airway constriction, dyspnea, and eventually suffocation. The procedure was considered an important palliative intervention. He was admitted to the hospital, and the surgical team performed a modified radical neck dissection, supracricoid laryngectomy with cricohyoidopexy, and tracheostomy as planned.

The team noted that the intraoperative course went fairly well. The tumor was removed, and the patient was hemodynamically stable. There were a few developments in the postoperative course, however, that had begun to complicate his recovery, resulting in the team consulting the psychiatry department.

The patient was initially intubated and sedated with midazolam and fentanyl. He received additional intermittent hydromorphone hydrochloride for pain. He was weaned off mechanical ventilation to a tracheostomy collar but developed respiratory distress and significant oxygen desaturation. This was thought to be secondary to pulmonary edema from congestive heart failure given his previous cardiac history and findings from his exam and diagnostic tests. His electrocardiogram (ECG) was unchanged compared with prior exams, his cardiac enzymes were unremarkable, and his white blood cell count and differential were unremarkable. His sputum was not purulent, and his chest X ray showed diffuse pulmonary infiltrates read by the radiologist and medical consultant as edema rather than a focal infiltrate suggestive of pneumonia. There was no unilateral lower leg edema noted, and he had been on sequential compression devices for deep venous thrombosis prophylaxis. He was treated with albuterol sulfate/ipratropium bromide via nebulizer and diuresed with furosemide at the recommendation of the internal medicine consulting service. His breathing and oxygen saturation improved, but shortly thereafter the patient became tachycardic in the 120–140 bpm range.

The patient's tachycardia was presumed by the primary team and medical consultant to be multifactorial, including an exacerbation of his atrial fibrillation in the setting of diuresis-induced hypovolemia, anemia with a hematocrit of 28, as well as "pain and anxiety." His ECG showed atrial fibrillation with a rate of 110 bpm but was otherwise not significantly changed. His QTc was 470 msec. Repeated assays of his cardiac troponin I and creatine kinase-MB were within normal limits. He was started on metoprolol, and his amlodipine, benazepril, aspirin, and atorvastatin were continued. His heart rate returned to the 90s to low 100s, and his blood pressure ranged in the previous 24 hours of our consultation from 124/80 to 136/90 mm Hg.

A percutaneous gastrostomy tube had been inserted, as the patient would need to remain on a nothing by mouth (NPO) regimen for several months as a result of the procedure performed. The patient developed abdominal pain with feeding through the tube and was taken back to the operating room for exploratory laparoscopy and replacement after peritoneal extravasation was noted with a contrast study. His medications were switched to intravenous equivalents wherever possible. After the tube was replaced, the patient was able to receive his medications and nutritional support via the gastrostomy tube. He continued to take omeprazole. He had bowel movements daily or every other day, and there was no evidence of impaction.

The patient was febrile on postoperative day 2 to 38.6°C despite receiving clindamycin, which was documented as being prescribed "for prophylaxis" during the surgery. His surgical site appeared unremarkable; his skin was examined and no pressure sores or ulcers were noted. His pulmonary exam and diagnostic tests, as described previously, were not felt to be consistent with pneumonia. Blood, sputum, and urine cultures were sent for analysis. Lumbar puncture was not performed. He was started on ciprofloxacin for what appeared possibly to be a consideration for peritonitis from the extravasation of the gastrostomy tube. On postoperative day 3 the ciprofloxacin was written as being prescribed for a presumed urinary tract infection as 2+ leukocyte esterase was noted on his urinalysis.

From a neurologic and psychiatric perspective, the patient was noted immediately postoperation to be heavily sedated with midazolam and fentanyl. He received additional intermittent hydromorphone hydrochloride for pain. His pain was documented as being "well controlled" and "0/10" in the nursing notes. On postoperative day 2 he was extubated, the midazolam was stopped, and he was started on patient-controlled analgesia with morphine. At that time he was documented to be "alert and oriented × 3" and to be "responding to commands" in the notes. His exam was documented as being "nonfocal." On postoperative day 3, however, he appeared to be "anxious," "depressed," and "tearful." The nurse informed the team that she felt the patient was growing increasingly "upset," possibly as a result of having to deal with several of the previously mentioned medical problems that were developing and were complicating his recovery.

He continued to be "oriented × 3" and "able to respond to commands" and continued to be described as "denies pain." In the evening before our consultation on postoperative day 3, the patient was noted as having become "increasingly tearful, upset, and anxious," gesticulating tremulously with his hands in a manner that appeared to the nursing staff to be insisting that he was "thirsty" and "wanted to drink water." He was receiving intravenous fluids as well as nutrition through his gastrostomy tube. He was NPO and had been instructed repeatedly not to drink. Despite this, he repeatedly reached for water on the nursing tray at the bedside that was intended to flush his gastrostomy tube. He attempted to drink this several times despite repeated instructions to remain NPO before the water was removed from the bedside by the nursing staff. He was tearful and was not consolable. Shortly afterward he was administered lorazepam and hydromorphone intravenously, and he became more sedate.

The nursing staff described feeling frustrated that he was acting in an "anxious and irrational" manner, which might complicate his recovery. He was described as being "restless" overnight and did not sleep well. He would not participate in the tracheostomy care and tube feeding training exercises recommended by his nursing staff the following day, and he appeared withdrawn from communication. On the same day he was later described as appearing "panicky" at times. The team, noting the anxiety that had been mentioned in the preoperative consultation notes, asked the patient if he was feeling depressed, and he seemed to nod "yes" in agreement to this and to questions about whether he felt like life was "not worth living anymore," although he would not elaborate. The psychiatry consult was then requested to better "assess the patient's worsening anxiety and depressed mood," which were "interfering with his ability to participate in tracheostomy and gastrostomy self-care instruction and training."

A specific question asked of the team was "should an antidepressant be initiated?"

Other Significant Findings From Assessment

Being called to assess a patient in a scenario similar to that presented previously is a relatively common and challenging task requested of the consultation-liaison team. This patient appeared to be "upset with his care" and to be suffering from "anxiety and depression" to the primary team. He was known to be in a chronic state of poor health and to have been admitted for treatment of his recurrent laryngeal cancer. He had suffered a series of complications after his procedure. He was unable to speak but appeared tearful and to endorse symptoms of depressed mood, anhedonia, and hopelessness. He appeared at times to be anxious and to have difficulty sleeping. He had thoughts of death and seemed to endorse that his life was not worth living. He initially appeared to be actively refusing reasonable interventions such as remaining NPO to improve his outcome and was then observed to be sullen and withdrawn and to refuse physical therapy and rehabilitation. The psychological stress and existential issues in dealing with severe medical illness and the complications of treatment were high. The medical team felt these symptoms were causing sufficient interference with his recovery and wondered whether an antidepressant should be initiated.

• Before we proceed further, take a moment to briefly write down three to five diagnoses you might consider in this patient. We will return to this later as an exercise in discussing hindsight bias (Bornstein and Emler 2001). Please write these down now.

Diagnosis

Importance of Assigning an Accurate, Reproducible Diagnosis

Clinicians assign diagnoses in their attempts to search for relevant past experiences that might permit them a better inductive forecast of the future and guide their decision making to improve patient outcomes. We see a patient today and consider how well their circumstances and pattern of symptoms might be conceptualized as part of one or more previously operationalized diagnostic syndromes. Our

knowledge and experience with these syndromes allow us to make educated guesses as to the options most likely to achieve optimal outcomes for our current patient. The more closely our clinical setting and diagnostic methods are to those of clinicians who have previously conducted carefully controlled clinical research trials on these syndromes, and the closer our patient's experiences are to the syndromes described within these trials, the more confidently we might be able to make inferences from the knowledge gained. Where these things are very dissimilar we are unlikely to be able to confidently forecast future outcomes. A person experiencing a depressive syndrome highly similar to the symptoms reported by persons described as having major depressive disorder in a high-quality randomized controlled trial conducted in a similar setting might benefit from the treatments that this research has found helpful. A person whose pattern of symptoms and signs are more similar, however, to those exhibited by the group whom we conceptualize as having bipolar depression might respond differently to these same interventions. Those whose depressive symptoms are associated with additional symptoms and signs suggesting profound hypothyroidism, or alcohol use or amphetamine withdrawal, or obstructive sleep apnea or hypoactive delirium, and so on, might respond differently still. Thus, where treatment options exist that might result differentially in better or worse outcomes for the patient, it is important to consider carefully the diagnostic process used to assign an accurate, reproducible diagnosis so that we can better guide our decision making (Pauker and Kassirer 1980).

Common Diagnostic Biases Leading to Errors in Assigning Diagnoses

The procedures that we use to assign a diagnosis vary. An approach often taken by clinicians is to assign a diagnosis based on the clinical gestalt suggested by the pattern of symptoms observed in examination of the patient. This has the advantage of being rapid and can be quite accurate when applied by experienced clinicians (Chunilal et al. 2003). There are situations, however, in which this approach is susceptible to a number of biases that can lead to assigning diagnoses very different from those using more optimal examination methods (Bornstein and Emler 2001). One of the most common biases that can occur resulting in assigning an incorrect diagnosis is failing to account for how common a given diagnosis might be in a given setting. This error of ignoring the pretest probability or base rate of a given diagnosis and being susceptible to being overly influenced by the patient's clinical presentation or test findings is a violation of a mathematical theorem of probabilistic reasoning called *Bayes theorem*. This bias, sometimes referred to as the *representativeness bias*, is a well-documented source of diagnostic error (Bornstein and Emler 2001; Casscells et al. 1978; Ghosh et al. 2004; Kahneman et al. 1982; Lyman and Balducci 1993, 1994). In medicine we use the phrase "when you hear hoofbeats, think of horses, not zebras" as a reminder to ourselves not to forget to incorporate the base rates of a given diagnosis in a particular setting. Applying this clinically, however, is challenging even with training (Steurer et al. 2002). Knowing how to combine estimates of the pretest probability of a given diagnosis in a particular setting together with the clinical features that distinguish this diagnosis from others in the differential is part of the art of practicing evidence-based medicine that we will illustrate with this case.

Differential Diagnosis

When Should a Differential Diagnosis and Further Diagnostic Testing Be Considered?

In psychiatry, our clinical trials most often use the procedures suggested by DSM-IV-TR (American Psychiatric Association 2000) to assign diagnoses. The patient in this case certainly did appear to have many symptoms similar to the pattern described as being present in a DSM major depressive episode.

This diagnosis appeared to be a good "snap fit" to the primary team. Would there be any point in generating a differential diagnosis? Major depressive disorder was certainly a possibility. The pattern was clearly not an exact match, but similar features certainly were present.

A second bias often affecting clinical decision making is called the *confirmation bias*. This occurs when we selectively gather and interpret evidence that confirms a diagnosis and ignore evidence that might disconfirm it. Another bias that often occurs affecting the validity of a diagnosis is called the *availability bias*. This bias occurs when we overestimate the probability of a diagnosis when instances of that diagnosis are relatively easy to recall. Generating a

differential diagnosis is a method that we use to combat these biases.

In this case, many diagnoses possibly were consistent with this patient's symptoms and circumstances. Numerous serious medical conditions were present, and multiple medications were being prescribed to this patient in the intensive care unit (ICU) in which the delirium syndrome is known to be quite prevalent (Ely et al. 2004). Delirium can present with profound anxiety and depressive symptoms and is often overlooked (Farrell and Ganzini 1995). Treatments for delirium would involve actively seeking and correcting the medical causes of these symptoms, and this would differ markedly from an approach recommended for major depressive disorder. Persons with preexisting dementia, anxiety disorders, mood disorders, or multiple other psychiatric conditions might have increased difficulty coping with the extreme stresses present in this case. We knew nothing of this patient's prior history and whether the symptoms observed were acute or chronic. Substance- and medication-related effects as well as their withdrawal could cause or exacerbate the symptoms exhibited. Any number or combination of factors potentially could be contributing to the symptoms that our patient was exhibiting.

A *diagnostic testing threshold* (Pauker and Kassirer 1980) had therefore been reached. The treatment recommendations varied widely for the conditions that could be present, and we were not convinced that major depressive disorder was the best or the only diagnosis consistent with this patient's symptoms. We had not yet crossed a *test–treatment threshold* in which we could feel confident in our making treating recommendations. This prompted us to expand the differential diagnosis beyond the diagnosis of a major depressive episode and to conduct further diagnostic assessment. In general, as per Pauker (Pauker and Kassirer 1980), treatment should be withheld if the probability of disease is smaller than the diagnostic testing threshold, and treatment should be given without further testing if the probability of disease is greater than the test–treatment threshold. Further diagnostic testing should be considered (with treatment depending on the test outcome) only if the probability of disease is between the two thresholds.

How might a differential diagnosis be generated? A final bias that must be considered in diagnostic decision making is called *regret bias*. This occurs when

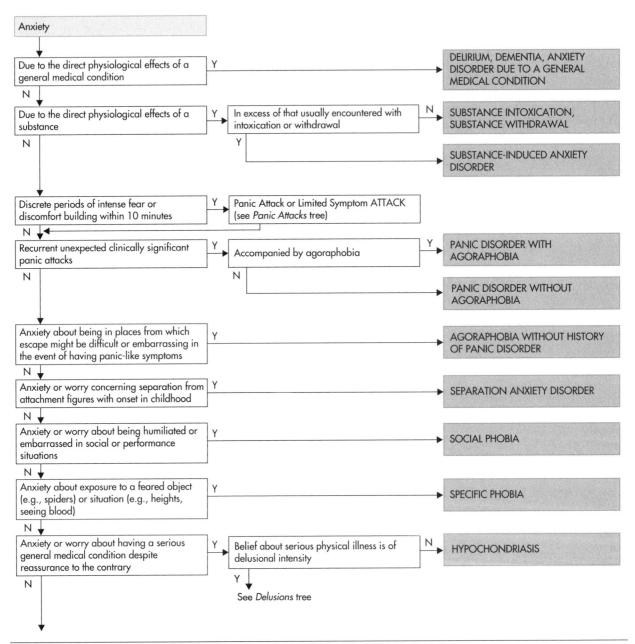

FIGURE 33–1.　DSM-IV-TR decision tree for differential diagnosis of anxiety.

Source.　First MB, Frances A, Pincus HA: *DSM-IV-TR Handbook of Differential Diagnosis.* Washington, DC, American Psychiatric Publishing, 2002, pp. 21–23. Copyright ©2002 American Psychiatric Publishing, Inc. Used with permission.

we overestimate the probability of a diagnosis with a severe possible outcome because of anticipated regret if such a diagnosis were missed (Bornstein and Emler 2001). We can consider an approach that borrows elements of several potential strategies that a reasonable clinician might use to form a differential diagnosis (Richardson et al. 1999) that minimizes the risks of the various biases introduced previously. We might consider a broad differential diagnosis (possibilistic approach) that weights more heavily

those causes that cannot be missed (prognostic approach) as well as those that are highly likely in that practice setting (probabilistic approach) that can be treated resulting in better patient outcomes (pragmatic approach).

The *DSM-IV-TR Handbook of Differential Diagnosis* (First et al. 2002) is a resource that we might consider consulting to help us form and focus our initial differential diagnosis. It includes decision trees (see Figure 33–1) that help the psychiatric clinician to use

FIGURE 33–1. DSM-IV-TR decision tree for differential diagnosis of anxiety (*continued*).

procedures to assign diagnoses consistent with those of the formal procedures described in the text of the DSM used in randomized controlled trials. It is organized somewhat consistently with the pragmatic strategy described previously, weighting those conditions such as disorders commonly caused by medical or substance-related etiologies as diagnoses to examine prior to assigning other diagnoses because these syndromes might have important treatment implications. The clinician must use this tool carefully because many nuanced factors must be considered together with this resource, as we will see.

Delirium, dementia, and anxiety secondary to a general medical condition or pharmacological substance intoxication/withdrawal are the diagnoses that appear at the top of the list from the *DSM-IV-TR Handbook of Differential Diagnosis*. Delirium is an extremely prevalent state of acutely altered mental status that occurs in patients who are seriously ill.

Occurrence rates of delirium in hospitalized medical patients range from 11% to 42% of all admitted patients (Siddiqi et al. 2006) on general medical units. Estimates are much higher for those in the ICU, where our patient consultation occurred. For example, a well-designed prospective study using validated methods for detecting delirium found that 81.7% of mechanically ventilated patients in the ICU were delirious (Ely et al. 2004). Despite the high prevalence rates, clinicians are often led astray by the clinical presentation of delirium. Delirious patients often endorse anxious and depressive symptoms, such as low mood (60%), worthlessness (68%), and frequent thoughts of death (52%) (Farrell and Ganzini 1995), as part of the delirium syndrome. Patients who are alert, easily aroused, able to make eye contact, and able to follow commands are often presumed by clinical staff to have normal cognitive functioning, but 40% of these patients have been found to be delirious when examined by more rigorous examination methods (Ely et al. 2001a). Acute changes in mental status in elderly patients in medical settings frequently are misattributed to primary psychological causes such as anxiety or depression (Boland et al. 1996; Farrell and Ganzini 1995; Nicholas and Lindsey 1995; Swigart et al. 2008), if they are diagnosed at all (Gustafson et al. 1991; Inouye 1998; Inouye et al. 2001). Delirium is an important risk factor for increased mortality in both general medical (Siddiqi et al. 2006) and ICU settings (Ely et al. 2004) and has very different treatment implications than the other diagnoses considered in the differential. Delirium can be a marker of serious substance withdrawal syndromes and other acutely unfolding medical conditions and thus became a very important diagnosis for us to consider in our differential diagnosis.

DSM-IV-TR diagnostic criteria for delirium appear in Table 33–1.

Narrowing the Differential

The patient at the time of our examination was unfortunately unable to speak to us as a result of his recent laryngectomy. There was little information available in the chart record about any past psychiatric history, cognitive impairment, dementia, or substance use, and no family members were present at the bedside. We did not know if the patient lived independently or in an assisted living facility or if he had caregivers at home. This is a common scenario that can make assessment more challenging. Often in these cases attempting to collect information from collateral historians and conducting a thorough physical and mental status exam are the only sources of information available.

DSM-IV-TR diagnostic criteria for delirium require that a preexisting dementia be excluded as being better able to account for the disturbances observed. Because delirium was the most critical diagnosis in our differential, evaluating for preexisting dementia thus became important. Treatment recommendations for agitation in dementia could be considerably different from those recommended for delirium, which focus much more intensely on identifying and primarily correcting underlying physiologic processes and secondarily on pharmacotherapies to help manage agitation. If the patient were delirious from alcohol or benzodiazepine withdrawal, for example, we would recommend a substantially

TABLE 33–1. **DSM-IV-TR diagnostic criteria for delirium due to multiple etiologies**

A. Disturbance of consciousness (i.e., reduced clarity of awareness of the environment) with reduced ability to focus, sustain, or shift attention.

B. A change in cognition (such as memory deficit, disorientation, language disturbance) or the development of a perceptual disturbance that is not better accounted for by a preexisting, established, or evolving dementia.

C. The disturbance develops over a short period of time (usually hours to days) and tends to fluctuate during the course of the day.

D. There is evidence from the history, physical examination, or laboratory findings that the delirium has more than one etiology (e.g., more than one etiological general medical condition, a general medical condition plus substance intoxication or medication side effect).

Source: American Psychiatric Association 2000, p. 147. Used with permission.

different treatment than we would for a patient agitated from Alzheimer's disease. Thus a diagnostic testing threshold had been reached to tease these apart. The absence of dementia would make our search for underlying reversible physiologic causes much more important. The presence of dementia of course would not exclude a delirium upon dementia and would result in a much more careful and detailed examination before we felt comfortable in excluding this possibility. Unfortunately, detection of dementia in clinical settings is difficult (Ardern et al. 1993; Boustani et al. 2003; Chodosh et al. 2004; Holsinger et al. 2007; Olafsdottir et al. 2000; Pisani et al. 2003b; Roca et al. 1984; Valcour et al. 2000). The absence of mention of dementia in the medical record was unlikely to exclude this as a diagnostic concern.

Distinguishing Dementia and Delirium From Other Diagnoses in the Differential

An Introduction to Likelihood Ratios, Pretest Probability, and Evidence-Based Diagnosis

In an ideal scenario, the clinical judgment of the experienced physician is informed by the pretest probabilities of some of the more important potential causes in the differential diagnosis that might occur in that specific practice setting (Richardson et al.

1999, 2000a, 2000b, 2003). Diagnostic procedures with operating characteristics derived from high-quality diagnostic studies conducted in similar settings (Bossuyt et al. 2003b) might be used to assist the clinician in sorting through the differential. *Likelihood ratios* are the operating characteristics of various clinical findings (including items in the history, physical exam, or diagnostic tests) that we use in combination with pretest probabilities to estimate the *posttest probability* of a given condition being present (Deeks and Altman 2004; Sackett 1992).

Rarely are these findings capable of ruling in or ruling out a diagnosis by themselves. Likelihood ratios are weighting factors that tell us how strongly the presence or absence of a given finding is in influencing our estimate of the probability of a given disorder being present. Understanding these operating characteristics is important in assisting us in overcoming representativeness bias. Several studies suggest that we often grossly overestimate the findings of the clinical presentation and diagnostic tests in our decision making (Ghosh et al. 2004; Lyman and Balducci 1993, 1994; Rothman and Kiviniemi 1999; Sackett 1992; Steurer et al. 2002; Streiner 2003). A likelihood ratio greater than 1 indicates that a given finding is associated with the presence of the disease, whereas a likelihood ratio less than 1 indicates that a given finding is associated with the absence of disease. The further likelihood ratios are from 1, the stronger the evidence for the presence or absence of disease. Likelihood ratios above 10 and below 0.1 are considered to provide strong evidence to rule in or rule out diagnoses, respectively, in most circumstances; however, the pretest probability must always be considered. Diagnostic procedures for which likelihood ratios are available include assessment of the symptoms endorsed in the patient's history, mental status exam, or conducting structured bedside assessment inventories such as the Folstein Mini-Mental State Examination (McGee 2007). Likelihood ratios are easily calculated from the same information used to calculate sensitivity and specificity. The Rational Clinical Exam series in *JAMA* (Sackett 1992) has dozens of articles dating back over a decade presenting likelihood ratios and pretest probabilities for many of the most common medical problems that we encounter clinically, although the quality of many of the available diagnostic studies remains an ongoing source of concern (*Bandolier* 2002; Richardson 2007).

Does the Patient Have Dementia?

We knew from a well-designed prospective study using validated methods for detecting delirium that more than 80% of mechanically ventilated patients in the ICU were delirious (Ely et al. 2004) The prevalence of dementia is not well studied in inpatient medical settings. Our previous exploration of the medical literature had yielded only one study that we felt provided a reasonable estimate of the prevalence rate of preexisting (nondelirious) cognitive impairment in the ICU (Pisani et al. 2003a). This study estimated the pretest probability to be 42%. If we make the assumption for the time being that this estimate was a reasonable one, we then are faced with the task of identifying and implementing further diagnostic procedures with known operating characteristics by which to modify our pretest probability estimates.

Examining a nonverbal patient in the ICU under medical duress for dementia is not an easy task. We hoped to find diagnostic procedures using collateral historians as informants to assist us in our task. Because this situation arises so often and has important diagnostic implications, we previously have conducted a focused search of the literature to find an answer to the PICO question below (see Chapter 3 of this volume and Richardson et al. 1995).

Ask

*P*atient/population: Medically ill elderly hospitalized patients suspected of having dementia.

*I*ntervention: Brief, structured, informant-based interview.

*C*omparison: Much more intensive "gold standard" reference examination integrating information from collateral historians, prehospital cognitive performance–based measures, and expert clinical evaluation.

*O*utcome: Accuracy—likelihood ratios (positive and negative) of the brief measure compared against the gold standard. Precision—measures of interrater reliability such as kappa or intraclass correlations.

Acquire

There are unfortunately no organized repositories of high-quality preappraised systematic reviews of the medical literature pertaining to diagnosis available for rapid clinical queries at the time of this writing. The Rational Clinical Examination series in *JAMA* contains a limited review of diagnostic methods for various clinical problems but does not have a rapidly accessible search interface. The Cochrane database is, at the time of this writing, still in the process of developing a series of systematic reviews pertaining to diagnostic studies. As a result we do not expect to conduct such a search at the bedside to find a rapid answer to our question. We instead do monthly searches and appraisals of articles pertaining to diagnosis as part of a journal club in which we present critically appraised topics (CATS) relevant to our clinical work, then save these to a Web site for easy access during future episodes of patient care (Mascola 2008; Sackett and Straus 1998). Previously we had searched the literature for high-quality systematic reviews addressing the topic in the PICO question described previously using the PubMed Clinical Queries filters and were unable to find any reviews focused on assessing hospitalized patients for dementia. We had found previously two systematic reviews of studies conducted in primary care settings that referenced a limited number of informant questionnaires for assessing for dementia in outpatient settings (Boustani et al. 2003; Holsinger et al. 2007).

The Informant Questionnaire on Cognitive Decline in the Elderly (IQCODE) was an instrument that appeared in these reviews to be brief, requiring only minutes to perform, that collects information from collateral historians. It appeared to have been validated against several more resource-intensive, performance-based criterion standards for dementia (Jorm 2004) in outpatient settings in which such validation would be more easily performed and also to have been used in prognosis studies in inpatients with delirium (McCusker et al. 2002). It had favorable operating characteristics in these settings relative to these gold standard examinations. We thus focused our search for trials in which this measure might have been validated in medically ill inpatients and found one study in which the measure had been used in a teaching hospital general medical unit (Harwood et al. 1997) and another in which it was used to assess patients in the ICU (Pisani et al. 2003a). We had selected these articles in previous months to appraise critically for validity and applicability in our practice setting because we felt they might affect our practices, and we had CATS and the measures accessible on our internal Web site.

Appraise

We often use the STARD (Standards for the Reporting of Diagnostic Accuracy Studies) checklist for the reporting of studies of diagnostic accuracy (Bossuyt et al. 2003a, 2003b) to appraise the diagnostic studies that we find for quality in writing up our CATS. The STARD checklist is meant for editors of medical journals to use in appraising studies of diagnostic accuracy for completeness of reporting and for common sources of bias that can invalidate the findings. It works nicely for our purposes. There are other instruments available to use to appraise studies of diagnostic accuracy for quality (Richardson et al. 1999; Whiting et al. 2006) that you might consider in your setting.

• The reader is encouraged to stop here and obtain the Harwood study (Harwood et al. 1997), if fortunate enough to have access to the full text. You can then use a copy of the STARD checklist as an exercise in appraising a diagnostic study. (You can obtain the checklist at www.stard-statement.org and the guide for its use from Bossuyt et al. 2003a.) You might consider taking 30 minutes or so to read through the study while completing the checklist using the how-to guide. You can then compare your appraisal of the quality of the Harwood study with our appraisal and determine whether you might consider using the IQ-CODE in the assessment of the patients you see in your setting. Continue reading after you have finished your appraisal.

The Harwood study estimated the IQCODE had an optimal post hoc sensitivity of 100% and specificity of 86% using a cutoff of >3.44 as positive for dementia. The reader can convert these sensitivities and specificities into likelihood ratios by using the following formulas (McGee 2007):

$$\text{LR+} = \text{sensitivity}/(1-\text{specificity}) \text{ and}$$
$$\text{LR--} = (1-\text{sensitivity})/\text{specificity}$$

These formulas are available on many of the online EBM calculator sites. Crunching the numbers yields a positive likelihood ratio (LR+) of 7.1 and a negative likelihood ratio (LR−) of 0.1 against a gold standard diagnosis made by detailed informant history together with clinical evaluation by an examiner using DSM criteria. This means that conducting a brief informant interview and obtaining a score above 3.44 on this instrument would modestly increase the probability of dementia being present, whereas scores

<3.44 on this instrument would be likely to greatly reduce the probability of a diagnosis of dementia in a patient being examined. These are impressive operating characteristics for a brief test conducted in a challenging clinical setting. We thus wanted to appraise the Harwood study to see if the estimates of these operating characteristics were likely to be valid and generalizable to our clinical setting.

In our critical appraisal we felt that this study fell short of optimal STARD criteria and included appreciable risk for bias, which could result in the test characteristics appearing much better than they might actually be at discriminating demented from nondemented patients. We present the most important concerns we had from our appraisal using STARD below. Our comments correspond to the item numbers on that checklist. We focus, because of space constraints, on those items that, to our read, conferred a significant risk for bias.

Items 8, 9, and 10 from the STARD checklist (Table 33–2) regarding the reference standard diagnosis were of concern to us. The final process by which the reference standard diagnosis (DSM diagnosis of dementia or clinical diagnosis of other cognitive impairment) was assigned in this study was difficult to determine. The qualifications, expertise, and training of the person executing and reading the index (IQCODE) and reference standard tests were not specified in the body of the manuscript. The qualifications of the author cited as doing the assessment could be searched on the Internet, and he appeared to be an accomplished authority in his field. One challenge, despite the authority of the author, was to understand the process that he used to come to the gold standard diagnosis so that we could understand how accurate the estimate of the test's performance in agreement with this diagnosis was likely to be. STARD reminds us that this process should be clearly specified and reproducible so that the results of the research are replicable and the procedures used to reach a gold standard diagnosis do not introduce bias into the estimate of test accuracy. The procedures used in the study listed the tests performed for the reference standard but included sources of history and procedures for gathering information that were poorly specified and would be difficult to reproduce with the potential for introducing significant bias.

For example, in appraising the study for STARD item 11 we felt the procedures used introduced the possibility of a form of bias referred to as *clinical review bias*, in which interpretations of diagnostic procedures become more accurate by providing additional clinical information to interpreters. The methods section of the study describes that a single person, the author mentioned previously, performed the Confusion Assessment Method (Inouye et al. 1990) to detect delirium, the Abbreviated Mental Test (Hodkinson 1972), and the 16-item version of the IQCODE as well as "further standard psychiatric assessment…[which] included further cognitive assessment, obtaining a history from the informant and/or nursing staff and scrutinizing clinical notes." The additional clinical information provided by each test was likely to influence the findings of the other tests performed.

The author stated that "all patients with some evidence of abnormal cognitive function—either a positive screening test or a note indicating abnormal cognitive status in the clinical records—were assigned a DSM-III-R diagnosis, or if not meeting DSM criteria, a clinical diagnosis of their cognitive impairment." It appeared from this description that results of the IQCODE influenced whether the gold standard diagnostic procedures were performed and whether a DSM-III-R or clinical diagnosis was assigned, a source of bias referred to as *verification bias* (item 16), that could increase the estimate of diagnostic accuracy (Bossuyt et al. 2003b). The person assigning the criterion standard diagnosis was not blinded (item 11) to the findings of the index test, which were included in the gold standard diagnosis reached. The same person was assigning both diagnoses. This results in both *test review bias* and *diagnostic review bias*, both of which are likely to inflate the estimates of diagnostic accuracy. No confidence intervals about the point estimates for sensitivity and specificity were provided (item 21), nor was a cross-tabulation of the results of the index tests by the results of the reference standard given (item 19). The operating characteristics provided used optimal post hoc estimates, which were unlikely to be replicated. However, cutoff points suggested by the authors as the maximally discriminative values obtained from previous outpatient validation studies of the test with more rigorous designs had similar accuracy (test score cutoff >3.38 had a sensitivity of 100%, specificity 84%). There were no estimates of the variability of diagnostic accuracy or reproducibility provided.

Overall we felt that further study of this test with respect to a gold standard test using a more rigor-

TABLE 33–2.   STARD checklist of studies of diagnostic accuracy

Section and topic	Item #		On page
TITLE/ABSTRACT/ KEYWORDS	1	Identify the article as a study of diagnostic accuracy (recommend MeSH heading "sensitivity and specificity").	
INTRODUCTION	2	State the research questions or study aims, such as estimating diagnostic accuracy or comparing accuracy between tests or across participant groups.	
METHODS		Describe:	
Participants	3	The study population: The inclusion and exclusion criteria, setting and locations where data were collected.	
	4	Participant recruitment: Was recruitment based on presenting symptoms, results from previous tests, or the fact that the participants had received the index tests or the reference standard?	
	5	Participant sampling: Was the study population a consecutive series of participants defined by the selection criteria in item 3 and 4? If not, specify how participants were further selected.	
	6	Data collection: Was data collection planned before the index test and reference standard were performed (prospective study) or after (retrospective study)?	
Test methods	7	The reference standard and its rationale.	
	8	Technical specifications of material and methods involved including how and when measurements were taken, and/or cite references for index tests and reference standard.	
	9	Definition of and rationale for the units, cut-offs and/or categories of the results of the index tests and the reference standard.	
	10	The number, training and expertise of the persons executing and reading the index tests and the reference standard.	
	11	Whether or not the readers of the index tests and reference standard were blind (masked) to the results of the other test and describe any other clinical information available to the readers.	
Statistical methods	12	Methods for calculating or comparing measures of diagnostic accuracy, and the statistical methods used to quantify uncertainty (e.g. 95% confidence intervals).	
	13	Methods for calculating test reproducibility, if done.	
RESULTS		Report:	
Participants	14	When study was performed, including beginning and end dates of recruitment.	
	15	Clinical and demographic characteristics of the study population (at least information on age, gender, spectrum of presenting symptoms).	
	16	The number of participants satisfying the criteria for inclusion who did or did not undergo the index tests and/or the reference standard; describe why participants failed to undergo either test (a flow diagram is strongly recommended).	
Test results	17	Time-interval between the index tests and the reference standard, and any treatment administered in between.	
	18	Distribution of severity of disease (define criteria) in those with the target condition; other diagnoses in participants without the target condition.	
	19	A cross tabulation of the results of the index tests (including indeterminate and missing results) by the results of the reference standard; for continuous results, the distribution of the test results by the results of the reference standard.	
	20	Any adverse events from performing the index tests or the reference standard.	
Estimates	21	Estimates of diagnostic accuracy and measures of statistical uncertainty (e.g. 95% confidence intervals).	
	22	How indeterminate results, missing data and outliers of the index tests were handled.	
	23	Estimates of variability of diagnostic accuracy between subgroups of participants, readers or centers, if done.	
	24	Estimates of test reproducibility, if done.	
DISCUSSION	25	Discuss the clinical applicability of the study findings.	

Note.   MeSH=Medical Subject Heading; STARD=Standards for Reporting of Diagnostic Accuracy.

Source.   Bossuyt et al. 2003a. Available at: http://www.stard-statement.org.

ously controlled design would be likely to result in a change in the estimate of diagnostic accuracy and that the estimate provided in this study was likely to be inflated. The study performed in the ICU to estimate the prevalence of preexisting cognitive impairment (Pisani et al. 2003a) indicated that there was substantial agreement between the IQCODE and the Modified Blessed Dementia Rating Scale—another informant interview validated in outpatient settings—with a kappa of 0.69. This study was limited by the difficulty in establishing a gold standard diagnosis against which to estimate the operating characteristics of the test.

Apply

These studies appeared to be the only recent studies looking at methods to determine whether a patient might have a preexisting, nondelirious form of cognitive impairment, such as dementia, in the setting in which we found our patient. For our purposes we decided that despite the limitations, the IQCODE remained the best-studied instrument available for our purpose and that the point estimates derived from this limited study would represent our best estimate as to this test's accuracy. We felt that the accuracy estimate was likely to be biased in favor of greater accuracy than was warranted, and thus we made a mental note of this in our interpretation.

We thus contacted the patient's family to obtain their impression of the patient's mental state at baseline prior to admission and to administer the IQCODE. The patient had been married for 53 years. His wife was in her early 70s and was a retired administrative assistant for the local technology company where the patient had worked for many years. She had been with the patient daily prior to the hospitalization. He also had a daughter in her mid-40s who was a schoolteacher in the local area. Both appeared to be good historians and had spent a minimum of 4 hours per week with the patient for at least 10 years as was suggested by the IQCODE procedure.

They were contacted for interview over the telephone. They informed us that they had just the left the hospital and were going to get something to eat after being at the bedside for many hours that day as they had each day since admission. They were quite concerned about the patient's mental state. They had never known the patient to be depressed or anxious previously, and he had never before seen a psychiatrist for any reason. His wife felt that he was in good

spirits prior to the admission and he seemed to be dealing fairly well with the knowledge that his cancer had returned. He had expressed hopefulness and confidence in the surgical approach recommended by his doctors, although he was anxious as to whether his heart would tolerate the procedure. After receiving the diagnosis he seemed to still be able to enjoy visiting with friends and family as he had before. He still paid the bills for the household and was quite active. He had been productively employed as an engineer at a local technology company until about 8 years before he was admitted. He had slowed down somewhat after his heart surgery in 1991, but he still managed to enjoy his activities and to manage his affairs without difficulty. Neither she nor her daughter had noticed any significant decline in his memory or ability to take care of things around the house in the years preceding his current admission. They described him as being "as sharp as ever" before his hospitalization. We went through each item on the 16-item IQCODE together, comparing his cognitive abilities 1 month prior to his admission to his performance 10 years before as was done in Pisani et al. (2003a). The final score was 3.1, which was a negative result using the cut point of 3.44 suggested by the authors.

Remember that the Bayes theorem tells us that the findings of the test must be considered together with the pretest probability of the condition before a diagnosis is assigned. Remember representativeness bias. This is the clinical error that occurs when we assume that test results rule in and rule out diagnoses without considering the probability of the diagnosis and the fact that each test has false positives and negatives and is not perfect. We use information from the pretest probability of dementia together with the negative findings of this test to estimate our posttest probability of dementia.

We assumed a pretest probability of dementia for hospitalized patients in the ICU of 42% from the best estimate we had available (Pisani et al. 2003a). We had an optimistic estimate of the operating characteristics of the IQCODE from the Harwood et al. (1997) study, which provided a negative likelihood ratio of 0.1. We combined these pieces of information to estimate the posttest probability of dementia using an adaptation of Fagan's nomogram (Fagan 1975; Glasziou 2001). See the introductory chapters from McGee (2007) or the article by Sackett (1992) for more on how to do this if this is confusing to you. This approach resulted in an estimate of the posttest

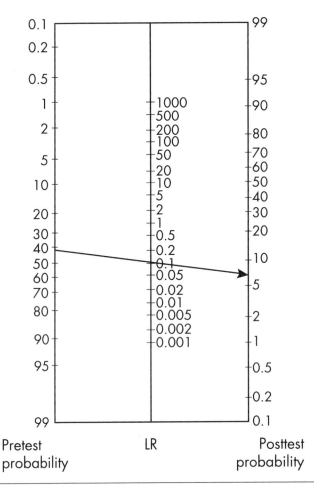

FIGURE 33–2.   Likelihood ratio (LR) nomogram for posttest probability of dementia.

probability of dementia as being fairly unlikely, in the range of 5%–10%, as plotted in Figure 33–2. (An online automated version of Fagan's nomogram can be found at www.cebm.net/index.aspx?o=1161.)

Because we had previously appraised this literature and had this information easily available to us, our rough estimate of the probability of dementia took less than 10 minutes to acquire, including our conversation with the patient's wife, which took the bulk of the time, and the previous calculations using the nomogram, which took approximately 10 seconds. While the precision of the quantitative estimate of the probability of dementia was somewhat uncertain given the biases likely to be present in the validation of the test, we were confident in our clinical judgment at this point that the history pointed to a much more acute change in the patient's mental status that would be much more consistent with delirium than with dementia. The results certainly had clinical face validity, and the focused questions in the

assessment included in the IQCODE were likely to have prompted us to consider more carefully symptoms that we might not otherwise have assessed for without a structured questionnaire. We decided to continue to investigate for the possibility of delirium being present in our patient.

Does the Patient Have Delirium?

Given the frequency with which we encounter delirium in our practice setting we also hoped to have a soundly validated procedure with known operating characteristics that we might use together with estimates of pretest probability to provide an accurate assessment of the probability of delirium being present in our patient. We had thus formed and sought an answer to the following PICO question.

Ask

*P*atient/population: Patients in intensive care unit settings.

*I*ntervention: Brief, bedside diagnostic methods for assessing for delirium.

*C*omparison: More extensive expert clinical consensus diagnosis using DSM criterion.

*O*utcome: Outcome measures as before—likelihood ratios positive and negative, estimates of interrater reliability such as kappa.

Acquire

In our previous searches of the medical literature we found a handful of studies addressing this question. One method developed for the ICU for assessing mechanically intubated, nonverbal patients is the Confusion Assessment Method for the Intensive Care Unit (CAM-ICU) (Ely et al. 2001a, 2001b).

• We encourage the reader to stop here and obtain a copy of the article in *JAMA* for the validation of this study (Ely et al. 2001a), if fortunate enough to have full-text access. Please also print out the STARD checklist and critically appraise this and see if you agree with our summary below. No peeking!

Appraise

The validation study for this instrument in our opinion was quite strong with respect to the STARD criteria (Ely et al. 2001a). By going through the checklist we detected very little risk for bias in the methods used. The validation study did exclude assessment of patients with a previous history of psychosis and neurologic disease (limited challenge bias), of which we made note. The study did not provide a cross-tabulation of the results of the index tests by the results of the reference standard, reporting the summary operating characteristics only. Overall, however, the study addressed each of the major threats to validity for studies of diagnostic accuracy. The use of the CAM-ICU appeared to be significantly more rapid (a mean of 2 minutes, with a standard deviation of 1 minute) than the gold standard assessment (30–45 minutes) using usual clinical methods of arriving at a DSM-IV-TR diagnosis. Overall our critical appraisal by the STARD criteria suggested future studies of this instrument would be unlikely to result in a significant change in the operating characteristics reported. The positive likelihood ratio for this test was quite strong, with point estimates for each assessor at 50 (95% confidence

interval [CI] 20–77) and >100 (95% CI 21 to >100). The negative likelihood ratio was not reported. Using the sensitivity and specificity data we estimated point estimates for the LR– to be 0 and 0.07, respectively. It had excellent interrater reliability, with a kappa of 0.96 (95% CI 0.92–0.99). We were more confident in the estimates provided by the validation report of this test than in those provided by the IQ-CODE as a result of the stronger design and reporting of the study.

Apply

Training information (www.icudelirium.org) was available that led our team to feel confident in our ability to use the CAM-ICU in our setting. We have thus adopted this instrument into our routine assessment of mechanically ventilated patients in the ICU for delirium, but do note that this test has not been validated in patients with preexisting cognitive or neurologic impairment and that its operating characteristics in these populations are likely to be significantly less strong.

The patient's wife and daughter described having visited with him daily since the operation. They noted that shortly after the surgery they had noticed a marked change in his emotions and behavior that were very troubling to them. At times the patient seemed to be frightened, suspicious, and confused. At other times he seemed to be very tearful. He was often inattentive and would nod off to sleep. He was "trembling" and "sweaty." They were quite concerned to see him crying and nodding his head when the doctors asked him if he was depressed and hopeless, because he had always been a very optimistic man. When they tried to console him and talk to him about how he was feeling they found that he seemed to be confused and agitated, which appeared very out of character for him. They had never previously noticed that he had any problems with his memory, but he seemed to be unable to recall important information or to be confused, although it was never easy to know because he was unable to speak.

The nursing staff from the night shift prior to our consultation had noted that the patient attempted to drink water at the bedside despite being NPO. The patient's wife and daughter described this behavior as being very out of character for him. The vigorousness of his attempts to obtain water and get out of bed had appeared to prompt his receiving lorazepam and hydrocodone. At other times, according to the records provided by the physical therapist, he appeared sullen, apathetic, and withdrawn.

In performing the CAM-ICU (Figure 33–3) we noted that the Richmond Agitation-Sedation Scale (RASS) score ranged between +3 on the evening prior to our examining the patient when he attempted to get out of bed and to obtain water to –1 at the time we initially came to see him in which he was drowsy but able to open his eyes to verbal stimulation and keep them open for more than 10 seconds. This, together with the history obtained by the patient's wife and daughter, satisfied the acute onset or fluctuating course criterion for us. He exhibited marked difficulty with attention and had markedly disorganized thinking on these items of the CAM-ICU, answering inappropriately to questions such as "Are there fish in the sea?" "Does a stone float on water?" "Can you use a hammer to pound a nail?" He also exhibited difficulty in following the command. Thus we felt the CAM-ICU overall was positive and we were then able to proceed to estimate a quantitative probability of delirium being present in this patient.

Pretest probability estimates of delirium in studies using the CAM-ICU excluding patients with neurologic illness and psychosis range between 22% and 87%, with most of the estimates being closer to the high end of the range (83%, 87%, 47%, 22%) (Devlin et al. 2007). Assuming even the most conservative pretest probability estimate of 22% and the more conservative of the two-point estimates of the likelihood ratio positive of 50, the posttest probability for delirium is >90% (Figure 33–4).

We thus felt that it was extremely likely that our patient was in fact delirious and that the cognitive, emotional, and behavioral symptoms should not at this time be assumed to be secondary to depression as the primary team had been considering prior to our consultation. We felt that the depressive symptoms were more likely to be those that are often displayed in conjunction with the delirium syndrome that had been previously reported (Boland et al. 1996; Farrell and Ganzini 1995; Nicholas and Lindsey 1995; Swigart et al. 2008).

What is the Differential Diagnosis of the Delirium Syndrome?

A recent guideline on delirium written consistently with the conventions established by AGREE (Appraisal of Guidelines Research and Evaluation;

AGREE Collaboration 2003) was consulted for guidance (British Geriatrics Society 2006). Our assessment process was not yet complete because the most important action for the management of delirium is the identification and treatment of potential underlying reversible causes (British Geriatrics Society 2006). The differential diagnosis of the many suspected causes of delirium is quite lengthy and poorly studied, and a detailed discussion is beyond the scope of the space we have. Many risk factors have been described for the development of delirium (mostly from non-ICU cohorts), although none has been proved with a strong association or definite causality (Devlin et al. 2007; Kraemer et al. 1997). The pretest probabilities of these risk factors are poorly defined, making workup challenging.

The underlying cause of delirium is often considered to be multifactorial. Common contributory medical causes of delirium include (British Geriatrics Society 2006):

- Infection (e.g., pneumonia, urinary tract infection)
- Cardiac illness (e.g., myocardial infarction, heart failure)
- Respiratory disorder (e.g., pulmonary embolus, hypoxia)
- Electrolyte imbalance (e.g., dehydration, renal failure, hyponatremia)
- Endocrine and metabolic disorder (e.g., cachexia, thiamine deficiency, thyroid dysfunction)
- Drugs (particularly those with anticholinergic side effects [e.g., tricyclic antidepressants, antiparkinsonian drugs, opiates, analgesics, steroids])
- Drug (especially benzodiazepine) and alcohol withdrawal
- Urinary retention
- Fecal impaction
- Severe pain
- Neurological problem (e.g., stroke, subdural hematoma, epilepsy, encephalitis)
- Multiple contributing causes

In Mr. C.K.'s case, several of these possible risk factors were known to be present. We anticipated that identification of a single culprit that caused his delirium might be unlikely, but we felt it could be important to see if potential causes could be identified, for which treatment had not been initiated, that if treated might reduce his risk for harm.

CAM-ICU Worksheet

	Positive	Negative
Feature 1: Acute Onset or Fluctuating Course Positive if you answer 'yes' to either 1A or 1B.	Positive	Negative
1A: Is the pt different than his/her baseline mental status? Or **1B:** Has the patient had any fluctuation in mental status in the past 24 hours as evidenced by fluctuation on a sedation scale (e.g. RASS), GCS, or previous delirium assessment?	Yes	No
Feature 2: Inattention Positive if either score for 2A or 2B is less than 8. Attempt the ASE Letters first. If pt is able to perform this test and the score is clear, record this score and move to Feature 3. If pt is unable to perform this test or the score is unclear, then perform the ASE Pictures. If you perform both tests, use the ASE Pictures' results to score the Feature.	Positive	Negative
2A: ASE Letters: record score (enter NT for not tested) <u>Directions:</u> Say to the patient, "I am going to read you a series of 10 letters. Whenever you hear the letter 'A,' indicate by squeezing my hand." Read letters from the following letter list in a normal tone. **S A V E A H A A R T** Scoring: Errors are counted when patient fails to squeeze on the letter "A" and when the patient squeezes on any letter other than "A."	Score (out of 10): _____	
2B: ASE Pictures: record score (enter NT for not tested) Directions are included on the picture packets.	Score (out of 10): _____	
Feature 3: Disorganized Thinking Positive if the combined score is less than 4	Positive	Negative
3A: Yes/No Questions (Use either Set A or Set B, alternate on consecutive days if necessary): **Set A** 1. Will a stone float on water? 2. Are there fish in the sea? 3. Does one pound weigh more than two pounds? 4. Can you use a hammer to pound a nail? **Set B** 1. Will a leaf float on water? 2. Are there elephants in the sea? 3. Do two pounds weigh more than one pound? 4. Can you use a hammer to cut wood? Score ___ (Patient earns 1 point for each correct answer out of 4) <u>3B: Command</u> Say to patient: "Hold up this many fingers" (Examiner holds two fingers in front of patient) "Now do the same thing with the other hand" (Not repeating the number of fingers). *If pt is unable to move both arms, for the second part of the command ask patient "Add one more finger." Score___ (Patient earns 1 point if able to successfully complete the entire command)	**Combined Score (3A+3B):** _____ (out of 5)	
Feature 4: Altered Level of Consciousness Positive if the Actual RASS score is anything other than "0" (zero)	Positive	Negative
Overall CAM-ICU (Features 1 and 2 and either Feature 3 or 4):	Positive	Negative

FIGURE 33–3. Worksheet from the Confusion Assessment Method for the Intensive Care Unit (CAM-ICU) training manual

ASE=Attention Screening Examination; GCS=Glasgow Coma Score; pt=patient; RASS=Richmond Agitation-Sedation Scale.

Source. Ely EW: *The Confusion Assessment Method for the Intensive Care Unit (CAM-ICU): Training Manual.* Copyright 2002, E. Wesley Ely, M.D., M.P.H. and Vanderbilt University, all rights reserved. Used with permission.

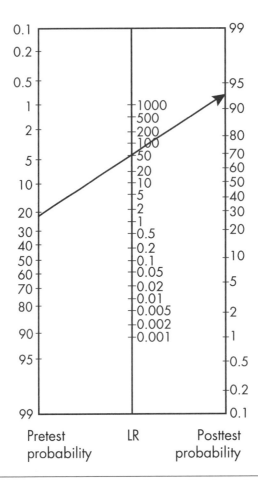

FIGURE 33–4.   Likelihood ratio (LR) nomogram for posttest probability of delirium.

The possibility of medication-induced mental status changes as a result of the opiates and intermittent benzodiazepines that he was receiving appeared likely. The possibility of alcohol use and withdrawal were especially of concern because his alcohol and substance use had not been well documented in the record, and he was noted to have been trembling and diaphoretic by his family. He had several possible reasons for tachycardia, but his pulse remained elevated despite correction of these factors and he continued to exhibit tremor and diaphoresis.

Worsening of his cardiac and respiratory function was a possible contributor, given his previous smoking history and known cardiac disease, the tachyarrythmias noted, and his pulmonary congestion. His atrial fibrillation was now more optimally rate controlled, his breathing and chest X ray were improved, and his ECG and cardiac enzymes were unremarkable. He had an echocardiogram performed, which had shown normal left ventricular (LV) size with LV systolic function at lower limits of normal

and inferior wall hypokinesis, and mildly thickened mitral valve with mild mitral regurgitation. The right ventricle was of normal size, with normal ejection fraction. Both atria were severely dilated. Findings were unchanged compared with the prior study from 6 months prior to admission. He was no longer tachypneic, his oxygen saturation and arterial blood gas were unremarkable. He had no unilateral lower extremity edema or pain with palpation of his deep leg veins, he had no hemoptysis, and his acute hypoxia seemed to be better accounted for by congestive heart failure than by a pulmonary embolus. However, he was recently immobilized and had surgery for his cancer, and he was tachycardic, which did indicate a moderate pretest probability by the simplified Wells criteria for a pulmonary embolus (Chunilal et al. 2003).

The possibility of infection was present given his recent fever. Several possible sites could be considered. He had recently had his procedure on his larynx, he also had complications of his gastrostomy tube extravasation into his peritoneal space, and he had respiratory difficulties and abnormal urinalysis. His fever, together with his having been ventilated, with new infiltrates on chest X ray, could suggest a pulmonary infection. The absence of a white count or shift and the absence of purulent sputum could not exclude the possibility of infection (Klompas 2007). He did have other reasons to have a pulmonary infiltrate and did seem to be responding well to treatment. The bladder catheter and central venous catheters were other possible sources of infection. Blood, sputum, and urine cultures had been sent to the lab, and the patient had been started on antibiotics.

A cerebrovascular accident was possible given his recent unanticoagulated atrial fibrillation; however, his neurologic exam was unremarkable, with the exception of his altered mental state, and a head computed tomographic image obtained prior to our consultation by the medical service was unremarkable. We felt this was less likely.

The patient's family denied he had any significant visual or hearing impairment or any history of depression, dementia, or other psychiatric illnesses.

The most important possibility that did not seem to have been adequately considered was alcohol withdrawal. We thus asked the family if the patient consumed alcohol, and they indicated that he did not like to talk about this because he knew the doctors did not approve of this given his throat cancer. They did acknowledge, when informed that this could have important and possibly life-threatening consequences, that he had consumed alcohol in addition to cigarettes for many years and that he continued up until the night prior to hospitalization to consume at least three to four cocktails every evening, and he was known at times to have more. This had not previously been noted in the history. The patient remained tachycardic, which had reasonably been attributed to the many factors cited previously plus postoperative pain and discomfort. His recent tremulousness and disturbance in mental state had been attributed to anxiety and emotional upset. Alcohol withdrawal delirium rose to be included as a possible contributing factor that would be likely to require a change in the management of the patient. We considered it difficult to determine, however, whether all of the symptoms of autonomic hyperarousal could be because of alcohol withdrawal but felt that the risk was high enough that it should be considered. The other factors were being carefully considered in the management of the patient, and treatment decisions were being made accordingly.

We discussed our impression with the team and the patient's family. The patient was assessed as lacking the capacity to understand his current condition, the treatment recommendations, and alternatives, including the consequences of not receiving treatment, and thus we felt he could not provide informed consent for his care. We thus recommended that the patient's wife act as a surrogate for her husband. We discussed the general guidelines suggested for the management of delirium (British Geriatrics Society 2006), noting that the patient was hyperactive at times and at risk for falls. Shortly after we were consulted he had attempted to pull out his intravenous lines. We felt that this hyperactive delirium and the risk for the complications of alcohol withdrawal were going to require pharmacological intervention. We advised this in addition to the environmental interventions suggested by the guideline. This guideline did not cover alcohol withdrawal, and thus treatment recommendations for the pharmacologic management of alcohol withdrawal were made in reference to a previously appraised systematic review of reasonable quality (Mayo-Smith et al. 2004) on alcohol withdrawal delirium. It was noted that injudicious use of symptom-triggered withdrawal protocols could be associated with harms in patients unable to communicate well who had alternative causes of their symptoms that might be consistent with those symptoms produced by alcohol withdrawal (Hecksel et al. 2008). Making treatment recommendations for this type of case is more challenging than for the typical alcohol withdrawal delirium case. The Clinical Institute Withdrawal Assessment for Alcohol was not considered an appropriate instrument for following the patient's progress given his inability to communicate well and was not recommended. Treatment of delirium with benzodiazepines has been considered to be a risk factor for worsening delirium by one small randomized controlled trial of modest quality in hospitalized AIDS patients (Breitbart et al. 1996) and is often cited as a possible causal risk factor based upon observational studies of varying quality in general medical patients (British Geriatrics Society 2006).

We opted to recommend that the team follow the patient's vital signs and CAM-ICU ratings each shift and to use intravenous lorazepam with the goal of attaining light sedation to the point of a Richmond

Agitation-Sedation Scale score of –1 during the day, with sleep the goal overnight, consistent with the recommendations in the systematic review by Mayo-Smith (Mayo-Smith et al. 2004). We felt that despite the CAM's dichotomous nature, the RASS score would be valuable along with the vital signs and other signs of autonomic hyperactivity in continuing to guide our approach, which was focused on reducing the risks of hyperactive delirium (line pulling, getting out of bed, taking things orally despite NPO status) and the effects of alcohol withdrawal. Because other possible causes of delirium were present, we discussed additional use of a neuroleptic agent (Lonergan et al. 2007) if the intervention with the benzodiazepine was ineffective and the patient remained severely agitated and at risk for pulling lines or falling from his bed. We opted for a watchful waiting approach given the patient's prolonged QTc of 470 msec (Ray et al. 2009) and opted to see if he might respond to the benzodiazepine protocol first. The patient's wife provided informed consent, and treatment along these lines was initiated.

The patient's course gradually improved. The remainder of his medical course was relatively unremarkable. He suffered no obvious motor seizures or worsening of his medical condition. He was intermittently hypoactively delirious by CAM-ICU criteria for several more days. He was no longer hyperactively delirious, however, and was significantly calmer, with markedly decreased agitation, tremor, diaphoresis, and tachycardia. He required no neuroleptics. His mental status improved significantly to being CAM-ICU negative consistently after 1 week, although residual cognitive symptoms remained at 2 weeks, at which time the patient had been completely titrated off of all benzodiazepines and had recovered medically sufficiently to be discharged from the hospital. We recommended that he be discharged home with additional in-home nursing support made available to him. We noted, on the basis of the limited literature in this area, that his prognosis could possibly include longer-term cognitive difficulties that might be significant and that might require continued supportive resources for him and his wife (Gordon et al. 2004).

• Now take a moment to review the list of three to five diagnoses that you wrote down at the start of the case presentation. *Hindsight bias* occurs when we overestimate the probability of a given diagnosis when that diagnosis has been established previously (Bornstein and Emler 2001). Things often appear quite obvious in looking backwards at a case. We hope that the previous case presentation was helpful in discussing some of the common biases affecting our judgment and decision making and that you find some things in the discussion of use in your practice.

Summary

- Selecting a treatment intervention strongly supported by high-quality randomized controlled trials is unlikely to benefit the patient and may cause harm if the diagnosis is incorrect. Treating this patient for major depressive disorder or even for delirium with a neuroleptic agent given his cardiac history, prolonged QTc, and likely alcohol withdrawal could have resulted in a poorer outcome.

- The EBM approach to diagnosis is still in its infancy. The literature is sparse, and there are not yet large repositories of systematic reviews of diagnostic accuracy or precision available to the clinician.

- Various approaches to generating a differential diagnosis can be considered. One might consider combining approaches to avoid common biases that result in diagnostic error: a broad differential diagnosis can be generated (possibilistic approach) that weights more heavily those causes that cannot be missed (prognostic approach) as well as those that are highly likely in that practice setting (probabilistic approach) that can be treated resulting in better patient outcomes (pragmatic approach).

- The *DSM-IV-TR Handbook of Differential Diagnosis* (First et al. 2002) can be used to quickly generate a differential diagnosis likely to be consistent with those considered in randomized controlled trials in psychiatry.

- Carefully considering estimates of the pretest probability of conditions that are pertinent in the differential diagnosis in the setting in which the patient is encountered is important in making a valid diagnosis and avoiding representativeness bias.

- Preappraisal of bedside diagnostic procedures important in clinical settings for the common diagnoses encountered may increase the speed and confidence in the diagnoses assigned in those settings.

- The STARD checklist or other structured appraisal tools for diagnostic quality can be used to assist practitioners in identifying and assembling a toolkit of valid and reliable appraisal instruments for approaching the common differential diagnoses occurring in their practice settings.

- The operating characteristics of various diagnostic tests can be considered together with the pretest probabilities of the conditions being considered to estimate the posttest probability of that condition being present, because tests are not perfect and representativeness bias can strike again.
- Good clinical judgment is necessary at every step.

References

AGREE Collaboration: Development and validation of an international appraisal instrument for assessing the quality of clinical practice guidelines: the AGREE project. Qual Saf Health Care 12:18–23, 2003

American Psychiatric Association: Diagnostic and Statistical Manual of Mental Disorders, 4th Edition, Text Revision. Washington, DC, American Psychiatric Association, 2000

Ardern M, Mayou R, Feldman E, et al: Cognitive impairment in the elderly medically ill: how often is it missed? Int J Geriatr Psychiatry 8:929–937, 1993

Bandolier: Evidence and diagnostics. February 2002. Available at: http://www.medicine.ox.ac.uk/bandolier/booth/diagnos/Diagessy.html. Accessed May 18, 2009

Boland RJ, Diaz S, Lamdan RM, et al: Overdiagnosis of depression in the general hospital. Gen Hosp Psychiatry 18:28–35, 1996

Bornstein BH, Emler AC: Rationality in medical decision making: a review of the literature on doctors' decision-making biases. J Eval Clin Pract 7:97–107, 2001

Bossuyt PM, Reitsma JB, Bruns DE, et al: The STARD statement for reporting studies of diagnostic accuracy: explanation and elaboration. Ann Intern Med 138:W1–W12, 2003a

Bossuyt PM, Reitsma JB, Bruns DE, et al: Towards complete and accurate reporting of studies of diagnostic accuracy: the STARD Initiative. Ann Intern Med 138:40–44, 2003b

Boustani M, Peterson B, Hanson L, et al: Screening for dementia in primary care: a summary of the evidence for the U.S. Preventive Services Task Force. Ann Intern Med 138:927–937, 2003

Breitbart W, Marotta R, Platt MM, et al: A double-blind trial of haloperidol, chlorpromazine, and lorazepam in the treatment of delirium in hospitalized AIDS patients. Am J Psychiatry 153:231–237, 1996

British Geriatrics Society: Guidelines for the prevention, diagnosis and management of delirium in older people: concise guidance to good practice series. January 2006. Available at: http://www.bgs.org.uk/Publications/Clini-cal%20Guidelines/clinical_1-2_fulldelirium.htm. Accessed May 28, 2009

Casscells W, Schoenberger A, Graboys TB: Interpretation by physicians of clinical laboratory results. N Engl J Med 299:999–1001, 1978

Chodosh J, Petitti DB, Elliott M, et al: Physician recognition of cognitive impairment: evaluating the need for improvement. J Am Geriatr Soc 52:1051–1059, 2004

Chunilal SD, Eikelboom JW, Attia J, et al: Does this patient have pulmonary embolism? JAMA 290:2849–2858, 2003

Deeks JJ, Altman DG: Diagnostic tests 4: likelihood ratios. BMJ 329:168–169, 2004

Devlin JW, Fong JJ, Fraser GL, et al: Delirium assessment in the critically ill. Intensive Care Med 33:929–940, 2007

Ely EW, Inouye SK, Bernard GR, et al: Delirium in mechanically ventilated patients: validity and reliability of the Confusion Assessment Method for the Intensive Care Unit (CAM-ICU). JAMA 286:2703–2710, 2001a

Ely EW, Margolin R, Francis J, et al: Evaluation of delirium in critically ill patients: validation of the Confusion Assessment Method for the Intensive Care Unit (CAM-ICU). Crit Care Med 29:1370–1379, 2001b

Ely EW, Shintani A, Truman B, et al: Delirium as a predictor of mortality in mechanically ventilated patients in the intensive care unit. JAMA 291:1753–1762, 2004

Fagan TJ: Nomogram for Bayes theorem (letter). N Engl J Med 293:257, 1975

Farrell KR, Ganzini L: Misdiagnosing delirium as depression in medically ill elderly patients. Arch Intern Med 155:2459–2464, 1995

First MB, Frances A, Pincus HA: DSM-IV-TR Handbook of Differential Diagnosis. Washington, DC, American Psychiatric Publishing, 2002

Ghosh AK, Ghosh K, Erwin PJ: Do medical students and physicians understand probability? QJM 97:53–55, 2004

Glasziou P: Which methods for bedside Bayes? Evid Based Med 6:164–166, 2001

Gordon SM, Jackson JC, Ely EW, et al: Clinical identification of cognitive impairment in ICU survivors: insights for intensivists. Intensive Care Med 30:1997–2008, 2004

Gustafson Y, Brännström B, Norberg A, et al: Underdiagnosis and poor documentation of acute confusional states in elderly hip fracture patients. J Am Geriatr Soc 39:760–765, 1991

Harwood DM, Hope T, Jacoby R: Cognitive impairment in medical inpatients. I: Screening for dementia—is history better than mental state? Age Ageing 26:31–35, 1997

Hecksel KA, Bostwick JM, Jaeger TM, et al: Inappropriate use of symptom-triggered therapy for alcohol withdrawal in the general hospital. Mayo Clin Proc 83:274–279, 2008

Hodkinson HM: Evaluation of a mental test score for assessment of mental impairment in the elderly. Age Ageing 1:233–238, 1972

Holsinger T, Deveau J, Boustani M, et al: Does this patient have dementia? JAMA 297:2391–2404, 2007

Inouye SK: Delirium in hospitalized older patients: recognition and risk factors. J Geriatr Psychiatry Neurol 11:118–125; discussion 157–158, 1998

Inouye SK, van Dyck CH, Alessi CA, et al: Clarifying confusion: the confusion assessment method. A new method for detection of delirium. Ann Intern Med 113:941–948, 1990

Inouye SK, Foreman MD, Mion LC, et al: Nurses' recognition of delirium and its symptoms: comparison of nurse and researcher ratings. Arch Intern Med 161:2467–2473, 2001

Jorm AF: The Informant Questionnaire on Cognitive Decline in the Elderly (IQCODE): a review. Int Psychogeriatr 16:275–293, 2004

Kahneman D, Slovic P, Tversky A (eds): Judgment Under Uncertainty: Heuristics and Biases. Cambridge, UK, Cambridge University Press, 1982

Klompas M: Does this patient have ventilator-associated pneumonia? JAMA 297:1583–1593, 2007

Kraemer HC, Kazdin AE, Offord DR, et al: Coming to terms with the terms of risk. Arch Gen Psychiatry 54:337–343, 1997

Lonergan E, Britton AM, Luxenberg J, et al: Antipsychotics for delirium. Cochrane Database Syst Rev (2):CD005594, 2007

Lyman GH, Balducci L: Overestimation of test effects in clinical judgment. J Cancer Educ 8:297–307, 1993

Lyman GH, Balducci L: The effect of changing disease risk on clinical reasoning. J Gen Intern Med 9:488–495, 1994

Mascola AJ: Guided mentorship in evidence-based medicine for psychiatry: a pilot cohort study supporting a promising method of real-time clinical instruction. Acad Psychiatry 32:475–483, 2008

Mayo-Smith MF, Beecher LH, Fischer TL, et al: Management of alcohol withdrawal delirium: an evidence-based practice guideline. Arch Intern Med 164:1405–1412, 2004

McCusker J, Cole M, Abrahamowicz M, et al: Delirium predicts 12-month mortality. Arch Intern Med 162:457–463, 2002

McGee S: Evidence-Based Physical Diagnosis. Philadelphia, PA, WB Saunders, 2007

Nicholas LM, Lindsey BA: Delirium presenting with symptoms of depression. Psychosomatics 36:471–479, 1995

Olafsdottir M, Skoog I, Marcusson J: Detection of dementia in primary care: the Linkoping study. Dement Geriatr Cogn Disord 11: 223–229, 2000

Pauker S, Kassirer J: The threshold approach to clinical decision making. N Engl J Med 302:1109–1117, 1980

Pisani MA, Inouye SK, McNicoll L, et al: Screening for preexisting cognitive impairment in older intensive care unit patients: use of proxy assessment. J Am Geriatr Soc 51:689–693, 2003a

Pisani MA, Redlich C, McNicoll L, et al: Underrecognition of preexisting cognitive impairment by physicians in older ICU patients. Chest 124:2267–2274, 2003b

Ray WA, Chung CP, Murray KT, et al: Atypical Antipsychotic Drugs and the Risk of Sudden Cardiac Death. N Engl J Med 360:225–235, 2009

Richardson WS: We should overcome the barriers to evidence-based clinical diagnosis! J Clin Epidemiol 60:217–227, 2007

Richardson WS, Wilson MC, Nishikawa J, et al: The well-built clinical question: a key to evidence-based decisions. ACP J Club 123:A12–A3, 1995

Richardson WS, Wilson MC, Guyatt GH, et al: Users' guides to the medical literature: XV. How to use an article about disease probability for differential diagnosis. Evidence-Based Medicine Working Group. JAMA 281:1214–1219, 1999

Richardson WS, Glasziou P, Polashenski WA, et al: A new arrival: evidence about differential diagnosis. ACP J Club, 133:A11–A12, 2000a

Richardson WS, Wilson MC, Williams JW Jr, et al: Users' guides to the medical literature: XXIV. How to use an article on the clinical manifestations of disease. Evidence-Based Medicine Working Group. JAMA 284:869–875, 2000b

Richardson WS, Polashenski WA, Robbins BW: Could our pretest probabilities become evidence based? A prospective survey of hospital practice. J Gen Intern Med 18:203–208, 2003

Roca RP, Klein LE, Kirby SM, et al: Recognition of dementia among medical patients. Arch Intern Med 144:73–75, 1984

Rothman AJ, Kiviniemi MT: Treating people with information: an analysis and review of approaches to communicating health risk information. J Natl Cancer Inst Monogr 25:44–51, 1999

Sackett DL: The rational clinical examination. A primer on the precision and accuracy of the clinical examination. JAMA 267:2638–2644, 1992

Sackett DL, Straus SE: Finding and applying evidence during clinical rounds: the "evidence cart." JAMA 280:1336–1338, 1998

Siddiqi N, House AO, Homes JD: Occurrence and outcome of delirium in medical in-patients: a systematic literature review. Age Ageing 35:350–364, 2006

Steurer J, Fischer JE, Bachmann LM, et al: Communicating accuracy of tests to general practitioners: a controlled study. BMJ 324: 824–826, 2002

Streiner DL: Diagnosing tests: using and misusing diagnostic and screening tests. J Pers Assess 81:209–219, 2003

Swigart SE, Kishi Y, Thurber S, et al: Misdiagnosed delirium in patient referrals to a university-based hospital psychiatry department. Psychosomatics 49:104–108, 2008

Valcour VG, Masaki KH, Curb JD, et al: The detection of dementia in the primary care setting. Arch Intern Med 160:2964–2968, 2000

Whiting PF, Weswood ME, Rutjes AW, et al: Evaluation of QUADAS, a tool for the quality assessment of diagnostic accuracy studies. BMC Med Res Methodol 6:9, 2006

Alcohol Dependence Treated by a Psychiatry Resident

Violeta Tan, M.D.

Setting

This patient was treated while I was on a 6-month rotation during my fourth year as an adult psychiatry resident in a university outpatient clinic. The clinic serves a mostly insured population with a broad ethnic diversity. The focus is on short-term therapies using a combination of psychotherapy and psychopharmacology.

Illustration

- Use of the American Psychiatric Association (APA) *Practice Guideline for the Treatment of Patients With Substance Use Disorders* (2006)
- Use of relapse prevention strategies
- Use of motivational interviewing principles
- Use of psychotherapy termination recommendations

Chief Complaint

Ms. M.T. is a 35-year-old divorced female engineer who presents with a chief complaint of depression.

Present Illness

Ms. M.T. had been seen by two previous adult psychiatry residents over a span of 8 months prior to my first meeting her. She initially presented to the clinic with worsening depressive symptoms following her discontinuation of citalopram. Psychosocial stressors included financial negotiations related to her divorce and her son's living with her ex-husband. She was restarted on citalopram, which was eventually augmented with bupropion.

She had been drinking approximately a quarter to a half of a bottle of wine per night over the past 3 years. She noted diminished effect with continued use of the same amount and admitted the amount had increased over a longer period than she had intended. Furthermore, she found herself often turning to alcohol instead of engaging in her usual recreational or social activities, losing touch with friends in the process. She reported feeling the need to cut down on her drinking, and, although her previous mental health care providers had encouraged her to stop drinking and to attend Alcoholics Anonymous (AA), she resisted their recommendations for months. However, the day after termination with her previous psychiatrist, before beginning therapy with me, the patient did attend AA and decided to abstain.

On our first meeting, Ms. M.T. was proud of herself for having attended AA. Yet she also admitted to feelings of grief and loss in not having alcohol available any longer. She shared that she often used alcohol as a coping mechanism to quell feelings of sadness and isolation. Further review of psychiatric symptoms revealed anhedonia, sleep disturbances with awakenings in the middle of the night, energy loss, and concentration difficulties. Her appetite was better than usual and she denied thoughts of self-harm. In addition to her current symptoms, she provided a clear past history of depression in the absence of substances. Ms. M.T. reported continuing depression over her failed marriage, financial burdens, and worries about future interactions with her ex-husband. She furthermore described a longing to return to her hometown on the East Coast where her family resided yet also felt obligated to remain in her current location for her 13-year-old son, who was in his last year of grade school.

Other Significant Findings From Assessment

Ms. M.T. denied tobacco use. She drank about two cups of a caffeinated beverage each day. She did not exercise regularly and was unsatisfied with her weight. Family history was significant for alcoholism and anxiety among her grandparents, parents, and siblings. Siblings and grandparents also suffered from depression.

DSM-IV-TR Diagnosis

Axis I   Major depressive disorder, recurrent
           Alcohol dependence
Axis II   None
Axis III   Asthma
Axis IV   Limited social support, strain with ex-husband, living circumstances, financial burden
Axis V   GAF score: 60

Treatment Plan Considerations

Problems

The patient's main problems were depression and alcohol dependence. In her medical history form, she had written that her main reasons for seeking treatment were "depression, wanting to make changes, and needing support." She also hoped to maintain abstinence but seemed more concerned with her mood and felt her drinking was under control.

Secondary issues were related to interpersonal relationships, which partly fueled her depressed mood. She felt isolated and longed to return to her family on the East Coast, yet was tied to her current residence for her son's benefit. Beyond her current interpersonal issues and future concerns, her past divorce haunted her.

Selecting a Guideline

My supervisor referred me to the APA *Practice Guideline for the Treatment of Patients With Substance Use Disorders* (2006). The general treatment principles are broken into eight steps followed by psychiatric management, each with detailed recommendations. By the time I first met the patient, I felt that several of the APA's recommended steps were already achieved by my predecessors. The goals of treatment, as suggested in the guideline, including motivating the patient to change, reducing substance use or achieving complete abstinence, and improving social functioning, were already under way. Because the patient was abstinent when I first met her and had started attending AA, I anticipated I would focus on the relapse prevention section of the guideline (Table 34–1). In reading about counseling for alcohol-related disorders, I knew much of the emphasis would be on how to build a lifestyle free of alcohol (Sadock and Sadock 2003). I expected to use relapse prevention strategies and motivational interviewing while also encouraging support groups such as AA.

To address her depression, I decided to monitor her mood and substance use weekly via general assessment charts provided by the clinic (Figures 34–1 through 34–3). Note that I began to use the Sequenced Treatment Alternatives to Relieve Depression (STAR*D) Quick Inventory of Depressive Symptomatology–Self-Report (QIDS-SR$_{16}$) (University of Pittsburgh Epidemiology Data Center 2009) for assessment later in the course of therapy.

With these considerations, I discussed an initial treatment plan and approach with the patient, outlined in Table 34–2.

I continued the patient's regimen of citalopram 60 mg every day (qd) and bupropion XL 300 mg qd. Ms. M.T. denied any side effects. I scheduled her follow-up visit in 1 week.

Course

Visit 2 (Week 2)

Ms. M.T. continued to abstain from alcohol, now 9 days sober, although she admitted to having some difficulty with cravings. She had not attended AA in the past week. I explained that I would begin monitoring her depression, drinking, and craving trends from this session onward. This day, she rated her depression at 7/10 (Figure 34–1). Her interpersonal

TABLE 34–1. Treatment strategy for alcohol dependence

Psychiatric treatment	Followed
Use relapse prevention strategies:	√
Help the patient anticipate and avoid drug-related cues (e.g., instruct the patient to avoid drug-using peers).	√
Decrease access to abusable substances.	√
Train the patient to self-monitor states associated with increased craving.	√
Use contingency contracting (e.g., set up positive and negative reinforcements in advance).	√
Teach desensitization and relaxation techniques to reduce the power of substance-related stimuli.	√
Help patients develop alternative, nonchemical coping responses.	√
Provide social skills training.	√
Provide positive feedback for the patient's successes, even if relapse does occur.	√
Analyze relapses and periods of sobriety from functional and behavioral standpoints and modify the treatment plan, including psychotherapy, accordingly.	√

Source. Adapted from American Psychiatric Association: *Practice Guideline for the Treatment of Patients With Substance Use Disorders.* 2006. Available at: http://www.psychiatryonline.com/pracGuide/loadGuidelinePdf.aspx?file=SUD2ePG_04-28-06. Accessed June 1, 2009.

stressors were related to forming a relationship with a man in the East and having concerns over sustaining it given the distance. Even more, Ms. M.T. felt her son disapproved of this developing bond. She was struggling with a desire to fulfill her own needs versus the needs of her son—wanting to move East where her family and new boyfriend were living yet feeling a responsibility to remain in California at least until her son completed the eighth grade. She revealed unmet fantasies of having more children to create the picture of a family she had envisioned with a stable marriage. During this session, I primarily used supportive and interpersonal therapy techniques in addressing her relationship issues. I recognized Ms. M.T.'s 9 days of sobriety and also encouraged her to attend AA.

TABLE 34–2. Initial treatment goals, measures, and methods of case

Treatment goal	Measure	Method
Mood improvement and stabilization	Weekly quantitative assessment of mood STAR*D QIDS-SR$_{16}$[a]	Pharmacotherapy Techniques from interpersonal therapy and supportive therapy
Reduce depressive symptoms by 50% by week 8	Weekly quantitative assessment of mood STAR*D QIDS-SR$_{16}$[a]	Pharmacotherapy Techniques from interpersonal therapy and supportive therapy
Abstain from alcohol	Self-report (episodes/week)	Relapse prevention Motivational interviewing Encourage attending Alcoholics Anonymous
Improved interpersonal relationships	Self-report (qualitative)	Techniques from interpersonal therapy and supportive therapy

Note. QIDS=Quick Inventory of Depressive Symptomatology–Self-Report (QIDS-SR$_{16}$); STAR*D=Sequenced Treatment Alternatives to Relieve Depression.

[a]Added at visit 10 (week 12).

In the past week, what was your average level of depression?
(1 = no symptoms to 10 = severe [and use of STAR*D QIDS-SR₁₆])

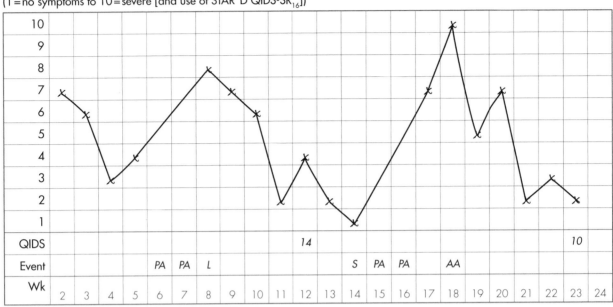

FIGURE 34–1.   Depression trends.

AA=author away and no appointment; L=lapse; PA=patient away and no appointment; S=session addressing alcohol as a problem. QIDS=Quick Inventory of Depressive Symptomatology–Self-Report (QIDS-SR₁₆); STAR*D=Sequenced Treatment Alternatives to Relieve Depression.

Visit 3 (Week 3)

Ms. M.T.'s mood remained relatively unchanged from her last visit, with depression rated at 6/10. She successfully abstained for yet another week, but described significant, strong cravings triggered by walking down a wine-filled aisle at the grocery store. Related to the APA guideline suggestion of anticipating and avoiding drug-related cues as a relapse prevention strategy, I recommended that she self-monitor states associated with increased craving. I spent much of this session gathering the patient's past alcohol history to better understand her present picture. This was also in line with the second step of

the general treatment principles of the APA guideline in assessing a patient (Table 34–3). Although assessment of the patient's history of use had been done in previous sessions by her prior therapists, I thought it important and worthwhile to conduct my own assessment—both to offer me a better understanding of the patient's current situation and for the patient to reassess her goals.

The patient described growing up in a household where alcohol was the norm, her parents drinking daily. She began drinking at the age of 13, often mixing drinks found in her and her friends' homes. Her drinking progressed into college and beyond, with

How often did you drink in the past week?
(1 = never, 2 = almost never, 3 = a few times a week, 4 = a few times a day)

FIGURE 34–2.   Alcohol use.

How severe were the cravings in the past week? (1 = no cravings to 10 = severe)

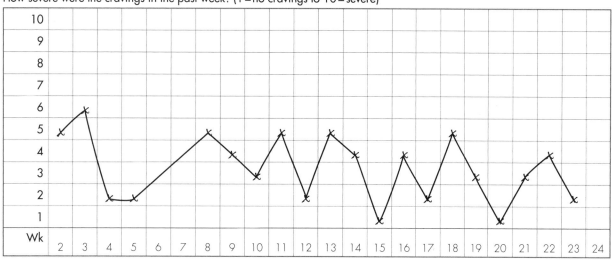

FIGURE 34–3. Cravings.

brief periods of abstinence. Her longest period of sobriety was about 7 years while she was with her ex-husband, who did not drink. After their separation, she began drinking off and on, oftentimes returning to alcohol under stress.

I focused on events that she could recall that led to her drinking, identifying her triggers in the process. In the past year, her drinking was motivated by a desire to numb out personal problems related to her ex-husband. By the end of this session, we had gathered a handful of triggers to be mindful of for the future, most notably including the sight of alcoholic beverages and periods of depression and isolation.

Ms. M.T. was preparing for a trip to the East Coast to visit family and expressed concerns of relapse in this familiar environment with many potential alcohol-related triggers. In following the relapse prevention strategies (Table 34–1), we discussed alternative, nonchemical coping responses, which included attending AA on the East Coast, informing family in advance about her goals, using nonalcoholic beer as a substitute, and finding alternate activities such as art. During this session, I utilized several of the APA's relapse prevention strategies (Table 34–1), with some points addressed or expanded on in future encounters.

Visits 4–5 (Weeks 4–5)

Ms. M.T.'s mood was notably improved the next couple visits, rated at 3–4/10. This was partly attrib-

uted to improved relations with her boyfriend and son. She had visited her boyfriend recently, which eased some of her loneliness. She also spoke with her son about her dilemma of wanting to return to the east yet not wanting to remove him from his comfortable California network of friends. Although there was no firm resolution with this issue, she was relieved after sharing her struggles with the individual she felt it would most affect.

She continued to successfully abstain from alcohol, finding support in her new boyfriend, who I discovered had a history of alcohol dependence and who was, at that time, abstaining. Ms. M.T.'s cravings were also diminished, rated at 2/10. We continued to discuss strategies for preventing relapse, particularly for her upcoming visit back home. Another trigger for cravings was identified—that of boredom leading to depressed mood. To prevent relapse, she engaged herself in various activities after work, including painting, piano, and swimming.

We reinforced the various strategies and coping skills for her to use during her 2-week trip to the East Coast. She was advised to seek AA while there and to return to the clinic when she arrived back in California.

Visit 6 (Week 8)

Ms. M.T. returned from her trip, where she had successfully remained sober. However, upon her return to California, she lapsed, experiencing loneliness and boredom, which led to her drinking leftover al-

TABLE 34–3.   Assessment of alcohol history strategy

Assessment	Followed
Obtain information from the patient and, with the patient's permission, from collateral sources (e.g., available family members, friends, current and past treaters, employers) as appropriate	√
Obtain detailed history of the patient's past and present use of substances, including:	
Types of substance used (including nicotine, caffeine, prescribed and over-the-counter medications) and whether multiple substances are used in combination	√
Mode of onset, quantity, frequency, duration, route of administration, and pattern and circumstances of substance use (e.g., where, with whom)	√
Timing and amount of most recent use	√
Degree of associated intoxication, withdrawal, and subjective effects of all substances used	√
History of prior substance use treatments (e.g., settings, context, modalities, duration, and adherence), efforts to stop substance use, and outcomes (e.g., duration of abstinence, subsequent substance use, reasons for relapse, social and occupational functioning achieved)	√
Current readiness to change, including:	
Awareness of substance use as a problem	√
Plans for ceasing substance use	√
Motivations for substance use, including desired effects	√
Barriers to treatment and to abstinence	√
Expectations and preferences for future treatment	√
Effects on cognitive, psychological, behavioral, social, occupational, and physiological functioning	√
General medical and psychiatric history and physical and mental status examination	√
Family history of substance use or psychiatric disorder	√
Social history (including family and peer relationships, financial problems, and legal problems) and psychosocial supports (including influence of close friends or other household members to support or undermine past efforts at abstinence)	√
Educational and occupational history, including school or vocational adjustment and identification of occupations at increased risk of substance use	√

Source.   Adapted from American Psychiatric Association: *Practice Guideline for the Treatment of Patients With Substance Use Disorders*, 2nd Edition. 2006. Available at: http://www.psychiatryonline.com/pracGuide/loadGuidelinePdf.aspx?file=SUD2ePG_04-28-06. Accessed June 1, 2009.

cohol in her home. Her depression was rated higher than when we first met. We discussed reasons for her lapse, and she identified missing her family and boyfriend. We agreed that we had planned adequately for her trip to the east but had not anticipated the difficulty she might have returning to California.

In addressing where to go at this point, Ms. M.T. was ambivalent. She expressed a desire to limit her drinking to weekends, giving up her goal of complete abstinence but also hoping to return to that goal eventually. Although I was already using motivational interviewing, I knew this clinical method would be especially relevant in exploring and resolving the pa-

tient's ambivalence. We set a goal for her to contact her former neighbor, who also was recovering from alcohol dependence, to attend AA with her.

After this lapse, I found myself searching for more in-depth relapse prevention guidelines. I logged onto the National Guideline Clearinghouse at www.guideline.gov, but the recommendations I did find were strategies I had already been using or more related to screening for substance use. Therefore, I turned to researching articles online and seeking advice from supervisors. I presented the case during a conference to a group of psychiatrists and psychologists, seeking their opinions. I also videotaped my sessions and showed them to my supervisor for input.

I came across an article online with suggestions on how to prevent a lapse from becoming a relapse, the main message being to view the lapse not as a failure but as a reminder flag to be vigilant about one's behavior—to learn from the lapse rather than using it as an excuse to relapse completely (Hunt 2007). From my last session with Ms. M.T., I feared she might already be viewing her lapse as an excuse to continue drinking—she was considering a new goal that would allow her to drink on weekends instead of completely abstaining. Hence, prior to her next visit, I called Ms. M.T., validating her efforts and achievements of the past several weeks and giving her affirmation that her lapse did not need to become a relapse. The online suggestion allowed me to present to Ms. M.T. another way of viewing her setback that aided in maintaining hope and self-esteem. Ms. M.T. expressed her appreciation for the call.

Visits 7–11 (Weeks 9–13)

Over the next several sessions, my patient continued to drink approximately two to three glasses of wine two to three times per week. Beyond using alcohol as a coping mechanism for depression and isolation, I recognized that she began to use it as a reward for accomplishing things such as exercising or even going to AA. During week 9, I discovered that she did not feel alcohol was that problematic for her, believing that she could control her use. I realized the initial steps in the APA guideline, which we had once gone through, needed to be reassessed, particularly with current readiness to change (Table 34–3). Ms. M.T. felt that because she had lapsed, she could indulge in alcohol before abstaining again. Further complicating the picture, her boyfriend, who had also lapsed, stayed with her for a period and encouraged her to drink to celebrate their reunion.

Throughout these sessions, we discussed alternate forms of reward, incorporating other activities into her life such as exercise, reading books, watching DVDs, and establishing other sources of support/contact. Each time we ended a session, she committed herself to beginning sobriety that day, but the pattern of drinking continued over a 5-week period. She admitted being reluctant to attend AA, feeling she needed a companion to attend at least at the outset. She identified the wine glasses in her

home as another trigger for her alcohol use and agreed to pack them away. Concerned that I needed to more carefully assess the extent of her depression and better monitor its relation to her drinking, I decided to incorporate the STAR*D QIDS-SR$_{16}$ questionnaire at week 12. She scored 14, in the moderate range, and could be considered for the next step in the STAR*D algorithm. However, given her general improvement in depression, I decided to wait before making further medication changes.

By week 13, she had incorporated some changes into her life including exercise, meditation, reading, contacting sources of support, and attending AA again. Despite these many achievements, she craved alcohol and continued to drink. She mentioned during this session that she disliked that in AA individuals usually say their name and announce "I am an alcoholic" before speaking. I wanted to probe further but instead found myself highlighting her accomplishments. I made a note to myself to address this next week. We agreed she would make a list of rewards to use instead of alcohol and to continue attending AA.

Visit 12 (Week 14)

The patient was abstinent for 1 week, an achievement she was clearly proud of. She continued to attend AA and to exercise. Although I recognized her achievements, I felt I needed to address the lingering issue of whether she viewed alcohol as a problem in her life. I began by addressing her hesitancy to say "I am an alcoholic" in AA. She first gave reasons for why alcohol might not be a problem for her but in the process realized her use of alcohol was not as controlled as it had been in the past. She then wanted to know if I thought she was an alcoholic. I responded first recognizing her accomplishments, then moved toward recognizing her struggles in trying to abstain, careful to avoid argumentation and expressing empathy throughout. In line with the principles of motivational interviewing, I also noted discrepancies between her continued use of alcohol and the goals she set for herself each week to stop (Table 34–4). Ultimately, I did say that I believed she was an alcoholic. She was saddened, realizing she could never drink again if this was true, and seemed regretful that she had been lenient with herself in returning to alcohol. We discussed other barriers to her viewing alcohol as a problem, including family who viewed alcohol favorably.

TABLE 34–4. Five general principles of motivational interviewing

Principle	Explanation	Followed
1. Avoid arguments	Counselor avoids arguing with clients. Counselor does not try to "break through" the denial, but works around it. Clients are not given diagnostic labels such as "alcoholic" or "addict." Persuasion is gentle and subtle.	√
2. Express empathy	Counselor sees the world through the client's eyes, thinking about things as the client thinks about them, feeling things as the client feels them, sharing in the client's experiences.	√
3. Support self-efficacy	Counselor focuses efforts on helping clients stay motivated by supporting clients' sense that change is possible.	√
4. Roll with resistance	Counselor does not fight client resistance, but "rolls with it" to further explore clients' views. Clients are encouraged to develop their own solutions to the problems that they themselves have defined.	√
5. Develop discrepancy	Counselor helps clients examine the discrepancies between their current behavior and future goals. When clients perceive that their current behaviors are not leading toward some important future goal, they become more motivated to make important life changes.	√

Source.   Adapted from U.S. Department of Health and Human Services, Substance Abuse and Mental Health Services Administration, Center for Substance Abuse Treatment: TIP 35: Enhancing motivation for change in substance abuse treatment. There are five general principles behind motivational interviewing. 2000. Available at: http://www.dawnfarm.org/pdf/MI_Principles.pdf. Accessed June 1, 2009.

I videotaped this session, which I played for my supervisor. This session, utilizing the five general principles of motivational interviewing (Table 34–4), propelled the patient to view her alcohol use in a different light. It made her step back and question how she had been handling her use. It also allowed her to contemplate the implications of being abstinent and how not drinking would influence various aspects of her life.

Visit 13 (Week 17)

Three weeks passed until my next session with Ms. M.T. She had been out of town visiting family. Despite a spike in depression attributed largely to stressors on her return home, her alcohol use had diminished; she had abstained in the week following our last session, then had one glass of wine on her return home. She had not been attending AA but was making use of relaxation techniques. Although I continued to encourage her to attend AA, what I had failed to do in this and previous sessions was explore why she was not going to AA in the first place. I asked her how she felt about our last session, and although she was ambivalent about accepting alcohol as a significant problem in her life, her cravings "disappeared" for a time after that session. I wondered, if she had not been out of town and if we had followed up sooner on our last session, would she have been more accepting of the things we discussed?

Visit 14 (Week 19)

Two weeks passed until my next session with Ms. M.T. because of my being away at a conference. In my absence, the patient's depression peaked to its highest, with a continuation of her prior stressors involving family strife and feelings of loneliness. For the first time since I had known her, she expressed death wishes, without suicidal intent or plan but more with a wish to release the emotional pain. I recognized the vicious cycle she was in of feeling depressed and drinking as a consequence to numb the pain. Although I had been careful to monitor her mood weekly, I realized that I may not have been addressing it sufficiently given my emphasis on her alcohol use. Ms. M.T. was not interested in commitments to abstain at this point, but she did feel that any changes in her alcohol use would be difficult to achieve unless her mood was better. I reviewed her antidepressant medications, which was a reasonable combination of two antidepressants at good doses. Although I considered increasing her bupropion, I decided to hold off making pharmacological changes, feeling her mood seemed most affected by current interpersonal stressors, which we spent the session processing.

Visits 15–16 (Weeks 20–21)

Patient's mood gradually improved over the next couple weeks, utilizing assertiveness skills, which worked well in her interpersonal relationships. She also began to exercise regularly, which she found enormously helpful. Despite significant improvements in her mood, her drinking persisted, increasing to the point of drinking daily.

I decided to reassess where she wanted to go with her alcohol use. I had reminded Ms. M.T. I would be leaving the clinic in about a month. In probing, she revealed that knowing that I would be leaving the clinic soon left her feeling unmotivated to quit alcohol. She admitted she was giving herself the allowance to drink. She felt an obligation toward me, regularly coming to the clinic despite the financial and scheduling burdens. And part of this obligation involved not wanting to disappoint me if she set a commitment to quit and failed. I felt another key moment in therapy where change might be possible, similar to our session when I addressed her awareness of alcohol as a problem. After sharing these feelings of needing to please me, she felt a weight lifted from her shoulders and readily set a commitment to stop drinking for a week and to attend AA.

This session encouraged me to look deeper into the process of psychotherapy termination. Although I had ensured that Ms. M.T. was fully informed from the beginning that my time in this resident clinic would be limited to 6 months, it was clear that my upcoming departure was influencing her life decisions in ways opposite to what we were trying to achieve. Not only did she verbally reflect this, but I also noticed spikes in her depression and drinking in the weeks when either she or I was away and unable to meet (Figures 34–1 and 34–2). I found that, in some ways, she was using my departure as a way to explain her continued drinking. I could find no evidence-based guidelines on psychotherapy termination, but I did find an article in the *Journal of Clinical Psychology* (Vasquez et al. 2008) via PubMed that discussed the consequences of inappropriate termination, ethical and clinical responsibilities of the therapist, and practice recommendations (Table 34–5). In this case, there was a strong therapeutic alliance between us,

and we agreed that the process was not finished but that I would not be available to continue in her care. The article provided a similar example, and stated that regression could be an unfortunate consequence. Ms. M.T. was toying with the idea of discontinuing therapy after I left, and after my research, I felt even stronger about encouraging her to continue. I made a note to myself to address this in the next session.

Visit 17 (Week 22)

The patient's mood remained stable, but despite her intended commitment to abstain, she had used alcohol every day in the past week and had not attended AA. Unanticipated celebrations and boredom led to her drinking, although she admitted to feelings of disappointment. We discussed her boyfriend's impending move and her concern that he could influence her if he continued drinking. She set goals to discuss this with her boyfriend and to attend AA. But the most significant goal she set for herself was quitting alcohol for "an extended period," recognizing that setting a commitment to quit for a limited period was not working. It was a movement toward closing the door of leniency she had given herself for years.

During this session, we continued with pretermination counseling. I wanted to readdress her plans after I left the clinic, concerned that she might decide to halt therapy and regress. My strategy was to use the content of this session and emphasize the many changes she was about to confront in the coming months and ask her how she felt about handling it on her own without a therapist. She admitted that it could be challenging and seemed to recognize the potential pitfalls of discontinuing. We discussed her reservations, namely that therapy was work on her end and that this termination was a chance to take a break before signing up with another therapist. I agreed with her that therapy was work but then noted that in the work she had done in this clinic, she had made tremendous progress. She agreed that what might be better was a therapist closer to her home, covered by her insurance, and one where continuity could be better ensured. The plan seemed to lift some of the burdens she had been feeling and removed the ambivalence she had with continuing in therapy.

Visit 18 (Week 23)

The patient's depression continued to steadily decline, her STAR*D QIDS-SR$_{16}$ score at 10. Accord-

TABLE 34–5.   Practice recommendations for psychotherapy termination

Recommendation	Followed
Provide patients with a complete description of the therapeutic process, including termination; obtain informed consent for this process at the beginning of treatment and provide reminders throughout treatment.	√
Ensure that the psychotherapist and client agree collaboratively on the goals for psychotherapy and the ending of psychotherapy.	√
Provide periodic progress updates that include discussions of termination and, toward the end of psychotherapy, provide pretermination counseling.	√
Offer a contract that provides patients with a plan in case the psychotherapist is suddenly unavailable (including death, or financial, employment, or insurance complications).	No
Help clients develop health and referral plans for posttermination life.	√
Make sure you understand termination, abandonment, and their potential effects on patients.	
Consider developing (and updating) your professional will to proactively address unexpected termination and abandonment, including the name(s) of colleagues who will contact current patients in the case of your sudden disability or death.	No
Contact clients who prematurely terminate via telephone or letters to express your concern and offer to assist them.	NA
Use the American Psychological Association Ethics Code (2002), your state practice regulations, and consultations with knowledgeable colleagues to help guide your understanding and behavior in regard to psychotherapy termination.	√
Review other ethics codes for discussions of abandonment. The American Counseling Association (http://www.counseling.org/Resources/CodeOfEthics/TP/Home/CT2.aspx) and the American Mental Health Counselors Association (http://www.amhca.org/code) contain prohibitions against abandonment.	√
Make the topic of termination a part of your regular continuing education or professional development.	√
Be vigilant in monitoring your clinical effectiveness and personal distress. Psychotherapists who self-monitor and practice effective self-care are less likely to have inappropriate terminations or clients who feel abandoned.	√

Note.   NA=not applicable.
Source.   Adapted from Vasquez et al. 2008.

ing to the QIDS-SR$_{16}$ scoring criteria (University of Pittsburgh Epidemiology Data Center 2009), this was an improvement from moderate depression at week 12 to mild depression. Her alcohol use decreased substantially as well—she had 2 drinking days in the past week, compared with her daily drinking during the previous couple of weeks. She also made courageous steps toward asking her boyfriend to not drink upon his move because of its likely influence on her. I recognized how her achievements seemed to make her feel positive, careful that my own commendations or expressions of pride could hasten any obligations she might feel toward me. This was a recommendation offered by other therapists when I

presented Ms. M.T. during a case conference. I decided to readdress how she viewed her alcohol use, and although she felt she was not dependent on alcohol, she believed there was a stronger "potential" for this and firmly stated she was not going to wait for it to get out of hand.

We continued with pretermination counseling, Ms. M.T. reflecting on and proud of the progress she had made in the last year. I validated her growth and strengths. She openly shared that transitioning to a new therapist might be difficult given how much she had revealed and how hard that had been for her. I recognized her feelings and was forthcoming that the termination would be difficult for me as well, acknowledging our strong therapeutic alliance. We again touched on her plans to find a therapist closer to her home to continue with after my departure. I offered to look over the list of providers covered under her insurance plan with my supervisor and provide her with recommendations. In inquiring what her future goals in therapy would be, she stated "Alcohol use, going to AA, and making sure I don't get off track"—a positive addition to her prior goals, which had primarily focused on addressing her mood.

Summary of Guideline Use

At the end of 23 weeks, I reviewed my use of the guidelines. I felt I had followed the APA *Practice Guideline for the Treatment of Patients With Substance Use Disorders* (Tables 34–1 and 34–3) relatively well and consistently. The few areas I did not carry out involved intensifying relapse prevention either through encouraging monitoring programs or obtaining more objective evidence of relapse. Both these approaches may have given the patient more accountability for her actions. Furthermore, my supervisor and I had considered medications for her cravings, but I did not pursue this, and I may have assumed prematurely she would have decided against this since she believed she had self-control of her alcohol use. A thorough discussion regarding her cravings and medications as an option could have offered her an alternate treatment route to consider.

The clinic charts (Figures 34–1 through 34–3) were excellent tools that allowed Ms. M.T. and me to view the trends of her mood as it related to her alcohol use and cravings. I would have liked to use the STAR*D assessments and guidelines more carefully and from the beginning of treatment.

Although I had had a few lectures in the course of residency on motivational interviewing, I plunged into the practice for the first time after Ms. M.T.'s initial lapse. Only later did I review the five general principles (see Table 34–4), which I felt I had covered sufficiently. The one recommendation I failed to follow was not to give clients a label such as "alcoholic." In answering Ms. M.T.'s question, I did state I believed she was an "alcoholic" which triggered her into viewing her use differently. Although I felt this was a pivotal and significant point in ther-

apy, perhaps the emphasis could have been less on the label and more on alcohol as a problem.

I also reviewed my use of the practice recommendations for psychotherapy termination, which I was satisfied I had followed. Despite following published guidelines and recommendations, this case demonstrated and affirmed for me the need to expand one's use of resources in caring for patients (i.e., conferences, supervision, articles, etc.), especially when no further guidelines exist.

The prevailing question I had for myself at the end of my time with Ms. M.T. was how successful I had been treating her alcohol use. What measure could I use as a gauge? In the COMBINE study, about 1,300 patients were enrolled in a study that compared nine different alcohol abuse treatments (Anton et al. 2006). In this study, the main outcomes were percentage of days abstinent over the 16 weeks of the study and time to first heavy drinking (five standard drinks per day for men, four for women). The mean percentage of days abstinent was about 65%, or 2 days out of 3, which was considered a minimal standard. Using this study's criteria, my patient did indeed achieve a level of abstinence above the minimal standard, at 68%.

Ways to Improve Practice

In reviewing my practice, although I had encouraged family therapy, I might have improved my care of Ms. M.T. by inviting her boyfriend and perhaps her son to one of our sessions because there were interpersonal stressors. This would have allowed me to gather collateral information, explore interpersonal dynamics, examine what understanding her family had of her drinking, and perhaps discuss ways in which they could assist with her goals. Second, I would have more carefully monitored and inquired about how our missed sessions were affecting her. Had I noticed this pattern earlier, I could have been more vigilant about checking in via telephone if we were unable to meet in person. Third, I might have been more aggressive with following the STAR*D algorithm. Her QIDS-SR$_{16}$ was still above the optimal level for remission at our last visit. Lastly, a consultation with experts in the field of substance use/addiction could have offered further guidance in helping my patient achieve abstinence for a sustained period.

References

American Psychiatric Association: American Psychiatric Association Practice Guidelines for the Treatment of Psychiatric Disorders 2004. Treating Substance Use Disorders: A Quick Reference Guide. 2006. Available at: http://www.psychiatryonline.com/pracGuide/pracGuideTopic_5.aspx. Accessed June 1, 2009

American Psychiatric Association: Practice Guideline for the Treatment of Patients With Substance Use Disorders, 2nd Edition. 2006. Available at: http://www.psychiatryonline.com/pracGuide/loadGuidelinePdf.aspx?file=SUD2ePG_04-28-06. Accessed June 1, 2009

American Psychological Association: Ethical principles of psychologists and code of conduct. Am Psychol 57:1060–1073, 2002

Anton RF, O'Malley SS, Ciraulo DA, et al: Combined pharmacotherapies and behavioral interventions for alcohol dependence. JAMA 295:2003–2017, 2006

Center for Substance Abuse Treatment: Substance abuse: clinical issues in intensive outpatient treatment. Rockville, MD, Subxstance Abuse and Mental Health Services Administration, 2006. Available at: http://www.guideline.gov. Accessed June 1, 2009

Hunt T: Prevent a lapse becoming a relapse. Bright Eye: Online Alcoholism and Addiction Counseling. 2007. Available at: http://www.brighteyecounselling.co.uk/alcohol-drugs/prevent-a-lapse-becoming-a-relapse. Accessed June 1, 2009

Michigan Quality Improvement Consortium: Screening, diagnosis and referral for substance use disorders. Southfield, MI, Michigan Quality Improvement Consortium, 2007. Available at: http://www.guideline.gov. Accessed June 1, 2009

Sadock BJ, Sadock VA: Kaplan and Sadock's Synopsis of Psychiatry, 9th Edition. Philadelphia, PA, Lippincott Williams & Wilkins, 2003, p 412

Scottish Intercollegiate Guidelines Network: The management of harmful drinking and alcohol dependence in primary care: a national clinical guideline. Edinburgh, Scottish Intercollegiate Guidelines Network, 2003. Available at: http://www.guideline.gov. Accessed June 1, 2009

University of Pittsburgh Epidemiology Data Center: Inventory of Depressive Symptomatology (IDS) and Quick Inventory of Depressive Symptomatology (QIDS)—Scoring. 2009. Available at: http://www.ids-qids.org/index2.html#SCORING. Accessed June 1, 2009

U.S. Department of Health and Human Services, Substance Abuse and Mental Health Services Administration, Center for Substance Abuse Treatment: TIP 35: Enhancing motivation for change in substance abuse treatment. There are five general principles behind motivational interviewing. 1999. Available at: http://www.dawnfarm.org/pdf/MI_Principles.pdf. Accessed June 1, 2009

Vasquez MJ, Bingham RP, Barnett JE: Psychotherapy termination: clinical and ethical responsibilities. J Clin Psychol 65:653–665, 2008

Glossary

absolute risk increase (ARI) Difference between experimental event rate (EER) and control event rate (CER) when a treatment increases the risk of a negative outcome.

absolute risk reduction (ARR) Difference between control event rate (CER) and experimental event rate (EER) when a treatment decreases the risk of a negative outcome.

allocation concealment Refers to whether the person making the allocation of a patient to either the experimental or control treatment in a randomized controlled trial is aware of the group to which the next patient will be assigned.

alpha (α) Probability of a type I error (i.e., falsely concluding that there is a difference between the experimental and control groups when such a difference is the result of chance alone).

attributable risk Difference in incidence rates between exposed and nonexposed cohorts; also known as *risk difference* (RD).

beta (β) Probability of a type II error (i.e., falsely concluding that there is no difference between the experimental and control groups when such a difference in fact exists).

bias Systematic deviation of the results from the truth.

blinded or blind Refers to whether patients, clinicians, raters, and data analysts are aware of which treatment a patient in a trial is receiving. Although terms like *single blind*, *double blind*, or *triple blind* are sometimes used, there is no consistent meaning to them, and it is better to specify which participants have been blinded.

case report Description of a single case.

case series Description of a series of cases.

case-control study Observational study in which exposure to a suspected risk factor is assessed in cases with the disease and in control subjects without the disease.

cohort A group of persons followed over time.

cohort study An observational study in which a cohort is followed over time and the number of cases of disease (or another outcome measure) is assessed. Typically, the cohort is divided into those who are exposed to a potential risk factor and those who are not exposed, and the difference or ratio of incidence rates is computed.

co-intervention Intervention other than the treatment under study that is applied differentially to the control and experimental groups.

confidence interval (CI) Range of values within which the true value most likely lies.

confounding variable Variable related to the outcome, which differs in frequency between the experimental (or exposed) and control (or nonexposed) groups. Confounding variables, not the variable under study, may be responsible for observed differences in the groups.

control event rate (CER) Rate of events in the control (nonexposed or nonexperimental) group. Typically expressed in terms of negative events.

cross-product ratio   Odds ratio.

cross-sectional survey   Observational study design in which exposures and outcomes are determined at the same point in time.

dichotomous outcome   Outcome that can take only two values (e.g., dead or alive).

effect size   Measure of the difference in outcomes between the control and experimental groups.

experimental event rate (EER)   Rate of events in the experimental (exposed) group. Typically expressed in terms of negative events.

Hawthorne effect   Performance improves when subjects know they are being studied.

inception cohort   Group of people assembled at a common point, early in the course of their illnesses.

incidence   Number of new cases of disease in a population in a given period of time.

intention-to-treat analysis   Statistical analysis that includes all patients assigned to a treatment group, regardless of whether they completed study.

Kaplan-Meier curve   Survival curve.

likelihood ratio (LR)   Relative likelihood of test results in those with disease, compared with those without disease.

meta-analysis   Statistical technique that pools results from more than one study to yield a summary result.

negative predictive value (NPV)   Proportion of negative test results that are true negatives.

number needed to harm (NNH)   Number of patients that must be treated with an experimental therapy to produce one additional bad outcome that would not have occurred on the control therapy. Inverse of *absolute risk increase*.

number needed to treat (NNT)   Number of patients that must be treated with an experimental therapy to prevent one bad outcome that would have occurred on the control therapy. Inverse of *absolute risk reduction*.

odds   Ratio of the probability of an event occurring to the probability of an event not occurring.

odds ratio (OR)   Ratio of odds of event in exposed group to odds of event in nonexposed group. In a case-control study, ratio of odds of exposure in cases to odds of exposure in control subjects; also known as *cross-product ratio*.

patient expected event rate   Expected risk of negative outcomes in patient if control treatment is administered.

positive predictive value (PPV)   Proportion of positive test results that are true positives.

posttest odds   Odds of disease in patient after results of test are known.

posttest probability   Probability of disease in patient after results of test are known.

pretest odds   Odds of disease in patient before results of test are known.

pretest probability   Probability of disease in patient before results of test are known.

prevalence   Proportion of persons in a population with disease of interest.

randomization   Allocation of subjects to groups by chance.

randomized controlled trial (RCT)   Clinical trial in which patients are randomly allocated to control or experimental treatment groups.

receiver operating characteristic curve (ROC)   Plot of false positive rate (1–specificity) versus true positive rate (sensitivity).

relative risk (RR)   In a cohort study, ratio of incidence of disease in exposed group to incidence in nonexposed group. In a randomized controlled trial, ratio of rate of negative events in experimental group (EER) to rate in control group (CER).

relative risk reduction (RRR)   In an randomized controlled trial, proportion of risk of negative outcome reduced by the experimental therapy. Calculated as 1–relative risk (RR).

reliability   Degree to which results are reproducible.

risk difference (RD)   Difference in incidence rates between exposed and nonexposed cohorts.

risk factor   Patient characteristic that increases risk of disease.

risk ratio   Relative risk.

sensitivity   Proportion of persons with a disease who are correctly identified by a diagnostic test.

specificity   Proportion of persons without a disease who are correctly identified by a diagnostic test.

survival analysis   Method of analyzing time-to-event data.

survival curve   Graphical display of proportion of individuals who have not had event occur, plotted over time.

systematic review   Literature review that involves comprehensive search for relevant articles, followed by critical appraisal and summarizing of articles that meet quality criteria.

type I error   Falsely concluding that there is a difference between experimental and control groups when such a difference is the result of chance alone.

type II error   Falsely concluding that there is no difference between experimental and control groups when such a difference in fact exists.

validity   Degree to which results of a study are unbiased.

Statistical Formulas and Tables

B–1: Confidence intervals (CIs) for number needed to treat and number needed to harm

B–2: Calculating patient-specific number needed to treat and number needed to harm estimates

B–3: Calculating the likelihood of being helped versus harmed by a therapy

B–4: Calculating number needed to treat and number needed to harm from the odds ratio

B–5: Interpreting standardized effect size

Bibliography

Altman DG: Confidence intervals for the number needed to treat. BMJ 317:1309–1312, 1998

Freemantle N, Geddes J: Understanding and interpreting systematic reviews and meta-analyses, II: meta-analyses. Evid Based Ment Health 1:102–104, 1998

Leung R: Appendix: calculations, in Users' Guides to the Medical Literature: A Manual for Evidence-Based Clinical Practice. Edited by Guyatt GH, Rennie D. Chicago, IL, AMA Press, 2002, pp 659–664

Sackett DL, Straus SE, Richardson WS, et al: Evidence-Based Medicine: How to Practice and Teach EBM, 2nd Edition. New York, Churchill Livingstone, 2000

TABLE B–1. **Confidence intervals (CIs) for number needed to treat and number needed to harm**

	Experimental treatment	Control treatment
Bad outcome	A	B
Good outcome	C	D
Total	n_1	n_2

Control event rate (CER)=B/n_2

Experimental event rate (EER)=A/n_1

If treatment leads to fewer bad outcomes:

Absolute risk reduction (ARR)=CER–EER

Number needed to treat (NNT)=1/ARR

Standard error of ARR (SE_{ARR})=
    $\{[(CER)(1-CER)/n_2]+[(EER)(1-EER)/n_1]\}^{1/2}$

Upper limit of 95% CI for ARR (U_{ARR})=ARR+1.96 SE_{ARR}

Lower limit of 95% CI for ARR (L_{ARR})=ARR–1.96 SE_{ARR}

Upper limit of 95% CI for NNT (U_{NNT})=1/L_{ARR}

Lower limit of 95% CI for NNT (L_{NNT})=1/U_{ARR}

If treatment leads to more bad outcomes:

Absolute risk increase (ARI)=EER–CER

Number needed to harm (NNH)=1/ARI

Standard error of ARI (SE_{ARI})=
    $\{[(CER)(1-CER)/n_2]+[(EER)(1-EER)/n_1]\}^{1/2}$

Upper limit of 95% CI for ARI (U_{ARI})=ARI+1.96 SE_{ARI}

Lower limit of 95% CI for ARI (L_{ARI})=ARI–1.96 SE_{ARI}

Upper limit of 95% CI for NNH (U_{NNH})=1/L_{ARI}

Lower limit of 95% CI for NNH (L_{NNH})=1/U_{ARI}

TABLE B–2. **Calculating patient-specific number needed to treat and number needed to harm estimates**

	Experimental treatment	Control treatment
Bad outcome	A	B
Good outcome	C	D
Total	n_1	n_2

Control event rate (CER)=B/n_2

Experimental event rate (EER)=A/n_1

Relative risk (RR)= EER/CER

Patient's expected event rate (PEER)=estimate of patient's
    risk of bad outcome on control treatment

If treatment leads to fewer bad outcomes:

Relative risk reduction (RRR)=1–RR

Patient's expected absolute risk reduction
    (PARR)=PEER×RRR

Patient-specific number needed to treat (PNNT)=1/PARR

If treatment leads to more bad outcomes:

Relative risk increase (RRI)=RR–1

Patient's absolute risk increase (PARI)=PEER×RRI

Patient-specific number needed to harm (PNNH)=1/PARI

TABLE B–3. Calculating the likelihood of being helped versus harmed by a therapy

Step 1

Calculate the patient-specific number needed to treat (PNNT) for the desired therapeutic effect and the patient-specific number needed to harm (PNNH) for the side effect of concern (Table B-2).

Step 2

Determine the patient's relative preference (RP) for the desired effect versus the side effect. For example, if a patient feels that it is twice as bad to gain 10 kg as it is to relapse, RP=1/2.

Step 3

Calculate the likelihood of being helped or harmed (LHH), using this formula:

$$LHH = PNNH/(PNNT \times RP)$$

The LHH is the relative likelihood of being helped versus harmed by a therapy, taking into account the patient's individualized risks and values.

TABLE B–4. Calculating number needed to treat and number needed to harm from the odds ratio

If treatment leads to fewer bad outcomes:

$$NNT = \frac{1 - (CER)(1 - OR)}{(CER)(1 - CER)(1 - OR)}$$

If treatment leads to more bad outcomes:

$$NNH = \frac{1 + (CER)(1 - OR)}{(CER)(1 - CER)(1 - OR)}$$

Note. NNT=number needed to treat; CER=estimated control event rate; OR=odds ratio; NNH=number needed to harm.

TABLE B–5. Interpreting standardized effect size

Standardized effect size (*d*) is a measure of the degree of overlap between experimental and control groups when there is a continuous outcome measure. To interpret *d*, use the chart below.

$d > 0$: The average (mean) response in the experimental group is greater than this percentage of responses in the control group.

$d < 0$: The average (mean) response in the experimental group is less than this percentage of responses in the control group.

d	Percentile
0	50
0.2	58
0.4	66
0.6	73
0.8	79
1.0	84
1.2	88
1.4	92
1.6	95
1.8	96
2.0	98
2.3	99

Index

Page numbers printed in **boldface** *type refer to tables or figures*

S0-ADS-351

THE NATIONAL EXPERIENCE

A HISTORY OF THE UNITED STATES

SIXTH EDITION

THE NATIONAL EXPERIENCE

A HISTORY OF THE UNITED STATES

SIXTH EDITION

John M. Blum
Yale University

Arthur M. Schlesinger, Jr.
The City University of New York

William S. McFeely
Mount Holyoke College

Kenneth M. Stampp
University of California, Berkeley

Edmund S. Morgan
Yale University

C. Vann Woodward
Yale University

Harcourt Brace Jovanovich, Publishers
San Diego   New York   Chicago   Atlanta   Washington, D.C.
London   Sydney   Toronto

Cover art: Geoff Gove, © 1984

Drawings by: Karl Nicholason

Preface

Men and women make history. Their ideas and their hopes, their goals and contrivances for reaching those goals, shape all experience, past and present. The Indians, the first Americans, had to decide, by deliberation or by default, how to use the continent and its extraordinary resources. So have the successors of the Indians and the children of those successors—the early European settlers, the English colonists, the men and women of the new United States, and the generations that have followed them. Each generation has committed the nation to a complex of policies, some the product of thought and debate, others of habit or inadvertence, still others of calculated or undiscerning indifference. As the nation has grown, as its population has diversified, its economy matured, and its responsibilities multiplied, questions of national policy have become more difficult to understand but no more troubling. It took long thought and hard debate to settle the issues of independence, of democratic reform, of expansion, of slavery, of union itself, of control of private economic power, of resistance to totalitarianism across two oceans. All those issues and many more have made up the national experience.

This book endeavors to recount and explain that experience. It examines both the aspirations (often contradictory among themselves) and the achievements (often less grand than the best hopes) of the American people. It examines, too, the ideas, the institutions, and the processes that fed hope and affected achievement. It focuses on the decisions, positive and negative, that reflected national goals and directed national purposes, and consequently it focuses continually on the men and women who made those decisions, on those who made history. The book emphasizes public policy, but the history of public policy perforce demands continuing discussion of the whole culture that influenced it.

The authors of this book believe that a history emphasizing public policy, so conceived, reveals the fabric and experience of the past more completely than does any other kind of history. They believe, too, that an emphasis on questions of public policy provides the most useful introduction to the history of the United States. In the light of those convictions they have agreed on the focus of this book, on its organization, and on the selection and interpretation of the data it contains. The structure of the separate parts and chapters is now chronological, now topical, depending on the form that seemed most suitable for the explanation of the period or the subject under discussion. The increasing complexity of public issues in the recent past, moreover, has persuaded the authors to devote half of this volume to the period since Reconstruction, indeed more than a third to the twentieth century.

The authors have elected, furthermore, to confine their work to one volume so as to permit instructors to make generous supplementary assignments from the abundance of excellent monographs, biographies, and "problems" books now readily available. Just as there are clear interpretations of the past in those books, so are there in this, for the authors without exception find meaning in history and feel obliged to say what they see. The authors also believe that, especially for the beginning student of history, literature is better read than read about. Consequently, in commenting on belles-lettres and the other arts, they have consciously stressed those expressions and aspects of the arts relevant to an understanding of public policy. Finally, they have arranged to choose the illustrations and the boxed selections from contemporary and other sources in order to enhance and supplement not only the text but its particular focus.

This is a collaborative book in which each of the six contributors has ordinarily written about a period in which he is a specialist. Yet each has also executed the general purpose of the whole book. Each section of the book has been read and criticized by several of the contributors. This revision has profited from the assistance of many historians who were kind enough to review portions of the book before it was revised. These include: Robert Abzug, University of Texas, Austin; Geoffrey Blodgett, Oberlin College; Eric Foner, The City University of New York; George M. Fredrickson, Northwestern University; John L. Gaddis, Ohio University; William H. Goetzmann, University of Texas, Austin; Christine Heyrman, Uni-

versity of California, Irvine; Reginald Horsman, University of Wisconsin; Pauline Maier, Massachusetts Institute of Technology; William L. O'Neill, Rutgers University; Michael Parrish, University of California, San Diego; Lawrence Powell, Tulane University; Robert V. Remini, University of Illinois, Chicago Circle; Peter E. Robinson, Jacksonville State University; Bernard Sinsheimer, University of Maryland, Paris, France; Alan Trachtenberg, Yale University; and Harold Woodman, Purdue University.

Not even a collaboration as easy and agreeable as this one has been can erase the individuality of the collaborators. Each section of this book displays the particular intellectual and literary style of its contributor; all the contributors have been permitted, indeed urged, to remain themselves. The ultimate as well as the original responsibility for prose, for historical accuracy, and for interpretation remains that of the author of each section of this book: Edmund S. Morgan, Chapters 1–6; Kenneth M. Stampp, Chapters 7–12; William S. McFeely, Chapters 13–15; C. Vann Woodward, Chapters 16–21; John M. Blum, Chapters 22–26; Arthur M. Schlesinger, Jr., Chapters 27–29, revised for this edition by John M. Blum; and Arthur M. Schlesinger, Jr., Chapters 30–35.

JOHN M. BLUM, *Editor*
New Haven, Connecticut

A Note On the Suggestions for Additional Readings

The lists of suggested readings that follow the chapters of this book are obviously and intentionally selective. They are obviously so because a reasonably complete bibliography of American history would fill a volume larger than this one. They are intentionally so because the authors of the various chapters have tried to suggest to students only those stimulating and useful works that they might profitably and enjoyably explore while studying this text. Consequently each list of suggested readings points to a relatively few significant and well-written books, and each list attempts to emphasize, in so far as possible, books available in inexpensive, paperback editions—books whose titles are marked by an asterisk.

Use of the suggested readings, then, permits a student to begin to range through the rich literature of American history, but interested and energetic students will want to go beyond the lists. They will profit from the bibliographies in many of the works listed. They should also consult the card catalogs in the libraries of their colleges and the invaluable bibliography in the *Harvard Guide to American History*, rev. ed. (Belknap). For critical comments about the titles they find, they should go on, when they can, to the reviews in such learned journals as the *American Historical Review*, the *Journal of American History*, the *Journal of Southern History*, and the *William and Mary Quarterly*.

Those students who want to acquire libraries of their own and who want also to economize by purchasing paperback editions will find the availability of titles in paperbacks at best uncertain. Every few months new titles are published and other titles go out of print. For the most recent information about paperbacks, students should consult *Paperbound Books in Print* (Bowker), which appears biannually.

The reading lists refer to very few articles, not because articles are unimportant, but because they are often rather inaccessible to undergraduates. There are, however, many useful collections of important selected articles, often available in inexpensive editions. So, too, students will have no difficulty in finding collections of contemporary historical documents that add depth and excitement to the study of history. A growing number of thoughtful books organize both contemporary and scholarly materials in units designed to facilitate the investigation of historical problems.

The problems books, documents books, and collections of articles will whet the appetite of engaged students for further reading in the fields of their interest. They can serve in their way, then, as can the lists of suggested readings in this volume, as avenues leading to the adventures of the mind and the development of the understanding that American history affords.

Contents

Beginnings to 1789   2

1   Making Use of a New World   6

2   The Pattern of Empire   32

7 Jeffersonian Republicanism 166

8 Nationalism and Economic Expansion 192

9 Politics for the Common Man 220

10 An Era of Reform 250

11 Expansion and Sectional Crisis 274

12 America at Mid-Century 302

16 The New South: Reunion and Readjustment 412

17 The New West: Empire Within a Nation 432

18 The Ordeal of Industrialization 452

19 The Urban Society 474

23 Progressivism: Retreat and Resurgence 574

24 War and its Sequel 598

25 A New Age of Business 630

29 The World in Flames   728

1945-1984   758

30 The Cold War   762

31 Consolidation and Conflict 788

32 Reform and Revolt 812

Maps

xxi

THE NATIONAL EXPERIENCE

A HISTORY OF THE UNITED STATES

SIXTH EDITION

Beginnings
to 1789
THE
NATIONAL
EXPERIENCE

America was not supposed to be there. Everyone knew that the world contained three parts: Europe, Asia, and Africa. The rest was water. When two continents turned up in the midst of the water, it took time for people in Europe to get used to the idea. Many saw the unexpected lands as a global nuisance, a barrier blocking ships from a new route to familiar trading grounds. Some explorers probed for a way through or around that barrier; others recognized a new world with new opportunities.

The Spanish, who were first on the scene, were also first to see and seize the opportunities. They had happened on the most thickly populated areas, located in the tropics, and they soon put the masses of people there to work for them, digging out the things that Europeans valued most: gold, silver, pearls, and precious stones. For more than a century hardly anyone paid much attention to the more northerly lands that were to become the United States. The Spanish looked them over and could have taken them but did not bother. It was left to the English to plant themselves there and begin to feel out the possibilities of life in the outsize forests and meadows along the Atlantic coast from present-day Maine to Georgia.

Before the first English landed they thought of doing what the Spanish had done: they would put the native Americans to work for them. But they would do it better, make the people love them, make them work willingly. It did not turn out that way. By the time the English came, the native population of the northern areas, never as large as in the tropics, had already been decimated by European diseases caught from earlier exploring parties. Those who were left showed no eagerness to work for the English, so the English swept them aside to plant their own kind.

The English men and women who made America theirs came with different dreams and different designs. They hoped for more food, more land, more money, more power, or for more holiness, more justice, more brotherly love, or for more fame, more adventure, more reason to stay alive. Up and down the coast they built their new worlds, improved models, they hoped, of the old, each a little different from the others.

At first England was content to let them go their separate ways. England's part of America might fill the needs of those who settled there, but it seemed unlikely to fill the coffers of the country they came from. There were none of the treasures the Spanish had found to the south. The only North American export of any consequence was the tobacco of the Chesapeake region, and that seemed a poor substitute for gold and silver. But before the end of the seventeenth century the colonists had begun to show a trait that made the English at home sit up and take notice: they were growing like Jack's beanstalk. At a time when the population of England and the rest of Europe had become nearly stationary and the native population of the New World had suffered a catastrophic decline, England's American colonists had begun to increase by geometric progression. They were doubling every twenty-five years.

At this rate the settlers would quickly fill up the continent that European diseases and European guns were emptying of its earlier inhabitants. North America might thus furnish a vast market for English manufactures and an endless source of agricultural and forest products as well as tobacco for English merchants to sell to the rest of Europe. To be sure, it seemed unlikely that so many people, occupying a whole continent, would remain subject forever to a small island across the ocean. But even at the rate the colonists were growing it would take them more than a century to overtake the mother country. Meanwhile, England should get what it could from them while the getting was good.

England accordingly drew in the slack reins of empire, and for better than a hundred years, roughly from 1660 to 1775, managed to monopolize most of the colonists' trade. The reins were never drawn tight enough to hurt. England was a good customer for colonial produce, and the colonists were good customers for English manufactures. The system worked. But it did not take account of the colonists' relentless expansion.

The end came in 1776, before anyone could have expected, but not before the colonists had grown more like one another, more American, than they had been in their first century. They were used to elbow room now and to opportunity, and they already showed an American impatience with officers and officials who stood in their way. They knew what it meant to be poor, and they could see with their own eyes what it meant to be a slave, for there were slaves in every colony; but they were as unfamiliar with beggars as they were with kings and courtiers. They still had their differences, and the very growth that strained and broke their ties with England had pitted them often enough against each other, East against West, generation against generation, colony against colony. But by the time they met together in the Continental Congress, they recognized that they were creatures of their continent and that they had a lot in common, not least, ironically, their fading devotion to the country they were now defying.

They recognized too that, without union, their defiance would be futile. As Benjamin Franklin put it to them, they had best hang together if they did not wish to hang (or be hanged) separately. To hang together they would have to settle their differences and build institutions that could contain their fearful growth and the conflicts that went with it. That was the problem they faced in 1776. That was the problem they faced again in the government they launched in 1789.

1
MAKING USE OF A NEW WORLD

The first American was an immigrant. Although anthropologists disagree about where man first appeared on earth, no one claims the honor for the Western Hemisphere, which had probably never been seen by human eyes until twenty or thirty or at most forty thousand years ago. Presumably the earliest immigrant came by way of the Bering Straits and was followed by hundreds, perhaps thousands, more who trickled slowly southward, spreading out across North America and funneling through Mexico into Central and South America, venturing across the water to the Caribbean islands and perhaps much farther to the South Pacific. The immigration may have gone on for centuries, and it probably included people from various parts of Asia, Africa, and Europe.

For these early arrivals America was no melting pot. The people we lump together as Indians, or Native Americans, were divided into hundreds of tribes, enormously varied in physical appearance, language, and civilization. Those who made their homes south of the present United States were unquestionably the most numerous and the most skillful in exploiting their territory. They were the inventors of Indian corn (maize), as efficient a method of transforming earth into food as has ever been devised. Corn is so civilized a plant, so highly bred, that botanists have only recently been able to track down the wild ancestors from which the Indian plant-breeders developed it. The early inhabitants of Mexico and South America

were skilled in other ways too. They built great cities of stone, richly carved and ornamented. They knew enough mathematics and astronomy to construct a calendar that required no leap year and to predict eclipses of the sun. And they knew enough political science to construct strong governments under which they worked out an advanced division of labor. In central Mexico their economy supported a population of several million and a city (Tenochtitlan, now Mexico City) that ranked in size with those of Europe.

By contrast, the Indians who lived north of Mexico were primitive. They made less effective use of the land, and it supported far fewer of them, probably not many more than ten million in the present area of the United States. They grew some corn and other vegetables but also relied on nuts and berries, game and fish, and starved when these were unavailable. In parts of the Southeast they organized governments with real authority, the Powhatan Confederacy in Virginia and the Creek Confederacy in the Gulf Plains. But most often they joined together only loosely in tribes or clans under leaders or chiefs whose authority depended on the respect that their fierceness in war and their wisdom in peace could elicit from the other members of the tribe. They had dignity in abundance, self-reliance, and self-control—it was rare for Indians to show anger or even to raise their voices. Indeed, they were so self-reliant, so individualistic, that even

Their greene corne.

Corne newly sprong.

Their sitting at meate.

The place of solemne prayer.

The honse wherin the Tombe of their Herounds standeth.

SECOTON

A Ceremony in their prayers w
strange iesturs and songs dansing
abowt posts carued on the topps
lyke mens faces.

John White, *The Village of Secoton*, c. 1585–87

in war it was apt to be every man for himself; and in peace they did not achieve the cooperation and organization, the division of labor, needed to make the most of the country's resources or to defend it against strangers better organized than they.

Exploration

Such strangers began to arrive shortly after 1492. There had been earlier visitors in the eleventh century, when some wandering Norsemen from Iceland, led by Leif Ericson, spent a winter in what they called Vinland, probably in Newfoundland. A few years later other Icelanders attempted to establish a settlement. But the Norsemen had no real need for this vast continent and went home, leaving behind only the ruins of their encampments to show that they had been there.

The rise of kings and commerce. If Columbus had sailed when the Norsemen did, his voyages would probably have had as little effect as theirs on the course of history. By 1492, however, Europeans were ready for new worlds. During the intervening centuries two important historical developments had prepared them. One was the rise of a large merchant class hungry for foreign trade. Spices, dyestuffs, and textiles from India and the Far East traveled overland by slow, expensive caravan through Asia or partly by sail through the Red Sea or the Persian Gulf, passing from one dealer to another along the way until they finally reached the marketplaces of Europe. The prices people were willing to pay for these exotic imports were enough to send fifteenth-century sailors in search of sea routes to the source of the treasures. A direct sea route would permit importation in greater volume at less expense and would net the importer a huge profit.

Portugal took the lead in maritime exploration with a new type of vessel, the caravel—faster, more maneuverable, more seaworthy than any formerly known. Portuguese explorers, encouraged by their kings and by Prince Henry the Navigator (1394–1460), discovered the Azores and pushed their caravels farther and farther south along the coast of Africa. At first they were probably seeking only new trading opportunities in Africa itself, but by the 1480s they were searching for a way around the continent to the greater riches of the Orient. In 1488 Bartholomeu Diaz rounded the Cape of Good Hope. Ten years later Vasco da Gama reached India.

The rise of kings was the second great development that prepared Europeans to use a new world. At the time of Leif Ericson's voyage Europe was divided into tiny principalities, usually owing nominal allegiance to a king but actually dominated by local magnates who levied tolls on all trade passing through their territories. Even towns and cities tended to be autonomous, bristling with local regulations that discouraged trade with the outside world. The rise of kings meant the reorganization of society into larger units, into national states more wealthy and more powerful than any one of the towns or cities or principalities of which they were composed. A state organized under a king had the power and resources to cut through the strangling web of local trade barriers, to sponsor exploration for new lands to trade with, and even to seize the lands and their riches when the natives were not strong enough to resist.

During most of the fifteenth century Portugal far outran the rest of Europe in pursuit of foreign trade and of new lands to conquer. Other countries were still too troubled by domestic feuds and foreign wars to offer much competition. The first to emerge as a serious rival was Portugal's neighbor, Spain. And, as luck had it, Spain was also first to find America and first to find a use for it.

Columbus and the Spanish. Christopher Columbus, the son of a Genoese weaver, was a man with a mission. He wanted to reach the Orient by sailing

Caravel—faster and more seaworthy

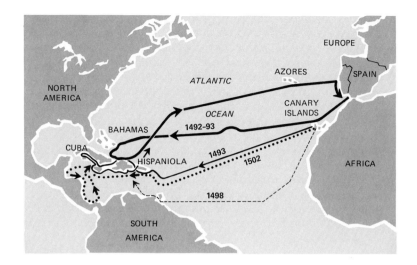

west, and he was convinced that the distance was no more than three or four thousand miles. Columbus was wrong, and when he tried to sell his idea the experts told him so. The experts had known for centuries that the world was round, and they had a much better notion of its size than Columbus did. The king of Portugal would have none of his scheme, and neither would anyone else until Queen Isabella of Spain, who was not an expert, decided to take a chance. In the very year that the consolidation of the Spanish monarchy was completed by the conquest of Granada from the Moors, she persuaded her husband, Ferdinand II, to pay for an expedition of three ships and to give Columbus authority, under Spain, over any lands he might discover on the way.

Armed with this commission and with a letter to the emperor of China, Columbus made his magnificent mistake. He failed to deliver the letter but found America (so named after his death for a later explorer, Amerigo Vespucci), at the island of San Salvador, on October 12, 1492. From here he threaded his way through the other Bahamas to Cuba and Hispaniola. By March 15, 1493, he was back in Spain. In succeeding years he explored the rest of the Caribbean area, still looking for China and Japan. Though he did not find them, he did find gold; and everyone in Europe knew what to do with that.

But for the gold, Europeans would probably have looked upon America as a mere obstacle on the route to the Orient. Even after Ferdinand Magellan carried out Columbus' original intention by sailing around the tip of South America (1519–22), explorers continued for two centuries to probe hopefully up American rivers in search of the Pacific. But the Spanish recognized at once that Columbus' substitute for China might have advantages surpassing the original. With

approval of Pope Alexander VI they joined the Portuguese in the Treaty of Tordesillas (1494), dividing the world by a line drawn north and south, 370 leagues west of the Cape Verde Islands (between the present forty-sixth and forty-seventh meridians): Spain was authorized to take possession of all the heathen lands it found to the west of the line; Portugal could do the same to the east. Thereafter the Spanish swarmed over the Caribbean islands and onto the mainland of North and South America.

By comparison with the natives, the invaders were few in number, but they were courageous, unscrupulous, and armed. They wanted gold, and they were ready to take what the natives had and make them dig for more. The Indians were no match for them. In the West Indies the first Spaniards killed or enslaved wherever they went, and slavery was only a slower form of killing. After working the Caribbean natives to death, they brought in black slaves purchased from the Portuguese, the beginning of an involuntary migration that ultimately carried nearly 10 million Africans to the New World. In the Caribbean islands the Africans died, too, but not before they had earned their purchase price many times over. When the supply of gold ran out, the Spanish turned them to planting sugar, which in the long run proved even more lucrative—and no less deadly—than digging for gold.

On the mainland, where the Indians were more numerous, small armies led by private adventurers, the conquistadors, subdued whole countries. Hernando Cortez with fifteen hundred men conquered Mexico (1519–21), and Francisco Pizarro with still fewer men conquered Peru (1531–35). The extraordinary conquests made by these small forces were possible because Spanish firearms and cavalry seemed irresistible to people who had never seen either guns or horses before—the Indians frequently took a man on horseback to be some superhuman quadruped. But even with this enormous advantage the Spanish could scarcely have subdued such large and populous areas if the Indians had not been divided among themselves and if most of them had not already been living as subject peoples. To many Indians the Spaniard was only a more powerful and exacting master than the Aztec or Inca ruler whom they had served before.

The conquistadors were quick to seize the gold and silver with which the native palaces abounded, but the people themselves were the greatest treasure of Spain's new possessions. Spain in the sixteenth century had a population of about 9 million. The native population of Spanish America probably amounted to many more than that, and they all could be put to work for Spain. In the course of the century, thousands of Spaniards came to the new land, most of them to profit from the immense supply of cheap labor that Columbus and the conquistadors had delivered to them.

The Spanish government did what it could, from a distance of three thousand miles, to protect the rights of its Indian subjects, and the Church sent countless priests, friars, and bishops to look after their souls. Devoted Spanish clerics never ceased to denounce the way in which their countrymen relentlessly overworked the Indians. But everyone agreed that they ought to work, and neither church nor state

Hernando Cortez

Broken spears lie in the roads;
we have torn our hair in our grief.
The houses are roofless now, and their walls
are red with blood.

Worms are swarming in the streets and plazas,
and the walls are splattered with gore.
The water has turned red, as if it were dyed,
and when we drink it,
it has the taste of brine.

We have pounded our hands in despair
against the adobe walls,
for our inheritance, our city, is lost and dead.
The shields of our warriors were its defense,
but they could not save it.

We have chewed dry twigs and salt grasses;
we have filled our mouths with dust and bits of adobe,
we have eaten lizards, rats and worms....

**Miguel Leon-Portilla, ed., _The Broken Spears:_
The Aztec Account of the Conquest of Mexico, 1521.**

was able to prevent the new lords of the land from exacting the utmost from every Indian who came within their reach.

Indians who resisted the Spanish advance were enslaved. Others, technically free, were parceled out in _encomiendas_, at first to the conquerors but later to nearly every Spaniard who appeared on the scene. From the Indians of his _encomienda_ the _encomendero_ could demand labor at token wages and also an annual tribute. When the government finally brought this form of exploitation under control in the middle of the century, the settlers devised other forms of forced labor.

The Spanish colonists made use of the Indians in mining the great deposits of silver ore that were discovered in both Mexico and Peru and in manning huge ranches and farms (haciendas). While the labor supply lasted, many settlers made fortunes, and the Spanish treasury welcomed the silver that poured in from its numerous taxes, which included a fifth of the proceeds of privately owned mines. But within a century the boom had ended, because overwork, despair, and disease destroyed the Spanish empire's basic resource. In the century after the conquest the native population of Mexico declined from several million (some scholars say 25 million) to little more than a million. A comparable decline is thought to have occurred in Peru.

**Cannons and crossbows against spears:
an Indian view of the Spanish Conquest**

The discovery of America, and that of a passage to the East Indies by the Cape of Good Hope, are the two greatest and most important events recorded in the history of mankind. Their consequences have already been very great; but in the short period of between two and three centuries which has elapsed since these discoveries were made, it is impossible that the whole extent of their consequences can have been seen. What benefits or what misfortunes to mankind may hereafter result from those great events, no human wisdom can foresee. By uniting, in some measure, the most distant parts of the world, by enabling them to relieve one another's wants, to increase one another's enjoyments, and to encourage one another's industry, their general tendency would seem to be beneficial. To the natives, however, both of the East and West Indies, all the commercial benefits which can have resulted from those events have been sunk and lost in the dreadful misfortunes which they have occasioned. These misfortunes, however, seem to have arisen rather from accident than from anything in the nature of those events themselves. At the particular time when these discoveries were made, the superiority of force happened to be so great on the side of the Europeans that they were enabled to commit with impunity every sort of injustice in those remote countries. Hereafter, perhaps, the natives of those countries may grow stronger, or those of Europe may grow weaker, and the inhabitants of all the different quarters of the world may arrive at that equality of courage and force which, by inspiring mutual fear, can alone overawe the injustice of independent nations into some sort of respect for the rights of one another.

From Adam Smith, *The Wealth of Nations*, 1776.

Of the acknowledged causes for this catastrophic loss, probably the most lethal was the unavoidable introduction of European diseases against which the Indians had no natural resistance. Many of those who did survive were of mixed ancestry, mestizos as they were called. They, together with the creoles (people of European descent born in Spanish America), the Africans, and the few remaining Indians, furnished a base from which Spanish America in succeeding centuries was to recover its population and perpetuate the new civilization that Spain had brought to the New World.

North of Mexico the Spanish at first found little to interest them. Ponce de León cruised along the shores of the Florida peninsula in 1513, and Pánfilo de Narváez and Hernando de Soto both explored the western side of the peninsula and the Gulf Plains before the middle of the sixteenth century. But there was no visible gold or silver about and no extensive population to exploit. Both expeditions marched on across the continent to Mexico without finding anything on the way that made them want to stay. In a futile search for seven legendary cities of gold, Francisco Vásquez de Coronado circled through present Arizona, New Mexico, Texas, Oklahoma, and Kansas (1540–42). He too thought the country not worth taking and returned to Mexico.

During the second half of the sixteenth century the Spanish began to take a more lasting interest in the northern areas. They established a fort at St. Augustine, Florida (1565), and carried on missionary activities as far north as Port Royal (South Carolina) and for a few years even up to Chesapeake Bay. By the end of the century they were settling into present New Mexico and Arizona, planting missions to benefit the peaceable natives and *presidios* (military outposts) to hold back hostile ones. The mission was an ambitious undertaking, a nucleus from which Spanish civilization might grow in the borderlands of the empire. The mission gathered Indians (often nomadic in this section) into settled communities where, under supervision of the Church, they were taught Christianity along with techniques of farming and handicrafts. During the seventeenth century Spain sowed missions in Texas and during the eighteenth in California. But long before this, the force of the Spanish thrust had spent itself, and other countries were ready to make use of the vast and lonely North American continent.

The Europeans in North America. Columbus never saw the shores of North America, nor do we know what European was the first to do so. Perhaps other sailors had happened on it just as the Norsemen had. There may even have been fishermen walking the streets of St. Malo or Bristol or Plymouth who could have told Columbus of a distant coast where pines were tall and codfish plentiful. If so, no chronicler set down their discoveries until in 1497 John Cabot, like Columbus a Genoese, sailed west for the king of England and returned to report a new land. Henry VII gave Cabot £10 and an annuity of £20. Cabot undertook another voyage the next year, but he and other Europeans thought of the new land as a barrier, not an opportunity.

In 1524 the king of France, Francis I, sent a Florentine navigator, Giovanni da Verrazano, along the Atlantic coast from North Carolina to Nova Scotia in search of a passage through the barrier to the Pacific. Ten years later the king sent Jacques Cartier on the same errand. Cartier, encouraged by the promisingly large entrance of the St. Lawrence River, sailed inland as far as the first rapids before giving up. He was sufficiently impressed by the surrounding country, however, to attempt a settlement there in 1541. Since Spain had found riches in the southern continent, it seemed reasonable to expect them in the north as well. When Canadian gold proved to be fool's gold, Canadian diamonds quartz, and Canadian winters terrible, the colonists returned home, and France forgot about North America for the rest of the century.

The first Europeans to find a lasting use for the continent were summer people, who liked the fishing there. Every spring in the ports of France, England, Portugal, and Spain fishermen piled aboard their precarious craft and headed for the Grand Banks, where the continental shelf of North America lies submerged at a depth that codfish find congenial. They set up docks and drying stages ashore and assembled knocked-down dories and other small boats carried in the holds of their ships. They killed a few auks or netted some minnows for bait, rowed far out to the deeper waters, and fished all day with hand lines. Each night they brought in their catch to be dried, salted, and packed for sale in the markets of Europe. Caring little for the doings of their remote monarchs, they lived together in little international communities in Newfoundland and Nova Scotia—sleeping aboard their ships or in rough cabins ashore, planting gardens, and visiting one another of an evening—until

Spanish and French explorations of North America

the approach of winter sent them and the cod to friendlier climates. None of them seems to have contemplated permanent residence.

As the years passed, more and more Europeans sailed west to cruise along the coasts of North America, catching its codfish, prying into bays and rivers, kidnaping an occasional Indian to show off at home. Gradually they became aware that the country had more to offer than fish and pine trees. Behind the coast lay rivers and lakes teeming with beaver, otter, and other fur-bearing animals, which the Indians were adept at trapping. When Indians and Europeans met, the Indians demanded metals, whose superiority to stone they were quick to recognize. The furs they offered in exchange brought a good price in Europe—especially beaver, which was turned into felt for hats.

Early in the seventeenth century the French, the Dutch, and the Swedes all set up permanent fur-trading posts in America. The great French explorer Samuel de Champlain, after reconnoitering the New England coast and the St. Lawrence region, founded Quebec in 1608. Henry Hudson, an Englishman working for a Dutch company, in 1609 sailed up the river he named for himself; the Dutch planted trading posts there in 1624, on the Delaware River in 1623, and on the Connecticut River in 1633. A Swedish company also maintained posts on the Delaware from 1638 until the Dutch seized them in 1655.

The French and the Dutch came to trade with the Indians, not to subjugate them. Neither in New France nor in New Netherland, as their settlements were called, did the Indians become slaves. Instead they lived on in their customary manner, roaming the woods they had roamed before, though trapping beaver in unaccustomed numbers. Contact with the Europeans inevitably meant new things for them: Christianity, comfort, progress, guns, hatchets, deadly drinks, deadlier diseases, sharper rivalry with other tribes, and a weakening of tribal customs. But the continent was still theirs. In the course of time both the French and the Dutch did try to transform their trading posts into larger settlements of Europeans, who would supplant rather than suppress or exploit the Indian, but this was only after the English had arrived on the continent and begun to fill it with their children.

Tudor England and the New World

Before England could turn its interests to America at all, before its merchants could support expensive and risky overseas expeditions, it had to experience the same political consolidation under a powerful king that Spain and Portugal had undergone a century earlier. Henry VII, who sent John Cabot to America in 1497, began the job; his son Henry VIII and his granddaughter Elizabeth I finished it. In the process they transformed England from a Catholic country into a Protestant one, a fact that would affect profoundly the land that John Cabot had found across the seas.

Henry VIII and the Reformation. Soon after Martin Luther launched the Reformation, which split the monolithic west-European Church into Protestant and Roman Catholic segments, Luther's teachings reached England. Perhaps no Englishman was less receptive to them than the king, Henry VIII, who demonstrated his devotion to Rome by writing a book against the German heretic. The pope rewarded Henry by conferring on him the title "Defender of the Faith."

Before many years passed Henry found himself, if no friendlier to Luther, a good deal less friendly to the pope. Henry was the most powerful king England had ever known. Only one set of men in England dared challenge his authority: the priests and bishops, the monks and abbots, who acknowledged a higher power than Henry not only in the heavens but on earth, in Rome. Moreover, the Church owned about one-fourth of England and collected a yearly income of more than £320,000, much of it from the rent of lands owned by monasteries. When Henry needed funds to meet the cost of England's new and growing governmental machinery, the wealth of the monasteries caught his eye. He soon found an opportunity to lay hold of it.

In 1509 Henry had married Catherine of Aragon, daughter of Ferdinand and Isabella, and in twenty years she bore him no son who lived. Henry desperately wanted an heir, and besides he had grown tired of Catherine. In 1529 he asked the pope for a divorce. When the pope refused, Henry defied him, married Anne Boleyn, severed England's ties with Rome, and made himself head of the English Church. By 1539 he had confiscated the monastic lands.

The results of Henry's break with Rome. Although Henry never showed the slightest interest in the New World, his divorce and his defiance of the pope had enormous consequences for both England and America.

The first and simplest consequence was that his new wife bore him a daughter, Elizabeth, who was to become England's greatest monarch. Elizabeth became queen in 1558 and ruled for forty-four glorious years—years in which the English triumphed on land, at sea, and in the human spirit. Under her direction England became strong enough to begin the building of a North American empire.

Second, by divorcing his Spanish queen, Henry touched off over a hundred years of intermittent hostility with Spain. Spain, the spearhead of Catholicism and the headquarters of the Inquisition, gradually became synonymous in Protestant England with the antichrist. Englishmen attacked the Spaniard most successfully at sea not only by outright war but by privateering against Spanish shipping. The English privateers (or sea dogs, as they came to be called)

Queen Elizabeth I: England's greatest monarch

resembled the earlier conquistadors in their daring, toughness, unscrupulousness, and flair for the spectacular and heroic. But the sea dogs operated on water rather than on land, scouring the Atlantic and the Caribbean for Spanish vessels laden with gold and silver from the New World. Under Queen Elizabeth privateering against Spain reached its height and drew England's attention to the riches of America.

Third, Henry's break with Rome gave impetus to a Protestant movement in England that had been covertly under way for some years. Its adherents interpreted Henry's defiance of the pope as a total repudiation of Roman hierarchy, ritual, and doctrine. Henry himself would have been content to serve as England's pope without substantially altering the internal organization or doctrines of the Church. But he could not wholly control the forces he had unleashed. The ideas of Luther and of the French reformer John Calvin became increasingly popular during the next 125 years; and, as their numbers grew, the extreme Calvinists—the Puritans—became increasingly discontent with the incomplete reformation of the English Church. Many of them would go to America with a view to completing the Reformation there.

Finally, Henry's confiscation of the monasteries set off a train of unexpected events that indirectly provided still more English men and women willing to people a new world. Henry, not content with the income from the lands he had confiscated, began to sell them; succeeding monarchs continued the process, selling other royal lands as well. They were led to do so partly by a steady rise in prices during the sixteenth and seventeenth centuries (the so-called Price Revolution) that was accelerated by the flow of Spanish gold and silver from America. Other people felt the pinch, especially landlords whose rents were fixed by custom and unalterable. They too began selling land to make ends meet. The turnover of so much real estate had widespread repercussions: in some places the rich got richer and the poor poorer, while in other places the rich were getting poor and the poor rich. The sale of monastic lands was certainly not wholly responsible for this upheaval, but it was a step in the chain of events that destroyed the social and economic security of large numbers of people and helped to make the fortunes of others, especially the merchants. Whoever lost from the rise of prices and the sale of lands, it was not they. As the sixteenth century wore on, they accumulated more and more capital, enough to finance overseas expeditions, while those who lost their homes, fortunes, and jobs began to think of regaining them, perhaps in another part of the world.

Gilbert finds a use for North America. The historical developments that were set in motion by Henry VIII's break with Rome became significant for America only gradually. After the voyage of John Cabot in 1497, the English showed very little interest in the New World until 1576, when the Cathay Company (Cathay was another name for China) was formed to trade with China by way of North America. The company sent Martin Frobisher to find a way through the continent. He probed the northern waters and found Baffin Land and Frobisher's Bay, where glittering gold-flecked rocks diverted his attention from further search. With the usual captive Indian and a case of ore samples, he hurried back to England. The assayers declared that the ore was indeed gold, and he returned to North America for more. When the twelve hundred tons he brought back turned out to be worthless, the Cathay Company folded. For years thereafter Englishmen with capital to invest were wary of risking it in America.

Although the Cathay Company had planned to establish a small permanent settlement in America, it was intended to serve merely as a supply station for voyages to the Orient. The first Englishman, possibly the first European, to have a glimmering of the northern continent's colonial future was a soldier of fortune named Humphrey Gilbert. Gilbert had served the queen in Ireland, where his skill in exterminating the natives won him a knighthood. While there he concocted a scheme for peopling Ireland with English settlers. But then his interest shifted. North America was a larger Ireland. Englishmen planted there could exploit the natives (the counterpart of the wild Irish), forestall Spanish settlement, catch codfish, and search for a passage to the Pacific. Until one was found, an American colony would serve as a base from which sea dogs could raid the Spanish treasure fleets that sailed every year from the Caribbean. In every way America was more attractive than Ireland.

Gilbert, impelled by greed and chauvinism, had vision: he was the first to see America as a place for the English to live. In 1578 he induced Queen Elizabeth to grant him a charter empowering him to settle a colony over which he would exercise absolute authority, provided he made no laws contrary to the Christian faith, and provided he gave the queen one-fifth of the gold and silver he mined (a provision generally inserted by subsequent monarchs in such charters).

Gilbert made two attempts to found his colony. The first attempt, in 1578, is a mystery. No one knows where he went or what he found. His second attempt, in 1583, was a larger undertaking, for by this time he had managed to sell his idea to others: noblemen who felt the pressure of inflated prices and the loss of lands and power their fathers had had; merchants who scented opportunities for trade in the new land; discontented religious minorities, privateers, pirates, paupers, and fools. Drawing men and money from these divergent sources, Gilbert got underway in June 1583 with two hundred sixty prospective settlers and five ships, one of which he stole from a pirate just before departing and took along, pirate crew and all.

In August the expedition reached Newfoundland, where Gilbert came upon a sizable international community of summer fishermen. He probably did not intend to establish his colony this far north (though it should be remembered that Newfoundland is south of England), but he made a great ceremony of taking possession of the settlement. The fishermen humored him and even agreed to pay rent for their fishing stages. They probably calculated, rightly, that no one would come to collect it.

After two weeks in Newfoundland, Gilbert cruised southward, filled with enthusiasm by the splendor of the uninhabited coast. Although two of his ships deserted him and another was lost on a reef, he was still confident of founding a colony when he turned his two remaining ships homeward for more supplies. In mid-ocean they ran into an alarmingly heavy sea, but Gilbert demonstrated his nonchalance by sitting on the afterdeck of his small vessel reading a book. At one point he shouted across to a friend in the

English explorations of the New World

other ship: "We are as near to heaven by sea as by land." That night, as the others watched, the lights of his vessel went out. No more was ever heard of the man who first envisaged England's American empire.

Raleigh and Roanoke. Although Gilbert's ventures accomplished nothing concrete, he had stirred the imagination of other Englishmen: the kind of men who backed him would back other expeditions to the New World. Before his last voyage, he had enlisted the talents of his younger half-brother, Sir Walter Raleigh. Raleigh equaled Gilbert in daring and exceeded him in polish. He was a favorite with Queen Elizabeth, who gave him nearly everything he asked for. After Gilbert's death, Raleigh asked her for a charter to found a colony in the New World.

Raleigh was as interested as Gilbert in piracy against Spanish treasure fleets, and like Gilbert he wanted his colony to be more than a base of opera-

tions. From the beginning he planned it as a permanent settlement, and he enlisted his friend Richard Hakluyt to write propaganda persuading people to emigrate. Hakluyt was already fascinated by the idea of colonization and developed into England's greatest advocate of overseas expansion.

Raleigh got his charter in 1584 and immediately sent out a reconnoitering force under Philip Amadas and Arthur Barlow. They made their landfall a couple of thousand miles south of Newfoundland—perhaps in order to be closer to the Spanish—and explored the coast south of Chesapeake Bay. When they returned with glowing descriptions of the region, Raleigh named it Virginia in honor of Elizabeth, the Virgin Queen.

In 1585 Raleigh fitted out an expedition to settle Roanoke Island, near the present boundary between Virginia and North Carolina. The group, under the command of Ralph Lane, included John White, an artist; Thomas Cavendish, who later sailed round the world; and Thomas Hariot, a noted mathematician. White made some excellent drawings of the American Indians, the best executed during the whole colonial period; Hariot took notes from which he later prepared the first detailed description in English of any part of the present United States. The settlers themselves, instead of digging in, spent their time searching Virginia's rivers unsuccessfully for the Pacific and its shores unsuccessfully for gold. In June 1586, when Sir Francis Drake called to visit them after searching successfully for gold in the Spanish fortresses of the West Indies, the settlers all climbed aboard with him and went home.

Raleigh tried again the next year, 1587, sending one hundred twenty persons under the command of John White. White spent a month getting the new Roanoke settlement started and then returned to England for supplies, leaving his daughter, her husband, and their new-born child with the settlers. A supply fleet commanded by Sir Richard Grenville was prepared, but the Spaniards chose this moment for an all-out attack on England (the great Spanish Armada), and Grenville and his ships were pressed into service for defense. Not until 1590 could White sail back to Roanoke, and when he got there his colonists had vanished. Someone had carved the name of a neighboring island, CROATOAN, on a post. But no trace of the colonists was ever found there. Presumably, hostile Indians had overwhelmed them, but to this day no real clue to their fate has been found.

Sir Francis Drake: knighted for his exploits

The sixteenth century closed without an English colony in North America. Raleigh turned his attention to South America. Richard Hakluyt sang the praises of England's explorers and published accounts of their great voyages in *The Principall Navigations, Voiages, and Discoveries of the English Nation* (1589). But no one else with the vision of a Gilbert or a Raleigh stepped forward to lead Englishmen to new homes.

Actually Gilbert and Raleigh were as wrong, in their way, as Columbus. He expected to find China and found America. They expected not only to settle North America but to make a profit out of it. They failed, and even if their settlements had succeeded there would almost certainly have been no profit, unless from piracy. But Gilbert and Raleigh were not the last to be mistaken about the New World. In 1606 another group of English investors risked their money, and lost it, in an enterprise from which in the fullness of time grew the United States.

The Founding of Virginia

While Elizabeth reigned, men of daring in England enjoyed risking their money and their lives for her by attacking Spain. Her successor, James I, was so different from the great queen that he has always suffered by comparison. Elizabeth knew everything about power and kept her own counsel. James knew everything about everything and told everybody. One of the things he knew was that the war with Spain had gone on long enough. In 1604, the year after his accession, he made a peace that lasted twenty years.

James was probably right in ending the war, but his subjects did not all love him for it, especially after he told them that raids on Spanish shipping must cease. During the sixteenth century the line between legitimate privateering and piracy had been left conveniently thin, and hijacked Spanish bullion had poured into England. Francis Drake alone picked up close to a million pesos (over £300,000) worth of loot from Spanish ships he met during his dramatic voyage around the globe (1577-80). Elizabeth knighted Drake for his exploits and cheerfully collected a share of the profits. But James forswore such profits for his subjects as well as himself. As a result, men with spare lives and money began to think again about getting gold where the Spanish got it. Efforts to find it in North America had so far been unsuccessful, but no one had tried very hard. Even if no gold was found, the continent might hold other things of value. After the Roanoke venture of 1586, Thomas Hariot had described some promising native commodities, including sassafras, a root that the Spanish were selling in Europe at high prices as a cure for syphilis. And piracy itself, now that the king had pledged his protection to Spanish shipping, might still be carried on from a base out of royal reach on the other side of the Atlantic. And so the tantalizing possibility of riches from America again lured Englishmen to try to plant a colony there.

Jamestown. In 1606 a number of noblemen, gentlemen, and merchants joined to petition the king for authority to establish colonies in America. Merchants had discovered a means of undertaking large and dangerous enterprises without risking financial ruin. Their scheme was the joint-stock company, in which participants profited or suffered in proportion to the number of shares they purchased. By investing modestly in a number of companies a man would gain only modest profits from successful ventures, but he would also avoid heavy losses from unsuccessful ones. In this way, through many small contributions, it was possible to accumulate the large amounts of capital necessary for undertakings that were beyond the range of private fortunes. The joint-stock company became the principal instrument of England's early overseas expansion.

The men who petitioned the king in 1606 were divided into two groups, one from London, the other from Plymouth; and the king gave them a charter incorporating two companies for the colonization of North America: the Virginia Company of Plymouth was to operate in the northern part of the continent, and the Virginia Company of London in the southern part. The companies planned to finance the emigration of settlers who would agree to relinquish the fruits of their labors to the investors for the first seven years; after that the settlers could enrich themselves. Those who paid their own passage were free to begin getting rich at once.

Both companies got off to a quick start. The Plymouth group dispatched an exploratory expedition in 1606 and in 1607 founded a colony at the mouth of the Sagadahoc River in Maine. The colony survived only one winter. The Virginia Company of London, in December 1606, sent over its first settlers, a hundred men and four boys crammed aboard three small ships, the *Susan Constant,* the *Godspeed,* and the *Discovery.* In May 1607 they sailed up a river they called the James and landed on a peninsula they called Jamestown. Swampy and forested, the site was well situated for defense but a haven for mosquitoes and microbes. The colonists made almost every possible mistake in their new environment, but they also corrected their mistakes; and they had the vision, the courage, or the foolhardiness to stick it out.

Their first big problem was leadership. In the charter granting authority to settle the colony, the king

Virginia and New England grants

had retained authority to govern the colony himself, and he exercised it through a council sitting in England. This council in turn acted through another sitting in Virginia. The Virginia council consisted of seven men with a president who presided over its meetings but who had no authority to give orders of his own and no power to enforce orders transmitted from the king's council in England. Government by council proved to be no government at all. The members of the council in the colony quarreled with one another; and the colonists, undisciplined and disorganized, neglected the elementary tasks of plowing, planting, and building.

Fortunately, one man had the nerve to take command. John Smith, twenty-seven years old, of humble background but no humility, was not popular with the other members of the council, all men of greater age, importance, and indecision. Smith had spent four years fighting the Turks in Hungary, where he had been captured, sold into slavery, and rescued by fair maidens. In Virginia, by his own account, when the other members of the council proved fools, knaves, or cowards he took control of the colony, explored it, mapped it, overawed the Indians (and was again rescued by a maiden, Pocahontas), and obtained from them the corn that kept the settlers from starving. He

Pocahontas

Ætatis suæ 21. A°.1616.

stopped the disorganized scramble for gold, built fortifications, planted Indian corn, and cut a cargo of cedar wood to send back to the investors as the first tangible evidence of the colony's worth. He later told about it with such relish for his own role that readers ever since have suspected his veracity. Nevertheless, wherever his account can be checked, it holds up. Moreover he prepared a surprisingly accurate map of the region—a map that could only have been the product of first-hand observation.

In London, however, the armchair colonizers were not pleased. Smith, they heard, was unkind to the Indians. He had failed to find either gold or the Pacific Ocean. And some of the other members of the Virginia council, returning to the mother country, described his leadership as tyranny. The company did recognize, however, that the colony needed stronger direction. In 1609 it obtained a new royal charter establishing a new governing council (resident in London) composed entirely of company members and empowered to appoint an all-powerful governor or governors in the colony. The council decided on a single governor, who should choose a council of Virginians to advise him. To prevent a repetition of the colony's earlier squabbles over leadership and to ensure that the governor's council understood that its function was limited to advice, the London council specified that the Virginia councilors "shall not have, single nor together, anie bindinge or negative voice or power." The post of governor went not to Smith but to a nobleman, Lord De La Warr.

Under the new charter the company launched an

elaborate campaign to sell Virginia to the English public. With the proceeds of stock sold at £12 10s. a share, it fitted out a fleet of nine vessels to carry some six hundred emigrants, the great majority of whom were men. Some paid their own way (passage was worth about £6) and received a share of stock as a bonus. The rest came as servants, having agreed to work for the company for seven years in return for their passage. But all would work together until 1616, at which time the servants would be freed, the profits would be divided among the shareholders both in England and in America, and every shareholder would receive at least a hundred acres of land.

The expedition set sail from Plymouth in June 1609. Though one of the ships was wrecked at Bermuda, at least four hundred settlers reached Virginia that summer. Unfortunately Lord De La Warr was not among them. His departure from England had been delayed, and his substitute, Sir Thomas Gates, was on the ship lost at Bermuda. John Smith, injured in a gunpowder explosion, returned to England in the fall of 1609, and from then until the arrival of Governor Thomas Dale in 1611 the colony was without effective government and fell into worse disorder than before. People starved; fortifications fell to ruins; at one point the entire colony had embarked, prepared to abandon the settlement, when a relief ship arrived. After 1611, Governor Dale and Governor Samuel Argall, who succeeded him, imposed rigorous disciplinary laws and resumed the course set by John Smith. Once again the colonists began to plant corn, erect and repair fortifications, and build houses.

But the men who left England for Virginia wanted more than corn bread and a place to lay their heads. To them survival was a means to an end, and they kept looking for a way to wealth, a way to live better in Virginia than they had in England. Since they had found no gold or silver, they had to find some other commodity of high value that they could produce in sufficient quantity and with sufficient ease to make the long voyage to English or European markets worthwhile. They tried cedar. They tried sassafras. But the market for both was quickly satisfied. The directors of the company had high hopes at different times for wines, silk, iron, tar. But in 1612, though they were not at once aware of it, the Virginians discovered their future—in smoke.

Tobacco was native to America. The Indians had taught the Spanish to use it, and the Spanish had taught the rest of Europe. At first it was valued only as a medicine, said to cure any affliction from the waist up. But by the end of the sixteenth century people were smoking for the fun of it, much to the distress of those who knew better, including King James, and much to the joy of Spanish tobacco merchants. The Indians of Virginia smoked a native variety, coarse and unpalatable. John Rolfe, who later gained greater fame by marrying Pocahontas, tried planting the West Indian species in 1612, just as other settlers were experimenting with other Spanish products. The West Indian variety grew extraordinarily well in Virginia, and the settlers turned enthusiastically to growing it. By 1617 they were able to ship twenty thousand pounds to England.

The Virginia Company's great effort. The stockholders of the Virginia Company were pleased to have their faltering confidence in the colony reconfirmed by the promising shipments of tobacco. Hitherto they had received nothing but a few tons of sassafras, cedar, and other trifles in return for an investment of approximately £50,000. In fact, when they sat down to divide up their profits in 1616, they had found nothing to divide except the land itself, and to many of them it hardly seemed worth dividing. Moreover, most of the servants they had sent over to work for the company had served out their time and had become free to work for themselves. To hire more men to produce so little would be to throw good money after bad.

Although the colonists' success with tobacco rekindled the expectations of the investors, they did not suppose that the colony could prosper with that product alone. But if Virginia could grow tobacco there must be other things it could produce too. They must keep the settlers experimenting until the right products were found, and then everyone could sit back and reap the profits of perseverance. While this new burst of enthusiasm was upon them, the members of the Virginia Company decided to revitalize and expand their venture by means of a reform program, which they inaugurated in 1618 under the leadership of Sir Edwin Sandys, a prominent figure in the English House of Commons. The program contained four points designed to entice more adventurers (investors), more planters (settlers), and more servants:

1. By overhauling its land policies the company made both investment and emigration more profitable. Henceforth anyone who paid the fare to Virginia for himself or anyone else received a "headright" of fifty acres on which he would pay a "quitrent" of a shilling a year to the company. Wealthy investors could thus acquire large tracts (called "particular plantations") simply by sending men to cultivate them on a sharecropping basis. The company in turn, with almost unlimited acreage at its disposal, would gain a perpetual income from quitrents.

2. To make life in Virginia more like life in England, the company relaxed the severity of its discipline and assured actual and potential settlers that henceforth the colony would be governed by English law and that the colonists would have the rights of Englishmen.

3. Even more important, the company decided to give the settlers a voice in the management of the colony. The planters were allowed to elect representatives to an assembly, which, along with the governor's appointed council, would have power to make laws for the colony. And to relieve the settlers of taxes, the cost of government was to be borne by assigning lands (and tenants to work them) to each government office.

4. The final point in the new program called for an all-out effort to diversify the colony's activities. The company itself took responsibility for sending over various craftsmen: vintners, ironworkers, brickmakers, glass-blowers. Somewhere among these skills, it was hoped, would be the right ones to give Virginia a healthy and profitable economy of which tobacco-growing would be only one part.

For five years and more, new settlers streamed into the colony. By the end of 1618 the population, which was only 400 in April of that year, had risen to 1,000. Between 1618 and 1624, about 4,000 more arrived. To judge by the number of ships landing passengers in Virginia, the colony was a success. To judge by the number of graves dug there, it was not. In spite of the heavy immigration, the population in 1625 stood at only 1,210 by official count. Some of the settlers had doubtless returned to England, but for most of them the colony had been a death trap. Sandys (who never set foot in Virginia) had sent shipload after shipload of settlers without supplies. Ill fed, ill clothed, and ill housed, they sickened and died. In 1622 the Indians rose up and killed 347.

Those who survived found themselves subjected to ruthless exploitation, unlike anything known in England. From 1618 until about 1629, Virginia tobacco brought prices ranging from a shilling to three shill-

People were smoking for fun, to the distress of those who knew better

ings a pound. Since a man could produce 500 to 1,000 pounds a year, his labor was worth at least £25 and might be worth over £100 a year. As a result, those who had the nerve, the strength, and the authority (legal or illegal) to control the labor of lesser men could make small fortunes in a short time. In the scramble for the servants and tenants who arrived each year, the governor and members of his council were among the most successful in laying hold of large numbers. As long as tobacco prices held up, they made handsome profits—but for themselves, not for the company. While they grew rich on the labors of the men the company sent, the company itself was going bankrupt; and rumors reached England that men and boys were sold back and forth in Virginia like horses. In 1624 when James I appointed a commission to investigate, the commissioners reported such shocking treatment of the settlers that the king dissolved the company and resumed control of the colony himself.

Thus ended the Virginia Company of London. At the cost of several thousand lives and perhaps £100,000 it had in the course of eighteen years established only twelve hundred settlers in America. But in spite of its wretched beginning, the colony was there to stay.

After the king took over, the population gradually rose as ships that came to carry away the tobacco every year continued to bring new supplies of men and some women. But, because English women were not used for field work, the planters imported many more men than women, giving Virginia a lopsided sex ratio throughout the century. Only a few of the newcomers were slaves brought from Africa (Virginia's shift to slave labor came later, as we shall see), but servants in Virginia continued to fare little better than slaves. Although the king may have aimed at curbing the exploitation of his Virginia subjects by unscrupulous masters, his authority at three thousand miles' distance was no greater obstacle to the local labor barons than the company's had been. But in 1630 tobacco dropped to a penny a pound and then, after a few wild fluctuations, settled for about twenty-five years at a little more than two pence a pound. At that price it still offered reasonable rewards but did not excite the kind of cupidity that had made Virginia in the 1620s a scene of misery, profiteering, and peculation. Men began to settle down and to think of the colony less as a labor camp and more as a home. They built houses, grew more corn, raised more cattle, imported wives, went to church, and stopped working each other quite so hard. But they kept on growing tobacco.

In the cultivation of tobacco the Virginians had found a way to use America. And, in spite of all efforts to turn them to other occupations, they persisted in growing tobacco. They demonstrated, in-deed, a certain headstrongness that England was to find characteristic of Englishmen living in America. In 1619 (before any other permanent English settlement had even been launched) Virginians met in their first representative assembly and passed their first laws. When James I took control of the colony in 1624 he did not provide for the continuance of a representative assembly; nor did his son Charles I, who became king in 1625. Charles was having enough difficulties with his own Parliament in England. But the governors he appointed found it impossible to rule Virginia without the help of Virginians. Though Charles refused them recognition until 1639, annual assemblies of representatives began making laws again in 1629 and have been doing so ever since.

The Founding of New England

James I stopped the Virginia Company but not the flow of colonists to America. The social, religious, and economic forces that had made their appearance in the time of Henry VIII were still at work, upsetting the lives of an increasing number of people. Prices were still rising; lands were changing hands; and sheep were grazing where men once drove their plows. To make matters worse, a depression settled over the woolens industry in the 1620s. It lasted through the next decade and was accompanied by a series of bad wheat harvests that sent food prices soaring. The land seemed "weary of her inhabitants," and the new king made it seem wearier by levying taxes without the consent of Parliament and by repressive measures against religious dissenters. The result was a large-scale exodus to the New World, mostly of young men in their teens and twenties, unable to find work at home. In the course of the century over three hundred thousand people left the British Isles to man the tobacco plantations of the Chesapeake and the first English sugar plantations of the West Indies. By 1640, despite catastrophic death rates, they had raised the Virginia population to 8,000 and had helped to people English colonies in Maryland, Bermuda, Barbados, St. Kitts, and other West Indian islands.

During the 1630s, while a host of young men embarked for the plantation colonies, some fifteen thousand people of a different character headed farther north in a "Great Migration" to New England. There were single men and women among them, but they came mainly in families, often many families from the same town, and they were looking for something more than a way to make a living. They were looking for a truly new and holier England.

After the failure of its Sagadahoc settlement in 1608, the Virginia Company of Plymouth had shown only sporadic interest in its territory. The company's most important action was to send Captain John Smith to explore the country in 1614. Smith named the place New England and first described its attractions. But his backers were not sufficiently impressed or not sufficiently affluent to support him in attempts to colonize it, and in 1620 they surrendered their rights to a more distinguished group of forty men who were impressed with New England but not with Smith.

The new group, made up of a duke, two marquises, six earls, a viscount, three barons, nineteen knights, the dean of a cathedral, and seven esquires, had visions of organizing feudal estates on a grand scale. Led by Sir Ferdinando Gorges, a Devonshire man who had also been the leading spirit of the Plymouth group, they gained from the king a charter establishing them as the Council for New England and granting them proprietary and governmental rights over the whole area from the fortieth to the forty-eighth parallels and from the Atlantic to the Pacific. In addition they were to have a monopoly of fishing in the offshore waters.

Cut up forty ways, the region would have provided each member of the council with a huge estate, a whole new England larger than the old. But the future of New England was to be less grand than gritty. In the very month in which the Council for New England was created, a band of humble but determined men and women put ashore below Cape Cod and began to use the country in their own way. Their way was called Puritanism.

Puritanism. Puritanism has come to mean prudishness, cruelty, fanaticism, superstition, Philistinism, and hypocrisy. Actually, the Puritan men and women who settled New England had no greater share of these human qualities than did their contemporaries or their descendants. What they did possess in stronger measure than others was John Calvin's belief that God is omnipotent and good and that all mankind are evil and helpless, predestined before they are born either to salvation or to eternal torment. Critics of this doctrine of predestination have always charged that it leads to moral indifference: if a man's present behavior does not affect his future salvation, why be good? But the facts belie the criticism: those who accept Calvin's doctrine have always outdone their neighbors in efforts to follow God's commandments as given in the Bible. The Puritan, knowing his efforts to be futile, nevertheless took a holy joy in them. They made him feel close to God's transcendent purpose. They also helped to ease his agonizing concern over whether he was headed for heaven or hell. Even though good behavior could not alter anyone's predestined fate, it was observable that religious conversion (a personal experience by which God let the

John Calvin (as drawn by one of his students)

saved know they were saved) often befell those who did try to live godly lives. Moreover, conversion manifested itself outwardly in renewed and intensified efforts to obey God's commands. A man's striving might thus be a sign that he was saved.

Not content with their own striving, the Puritans also felt responsible for their fellow men. Indeed, they were certain that any society that failed to honor God by punishing infractions of his commands would meet with his sudden wrath, not in the next world but here and now. Governments, they thought, existed for the purpose of enforcing obedience to God.

The Puritans' ideas of what God required were less rigorous than many people have supposed. God did *not* require his people to wear drab clothes, live in drab houses, or drink water when something stronger was available. He *did* require that they refrain from drunkenness, theft, murder, adultery, and breaches of the Sabbath. Puritans were vastly uneasy about the English government's indifference to these evils. They were even more concerned because the Church of England—supported by the government—retained corrupt practices inherited from Rome and not sanctioned by God in the Bible. They thought the Church should abolish bishops and ecclesiastical courts and such other relics of Catholicism as kneeling and the use of priestly vestments and altars.

Puritans all agreed on what was wrong with the English Church, but they disagreed on how to make it right. Though they all relied on the Bible for guidance, they extracted different opinions from it about how God wanted his churches to be run. Those who settled New England belonged to a group that came to be known as Congregationalists. They differed from the other principal group of Puritans, the Presbyteri-

Elizabeth and Mary Freake: Puritans, circa 1670

ans, in two beliefs: first, that there should be no general church organization with authority over individual churches; second, that a church should admit to membership only those who gave visible evidence of their Christian beliefs. Persons who openly flouted the laws of God should be excluded or expelled. Congregationalists wanted to change the structure and practices of the Church to conform with these beliefs.

Their dissatisfaction with the Church of England led them to the problem of all reformers: whether to remain inside a corrupt institution and try to reform it from within or to separate from it and start a pure new one. In 1583 an early Congregational leader, Robert Browne, advocated the latter course in a pamphlet appropriately titled *Reformation without Tarrying for any.* His followers, known as Separatists, deserted the English Church to meet in little churches of their own—of necessity in secret because the government did not acknowledge or permit any church other than the established one. But most Congregationalists were not Separatists. They did not think the Church of England was a hopeless case, and they believed the chances of reforming it were better from within than from without.

The Pilgrims. The men and women who began the settlement of New England at Plymouth in 1620 were Separatists, part of a group that originated in 1607 at the village of Scrooby in Nottinghamshire. The English government did not look with favor on Separatists. Under Elizabeth two had been executed and

many more imprisoned for long periods. Although the members of the Scrooby group were not seriously molested, they were distressed by the hostility of the government and the contempt of their neighbors. In 1608–09 they made their way, not without many hardships, to Holland, where the Dutch were known to be more tolerant. But as the years passed in Leyden they were still unhappy: their children were becoming Dutch; the only work they could get was day labor, poorly paid; and the weak among them were being tempted by the other religions that flourished under Dutch tolerance. They thought of Virginia, a place where they might remain English and work for themselves, a place isolated from contagious heretical religions and far enough from government control so that they could have a church of their own design.

Since they were poor people, without funds to finance their passage, they proposed to set up a "particular plantation" in Virginia for a group of English merchants. As in other such ventures, they would work together for seven years as a community, and then the profits would be divided between them and their sponsors. They evidently intended to establish themselves some distance north of the other settlements (the claims of the Virginia Company extended as far north as the present site of New York City) and at one point even considered seeking a grant from the Council for New England, which was then being formed. In the end, one hundred two persons boarded the *Mayflower,* bound for Virginia. But after making their landfall at Cape Cod and exploring the coast, they decided to stay. In late December 1620 they began a settlement, which they named Plymouth after the English port from which they had embarked.

These "Pilgrims" as Americans have come to call them, were as poorly equipped in everything but courage as any group that ever landed in America. They had guns but knew little about shooting. They planned to become fishermen but knew nothing about fishing. They expected to settle in Virginia but landed in New England without enough supplies to last the winter. Like their predecessors and contemporaries in Virginia, many of them sickened and died. But the living stuck it out and justified their own estimate of themselves: three years earlier they had written to the men they hoped would sponsor their emigration, "It is not with us as with other men, whom small things can discourage, or small discontentments cause to wish themselves at home again." Since New England was outside the jurisdiction of Virginia's government, the Pilgrims established a government of their own by the *Mayflower* Compact, which forty-one adult males subscribed before going ashore. For governor they elected John Carver; and upon his death in 1621 they chose William Bradford, who recorded the colony's struggles in an eloquent history and was reelected nearly every year from 1621 to his death in 1657. Under his leadership the Pilgrims liquidated their debt to the English merchants (who had failed to send them the supplies they expected) and established for themselves a self-supporting community.

The Pilgrim settlement was important as a demonstration that men and women could live in New England. It remained, however, a small and humble community, attracting few immigrants. The great Puritan exodus did not begin until ten years after the landing of the Pilgrims. It engulfed, but did not greatly expand, the Plymouth colony.

The Massachusetts Bay Company. While the Pilgrims went their way outside the Church of England first in Holland and then in America, other Puritans, both Congregational and Presbyterian, continued the struggle to reform the Church from within. While James I reigned, the struggle did not seem hopeless. Although James scolded them, and even married his son to a Catholic princess, he did not "harry them out of the land," as he once threatened to do. If he had tried, they would have had enough strength in Parliament to stop him. But when Charles I became king in 1625, he quarreled incessantly with Parliament and finally announced in 1629 that he intended to rule henceforth without it. At the same time he befriended a group of aspiring churchmen who were as eager to suppress Puritanism as the Puritans were to make it prevail. Under the leadership of William Laud, whom Charles made Bishop of London in 1628 and Archbishop of Canterbury in 1633, these friends of the king deprived Puritan ministers of their pulpits and moved the Church of England ever closer to Rome in its ceremonies, vestments, and doctrines.

As the prospects of reform grew dim and the sins of the land grew heavy, the Puritans feared that God was preparing England for some great purging catastrophe. In despair and hope they, too, turned their thoughts to America, where they might worship in purity and escape the wrath both of God and of the king.

In 1628 a number of prominent congregational Puritans bought their way into a commercial company that was being organized in London. Called the New England Company, it took over the rights of a defunct group, the Dorchester Adventurers, which in 1623 had tried to plant a farming and fishing settlement at Cape Ann. From the Council for New England, the new company obtained a charter authorizing settlement in the area known as Massachusetts Bay, to the north of Plymouth. A year later, on March 4, 1629, the New England Company reorganized as the Massachusetts Bay Company and had its proprietary and governmental rights confirmed by a new charter obtained directly from the king.

In the shuffle the Puritan stockholders gained control of the company, and they had something more than commerce in mind. The royal charter bestowed on the company full authority to govern its own territory and made no mention of where company meetings were to be held. In 1629 the Puritans simply voted to transfer the company to Massachusetts. This meant that if Puritan company members emigrated, they would have full control of the government under which they would live. Thus in one bold stroke the Puritans won for themselves the opportunity to do in Massachusetts what Puritans for nearly a century had been yearning to do in England.

To act as governor, the company elected a solid Puritan squire, John Winthrop of Groton Manor, Suffolk. He and perhaps a dozen other company members, all Puritans, crossed the ocean in 1630, accompanied by a thousand like-minded men and women, who preferred a wilderness governed by Puritans to a civilized land governed by Charles I. Before the year was over they had planted settlements around Massachusetts Bay at Dorchester, Roxbury, Watertown, Newtown (Cambridge), Charlestown, and Boston. During the next ten years, as Charles ruled without Parliament and Laud grew increasingly powerful, fifteen or twenty thousand more followed and their towns stretched out in all directions.

Winthrop and the handful of other company members had authority from the king's charter to govern this whole body of settlers. But Winthrop and his friends wanted a broader base for their government. And so, shortly after their arrival in New England, they transformed the Massachusetts Bay Company from a trading company into a commonwealth. In 1631 they admitted more than a hundred adult males as members, or "freemen," of the company eligible to vote at its meetings. The term "freeman" in seventeenth-century England generally meant a voting member of a business corporation or of an incorporated city or borough. In America the word came to mean a man who had the right to vote for representatives to the assembly in his colony. In Massachusetts, when the company and colony were blended, the freemen of the company became the freemen of the colony. The increase in their numbers did not remove the colony from Puritan control, because most of the new freemen (who must have been a majority of the heads of families then in the colony) were probably Puritans; moreover, it was specified that, in the future, members of Puritan congregational churches (and only such) should be eligible to become freemen.

The charter, which had envisaged only a trading company with limited membership, provided that company members assemble as a General Court four times a year to make laws. Between the meetings of the General Court a governor (or his second in command, a deputy governor) and a council of eighteen "assistants," elected annually, were to manage the company. When Winthrop and his associates opened freemanship to all church members, they foresaw that the number of freemen would soon become too large to assemble and work together as a legislature; and they decided to leave lawmaking to the council of assistants, who were still to be elected annually by all the freemen. But in 1634 the freemen insisted that the lawmaking powers assigned to them by the charter be delegated to "deputies" elected from each settlement. Henceforth the General Court consisted of the governor, the deputy governor, the executive council of assistants, and a body of deputies, or representatives. All were elected annually by the freemen. Since the company had power to govern the colony, this General Court was in reality both the legislature and the supreme court of the colony. Here, in truth, was a self-governing commonwealth, a Puritan republic.

Puritan New England. The freedom to do as they pleased posed many new problems to men who had not hitherto wielded the powers of government. Reformers and idealists are notoriously prone to dissipate their energies wrangling with one another. And there were disagreements in New England, though not so numerous or severe as has sometimes been suggested. The New England Puritans agreed on a great deal. They wanted congregational churches. They did not want bishops, church courts, or hierarchy. They wanted a government that would take seriously its obligation to enforce God's commandments and to support pure religion. Accordingly they confined voting to church members and levied taxes to pay ministers' salaries. But, contrary to common assumption, they did not want their clergy to take part in government. For a minister to exercise political authority of any kind seemed to the Puritans a dangerous step toward Roman Catholicism. Compared to the clergy

of England and Europe the New England minister, though highly influential, had little authority even within his own church. He taught, prayed, preached, and admonished; he commanded respect—else he lost his job—but he did not rule his church. Admissions to membership, censures, pardons, and excommunications were all decided by vote of the church members.

Neither the leaders of the Massachusetts Bay Colony nor the great majority of settlers were Separatists. Though they organized their own churches in the congregational manner, they took pains to affirm their love and friendship for the churches of England. Some

John Winthrop

But hear I cannot but stay and make a pause, and stand half amazed at this poore peoples presente condition; and so I thinke will the reader too, when he well considers the same. Being thus passed the vast ocean, and a sea of troubles before in their preparation..., they had now no freinds to wellcome them, nor inns to entertaine or refresh their weatherbeaten bodys, no houses or much less townes to repaire too, to seeke for succoure. It is recorded in scripture as a mercie to the apostle and his shipwraked company, that the barbarians shewed them no smale kindnes in refreshing them, but these savage barbarians, when they mette with them ... were readier to fill their sides full of arrows then other wise. And for the season it was winter, and they that know the winters of that cuntrie know them to be sharp and violent, and subjecte to cruell and feirce stormes, deangerous to travill to known places, much more to serch an unknown coast. Besides, what could they see but a hidious and desolate wildernes, full of wild beasts and willd men? and what multitudes ther might be of them they knew not. ... What could now sustaine them but the spirite of God and his grace? May not and ought not the children of these fathers rightly say: Our faithers were English men which came over this great ocean, and were ready to perish in this willdernes, but they cried unto the Lord, and he heard their voyce, and looked on their adversitie, etc. Let them therfore praise the Lord, because he is good, and his mercies endure for ever. Yea, let them which have been redeemed of the Lord, shew how he hath delivered them from the hand of the oppressour. When they wandered in the deserte [and] willdernes out of the way, and found no citie to dwell in, both hungrie, and thirstie, their sowle was overwhelmed in them. Let them confess before the Lord his loving kindnes, and his wonderfull works before the sons of men.

From William Bradford, *Of Plymouth Plantation*, c. 1630.

even thought that the churches of Rome were not beyond redemption. But among the thousands who stepped ashore at Boston every year were substantial numbers of Separatists and other extremists, full of zeal and eloquence, full of impatience with anyone who disagreed with them. John Winthrop, whom the freemen elected governor year after year during most of his life, was good at turning away wrath and directing zeal to constructive ends. But during the three years from 1634 to 1637, when lesser men sat in the governor's chair, Massachusetts all but succumbed to the denunciations of a brilliant, saintlike, intractable man and a brilliant, proud, magnetic woman.

Roger Williams, who arrived in 1631, was a Separatist. He wanted everyone to repudiate the wicked churches of England. Moreover, he insisted that the royal charter of Massachusetts contained a lie (in claiming that England first discovered the region) and that the king had had no right to grant the charter or the people to accept it without first purchasing the land from the natives. If word got back to England that the Massachusetts government allowed the expression of such subversive ideas, the king might be prompted to take control of the colony and end the Puritan republic. Williams also tried to persuade peo-

ple that no government had authority over religious matters, not even the right to punish breaches of the Sabbath. In a community believing that the prime purpose of government was to enforce God's commandments, Williams' teachings were rank sedition.

Williams was a man whom everyone loved on sight; even John Winthrop became his good friend. But he propagated his inflammatory ideas so insistently, first as assistant to the minister and then as minister of the church at Salem, that the unity of the colony was endangered and the government finally felt obliged to banish him in 1636. He went to Rhode Island, where he was joined by those who believed him. There, while retaining his conviction that the state had no authority over religious matters, he reached the conclusion that in the existing phase of human history God authorized no organized churches at all. In spite of this view, which few of his followers could share, he retained the love and respect of his neighbors and lived out a long and useful life as the leading citizen of the new colony.

Scarcely had Williams been banished when a new threat to the civil and religious security of Massachusetts appeared: Anne Hutchinson, the wife of a merchant whom Winthrop described as "a man of a very mild temper and weak parts, and wholly guided by his wife." An amateur theologian, Mrs. Hutchinson took to elucidating her minister's Sunday sermons in informal gatherings of her neighbors. As the circle of her listeners steadily widened, her discourses became more original, for her keen and imaginative mind could not be contained within the standard doctrines of Puritanism. Starting from the accepted principle that God grants salvation without regard to human merit, she denied (what other Puritans affirmed) that good conduct could be a sign of salvation and affirmed (what other Puritans denied) that the Holy Spirit in the hearts of true believers relieved them of responsibility to obey the laws of God. So, at least, her enemies charged, and she gave substance to their accusation by asserting that all the New England ministers except her favorite, John Cotton, and her brother-in-law, John Wheelwright, were preaching unsound doctrines. By emphasizing morality, she said, they were deluding their congregations into the false assumption that good deeds would get them into heaven. The clergymen hotly denied what was virtually a charge of heresy, and Mrs. Hutchinson herself protested that she had intended no insult. Nevertheless, a host of devoted Bostonians hung on every word she uttered and refused to conceal their contempt for her opponents. The colony split into hostile camps, and finally Mrs. Hutchinson was brought before the authorities. After they had cross-examined her for two days, she made the mistake of claiming that she had received an immediate revelation from God. To Puritan ears, this was blasphemy. So Mrs. Hutchinson too was banished and went to Rhode Island, which thus became the refuge for Puritans with too much originality.

After Charles I was forced to resummon Parliament in 1640, Roger Williams applied to that body (which was overwhelmingly Puritan) for a charter for his colony. The charter, granted in 1644, gave the Rhode Islanders a government much like that of the colony from which they had been expelled: they elected annually a representative assembly, a council of assistants, and a governor (at first called a president), but they did not confine voting to church members or collect taxes to support the clergy. In 1663 the existing government was confirmed by a royal charter that also guaranteed the "liberty in religious concernments" which had been the colony's distinction from the beginning.

Meanwhile another part of New England was filling up with Puritans who differed from those of Massachusetts primarily in their desire for more elbow room. In 1636 Thomas Hooker, the minister of Newtown (Cambridge), led an exodus overland to the fertile Connecticut Valley, where the small garrison of a Dutch trading post at Fort Hope (Hartford) was unable to prevent them from settling. They formed a government by a simple agreement among themselves (called the Fundamental Orders). The model, once again, was Massachusetts (but voting was not confined to church members), and again the existing arrangement was confirmed by royal charter (1662). The charter also joined to Connecticut the colony of New Haven, initiated in 1638 by a group of Londoners who could find no lands in Massachusetts to suit them.

The settlers of New Haven, beginning with a good supply of capital, had been disappointed in their expectations of a thriving commerce; but they had succeeded in establishing a somewhat stricter government than existed elsewhere in New England, and they were not altogether happy about the union with Connecticut.

There was, nevertheless, no serious difference between New Haven and the rest of New England. In New Haven as in Plymouth, Massachusetts, Rhode Island, and Connecticut, the population was predominantly Puritan. Puritans directed public policy, and the only serious resistance came from other Puritans. Although some of the inhabitants may have been indifferent or hostile to Puritanism, they were never strong enough or discontented enough to challenge Puritan control.

Settlers who wanted nothing more from the New World than an opportunity to make their fortunes or to live more comfortably than in England had little reason to object to Puritan control anyway. The government frowned on private cupidity when it threatened the public welfare, but Puritans saw no virtue in poverty. They had not traveled three thousand miles simply to starve in a holier manner than in England. They had come in order to build a society that would win God's favor, and they meant it to be a success, economically as well as religiously.

So long as the Great Migration lasted, the colonists prospered by selling cattle and provisions to the newcomers each year. When Charles I recalled Parliament in 1640, his first since 1629, English Puritans saw an opportunity to set things right at home. The migration to New England accordingly came to an end, and New England farmers, thus deprived of customers, suffered their first depression. The leaders looked hard for some native product they could sell to the outside world. Fortunately for them, they found no single product such as the Virginians' tobacco, and they consequently developed a more balanced economy. They caught fish, raised corn and wheat, bred cattle, cut lumber, and built ships. Before many years had passed, New England vessels were prowling the Caribbean and the Mediterranean, peddling their assorted wares, transporting other people's, and bringing home the profits. By the middle of the seventeenth century New England had laid down its economic as well as its religious foundations.

Proprietary Ventures

During the years that Puritans were building their republics in New England, non-Puritans were trying to establish private domains there and elsewhere. Three years after the Pilgrims landed, Sir Ferdinando Gorges, the most active member of the Council for New England, had backed a settlement at Wessagusset (Weymouth) in the Massachusetts Bay region, but it broke up after a year. Its failure discouraged the rest of the council from further efforts, and they apparently raised no serious objections in 1628 when the Earl of Warwick, president of the council, took it upon himself to grant the Puritans permission to settle the Bay area. In 1637 the Council for New England finally dissolved, leaving behind a host of shadowy claims. Only one claim was perfected: that of Ferdinando Gorges to the region north of the Merrimac River. Gorges divided the area with another would-be New England lord, John Mason, and in 1639 obtained a separate royal charter for his own share. He died in 1647, with no feudal retainers in his New World barony except a few hardy fishermen who pledged allegiance to no one. Massachusetts annexed the whole region in 1651.

The king authorized other ambitious gentlemen to colonize Newfoundland, Nova Scotia, and the Carolinas, but to no effect. The first English nobleman to realize the aristocrat's dream of founding a New World domain for his family was George Calvert, Lord Baltimore. A notable figure in the court of James I, Calvert had become interested in America first as a member of the Virginia Company and later as a member of the Council for New England. In 1620 he purchased rights in southeastern Newfoundland from another noble dreamer and started a settlement there. When he visited the place himself, he found that "from the middle of October to the middst of May there is a sadd face of wynter upon all this land." Deciding to leave Newfoundland to the fishermen, he asked the king for a grant farther south. The charter, which was in the making when Calvert died in 1632, was finally issued to his son Cecilius. It conveyed to him 10 million acres on Chesapeake Bay, where the Calvert family was to have complete powers of government. The colony was to be known as Maryland, in honor of the queen of Charles I.

The name was appropriate, for both the queen and the Calverts were Catholics. Maryland was to be a feudal seigniory and at the same time a religious refuge. As a feudal seigniory it came nearer to success than any other attempted in America. Though the Calverts did not live there, they governed the colony (sometimes through a younger son), owned all the public lands, granted small estates or "manors" to their friends, and collected rents from the settlers. Because Virginia, Plymouth, and Massachusetts lent a hand, the settlers of Maryland were spared the early days of starvation that had been suffered by other colonists. Tobacco grew as readily in Maryland as in Virginia, and the two colonies became identical in their economic pursuits and interests.

As a religious refuge Maryland also succeeded, at least for a time. Although official hostility to Catholicism had relaxed in England under Charles, Catholics were still required by law to take oaths and to attend religious services that conflicted with their beliefs. In

Maryland they would be free to worship as they chose, and so would other Christians. As it turned out, more Puritans came to the colony than Catholics. The Calverts welcomed both, and from the time of the first settlement in 1634 tried to prevent either group from oppressing the other. When the Jesuits threatened to become too powerful, Baltimore, in 1641, forbade them to hold land in Maryland. The Puritans were harder to handle, especially after 1640, when their friends gained the upper hand in England, but Baltimore did his best to restrain them. By the terms of his charter he was obliged to obtain the consent of the "freemen" (presumably in this case the term meant all adult males not bound as servants) to all legislation. As the population increased, the freemen deputed a few individuals to act for them, and thus arose a representative assembly similar to those which developed in the other colonies. This assembly in 1649 consented to the famous Maryland Toleration Act, securing freedom of worship for all Christians, whether Protestant or Catholic, who believed in the Trinity. Although later assemblies restricted the rights of Catholics, the act pointed toward the pluralism in religion that would ultimately characterize society in America.

By the middle of the seventeenth century England had seeded North America. Many more immigrants were to come, from England and elsewhere, but the future was already visible on the coasts of New England and of Chesapeake Bay. The English had moved in, and whether they favored toleration, as in Maryland and Rhode Island, or intolerance, as in Massachusetts, whether they caught fish or grew tobacco, the continent was effectively theirs.

Suggestions for Reading

A good account of the American Indians before the coming of the white man is Kenneth MacGowan and J. A. Hester, Jr., *Early Man in the New World** (1950). H. E. Driver, *Indians of North America** (2d ed., 1970), is more comprehensive. W. E. Washburn, *The Indian in America** (1975), incorporates new anthropological data and insights. G. B. Nash, *Red, White, and Black: The Peoples of Early America** (1974), surveys the development and relationships of all three races during the colonial period. And A. W. Crosby, Jr., *The Columbian Exchange: Biological and Cultural Consequences of 1492** (1972), traces some of the consequences of the discovery of America for the peoples of both the Old World and the New.

Anyone interested in the age of exploration should give first attention to S. E. Morison's great biography of Columbus, *Admiral of the Ocean Sea* (1942), and to his lively and authoritative *European Discovery of America: The Northern Voyages, 500–1600* (1971), and *The Southern Voyages, 1492–1616* (1974). J. H. Parry, *The Age of Reconnaissance** (1963), covers voyages to all the continents. A penetrating and succinct study of Spanish exploits and problems is Charles Gibson, *Spain in America** (1966), which contains a good bibliography of the subject. On the English voyages there is no substitute for Richard Hakluyt's collection of first-hand accounts, *The Principall Navigations, Voiages, and Discoveries of the English Nation* (1589, 1599), reprinted in Everyman's Library, *Hakluyt's Voyages*, 8 vols. Hakluyt's work has been carried on in the voluminous publications of the Hakluyt Society. Among these, see especially the volumes edited by D. B. Quinn, *Voyages and Colonising Enterprises of Sir Humphrey Gilbert*, 2 vols. (1940), and *The Roanoke Voyages, 1584–1590*, 2 vols. (1955). In *England and the Discovery of America, 1481–1620* (1974) and *North America from Earliest Discovery to First Settlements** (1977), Quinn summarizes a lifetime of work on the subject.

M. M. Knappen, *Tudor Puritanism** (1939), and Patrick Collinson, *The Elizabethan Puritan Movement* (1967), are the best accounts of early Puritanism. Two challenging interpretations are C. H. and Katherine George, *The Protestant Mind of the English Reformation* (1961), and Michael Walzer, *The Revolution of the Saints** (1965). For social conditions in England see Carl Bridenbaugh, *Vexed and Troubled Englishmen, 1590–1642** (1968), and Peter Laslett, *The World We Have Lost** (1965); for economic conditions, Joan Thirsk, ed., *The Agrarian History of England and Wales, 1500–1640* (1967); for political and legal institutions, Wallace Notestein, *The English People on the Eve of Colonization, 1603–1630** (1954). Keith Thomas, *Religion and the Decline of Magic** (1971), is a massive study of English folk religion and beliefs in the sixteenth and seventeenth centuries. Mildred Campbell, *The English Yeoman under Elizabeth and the Early Stuarts* (1942), is well matched by Lawrence Stone's monumental *Crisis of the Aristocracy** (1965).

On the first permanent English settlements in America, the most convenient and the most authoritative account is still C. M. Andrews, *The Colonial Period of American History*, Vols. I–III* (1934–37). For the Southern colonies this should be supplemented by W. F. Craven, *The Southern Colonies in the*

*Seventeenth Century** (1949). J. E. Pomfret and F. M. Shumway, *Founding the American Colonies* (1970), incorporates recent research. Captain John Smith tells his own story in *Travels and Works of Captain John Smith*, 2 vols. (1910), ed. by Edward Arber and A. G. Bradley. The fullest modern account is P. L. Barbour, *The Three Worlds of Captain John Smith* (1964), but Alden Vaughan, *American Genesis: Captain John Smith and the Founding of Virginia** (1975), is a perceptive shorter biography. W. F. Craven, *The Dissolution of the Virginia Company* (1932), is a masterful study of the internal divisions that impaired the company's efforts in America. E. S. Morgan, *American Slavery American Freedom: The Ordeal of Colonial Virginia** (1975), shows how experience in Virginia eroded the original intentions of the founders.

The New England Puritans have been subjected to the scrutiny of historians, sympathetic and unsympathetic, from the time the settlers first stepped ashore. William Bradford, governor of the Plymouth Colony, told the story of the Pilgrims in *Of Plymouth Plantation*, an American classic that can best be read in S. E. Morison's edition (1952). A thorough history by a modern scholar is George Langdon, *Pilgrim Colony: A History of New Plymouth, 1620–1691** (1966). In his *Journal* (1853, 1908) Governor John Winthrop did for Massachusetts Bay what Bradford did for Plymouth. For a contrast with Bradford and Winthrop, read Thomas Morton, *New English Canaan* (1637, 1883).

S. E. Morison, *Builders of the Bay Colony** (1930), is by all odds the best modern introduction to the history of New England. Morison continued his study of the Puritans in his works on Harvard, *The Founding of Harvard College* (1935) and *Harvard in the Seventeenth Century*, 2 vols. (1936).

New England Puritanism is also the subject of the most profound study of intellectual history yet written by an American, Perry Miller, *The New England Mind: The Seventeenth Century** (1939) and *The New England Mind: From Colony to Province** (1953). These volumes were preceded by his briefer study, *Orthodoxy in Massachusetts, 1630–1650* (1933), the subject of which falls chronologically between the two. He explores other aspects of New England history in a brilliant collection of essays, *Errand into the Wilderness** (1956). Some of Miller's conclusions are modified in Robert Middlekauff's sensitive study, *The Mathers** (1971), and by David Hall's examination of the New England ministry in *The Faithful Shepherd** (1972), and by Sacvan Bercovitch, *The American Jeremiad** (1978). Puritan domestic life and social relations are examined in E. S. Morgan, *The Puritan Family** (1966), in John Demos, *A Little Commonwealth** (1970), and in D. H. Flaherty, *Privacy in Colonial New England* (1972). The best study of women in early New England is L. T. Ulrich, *Good Wives** (1982). David Stannard, *The Puritan Way of Death** (1977), places the subject in an anthropological perspective. P. J. Greven, *Four Generations** (1969), traces the demographic changes over a century among the families that founded Andover, Massachusetts. Greven discusses patterns of child-rearing in *The Protestant Temperament** (1977). John Demos, *Entertaining Satan** (1982), offers a major analysis of New England social relations in discussing early witchcraft trials. Stephen Foster analyzes Puritan social thought in *Their Solitary Way* (1971). The conduct of church affairs is treated in Ola Winslow, *Meetinghouse Hill** (1952); the Puritan conception of the church in E. S. Morgan, *Visible Saints** (1963), and in R. G. Pope, *The Half-Way Covenant* (1969). The best biography of Roger Williams is Ola Winslow, *Master Roger Williams* (1957). E. S. Morgan, *Roger Williams: The Church and the State* (1967), analyzes Williams' ideas. Emery Battis, *Saints and Sectaries* (1962), gives a provocative psychological interpretation of Anne Hutchinson, and Kai Erikson gives a sociological interpretation in *Wayward Puritans** (1966). W. K. B. Stoever reassesses the theological implications of Hutchinson's challenge in *A Faire and Easie Way to Heaven* (1978). C. E. Hambrick-Stowe analyzes Puritan day-to-day devotional practices in *The Practice of Piety* (1982).

For early New England economic history see Bernard Bailyn, *The New England Merchants in the Seventeenth Century** (1955). E. S. Morgan has dealt with some of the political problems faced by the founders of Massachusetts in *The Puritan Dilemma: The Story of John Winthrop** (1958). R. E. Wall, *Massachusetts Bay: The Crucial Decade, 1640–1650* (1972), stresses the rivalry of magistrates and deputies. Later Puritan problems as exemplified in the Winthrop family are treated in R. S. Dunn, *Puritans and Yankees: The Winthrop Dynasty of New England** (1962). G. L. Haskins, *Law and Authority in Early Massachusetts** (1960), describes political and social as well as legal institutions while David Konig, *Law and Society in Puritan Massachusetts* (1979), stresses the growth of litigation. T. H. Breen, *The Character of the Good Ruler** (1970), treats the development of Puritan political thought during the first century of settlement.

*Available in a paperback edition.

2
THE PATTERN
OF EMPIRE

The first settlements in America, which cost the English people dearly in lives and money, cost the English government nothing. But in authorizing settlement the government did expect to gain something more than an outlet for disgruntled Puritans, misguided merchants, and adventurous fortune-seekers. Every European government, during the sixteenth, seventeenth, and eighteenth centuries, followed an economic policy that has been known since 1776, when Adam Smith coined the word, as mercantilism.

Mercantilism

Mercantilism meant that the state directed all economic activities within its borders, subordinating private profit to public good. In particular, the government sought to increase national wealth by discouraging imports and encouraging exports. The English government let its subjects go to America because it was persuaded that their presence there would further this end.

Long before the settlement of Jamestown, Richard Hakluyt had explained how the mother country could profit from American colonies: they would furnish England with supplies such as lumber, tar, and hemp, which it was buying from other countries, and

they would offer a market for the woolens that were England's principal export. "It behooves this realm," Hakluyt wrote in 1584, "if it mean . . . not negligently and sleepingly to slide into beggary, to foresee and plant [a colony] at Norumbega [a name for northern North America] or some like place, were it not for anything else but for the hope of the sale of our wool." What England wanted from America was what Hakluyt said it would get: a market for its woolen cloth and other manufactures and a source of supply for raw materials that it had to import from other countries.

What England wanted was not incompatible with what the colonists wanted: a ready market for the raw materials they had to sell and a cheap source for the manufactures they had to buy. During the years of settlement, the shortage of labor in North America made manufacturing unfeasible. England, on the other hand, had a surplus of labor and a low wage scale that made for cheap manufactured goods. It was mutually advantageous for the colonies to buy manufactures from the mother country and for the mother country to buy raw materials from the colonies.

The British empire in America was based on this compatibility of interests. But, while the interests were compatible, they required guidance to make them coincide. Left to themselves, the colonies might peddle their produce in France or Holland instead of England and take home French textiles instead of

William Penn's treaty with the Indians.

English ones, or they might produce materials not needed in England. In order to make the system work, it was necessary for the mother country to maintain continuous supervision and control over the economic activities of the settlers just as it did over the activities of Englishmen at home. The English government never doubted its right to exercise such control, but it was slow to develop consistent directives or effective machinery for carrying them out.

England's imperial delay. In the early years, before the colonies began to fulfill Hakluyt's glowing predictions, economic regulation probably did not

Charles I: he needed Parliament to pay his bills

seem urgent. Although the English government in 1621 ordered all Virginia tobacco to be brought to England, the order was not enforced, perhaps because English authorities considered it a mixed blessing for the nation to have its own private supply of smoke. But other regulations, adopted from time to time, also went unenforced. One reason was distance. Three thousand miles of ocean made a formidable barrier in the seventeenth century. Although it was faster and easier to travel long distances by water than by land, even over water three thousand miles was space enough in which to lose messages, orders, and interest.

A more serious obstacle to English control than either the distance or the seeming unimportance of the colonies was politics. During the seventeenth century, when most of its American colonies were founded, England was torn by a struggle for power between king and Parliament. In the 1630s Charles I ruled without Parliament, but by 1640 he needed it to pay his bills. He called it, dismissed it, called it again, and then found that he could not dismiss it any more. In 1642 the members raised an army to make war on him; in 1649 they cut off his head, and for eleven years England had no king. In his place from 1649 to 1658 stood Oliver Cromwell, the soldier who had defeated him.

When Charles II, son of the old king, was placed on the throne in 1660, the acts passed by Parliament in the preceding eleven years were declared null and void. But Charles had the good sense to realize that English kings henceforth must work with Parliament or not at all. His brother and successor, James II, had no sense, and within three years of his accession in 1685 he had to flee the country. Parliament quietly

Boston, New England, February 26, 1743

... there has lately been carried on here a large illicit trade (Distructive to the interest of Great Britain in her trade to her own plantations, and contrary to the main intent of all her laws made to regulate that trade) by importing into this province large quantities of European goods of almost all sorts from diverse parts of Europe, some of which are by the laws wholly prohibited to be imported into the Plantations, and the rest are prohibited to be imported there unless brought directly from Great Britain. ... one of these illicit traders, lately departed hence for Holland, proposed to one of the greatest sellers of Broad Cloths here (and to how many others I can't say) to supply him with Black Cloths from thence, saying that this country might be better and cheaper supply'd with Broad Cloths of that colour from Holland than from England; But to prevent or rather increase your Lordships' surprize on this head I need only to acquaint you that I write this clad in a superfine French Cloth, which I bought on purpose that I might wear about the evidence of these illegal traders having already begun to destroy the vital parts of the British commerce; and to use as a memento to myself and the Customhouse Officers to do everything in our power towards cutting off this trade so very pernicious to the British nation.

From a letter of William Bollan, advocate general, to the Board of Trade in London.

replaced him with William and Mary in the bloodless Revolution of 1688. After 1688 the king was still no cipher in government, but everyone understood that he was subordinate to Parliament.

All but one (Georgia) of the thirteen colonies that later became the United States were founded before 1688, during the years when the ultimate location of sovereignty in England was uncertain. They were all founded under authority of the king, and their relationship to Parliament remained ambiguous. Parliament sometimes passed legislation affecting them, but even after 1688 it did not do so regularly. Yet if the king had denied the authority of Parliament in the colonies, Parliament would doubtless have brought him up short.

Distance, indifference, and the uncertain location of authority in England conspired to delay the development of a consistent and continuous colonial policy. From the founding of Virginia in 1607 until the middle of the seventeenth century the colonies interested king and Parliament only as a minor prize in the contest for sovereignty. In 1633, when Charles I was trying to rule without Parliament, he appointed a commission headed by Archbishop William Laud to govern the colonies. But the commissioners were too busy in England to do anything about America. During the English civil wars of the 1640s, Parliament and king both claimed authority over the colonies, but neither was able to exercise it.

Oliver Cromwell was the first ruler of England sure enough of his position at home to think seriously about fitting the colonies into a general imperial scheme. In 1650 and 1651 he secured legislation to keep foreign shipping out of the colonies. He also planned a great expansion of the empire in the Caribbean and tried to persuade New Englanders to move to the West Indies, where the cultivation of sugar and other tropical products promised rich rewards. But his legislation against foreign shipping led to war with the uncooperative Dutch; his large military and naval expedition to the West Indies in 1655 captured only Jamaica; and his powers of persuasion proved insufficient to lure New Englanders from their rocky soil. They suspected, perhaps, that Puritanism would not work well in the tropics.

The Navigation Acts. When Charles II came to the throne in 1660, the colonies, in spite of Cromwell's failures, had grown enough to require attention. Virginia and Maryland were exporting over 7 million pounds of tobacco yearly, much of which never reached England, and New England harbored a group of merchants whose ships were already familiar in the markets of the world. English merchants, awakened to the potentialities of colonial trade, pressed the government for measures to prevent the profits from leaking into the pockets of foreign rivals. What they wanted was not merely to exclude foreign shipping from the colonies (as Cromwell had attempted in the acts of 1650 and 1651) but to direct colonial trade into channels profitable to the mother country. King and Parliament, in the first flush of Restoration harmony, agreed on two acts to take care of the matter.

These so-called Navigation Acts (1660 and 1663) were modified from time to time during the ensuing century, but their basic principles remained the same: (1) they forbade all trade with the colonies except in ships owned and constructed there or in England and manned by crews of which at least three-quarters were English or colonial; (2) they forbade the transportation *from* the colonies *to* any place except England or another English colony of certain "enumerated commodities," namely sugar, cotton, indigo, dyewoods, ginger, and tobacco; and (3) with a few exceptions they forbade the transportation of European and Asiatic goods *to* the colonies *from* any place except England.

Subsequent modification of the Navigation Acts consisted mainly of additions to the list of enumerated commodities (rice in 1704, naval stores in 1705, copper and furs in 1721) or specific limitations on, or encouragement of, colonial products. The act of 1705 that enumerated naval stores (pitch, tar, turpentine, masts, spars) also placed bounties on their production. The Wool Act (1699) forbade export from the colonies of certain textiles manufactured there. The Hat Act (1732) forbade export of colonial-made hats. The Iron Act (1750) removed all duties on English imports of colonial pig and bar iron (thus encouraging their production) but forbade the erection of any new colonial iron mills for manufacturing raw iron into finished products.

The Navigation Acts were ostensibly intended to ensure that the mother country would benefit from the economic activities of the colonies. But, in passing the original acts and in modifying them over the years, Parliament was not immune to the wishes of special groups. Adam Smith, in coining the very name "mercantilism," was charging that English policies were dictated by merchants at the expense of the rest of the community. And indeed particular acts were often opposed by one group as much as they were favored by another. The Iron Act, for example, represented a victory of English iron-manufacturers over English iron-miners and smelters; and in 1733 the Molasses Act, which placed a heavy duty on foreign molasses imported into North America, was a victory for one group of colonists, the West Indian sugar-planters, over another, the New Englanders who distilled molasses into rum.

Besides serving such private interests, and besides subordinating colonial trade to English trade, the Navigation Acts aimed at increasing the revenue of the English government, at least indirectly. Although the acts of 1660 and 1663 levied no taxes, the government from the beginning had collected duties in England on imports from the colonies. By requiring enumerated commodities to be brought only to England, the government expected to step up the volume of dutiable goods. The expectation was not unrealistic.

New Englanders away from home: *Sea Captains at Surinam,* **by John Greenwood**

Revenue obtained from duties on tobacco imports alone may have amounted in the 1660s to as much as £100,000 annually, which was more than the planters themselves made from the crop.

The Navigation Acts transformed the hopeful predictions of Hakluyt into specific legislation that told the colonists what they could and could not make, where and how they could trade. But the colonies were still three thousand miles from the lawmakers. If England was to receive the full benefit of the acts, they had to be enforced against foreign nations on the one hand and against refractory colonists on the other.

The Dutch. The principal foreign threat to England's emerging mercantilist empire in the seventeenth century came from the Dutch. This was their century; they seemed on the way to running the world. After shaking off Spanish domination, they built the largest merchant fleet yet known. Dutch captains nosed out rival vessels everywhere, took over most of the Portuguese empire in the East Indies, opened trade with Japan. Dutch privateers led the pack in raiding Spanish treasure fleets. Dutch merchants controlled the lumber trade from the Baltic and made Amsterdam the sawmill of Europe. Dutch fishermen dominated the North Sea. Dutch textile-workers finished and resold woolen cloth imported raw from England. When England tried to stop the export and save the valuable finishing process for its own workers, the Dutch simply boycotted English cloth, and depression settled over the whole English woolens industry. This was the century of Rembrandt, Vermeer, Hals, Hobbema, DeHooch, the century of Huygens and Spinoza. Man for man, no people has ever surpassed the seventeenth-century achievement of the Dutch.

In North America the Dutch had not extended themselves with the vigor they showed elsewhere, probably because North America offered fewer prospects of immediate reward. Nevertheless, Dutch ships every year appeared in Virginia's great rivers to carry tobacco to Holland instead of England. Dutch textiles were sold in the shops of Boston. And the region that the Dutch had chosen for their settlements and trading posts in North America was strategically and economically the most important on the continent. The Hudson River commanded access to the interior by the only water-level route through the Appalachian Mountains. From the Hudson, it was possible to reach the Mississippi Valley along the Mohawk River Valley (or with greater difficulty by Lake George, Lake Champlain, and the St. Lawrence). Economically the Hudson River was the principal outlet of the fur trade south of the St. Lawrence; strategically it was an avenue along which an ambitious nation could strike for control of the inner continent. The Dutch were not that ambitious, but they did find New Netherland a convenient base from which to drain off the continent's fur supply, and collect profit from England's settlements to the north and south. They used their colonies in the West Indies similarly to annex much of the trade of the English sugar planters there.

When Charles II set about enforcing the Navigation Acts, he took care of the Dutch problem in North America in the simplest possible way. He made a gift of the Dutch territories to his brother James, the Duke of York. To the seemingly formidable task of delivering the gift he assigned four commissioners, with four frigates and four hundred men. The commissioners arrived in 1664, a time when the Dutch settlers had been demoralized by arbitrary and incompetent governors. To everyone's surprise, the colony surrendered without resistance, and the commissioners took possession for the duke of the entire region from Maryland to Connecticut.

The Dutch in Holland, already at odds with England, declared war and continued to violate the Navigation Acts wherever willing colonists and the absence of the British navy made it possible. In the long run, the problem of enforcement could be solved not by foreign war but only by effective administrative machinery within the colonies themselves. That problem became at once more difficult and more urgent as a new burst of colonizing activity increased the dimensions of the empire.

The Restoration Colonies

The colonies founded in the second half of the seventeenth century were "proprietary," that is, they were founded by proprietors who exercised government over them and initially owned all the land in them. The proprietors, generally friends or relatives of the king, hoped to grow rich from the sale of their lands and from the annual fees, or quitrents (usually a shilling per fifty acres), that they charged the settlers. They kept the quitrents low enough not to deter prospective immigrants but high enough to guarantee themselves a tidy permanent income when the colony should be fully populated.

The new colonies all resembled Maryland in their proprietary origin (see p. 29); they differed from Maryland and the other old colonies in the sources from which they drew their actual settlers: comparatively few came directly from England. Some were on the spot already, like the Dutch and Swedish settlers in New Netherland. More came from Scotland, Ireland, Wales, France, and Germany. Still more came from America itself, men and women who had grown

New York harbor

discontented with the part of the New World they already occupied and wanted to try a new place.

This search for greener pastures was to become one of the abiding characteristics of American life. Once uprooted, people might wander long before they found a spot where they could remain content. After a few months or years in a new home, one morning they would turn their backs on surroundings that had scarcely become familiar and be off to the promised land beyond the horizon. From this restless breed the new proprietors hoped to draw tenants for their feudal domains. Tenants less likely to pay feudal rents would have been hard to find, but that fact was not immediately apparent.

New York. The most important of the new colonies was New York, whose settlers and problems the Duke of York had inherited from the Dutch. New Netherland had been primarily a series of riverside trading posts, located at Swaanendael (Lewes), Fort Nassau (Newcastle), and Fort Casimir (in Gloucester County, New Jersey) on the Delaware, and at Fort Orange (Albany) and Esopus (Kingston) on the Hudson. But New Amsterdam (New York City) at the mouth of the Hudson and a few other areas had more advanced settlements. The merchants of New Amsterdam were no longer mere Indian traders, and their flourishing overseas business supported a sizable and diversified community. In the Hudson Valley a number of well-to-do Dutchmen had tried to found agricultural settlements, known as patroonships, of the very kind that English proprietors were hoping to establish. One of these, belonging to Kiliaen van Rensselaer, had approached success. Though Rensselaer himself had gained little profit from it, his tenants still occupied the lands. On Manhattan, on the western end of Long

Island, and in the lower Hudson Valley there were a few villages of Dutch farmers; and in eastern Long Island a number of New England Puritans had transplanted themselves and their way of life. The Dutch, finding them difficult to cope with, had left them much to themselves.

The Dutch West India Company had governed these sprawling settlements (probably totaling no more than seven or eight thousand persons at the end) through a director-general. Of the men who held the post, Wouter van Twiller (1633–38) and Willem Kieft (1638–47) had been disastrously foolish; and Peter Stuyvesant (1647–64), who surrendered the colony to the English, was little better. All had governed without benefit of a popular assembly. English rule brought no immediate changes, except in the quality of the governors. The terms of surrender confirmed the old settlers in their property rights. The Duke of York, by the charter that conveyed the area to him, was given full authority to govern as he saw fit. Since the duke had no fondness for representative assemblies, he appointed a governor to rule in the same manner as the old director-general.

The Dutch colonists were not happy about English rule and welcomed their country's reconquest of New York in 1673. But the Dutch authorities still attached no great value to the place and handed it back to the English when they made peace the next year. The American Dutch swallowed their pride and submitted peacefully to the governors sent by the Duke of York: Richard Nicolls (1664–68), Francis Lovelace (1668–73), Edmund Andros (1674–81), and Thomas Dongan (1683–88). The New Englanders on Long Island were less docile. They showed the familiar unfriendliness of Englishmen toward governments in which the governed had no representation. Governor Nicolls tried to appease them at the outset by compiling a special set of laws for them, drawn in part from the New England laws, which they presumably liked. This code, known as the Duke's Laws, was presented to a meeting of representatives from seventeen towns in 1665, but the meeting was not allowed to alter or add to it. The inhabitants accepted it, but not gratefully. During the ensuing years they objected continually to paying taxes without representation and, instead of being happy about their rescue from the Dutch, complained that they were now "inslav'd under an Arbitrary Power."

Perhaps because of the noisy discontent of these New Englanders, New York attracted comparatively few new settlers. There was consequently little profit from rents for the Duke of York. His governors told him of the demand for a representative assembly and hinted that the colony might be easier to govern with one than without. In 1683 he gave way, and on October 17 the first assembly was held at New York with eighteen representatives elected from the various areas of the duke's propriety. One of the assembly's first actions was to pass a Charter of Liberties stating the right of the inhabitants to all the traditional English political and civil liberties, such as trial by jury and representative government. Though this charter received the duke's assent, he repudiated it in 1686, after New York had been transformed from a proprietary to a royal colony by his accession (1685) to the throne of England as James II.

Routes to the interior of North America

New Jersey. New York in 1685 was not as large as New Netherland had been. Three and a half months after receiving his grant of the area, James had transferred the part later called New Jersey to two friends: John, Lord Berkeley, a privy councillor much interested in naval affairs, and Sir George Carteret, Vice-Chamberlain of the Royal Household and Treasurer of the Navy (James himself was Lord High Admiral, in charge of the navy). There followed a comedy of errors that was never entirely straightened out.

James' governor in New York, Richard Nicolls, did not learn of the transfer to Berkeley and Carteret until after he himself had granted lands in the New Jersey region to a number of New England Puritans from eastern Long Island. Nicolls, who was anxious to get the land settled and producing revenue, offered the Puritans the right to govern themselves through their own assembly. They in turn agreed to pay quitrents to James. Nicolls actually had no authority to offer such terms, but the Puritans accepted them and moved in.

When Berkeley and Carteret gained possession, they too offered liberal terms to settlers. They too wanted quitrents and promised a representative assembly to make laws. More Puritans, this time from New Haven, accepted the offer and moved in.

James, in transferring New Jersey to Berkeley and Carteret, gave them only property rights over the colony. His own governmental authority was not transferable. Berkeley and Carteret, therefore, had no authority either to hold a representative assembly or to appoint a governor. Yet they did both, and neither James nor his brother the king objected.

But the cantankerous transplanted New Englanders, who had accepted grants from Nicolls, did object. They held their own assembly and refused to accept the authority of the government established by the proprietors. The vehemence of their protests and their carelessness in paying rents were not diminished by subsequent developments. Berkeley and Carteret divided the province in two in 1674. Berkeley, who had taken the western half, sold it that same year to a Quaker, who resold shares to other Quakers. In 1680, after Carteret died, the eastern half, where both groups of Puritans were located, was sold at auction to another group of Quakers. Quakers were dissenters from the Church of England who carried a number of Puritan doctrines much farther than the Puritans did, and who thereby earned the anger and contempt of Anglican and Puritan alike. The fact that the proprietors were now Quakers did not endear proprietary government to the Puritan settlers. They continued to protest until the English government awoke to the fact that the government of New Jersey rested on a false assumption of power by the original proprietors. In 1702 East and West New Jersey were united as a royal colony with a single representative assembly and with the proprietors retaining only their property rights.

The Carolinas.

Before Berkeley and Carteret received the grant of New Jersey, they had already become involved with several highly placed friends in a project for another colony in the region directly south of Virginia, known as Carolina. The moving spirit in this enterprise was probably Sir John Colleton, an old royalist soldier. After Charles I lost his head in 1649, Colleton had gone to Barbados. There he found that the earlier exodus from England had deposited thousands of hopeful immigrants, who had carved the island into small farms. After 1640, however, as sugar gradually became the dominant crop, the land was absorbed into ever larger plantations worked by increasing numbers of imported black slaves. Many of the settlers had been squeezed off their farms and were now ready to move to the continent, where land was more plentiful.

When Colleton returned to England in 1660, he realized that this ready-made population for a new colony lay waiting, and he was probably already interested in the Carolina region. In London he met Sir William Berkeley (brother of John), the royal governor of Virginia (1641–52 and 1660–77). The governor knew that the Virginians had occupied much of their own tidewater land and were ready to expand down the coast into Carolina. Before long, he and Colleton had assembled a blue-ribbon board of would-be proprietors for the new colony. Besides themselves there were Berkeley's brother John; Sir George Carteret; Anthony Ashley Cooper, later Earl of Shaftesbury; George Monck, Duke of Albemarle (who had engi-neered Charles II's return to the throne); William, Earl of Craven; and Edward Hyde, Earl of Clarendon. To such men the king could not say no even though they were asking for the whole area extending from the present Atlantic border of the states of North Carolina, South Carolina, and Georgia westward to the Pacific.

The proprietors received the territory by royal charter on March 24, 1663, and they moved at once to fill it with footloose farmers from Virginia, New England, and Barbados. From the beginning they proposed two distinct centers for settlement. The region of Albemarle Sound in the northernmost part of their grant was already sparsely occupied by settlers who had drifted in from Virginia. The proprietors gave them a governor in 1664; a popularly elected assembly met for the first time by June 1665. At the end of the century this colony of North Carolina had a population of four or five thousand. They engaged in subsistence farming and also grew enough tobacco to prompt enterprising New England merchants to go after it every year with shallow-draft vessels that could clear the shoals of the area.

Farther south, where the Cape Fear River offered a better harbor than did Albemarle Sound, the proprietors intended to plant a second colony. New Englanders had already tried living here without authorization from England but had pulled out after tacking up a sign at the mouth of the river, warning future settlers that the country was not worth occupying. This may have been an early piece of Yankee shrewdness, for the proprietors found a continuing interest in the region among New Englanders—not enough, however, to induce many Puritans to move there and

**Charles Town
grew into a city**

pay quitrents to absentee proprietors (there were no quitrents in New England). The first authorized colonists were mainly Barbadians, who came in 1665 and dispersed in 1667—to Virginia, to the Albemarle region, to New England, or back to Barbados. A successful settlement, sponsored primarily by Anthony Ashley Cooper, was finally made farther south. Well equipped with provisions, an expedition set out from England in 1669 and picked up reinforcements at Barbados and other islands en route. The settlers located themselves at first on the south bank of the Ashley River about twenty-five miles from the sea. In 1680 they moved to the present site of Charleston (called Charles Town until 1783), where, as later Carolinians would have it, the Ashley and Cooper rivers join to form the Atlantic Ocean.

The proprietors had provided the settlers with a constitution designed to strike a balance between aristocracy and democracy. Drafted presumably by Cooper's secretary, John Locke, the Fundamental Constitutions of Carolina were based more on the political philosophy of James Harrington than on the philosophy for which Locke himself was to become famous (see p. 77). Harrington believed that the structure of government should match the distribution of property among the governed. The proprietors proposed to people three-fifths of their property with ordinary settlers (who would pay an annual quitrent) and to keep the rest in seigneurial and manorial estates for a hereditary nobility. The government was to consist of a governor appointed by the proprietors and a legislature in which the upper house would represent the nobility, the lower the commoners. The upper house was to have the sole right to initiate legislation (another idea of Harrington's).

The settlers of South Carolina, by accretions of Barbadians, Huguenots (who were the French equiva-

lent of Puritans), New Englanders, Englishmen, Scots, and black slaves, increased to eight or ten thousand by the end of the century. They worked at turning the pines of the area into pitch and tar and turpentine (naval stores) and in producing rice. It was probably the slaves who taught the Carolina planters to grow rice, which was a familiar crop in Africa but not found in the areas from which the other settlers had come. Eventually it became South Carolina's most valuable export, cultivated extensively in the lowlands around Charles Town. Beyond the rice plantations frontiersmen outflanked the Appalachian Mountains, pushed back Spanish missions, and penetrated the interior of the continent to open a brisk trade with the Indians in deerskins and in slaves captured from other tribes. Charles Town grew into a city, the only one in the South. In spite of hurricanes, Indian attacks, and internal quarrels, South Carolina succeeded.

The Fundamental Constitutions did not. As in other colonies, the representative assembly—the lower house of the legislature—was impatient of restrictions: it claimed and took the right to initiate legislation, quarreled with the governor and the upper house, and generally got its way. By 1700 the Fundamental Constitutions were a dead letter, and proprietary rule was faltering. In 1719 a rebellion in Charles Town overthrew the last proprietary governor, and two years later a provisional royal government was organized in the colony. The proprietors finally surrendered their charter in 1729, and royal governments were provided for both North and South Carolina, each with a governor and council appointed by the king and an assembly elected by the landowners.

William Penn's holy experiment. The last English colony to be founded in the seventeenth century was also the private property of a friend of the king. It would be hard to imagine a more unlikely friend for Charles II than William Penn, Quaker, commoner, and enemy of royal prerogative. The association, a tribute to breadth of character in both men, began in the career of Penn's father, who was no Quaker. William Penn the elder started life as a seaman and by sheer ability worked his way to the rank of admiral. He was in charge of naval operations in Cromwell's grandiose expedition to the West Indies. When the expedition captured nothing but Jamaica, the admiral retired in disgrace to Ireland, where he remained until Charles II took the throne.

Disgrace under Cromwell was no bar to preferment under Charles. Admiral Penn was on hand to see the new king crowned in 1660 and took the occasion to present his son, then aged sixteen. In the ensuing years, while the father headed the navy office under the Duke of York, young Penn did the things that sons of gentlemen were expected to do. It was conventional that he should attend Oxford and almost conventional that he be expelled after two years and sent on the grand tour of the Continent by a worried father. It was conventional, too, that he should spend some time at the Inns of Court studying law, but without becoming a barrister. As he reached maturity, Penn had the standard qualifications of a young courtier: high spirits, ready wit, skill as a swordsman. He cut a dashing figure at the court of the king. But he had one quality that was not quite conventional, one that kings, courtiers, and fathers of young gentlemen have often found embarrassing: he took ideas seriously.

What was worse, the ideas he took most seriously were of the most embarrassing kind: radical, offbeat, faintly ridiculous. The early Quakers (later called Friends) were drawn from a wide spectrum of English society, including a substantial number of gentry and merchants, but they seemed to be the lunatic fringe of the Puritan movement. They heard voices; they insulted their betters; they appeared naked in church. One of them, James Nayler, thought he was Jesus Christ and entered the city of Bristol riding on an ass, with his admirers singing holy, holy, holy before him.

The authorities dealt with Nayler: they bored his tongue with a hot iron, cut off his ears, and branded his forehead with the letter *B* for blasphemer—thereby demonstrating what might have happened to Christ if he *had* reappeared. Respectable people thought that madmen like Nayler were typical of Quakerism. But by the 1660s, Quakers had shaken free of these eccentricities and were challenging the world by practicing what they preached.

What they preached was not far different from what other Christians had always preached. What others had variously called conscience, revelation, or saving grace, Quakers called the Inner Light. The Inner Light, they said, glowed in every human being. One had only to live by it in order to be saved. Quakers tried to live by it.

All Christians believed that humility is a virtue. But the Quakers studiously, almost fanatically, avoided pride and the institutions that pride erected: they wore conspicuously plain and out-of-date clothes; they refused to honor one another—or anyone else—by bowing or kneeling or taking off their hats, or by using the second person plural when addressing an individual (ultimately they forgot the nominative and used only "thee"). All Christians professed brotherly love; but the Quakers refused to make war. They also refused to give or take oaths, partly because they believed the imposition of an oath implied distrust of one's fellow men.

Ideas of this kind first infected William Penn as a

student at Oxford and may have been responsible for his expulsion. One reason for the grand tour was to get them out of his head and something more fashionable into it. The tour worked, too, but only until Penn encountered a Quaker named Thomas Loe, whom he may have known earlier. In 1667 Samuel Pepys, a diarist who worked in the navy office, recorded the sad fact that Sir William Penn's son was "a Quaker again, or some very melancholy thing."

From this time forward, Penn was Quakerism's most energetic and effective supporter. He knew enough theology to argue with priests, enough law to argue with judges. He was so friendly with the king that no one dared ignore him, and he had such courage that he never allowed his friendship to weaken his arguments against the king's policies. He fought not only for Quakerism but for the right of all English subjects to worship as they pleased and to run their own government.

The "golden days of good King Charles" were nevertheless hard times for Quakers. The Anglican Church was doing its best to limit and control dissent. Quakers, because they refused to hold their meetings in secret, spent more time in jail than other Dissenters. Penn joined with other Quakers in the purchase of New Jersey, which for a time served as a Quaker refuge. But eastern New Jersey was full of Puritans, always unfriendly to Quakers, and western New Jersey had poor soil. Penn heard that the land across the Delaware was better and that no one was there but wild Indians, who would be easier to live with than English bishops or New Jersey Puritans. The king owed him £16,000, a debt contracted to his father (who died in 1670) for back pay and loans to the royal exchequer. In 1680 Penn asked the king for the land and, after many protests from the king's advisers, got it. Charles named it Pennsylvania after the admiral. In addition,

Penn later laid claim successfully to the region that is now the state of Delaware, which was already populated by a few Dutch and Swedish settlers.

According to the terms of his charter, issued in March 1681, Penn was specifically required to enforce the Navigation Acts, to submit laws to the king for approval, to allow appeals to the king from Pennsylvania courts, and to provide an Anglican minister whenever twenty or more colonists asked for one. He was also required to obtain the approval of the freeholders (the male owners of land) for any laws that he imposed. Otherwise he had a free hand to govern the colony as he saw fit.

Penn saw fit to govern in a manner that he hoped would demonstrate the virtues of Quakerism and of political and religious liberty. Though, like other proprietors, he hoped to profit from his colony by quitrents on land, his primary purpose was to conduct a holy experiment in popular government and Christian living. He served as governor when in the province and appointed a deputy when absent, but neither for himself nor for his deputy did he retain extensive powers. The people, he made plain in a statement issued a month after he received the charter, "would be allowed to shape their own laws." In the Frame of Government that he worked out to embody this principle, Penn placed the legislative power in a council and an assembly, both elected by the freeholders. He probably assumed, however, that the freeholders would choose the more successful and well-to-do among them to the council, while the assembly would be composed of more ordinary folk. And Penn, who retained some traditional ideas about the prerogatives of the well-to-do, made the council the more powerful of the two bodies, with the sole right to initiate legislation.

Attracted by the prospect of good land, free government, and religious liberty, English, Irish, Welsh, Dutch, and German Quakers flocked to the colony. It prospered from the start and attracted many non-Quakers as well, partly because Penn advertised its advantages in pamphlets that were circulated widely. By the end of the century the total population was close to twenty thousand. Penn himself went to the colony in 1682 but had to return to England in less than two years to defend his southern boundary in a legal dispute with Lord Baltimore. The dispute was not fully settled until the 1760s, when Charles Mason and Jeremiah Dixon surveyed their famous line. Litigation, losses, and revolution kept Penn in England for fifteen years. During that time his friend King Charles died and his friend the Duke of York ascended the throne, only to flee from it in 1688.

In Pennsylvania, Quakerism in power fulfilled many but not all of Penn's anticipations. It brought religious peace (other sects found complete freedom), economic prosperity, and political quarrels. Although the council, where power was concentrated, was elected by the same people who elected the assembly,

just as the United States Senate and House of Representatives are today, the assembly acted as though its lack of the right to initiate legislation was a denial of popular rights. The council and the assembly joined in attacking the governors whom Penn sent over, even though the executive power in Pennsylvania was weaker than in any other colony. It is true that Penn, who could never believe ill of anyone, often sent incompetent, or at least inappropriate, governors, such as the old Cromwellian soldier, John Blackwell. Blackwell left the province saying that Quakers prayed for their neighbors on Sundays and preyed on them the other six days of the week.

After the fall of James II, Penn was for a while suspect in England because of their long-standing friendship. His province was temporarily taken from him and, from 1692 to 1694, was under a royal government, which gave the assembly the right to initiate legislation. Upon recovering the colony, Penn recognized that right, but by then the assembly was in pursuit of still larger powers. In 1699 he finally returned to the province and told the members of the

Quakers: an eighteenth-century meeting

assembly, since they did not like his plan of government, to draft one of their own. They did so, eliminating the legislative authority of the council altogether (it retained only the function of advising the governor), and leaving the proprietor with only the ownership of ungranted land and a veto power over legislation, normally exercised through his appointed governor.

The new plan, known as the Charter of Privileges, was established in 1701, with Penn's approval, by an act of the assembly. Pennsylvania thus became the only colony with a unicameral legislature. The same Charter of Privileges gave the counties of Newcastle, Sussex, and Kent (later the state of Delaware) a separate representative assembly, though they retained the same governor as Pennsylvania. In 1701 Penn returned to England, where bad planning and good nature eventually landed him in debtor's prison, an institution he had tried to eliminate in his colony. No quitrents arrived from Pennsylvania to extricate him. He died in 1718.

Problems of Enforcement

The settlement of Pennsylvania completed English occupation of the Atlantic coast from Spanish Florida to French Canada. All the colonies had been founded under authority of the king, but without his active participation or financial support. The government of each had been uniquely shaped by the varying purposes of the founders and settlers, not by an overall imperial policy. When, with the Navigation Acts of the 1660s, the king and his Parliament began to apply an imperial policy to America, they found that most of the machinery of colonial government by which the acts might have been enforced lay beyond their immediate control. Only in Virginia (through the royally appointed governor and council) did England exercise any voice in colonial government.

Even as the Navigation Acts were passed, Charles II was furthering this dispersion of power. In 1663 he gave Rhode Island a royal charter (to replace a similar parliamentary charter of 1644), authorizing the settlers to choose their own governmental officers. In 1662 he had given the same charter privilege to Connecticut (including New Haven, which would have preferred a separate charter). By these charters and by the others he granted, Charles, perhaps thoughtlessly, distributed authority that might have been used to enforce imperial policies.

At the same time, Charles strengthened another element in colonial government that was to make imperial control difficult. In each of his charters, except the one given to the Duke of York, he required

the consent of the settlers to local legislation. The requirement was met by popularly elected representative assemblies like those already existing in older colonies. Assemblies had demonstrated their usefulness: to operate effectively, a colonial government had to obtain the advice and cooperation of the actual settlers, especially where they were English, used to having their laws made by their representatives. But the assemblies had also demonstrated a truculence, not unlike that of Parliament in England, which promised trouble for policies imposed from above. Nowhere was the threat greater than in New England.

Recalcitrant colonists. New England, of all the regions in the empire, fitted least well into the mercantilist scheme of supplying needed raw materials to the mother country. Its farmers and fishermen produced enough provisions to help feed the West Indies sugar plantations. But it had nothing in quantity that the mother country wanted. Since furs from the interior of the continent came out by way of the Hudson or the St. Lawrence, the New England fur trade lasted only until the local animals had been depleted. Lumber and lumber products, such as pitch and tar, were a minor resource. But mostly New England grew rocks, and even these contained no valuable minerals or ores. Because their resources were limited, New Englanders went into the business of distributing what the rest of the world produced. In plying their trade wherever the best price was offered, they competed—all too successfully—with the merchants of the mother country.

They could still have carried on a successful trade in obedience to the Navigation Acts, but disobedience was more profitable. The merchant who bought French silks and laces in France and carried them directly to Boston could undersell one who bought the same goods in England, because English prices included the extra cost of English duties and of transportation from France to England. The same advantage accrued to a merchant or captain who illegally carried enumerated commodities, such as sugar or tobacco, directly from the colonies to Europe.

New Englanders, therefore, had good economic reasons for resisting or evading directions from England. And, as was often the case in New England, economic interest coincided with religious interest. The New Englanders were Puritans, and they had come to New England to live as Puritans. Charles II, whatever else he may have been, was notoriously not a Puritan. New Englanders consequently looked with suspicion on his government and were wary of any move to bring them under its control. The founders of New England had struck this defensive attitude almost as soon as they set foot there. According to Governor Winthrop, the Puritans had "hastened"

The day after, I went to visit the governour at his house, and among other discourse I told him I tooke notice of severall ships that were arrived at Boston, some since my being there, from Spain, France, Streights, Canaries and other parts of Europe, contrary to your Majesties lawes for encouraging navigation, and regulating the trade of the plantations. He freely declared to me that the lawes made by your Majestie and your parliament obligeth them in nothing but what consists with the interest of that colony, that the legislative power is and abides in them solely to act and make lawes by virtue of a charter from your Majesties royall father, and that all matters in difference are to be concluded by their finall determination, without any appeal to your Majestie, and that your Majestie ought not to retrench their liberties, but may enlarge them if your Majestie please, and said ... that your Majesty could doe no lesse in reason than let them enjoy their liberties and trade, they having upon their own charge and without any contribution from the crown made so large plantation in the wildernesse ... and that notwithstanding the colony had many enemies, yet they did believe your Majestie to be their very good friend, for that your Majestie had by severall letters expressed your kindnesse to them....

From Edward Randolph, Letter to the King of England, 1676.

their fortifications in 1633 when they heard that Charles I had appointed a commission under Archbishop Laud to govern them. Fortunately the fortifications did not have to be manned against the archbishop. Thereafter New Englanders had easily withstood the halfhearted efforts at control made by Parliament and by Oliver Cromwell. When Charles II came to the throne, they still had the royal charter of Massachusetts intact and did not hesitate to remind the new king of the privileges granted by his father (even though they were secretly harboring the men who had passed the death sentence on Charles I).

Charles II knew that New England was full of Puritans, whom he abhorred, and that Massachusetts in particular had passed laws that did not fully satisfy the requirement, stated in its charter (as in other colonial charters), that all laws conform to those of England. In 1662 he sent a letter commanding revisions. The assembly ignored it. And so, in 1664, when Charles sent his commission of four to capture New Netherland from the Dutch, he assigned them the additional task of investigating New England. They were empowered to adjust boundaries, hear appeals from colonial courts, redress grievances against colonial governments, and report to the king on how well New England was obeying the Navigation Acts.

The commissioners, who went to New England fresh from their triumph over the Dutch, made a discovery that was to be repeated often in the history of the British empire: England could govern the Dutch (and the French, the Spanish, the Egyptians, the Indians, and the Chinese) more easily than it could govern Englishmen. The commissioners were treated well enough in Rhode Island, Connecticut, and Plymouth, all of which were looking for improvements in their boundaries. Plymouth had no charter and perhaps hoped to get one by good behavior. But when the commissioners appeared in Boston they met with a reception the coolness of which has seldom been matched even in that city. The officers of government referred them to the charter of 1629 and ostentatiously refused to recognize their authority. A herald appeared before the house where the commissioners were staying and, after a blast from his trumpet, in the name of the king formally forbade anyone to appear before them. Frustrated at every turn, they went back to England to report that the Massachusetts government was making no effort to enforce the Navigation Acts. They also recommended to the king that he revoke the Massachusetts charter, a suggestion echoed by every royal official to visit the colony in the next twenty years.

The king could not revoke the charter at will. It was a contract, binding both grantor and grantee. But the terms required that Massachusetts make no laws contrary to those of England. If it could be shown that Massachusetts had done so, a court of law would declare the charter void, and the king would recover all governmental powers.

After the experience of his commissioners, Charles decided to continue the investigation in England and demanded that Massachusetts send agents to account for its behavior. The General Court (as the Massachusetts assembly was called) sent masts for the king's navy, money for the sufferers in the great fire of London, provisions for the fleet, but no agents. The

As long as Plum Island *shall faithfully keep the commanded Post; Notwithstanding all the hectoring Words, and hard Blows of the proud and boisterous Ocean; As long as any Salmon, or Sturgeon shall swim in the streams of* Merrimack; *or any Perch, or Pickeril, in* Crane-Pond; *As long as the Sea-Fowl shall know the Time of their coming, and not neglect seasonably to visit the Places of their Acquaintance; As long as any Cattel shall be fed with the Grass growing in the Medows, which do humbly bow down themselves before* Turkie-Hill; *As long as any Sheep shall walk upon Old Town Hills, and shall from thence pleasantly look down upon the River* Parker, *and the fruitfull Marishes lying beneath; As long as any free and harmless Doves shall find a White Oak, or other Tree within the Township, to perch, or feed, or build a careless Nest upon; and shall voluntarily present themselves to perform the office of Gleaners after Barley-Harvest; As long as Nature shall not grow Old and dote; but shall constantly remember to give the rows of Indian Corn their education, by Pairs; So long shall Christians be born there; and being first made meet, shall from thence be Translated, to be made partakers of the Inheritance of the Saints in Light.*

From Samuel Sewall, *Phaenomena*, 1697.

New England: a New Englander's view

leaders of Massachusetts knew that many of their laws did violate England's, especially their laws about religion. It was precisely these laws that they wished to keep, even more than they wished to escape the Navigation Acts. So they tried every means to avoid a showdown, relying heavily on distance to support them in one delaying action after another. For ten years they got away with it and grew ever more prosperous and powerful.

In England the king paid only sporadic attention to them and made no effective move against them. But Parliament, in 1673, passed an act to make smuggling to foreign countries less profitable. It levied export duties, known as "plantations duties," on any enumerated commodity shipped to another colony instead of to England. Now, if a shipper pretended to be taking tobacco from Virginia to Boston but took it instead to Holland, he would already have paid a tax equivalent to that levied in England, and he would be unable to sell his cargo in Holland at a price much lower than that of tobacco reshipped legitimately from England. The act of 1673 made smuggling more difficult but did not stop it. As before, the most persistent evaders were the New Englanders, and the governors of other colonies complained that the example of Massachusetts undermined their own attempts to enforce the Navigation Acts.

The main reason why Charles II failed to act decisively against Massachusetts during these years was that he had no administrative body devoted primarily to colonial affairs. At last, in 1675, he appointed a special committee of the Privy Council known as the Lords of Trade, which set about pulling together the

strings of empire. The members quickly realized that they could not rely on the colonial governments to enforce the policies of the English government. England must have its own means of enforcement in the colonies. The first step, the Lords of Trade decided, was for the king to take a hand in governing them.

The earliest opportunity came in New Hampshire, into which Massachusetts had extended its authority beyond the boundaries set by its charter. Robert Mason, who had inherited a claim to the region from the Council for New England, complained to the king about this encroachment, and in 1679 Charles took New Hampshire away from Massachusetts and gave it a royal government. Massachusetts was in danger of losing Maine as well, after an English court had declared its title to that area invalid. But Massachusetts managed to purchase the title of the counterclaimant, Ferdinando Gorges (who was the heir of the original Ferdinando), before the king could act.

The Lords of Trade took over Charles' fight against the Massachusetts charter by renewing the demand that the colony send agents to London. The General Court finally did so, but it gave them no authority to answer the questions the Lords wanted answered. The Lords insisted that the Massachusetts government enforce the Navigation Acts. The General Court, hardened by thirty years of ignoring and defying orders from England, loftily retorted that it was legally endowed by the king's own charter with full powers to govern the province and that therefore Parliament had no authority to pass laws affecting Massachusetts. But, in order to avoid a head-on collision, the General Court formally ordered enforcement of the Navigation Acts. Without waiting to see if Massachusetts would actually carry out the order, the Lords sent an imperial customs officer, Edward Randolph, to do the job; the General Court refused to recognize his commission, set up its own customs office, and imprisoned the deputies appointed by Randolph. The Lords demanded that Massachusetts show cause why its charter should not be revoked; again the General Court sent agents with insufficient powers and inadequate answers. In 1683 legal proceedings were begun, and in 1684 the charter was revoked. In 1685 the Duke of York became King James II.

The Dominion of New England. The accession of James II, which made New York a royal colony, together with the revocation of the Massachusetts charter, cleared the way for a scheme the Lords of Trade had long had in mind: a reconstruction of the American empire from New Jersey northward. The scheme shows that they had identified clearly the immediate sources of trouble; it also shows that they had learned little about political realities in either England or America. They proposed to place New Jersey, New York, Connecticut, Rhode Island, Plymouth, Massachusetts, New Hampshire, and Maine under one governor. And in this whole area, to be called the Dominion of New England, there would be no troublesome representative assembly. The royally appointed governor would be assisted by a council whose members would also be appointed by the king. It apparently did not occur to their lordships that the people, deprived of any share in their own government, might prove more troublesome than the assemblies had been.

When news reached Boston that the Massachusetts charter had been revoked, men talked of resistance, as their fathers had fifty years before when threatened with the rule of Archbishop Laud. But their fathers had never been put to the test and had had less to lose in ships, houses, and money than the Bostonians of 1685. Boston was no longer a mere beachhead on an unsettled coast. It was a prosperous city of some seven thousand people with a fleet rivaling that of any English city except London. Most Bostonians held to the faith of their fathers, but they and other New Englanders were perhaps a little more prosperous than Puritan. They allowed their General Court to be dissolved and submitted reluctantly to the interim government of a council appointed by the king. In 1686, when Sir Edmund Andros arrived to establish the Dominion of New England, he faced hard looks and sullen words but no manned fortifications. Although the charters of Rhode Island and Connecticut had not been revoked, Andros extended

The Dominion of New England

James Martin:

I received a wrighting from you by Mr. Shippin wherein you say you have a message from god to deliver to the people of Boston. Well, were it soe indeed, it is meete you should be heard: but for as much as I beleeve the contrary and that it is but a delution or suggestion of satan their is noe reason for me to grant your request for by your behaviour and wrighting you seame to be a professed Quaker and in reason to be thought to be of the same principals and perswations of the cheefe of the Leaders som of whose boocks I have seane and Red and Judg such to be as pernitious hereticks as ever was whose cheaf if not only rule for life and maners is imediate revelation and denying the trew Christian faith and salvation by believing in the Lord Jesus Christ god man and soe no cristians and theirfore that which you call Reasonable I conseave most unreasonable and unsafe and unlawfull as to permit a Jesuit or popish preest to preach or prate to the people and theirfore doe advise and Require you forthwith to depart out of this towne and jurisdiction without giving us any further trouble or disturbance.

From Simon Bradstreet, Governor of Massachusetts, Letter to James Martin, March 27, 1683.

The rights of Quakers: Massachusetts, 1683

his government over them without difficulty and in 1688 completed his domain by taking over New York and New Jersey, which he ruled thereafter through a lieutenant-governor. In each colony he dissolved the assembly.

Andros was not a happy choice to inaugurate the new system. An experienced administrator, he had already served as governor of New York and would, in the years ahead, serve as governor of Virginia. But the present task called for diplomacy and tact as well as administrative skill. A blunt, outspoken man, Andros made decisions more easily than he made friends. He and the Lords of Trade believed, not without reason, that in order to establish imperial authority in New England the grip of the Puritan leaders must be broken and room made for a party of moderation. But it would have required a man of moderate temper and winning ways to organize and lead such a party.

The Lords of Trade, encouraged by the reports of Edward Randolph, supposed that the Puritans were a minority and that the majority of the population was tired of Puritan intolerance toward Quakers, Baptists, Anglicans, and customs officers. Nothing could have been further from the truth. Enemies of the old government were few, and Andros, by following the instructions of his superiors in England, succeeded in alienating what few there were. He levied taxes for the support of government, necessarily without the consent of a representative assembly. And when the inhabitants objected and pleaded their rights as English subjects, he told them they had no rights. Massachusetts had parceled out lands to individuals through the agency of incorporated towns; Andros maintained that the Massachusetts Bay Company had no authority to create corporations and that all titles to land granted by towns were therefore invalid. Anyone who wanted to own the land that he or his fathers had carved out of the wilderness had to ask for a new deed from the governor, pay a fee for it, and agree to pay quitrents ever after.

Andros, with the help of customs officers sent from England, enforced the Navigation Acts, and Randolph later claimed that this was the real cause of opposition to him. But the fact was that the Lords of Trade, in their zeal to establish imperial authority, had assigned Andros an impossible task. They required him to violate long-established rights and privileges and, without the support of an army, a police force, or a political party, to rule arbitrarily over a people who for more than fifty years had ruled themselves. Whether Puritan, non-Puritan, or anti-Puritan they could not be expected to like it. As Andros spelled out the dimensions of his immense authority, they began to have second thoughts about the wisdom of their submission.

The Revolution of 1688. Fortunately for New England, the rule of Andros coincided with the reign of James II. Although James could not dispense with Parliament as he had with the New England assemblies, he made it appear that he would have liked to. By exercising his power of pardon he effectively suspended the operation of many parliamentary enactments. He was, besides, a Catholic and made no secret of it. The political patience of the English was as thin in old as in New England. In 1688 they welcomed William of Orange (who had married James's Protestant daughter Mary) and chased James out of the country.

In Boston the Puritans did not wait for the fall of James to liquidate the Dominion of New England. After they had heard of William's landing in England, but before they had learned of his success in ousting James, they carried out a tidy, bloodless revolution of their own. Spurred by rumors that Andros and James were plotting to hand New England over to the pope, the inhabitants of Boston seized and imprisoned the governor and his council, restored the old government, and waited to hear how William was faring in England. The colony's most eminent minister, Increase Mather, had gone to London the year before to plead the colony's cause against Andros. Mather did his best to persuade the new monarchs, William and Mary, that the Dominion of New England was part and parcel of James' tyrannical policies in England and that the Glorious Revolution ought to include a glorious restitution of the Massachusetts charter. William gave orders for the recall of Andros and authorized Massachusetts to proceed temporarily under its old government, but he refused to restore the charter until he and his advisers should have time to investigate the situation.

Plymouth, Rhode Island, and Connecticut quietly resumed their old governments, and New Jersey returned to anarchy. But New York had its own revolution, which was not entirely bloodless. Andros' lieutenant-governor there, Francis Nicholson, was left in an anomalous position as the appointee of a deposed officer who was in turn the appointee of a deposed king. Nicholson was, besides, young and headstrong, a professional military officer with an unconcealed scorn for popular rights and liberties. When rumors of popish plots alarmed the population, he did nothing to quiet them.

At the end of May 1689 a party of local militia seized the fort that commanded New York harbor and took control of the government. The party was led by Jacob Leisler, a successful German immigrant who had married into a prominent Dutch family. After Nicholson departed for England in June 1689, a meeting of delegates from different parts of the province chose a committee of safety, which in turn named Leisler as commander in chief of the province. Leisler proclaimed the accession of William, and when ambiguously addressed letters arrived from the new king authorizing a continuation of government, Leisler claimed them.

Basing his authority on the letters, Leisler governed the colony arbitrarily but effectively for nearly two years. New York, thinly settled by people of differing nationalities and religions living in widely differing circumstances, was a long way from political maturity. To maintain order, Leisler had to rely heavily on his followers among the militia. When King William finally got around to appointing a regular

Increase Mather: eminent minister

governor in 1691, Leisler hesitated before surrendering authority to him and thereby gave the new appointee the pretext for an accusation of treason. Leisler and his son-in-law, Jacob Milborne, were convicted and hanged on May 16, 1691. Four years later Parliament reversed the sentence.

The reorganization of 1696. The downfall of the Dominion of New England, together with the revolution in England, brought to a halt the efforts to consolidate the empire. After William mounted the throne, he was kept busy defending England in war against France and trying to shore up what was left of the royal prerogative. The new men he appointed to the Privy Council were unfamiliar with colonial problems, and the Lords of Trade had been turned into a committee of the whole, charged with new and broader functions. Once again nobody in the government devoted himself exclusively to colonial policy. The result was seven years of neglect.

In the colonies merchants and shippers ignored the Navigation Acts, and pirates brazenly pursued their prey in and out of harbors. Edward Randolph, now trying to enforce the acts in Maryland, found himself again thwarted by New Englanders who were buying tobacco from the planters and taking it to Scotland instead of England. Though Scotland had the same king as England, the two countries remained separate until 1707. Under the Navigation Acts, Scotland, like nations on the Continent, was excluded from the benefits of trade with England's colonies.

Scottish competition for the tobacco trade raised such a howl of protest from English merchants that the king and Parliament were driven to act. In 1696, guided by Edward Randolph, Parliament in one extensive enactment constructed machinery for enforcing the Navigation Acts. Henceforth the governors of all colonies, whether royal, proprietary, or corporate (Rhode Island and Connecticut), were to take an oath to enforce the acts. Failure to do so meant forfeiture of office. In place of the occasional peripatetic customs officer, a regular customs service subject to the English Treasury was established in each colony. The customs officers were authorized to take out "writs of assistance" from local courts entitling them to open buildings by force in search of smuggled goods. The officers were also empowered to prosecute violators of the Navigation Acts in admiralty courts, which the Privy Council ordered to be established in the colonies. Admiralty courts operated without juries, and it was expected that the judges, who held office only as long as they pleased the crown, would give short shrift to colonial offenders.

While Parliament was passing this measure, it also considered, and then rejected, a bill to create a council of trade and plantations to develop and administer colonial policy. The Privy Council, which had already planned a similar body, now swung into action to keep control of colonial policy under the king. In May 1696, by royal order, a new bureau was established to replace the old Lords of Trade. The Lords Commissioners of Trade and Plantations, as it was called, or more simply the Board of Trade, resembled a national chamber of commerce. It was appointed by the king and was charged to furnish him with information and advice on all colonial matters. Although the board included some members of the Privy Council, ex officio, the eight working members were not councilors and had no authority to issue orders. Their function was purely advisory. But, since they constituted the only body directly concerned with the colonies, their advice was seldom ignored.

Although the king retained control of colonial policy and administration, the circumstances of William's accession affected the kind of control that he and his successors were able to exert in the colonies. After the unhappy experience with James II, Parliament would have looked with suspicion on any move by the king to do away with a representative assembly, even in America. Parliament did not object, however, to the introduction of royal governors in colonies that had not formerly had them. Nor was there serious objection from the settlers, for in almost every case the advent of royal government relieved an in-

tolerable internal situation. Maryland was converted to royal government in 1689, after a local rebellion against the proprietor. (It returned to proprietary government in 1715 after the fourth Lord Baltimore turned Anglican.) As we have seen, New Jersey became a royal colony in 1702 (see pp. 39–40), South Carolina and North Carolina in 1729 (p. 41). In the new charter that William granted Massachusetts in 1691 (which incorporated Plymouth and Maine as parts of Massachusetts), the king retained power to appoint the governor. Thus most of the colonies reverted eventually to the king.

Wherever a royal government was introduced, the king gained more direct control over his subjects. He appointed the governor, and he appointed the governor's council (except in Massachusetts). Although in each royal colony a representative assembly of freeholders retained legislative authority, the governor's council served as the upper house of the legislature, and its approval was necessary before any act passed by the lower house became law. Even an act passed by both houses was subject to veto by the governor, and even an act approved by the governor might be disallowed by the king. During the eighteenth century, usually on the advice of the Board of Trade, some 5½ percent of the acts passed by colonial assemblies were disallowed by the king, though no act of Parliament was ever vetoed after 1708. Moreover, in the eyes of the mother country the king's instructions to his governors were supposed to bind the assembly as well as the governor. But in spite of royal theories the popularly elected lower house of the assembly remained the most powerful branch of government in every colony. It enjoyed sole authority to levy taxes, and by threatening to withhold them it was often able to get its own way against both king and governor.

The Old Colonial System. Of the three agencies England now had for enforcement of the Navigation Acts, the admiralty courts proved unable to exercise jurisdiction because of ambiguities in the act of 1696; the customs service was ill paid and susceptible to bribes and could not operate effectively without the support of the local government. England's control of its colonies depended most heavily on the success of its royal governors in working with the colonial assemblies. Since every legislative act required the assent of both the governor and the assembly, the needs of neither the mother country nor the colonies could be satisfied if the two refused to cooperate.

Thus in the last analysis the Old Colonial System (embodied in the Navigation Acts and in the act of 1696) rested on the harmony of English and colonial interests. Although occasional discord developed, especially at points of contact between royal governors and assemblies, the harmony was real and the

New England: woodcut, 1677

system worked. Enriched by its colonies, England grew to be the world's most powerful nation.

The Contest for the Continent

Protected by England, the American colonies also grew, their population doubling every twenty-five years. As they thrust outward from their coastal beachheads, they came into conflict with other peoples—Indians, French, and Spanish—who had found their way to the American continent and who had their own uses for the lands into which the burgeoning English settlers were pressing. The result was a contest for the continent that became one of the persistent facts of life for colonial Americans.

UNITS STATES POPULATION GROWTH, 1620–1860*			
1620	2,000	1750	1,171,000
1630	5,000	1760	1,594,000
1640	27,000	1770	2,148,000
1650	50,000	1780	2,780,000
1660	75,000	1790	3,929,000
1670	112,000	1800	5,297,000
1680	152,000	1810	7,224,000
1690	210,000	1820	9,618,000
1700	251,000	1830	12,901,000
1710	332,000	1840	17,120,000
1720	466,000	1850	23,261,000
1730	629,000	1860	31,513,000
1740	906,000		

*Figures rounded to the nearest thousand.
From *Historical Statistics of the United States: Colonial Times to 1957*, Series A 1–3, Z 1–19.

Indian warfare. The Indians of eastern North America were slow to perceive that their way of life was incompatible with that of the English. They often sold their land or gave it away without realizing that it would no longer be theirs too. They used the land mainly for hunting and were willing to let the English hunt on it with them. But the English taking possession cut the trees, drove out the game, and evicted the Indians. Before the Indians realized what was happening, they were outnumbered.

They could probably have done nothing to stem the English advance anyhow. They were many people, not one, and they made war on one another as often as they did on the white invaders. Indeed, they often welcomed the white man for the assistance they hoped he would offer in quarrels with their neighbors. But, except when directed and organized by the French or Spanish, they were not formidable military opponents for the English. Superior woodsmanship gave them some advantage, especially when they were armed with the white man's weapons, and they posed a constant threat to the isolated frontier farmer. But they were too independent, too individualistic, to submit for long to military discipline. They might gather for a surprise assault, but they could not stick together long enough to take advantage of their success.

The colonists, if not more warlike, were better armed, better organized, and more systematic about killing. Indians of the Powhatan Confederacy in Virginia massacred 347 settlers in a surprise attack in 1622 (Indian victories in American history are generally known as massacres), but from that time on the Virginians pursued a policy of extermination that gradually eliminated the Indian menace in the tidewater area. In 1637 the Puritans, acting in support of a group of tribes, broke the power of the one most dangerous New England tribe, the Pequots. An army led by John Mason surprised their main village at night, set fire to it, and shot men, women, and children as they ran to escape the flames. Thereafter New England suffered no serious Indian attack until 1675, when the Wampanoag chieftain Metacomet, known to the English as King Philip, undertook a war that lasted longer than usual but ended with the usual result.

Rivalry with France and Spain. After 1676 the surviving Indians east of the Appalachians were too few in number to menace the English settlers. But those farther west, led by the French, stood ready to halt English expansion at the mountains. The French in Canada, from the time of Champlain's founding of Quebec in 1608, had taken an acquisitive interest in the interior of North America. Missionaries in search of souls and *coureurs de bois* in search of furs traveled up and down the Mississippi and through the wilder-

The extension of settlement, 1660–1760

ness of its eastern tributaries. The *coureurs* were as good woodsmen as the Indians and as casual with their lives as the old English sea dogs. One of them, Louis Jolliet, together with the Jesuit Father Marquette, descended the Mississippi to the Arkansas as early as 1673. Robert Cavelier, Sieur de la Salle, reached the mouth of the Mississippi in 1682, and seventeen years later the French took possession of Louisiana by planting a settlement at Biloxi. In 1702 they started another one at Mobile. They also set up forts and trading posts in the Illinois country at Kaskaskia, Cahokia, and Vincennes, way stations between the St. Lawrence and the Mississippi, the two main arteries into the heart of North America.

In the competition for Indian furs, the French outdid the English. They also did a better job of winning the Indians' friendship. Instead of evicting the Indians from their land, the Frenchmen lived in their wigwams, occasionally married their daughters, and taught them to like Catholicism and hate the English.

The French government during the seventeenth century did not appreciate the exploits of its wandering subjects. In 1663 the king had taken New France from a French trading company, and thereafter the colony was governed by royal decrees (executed through a governor and an intendant, with no representative assembly). The king consistently discouraged the activities of the *coureurs*. He rejected, for example, the scheme of two *coureurs*, Pierre Radisson and Médart Chouart, Sieur de Groseilliers, who proposed a trading company to reach the northern fur supply by sea instead of by land; as a result, in 1672 they formed the Hudson's Bay Company in England instead of France.

Louis XIV was not interested in the wastes of Hudson Bay. Guided by his great minister Colbert, he wanted New France to be populated with hard-working, docile farmers. He sent women to entice the wild *coureurs* into a more settled life; he placed a bounty on large families. He forbade all but a few privileged individuals to engage in the fur trade. He even enlisted the Church in the cause: men who left their farms without permission were liable to excommunication. But all Louis' efforts produced only a meager scattering of agricultural settlements in Nova Scotia, along the St. Lawrence River, and later in Louisiana and in the Illinois country. Immigrants were few, and the total population remained small, no more than fifty or sixty thousand by the middle of the eighteenth century.

Fifty thousand Frenchmen proved formidable to a million and a half Englishmen only because Louis' governors in Canada had not enforced his decrees. Count Frontenac (who governed during most of the period from 1672 to 1698), perceived the strategic importance of what the *coureurs* were doing and disregarded instructions to halt them. Frontenac's vision was justified in the next century when war between England and France gave the *coureurs* a new strategic importance. Again and again they led their Indian friends in raids on outlying English settlements in New England and New York. The English protected themselves by an uneasy alliance with the Iroquois. The Iroquois controlled the Mohawk Valley, which, in combination with the Hudson Valley, Lake George, and Lake Champlain, was the only easy invasion route through the mountains that stretched from New England to the Carolinas.

From 1689 to 1713 warfare between England and France was almost continuous, in the War of the League of Augsburg (1689–97) and the War of the Spanish Succession (1702–13), known in the colonies as King William's War and Queen Anne's War. At this time neither France nor England considered America worth the expenditure of royal troops. But the settlers, aware of how much was at stake, carried on their own warfare. The French sent their Indians to raid Schenectady and Deerfield and the thinly populated villages in Maine. The New Englanders in turn captured Port Royal in Nova Scotia in 1690, saw it returned to France at the Peace of Ryswick in 1697, and recaptured it in 1710. The Treaty of Utrecht in 1713, besides recognizing England's claim to Hudson Bay, gave England Nova Scotia with its population of more than a thousand French farmers; it left Cape Breton Island, unpopulated but strategically located at the mouth of the St. Lawrence, to the French.

In the South, where the Appalachian barrier ended, both sides had carried on their warfare largely through Indians. South Carolina fur-traders rivaled the French in their skillful handling of Indian tribes. Ranging as far as the Mississippi in search of deerskins, they gradually gained the allegiance of the Yamasee and of most of the tribes forming the great Creek Confederacy of the Southeast. With Indian assistance they pushed back the Spanish in Florida and threatened the French in Louisiana. Two years after Queen Anne's War ended, however, the Creeks

Major Indian tribes in the East

CAPE BRETON I.

Louisburg ★

ACADIA
(NOVA SCOTIA)

★ Port Royal

● Quebec

Montreal ●

St. Lawrence R.

L. Champlain

L. George ★

Mohawk R.

Deerfield ●

Schenectady ●

L. Ontario

NEW FRANCE

L. Superior

★ IROQUOIS

L. Huron

Marquette and Joliet 1673

La Salle 1681–82

L. Erie

Hudson R.

APPALACHIAN MOUNTAINS

BRITISH COLONIES

ATLANTIC
OCEAN

Wisconsin R.

Fox R.

L. Michigan

Ohio R.

Mississippi R.

Illinois R.

★ Vincennes

Missouri R.

Cahokia ★
Kaskaskia ★

★ French Posts

Arkansas R.

FLORIDA (Spanish)

La Salle

Mobile ●
★

Biloxi ●
★

LOUISIANA

● New Orleans

GULF OF MEXICO

and Yamasee turned and attacked their English allies. But for the loyalty of the Cherokee, South Carolina might have suffered disaster.

After their assault failed, the Creeks moved westward and the Yamasee southward. Spain had always claimed the area they vacated and now threatened to recover it. When England's countermove, the planting of Fort King George on the Altamaha River in 1721, proved ineffective, the English turned to a more familiar method of holding the territory. Forts and missions and Indian diplomacy were a Spanish and French specialty. The English way of occupying America had always been to live in it. English settlers had striven not so much to exploit the Indians as to displace them entirely. And in 1732 the English prepared to move their homes into the area deserted by the Creeks and Yamasee.

The founding of Georgia.

During the quarter-century of peace following the Treaty of Utrecht, the population of the English colonies passed the million mark. The expansion took place east of the mountains, within the bounds of the old colonies. But one new colony, Georgia, was organized in the exposed region of South Carolina.

Like most of the original colonies, Georgia was founded for two purposes, one worldly and realistic, the other altruistic and hopeful. In order to defend its southern flank in America, England needed settlers. At the same time, an English gentleman with military experience and philanthropic motives wanted to do something for the poor. General James Oglethorpe, while serving on a parliamentary committee, had looked into the appalling condition of English debtors and paupers who frequently wound up in jail through no fault of their own.

General Oglethorpe organized other philanthropic gentlemen to seek a charter for a colony in which the unfortunate but deserving poor might rehabilitate themselves. The English government was glad to get people out of trouble at home and into the firing line on the southern frontier of the Carolinas, but it did not propose to let them get out of hand. In 1732 a royal charter gave Oglethorpe and his friends authority as trustees for twenty-one years, after which the colony would revert to the king.

The trustees collected enough capital to get the enterprise off to a strong start. The area had been pictured in English tracts as a paradise compared to which the Garden of Eden was "at most but equal," and settlers eager to pay their own way appeared from Scotland, Germany, and New England as well as from England. The trustees gave them their blessing and rounded up deserving paupers to go with them. In Georgia, Oglethorpe himself saw that each immigrant got fifty acres of land (those who paid their own way might get up to five hundred acres), tools to work it with, and enough supplies for the first year.

The trustees did their best to bar sin and temptation from the new paradise. To keep the rehabilitated colonist sober they forbade rum. To keep him industrious they forbade slavery. To ensure his livelihood they forbade land sales without their permission. But the zeal was only on the part of the trustees. Georgia proved, after all, to be somewhat less attractive than paradise, and the Georgians thought they deserved at least the compensation of sinning like other men. In 1751 the trustees conceded defeat, allowed slavery and rum, and in 1752, a year before their charter expired, turned their fallen colony over to the king. Thereafter it began to fill up with Americans from other colonies, especially South Carolinians, who were more interested in raising rice than in redeeming paupers.

The trustees had been scarcely more successful in attaining the colony's military objectives. Although Oglethorpe conducted an expedition against Spanish Florida during the War of Jenkins' Ear between England and Spain (1739–42), his troops came mostly from England and South Carolina and accomplished nothing. Georgia never became a military stronghold.

Fortunately, when the European conflict broadened into the War of the Austrian Succession (1740–48), known in the colonies as King George's War, the action shifted to the Northern colonies. There, New Englanders got up an expedition under William Pepperell, a merchant from Maine, to attack the French fortress of Louisburg on Cape Breton Island. The colonists' capture of Louisburg was England's only real success on any front during the war. Although the Treaty of Aix-la-Chapelle (1748) restored the status quo and thus gave Louisburg back to France, its capture had focused the attention of both countries on the increasing strength and importance of England's American subjects.

They were a million-and-a-half now, and the majority of them had never seen the shores of Great Britain. Though Britain directed their trade and supervised their government, though they took pride in being British subjects, they had also become Americans. And as Americans they had begun to have their own ideas about a number of things, ideas that set them apart from their brethren in England on the one hand and from their French and Spanish rivals in North America on the other.

Suggestions for Reading   Eli Heckscher in *Mercantilism*, 2 vols. (1935), sets the economic policies of the seventeenth and eighteenth centuries in historical perspective and thus furnishes the best introduction to an understanding of the Navigation Acts. For the acts themselves and the thinking behind them, the pioneering works of G. L. Beer are still valuable: *The Origins of the British Colonial System* (1908) and *The Old Colonial System*, 2 vols. (1912). On the administration and interpretation of the acts, see L. A. Harper,

The English Navigation Laws (1939), C. M. Andrews, *The Colonial Period of American History*, Vol. IV* (1938), and T. C. Barrow, *Trade and Empire* (1967). Special aspects of British policy are well treated in Curtis Nettels, *The Money Supply of the American Colonies Before 1720* (1934), L. V. Brock, *The Currency of the American Colonies, 1700–1764* (1975), and A. C. Bining, *British Regulation of the Colonial Iron Industry* (1933). A. G. Olson, *Anglo-American Politics, 1660–1775* (1973), traces the effect of party politics on colonial administration. In *The Governors-General* (1979) Stephen S. Webb argues vigorously but not always convincingly that military rather than commercial considerations dominated England's colonial policy in the seventeenth century. J. M. Sosin, *English America and the Restoration Monarchy of Charles II* (1980) and *English America and the Revolution of 1688* (1982), stresses the local difficulties encountered by England in bringing her widely diverse colonies within an imperial administration.

On New Netherland and on the Restoration colonies a good general account is again C. M. Andrews, *The Colonial Period of American History*, Vols. II and III*. W. F. Craven, *The Colonies in Transition, 1660–1713** (1968), incorporates more recent research. J. E. Pomfret, *Colonial New Jersey: A History* (1973), has untangled much of New Jersey's early history. For the Carolinas see Verner Crane, *The Southern Frontier, 1670–1732* (1929), M. E. Sirmans, *Colonial South Carolina* (1966), and C. L. Ver Steeg, *Origins of a Southern Mosaic* (1975).

There is no definitive biography of William Penn, but C. O. Peare, *William Penn* (1956), and H. E. Wildes, *William Penn* (1974), are adequate. M. M. Dunn has made a scholarly study of his activities in *William Penn: Politics and Conscience* (1967), and M. B. Endy of his religious ideas in *William Penn and Early Quakerism* (1973). J. E. Illick, *William Penn the Politician* (1965), treats his relations with the English government. Rufus Jones, *Quakers in the American Colonies** (1911), is a standard work, but see also F. B. Tolles' eloquent essays in *Quakers and the Atlantic Culture* (1960). The early history of Pennsylvania is treated in F. B. Tolles, *James Logan and the Culture of Provincial America* (1957), G. B. Nash, *Quakers and Politics: Pennsylvania, 1681–1726* (1968), and Alan Tully, *William Penn's Legacy* (1977).

Efforts of England to enforce the Navigation Acts are dealt with in Michael Hall, *Edward Randolph and the American Colonies, 1676–1703** (1960). Viola Barnes, *The Dominion of New England: A Study in British Colony Policy* (1923), is the classic account of that episode, exonerating Andros of blame. Richard R. Johnson, *Adjustment to Empire* (1981), treats the Dominion in the context of long-range developments in both old and New England. The long-range causes and consequences of Leisler's Rebellion are discussed in Robert C. Ritchie, *The Duke's Province: A Study of New York Politics and Society, 1664–1691* (1977), and in L. H. Leder, *Robert Livingston and the Politics of Colonial New York, 1654–1728* (1961). A good general study of the colony is Michael Kammen, *Colonial New York: A History** (1975). David S. Lovejoy, *The Glorious Revolution in America** (1972), is the best overall view of that subject.

On the reorganization of colonial administration in 1696, see again C. M. Andrews, *The Colonial Period of American History*, Vol. IV*, and I. K. Steele, *Politics of Colonial Policy: The Board of Trade in Colonial Administration, 1696–1720* (1968). The standard works on the Board of Trade are O. M. Dickerson, *American Colonial Government, 1696–1765* (1912), and A. H. Basye, *The Lords Commissioners of Trade and Plantations, 1748–1782* (1925). On the activities of the board in securing the disallowance of colonial acts of legislation, see E. B. Russell, *The Review of American Colonial Legislation by the King in Council* (1915). The role of colonial governors in administering British policy is the subject of L. W. Labaree, *Royal Government in America: A Study of the British Colonial System Before 1783* (1930). Finally, Lawrence Gipson, in fifteen volumes, surveys *The British Empire Before the American Revolution* (1936–1970).

*Available in a paperback edition.

3

THE FIRST AMERICAN WAY OF LIFE

Americans moving across their continent have faced three questions again and again: how to live, how to live with one another, how to live with the outside world. They first learned how to live by tobacco, rice, furs, and fish. England told them, in the Navigation Acts, how they must live with the outside world. How did they live with one another?

A few simply did not. When the Puritans explored Boston harbor, they came upon an Englishman at Beacon Hill living alone among the blueberries. William Blackstone was company enough for himself. After the Puritans moved in, he moved out. For nearly three centuries the continent afforded room for men like Blackstone, American hermits who felt crowded when they could see the smoke from their neighbor's campfire.

Patterns of Existence

Most Americans have been more gregarious. They have asked *how*, rather than whether, to live together, and they have answered partly from the heritage of ideas and institutions carried from Europe, partly from their own ideas evoked by the opportunities and limitations of their strange new environment. Each generation has solved the problem a little differently from the preceding one, but the first settlers, moving from an old established world to an empty new one,

had the biggest problem and made the biggest change. Many of them came to America primarily for a chance to live together in a new and, they hoped, a better way. All of them had to adapt ideas made in Europe to existence in America. The results differed from time to time and from place to place. But before the end of the colonial period most Americans were living together in one of four distinct patterns: the Southern plantation, the New England town, the loose collection of individual farms, or the coastal city.

The plantation. Plantations developed in colonies where the majority of people lived by growing a single crop for export: tobacco in Virginia and Maryland, rice or indigo in South Carolina, sugar in the West Indies. Originally "planter" meant simply a settler, and "plantation" a settlement—Jamestown was the London Company's plantation. Gradually the term "plantation" came to be attached to individual holdings and then to holdings where substantial numbers of people worked for the owner. Gradually too the term came to imply that the workers were slaves, the property of the person for whom they worked.

The plantation manned by slaves originated in the West Indies, but within the present United States it developed first in Virginia. It was the most novel way of living that colonial Americans devised for themselves. It was also the most productive, if we may judge by the exports of the thirteen colonies. And it was the most violent and oppressive, a way of living

Pennsylvania farm, 1757

Mulberry Plantation

that required the continuous coercion of unwilling and unrewarded labor. In order to understand the role it played in American life, we shall have to look into its beginnings.

The first steps were taken during Virginia's tobacco boom of the 1620s, when everyone was scrambling for labor. A number of successful Virginians at this time were able to gather crews of ten, twenty, even thirty-odd men to grow tobacco for them. The men were mostly Englishmen who had agreed to serve for up to seven years in return for passage across the ocean to the new land of opportunity. They themselves constituted an opportunity for the planters who bought them, sold them, traded them, and even won or lost them in card games. The planters would buy the labor of any man delivered to them, and Dutch traders delivered a few from Africa bound to serve for a lifetime. But the plantation labor force remained overwhelmingly English for many years, because you could buy an Englishman for seven years cheaper than you could buy an African for life; and in early Virginia seven years was more than most immigrants, black or white, were likely to live.

The death rate was comparable to that reached in England during years of the plague. The cause is not clear. Probably it was a combination of malnutrition with malaria and typhoid fever. Between 1625 and 1640 some fifteen thousand immigrants increased the population of the colony from around thirteen hundred to only seven or eight thousand. Most of them arrived as servants, and most of them were male. Since women were not used for fieldwork, the planters needed few of them. One woman would cook and wash for a sizable crew of men.

In spite of the colony's heavy death rate, servants were cheap enough to be worth importing even after the price of tobacco dropped to around 20 shillings a hundred pounds (2.4 pence per pound) in the 1640s and 1650s. By then the Virginians' increasing skill with the crop enabled a man to grow from one to two thousand pounds of tobacco a year, together with enough corn to feed himself. At that rate his output was still worth between £10 and £20—while he lived. And beginning somewhere around the middle of the century people in Virginia evidently started living longer. The population rose to about fifteen thousand by 1653 and about twenty-five thousand by 1660.

As more and more men lived to complete their term of servitude, the added years of labor meant added profits to their masters (who could thus acquire still more servants to operate still larger plantations). And the ex-servants ("freedmen") could at long last begin to enjoy the opportunities they had been helping to bring to others. They could start small plantations, grow tobacco for export, and import servants of their own.

For a number of reasons the opportunities diminished sharply after 1660. The increase in population brought an increase in the labor force and a consequent increase in the production of tobacco. Since the rise in production was accompanied by passage of the Navigation Act of 1660, restricting the market for Virginia and Maryland tobacco, the price fell to a penny a pound and sometimes less. At the same time the cost of production went up, especially for beginners, because land was more in demand and hence more valuable. Farsighted planters began acquiring huge tracts and by the 1670s had engrossed most of the best land in the tidewater, the area cut by great rivers and bays along which ocean-going ships could collect tobacco as much as a hundred miles inland. A new freedman looking for a place to plant either had to rent from the big owners or else settle for a location in the interior, cut off from river transportation, or far up one of the rivers, where he would be exposed to Indian attack.

As a result Virginia and Maryland (where the same conditions prevailed) acquired a growing class of indigent freedmen. They wandered from county to county, living from hand to mouth, dodging the tax collector, renting a bit of land here, squatting there, sometimes working for wages, sometimes trying to live from the land, hunting, stealing hogs, and enticing servants to run away with them. They were mostly young, because planters imported young servants; they were mostly single, because planters imported far more men than women; and they were mostly armed, because guns were a necessity of life in Virginia and Maryland, where dwellings were widely separated and a man had to be ready to shoot it out if attacked by Indians.

The established planters became increasingly uneasy about the band of wild bachelors in their midst. William Berkeley, who had been governor of the colony from 1641 to 1652 and became governor again in 1660, clearly saw danger ahead. When the Dutch made war against England and raided the James River in 1673, Berkeley led the militia against them with considerable trepidation, for he estimated that a large percentage of the men at his back were poverty-stricken freedmen, who "upon any small advantage the Enemy may gaine upon us, would revolt to them in hopes of bettering their condition by Shareing the Plunder of the Country with them."

Berkeley's fears were justified. Three years later, sparked by an Indian attack on the frontiers, a band of self-appointed Indian-fighters turned from an unsuccessful pursuit of the elusive enemy to attack their much less elusive rulers. Led by Nathaniel Bacon, a well-to-do sympathizer, the freedmen of the frontier found ready allies in nearly every part of the colony. In the largest popular uprising before the American Revolution they burned the capital settlement at Jamestown and drove the governor and his friends in flight to the Eastern Shore, the only loyal stronghold in the colony. Before it was over, the rebellion had swept up servants as well as freedmen in plundering forays against everyone who offered resistance.

Then, after they had redistributed as much of the wealth as they could lay their hands on, the rebels gave up as quickly as they had risen. Their leader, Bacon, had died of a fever; and he left them with no long-range solution to the problems that faced them, no revolutionary program, not even any revolutionary slogans. Old Governor Berkeley exacted a savage revenge by hanging the remaining leaders, though the king had sent a general pardon. For the rest of the century Virginians continued to eye one another uneasily, alert for new Bacons in their midst. Though the rebellion had subsided, its causes had not. Servants were still arriving every year to man the plantations; they were still becoming free every year in large numbers; and they still could not afford the land on which to sustain their freedom. They had crossed the ocean to a wilderness and sold away several years of their lives only to face the prospect of working out the remainder on another man's plantation. Their continuing discontent posed a real and present danger to the established planters.

The tidewater and the piedmont

It was under these circumstances that the traders who had been supplying the West Indies with slaves began delivering them in larger numbers to the tobacco colonies. A slave cost only about twice as much as a servant, around £20 instead of £10 at the close of the seventeenth century. With the decline in Virginia's death rate, slaves became a more profitable investment than servants, and for that reason alone the planters bought all the traders could bring. But the unsought social benefits to Virginia's big planters were larger than the economic benefits. Although every planter worried about taking into his household men and women who had good reason to hate him, slaves proved to be less dangerous than servants who had become free. No slave rebellion in American history ever approached the success of Bacon's Rebellion.

Slaves remained permanently under the control of their masters. They could safely be denied rights that the English, servant or free, could legally demand. They could be subjected to harsh punishments without recourse to the courts. They could be kept unarmed, unorganized, helpless to resist. And the fact that they happened to be black announced their probable status and made escape difficult.

By importing permanent black slaves instead of temporary white servants for their plantations, Virginians ceased to add to the band of indigent freedmen, which gradually diminished. As the competition for land stopped escalating and the interior became safer for settlement, a man could once again get a foothold on the ladder that led up in the world. Slavery enabled the planters to go on growing ever larger crops without, on the one hand, creating a dangerous class of poor and discontented freedmen or, on the other hand, reducing those freedmen to some new sort of bondage that would shackle their discontent. Bondage was reserved for blacks, who accounted for most of the tobacco and rice produced in the colonies by the middle of the eighteenth century.

The English recognized slavery as the ultimate degradation to which human beings could be subjected, but they showed surprisingly little hesitation in imposing that degradation on peoples of darker complexion than their own. Though slavery had no place in English law, English colonists from the beginning had enslaved Indians who made unsuccessful war on them. The theory was that the lives of captives taken in just wars belonged to the captors; but history records no war acknowledged by the victors to have been unjust, and the English had not been in the habit of enslaving prisoners taken in their European wars. Making slaves of Indians and later of Africans (allegedly purchased from the victors in righteous tribal wars) was somehow different from making slaves of, say, the French or the Germans.

The difference, of course, was race. Although not all blacks were slaves—from the beginning a substantial minority even in the plantation colonies were free—all slaves were either blacks or Indians. Slavery became the dominant form of relationship between whites and other races and was recognized by law in every colony. North of Maryland race relations concerned relatively few people; from Maryland south they concerned most people. Though the plantation had begun with a free or semifree white labor force, it became in the eighteenth century the meeting place of black and white, the primary community in which free and enslaved Americans lived together.

Although the Southern plantation resembled similar establishments in the West Indies and South America, it had distinctive features that were to affect the way Americans of different races lived together after slavery ended. Of first importance was the fact that Southern slave owners, especially in the tobacco

The rights of Africans and Indians: Virginia, 1705

From W. W. Hening, *The Statutes at Large; Being a Collection of All the Laws of Virginia*, 1823.

colonies, did not make a policy of working their slaves to death. Whether because tobacco required less strenuous labor than sugar, or for other reasons, a slave on a Southern plantation had a longer and less arduous life than a slave on a sugar plantation in the West Indies, where planters counted on replacing a percentage of their worn-out and dying labor force annually by new purchases. The slave women of the West Indies could not or would not raise enough children to match the awful death rate. In the American South, while the planters continued to import

A slave ship

slaves throughout the colonial period, the numbers also increased naturally. Though black women, as in the West Indies, worked beside their men in the fields, they were able at the same time to raise children. Southern slaves could thus enjoy some semblance of family life.

The children, like their mothers and fathers, were the property of the master, and he could break up a family by selling any one of them. But so long as they were together slave families could in some measure—at night, on Sundays, and usually on Saturday afternoons—live lives of their own. The planters' policy of doling out the meagerest of rations and obliging the slaves to grow what more they wanted in plots adjoining their cabins even encouraged a close family relationship as father, mother, and children worked together, for themselves, in their own garden. In the rice plantations of Carolina slaves gained a further measure of independence through the task system. In this system slaves were assigned a certain amount of work per day, whether of hoeing, ditching, or harvesting, after which they were free to work for themselves.

As more and more slaves were native-born, speaking a common language (albeit the language of their masters), their ability to resist exploitation grew. Although concerted rebellion among them was uncommon and readily suppressed, slaves could often run away for substantial lengths of time, sheltering in the woods, and thus deprive the master of their services. As a result, a master might find that treating his slaves humanely was more productive than employing the severity that the law allowed.

Under these circumstances slaves on Southern plantations raised nearly as many children as free Southerners did. And while the colonies that later formed the United States received only 4½ percent of all the slaves imported into the New World, the de-

A community in itself: a tidewater plantation

scendants of that 4½ percent today constitute over 30 percent of the New World's inhabitants with African ancestry. The slave family was not responsible for all of them: the different shades of color among the children in the slave quarters testified to the fact that black women were not reserved for black men. But miscegenation was probably less than in other slave societies and racial prejudice was correspondingly stronger.

On the other hand the estrangement of black and white was in some measure limited by the circumscribed environment in which they coexisted. Since the largest effective unit of tobacco production was a thousand acres (including uncleared and exhausted land), few tobacco plantations had as many as a hundred slaves. A smaller area, with no more than thirty slaves, was the most efficient unit for rice.

The plantation often constituted a small community in itself. At the center lay a great house, normally facing a navigable river, and surrounded by trees and shrubs. Arranged symmetrically around it were attendant buildings: laundry, smokehouse, kitchen, and perhaps a schoolhouse, where a hired tutor taught the planter's children—or at least his free children. At some distance lay the barns and the cabins of the slaves.

In addition to field hands, the community included a small army of household slaves and skilled artisans—carpenter, blacksmith, tailor, cobbler—who might be either indentured white servants (bound by a contract to serve a specific number of years) or slaves educated for the purpose. With its own permanent labor force and with ready access to ocean-going ships, the riverside plantation needed little from its neighbors. What could not be made on the premises was imported directly from London.

And yet the planter and his family were not isolated. The river was a highway to the world by which he kept in touch not only with London but with other planters. His children often went to stay for several weeks at other plantations, and his own home was seldom without guests. Sometimes he gave a ball for friends who came from miles around and stayed for three or four days. Or he might attend the representative assembly in Williamsburg or Charles Town and take the family with him.

In the assembly and in the local county court the planter directed the lives of his lesser neighbors, the small farmers who made up the majority of the population even in the plantation colonies. They worked for themselves, but he dominated the society, buying and selling their surplus crops, sometimes renting them their lands, lending them money, selling them manufactures, and perhaps commanding their votes.

His command of their votes was by no means automatic, however. The deference his neighbors paid him was the voluntary tribute that success has generally exacted in a free society. It took the votes of free men to place him in the representative assembly, and votes were withheld often enough to remind him that he represented free men.

By officiating in the assembly, the county court, and the vestry of his church, and by managing his plantation, the planter learned to deal with men both free and unfree. And the ships that arrived at his wharf brought him regular news of the way men were dealing with one another across the water. In their writings he learned that they thought slavery the worst fate that could befall a people. From a closer knowledge than theirs he could agree; and he would, as the years passed, increasingly value and protect his own freedom.

The New England town.   Rivers, tobacco, and slavery made the plantation. Puritanism and past experience made the New England town, an institution that also appeared in the parts of New York and New Jersey settled by New Englanders. The past experience of New Englanders (as of other English colonists) included at least three English types of community: the borough, the village, and the parish.

The English borough was a town that normally possessed a charter of incorporation from the king entitling it to send two members to Parliament and to exercise a degree of local governmental independence. The freemen (or burgesses) of the borough, usually a very small proportion of the population, elected its members of Parliament as well as a mayor or a set of aldermen to handle local affairs. In many boroughs the aldermen had become so powerful that they were bypassing the freemen and were filling vacancies in their ranks by themselves.

The English village was not a formal political institution like the borough. It was simply a cluster of houses inhabited by people who cultivated the surrounding lands according to customs prescribed by earlier generations. All the village's arable land was laid out in three or four large fields, and every householder had strips of land scattered through all of them. No strips were fenced off from those adjoining; and everyone worked together at plowing (and subsequently at sowing, tilling, and harvesting) one field before moving on to the next. Thus everyone would get part of the crop early, part of it late. By the time the settlers left England, this open-field system was giving way to individual farms, but it still existed in many places.

Every Englishman, whether living in a borough or a village, belonged to a parish. Originally the parish was simply the area served by a single church, but it had gradually taken on, outside the boroughs, many of the functions of local government. In most villages a vestry made up of some ten or twenty of the more substantial inhabitants exercised the powers of the parish or chose two or three churchwardens to do so. The churchwardens or vestrymen not only maintained the church and managed its property but provided for the poor, required fathers to support their children, levied taxes, and sometimes acted as a kind of grand jury.

In creating their towns New Englanders drew something from the parish, the village, and the borough; but they also rejected parts of this institutional heritage because of their Puritan ideas about how people ought to live with one another. Puritans generally "gathered" a church before, or about the same time as, they established a town. The two usually covered the same territory, as was true of the English village and parish. But in New England the church and its officers were entirely distinct from the town and its officers. The church owned no property, not even a church building. People worshiped in a meetinghouse, which was owned by the town and used for any community meeting. It was not regarded as sacred. Nor did the church exercise any temporal, political powers. There was no vestry and no churchwarden. The church might elect ruling elders to reprimand erring members or to report them to the church, but neither elders nor church enjoyed coercive authority. The church was a spiritual association; its severest penalty was excommunication, which could be pronounced only by unanimous vote of the members. Excommunication deprived a person of church membership but carried no civil or political disabilities. Once a church assumed temporal powers, Puritans believed, it was on the wicked road to Rome. In New England, therefore, they assigned to the town both the duties of local government, performed in the English borough by the mayor and aldermen, and the secular duties exercised in the English parish by church officers.

New England towns and their governments were created under the authority of the colony's General Court (the legislature). A group of men, perhaps already gathered in a church, approached the court and requested a tract of land, usually adjoining some established town. If the court approved, it had the area surveyed and then incorporated the applicants as proprietors of the town of Concord, Sudbury, or whatever name they chose. The proprietors then moved to their new home and laid out the land in a pattern similar to that of an English village. Every man got a house lot in the center of town, where space was also set aside for a meetinghouse, a village green, and perhaps a school. Each man also received one or more parcels of arable land, a parcel of meadow for pasturage, and a parcel of woodland for fuel, all located in different parts of the town. In a few cases there seems to have been an attempt (quickly abandoned) to practice the open-field system. When the land of a town was originally apportioned, most of it was left undivided to meet the anticipated growth in population. The undistributed land, or commons, belonged to the proprietors jointly until they converted it into their private property through subsequent land divisions. A new settler moving into town might buy land from a proprietor's private holdings or might be granted or sold parts of the commons, but he did not necessarily become a proprietor with a share in the ownership of the remaining commons.

The power of the proprietors was limited to control over the commons; government of the town rested in a town meeting, in which they had no greater voice than other inhabitants. The town meeting acted on matters that intimately concerned the inhabitants: repairing roads, building a meetinghouse, hiring a schoolmaster, or deciding whether hogs should be fenced into pens or fenced out of gardens. The meeting also elected representatives to the colonial assembly and town officials of all kinds, including selectmen, who administered the rules made by the meeting. There was some attempt in early Massachusetts to confine voting in town meetings to the freemen, who it will be remembered had to be church members. After 1648, however, and probably before then in many towns, other free adult males, if approved by the freemen, were allowed to vote on all questions except the choice of representatives. Until 1685, representatives continued to be elected only by the freemen.

In the early years of a town's existence there was no conflict of interest between town meeting and proprietors, because all or most of the free adult males were also proprietors. And the inhabitants frequently felt a strong sense of duty to the community, a sense carried over from the religious purposes that guided the settlement. They sought to sustain their brotherhood in the political as well as the spiritual world by talking out any disputes that arose among them and by keeping out any newcomers who appeared likely to disturb their solidarity.

By the opening of the eighteenth century, with the passing of the founders, the waning of the high resolve that had moved them, and the dwindling away of the common lands, the towns began to take on a different character. Fathers could not or would not give their sons the amount of land they needed, and the young began to go west in search of greener pastures. Latecomers quarreled with the proprietors over the remaining common lands. Religious dissent appeared in forms that could not be talked down.

At the same time new towns were being formed by men without the spirit that had moved the first generation. Colonial governments, instead of granting townships gratis to groups of settlers, auctioned them off to groups assembled simply for the purpose of investing in real estate. These proprietors were sometimes not even residents of the towns they founded, and they sold land to settlers with more attention to private profit than to establishing a successful community. The settlers themselves were also less devoted to the community. Instead of living close to the meetinghouse and having their landholdings scattered about the countryside, they scattered their houses and tried to consolidate their land in one piece around the house.

Nevertheless, the New England town remained in the eighteenth century, if not as closely knit as in the seventeenth, remarkably homogeneous and neighborly. People still rubbed elbows often and tried to work out their differences peaceably. On Sunday everyone gathered in the meetinghouse, where the position of a man's pew indicated his place in the community and whether he must be addressed as "Mister," as "Goodman," or by no title at all. In general, the closer he sat to the pulpit, the higher his social rank. But proximity to God's minister was no sign of proximity to God. Though the law required that everyone attend church, only a minority of the town's inhabitants were "members," and membership in itself carried no social prestige. A slave might belong and a gentleman not. During the eighteenth century church membership became increasingly feminine, with women outnumbering men by more than two to one. But members or not, New Englanders went to church, were taxed for the minister's salary, and had a voice in selecting him.

The men of the town met not only at church and town meeting but on training day when the militia exercised. In frontier settlements, under constant threat of Indian attack, this was a serious business; in the older coastal towns it was likely to require more rum than gunpowder. Rum and hard cider lubricated most community activities in New England, whether marrying or burying, raising a meetinghouse or bringing home a harvest. The tavern, originally intended for the convenience of travelers, became another meeting place where men of the neighborhood lifted a glass of an evening and where, according to John Adams, "vicious habits, bastards, and legislators" were frequently begotten.

In tavern, school, and church, at town meeting and militia drill, the New Englander measured out the distance between himself and his fellow men. The distance was small, but it was enough to give him an independence of spirit for which he became famous. For those who needed more room, America offered another way of life.

The farm. In the colonies from New England southward, most Americans lived lonely lives. Men made a living from the land, as their fathers had done in Europe. But in the great emptiness of the New World, sheer space separated families from their neighbors in a way that few Europeans knew. A farm might lie miles from any other occupied land, because settlers chose lands, not for neighborliness, but for water supply, for the evenness of the ground, and above all for fertility (frequently indicated by a stand of hardwood).

The size of an American farm also tended to isolate the farmer. Because of the way he used the land, he needed a large tract. It was common practice to clear a plot, crop it for several years until its fertility was exhausted, and then clear another, allowing the first to lie fallow for five, ten, even twenty or thirty years. Clearing often meant no more than girdling the trees at the base to kill them, planting crops between the lifeless trunks, and then disposing of the trunks as they rotted away. By that time, however, the plot might be ready to abandon anyhow. It would gradually recover its fertility (and perhaps its forest) and could be cleared again in the same way.

To European visitors the practice seemed slovenly and shiftless, but it was actually the way to get the maximum in crops for the minimum of labor. It is still common practice wherever land is abundant and people scarce. The first settlers in most colonies probably learned it from the Indians, though a small group of Finnish settlers on the Delaware River may already have been familiar with it (they also introduced the technique of building log cabins, perhaps the easiest way to turn trees into houses). But however effective this kind of farming may have been, it did mean that a farm had to be large, with much of the land under forest or scrub most of the time.

Though most farmers owned the land they lived on, farm tenancy became common in some areas where the soil was fertile enough to support both a landlord and a tenant. In New York's Hudson Valley, for example, some landlords exacted high rents and feudal services. In Virginia's tidewater, tenants took farms and even plantations as sharecroppers, paying the owner a proportion of the crop as rent. Even in the uncleared back country it was not always easy for a farmer to obtain title to land in the most fertile areas, because speculators often acquired such lands in advance of actual settlers. By the eighteenth century the headright system (practiced earlier in most of the colonies south of New England) had become a mere form. Speculators could obtain title to as much land as they could afford simply by paying a fee (usually 5 shillings per hundred acres) to the colony's secretary or land office. Later they could rent the land to a bona fide settler or else sell it for a good deal more than the original price. Not all speculators were rich. Many farmers, tradesmen, and even parsons invested their small earnings in real estate, for everyone knew that land values would rise as population increased, and everyone could see that population was increasing rapidly.

In New England most of the increase came from natural growth of the old stock who, unlike the early Virginia immigrants, arrived primarily in family groups and began multiplying at once. Also unlike Virginians, New Englanders seem to have lived ten or twenty years longer than their contemporaries in England; and they had far more children. Although women married at a later age than is usually supposed (probably at an average of about twenty-three in the seventeenth century and around twenty-one in the eighteenth), they commonly had five or six children. In spite of the heavy toll taken by smallpox, diphtheria, scarlet fever, and childbirth, the population kept growing at rates unheard of in the Old World. In the Southern colonies a shortage of women and a very heavy death rate held down the natural increase during most of the seventeenth century; but the importation of servants, and later of slaves, kept the population growing rapidly nevertheless. After the sex ratio evened out and the mortality rate diminished, natural increase joined with heavy immigration to send the population soaring in the eighteenth century.

The largest ethnic group of immigrants in the eighteenth century came involuntarily from Africa to man the plantations of Virginia, Maryland, and South Carolina. But the Middle colonies, especially Pennsylvania, welcomed a flood of voluntary immigrants, mainly from northern Ireland and Germany, most of whom became independent farmers. After landing in the New World, usually at Philadelphia, they traveled west to the Appalachian valleys and spilled down into the hinterland of Maryland, Virginia, and the Carolinas.

At crossroads in the farming areas, storekeepers traded hardware, clothing, and gossip for crops. But there was no real community, no local nucleus of political, social, and religious life. Even the churches responded slowly to the needs of the farmer. In colonies where the Anglican Church was supported by taxation (New York, Maryland, Virginia, and the Carolinas) it organized parishes to keep pace with the westward advance, but they were too large in area to serve the widely scattered farmers, many of whom were not Anglicans anyhow. The parish had been designed for more densely populated areas, where enough people to support a minister lived within Sunday traveling distance of his sermons. By the middle of the eighteenth century some denominations, especially Baptists, Presbyterians and Methodists, were sending itinerant missionaries through the back country. The circuit-riders, as the missionaries were called, often encountered families whose children had never seen a minister.

In the absence of village or town, colonial farmers relied heavily on a looser and larger community, the county. Every colony was divided into counties, and everywhere the county court was an important arm of government. Even in New England the county judges (appointed as elsewhere by the colonial governments) decided administrative as well as judicial questions, questions as important as where to build new roads. Outside New England, the county court took over the

duties of the town and sometimes of the parish. Besides trying cases, both civil and criminal, it might record wills and deeds, take charge of orphans and the poor, register births, marriages, and deaths, collect taxes, license taverns, authorize the establishment of ferries, and pay bounties for wolves' heads. On days when the court was in session, usually once a month, farmers from near and far would gather to sue one another for small sums, to exercise in the militia, to elect a representative to the colony's assembly, or simply to watch the proceedings, learn the news, and share talk and a bottle with distant neighbors.

The thinness of community life put a heavy burden on the family. Everywhere during the colonial period the family fulfilled many more functions than it does today, but among farmers it was everything—factory, church, school, hospital, and tavern. Unless a man held especially rich land and had ready access to a market, his crops went to feed his family, with little left over for sale. He and his wife had to make everything they could not buy, which might be most of their clothing and furniture. Without a school, they had to teach their children to read; without a church, to worship at home; without a tavern, to entertain passing strangers; without a doctor, to care for their sick. Children were plentiful and made more hands to do the endless work. Some might take over the farm as their parents grew old, but most of them would eventually leave to carve new farms out of the empty land. The family with three generations under one roof was exceptional everywhere in America, as it was in England.

The farmer, isolated from his neighbors and living a self-sufficient life within his own family, was the typical eighteenth-century American—even the townsman of western New England resembled him. But as farmers spread out through the interior a significant minority of Americans piled up in five cities and several large towns along the coast.

The city. The colonial farmer riding into a city for the first time left a road that was only a ribbon of stumps and mud and came upon streets of gravel or cobblestones, where a bewildering activity surrounded him. Swine roamed everywhere, feeding on the refuse; drovers herded sheep and cattle to the butchers. Elegant carriages rolled impatiently behind lumbering wagons as great packs of barking dogs worried the horses. Sailors reeled out of taverns, and over the roofs of the houses could be seen the swaying masts and spars of their ships. The farmer had been told that the city was a nursery of vice and prodigality. He now saw that it was so. Every shop had wares to catch his eye: exquisite fabrics, delicate chinaware, silver buckles, looking glasses, and other imported luxuries that never reached the crossroads store. Putting up at the tavern, he found himself drinking too much rum. And there were willing girls, he heard, who had lost their virtue and would be glad to help him lose his. Usually he returned to the farm to warn his children as he had been warned. He seldom understood that the vice of the city, if not its prodigality, was mainly for transients like himself. Permanent residents had work to do.

The key men in the community were the merchants, for colonial cities were built on trade. Merchants bought corn, wheat, cattle, and horses from thousands of farms and fish from hundreds of fishermen and shipped them to the West Indies. The planters there could not waste their valuable sugar lands growing corn, but they needed food for their slaves and horses to turn their sugar mills. Colonial merchants supplied them and brought back molasses, a by-product of sugar-making. Distilleries turned it into rum, which became a standard item in the diet of soldiers and sailors and men who toiled at heavy labor out of doors. Some rum went to the coasts of Africa in exchange for slaves (though, contrary to popular impression, few colonial merchants were heavily involved in the slave trade). The merchants also bought beaver and deerskins from Indian traders and huge pine trunks from lumbermen to send to England for masts. From England they brought back woolens and hardware, which the mother country made better and cheaper than the colonists could. Without the merchants there would have been no cities.

Many of the other city-dwellers depended on the merchants for a living. Besides the rum-distillers, there were shipwrights who turned out ships at a lower price than English ones. Workers in ropewalks and sail lofts rigged them. Instrument-makers fitted them with quadrants, telescopes, and clocks. Retail traders helped to distribute the goods imported from abroad. Millers ground wheat and corn into flour, and coopers built barrels to ship it in.

But cities accumulate people by a magic of their own, and many colonists found jobs that had no direct connection with the overseas trade. Schoolmasters were better trained and more plentiful than in the country. Dancing masters taught ladies and gentlemen the newest steps; stay-makers laced them into the newest shapes. Barbers cut their hair; wig-makers put it on again. And dozens of skilled craftsmen offered American-made copies of the latest English fashions in wearing apparel, furniture, and houses.

For all the glamour and excitement of their environment, city-dwellers had problems that other Americans had not yet faced: city opulence bred thieves and vice of all kinds; city filth necessitated sewers and sanitation laws; city traffic required paved streets and lights; and the city's closely packed wooden houses and shops invited fires that might, and repeatedly did, destroy vast areas. City-dwellers also came face-to-face, more often than other Americans, with poverty. So many of the jobs in a city depended on the prosperity of overseas trade that when trade was bad jobs disappeared, and the men and women who lived by them had no place to turn.

Boston, circa 1725

Baltimore in 1752, just beginning to grow

As cities grew, so did the numbers of the poor and unemployed who had to be cared for. In Boston, where the problem was most acute, a measure of the misery that city life could bring may be seen in the fact that the annual cost of caring for the poor rose from less than £200 sterling at the beginning of the eighteenth century to nearly £2,500 by the 1770s, though the total population increased only from 8,000 to 16,000.

To cope with their manifold problems, citizens relied both on voluntary associations, such as fire companies, and on their city governments. Boston and Newport were governed by selectmen and town meetings, New York (after 1731) by a popularly elected city corporation. In all three, city officials, under direct control of the citizens, were responsive to their needs. In Philadelphia and Charles Town, on the other hand, the citizens had no voice in their local government. Philadelphia was badly governed by a self-perpetuating closed corporation, and Charles Town just as badly by the South Carolina assembly.

By contemporary standards these were all substantial cities. Though small compared with London, by the middle of the eighteenth century they were larger than most English cities. Boston, which reached seventeen thousand in 1740, was at that time the largest, but it had already begun a decline that lasted for the rest of the colonial period. In the seventeenth century it had served as the shipping center for most of the mainland colonies, and it continued to serve as New England's major port. But other New England towns were cutting into its business, most notably Newport, which grew to urban dimensions in the eighteenth century.

New York City was the natural outlet and supply point for farmers in the Hudson Valley and adjoining regions of Connecticut and New Jersey; Philadelphia served not only Pennsylvania and the Delaware Valley and Bay but also the Southern back country. From the Carolinas, Virginia, and Maryland, farmers drove their wagons and cattle north along the great Appa-lachian valleys to the Philadelphia market. Although Baltimore began to drain off some of this trade after about 1750, Philadelphia continued to grow so rapidly that by the 1770s, with twenty-eight thousand people, it was one of the larger cities in the English-speaking world. South of Baltimore the tobacco-planters dealt directly with London and needed no cities; but in the 1760s and 1770s many planters and farmers were turning to wheat. They sold it to grain merchants in towns that sprang up along the coast and at crossroads in the back country. As a result, Norfolk, Virginia, for example, doubled in size, from 3,000 to 6,000 in the 1770s. In South Carolina the rice- and indigo-planters shipped their produce by way of Charles Town, as did the Indian traders who trekked around the southern limit of the Appalachians and brought deerskins from the lower Mississippi Valley.

ESTIMATED POPULATION OF COLONIAL URBAN CENTERS IN THE 1770s*			
Primary Colonial Cities		**Secondary Colonial Cities**	
Philadelphia	35,000	New Haven	8,000
New York	25,000	Norwich	7,000
Boston	16,000	Norfolk	6,000
Charles Town	12,000	Baltimore	6,000
Newport	11,000	New London	5,000
		Salem, Mass.	5,000
		Lancaster, Pa.	5,000
		Hartford	5,000
		Middletown	5,000
		Portsmouth	5,000
		Marblehead	4,000
		Providence	4,000
		Albany	4,000
		Annapolis	4,000
		Savannah	3,000

*Figures rounded to the nearest thousand.
Figures found in tables on pages 216–17 of *Cities in Revolt* by Carl Bridenbaugh. Copyright © 1955 by Carl Bridenbaugh. Figure for Philadelphia revised. Used with permission of Alfred A. Knopf, Inc.

Overseas trade gave city-dwellers and plantation-owners communication with the larger world that was denied to most other Americans, and for that matter to most Englishmen and Europeans. Boston and Philadelphia, with hundreds of ships coming and going, were in closer contact with London than many English cities were. The ships carried ideas as well as goods, and colonial cities were as well equipped to distribute one as the other. Every city had at least one newspaper by the middle of the eighteenth century, with every issue devoted largely to news from England and Europe. Through the columns of the newspapers and through the books imported from abroad and sometimes reprinted locally, the city-dweller kept up with the times. Although the cities held less than 5 percent of the colonial population, it was the best-informed and most-influential 5 percent.

The Emerging American Mind

Before the middle of the eighteenth century, Americans had little occasion to think of themselves as a distinct people. They had no opportunity at all to act as one. There was no American government, no single political organization in which all the colonies joined to manage their common concerns. There was not even a wish for such an organization except among a few eccentric individuals. America, to the people who lived in it, was still a geographical region, not a frame of mind.

Asked for his nationality, the average American in 1750 would have said English or British. In spite of substantial numbers of Dutch, Germans, and Scotch-Irish, Englishmen and English institutions prevailed in every colony, and most colonists spoke of England as home even though they had never been there. Yet none of their institutions was quite like its English counterpart; the heritage of English ideas that went with the institutions was so rich and varied that Americans were able to select and develop those that best suited their situation and forget others that meanwhile were growing prominent in the mother country. Some of the differences were local: the New England town, for example, and the Puritanism that went with it, set New Englanders off not only from people in old England but from Virginians. But some ideas, institutions, and attitudes became common in all the colonies and remained uncommon in England. Although American Englishmen were not yet aware that they shared these "Americanisms" with one another or that the English at home did not share them, many of the characteristic ideas and attitudes that later distinguished American nationalism were already present by mid-century.

Responsible representative government. The English brought with them to the New World the political ideas that still give English and American government a close resemblance. But Americans very early developed conceptions of representative government that differed from those prevailing in England during the colonial period. Representative government in England originated in the Middle Ages, when the king called for men to advise him. They were chosen by their neighbors and informed the king of his subjects' wishes. Eventually their advice became so compelling that the king could not reject it, and the representatives of the people, organized as the House of Commons, became the most powerful branch of the English government.

At first the House of Commons consisted of representatives from each county, or shire, and from selected boroughs. Over the centuries many of these boroughs became ghost towns with only a handful of inhabitants, and great towns sprang up where none had existed before. Yet the old boroughs continued to send members to Parliament, and the new towns sent none. Moreover, only a small fraction of the English population participated in choosing their representatives. It was not that the right to vote was severely restricted. In some boroughs all the free adult males could vote, and to vote for representatives of a county a man had to have only enough property to yield forty shillings' worth of produce or rent a year. One way or another, probably as much as a quarter or a third of all English adult males could vote. But in most elections the voters had no choice. The big men of the county or borough agreed in advance on which of them should be representatives, and the voters' role was reduced to a ritual shout of approval by whoever was standing about the polling place at election time. It was only when the local magnates were themselves divided that the voters had the opportunity to choose among them.

A number of Englishmen thought the electoral situation absurd, especially the continued representation of empty boroughs and the denial of representation to burgeoning new towns. But nothing was done to eliminate the absurdity. Instead, a theory was devised to justify it. A member of the House of Commons, it was said, represented not the people who chose him, but the whole country, and he was not responsible to any particular constituency. Not all English subjects could vote for representatives, but all were "virtually" represented by every member of the Commons.

Colonial assemblies were far more representative than the House of Commons. Although every colony had property qualifications for voting, probably the great majority of adult white males owned enough land to meet them. Then, as now, many who were qualified to vote did not bother to. But uncontested elections, where the voters had no choice between candidates, were far fewer than in England, and the apportionment of representatives was more rational. The New England colonies gave every town the right to send delegates to the assembly. Outside New England, the unit of representation was usually the county. The political organization of new counties and the extension of representation seldom kept pace with the rapid advance of settlement westward, but nowhere was representation so uneven as in England.

American colonists knew nothing of "virtual" representation; to them, representation was a means of acquainting the government with their needs and demands and with the amount and method of taxation they could most easily bear. A colonial assemblyman was supposed to be the agent of the people who chose him. In the large counties, of course, it was seldom possible, except on election day, for voters to gather in one place and express their opinions. But elections came every two or three years (annually in New England and Pennsylvania), and a representative was unlikely to stray far from his constituents' wishes in so short a time. In New England, where town meetings could be called any time, people often gathered to tell their delegate how to vote on a particular issue. He was supposed to look after their interests first, those of the colony second.

In America, therefore, representative government meant something different from what it did in England. Government existed to do a job, and it had to be kept responsible to its employers. While "virtual" representatives in Parliament created offices whose only purpose was to enrich the men who filled them, colonial assemblymen, watched closely by their constituents, had comparatively little opportunity to dip into the public purse.

Clergy and laity. Americans looked on their clergymen as they did on their elected representatives. They wanted the clergy to serve, not rule, them. The attitude had its roots in the English Reformation, and most Englishmen were sufficiently Protestant to share it in some degree; English Dissenters shared it wholeheartedly. But the Anglican Church held great powers in England: it was the only church supported by state taxation; during much of the colonial period only its members could hold public office; and its bishops enjoyed an authority that reached far beyond the realm of the spirit. As ex officio members of the House of Lords they voted on every act of Parliament, and as presiding judges in courts with jurisdiction over probate of wills and breaches of morality they could impose sentence of excommunication on offenders. Since excommunication cut a man off from political rights and from intercourse with his neighbors, it could

mean economic ruin as well as social ostracism. An offender could get the sentence lifted only by paying a heavy fee.

In the colonies, churchmen had no such powers. Except in Rhode Island, Delaware, Pennsylvania, and New Jersey, the assemblies did levy taxes in support of churches, favoring the Congregational churches in New England, the Anglican elsewhere. But this was the only connection between church and state that most Americans would tolerate. The Massachusetts rule that only church members could vote had ended with the revocation of the colony's charter in 1684.

In New England, the old Puritan hostility to clerical authority persisted into the eighteenth century. Ministers were influential and highly respected; a few were even elected as representatives to colonial assemblies. But no minister enjoyed temporal authority by virtue of being a minister.

The Anglicans in America also kept their clergymen on short leash. Because England never sent a bishop to the colonies (and without a bishop there could be no ecclesiastical court), the Anglican Church lost most of its temporal powers when it was transplanted to America. In the Northern colonies, Anglicans, who were a small minority of the population, repeatedly asked for a bishop—much to the annoyance of Congregationalists and Presbyterians. In the Southern colonies, where the Anglican Church was the established church, its members were cool to the proposal. The Southerners, acting through their vestries, ran their churches and hired and fired their ministers almost as independently as any New England Puritan congregation. The minister, unless he had been formally inducted into office (a ceremony performed by the governor at the request of the vestry), could be dismissed at any time. With no bishop at hand to insist on induction, a church could simply omit the ceremony.

Probably one reason for the failure of the Anglican Church to send a bishop was the fear of resistance from non-Anglicans, who multiplied rapidly during the eighteenth century. Besides Congregationalists and Presbyterians, there were Baptists, Quakers, Dutch Reformed, Lutherans, Mennonites, and a host of minor sects. This diversity of religious groups, each growing as population grew, made it increasingly difficult for any one of them to dominate the rest and made the extension of religious authority in America ever more unlikely. Even in New England, where the Congregationalists remained a majority, they ceased after the seventeenth century to persecute Quakers and allowed persons of all denominations to support their own ministers through public taxation.

The Great Awakening. In the 1740s the number of religious groups was expanded by a rash of schisms

George Whitefield

that followed a religious revival. The Great Awakening was touched off in 1740 by a traveling English preacher who combined Calvinism and showmanship. George Whitefield, only twenty-seven at the time, was no theologian. But he had perfected a technique of preaching that brought remarkable results: he frightened his audience by depicting in vivid detail the pain awaiting sinners in Hell. He dramatized the scene for them, playing all the parts himself. Now he was an angry God booming out fearful judgments, now a damned soul weeping in anguish. He strained to bring his audience to the point of hysterical despair. He wanted them to writhe in agony, for he had found that thorough "conviction"—of their own sinfulness, helplessness, and utter dependence on Christ for salvation—was usually followed by "conversion," the feeling that they actually had been saved. As Whitefield journeyed from the Carolinas to New England, preaching indoors and out, Sundays and weekdays, he wrought conversions by the hundreds, among old and young, rich and poor, educated and ignorant.

His technique, requiring only a flair for the dramatic, was not hard to imitate. In his wake other self-appointed messengers of Christ traveled about the country, outdoing him in the sound and fury of their preaching. Gilbert Tennent, a Pennsylvania Presbyterian, made a specialty of laughing loud and long at sinners in the throes of conviction. James Davenport, an itinerant Congregationalist, was at his best at night, when smoking torches revealed him half naked, jump-ing up and down to stamp on the devil.

In spite of these excesses, the Awakening brought religious experiences to thousands of people in every rank of society. One of its staunchest defenders was Jonathan Edwards, minister of Northampton, Massachusetts, who had himself inspired a local revival in 1735. Edwards was the most talented theologian America ever produced. He preached a stricter Calvinism than New England had ever heard, and he recast Calvinist doctrines to give a primary place to the emotions. Although his own manner in the pulpit was an austere contrast to Whitefield's, his doctrines emphasized the emotional impact of an omnipotent God on impotent man. Both conviction and conversion, Edwards insisted, were such overwhelming emotional experiences that the human frame could scarcely contain them. If occasionally someone fell to the ground or cried out in the grip of such powerful experiences, this was no reason to doubt that the spirit of God was the moving cause. Edwards' theology commanded respect in Europe as well as America and furnished the Awakening with an intellectual foundation that Whitefield could not have provided.

But not everyone agreed with Edwards. Many ministers thought that the new method of preaching provoked more hysteria than holiness. They were shocked by the sight of masses of people wallowing in terror or ecstasy on the cue of an ignorant man screaming damnation. They were offended when itinerants entered their churches unbidden and wrung from a hitherto sane congregation a chorus of shrieks and groans and hallelujahs. After listening to an itinerant preacher, people sometimes decided their own minister was worthless, and the most enthusiastic followers of the Awakening deserted their old churches to form new ones with more rigorous doctrines and standards of admission.

Once the shrieking had subsided, it became apparent that the Awakening had seriously undermined the position of the clergy. In every denomination, but especially in the Calvinist ones, ministers had been forced to take sides in favor of the revival (New Light) or against it (Old Light). And those who opposed it were not reconciled by the less exuberant expressions of piety that followed the initial madness. "Nay han't it been common," asked the Boston minister Charles Chauncy, "in some Parts of the Land, and among some Sorts of People, to express their religious Joy, by singing through the Streets, and in Ferry Boats?" The Old Lights, having set themselves against emotional "enthusiasm," prided themselves on a cool rationality. In this mood they reexamined Calvinist dogma and found it wanting. It was absurd, Chauncy decided, that men should suffer eternally by divine predestination: a rational God would allow some merit in human effort. The Old Lights took the road that led

The Great Awakening: New Light conviction

Now it pleased God to send Mr. Whitefield into this land ... I longed to see and hear him, and wished he would come this way ... then on a Sudden, in the morning about 8 or 9 of the Clock there came a messenger and said Mr. Whitefield preached at Hartford and Weathersfield yesterday and is to preach at Middletown this morning at ten of the Clock, I was in my field at Work, I ... ran home to my wife telling her to make ready quickly to go and hear Mr. Whitefield preach at Middletown, then run to my pasture for my horse with all my might.... when we came within about half a mile or a mile of the Road that comes down from Hartford Weathersfield and Stepney to Middletown; on high land I saw before me a Cloud or fogg rising: I first thought it came from the great River, but as I came nearer the Road, I heard a noise something like a low rumbling thunder and presently found it was the noise of Horses feet coming down the Road and this Cloud was a Cloud of dust made by the Horses feet; it arose some Rods into the air over the tops of Hills and trees and when I came within about 20 rods of the Road, I could see men and horses Sliping along in the Cloud like shadows and as I drew nearer it seemed like a steady Stream of horses and their riders, scarcely a horse more than his length behind another, all of a Lather and foam with sweat, their breath rolling out of their nostrils every Jump; every horse seemed to go with all his might to carry his rider to hear news from heaven for the saving of Souls, it made me tremble to see the Sight, how the world was in a Struggle ... and when we got to Middletown old meeting house there was a great Multitude it was said to be 3 or 4000 of people Assembled together.... When I saw Mr. Whitefield come upon the Scaffold he lookt almost Angelical; a young, Slim, slender youth before some thousands of people with a bold undaunted Countenance, and my hearing how God was with him every where as he came along it Solemnized my mind; and put me into a trembling fear before he began to preach; for he looked as if he was Cloathed with Authority from the Great God; and a sweet sollome solemnity sat upon his brow And my hearing him preach, gave me a heart wound; By Gods blessing: my old Foundation was broken up, and I saw that my righteousness would not save me.

From Nathan Cole, "Spiritual Travels," October 23, 1740.

ultimately to Unitarianism, Universalism, and deism, to a world in which there was little need either for Christ or for clergymen. Not many Americans went the whole length of that road in the eighteenth century, but many of the best educated traveled it for some distance.

The New Lights undermined the position of the clergy in a more direct manner by teaching congregations to be bold in judging ministers. Itinerant preachers often pronounced local ministers unregenerate and made much of the idea that a minister could not be God's instrument in bringing salvation to others unless he himself was saved. With this principle in mind, the New Lights in a church did not hesitate to interrogate the minister and then declare him saved or damned. The minister's learning, which had once won him respect, suddenly became a handicap, for many itinerants, uneducated and uneducable, dismissed religious erudition as an impediment to saving grace.

Ironically, in the decades that followed the Great Awakening, the New Light clergy of New England involved themselves so deeply in learned pursuit of Edwards' Calvinist theology that they in turn alienated their congregations. Edwards was not easily understood at best, but his disciples drew out his doctrines in subtle elaborations that scarcely anyone understood but themselves. The New Divinity it was called, and among many bright young men of the day it became the prevailing intellectual fashion. Entering the ministry, they uttered its complexities in sermons addressed more to one another than to their audience. The passionate preaching of the Awakening was forgotten, and the New Divinity grew into a recondite

The Question is, whether it be'nt a plain, stubborn Fact, that the Passions have, generally, in these Times, been apply'd to, as though the main Thing in Religion was to throw them into Disturbance? Can it be denied, that the Preachers, who have been the Instruments of the Commotions in the Land, have endeavoured, by all Manner of Arts, and in all Manner of Ways, to raise the Passions of their Hearers to such a Height, as really to unfit them, for the present, for the Exercise of their reasonable Powers? Nay, in order to alarm Men's Fears, has it not been common, among some Sort of Preachers, to speak and act after such a wild Manner, as is adapted to affrighten People out of their Wits, rather than possess their Minds of such a Conviction of Truth, as is proper to Men, who are endow'd with Reason and Understanding? And under the Notion of speaking to the Affections, were the Things of God and another World ever preached with more Confusion of Thought; with greater Incoherence; with the undue Mixture of more rash, crude, unguarded Expressions; or with Conceit to a higher Degree, appearing in fulsome Self-Applauses, as well as unheard of Contempt of others? These are Things of too publick a Nature to be denied: They have been too often practised, and in Places of too great Concourse, to admit of Debate.

From Charles Chauncy, *Seasonable Thoughts on the State of Religion in New England,*
1743.

game for clergymen.

Congregations reacted with the boldness they had been taught by deserting the preachers who seemed to have deserted them. By the third quarter of the eighteenth century the diversity of denominations allowed a man to shop around for a preacher and a religion that suited him. An American minister was expected to serve his people. When they thought he was failing to do so, they dismissed him or left him.

Education. If the American colonist stood in no awe of his ministers and government officials, it was because the workings of church and state held no mysteries for him. He understood them better than the average European, not only because he had a large share in operating them but because he was better educated. Europeans were fond of picturing Americans as children of nature who learned wisdom from the trees and flowers but not from books. Actually, in spite of their wilderness life, or perhaps because of it, colonial Americans were a bookish lot.

Most of them were Protestants, and Protestants believed that religious truth was incomprehensible to those who did not read the Scriptures. They wanted to read; they wanted their children to read. And their desire was sharpened by the sight of the real children of nature, the Indians, naked, savage, and ignorant. In Massachusetts the law directed every town of fifty families to maintain a schoolmaster and every town of one hundred families to maintain one who could teach Greek and Latin. Other New England colonies

had similar requirements. The laws were not always enforced, but the rate of literacy in New England exceeded that of England from the beginning and rose rapidly in the eighteenth century until nearly all adult males could read and write. Other colonial regions lagged behind. In the Southern colonies, laws forbade teaching slaves to read or write, but the free population enjoyed a literacy rate somewhat above the estimated 50 percent rate among adult males in England.

By the middle of the eighteenth century, nearly every colony had at least one printing press, and the printer usually produced a weekly newspaper, devoted mainly to news from abroad and from other colonies—everybody knew the local news—and to literary and political essays and verse, much of which was culled from English newspapers. The printers also turned out broadsides, almanacs, pamphlets, and books. Though the clergy were the most prolific colonial authors and sermons the most popular reading matter, local political issues were often discussed in print. There were even some efforts at verse. The best of these, the meditative poems of Edward Taylor, minister of Westfield, Massachusetts, were not published until the present century, but colonial readers bought another minister's versified account of the Last Judgment (*The Day of Doom* by Michael Wigglesworth) in such numbers that it went through five editions between 1662 and 1701.

The colonists made early provision for higher education. In 1636, only six years after the Puritans came to Massachusetts, they founded the college that later took the name of its first benefactor, John Harvard. Although the founders' purpose was to furnish the colony with a learned ministry, Harvard was no mere theological seminary. From the beginning, its students followed the traditional curriculum of the liberal arts taught in European universities: they studied grammar (Latin, Greek, and Hebrew), rhetoric, logic, mathematics, astronomy, physics, metaphysics, and moral philosophy. Only once a week, on Saturdays, did they turn to theology. Those who intended to become ministers received their professional training after they graduated, not before. But many Harvard graduates, the majority after the seventeenth century, went into professions other than the ministry.

The same was true of most other colonial colleges: William and Mary, chartered in 1693, remained for some years little more than a grammar school, but Yale (1701) offered a program similar to Harvard's, and so did Princeton (1746), Columbia (1754), Pennsylvania (1755), Brown (1764), Rutgers (1766), and Dartmouth (1769). It was not simply the children of the well-to-do who attended these colleges. Tuition rates were low, and every class contained boys fresh from the farm. Education even at the college level was widely diffused by comparison with that of England.

The fact that New Englanders fell victim to hysteria over witchcraft has often been cited as evidence of the shallowness of their education. How could educated people be so superstitious? The answer is that educated people everywhere believed in witchcraft. In 1692 twenty persons were hanged as witches in Massachusetts, and hundreds more had been accused when the ministers' objections to the unfairness of the trials induced the government to stop

them. No subsequent execution for witchcraft is recorded in America, but in Europe thousands were executed in the seventeenth century, and the executions continued into the eighteenth.

The Enlightenment. The ideas that conquered man's belief in witchcraft were originated, not by Americans, but by a succession of Europeans who had the imagination and daring to take the measure of God's world for themselves. During the sixteenth and seventeenth centuries, Copernicus, Galileo, and Kepler had studied the motions of the planets and accumulated evidence to show that they revolved around the sun. Sir Isaac Newton, building on their work, discovered the laws of motion, the "natural laws" by which God governed the movement of the planets. He also studied light and learned to break it into its different colors and to bend it with mirrors and lenses. Newton's success convinced his contemporaries that human reason was capable of exploring the universe and of ascertaining by observation and experiment the principles by which God governed it. Men who had been taught that reason was a feeble instrument, all but destroyed by Adam's original sin, now turned inquiring eyes on the world around them. They wanted to measure everything, to see how the world worked.

In looking so closely at God's world, men formed a new image of God himself. Where he had formerly been an arbitrary monarch, who glorified himself in the damnation of sinners and the salvation of saints, he now became a divine craftsman whose glory lay in his craftsmanship, a celestial watchmaker whose intricate and orderly handiwork lay everywhere visible to the eyes that reason directed toward it. The new God appeared more reasonable than the old, but also more remote and indifferent, a watchmaker who wound up his universe and then left it to run itself. He seemed, in fact, so reasonable that some men decided he was reason itself, or at least that reason was an adequate substitute for him.

Though few went this far, the eighteenth century earned the title of the Age of Reason. And the English philosopher John Locke furnished the century with a theory about reason that gradually won acceptance and further encouraged the pursuit of experiment and observation. In *An Essay concerning Human Understanding* (1690) Locke concluded that the human mind at birth was not the repository of any innate ideas placed there by the Creator. Rather, it was a complete blank and only gradually accumulated knowledge from the experience of the five senses attached to it. He who would grow in knowledge, therefore, must devote himself not simply to books, perhaps not even to the Bible, nor to abstract contemplation, but to seeing, hearing, feeling, tasting—in a

Harvard, 1726

A Prospect of the Colledges in Cambridge in New England

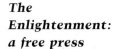
Printers are educated in the Belief, that when Men differ in Opinion, both Sides ought equally to have the Advantage of being heard by the Publick; and that when Truth and Error have fair Play, the former is always an overmatch for the latter: Hence they chearfully serve all contending Writers that pay them well, without regarding on which side they are of the Question in Dispute....

That it is unreasonable to imagine Printers approve of every thing they print, and to censure them on any particular thing accordingly; since in the way of their Business they print such great variety of things opposite and contradictory. It is likewise as unreasonable what some assert, "That Printers ought not to print any Thing but what they approve;" since if all of that Business should make such a Resolution, and abide by it, an End would thereby be put to Free Writing, and the World would afterwards have nothing to read but what happen'd to be the Opinions of Printers.

From Benjamin Franklin, "Apology for Printers," 1731.

word, to observation and experiment.

With man himself a fair subject for observation, Locke observed him and concluded that God had provided natural laws to make the human world run as smoothly as the physical world, but that he had left the enforcement of these natural laws of society to man. In two treatises on civil government (published in 1689 and 1690 but written earlier) Locke explained that men had voluntarily left the free state of nature (in which they were born and originally lived) and had, by mutual agreement, instituted civil government for the purpose of enforcing natural laws. The most important natural law was that no man should take away the life, liberty, or property of another (these were "natural rights" of man). A government that failed to protect life, liberty, and property lost its reason for existence and deserved to be altered or overthrown by the people it governed.

Reason led Locke to condemn absolute government, whether in church or state. It led others to advocate free trade, free speech, free thought. Together, Locke and Newton gave men confidence that all the world's evils as well as its mysteries would yield to the persistent application of human reason.

This confidence in reason, which animated the European philosophers of the eighteenth century, came to be known as the Enlightenment. Although the Enlightenment originated in Europe, its doctrines penetrated society more widely in America. Students in American colleges learned Newton's physics and Locke's psychology. Ministers, whether Old Light or New, adapted their theology to the new ideas and welcomed the discoveries of reason as an aid to revelation, a means to improve their understanding of God's creation. Politicians cited Locke to support their arguments. Gentlemen formed clubs to discuss

philosophy. Men awakened to the newness of the New World and turned amateur scientists; they described American plants and animals and made astronomical observations of the American skies to swell the growing body of scientific information that might provide answers to the limitless questions reason could now ask. In Boston the Reverend Cotton Mather and Dr. Zabdiel Boylston demonstrated by experiment the efficacy of inoculation against smallpox. In Philadelphia David Rittenhouse built the first American orrery, a mechanical model that reproduced the motions of the solar system.

In America even the common man, who never himself read Locke or Newton, was receptive to their philosophy. To the European peasant, following the footsteps of his ancestors, unable to read or write, with no voice in church or state, the Enlightenment meant little. But the ordinary American colonist had constantly to apply his reason to new situations, whether in field or forest, church or state. The Enlightenment made a virtue of his necessity and encouraged him to lift his voice against unreasonableness wherever he met it.

It is perhaps no accident that the man who best exemplified the Enlightenment both to his countrymen and to foreigners was not only an American but an American who came from the ranks of common men and never lost touch with them. Benjamin Franklin (1706–90) was born in Boston, made his fortune in Philadelphia, and then spent much of the remainder of his life in England and France on political missions for the American people. His genius brought him success in everything he tried, whether it was running a Philadelphia newspaper in his youth or wooing the ladies of Paris in his old age. The Enlightenment sang the praises of intellectual freedom;

Franklin as a printer defended his right to publish what he pleased. The Enlightenment called for freedom of trade; Franklin worked as a diplomat to achieve that freedom. The Enlightenment encouraged scientific experiment. Franklin made significant observations on a wide variety of scientific subjects (from ocean currents to the theory of heat); he was a prolific inventor (a stove, a clock, a musical instrument); and, as one of the first experimenters with electricity, he made major contributions to both the theory of the subject (positive and negative charges) and to its application (lightning rods).

As a son of the Enlightenment, Franklin was at home anywhere in the world, yet everywhere people recognized him as a typical American. Even without the fur cap he wore to emphasize it, no one could miss his American style, his down-to-earth insistence on doing things his own way and finding out for himself. Franklin's insistence on results in everything he undertook accorded with his countrymen's insistence that their governments and churches perform what was expected of them.

Social structure. In describing America for Europeans, Franklin advised no one to go there unless he had more to recommend him than high birth, for Americans, he said, "do not inquire concerning a Stranger, *What is he?* but, *What can he do?*" Franklin wrote these words after the period we are considering—probably in 1782. But by mid-century it had already become clear that high birth meant less in America than in Europe.

Europeans learned at an early age that God made men unequal. To some he gave riches beyond measure, to others nothing. Riches brought dignity. It might take more than one generation for a wealthy family to climb to the top of the social ladder, but once there its members enjoyed the security of a title—count, duke, earl, marquis—that passed in perpetuity from father to son. In Europe, men of title generally had a voice in government. In England, even though the House of Commons became the dominant branch of Parliament its members were drawn from the higher ranks of English society, and they could still pass no law without the consent of the highest ranks, assembled in the House of Lords.

Although the eighteenth-century American was taught that God assigned men to different ranks in society, the idea did not have quite the same meaning as in Europe. The American could see plainly that merchants and planters had more wealth and dignity than other men. And in the older settlements, by the middle of the eighteenth century, a larger share of the wealth was concentrated in the hands of a few than had been the case in the seventeenth century. But America was still the land of opportunity; with hard work and luck people of humble origins could better themselves. The top of the social ladder was lower than in Europe and easier to reach but at the same time more difficult to hang on to. Mobility, not nobility, determined the ranks of American aristocrats, who had no titles and no place of their own in the government. They were always having to make room at the top for new arrivals; and, if they wanted to gain

Merchants and planters had more wealth and dignity

and keep the power that came naturally to their European counterparts, they had continually to please other people. American voters commonly recognized the socially and economically successful by electing them to representative assemblies, and governors commonly selected the most successful for seats on the council. But the voters would drop a man who did not suit them as quickly as the governor would. No one could claim a place in the government simply by virtue of his birth or social position.

If the highest born had fewer rights in America than in England, so did the lowest born. No one in England was born a slave. And though the slave on a tobacco plantation might have the kind of security enjoyed by a fine horse, though he might live longer than the slave on a sugar plantation in the West Indies, he had virtually none of the rights that Englishmen had attained for themselves over the centuries. By the end of the colonial period 20 percent of the colonial population was in this position. And though most of them lived in the southern colonies, the northern cities also held large numbers. In 1746 they made up 21 percent of the population of New York City. Overall, slaves probably constituted a majority of the colonial labor force, of persons, that is, who worked for another rather than for themselves. And they had no hope of becoming anything else. Nobody asked either "What are they?" or "What can they do?" Everybody knew.

The remainder of the American population was far better off than the bulk of the English or European population. A small proportion, perhaps 6 or 7 percent of the total adult males, were artisans or laborers of one sort or another who spent their lives working for other men. Most worked for themselves on land or in workshops of their own. The average American, neither slave nor slave owner, enjoyed the economic and political independence that everyone in the eight-eenth century associated with the ownership of land. If there was not enough land where he was born and raised, a man could find more a little farther west. Standing on his own ground, raising his own food, he could bid defiance to landlords, merchants, and politicians alike. Moreover, he was likely to have in hand an instrument of defiance with which few European peasants were familiar—a gun. It was not safe to push him very hard.

In a number of ways, then, the eighteenth-century American differed from the Englishman or the European. Unless he was a slave, he was better educated and therefore less in awe of his superiors, who were in any case not far above him. He had more control over his government and over his clergymen. He had a greater opportunity to mold his own life. He used whatever tools might serve him to do it, whether ax, plow, musket, or vote; and he got results, from governments as well as from forest and field. He did not yet know it, but he was becoming a new kind of man.

Busy Americans

Suggestions for Reading   In many ways the most challenging problem of American history has been to discover in colonial America those institutions, attitudes, and events that found fruition in the later American way of life. George Bancroft first made the attempt on a large scale in his *History of the United States*, 10 vols.* (1834–74), in which he saw divine providence guiding the colonists toward independence. F. J. Turner searched for the answer along the frontier in *The Frontier in American History** (1920), and V. L. Parrington traced a conflict between the common man and the would-be aristocrat in *Main Currents in American Thought*, Vol. 1: *The Colonial Mind** (1927). These men were giants, and their works are too lightly dismissed today. A more recent attempt to discern the abiding meaning of the colonial past is D. J. Boorstin, *The Americans: The Colonial Experience** (1958).

Much recent scholarship has been concerned with labor relations in the colonies. The character of white servitude is analyzed in A. E. Smith, *Colonists in Bondage* (1947), and David Galenson, *White Servitude in Colonial America* (1982). The origins of modern slavery are discussed in D. B. Davis, *The Problem of Slavery in Western Culture* (1966), and in W. D. Jordan, *White over Black* (1968). E. S. Morgan, *American Slavery American Freedom** (1975), treats at length some of the developments described in this chapter; and Peter Wood, *Black Majority** (1974), deals with the beginnings of slavery in South Carolina. G. W. Mullin, *Flight and Rebellion** (1972), discusses slave resistance in Virginia; and T. H. Breen and Stephen Innes, *Myne Owne Ground* (1980), examine the condition of free blacks. Three valuable works give quantitative analyses of society in the Chesapeake area : T. W. Tate and D. L. Ammerman, eds., *The Chesapeake in the Seventeenth Century** (1979); A. C. Land et al., *Law, Society, and Politics in Early Maryland* (1977); and Gloria L. Main, *Tobacco Colony* (1982).

The best overall account of plantation agriculture is L. C. Gray, *History of Agriculture in the Southern United States to 1860*, 2 vols. (1933). On the Virginia plantation in the mid-eighteenth century, Louis Morton, *Robert Carter of Nomini Hall* (1941), offers a close-up view. L. B. Wright, *The First Gentlemen of Virginia* (1940), does the same for a number of earlier planters. On domestic life in the South see E. S. Morgan, *Virginians at Home* (1952); Julia Spruill, *Women's Life and Work in the Southern Colonies* (1938); and Daniel B. Smith, *Inside the Great House* (1980). Carl Bridenbaugh, *Myths and Realities: Societies of the Colonial South* (1952), challenges many conventional ideas about Southern society. Rhys Isaac, *The Transformation of Virginia, 1740–1790* (1982), stresses the role of evangelical sects. James Essig, *The Bonds of Wickedness* (1982), examines the attitude of the sects toward slavery.

The New England town has been a subject of lively interest among social historians. A pioneering case study of a single town (Sudbury) and its English origins is Sumner Powell, *Puritan Village* (1963). D. G. Allen, *In English Ways* (1981), traces the origins of institutions in several towns. Darrett Rutman has analyzed social changes in *Winthrop's Boston* (1965). Stephen Innes, *Labor in a New Land* (1983), describes the ascendancy of a single family in early Springfield. K. A. Lockridge, *A New England Town* (1970), discusses social and cultural changes in Dedham's first century. C. M. Jedrey, *The World of John Cleaveland** (1979), and Christine Heyrman, *Commerce and Culture* (1984), give a different view of social changes over time in some other towns. Michael Zuckerman, *Peaceable Kingdoms** (1970), stresses the forces making for consensus in eighteenth-century towns, while Paul Boyer and Stephen Nissenbaum, *Salem Possessed** (1974), analyze the social conflicts in Salem Village that preceded the witchcraft episode there. Charles Grant describes a single eighteenth-century town in *Democracy in the Connecticut Frontier Town of Kent* (1961). Much valuable information about town affairs is contained in Ola Winslow, *Meetinghouse Hill* (1952). E. M. Cook, Jr. *The Fathers of the Towns* (1976), analyzes social structure in relation to office-holding in eighteenth-century towns.

There is no good study of the American farm in the colonial period, but the anonymous *American Husbandry*, H. J. Carman, ed. (1775, reprinted 1939), offers a wealth of information; and a number of works discussing farming and other human ways of exploiting the land have arisen out of a revived interest in historical geography: C. F. Carroll, *The Timber Economy of Puritan New England* (1973); Carl Bridenbaugh, *Fat Mutton and Liberty of Conscience** (1975) (Rhode Island); J. T. Lemon, *The Best Poor Man's Country** (1972) (Pennsylvania); H. R. Merrens, *Colonial North Carolina in the Eighteenth Century* (1964); P. O. Wacker, *Land and People* (1975) (New Jersey); C. V. Earle, *The Evolution of a Tidewater Settlement System** (1975) (Maryland); and Sung Bok Kim, *Landlord and Tenant in Colonial New York* (1978). William Cronon surveys ecological changes in early New England in *Changes in the Land* (1983).

On the colonial cities the works of Carl Bridenbaugh are outstanding: *Cities in the Wilderness, 1625–1742** (1938); *Cities in Revolt, 1743–1776** (1955); *The Colonial Craftsman** (1950); and, with Jessica Bridenbaugh, *Rebels and Gentlemen** (1942). The last is a study of Philadelphia in the age of Franklin. Gary Nash, *The Urban Crucible* (1979), the first major study of colonial cities since Bridenbaugh, emphasizes economic growth and popular discontent. A valuable history of a colonial merchant firm is J. B. Hedges, *The Browns of Providence Plantation: Vol. I, Colonial Years* (1952). Stuart Bruchey in *The Colonial Merchant** (1966) offers a well-selected collection of source materials. J. F. Shepherd and G. M. Walton, *Shipping, Maritime Trade, and the Economic Development of Colonial North America* (1972), gives a quantitative analysis. The same authors offer a more comprehensive overview in *The Economic Rise of Early America* (1979).

The rise of American representative government is dealt with in L. W. Labaree, *Royal Government in America* (1930), and in J. R. Pole, *Political Representation in England and the Origins of the American Republic** (1966). J. P. Greene, *The Quest for Power** (1963), traces the rising power of the lower houses of assembly in the Southern colonies. Chilton Williamson, *American Suffrage: From Property to Democracy, 1760–1860** (1960), shows that the right to vote was enjoyed by the majority of adult males in all the colonies. A sophisticated approach to the distribution of political power is found in Robert Zemsky's analysis of Massachusetts politics, *Merchants, Farmers, and River Gods* (1971), and in Bernard Bailyn, *The Origins of American Politics** (1968). A sensitive study of social change is Richard Bushman, *From Puritan to Yankee: Character and Social Order in Connecticut, 1690–1765** (1967).

The best general survey of colonial social and intellectual history before the Revolution is L. B. Wright, *The Cultural Life of the American Colonies: 1607–1763** (1957). Henry May, *The Enlightenment in America** (1976), is a comprehensive treatment of that subject. R. B. Davis, *Intellectual Life in the Colonial South* (1978), is encyclopedic. E. S. Morgan, *The Gentle Puritan: A Life of Ezra Stiles, 1727–1795** (1962), shows how the various social and intellectual forces discussed in this chapter propelled one New Englander toward Americanism, republicanism, and democracy. Joseph Ellis, *The New England Mind in Transition: Samuel Johnson of Connecticut, 1696–1772*, (1973), traces another New Englander's odyssey from Puritanism to Anglicanism. The best biography of Franklin is still Carl Van Doren, *Benjamin Franklin* (1941).

Franklin's contributions to science are treated in I. B. Cohen, *Benjamin Franklin's Experiments* (1941) and *Franklin and Newton* (1956). Brooke Hindle, *The Pursuit of Science in Revolutionary America, 1735-1798** (1956), concentrates on the organization of scientific investigation in this period. R. P. Stearns, *Science in the British Colonies of America* (1970), is a more comprehensive account.

W. W. Sweet, *Religion in Colonial America* (1942), is more concerned with church history than with religion itself. The subject is treated more comprehensively in S. E. Ahlstrom, *A Religious History of the American People** (1972). On the Great Awakening, see E. S. Gaustad, *The Great Awakening in New England** (1957), and L. J. Trinterud, *The Forming of an American Tradition* (1949). Ola Winslow, *Jonathan Edwards, 1703–1758** (1940), is the best biography; Perry Miller, *Jonathan Edwards** (1949), is a brilliant interpretation of Edwards' thought. Joseph Haroutunian, *Piety Versus Moralism: The Passing of New England Theology** (1932), traces the development of Edwards' theology into the New Divinity, while Conrad Wright, *The Beginnings of Unitarianism in America** (1955), shows how a liberal theology developed among the opponents of the Awakening. W. G. McLoughlin, *New England Dissent, 1630–1833*, 2 vols. (1971), is authoritative on the role of the Baptists. J. W. Davidson, *The Logic of Millennial Thought* (1977), and N. O. Hatch, *The Sacred Cause of Liberty* (1977), analyze the impact on eighteenth-century Americans and American society of belief in the millennium.

In *American Education: The Colonial Experience** (1970), L. A. Cremin has written a broadly conceived and brilliantly executed treatment of the subject. The history of Harvard College through the seventeenth century has been written by a master in S. E. Morison, *The Founding of Harvard College* (1935) and *Harvard College in the Seventeenth Century*, 2 vols. (1936). Richard Warch has covered the first forty years of Yale College in *School of the Prophets* (1973). Secondary education in New England is ably treated in Robert Middlekauff, *Ancients and Axioms* (1963), and in James Axtell, *The School upon a Hill** (1974).

Francis Parkman made a study of the conflict between England and France in North America his life work, and all his writings are worth careful reading. Recent studies have focused on the conflict of the English with the Indians. Alden Vaughan defends the Puritans' treatment of the Indians in *New England Frontier: Puritans and Indians, 1620–1675** (1965). Francis Jennings attacks it in *The Invasion of America** (1975), as does Neal Salisbury in *Manitou and Providence* (1982). Later New England relations with the Indians are treated in Douglas Leach, *Flintlock and Tomahawk: New England in King Philip's War** (1958) and *The Northern Colonial Frontier, 1607–1763** (1966). C. E. Clark, *The Eastern Frontier: The Settlement of Northern New England, 1610–1763* (1970), emphasizes social history. Some new perspectives on early Indian-White relations are offered in James Axtell, *The European and the Indian** (1981). A. F. C. Wallace, *The Death and Rebirth of the Seneca** (1970), is an outstanding study of the culture of one Indian group. French institutions in the Mississippi Valley are described in C. E. O'Neill, *Church and State in French Colonial Louisiana* (1966).

*Available in a paperback edition.

4

THE SECOND DISCOVERY OF AMERICA

By the middle of the eighteenth century, while England's colonists were beginning to recognize their separate identity, the mother country was beginning to recognize their importance. A population that already amounted to a million and a half and that doubled every twenty-five years was going to be of some consequence in the world—and soon. Benjamin Franklin pointed out in 1751 that Americans would exceed the British in numbers within a century. As Britain and France continued their contest for empire, their statesmen turned eyes westward.

The Peace of Aix-la-Chapelle, which ended the War of the Austrian Succession in 1748, was recognized everywhere in Europe as more a truce than a treaty. It restored the status quo, returned Louisburg to France, took away French conquests in the Austrian Netherlands, but left French power unbroken. France set about at once to ensure that its position in America would be stronger in the next war. Not only did the French refortify Louisburg, but in a more ominous move they sent their agents along the western slope of the Appalachians to build forts, to cement alliances with the Indians, to claim the region for the king of France.

Contest for Empire

The Albany Congress. The English Board of Trade and the Privy Council, in order to bolster the loyalty of their own allies, called on the colonies from Virginia northward to send representatives to a meeting with the Iroquois at Albany. Virginia and New Jersey ignored the summons; but in June 1754 nineteen delegates from New Hampshire, Massachusetts, Connecticut, Rhode Island, Pennsylvania, and Maryland, together with the lieutenant-governor of New York and four gentlemen of his council, rode into Albany to confer with Iroquois chieftains who had slipped down the Mohawk Valley in response to a similar summons. As the Iroquois listened, the white men went through the formalities that Indians demanded in all negotiations: the grandiloquent declarations of esteem, the ceremonial presentation of gifts—scarlet coats, silver buttons, axes, scissors, guns. But the Iroquois had just been watching the French at work on fortifications in the interior, and they found English talk and English gifts less impressive than French action. They departed with the gifts but without offering the hoped-for assurance that they would help when the fighting began.

While in Albany the twenty-four colonial delegates discussed a scheme that had been talked of before: the formation of a permanent intercolonial union to conduct Indian relations. Benjamin Franklin, as he rode north from Philadelphia, had thought out a plan, which he presented at the beginning of the congress. By the time the congress ended, the delegates had agreed to propose to the colonial assemblies a grand council with authority over matters of defense, westward expansion, and Indian relations. The

Text visible in image: "AMERI CA, INDE PEND ANT. 1776"

Public reading of the Declaration of Independence

council would handle purchases of land from friendly Indians and the planting of new settlements. It would raise armies and build forts and warships. And it would pay its own expenses by levying taxes. Its presiding officer, appointed by the king, would have veto power over all its actions.

When the plan reached the assemblies, their reaction was cool—some rejected it, others ignored it. Experience had shown them that the power to tax was father to every other governmental power. They often used it to get their own way in legislative conflicts with royal governors, and they did not propose to share it with any intercolonial council. Nor did they wish to be deprived of the chance to beat their neighbors in the race for Indian lands.

The assemblies' rejection of the Albany plan spared the English government the embarrassment of having to veto it. England wanted a unified direction of Indian affairs, not a permanent colonial union that might prove more difficult to deal with than the separate assemblies. Failure of the plan suggested that England need not worry about a union: the assemblies were apparently more uncooperative in dealing with one another than with England. No one stopped to think that Indian relations and Western policy had always been the most divisive issues in colonial politics. How to use the unsettled land in the West and how to deal with its Indian inhabitants were questions that divided coast from interior, farmer from fur-trader, merchant from landowner, colony from colony. On other questions the colonists were more united than either they or England knew.

English defeats.   As the gentlemen at Albany were conducting their elaborate and unsuccessful courtship of the Iroquois, a younger gentleman was already firing on the French in the Ohio country. Virginia, instead of sending delegates to Albany, had sent a twenty-two-year-old colonel of the militia, George Washington, to help construct a fort at the forks of the Ohio (where the Monongahela and Allegheny rivers join). When Washington arrived in the Ohio country, the French were already in possession of the forks and hard at work on their own Fort Duquesne. He built a crude stockade, which he called Fort Necessity, at Great Meadows, fifty miles south, but was obliged to surrender it to a superior French force on July 3, 1754. Then the French let Washington march his men home to report that the land over the mountains belonged to France.

Washington's defeat was bad news to his fellow Virginians, for many reasons: as Englishmen they disliked Frenchmen; as Protestants they disliked Catholics; as Virginians they disliked anybody who invaded their empire. On the basis of their 1609 charter, Virginians claimed all land to the west and north-

The Ohio country

west of their colony, and they were jealous of encroachments on their territory. Reluctance to admit that other colonies should have any voice in dealing with the great Virginian West may have been behind Virginia's absence from the Albany Congress.

One group of Virginians in particular regarded the Ohio country as private property. In 1747 a number of prominent planters, including George Washington's half-brothers, Lawrence and Augustine, had organized the Ohio Company to trade with the Western Indians and to speculate in Western lands. In 1749, with the approval of the Privy Council, the government of Virginia gave the company 200,000 acres between the Monongahela and the Great Kanawha rivers, and followed this by other grants of Western lands to other speculators. By 1751, when Robert Dinwiddie became governor, many Virginians were looking to the lands of the trans-Appalachian West to make their fortunes, and Dinwiddie himself became a member of the Ohio Company.

Dinwiddie had arranged Washington's expedition in order to hold the Ohio Valley for England, for Virginia, and for the Ohio Company. Upon Washington's return, it was apparent that the job was too big for either the Ohio Company or Virginia, and Dinwiddie signaled for help from England. Although officially England and France remained at peace, the home government recognized that the new war was beginning, and it dispatched General Edward Braddock with two regiments.

Braddock, arriving in Virginia early in 1755, expected to increase his force by a large number of colonists and Indians and then to march on Fort Duquesne and teach the French that the Ohio Valley belonged to England. But Virginia had no wilderness diplomats to furnish the general with Indian braves. South Carolina could have delivered them, but Virginians were wary of letting Carolinians into the affairs of the Ohio country. Some Pennsylvania fur-traders showed up with their own Indian friends, who executed an impressive war dance for the general but disappeared when it came time to march. In the end, Braddock set off with only 8 Indians and about 1,200 colonial militia to supplement his 1,500 regulars. He took them successfully over the mountains, along with enough cannon to pound Fort Duquesne to dust. But as they were approaching the fort on July 9 the French surprised them and turned the march into a disastrous rout. Braddock himself was fatally wounded, and 976 of his men were killed or wounded.

The Indians of the area concluded that the English were finished, and for the next two years it looked as though they were. The colonists, despite their numerical strength, seemed more interested in scoring against one another than in defeating the French; and the English government was occupied with its European involvements. England gave Governor William Shirley of Massachusetts the title of commander in chief but left him to collect most of his men and money from the colonists. Shirley was an able man, the most popular of the royal governors, but his abilities were no match for the jealous intrigues of the other governors, the recalcitrance of the colonial assemblies, or the firepower of the French. While the assemblies dallied over raising troops, Shirley's ill-supported expeditions in 1755 against Fort Niagara and Crown Point both failed, but he did manage to build Fort William Henry at the southern end of Lake George.

Fear that France might try to regain Nova Scotia (or Acadia) led the British government in 1755 to deport several thousand French inhabitants from the province. The Acadians had lived under English rule since 1713, but they had never lost their affection for France and conscientiously passed it on to their children. Governor Shirley, recognizing that in case of a French invasion they were likely to side with the enemy, had suggested their deportation as early as 1747. In 1755 the British dispersed them through the other English colonies instead of sending them off to Canada, where they would have augmented the French forces. The circumstances of the deportations and the treatment of the refugees by the English colonists were unnecessarily cruel. But Nova Scotia was made more secure.

In 1756, after gaining the support of Prussia, England finally resolved on a full-scale conflict and declared war. It lasted for seven more years and so earned in Europe the title of the Seven Years' War. In America it was the French and Indian War. The formal declaration of war did nothing to break England's losing streak, for immediately the French defeated the English fleet in the Mediterranean and captured Minorca. In America a new commander in chief, Lord Loudoun, was given military authority over the colonial governors in order to unite the colonies in their own defense. But the colonial assemblies, holding fast the purse strings, regarded Loudoun's authority with suspicion and complied only casually with his requests for men and supplies. Nor did he achieve success with the troops, regular or colonial, that he did get. Shortly after he assumed command, the French captured Fort Oswego; in the following year they took the new Fort William Henry.

e war in the North, 1758–60

William Pitt: he knew he could save the country

Victory under Pitt. In 1757 the English at last found a statesman to bring their real strength into play. William Pitt had never doubted England's need for him. "I am sure," he said, "that I can save the country, and that no one else can." Pitt's assurance rested on a view of the war and of England's imperial future unlike that of earlier leaders. Hitherto the war in America had been regarded as an incidental part of a traditional European war. The fighting, it was hoped, would facilitate the continued expansion of colonial population, but English statesmen weighed American victories and defeats on a European scale, for their effect on the balance of power. When Pitt took office, English policy underwent a radical change. Pitt's object was not simply to reduce French power in the European balance or to facilitate colonial expansion. He proposed instead to make England master of all North America and perhaps of the rest of the world too.

In Pitt's vision of empire, Europe loomed less large than America and India. Accordingly, he paid Frederick of Prussia to wage the European war and threw England's weight into a campaign of violent aggression abroad. Territory was his object, and he dipped into the national treasury with a lavish hand to pay the men who would seize it for him. Rather than waste time bickering with colonial assemblies over the cost, he promised them reimbursement for a large part of their expenses in raising troops. The national debt went soaring, but so did colonial enlistments.

To drive France from the New World, Pitt needed not only men and money but military talent. He got it, as statesmen frequently have, by jumping young men over the heads of their elders. His greatest find was a gangly, hollow-chested boy of thirty, with a receding chin and a vile temper. James Wolfe was a prig and a martinet, but Pitt sensed his talent. Pitt also promoted Lieutenant Colonel Jeffrey Amherst, who at the age of forty had been in the army twenty-two years without ever holding an independent command, to the rank of major general and put him in charge of a large-scale expedition against Louisburg. With Wolfe supervising the landing operations, Amherst took the fortress on July 26, 1758, giving England its first great victory of the war.

The capture of Louisburg destroyed French power at the mouth of the St. Lawrence and jeopardized communications between New and old France. A month later Lieutenant Colonel John Bradstreet captured Fort Frontenac, which guarded the other end of the St. Lawrence on the shores of Lake Ontario. Now the French in Canada were cut off from the Mississippi Valley and had to give up Fort Duquesne, which the British renamed Fort Pitt (later Pittsburgh).

At last Pitt was ready for his grand strategy, a pincers move on Quebec and Montreal, with troops approaching from the north by the St. Lawrence and from the south by the Hudson River, Lake George, and Lake Champlain. Amherst was to operate from the south, Wolfe from the north. Wolfe sailed up the St. Lawrence with nine thousand men and on September 12, 1759, made a surprise night attack up one of the steep gullies in the cliffs that protect Quebec. In the battle that then took place on the Plains of Abra-

General James Wolfe: a martinet with talent

British attack on Cape Breton, 1758

ham the British were victorious, but both Wolfe and the French commander, the Marquis de Montcalm, received fatal wounds.

With the capture of Quebec, English victory in North America was only a matter of time. The French immediately laid siege to the city, but, when spring opened the ice-choked river and a British fleet appeared, the French withdrew. During the late summer, the expected troops from the south and a force from Quebec converged on Montreal for the final campaign. On September 8, 1760, the French gave up the city and all Canada with it. The war did not end until 1763, but in its final phases the action shifted from North America to the Caribbean, India, and the Philippines, as England plucked the overseas empires of its European rivals.

George III. Six weeks after the fall of Montreal, King George II died. Between them, George II and his father, George I, had ruled England since 1714, when the latter had been summoned to the throne from the quiet German principality of Hanover. Neither was distinguished in intelligence or character, but George II was the more energetic and enjoyed leading the army, which knew him affectionately as the Little Captain. Though George II took an active part in selecting his ministers, the English government during his reign and his father's fell more and more into the hands of a powerful group of private families. They called themselves Whigs, in memory of the Revolution of 1688, from which they liked to date their ascendancy. Though they made an occasional bow to the principles of liberty, there was nothing revolutionary about them. Comfortable and wealthy, they entered politics to get wealthier and organized small groups or factions to juggle the spoils of office.

George II outlived his eldest son Frederick (whose death in 1751 was attributed to a blow from a tennis ball); George III, who ascended the throne in 1760, was the old king's grandson. At twenty-two George III had a mind, such as it was, of his own and no intention of letting the great Whig families run *his* government. Under the tutelage of a Scottish peer, the Earl of Bute, he had learned to dislike vice, to distrust talent, and to love patriotism, barley water, and the Earl of Bute. As a Scot, Bute had no seat in the House of Lords, and as a lord he was disqualified from the House of Commons. But the new king gave him at once a place in the inner "Cabinet Council," which was taking the place of the larger Privy Council in conducting the executive branch of government. Together, George and the Earl of Bute set about reforming the wicked ways of English politics.

The politicians shared neither the king's aversion

to vice nor his fondness for Bute, and they were not interested in reform. Lacking any party organization, they could not present a united front against the king, but he and they both knew that he could not run the government without their help, and they made him pay dearly for it. For ten years George appointed and dismissed members of the council at a bewildering rate. Ministers responsible for colonial affairs came and went and came again as the king sparred with politicians over issues that usually had nothing to do with the colonies. Consequently, English colonial policy in this crucial decade was inconsistent and incoherent, not to say capricious.

When George took the throne, Pitt was running the war and the government. Trouble broke out almost immediately. Tormented by gout, hobbling about on crutches, Pitt snapped at everyone who disagreed with him and did not gladly suffer the many fools he had to deal with. The politicians liked him as little as they liked Bute. With the fall of Canada and the subsequent British successes in the rest of the world, they were ready to make peace with France and rid themselves of the tyranny of this ailing genius.

Pitt was ready for peace too, provided he could strip France of all its overseas possessions. France, however, though defeated abroad, was still a formidable power in Europe and was courting the support of Spain. Pitt, hearing of the negotiations, stopped talking peace and demanded instead that England declare war at once against Spain—Pitt always preferred to attack. No one had dared oppose Pitt while England was underdog in the war with France. But he had made England strong enough to do without him, and now his colleagues would not agree to take on a new enemy. When he could not have his way, Pitt resigned the ministry.

The Peace of Paris. With Pitt's resignation in 1761, the king's "dearest friend" became the leading figure in the council and the most unpopular man in England. Bute did not enjoy either role and retired from politics in 1763, but not until he had dictated the terms of the treaty that ended England's most successful war. The momentum of victory generated under Pitt carried the country through the final year of war without him. As he had foreseen, England ultimately had to add Spain to its list of enemies, but after crushing defeats at Manila and Havana, Spain was ready to call a halt. When Bute made peace in 1763, he took the whole of North America east of the Mississippi (Florida from Spain, Canada from France), and also took back Minorca, carved up the French possessions in India, and extricated England from its commitments in Germany. But Bute was schooled in the traditional diplomacy of balancing European powers against one another, and he was unmoved by Pitt's imperial ambitions. He gave Cuba and the Philippines back to Spain and let France give Louisiana to Spain. He returned Guadeloupe and Martinique to France and allowed it to keep the two tiny islands of St. Pierre and Miquelon as fishing bases.

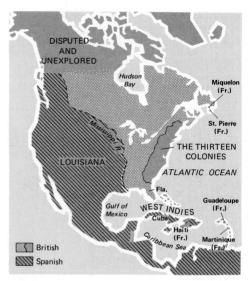

North America in 1763

Pitt was outraged by Bute's liberality toward France and Spain, and some of the colonists shared his view. But most of the English, both in England itself and in the colonies, welcomed the treaty even while they denounced its maker and glorified Pitt. For the colonists it meant the end of a threat that had been hanging over them for as long as anyone could remember. Now, as their children grew up and went looking for new homes, they could trek over the mountains into the lush Ohio Valley, into bluegrass lands they would name Kentucky and Tennessee, into the prairies of the Illinois country. The Indians, without the French to organize and direct them, could offer no serious obstacle to the settlement of the interior by the English.

A New Empire and New Ideas

The English looked with pride at their new territories. America was still the spearhead of European growth, and the conquest of New France conjured up the vision of a Mississippi Valley filled with people who spoke English and talked fondly of a small island across the ocean as "home." Englishmen had been the first Europeans to think of North America as a place to live. Now their perception was rewarded with an empire that promised to cover the continent.

The question of imperial authority. With the coming of peace a few men sensed that the government of the empire again needed overhauling, for it was clearly inadequate for a population of 2 million about to advance into the immense interior of North America. Several colonial governors, who had seen America at first hand, wrote urgently on the subject. From Massachusetts, for example, Francis Bernard warned his superiors in England that this was "the proper and critical time to reform the American governments upon a general, constitutional, firm, and durable plan; and if it is not done now, it will probably every day grow more difficult, till at last it becomes impracticable."

Bernard's sense of urgency was justified. Most of the colonies had been founded before the supremacy of Parliament in England had been firmly established. Even after the question of supremacy was settled Parliament concerned itself little with them. But now that America had grown important to England, Parliament would be giving it more attention. That attention (as Bernard foresaw) might not be welcomed by the colonies; for, since the time of their founding, they had regularly dealt with the mother country through the king, his councils, his governors. Before Parliament began making laws for them or levying taxes on them it needed to establish its own authority over them by reorganizing their governments.

Bernard thought that all the colonial governments should be given identical constitutions by act of Parliament, with governors appointed by the king. He recognized that the colonists, like other Englishmen, expected a share in their government, and he suggested that they be represented in Parliament. He did not think that they had any right to such representation, but he felt that it would be good politics to give them a voice in the decisions that Parliament would doubtless be making about them.

Francis Bernard was an ambitious man, and his superiors probably smiled at his advice. They realized that the empire needed repair, but Bernard's far-reaching plans seemed grandiloquent and prompted as much by a desire for promotion as by the actual needs of the situation. At the moment more immediate and pressing problems demanded their attention. For the next thirteen years a succession of shortsighted politicians and an industriously dull king kept their minds on a succession of immediate and pressing problems. By so doing, they inadvertently and unintentionally taught the colonists that Americans had more in common with one another than with Englishmen.

Trouble in the West. After the war England decided to station several thousand troops permanently in America. So much blood and money had been spent winning the continent that it seemed only proper to guard it, and the presence of troops would also help to restrain any possible insubordination on the part of the colonists and discourage France from trying to regain its losses. Almost at once the troops were called into action, not against France but against its former allies, the Indians, for whom the coming of peace presaged another westward surge of English colonists. The Indians of all tribes had been restive ever since the fall of New France, and the contemptuous and shortsighted policies of General Amherst toward them gave them a foretaste of what English rule of the continent would mean. When the Ottawas, led by their chieftain Pontiac, attacked Detroit in the spring of 1763, other tribes, following his lead, fell upon the English forts and settlements from the Great Lakes to the back country of Pennsylvania, Maryland, and Virginia. Since the British troops were not well located to protect the frontiers, the outlying settlers suffered heavily before the attacks could be stopped.

Pontiac's Rebellion had the divisive effect that Western problems usually produced among Americans. Easterners were reluctant to take it seriously. Westerners blamed the Easterners for the loss of farms and the death of wives, husbands, children, and friends. In western Pennsylvania a group of outraged pioneers known as the Paxton boys fell upon a village of peaceful Indians, massacred them, and marched on Philadelphia to get some action out of the government. They were halted by the Philadelphians, who evidently feared other Pennsylvanians more than Indians.

English statesmen could easily conclude that the Americans were a hopelessly uncooperative and cowardly lot, unwilling to help one another and unable to protect themselves against savages. During the preceding French and Indian War British officers had sent back disparaging reports of colonial troops. General Wolfe himself had characterized his four companies of American rangers at Quebec as "the worst soldiers in the Universe." Now, once again, it seemed, the colonists had demonstrated their weakness—and the British proceeded to demonstrate theirs.

When Bute took the Mississippi Valley from France and returned the islands of Guadeloupe and Martinique, the decision was widely justified on the grounds that the valley was potentially more valuable than the West Indies. But if its potential was to be realized, the area would have to be settled and exploited by the English, not kept as a giant game preserve. British politicians recognized this fact, but most of them saw no need to hurry settlers into the great emptiness beyond the mountains, where they would be less accessible to British control. Moreover, westward expansion would aggravate the most pressing colonial problem—the Indian resistance. While their troops crushed Pontiac's warriors, the politicians drafted a solution to the problem of Indian warfare: keep the colonists out of Indian territory. They had the king issue a proclamation forbidding settlement beyond the crest of the Appalachian Mountains and advising settlers in search of homes to go to Nova Scotia or Florida, for which England now provided governments.

The proclamation had little effect on American westward expansion, for the colonists took little notice of it. But it showed that the British were incapable of grasping the desperate speed of American growth. They thought they could take their time about developing the West, that they could deflect the expanding population by issuing a proclamation.

George Grenville's search for revenue.

While the king was erecting his paper fence along the crest of the Appalachians, one of his ministers was occupied with a matter closer to home, the enormous national debt that England had piled up in acquiring Canada and the Mississippi Valley. George Grenville, First Lord of the Treasury, knew his pounds, shillings, and pence. With the end of the French and Indian War and the retirement of Bute, the king turned to him as the man best qualified to put England's finances in order. Grenville was not impressed with a continent full of naked savages, impecunious Frenchmen, and wild beaver; he was impressed with a national debt that had doubled since 1754; and he was still more impressed with the cost of keeping troops under arms to protect England's new possessions. He did not question the need for the troops. That was beyond his concern. But he had to find the money to pay them, as well as the money to pay the interest on the national debt.

Soon after he took office in April 1763 Grenville came upon a remarkable fact: the American customs service was costing the government nearly £8,000 a year in salaries but was collecting less than £2,000 in duties. Everyone knew that the colonists were importing large quantities of molasses from the French West Indies, on which the Molasses Act of 1733 required them to pay a duty of sixpence a gallon. Obviously they were evading the duty. In October 1763 Grenville issued a sharp directive for its collection and ordered the British navy to patrol American waters for smugglers.

Grenville had another grievance against the colonists: they alleviated their perpetual currency shortage (resulting from their unfavorable balance of trade with the mother country) by issuing paper money. Although the money served an essential purpose and showed little depreciation in most colonies, its value was less than that of English sterling coin. English creditors feared that the colonists might manipulate the rate of exchange between their currency and ster-

ling and try to pay their English debts at an artificially low rate. As a result of complaints by creditors, the New England colonies had been forbidden in 1751 to make their paper money legal tender. By the Currency Act of April 1764, Grenville extended the prohibition to all the colonies.

In the same month Grenville directed through Parliament an act (later known as the Sugar Act) revising American customs duties and regulations. With good reason he reduced the duty on foreign molasses from sixpence a gallon to threepence. The purpose of the original levy had been to induce the colonists to buy their molasses from the British West Indies, where they could get it duty free (though higher priced). But colonial rum-distillers balked at paying premium prices for British molasses or the sixpence duty for French. To have done so, they claimed, would have raised the price of their rum to the point where it could not be sold in competition with other spirits. So the colonial importers simply bribed the customs officials (from a halfpenny to a penny and a half per gallon) not to collect the duty. Grenville accepted the fact that the sixpence duty was too high, but he believed that if the merchants could afford to pay bribes, they could afford, instead, a three-pence duty.

The Sugar Act also imposed new duties on colonial imports of sugar, indigo, coffee, pimento, wine, and textiles. To discourage smuggling, it required that elaborate official papers be filed for every ship entering or leaving a colonial port. Finally, it provided that violators of the customs regulations could be tried in admiralty courts, which operated under royally appointed judges acting without juries (in the common-law courts juries made up of local residents were inclined to sympathize with offenders). The colonists had been subject to such an enactment since 1696, but ambiguities in it had often enabled smugglers to avoid admiralty jurisdiction.

The stated purpose of the Sugar Act was to help defray the expenses England would incur in protecting its new American possessions. Grenville did not expect to raise the whole amount from the colonists, but he did expect more than the new duties were likely to yield; and in introducing the bill for the Sugar Act to Parliament he announced that he might levy a stamp tax on the colonies.

There was nothing novel in the idea of stamp taxes. The English at home had been paying them ever since the reign of King William, and there had already been suggestions that Parliament impose such taxes on the colonies. Massachusetts had even tried a stamp tax of its own in 1755. By February 1765 Grenville had completed his study of taxable items being used in the colonies and was ready to introduce his Stamp Act to Parliament. It called for taxes on every type of legal document and on newspapers, almanacs, playing cards, and dice (all of which had to bear a stamp, signifying that the tax was paid). As in the case of the Sugar Act, violators would be prosecuted in admiralty courts. A few members of Parliament raised objections to taxing the colonists. Colonel Isaac Barré, who had served under Wolfe in North America, warned that the Americans would resist. But the act passed both houses and was signed by the king on March 22, 1765, to take effect November 1.

In May 1765 Grenville put through a third measure, the Quartering Act, to help support English troops in America. This act provided that any colony in which troops were stationed must furnish them with living quarters and with fire, candles, vinegar, salt, bedding, and beer, cider, or rum.

Colonial suspicions. The colonists were stunned by Grenville's actions. In 1763 colonial merchants felt sure that his order calling for the strict collection of molasses duties would ruin the rum trade and the whole New England economy with it. Nor did they welcome the reduction in duties provided by the Sugar Act, for they believed that even a threepence duty would drive their rum out of the market. Moreover, the act established customs procedures so strict and complicated that all kinds of trade would be hampered. The currency restriction made matters still worse. With silver in short supply and with paper money no longer legal tender, merchants had no medium of exchange and were sometimes reduced to barter. When economic depression followed the acts, Americans blamed Grenville.

But the most shocking aspect of Grenville's measures was that they seemed to embody a new policy—a deliberate aim to disinherit the colonists by denying them the rights of Englishmen. The Americans believed that it was their right as Englishmen not to be taxed except by their own elected representatives; but Parliament had taxed them directly in the Stamp Act, indirectly in the Sugar Act and the Quartering Act. They believed that it was their right as Englishmen to be tried by juries of their peers; but Parliament had made infringement of the Sugar and Stamp acts punishable in admiralty courts. These courts were objectionable not only because they violated the right to trial by jury but because they put the burden of proof on the defendant, assuming that he was guilty until he proved himself innocent. Furthermore, in England admiralty courts tried only cases arising on the high seas. By giving the courts a wider jurisdiction in the colonies, the Sugar and Stamp acts suggested that England thought Americans not entitled to rights long recognized in the mother country.

Further evidence of some sinister design seemed apparent in the announced purpose of the acts: to

The Stamp: the Americans would resist

support troops in America. Why, the colonists wondered, did England want to keep armed soldiers in their midst? The troops had helped, to be sure, in crushing Pontiac's Rebellion, which the rash actions of their commander, General Amherst, had actually helped to bring on. But protection against Indians was patently not the purpose of keeping troops in America. Before 1754, while the French were sending their Indian allies to attack the colonists from Maine to Carolina, England had maintained scarcely any military garrison in America. Now, with the danger gone, with the French crushed and the Spanish pushed beyond the Mississippi, England insisted on keeping several thousand men on hand. Why? Perhaps, it was whispered, England intended to use the army not to protect but to suppress the colonists. There is evidence in British documents that such an intention did in fact exist, but the evidence was not known to the colonists. Grenville's acts, however, were sufficient in themselves to prompt suspicions.

Colonial convictions. The British statesmen who started Americans talking of standing armies, taxation without representation, and trials without juries would have done well to consider the origin and history of the colonies. New England and many other parts of America had been founded by Puritans who carried to America the ideas that shortly led to Oliver Cromwell's commonwealth in England. After that commonwealth ended with the restoration of the monarchy in 1660, many more Dissenters joined the exodus to America, and their descendants could talk of Hampden and Pym and other heroes of the struggle against Charles I with a familiarity that might have struck some Englishmen as quaint. Though loyal to the House of Hanover, the colonists admired much in the writings of James Harrington, the advocate of republican government, of Algernon Sidney, and of John Locke. They also admired England's latter-day republicans, the so-called eighteenth-century commonwealthmen whose writings (especially *Cato's Letters* by John Trenchard and Thomas Gordon) had argued for greater popular control of government.

Neither the eighteenth-century commonwealthmen nor their colonial admirers thought of themselves as advocating anything different from what their ancestors had fought for. All Englishmen believed that the course of their history had been a struggle to achieve a government that would protect life, liberty, and property. They believed that they had at last achieved such a government with the overthrow of James II in 1688 and the establishment of the House of Hanover in 1714. The colonists shared this belief, and they were proud to be members of the nation whose government, whatever its shortcomings, stood foremost in the world in protecting the natural rights of its subjects.

Like other Englishmen the colonists regarded the representative nature of English government as the most important guarantee of continued protection. They rejoiced in Parliament's supremacy in England and in the supremacy of their own assemblies in America. In each the elected representatives of the people guarded the rights of Englishmen, and the most precious right they guarded was the right of property, without which neither life nor liberty could be secure. Since the power to tax was a power to take away property, no man could call himself free if he was taxed without his own consent, given either personally or by his representative. The right to be taxed in this way, and in no other, was a hard-won principle of the British constitution. In England only the representative branch of Parliament, the House of Commons, could initiate tax bills; and in the colonies the representative assemblies claimed the same exclusive privilege. It therefore seemed monstrous to Americans that, in the Sugar Act and the Stamp Act, Parliament, a body in which they had no representative, had presumed to tax them. If Parliament could levy these taxes it could levy others. Once the precedent was set, the colonists would be as badly off as England had been before the rise of Parliament. They would, ironically, be oppressed by the very body that had rescued England from the same kind of tyranny.

As the colonists measured acts of Parliament against their own ideas of right, they faced the question that Governor Bernard had wished to settle earlier, the question of Parliament's authority in America. Their decision was different from Bernard's. Parliament, they believed, had some right to legislate for them; but it had no right to tax them. It was the central legislative body for matters of common concern to the entire empire, and as such it could regulate their commerce, even by imposing duties to discourage certain kinds of trade that it believed prejudicial to the good of the empire as a whole. But it

had no right to levy duties to raise money; such duties were taxes, and Parliament had no right to tax the colonies in any manner. Its members could not grant the property of people whom they did not represent.

The American colonists in 1764 and 1765 were remarkably unanimous in adopting this distinction between taxation and legislation. They began to affirm it in pamphlets and newspaper articles as soon as the Sugar Act was passed. New York and Virginia expressed it officially in petitions to Parliament. By the time the Stamp Act was passed, people in every colony were discussing the limits of Parliament's authority, and during the summer and fall of 1765 colonial assemblies passed resolutions setting forth those limits.

The Stamp Act crisis. The Stamp Act was to go into effect on November 1. In the May session of the Virginia assembly, Patrick Henry, a young lawyer, presented a series of resolutions declaring that only the House of Burgesses had the right to tax Virginians. The Burgesses adopted the resolutions but rejected some additional ones calling for outright resistance if England should try to collect the stamp tax. The other colonial assemblies rapidly followed Virginia's example, modeling their own resolutions on its. Although

Demonstration against the Stamp Act

the newspapers had printed Henry's rejected resolutions as though they had actually been passed, thus creating the impression that Virginia had acted more radically than was the case, nevertheless most of the other assemblies stopped where Virginia did, with a simple denial of Parliament's right to tax the colonies.

In addition to the resolutions of their individual assemblies, the colonies prepared a joint statement of their position. In June, before the colonial consensus had become apparent, Massachusetts proposed that all the colonies send delegates to a general meeting for the purpose of concerting their opposition to Parliamentary taxes. Nine assemblies complied: in October 1765 the Stamp Act Congress met at New York. After avowing "all due subordination" to Parliament, the delegates resolved that colonial subordination did not include acceptance of Parliamentary taxation or of admiralty courts operating beyond their traditional limits. They also sent petitions to king and Parliament demanding repeal of the Sugar and Stamp acts.

In objecting to taxation by Parliament, the colonists believed that they had common sense, natural law, and the British constitution all on their side. It was common sense that they already contributed to the wealth of the mother country by submitting to the Navigation Acts. If a more direct contribution was required, it ought to be made by the colonists' own representatives, who alone could know, as the Virginia resolves said, "what Taxes the People are able to bear, or the easiest Method of raising them, and must themselves be affected by every Tax laid on the People." If the members of Parliament could establish their authority to tax the colonies, they would have an all but irresistible motive to shift their own burdens and those of their constituents to America. Every penny collected in the colonies would be a penny less to take from English pockets. It was common sense that such a situation spelled tyranny.

It was also a violation of the British constitution and of the laws of nature by which every free people should be governed. The people's right to be taxed only by their own representatives was "the grand Principle of every free State . . . the natural Right of Mankind," proclaimed the members of the New York assembly. The Massachusetts assembly, in the same vein, announced that "there are certain essential Rights of the British Constitution of Government, which are founded in the Law of God and Nature, and are the common Rights of Mankind." Among those rights was "that no man can justly take the Property of another without his Consent."

Besides informing Parliament and posterity of what was right, the colonists took practical steps to see that right prevailed. Merchants in New York, Philadelphia, and Boston agreed to stop importing British goods, hoping by economic pressure to enlist British

merchants and manufacturers against the Stamp Act. Other Americans, too impatient to wait for repeal, were determined to prevent the Stamp Act from taking effect. On the night of August 14, a Boston mob stormed the house of Andrew Oliver, the local stamp-distributor. They broke the doors and windows and roamed through the house calling for the owner's head. Oliver resigned his office the next day. Stamp-distributors in other colonies hastened to follow Oliver's example. Mobs helped those who hesitated to make up their minds. On November 1, when the act was scheduled to go into effect, there was no one to distribute the stamps.

In every colony the violence that forced the resignation of the distributors had been carefully engineered by a group of conspirators. These men now organized under the name of Sons of Liberty and prepared to resist "to the last extremity" any efforts to enforce the Stamp Act. They had learned from John Locke that a people could alter or overthrow a government that exceeded its authority; and they repeated Locke's precepts to their countrymen in resolves, like those adopted at New London on December 10, 1765, declaring that "the People have a Right to reassume the exercise of that Authority which by Nature they had, before they delegated it to Individuals."

The total overthrow of government did not prove necessary. For a few weeks after November 1, people in most colonies simply refrained from doing any business that required stamps. Then newspapers began to appear without them. By threatening mob action, the Sons of Liberty soon persuaded judges to try cases and customs officers to clear ships with unstamped bonds and clearance papers. In less than three months the Stamp Act had been effectively nullified.

English response to colonial defiance was not what it might have been had Grenville remained in power. George III, for reasons that had nothing to do with the colonies, dismissed Grenville in July 1765 and in his place named the Marquis of Rockingham as first minister. Rockingham and the men he brought into the administration with him had opposed the Stamp Act in the first place and wanted nothing more than to escape the embarrassment of trying to enforce it. English merchants, stung by the American boycott, backed Rockingham's determination to wipe the act off the books, and he enthusiastically favored a repeal bill in Parliament.

But the spate of resolutions and riots in the colonies made members of Parliament reluctant to back down, especially after William Pitt, with his usual tactlessness, publicly rejoiced at American resistance and endorsed the colonists' definition of the limits of Parliament's authority. Taxation, he said, was "no part of the governing or legislative power."

The Fact is, that the Inhabitants of the Colonies are represented in Parliament: they do not indeed chuse the Members of that Assembly; neither are Nine Tenths of the People of Britain Electors; for the Right of Election is annexed to certain Species of Property, to peculiar Franchises, and to Inhabitancy in some particular Places; but these Descriptions comprehend only a very small Part of the Land, the Property, and the People of this Island....

The Colonies are in exactly the same Situation: All British Subjects are really in the same; none are actually, all are virtually represented in Parliament; for every Member of Parliament sits in the House, not as Representative of his own Constituents, but as one of that august Assembly by which all the Commons of Great Britain are represented. Their Rights and their Interests, however his own Borough may be affected by general Dispositions, ought to be the great Objects of his Attention, and the only Rules for his Conduct; and to sacrifice these to a partial Advantage in favour of the Place where he was chosen, would be a Departure from his Duty; if it were otherwise, Old Sarum would enjoy Privileges essential to Liberty, which are denied to Birmingham and to Manchester; but as it is, they and the Colonies and all British Subjects whatever, have an equal Share in the general Representation of the Commons of Great Britain, and are bound by the Consent of the Majority of that House, whether their own particular Representatives consented to or opposed the Measures there taken, or whether they had or had not particular Representatives there.

From Thomas Whately, *The Regulations Lately Made...*, 1765.

Other members were baffled by the distinction between taxation and legislation. Grenville declared it absurd. But in March 1766 Parliament repealed the act after first passing a Declaratory Act, which deliberately skirted the distinction and simply affirmed the authority of Parliament to "make laws and statutes of sufficient force and validity to bind the colonies and people of America . . . in all cases whatsoever." Precisely what that meant Americans were to find out later. For the moment they rejoiced in the end of the contest that had led them to the brink of war with the mother country. Repeal of the Stamp Act seemed to signal a return to the Old Colonial System under which England and its colonies had alike enjoyed freedom, prosperity, and harmony.

Commemorative teapot, 1766

Colonial discoveries. Nevertheless, as the colonists joined their English friends in celebrating repeal, they could reflect on their discoveries of the preceding two years. They had already found out more than England could have wished. A decade earlier, when the Albany Congress proposed a union against a danger in the West, they had unanimously declined. This time, when the danger came from the East, they had spontaneously joined to boycott British goods, to prevent the distribution of stamps, to define the limits of Parliament's authority. Indian tomahawks and French guns had revealed nothing but discord; the threat of tyranny had revealed fundamental agreement. The definition of Parliament's authority that the Stamp Act Congress had formulated was no compromise measure reluctantly agreed to under the pressure of circumstance. The congress merely reiterated principles already familiar in newspapers and pamphlets, principles that the colonial assemblies themselves had embodied in their resolutions. It nevertheless surprised the Americans to find themselves agreeing so readily. "The Colonies until now were ever at variance and foolishly jealous of each other," Joseph Warren of Massachusetts wrote to a friend, "they are now . . . united . . . nor will they soon forget the weight which this close union gives them."

In defending their rights the colonists also discovered that the ideas which united them and which they thought inherent in the British constitution were not shared by most Englishmen. Men in England had

To infer, my lord, that the British *members [of Parliament] actually represent the colonies, who are not permitted to do the least act towards their appointment, because Britain is unequally represented, although every man in the kingdom, who hath certain legal qualifications can vote for some one to represent him, is such a piece of sophistry that I had half a mind to pass by the cobweb without blowing it to pieces. Is there no difference between a country's having a privilege to choose 558 members to represent them in parliament, though in unequal proportions to the several districts, which cannot be avoided, and not having liberty to choose any? To turn the tables,—if the* Americans *only had leave to send members to parliament, could such sophistry ever persuade the people of* Britain *that they were represented and had a share in the national councils?... Suppose none of the 558 members were chosen by the people, but enjoyed the right of sitting in parliament by hereditary descent; could the common people be said to share in the national councils? How trifling then is the supposition, that we in* America *virtually have such share in the national councils, by those members whom we never chose? If we are not their constituents, they are not our representatives.... It is really a piece of mockery to tell us that a country, detached from Britain, by an ocean of immense breadth, and which is so extensive and populous, should be represented by the British members, or that we can have any interest in the house of commons.*

From the Providence *Gazette*, May 11, 1765.

denied not only the colonists' distinction between taxation and legislation but their conception of representation. At the outset of the tax controversy Grenville and his backers, admitting that English subjects had a right to representation in the body that governed them, had claimed that the colonists *were* represented—not actually but virtually. A member of Parliament, Grenville maintained, represented not only the men who elected him, but the whole empire. The concept of virtual representation was as yet not widely accepted even in England, and it was nonsense to Americans, who thought that a representative should be directly responsible to his constituents. By Grenville's reasoning, they said, Parliament could equally well claim an authority to tax the whole world.

Although a few suggestions had been made, like Governor Bernard's, that England should allow the colonies to send representatives to Parliament, the colonists did not take to the idea. It would be impractical, they thought, because of the great distance. Colonial representatives in London would lose contact with their constituents; it would cost too much to send them back and forth and to pay for their keep; they would be corrupted by the metropolis. But most important, there would be too few of them to have any real effect on the decisions of empire, yet their presence could be used to justify Parliamentary taxation of America.

These objections were serious, but not insupera-

ble had either England or the colonies wanted to resolve them. But the plain fact was that the colonists did not want representation in Parliament. Perhaps they were unconsciously influenced by a new attitude that had been taking shape in the colonial mind but that few yet recognized. England, by treating the colonists differently from Englishmen at home, was teaching them what it should have done its best to conceal: that they actually *were* different, and perhaps even wanted to be.

Though England had no way of knowing it, the men in whom this attitude first took hold included several of extraordinary ability. In Massachusetts three emerged as leaders of the opposition to Parliamentary taxation: James Otis, Samuel Adams, and John Adams. Otis, a lawyer, was volatile, unpredictable, and unbalanced, but powerful in argument and very influential among the people of Boston. Samuel Adams, a failure at everything else he tried, was a brilliant politician, gifted in organizing popular support for any measure. In the years to come, as Otis became more erratic and finally went insane, Adams would guide Boston toward revolution. John Adams, whose gifts were more those of a statesman than of a politician, was as ardent as his cousin Samuel in hostility to Parliament. Despising everyone who sought political office by royal appointment, he searched out opportunities to advance the interests of America and Americans.

In Virginia the Stamp Act had alerted another

The horse *America* throwing Lord North

trio of men whose names would likewise become unpleasantly familiar in London. Patrick Henry, as eloquent and almost as erratic as James Otis, gained instant fame by sponsoring Virginia's resolutions against the Stamp Act. George Washington, known to at least a few outside Virginia for his service in the late war, was more given to actions than to resolutions. He was at the House of Burgesses and may have voted for Henry's resolutions, but his thoughts went more toward home manufactures and new crops as a means of shaking off America's economic dependence on Great Britain. Thomas Jefferson, a twenty-two-year-old law student, was too young for politics in 1765. But he stood at the door of the House of Burgesses and listened to Henry's "torrents of sublime eloquence." Later Jefferson would show a certain eloquence himself.

Townshend's folly. The repeal of the Stamp Act set the bells ringing in England and America. But the Marquis of Rockingham, who had engineered the happy event, found himself unable to please either king or Parliament. In July 1766 he went the way of Grenville, and George III gave the government once again to William Pitt, now Earl of Chatham. Unfortunately, bad health made Pitt a mere figurehead, and the new government fell under the influence of the headstrong and irresponsible Chancellor of the Exchequer, Charles Townshend.

In taking up the search for revenue, Townshend, like Grenville, looked to the colonies. Fastening on their reviving trade as the likeliest source of new income, he persuaded Parliament in 1767 to pass an ill-considered act levying duties on colonial imports of lead, paint, paper, glass, and tea. Since these items could be legally imported only from England, the new taxes would actually discourage purchases from the mother country and encourage the manufacture of taxable goods in the colonies, thus violating every principle that British economic policy had hitherto supported. The taxes also violated the colonists' expressed views on the limits of Parliament's authority. And what was worse, the expressed intention of the duties was to pay the salaries of royal officials in the colonies, hitherto dependent on grants from the colonial assemblies. Without that dependence, the assemblies would lose their controlling position in government.

The colonial assemblies were at this time registering their unabated disapproval of Parliamentary taxes by resisting Grenville's Quartering Act, which they regarded as a form of taxation. To demonstrate their own superior authority, they voted to supply only part of the provisions that the act specified. Yet Townshend believed, mistakenly, that the colonists were becoming more amenable to taxation, especially to taxes on trade, because they were paying the duty on molasses. In 1766 the duty had been reduced to a penny a gallon, which approximated the cost of a bribe; it had also been extended to include molasses of British production. This new duty was clearly a tax and not a regulation of trade. Encouraged by the colonists' seeming compliance, Townshend decided that, if he but acted boldly, he could now settle the question of Parliament's authority in America for good and all.

To cow the assemblies into obeying the Quartering Act, he made an example of New York, one of the principal offenders: in 1767, at his bidding, Parliament declared all acts of the New York assembly to be void until the colony furnished full supplies for the troops quartered there. To ensure collection of his new taxes on trade and of older regulatory duties as well, Townshend directed a reorganization of the American customs service under a special board of commissioners residing in Boston, the center alike of colonial smuggling and of open resistance to taxation.

Americans did greet the Townshend Acts less violently than they had the Stamp Act, but they made it clear that they were still determined to rid themselves of Parliamentary taxation. In a series of eloquent newspaper letters, John Dickinson, a Philadelphia lawyer who had played a leading role in the Stamp Act Congress, repeated the arguments offered against the Stamp Act and showed that they applied equally to the Townshend Acts. Dickinson's "Letters from a Farmer" were printed and reprinted by virtually all the colonial newspapers. And the representative assemblies, stiffened by Dickinson's eloquence and by a circular letter from Massachusetts, again denied the authority of Parliament to tax the colonies. Under prodding from the Sons of Liberty, merchants again joined in nonimportation agreements, and again violators suffered popular indignation.

The new customs commissioners were as unpopular as the new duties. They were regarded as superfluous bureaucrats sent by a corrupt ministry to fatten on the toil of Americans. And, it was feared, they were only the first of many to come; soon the colonist would have to support as many functionless officeholders as the taxpayer in England did.

The commissioners lost no time in exceeding everyone's worst expectations. The procedures prescribed by the Sugar Act were immensely complicated; and it was easy for a merchant to make an unintentional mistake in carrying them out. By insisting on technicalities, an unscrupulous commissioner could usually find a pretext for seizing a ship and its cargo of goods. Rather than take the risk, most merchants were willing to grease the commissioners' palms. Anyone who refused to play the game was likely to have his ship condemned in an admiralty court: unless he could prove that he had fulfilled every provision of the law, the court would order his ship and cargo sold. One-third of the proceeds went to the English Treasury, one-third to the governor of the colony, and one-third to the customs officers prosecuting the case.

The officers had nothing to lose—except perhaps their lives. Even that danger was reduced when the commissioners persuaded the authorities in England to provide special protection against the hazards of their occupation. In September 1768 two regiments of troops were sent to Boston.

England's readiness to send the troops indicated how far its relations with the colonies had deteriorated and what caliber of men had taken over the empire. In 1768 Lord Hillsborough had just been made Secretary of State for the Colonies, a post created to handle the increasingly complex colonial business. His decision to send the troops to Boston may have sprung from ignorance of the situation there, but it was one of a series of blunders that prompted Benjamin Franklin to characterize his conduct in office as "perverse and senseless."

Other Americans had worse things to say. At the time of the Stamp Act the most radical objectors had suspected that it was only the first step in a design of the English ministry to reduce the colonists to absolute subjection, indeed to slavery. Resistance to the Stamp Act had thwarted the plan for the moment, but the measures that followed under Townshend seemed to be proof that the ministry had not given up. The sending of troops argued that they were putting the plan into full operation, for a standing army was the classic method by which would-be tyrants crushed resistance to their illegal and unconstitutional schemes.

When the troops arrived in Boston, therefore, Samuel Adams called for resistance. But few men were as yet ready to believe in a ministerial conspiracy. At the time the troops landed, the Massachusetts assembly was under suspension for refusing to rescind its circular letter against the Townshend Acts, and the extralegal convention that Adams organized in its place was unwilling to act on his radical demand.

The presence of the soldiers in Boston nevertheless spelled tyranny to Americans everywhere and showed again that the English ministry, if not bent on all-out tyranny, regarded Americans as not quite English. The soldiers themselves contributed to the impression by their arrogance. Even during the French and Indian War, when British and colonial troops were fighting side by side, the regulars had never disguised their contempt for the Americans. Now the feeling was returned with interest.

For a year and a half the soldiers lived in Boston, suffering icy stares, open taunts, and all the subtle harassments the citizens could devise. Hostility was steadily aggravated by the inflammatory speeches and publications of the indefatigable Samuel Adams on the one side and by the rapacity of the customs commissioners on the other. But there was no real violence until March 5, 1770. On that day a crowd looking for trouble found it in front of the Boston customhouse. They jeered the ten soldiers who stood guard before it, pelted them with oyster shells, snowballs, and sticks of wood, dared them to fire. The soldiers did fire, and eleven of the unarmed rioters were hit, five of them fatally. The massacre, as the Bostonians called it, roused such hostility to the troops that Lieutenant-

British troops quartered on the Boston Commons in 1768

Governor Thomas Hutchinson ordered them to Castle Island in the harbor. There they sat for the next four years.

Meanwhile a movement to repeal Charles Townshend's taxes was growing in England. Townshend died shortly after his acts were passed, and almost at once the English began to realize that the Townshend duties were a mistake. Even without the pressure of colonial nonimportation agreements, English merchants would have protested against taxes that encouraged colonial manufacturing. Many members of the king's council favored outright repeal of the duties, but once again the government was reluctant to back down in the face of colonial defiance. The new First Lord of the Treasury, Lord North, who took office January 31, 1770, suggested that all the duties that encouraged colonial manufactures be repealed and that only the duty on tea, which could not be grown in America, be retained. Since Americans were inordinately fond of tea, they were importing substantial quantities of it in spite of the duty. By keeping the duty in force, England would preserve an annual revenue of ten or twelve thousand pounds and would also sustain its authority.

Parliament adopted North's solution, and the king was pleased. North was the kind of politician George had been looking for—a plodding, dogged, industrious man, neither a fool nor a genius, much like the king himself. For the next twelve years, despite the opposition of abler men, he remained at the head of the government.

Toward Independence

North's repeal of all the Townshend duties except the one on tea was well calculated. In England it mollified both the merchants and the Parliamentary critics of the administration. In America it brought a revival of good feeling for the mother country. The Sons of Liberty met defeat when they demanded perseverance in the boycott of British goods until the tax on tea should be repealed. Merchants began importing, and trade boomed. Royal governors reported that only a factious few continued to object to British policies.

Discord and concord. As good will toward the mother country rose, the recent harmony among the colonists themselves gave way to new quarrels, from which England concluded, too hastily, that American unity was a fiction. Anglicans in the Northern colonies petitioned for the appointment of an American bishop; most Anglicans in the Southern colonies opposed such an appointment; Congregationalists and Presbyterians everywhere were horrified at the prospect but were unable to cement an effective union amongst themselves to work against it.

The West was also a source of friction again. In both North and South Carolina settlers in the back country complained that taxes were too high, court fees exorbitant, lawyers and government officers corrupt. In 1771 a large force of Westerners calling themselves Regulators rose against the government of North Carolina. An army of Easterners defeated them easily at the Battle of Alamance, but the clash left an enduring bitterness.

In other colonies disputes arose over the control of western lands. Connecticut claimed land on the Susquehanna River in northeastern Pennsylvania and even organized a county there. In England Connecticut agents pressed for official recognition of their claim and Pennsylvania agents for its rejection. Meanwhile Pennsylvanians and Virginians were squabbling over lands in the Ohio Valley.

England still adhered to the land policy outlined in the Proclamation of 1763—namely, that a boundary line should be maintained between settlers and Indians. But now, instead of following the crest of the Appalachians, the line was set farther west by treaties with various Indian tribes (with the Iroquois at Fort Stanwix in 1768, with the Cherokee at Hard Labor in 1768 and at Lochaber in 1770). Americans, however, were still competing vigorously for land beyond the line. A group of speculators from the middle colonies kept agents in England lobbying for the creation of a colony, to be known as Vandalia, south of the Ohio River. The site of the proposed colony was in territory claimed by Virginia, and the speculators of the Ohio Company angrily protested the scheme. The company was also quarreling with other Virginia speculators. Hillsborough refused to authorize the new colony.

To British politicians all these disagreements seemed more serious than they were, and colonial good will toward England seemed stronger than it was. The good will, though real, rested on the hope that Parliament was retreating from its new policies. American hostility to those policies was by no means extinguished, nor was it likely to be, so long as customs commissioners sat in Boston, the British navy patrolled American waters, and admiralty courts condemned American vessels without jury trial. Men like Samuel Adams were able to keep the colonists talking about colonial rights and Parliamentary tyranny by seeing to it that every new affront committed by the British was given wide publicity in the newspapers. And then, in 1772, at Adams' instigation the towns of Massachusetts appointed committees to formulate statements of American rights and grievances and to

The West: Indian treaties and speculative claims

correspond with one another on the subject. From Massachusetts the idea spread through the rest of New England; and in 1773, as a result of the *Gaspee* affair, it was taken up on an intercolonial basis.

The *Gaspee* was a British naval vessel, which, in 1772, patrolled Narragansett Bay and inflicted daily outrages upon the inhabitants: her commander seized small boats engaged in local traffic; her sailors cut orchards for firewood and helped themselves to livestock. When the *Gaspee* ran aground on one of her missions, the people of Providence came out after dark and burned her. It was a daring action and not the first of its kind. England decided to make an example of the colony. Suspecting that Rhode Island courts would make no serious effort to uncover the culprits, England appointed a special commission to investigate the incident. But Rhode Islanders would give no helpful testimony, and the commissioners never discovered the guilty parties.

The *Gaspee* commission attracted attention throughout America. Because it bypassed the Rhode Island courts, the colonists regarded it as an infringement of common-law procedures and consequently of the rights of Englishmen. In Virginia the assembly felt incited to establish a committee of correspondence for the whole colony (Patrick Henry was a member) and to propose that each of the other colonies appoint a committee of its own. When the proposal was accepted, Americans gained the machinery for coordinating their views and actions on any question affecting their common interests.

The Intolerable Acts. While men like Adams and Henry were laying the foundations of American union, Lord North was worrying over another immediate and pressing problem. England had left the administration of its empire in the East largely in the hands of a giant trading corporation, the East India Company; and the company was in serious financial trouble. After bringing it under more direct supervision of the British government, Lord North secured legislation to increase the company's profits from tea-drinking Americans.

The Tea Act of May 1773 relieved the company of various taxes in England and empowered it to export tea directly from its English warehouses to America, where it would be distributed by company agents. Hitherto the company had been required to sell its tea only by auction to English wholesale merchants, who sold it to American merchants, who in turn sold it to retailers. By eliminating the middlemen's profits and the company's taxes, North hoped to lower tea prices in America so sharply that the colonists would step up their purchases and put the East India Company back on its feet. The Americans would still have to pay the tax imposed by the Townshend Act, but even so they would be able to buy tea cheaper than ever before.

North, it soon became apparent, had misjudged the colonists. By the Tea Act he lost whatever ground he had won in America by repealing the other Townshend duties. Merchants who had been importing tea themselves resented being shut out of the competitive market by a powerful, privileged company. Even the consumers, who would have benefited

by the act, were hostile to it. Political leaders warned that the scheme was a trap to make Americans accept Parliamentary taxation. When the first shipments from London arrived in colonial ports, angry citizens forced the ships to return without unloading or stored the tea in warehouses from which no East India man dared remove it. In Boston, where Governor Hutchinson ruled that the ships could not depart without unloading their cargoes, a well-organized mob boarded the ships and pitched the tea into the harbor.

Lord North, who had had enough trouble with Boston, decided to punish the town with another demonstration of authority. Assisted by a new Secretary of State for the Colonies, Lord Dartmouth (Hillsborough had resigned in August 1772), he drafted the Boston Port Act, which ordered the port closed to shipping until the town made restitution for the tea. Parliament readily passed the act. North and Dartmouth might have been willing to stop there, but their fellow ministers insisted on proving Parliament's authority with three more acts (1774).

The Massachusetts Government Act altered the old constitution established by the charter of 1691 (see p. 51): henceforth the governor's council would be appointed by the king (rather than elected by the legislature) and town meetings would be held only once a year except by express permission of the governor. The Administration of Justice Act provided that any government or customs officer indicted for murder could be tried in England, beyond the control of local juries. A new Quartering Act authorized the quartering of troops within a town (instead of in the barracks provided by a colony) whenever their com-

The Boston Tea Party

manding officer thought it desirable. To underline the meaning of this act the British troops, with heavy reinforcements, were brought back into Boston from the fort in the harbor; and General Thomas Gage, the commander in chief of all the North American troops, was sent to act also as governor of the colony.

The colonists promptly dubbed these new measures the Intolerable Acts. They were followed by the Quebec Act, which had no punitive intention but which the colonists thought as outrageous as the others. Canada, since its acquisition in 1763, had been provisionally in the hands of a military governor; the Quebec Act gave the province a permanent government with no representative assembly, established French civil law, and offered special protection to the Catholic Church. Although Canada as a French colony had never had a representative assembly, Americans thought it ominous that Parliament had failed to establish one now that it was an English colony. It disturbed them even more that the act ignored colonial territorial claims by annexing the whole region west of the Appalachians and north of the Ohio to the province of Quebec. Now when settlers moved west they would have to live under Canada's autocratic government.

The Quebec Act and the Intolerable Acts were not the result of hasty or capricious decisions. The Quebec Act had been drafted only after lengthy discussions with officials who had been in Canada, and the Intolerable Acts incorporated certain changes that had often been recommended by royal governors and customs officers. The redesigning of the Massachusetts government in particular was a long-awaited assertion of Parliament's authority over colonial governments. It came, however, as Governor Bernard had feared it would, too late. By subjecting Massachusetts to direct Parliamentary control and by backing up that control with an army, Lord North and his colleagues thought they could teach Americans to respect the supremacy of Parliament. But the lesson the colonists learned was that the supremacy of Parliament meant an end to the power of their own representative assemblies and courts, an end to the right to trial by jury, an end to every political principle they held dear.

The committees of correspondence went into action immediately. Boston had once been known, and not loved, throughout the colonies for the hard bargaining of its merchants and the riotous behavior of its inhabitants. Now the town received universal admiration and sympathy. It was deluged with gifts of rice from the Carolinas, flour from Pennsylvania, and pledges of support from everywhere. To help carry out the pledges and to coordinate action against the Intolerable Acts, the committees of correspondence arranged for an intercolonial congress to meet in September.

The Quebec Act, 1774

The First Continental Congress. Fifty-five delegates from twelve colonies (Georgia sent none) assembled at Philadelphia in September 1774. As soon as the sessions began, it became apparent that the members were virtually unanimous in support of Massachusetts and ready to employ every sanction short of war to secure relief. Samuel Adams presented a set of resolutions that had just been passed by a convention in Suffolk County, Massachusetts, recommending outright resistance to the Intolerable Acts. The Congress unanimously adopted these Suffolk Resolves and went on to adopt, also unanimously, a nonimportation, nonexportation, and nonconsumption agreement, called "The Association," against trade of any kind with Great Britain, Ireland, and the West Indies.

In adopting the Association, Congress assumed an authority over the economic life of every American. To make that authority felt, it authorized the election of local committees "in every county, city, and town" throughout the colonies. The committees would search out violators of the agreement and publish their names, "to the end, that all such foes to the rights of British America may be publicly known, and universally condemned."

The members of Congress were clearly agreed that the Intolerable Acts must be resisted as a threat to American rights. But when they tried to formulate a statement of those rights and of the precise limits of Parliament's authority in America, they found themselves divided. In their disagreement, Joseph Galloway of Pennsylvania, perhaps the most conservative delegate, saw an opportunity for accommodation with England. He proposed a plan for imperial reorganization, which he wanted the congress to present to the king and Parliament. Galloway's plan called for a grand council of the colonies along the lines projected at the Albany Congress (see p. 82). Enactments of the council would be subject to Parliamentary review and veto; acts of Parliament affecting the colonies would likewise have to receive the approval of the grand council. But Galloway could not persuade the dele-

I know of no line that can be drawn between the supreme authority of Parliament and the total independence of the colonies: it is impossible there should be two independent Legislatures in one and the same state; for, although there may be but one head, the King, yet the two Legislative bodies will make two governments as distinct as the kingdoms of England and Scotland before the union. If we might be suffered to be altogether independent of Great Britain, could we have any claim to the protection of that government, of which we are no longer a part? Without this protection, should we not become the prey of one or the other powers of Europe, such as should first seize upon us? Is there anything which we have more reason to dread than independence? I hope it never will be our misfortune to know, by experience, the difference between the liberties of an English colonist, and those of the Spanish, French, or Dutch.

From Governor Thomas Hutchinson, Speech to the Council and House of Representatives of Massachusetts, 1773.

gates to subordinate their union to Parliament. In the years since the Stamp Act crisis they had had time and provocation to think further about their relationship to that body.

In 1765 the colonists had categorically denied that Parliament had the authority to tax them; and they had acquiesced in its general legislative authority over the whole empire, mentioning specifically only trade regulation and amendment of the common law as examples of what kind of legislation they thought acceptable. Apart from an unexplained stipulation in some of their resolutions that Parliament should not alter their "internal polity" (as it finally did in the Massachusetts Government Act of 1774), they had not defined the limits of Parliament's legislative authority over them.

Since 1765 many of them had decided that Parliament had no more right to make laws concerning them than it did to tax them. This idea had few adherents until the punishment of the New York assembly, the *Gaspee* commission, and the Intolerable Acts clearly demonstrated that Parliament could destroy men's rights as readily by legislation as by taxation. Thereafter the idea spread rapidly. Samuel Adams led the Massachusetts assembly in affirming it to Governor Hutchinson in 1773. In the summer of 1774 prospective members of the coming congress could read powerful demonstrations of it in two pamphlets. In *Considerations on the . . . Authority of the British Parliament*, James Wilson, a Pennsylvania lawyer, pointed out that all the familiar arguments against Parliamentary taxation applied equally well against Parliamentary legislation. Jefferson took the same position in *A Summary View of the Rights of British America*.

Neither Jefferson nor Wilson was present at the First Continental Congress, but enough of the dele-

gates agreed with them to defeat Galloway's plan. The radicals were unable, however, to bring the Congress to repudiate all colonial ties with Parliament. Of those who were no longer willing to admit that Parliament had any authority in the colonies, some still believed that it should be allowed to regulate colonial trade as a just compensation for the British navy's protection of colonial shipping. When the delegates came to framing a statement of colonial rights and grievances, John Adams finally got them to compromise on a resolution, drafted mostly by James Duane, that denied Parliament any authority over the colonies but agreed—as a matter of fairness and expediency—to submit to its acts for regulation of trade.

The Congress was inviting Parliament to return to the same supervisory role it had exercised in the colonies before 1763. Had Parliament been willing to do so, the breach, instead of widening, might have closed. The Earl of Chatham (William Pitt) and Edmund Burke both recognized the opportunity, but neither could muster more than a few votes for proposals to repeal the Intolerable Acts and renounce American taxation. Lord North, however, did secure passage in February 1775 of what he regarded as a conciliatory measure proposing to withhold Parliamentary taxation of any colony whose inhabitants taxed themselves "for contributing their proportion to the common defence." The proposal gave no indication of how much each colony's "proportion" might be or how large a total contribution would be required, and it was silent on the other issues raised by the Intolerable Acts and by the declarations of the Continental Congress. To Americans it appeared to be only an insidious attempt by the ministry to draw away individual colonies from the new union.

But English statesmen were in no mood for softer measures. Most of them were convinced that Samuel

Adams and his tribe were leading the colonists toward independence and that the march could be halted only by more forceful demonstrations of Parliamentary supremacy. The session that passed Lord North's conciliatory resolve also passed an act excluding New Englanders from the Newfoundland fisheries and prohibiting them from all trade except with the mother country and the British West Indies. At the same time the ministry took steps to prevent exportation of arms and ammunition to the colonies. Even the king expected the worst. "The New England Governments are in a State of Rebellion," he had told Lord North in November 1774. "Blows," he added, "must decide whether they are to be subject to this Country or Independent."

England clearly anticipated war, but its leaders had no conception of the size of the enemy. In spite of the increasingly obvious signs of colonial unity, Lord North and his colleagues persisted in regarding the enemy as Massachusetts alone. General Gage, sitting uneasily in the governor's chair in Massachusetts, did his best to disillusion them. The Americans, he reported, were as ready for blows as the English; to enforce Parliament's authority he would need twenty thousand men. Until England was prepared to send that many, he said, it would be well to suspend the Intolerable Acts.

George III thought Gage's dispatches absurd; Lord North turned from them to ask Parliament for a reduction in the size of Britain's armed forces. Gage was allowed about thirty-five hundred, and by the spring of 1775 he was himself persuaded that it was time to use them.

From Lexington to Bunker Hill. The general knew from his informers that the colonial militia were assembling arms and ammunition at strategic points. In Portsmouth, New Hampshire, they carried off a hundred barrels of powder belonging to the crown. Gage did not dare detach any part of his small force to recover the royal gunpowder, but occasionally he marched sizable columns for a few miles into the country around Boston, hoping by this show of strength to overawe incipient rebels. On April 14 he received instructions from Lord Dartmouth to take the offensive against the rebellious colonists, and on April 19 he sent seven hundred men to Concord to seize a supply of arms reportedly stored there.

Although the force got started in the dark of early

Lexington and Concord, April 19, 1775

morning, the tolling of alarm bells and the firing of signal guns showed that its errand was no secret. Anticipating trouble, the commanding officer sent back for reinforcements but ordered six companies under Major John Pitcairn to proceed. At Lexington, Pitcairn found colonial militia drawn up on the village green. At his command, they began to disperse. Then suddenly a shot rang out. Whether British or American, musket or pistol, accidental or deliberate, was not apparent; but when they heard the shot, the British soldiers fired a volley into the departing militiamen, killing eight of them and wounding ten.

This episode delayed the troops for only fifteen minutes, and by eight o'clock they were entering Concord. The Americans had already removed most of the military stores they had assembled there, but the British burned a few gun carriages and repulsed a group of militiamen who tried to drive them off. Two colonials and three British were killed in the skirmish. By noon the "battles" of Lexington and Concord were over, and the British troops started back to Boston.

Now a real battle began, a battle unlike any the troops had ever seen. Colonial militiamen for miles around had been alerted by a system of riders organized for just such an emergency, and the seven hundred British regulars were obliged to run a gauntlet of fire from three or four thousand Americans. At Lexington the returning troops were joined by nine hundred reinforcements, but still the Americans fired from rock and tree at the massed target of moving redcoats.

The total casualties on both sides were not large: the British lost 73 killed, 192 wounded, and 22 captured, the Americans, 49 killed, 39 wounded. But Gage's earlier fears had been justified: his offensive had turned into a rout. That night, as haggard British soldiers dragged themselves into Boston, watch fires dotted the landscape around the city: militia were beginning to move in from all over New England. Boston was already under siege by a people who had no proper army, no system of command, no regular government.

On June 17, less than two months later, Gage found how tightly he was held. Reinforced by sea with 1,100 troops and 3 major generals (William Howe, John Burgoyne, and Henry Clinton), he decided to roll back the siege. On the night of June 16, the Americans, forewarned of his plans, marched 1,200 men to Breed's Hill (just south of Bunker Hill, from which the ensuing action, for no good reason, received its name), overlooking Boston from the north. By morning, when 400 more joined them, they had dug a formidable redoubt.

That afternoon General Howe set out with 2,200 men to displace the rebels from their position. Since Breed's Hill was on a peninsula, Howe could have cut the Americans off by landing a force at their rear. Instead, he bombarded nearby Charlestown at the end of the peninsula and launched a frontal assault. The Americans inside the redoubt held their fire as the enemy, firing regularly and harmlessly, marched coolly up the hill. When the Americans returned the fire, the British went down in rows.

Howe regrouped his forces and tried again, with the same result. But now the Americans were low on ammunition, and the British regulars, reinforced by 600 men, finally charged the redoubt with bayonets. The Americans, clubbing their muskets, retreated slowly, leaving 140 of their men dead, 271 wounded, and 30 captured. Howe's victory had cost him 226 killed and 828 wounded. Another such victory, wrote Clinton ruefully, "would have ruined us." It had now

Boston and Charlestown, June 17, 1775

In 1827 Judge Mellen Chamberlain, then twenty-one, interviewed Captain Levi Preston of Danvers, then ninety-one and a veteran of the assault on the British retreating from Concord on April 19, 1775. The following dialogue ensued:

M. C. Captain Preston, why did you go to the Concord Fight, the 19th of April, 1775?

L. P. Why did I go?

M. C. Yes, my histories tell me that you men of the Revolution took up arms against "intolerable oppressions."

L. P. What were they? Oppressions? I didn't feel them.

M. C. What, were you not oppressed by the Stamp Act?

L. P. I never saw one of those stamps, and always understood that Governor Bernard put them all in Castle William. I am certain I never paid a penny for one of them.

M. C. Well, what then about the tea-tax?

L. P. Tea-tax! I never drank a drop of the stuff; the boys threw it all overboard.

M. C. Then I suppose you had been reading Harrington or Sidney and Locke about the eternal principles of liberty.

L. P. Never heard of 'em. We read only the Bible, the Catechism, Watt's Psalms and Hymns, and the Almanack.

M. C. Well, then, what was the matter? and what did you mean in going to the fight?

L. P. Young man, what we meant in going for those red-coats was this: we always had governed ourselves, and we always meant to. They didn't mean we should.

From Mellen Chamberlain, John Adams: the Statesman of the American Revolution, with other Essays and Addresses, Historical and Literary.

been demonstrated beyond dispute that Americans with guns were dangerous. The British never again underestimated the enemy they were fighting.

One people. While sixteen thousand colonial militia pinned down the British forces in Boston, other Americans were taking the necessary steps to support the war. Royal governors everywhere watched their authority collapse, as surely as Gage's had collapsed outside Boston. A few tried to organize loyalist support to combat the rebellion, but sooner or later they all gave up and fled to the safety of British warships. The colonial assemblies, which had hitherto met under royal authorization, now gathered as extralegal provincial congresses and began to act as independent governments, raising troops and issuing forbidden paper money to pay them. The transition in government presented no serious difficulty, because many representatives to the provincial congresses were former assemblymen and they simply carried on with their usual business.

A more extraordinary task faced the delegates who, in May 1775, assembled at Philadelphia for the Second Continental Congress (which had been arranged by the First Congress). Previous intercolonial meetings, the Albany Congress, the Stamp Act Congress, and the First Continental Congress, had devoted themselves to hammering out agreements of principle. But by the time the Second Congress met, the colonists were already deeply committed to common principles and a common cause. Fighting had just begun, and the delegates, instead of conducting another debating council, found themselves conducting America's first central government: they assumed responsibility for the provincial militia besieging Boston, ordered their transformation into a Continental Army, named George Washington as commander, issued paper money to support the troops, and appointed a committee to negotiate with foreign countries.

Although in taking these actions the Congress assumed many of the powers of an independent government, the members still did not intend to establish an independent nation. Delegates from the middle colonies, led by John Dickinson, were very reluctant to take any steps in that direction. Repudiation of Parliament was not repudiation of England, and the Congress did not see why Englishmen in America and in England should not retain their brotherhood in loyalty to a common king. In July they appealed to their fellow subjects in Great Britain and also laid their cause at the feet of the king with a petition asking him personally to promote repeal of the oppressive measures. Significantly they placed the blame for those measures on the ministry—"those artful and cruel enemies who abuse your royal confidence and authority for the purpose of effecting our destruction." They issued at the same time a "Declaration of the causes and necessity for taking up arms," in which they explained that they were "reduced to the alternative of choosing an unconditional submission to the tyranny of irritated ministers, or resistance by force." In choosing resistance, they said, they had no "ambitious designs of separating from Great Britain, and establishing independent states." As soon as England acknowledged their rights, they would lay down their arms.

Although some Americans had already begun to think of independence, the declarations of the Congress were made in good faith. Even at this date the repeal of the Intolerable Acts and the restriction of Parliamentary legislation to the regulation of trade might have kept the colonists in the empire. They still thought of their rights as the rights of Englishmen and of their union as a means of protecting those rights. But George III and Lord North were bent on subjecting the colonists to a Parliament in which they elected no representative. The king did not answer their petition; Parliament did, however, answer their "declaration"—by voting to send twenty-five thousand more troops against them. The addition would bring British military strength in America to forty thousand. In August the king issued a proclamation declaring the colonies in a state of rebellion, and in December Parliament passed an act outlawing all their trade and subjecting their ships and goods to confiscation.

Each British action weakened the colonists' emotional attachment to England. The principal ingredient in their national feeling had been admiration for the British form of government, which better than any other guaranteed the human rights of its subjects. When their admiration for Parliament crumbled, they had fastened the last shreds of their loyalty on the king alone. But he had enthusiastically supported Parliament against them. If the whole English government was determined to destroy the rights of its subjects, then it was a dubious privilege to be English.

In January 1776 the new image of George III as a tyrant was presented to the colonists with biting eloquence in a publication called simply *Common Sense.* The author, Thomas Paine, an Englishman who had arrived in America only in 1774, argued that it was foolish for Americans to stake their lives and fortunes simply to obtain a repeal of Parliamentary laws. "The object contended for," he said, "ought always to bear some just proportion to the expence. . . . Dearly, dearly, do we pay for the repeal of the acts, if that is all we fight for." Common sense forbade that Americans should remain loyal to a king who sanctioned the spilling of their blood. In fact monarchy itself was an absurdity, a form of government that had laid the world in blood and ashes. "Of more worth," declared Paine, "is one honest man to society and in the sight of God, than all the crowned ruffians that ever lived." Here Paine struck a responsive chord. Since the days of Cromwell republican government had never ceased to have its devotees both in Great Britain and in America, and the old distrust of kings had never entirely died out. The colonists' very devotion to the House of Hanover was in part an expression of this distrust, an oblique way of denouncing the House of Stuart (which the Hanoverians had replaced) and of affirming the right of a people to change kings. By calling on Americans to cast off kings altogether, Thomas Paine kindled a latent enthusiasm for republican government.

In the six months that followed the publication of *Common Sense,* sentiment in favor of independence and republicanism grew rapidly. Many who hoped that George III would save American liberty had been convinced by Paine that no king could help them. Many who had considered independence impossible to attain now began to change their minds. Ever since Lexington, American forces throughout the colonies had been fighting the British, and with every shot fired the likelihood of reconciliation diminished. As men thought beyond the mere repeal of Parliamentary laws, they began to cut their ties with England and England's king. The provincial congress of South Carolina established a republican constitution in March, and in May the Rhode Island congress repealed the law requiring allegiance to the king. North Carolina in April and Virginia in May instructed their delegates in the Continental Congress to vote for independence.

The Continental Congress, with representatives from thirteen colonies (delegates from Georgia had arrived in September 1775), was itself behaving more and more like an independent national government. In March it authorized privateering against British ships. In April it forbade the further importation of slaves and declared other trade open to all the world except Great Britain. In May, urged by John Adams, it even recommended that any member colonies who had not already done so should suppress all vestiges of royal authority within their borders and establish governments resting on popular consent.

By this time Adams and many other delegates from New England and the Southern colonies were prepared to make an outright declaration of independence. They were restrained only by the reluctant rebels of the middle colonies. Although virtually the whole Congress had by now concluded that Parliament had no constitutional authority at all in America, some Americans still felt bound to England by a lingering loyalty to the king and a sentimental attachment to the English people. By the end of June the continuing war had worn both feelings thin. Independence was becoming more and more attractive and a declaration of it perhaps necessary to show foreign countries that Americans were playing for keeps. To sustain the war, the colonists needed help—arms and ammunition and maybe men—from England's European enemies. But England was powerful, and no one wished to be exposed to its wrath by subsidizing a rebellion that might collapse into a reconciliation. When rumors mounted that England was engaged in a

John Adams, Roger Sherman, Robert Livingston, Thomas Jefferson, and Benjamin Franklin present their handiwork to the Congress in John Trumbull's _Declaration of Independence_

Machiavellian maneuver to forestall foreign assistance to the colonies and was proposing to France and Spain that they partition the North American continent among the three of them, it seemed high time for Americans to come to a decision. On July 2, the Congress finally agreed to a motion that had been introduced by Richard Henry Lee of Virginia nearly a month before: "That these United Colonies are, and of right ought to be free and independent states." Thomas Jefferson, assisted by Franklin and John Adams, expanded the resolution into the famous declaration that was adopted on July 4.

Jefferson's declaration was an eloquent application of the ideas made familiar by John Locke and by a century and a half of American experience. It affirmed the origin of government in the consent of the governed, its obligation to protect natural rights, and the duty of a people to alter or abolish a government that failed to fulfill its obligation. That the British government had failed was demonstrated by a long list of misdeeds. These were attributed not to Parliament, whose authority the colonists had already denied, but to the king, the only remaining link between the colonies and England. Every grievance suffered by Americans since 1763 was laid at his door. The indictment was not altogether realistic, but it effectively expressed the American rejection not only of George III but of monarchy itself. Embedded in the preamble was evidence that the colonists had learned the lesson England had taught: "When in the course of human events, it becomes necessary for one people to dissolve the political bands which have connected them with another. . . ." The English were "another" people; and the colonists, who twenty-two years before had rejected the union proposed at Albany, now spoke of themselves as "one people."

Suggestions for Reading

The period covered by this chapter was first treated in the grand manner by George Bancroft in Vols. IV–VII of his *History of the United States*, 10 vols. (1834–74); Bancroft is still grand reading. Although subsequent historians have been able to correct him on many points, few if any have matched him in comprehensive knowledge of the sources. Where Bancroft saw events with the future of the United States always in mind, G. L. Beer, in *British Colonial Policy, 1754–1765* (1907), viewed the French and Indian War from a British point of view. L. H. Gipson sees events in America in relation to Britain's imperial problems throughout the world in *The British Empire Before the American Revolution*, 15 vols. (1936–70). Vols. V–VIII deal with the French and Indian War, renamed "The Great War for the Empire." Vols. IX–XII cover the years from 1763 to 1776.

The understanding of British politics in the 1760s and 1770s has been considerably altered since Bancroft's time. The older views were well expressed in G. O. Trevelyan's magnificently written *The American Revolution*, 4 vols. (1898–1907, reprinted 1964). L. B. Namier, in *The Structure of Politics at the Accession of George III*, 2 vols. (1929), and *England in the Age of the American Revolution* (1930), argued that the party system assumed by Trevelyan did not yet exist and that George III was a better monarch than anyone had supposed. Bernard Donoughue, *British Politics and the American Revolution: The Path to War, 1773–75* (1965), spells out the implications of Namier's views, as does John Brooke, *King George III** (1972), a well-informed biography of the king. Namier's approach is now giving way to one that stresses the rise of popular participation in politics, as in John Brewer, *Party Ideology and Popular Politics at the Accession of George III** (1976). A valuable study of the radical political tradition in England is Caroline Robbins, *The Eighteenth-Century Commonwealthman* (1959).

Clarence Alvord, *The Mississippi Valley in British Politics*, 2 vols. (1916), is a classic study of British policy toward the American West. This should be supplemented by T. P. Abernethy, *Western Lands and the American Revolution* (1937), and J. M. Sosin, *Whitehall and the Wilderness: The Middle West in British Colonial Policy, 1760–1775* (1961).

The best overall history of the Revolution is Robert Middlekauff, *The Glorious Cause* (1982). A fuller account of the years 1763–76, stressing political history, is Merrill Jensen, *The Founding of a Nation* (1968). E. S. Morgan, *The Birth of the Republic** (1956), is a brief account of the period 1763–89. There are numerous specialized studies of particular developments that contributed to the Revolution. J. A.

Ernst, *Money and Politics in America, 1755–1775* (1973), deals with British fiscal policy, especially the Currency Act of 1764. O. M. Dickerson, *The Navigation Acts and the American Revolution** (1951), argues that the Navigation Acts were not a cause of the Revolution. A. M. Schlesinger, *The Colonial Merchants and the American Revolution, 1763–1776** (1917), shows how the merchants initially took the lead in opposition to England but became wary as popular feeling seemed to threaten their own position. John Shy, *Toward Lexington** (1965), traces the role of the British troops in bringing on the Revolution. B. W. Labaree, *The Boston Tea Party** (1964), shows how this event precipitated the crisis. H. B. Zobel, *The Boston Massacre** (1970), emphasizes the provocations that led the British to fire. A contemporary Tory view of the coming of the Revolution, pungently expressed, is Peter Oliver, *Origin and Progress of the American Rebellion**, Douglas Adair and John Schutz, eds. (1961). David Ammerman, *In the Common Cause** (1974), is a fresh analysis of American response to the Coercive Acts. Jay Fliegelman, *Prodigals and Pilgrims* (1982), places the Revolution in the context of eighteenth-century attitudes toward patriarchal authority.

Several books discuss the political and constitutional principles developed by the colonists before 1776. E. S. and H. M. Morgan, *The Stamp Act Crisis: Prologue to Revolution** (1953), describes the events and ideas of the years 1764–66; and E. S. Morgan, *Prologue to Revolution: Sources and Documents on The Stamp Act Crisis, 1764–1766** (1959), reprints many of the resolutions, petitions, newspaper articles, and pamphlets in which the colonists expressed their views. Later development of colonial opinion is treated in Carl Becker, *The Declaration of Independence** (1922), and R. G. Adams, *The Political Ideas of the American Revolution** (1922). J. P. Reid, *In a Defiant Stance* (1977) and *In Defiance of the Law* (1981), gives new perspectives on the legal and constitutional issues. Two works offer fresh and challenging interpretations of the Declaration of Independence: Garry Wills, *Inventing America** (1978), and Morton White, *The Philosophy of the American Revolution* (1978). Bernard Bailyn, ed., *The Pamphlets of the American Revolution, 1750–1776* (1965), reprints the most important tracts on the American side, with an important introduction analyzing the arguments, printed separately as *The Ideological Origins of the American Revolution** (1967). Richard Merritt employs techniques of modern political science to trace the rise of American nationalism in *Symbols of American Community, 1735–1775* (1966). Pauline Maier, *From Resistance to Revolution: Colonial Radicals and the Development of American Opposition to Britain, 1765–1776** (1972), traces the evolution of popular hostility to England.

A number of able books describe the internal developments within different colonies in the years preceding independence. R. E. Brown, *Middle-Class Democracy and the Revolution in Massachusetts, 1691–1780** (1955), stresses the absence of internal class conflict, but R. J. Taylor finds more evidence of such conflict in the West in *Western Massachusetts in the Revolution* (1954), as does S. E. Patterson, *Political Parties in Revolutionary Massachusetts* (1973). A good close-up of Boston is found in G. B. Warden, *Boston, 1689–1776* (1970). David Lovejoy, *Rhode Island Politics and the American Revolution, 1760–1776* (1958), traces political divisions and shows that all sides in Rhode Island were united against the British. Carl Becker, *The History of Political Parties in the Province of New York, 1760–1776** (1909), shows that in New York the Revolution was a contest not only about home rule but also about "who should rule at home." Becker's views are modified in P. U. Bonomi, *A Factious People** (1971) and extended in Edward Countryman, *A People in Revolution* (1981). Similar studies for other states are Theodore Thayer, *Pennsylvania Politics and the Growth of Democracy, 1740–1776* (1953); J. H. Hutson, *Pennsylvania Politics, 1746–1770* (1972); R. A. Ryerson, *The Revolution Is Now Begun* (1978); C. A. Barker, *The Background of the Revolution in Maryland* (1940); Ronald Hoffman, *A Spirit of Dissension: Economics, Politics, and the Revolution in Maryland* (1973); D. C. Skaggs, *Roots of Maryland Democracy, 1753–1776* (1973); R. E. and B. K. Brown, *Virginia 1705–1786: Democracy or Aristocracy* (1964); C. S. Sydnor, *Gentlemen Freeholders* (1952); Carl Bridenbaugh, *Seat of Empire: The Political Role of Eighteenth Century Williamsburg* (1950); Rhys Isaac, *The Transformation of Virginia* (1982); A. R. Ekrich, *Poor Carolina* (1981); and Oscar Zeichner, *Connecticut's Years of Controversy, 1750–1776* (1950). An important volume of essays discussing internal class conflicts in several different states is Alfred Young, ed., *The American Revolution: Explorations in the History of American Radicalism** (1976).

*Available in a paperback edition.

5
AN AMERICAN
PEOPLE

Although the colonists had moved slowly and reluctantly toward declaring independence, once the deed was done most of them had no regrets. There were, of course, loyalists, whose sympathies remained with England. They varied in number from place to place, but the best modern estimates put the total at no more than a fifth or sixth of the colonial population. Many of the most ardent left for Canada or England. Of those who remained, some were ready to fight their countrymen for their king—some, but never enough to win. There were also men indifferent to who ruled them and willing to sell supplies to either side, depending on the price offered. But in every colony that joined in the Declaration of Independence, the patriots were sufficiently numerous, vociferous, and aggressive to outweigh the loyalists and the indifferent. Once the royal governments collapsed, it proved impossible to revive British authority except in the immediate vicinity of British guns.

The Winning of Independence

The rebel army. Perhaps because they could over-awe the loyalists, the patriots counted too easily on doing the same to the British armies. After the rout on April 19 and the slaughter on June 17 (see pp. 103–105), they were inclined to believe that their militia could handle any force the British sent against them. George Washington knew better; the men encamped

around Boston did have spirit, courage, and marks-manship, but they were not an army. To make them into one was Washington's first concern after taking command at Cambridge on July 3, 1775.

It was not simply a matter of instruction and training in the art of war. Militia units had to be reorganized under a corps of officers appointed from above. In the process, many of the old officers lost rank and stalked off in a huff. Furthermore, many of the militia who had come to besiege Boston had elected their own officers and were touchy about taking orders from higher up. They were also used to short terms of service (for a local emergency or a particular campaign) and eager to get home to their crops. Wherever the enemy appeared, Americans from miles around would turn out to fight him; but they did not want to join the army. To join the army was to desert one's family for danger, discomfort, and disease hundreds of miles from home. The pay was low, and no pension system existed to compensate a man or his family for the loss of life or limb. It therefore took all of Washington's diplomacy and tact to persuade ten thousand militiamen to enlist until the end of 1776 as regular soldiers in the Continental Army. In addition the provincial governments supplied him with about seven thousand short-term militiamen.

The total was much smaller than Washington had hoped for. Throughout the war Congress was able to provide him with an ample army of men on paper. But men with arms, legs, heads, and guns remained in short supply. Since Congress had no power either to

The surrender of Cornwallis

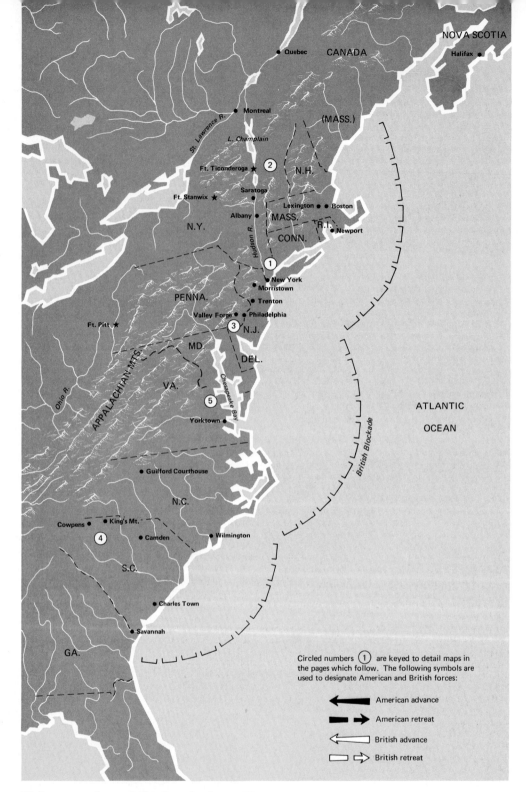

Major campaigns of the Revolutionay War

raise money or to draft men, it was dependent on requisitions to the states for both; and when the states lagged in supplying their assigned quotas, Congress could do nothing to coerce them. Supplies were as hard to come by as men; Washington had to spend much of his time pleading for both, and he had to fight the war with an army that was constantly in danger of dissolution.

The new army's first venture away from Boston began while Boston was still under siege, before independence was declared. Congress had invited the people of Canada to join their union, and, though the Canadians had failed to respond, some reports suggested that they would welcome an invading army. In any case, it was desirable to strike at the British in Quebec and Montreal in order to forestall an attack from that direction. After a grueling winter march, the effective forces that converged on Quebec amounted to only a thousand men, and the Canadians showed no disposition to help them. Colonel Benedict Arnold and General Richard Montgomery, who had already taken Montreal on his way north, besieged the city through the winter; but smallpox, hunger, cold, and an unsuccessful assault so thinned their ranks that in the spring they retreated to Ticonderoga. The colonists made no further military effort to draw Canada into their union.

In the South the Americans fared better. In June 1776, when Generals Henry Clinton and Charles, Lord Cornwallis, and Admiral Sir Peter Parker arrived at Charles Town, South Carolina, with fifty ships and an army of three thousand men, they made every mistake possible and were turned back by fire from a single fort constructed of palmetto logs and dirt. After a ten-hour duel the British withdrew and left Charles Town alone for the next four years.

In Massachusetts, Washington had meanwhile built a force strong enough to close in on Boston. He began by occupying and fortifying Dorchester Heights, which overlooked the city on the south as Breed's Hill did on the north. This time the British did not try to storm the hills. Instead, on March 17,

① **Washington's moves in New York and New Jersey, 1776–77**

Sir William Howe

1776, they departed by sea for Halifax, Nova Scotia, taking over a thousand loyalists with them.

A few months after the British evacuation of Boston, when Americans declared their independence, they appeared to be in a strong position. Although they were challenging the world's greatest military and naval power and had failed to win Canada to their cause, they had overpowered the British army in the march from Concord, withstood its assaults at Breed's Hill, forced its withdrawal from Boston, and fought off the British navy at Charles Town. But the British war machine, always a slow starter, was now grinding into action. Parliament had authorized an army of fifty-five thousand, and, when recruitment lagged in England, the government hired thirty thousand German mercenaries, seventeen thousand of them from Hesse-Cassel (hence the name Hessians). General William Howe and his brother, Admiral Richard Lord Howe, were given command.

The Howes were authorized to end the war as soon as the colonists submitted. Hoping to end it before they began, they addressed a conciliatory letter to "George Washington, Esq." (thus ignoring his military status). But General Washington was not receiving letters for George Washington, Esq., letters that denied American independence even in the address. The Howes therefore proceeded according to plan. On August 12, 1776, they arrived in New York harbor with thirty-two thousand troops and ten thousand seamen (the city's normal population was twenty-five thousand) aboard four hundred transports and thirty warships. Ten days later twenty thousand of the troops landed on Long Island near Brooklyn.

Washington had twenty-three thousand men in the New York area, but most of them were inexperienced local militia. When Howe, with plenty of men to spare, launched both frontal and flank attacks, Washington was forced to withdraw to Manhattan with heavy losses. Thinking that this taste of British power might have chastened the Americans, Howe offered to confer about a settlement before any more blows were struck. Congress sent Franklin, John Adams, and Edward Rutledge to deal with him, but the resulting conference broke off when it turned out, as Washington had suspected, that Howe was empowered to negotiate only with submissive colonists, not with the proud representatives of an independent nation. In September the British drove Washington off Manhattan Island; and by November the Continental Army, depleted by captures and desertions, was in full retreat across New Jersey.

Washington crossed the Delaware River into Pennsylvania on December 7. Now, with the river between him and the enemy, he planned his next move. The outlook was bleak. While pursuing him across New Jersey, the British had been able simultaneously to send a large force to Rhode Island, where on December 8 they occupied Newport. Washington's force was down to fewer than eight thousand effective fighting men, all of them dispirited, exhausted, ready to quit. By the end of the month all but fifteen hundred would have completed their term of enlistment, and with winter coming on they would sling their packs, head for home, and let someone else fight the war. While he still had them, Washington attacked. On the night of December 25, 1776, in high, freezing winds, he shuttled his men back across the river, marched them nine miles to Trenton, and caught the enemy asleep and befuddled. With a loss of only four men he took nine hundred prisoners. The brilliant reversal so cheered the troops that Washington was able to persuade many of them to reenlist. A few days later at Princeton he dealt the British another smashing blow, and they pulled back to New Brunswick for the winter. With spirits high again, the Continental Army moved into winter quarters at Morristown.

General Howe, contemplating the reverses that Washington had dealt him, had difficulty making up his mind about what to do when spring should come. After changing plans several times he finally decided to storm the rebel capital of Philadelphia, which, like New York, contained a large loyalist population. In July he took fifteen thousand men by sea from New York to the head of Chesapeake Bay. From there they marched north toward Philadelphia, the Hessians helping themselves to food, furniture, and women along the way. Washington intercepted them at Brandywine Creek; but, as on Long Island, Howe won the pitched battle and entered Philadelphia on September 26, 1777. When Washington challenged him

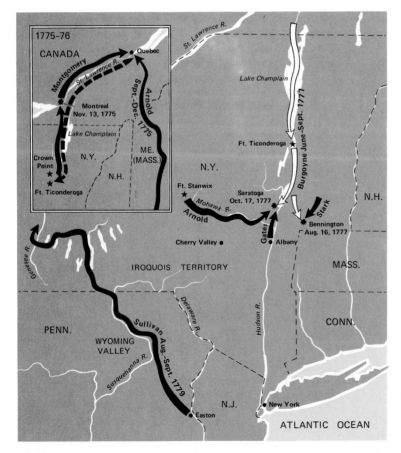

② **The war in the North, 1775-79**

The Battle of Princeton by William Mercer

a week later at Germantown, where most of the British troops were quartered, foggy weather broke up a powerful American attack, and Howe again was victorious.

These defeats discouraged the colonists, but actually Howe's success was hollow. Though he had captured America's largest cities and repeatedly defeated its generals, he had captured no armies and controlled only a small portion of American territory. And to the north of him disaster was brewing. General John Burgoyne had been authorized by the high

British view of the American soldier

command in England to mount an expedition for a march south from Canada by the Lake Champlain route. He set out from Fort St. John's in June with four thousand British, three thousand Germans, fourteen hundred Indians, and a pleasing mistress to cheer him along. Everything went swimmingly for a time. But American forces, under Horatio Gates and Benedict Arnold, gathered ever stronger before him, and each time they clashed Burgoyne lost several hundred men. On October 17, 1777, he finally surrendered at Saratoga.

The French alliance. Saratoga was one of the turning points of history, but not because it turned back any threat to the American armies. Burgoyne's march, if successful, would have signified little in a military sense; his surrender did not seriously reduce the British margin of superiority in troops and equipment. Saratoga had its great effect, not in New York or Philadelphia, but in London and Paris.

In London a complacent Parliament began to sense the possibility that England might lose the war. Better make peace, the ministry decided, and it authorized a commission headed by Lord Carlisle to offer the Americans virtually everything they had previously demanded: renunciation of Parliamentary taxation, repeal of the Intolerable Acts, and suspension of every other objectionable act passed since 1763. Two years earlier such concessions would probably have kept the colonies within the empire. But by now the rebels found independence exhilarating. England's eagerness to have them back merely furnished them with the final weapon they needed to make their independence last: the recognition and assistance of France.

From the outset the Americans had been hoping for help from England's traditional enemy, and on

Franklin played the role to the hilt

The three men constituted a commission with power to make treaties of amity and commerce.

The French at this time envisaged America as an Arcadia peopled by noble savages and almost equally noble farmers, rich in nature's wisdom; Franklin, seeing what was expected, donned his fur cap and played the role to the hilt. Completely enchanted, the Parisians showered the arch-American with favors, but Vergennes and his royal master remained cautious. Besides furnishing supplies to the colonists, they sometimes allowed American privateers the use of French harbors. They hesitated, however, to join in open war on England when the British armies, with the capture of New York, appeared to be winning.

As American military fortunes declined, Congress instructed the commissioners to go beyond their request for French assistance and to seek the deeper commitment of an alliance. All Franklin's charm was insufficient to win it. Vergennes wanted Spain by his side before he took on the British lion, and Spain was unwilling. Spain feared even to give open assistance to the Americans lest it encourage its own colonies to revolt.

Vergennes nevertheless prepared for war, with or without Spanish assistance, and was already moving toward a decision when news of Saratoga reached Paris on December 3, 1777. Vergennes perceived at once that the American victory might produce a conciliatory temper in England, and the last thing he wanted was to see the rebellious colonies reconciled to the mother country. Franklin played on his fears, and Vergennes sent frantic messages to Spain. When Spain remained immovable, he finally told the commissioners that France was ready to enter into a treaty of commerce and amity and a treaty of alliance with the Americans. He indeed required an alliance before entering the war, in order to prevent the United States from making peace before England was humbled.

The terms of the alliance, signed on February 6, 1778, were all that the United States could have wished for. The stated purpose of both parties was to maintain the independence of the United States. In case of war between France and England (which the signing of the treaty made inevitable), neither France nor the United States was to make peace without the consent of the other. France renounced all future claims to English territory on the continent of North America and agreed that any such territory captured in the war would go to the United States. These generous terms were less the result of American diplomatic skill than of French determination to weaken England and French distaste for further colonizing in the New World.

Even before the alliance the Americans had depended heavily on aid from France. The victory at Saratoga, for example, would have been impossible

November 29, 1775, Congress had appointed a secret committee to seek foreign aid. Louis XVI, delighted by the rebellion of England's colonies, had sent Achard de Bonvouloir to observe the situation in America. With Bonvouloir's encouragement the committee dispatched Silas Deane, a shrewd and sophisticated Yankee, to negotiate with France. Deane arrived in Paris on July 7, 1776, to find that the French foreign minister, the Comte de Vergennes, had already persuaded the king to help the American rebellion with a million livres' worth of munitions and supplies. Furthermore, Spain had matched the amount. The goods were to be dispensed secretly through a fake trading company run by Pierre Beaumarchais (author of *The Barber of Seville*). They were Deane's for the asking, though whether as a gift or as a loan remained uncertain.

Deane's negotiations took place before news of the Declaration of Independence reached France, when secret assistance was all the Americans dared ask for. Once the declaration had been announced, they hoped that France would recognize their independence and offer open assistance. To help Deane push these more ambitious requests, Congress sent Arthur Lee, a Virginian who had been serving the American cause in London, and Benjamin Franklin, who arrived from Philadelphia in December 1776.

without French supplies. And French financial support helped to bolster American credit at a time when Congress, with no authority to tax, was financing the war with money begged from the states or manufactured by the printing presses. With the signing of the alliance the hopes of the Americans soared, for France was the first nation to recognize them as "one people," and France had the military and naval power to make that recognition meaningful.

From Saratoga to Yorktown. After the battle of Saratoga the British fought a cautious war, their dreams of easy victory gone. Howe, snug in Philadelphia during the winter of 1777–78, did not even try to attack Washington's wretched forces, who were starving and freezing in their winter quarters at nearby Valley Forge. In the spring Howe was replaced by Sir Henry Clinton, who was to prove somewhat less languid though no bolder. The spring of 1778 also brought France's entry into the war and American refusal of the Carlisle Commission's peace overtures (see p. 115). Uncertain of where France would throw its weight, the British high command decided to play safe and ordered Clinton to withdraw from Philadelphia to New York. There he should plan a major campaign in the South, where—according to the strategists—loyalists would lend a decisive hand.

③ **Central campaigns, 1777–79**

At Valley Forge, as mild weather came on, Washington's forces thawed out and were drilled with Prussian precision by Baron Friedrich von Steuben, an idealist from the Old World who had come to help usher in the independence of the New. By June he and a good supply of provisions had turned the haggard men into a hard and maneuverable army. When Clinton pulled out of Philadelphia to march across New Jersey to New York, Washington kept pace with him on a parallel route and watched for a chance to strike. But the only opportunity that came (the Battle of Monmouth Courthouse on June 28) was badly bungled by General Charles Lee, and the main body of Clinton's troops arrived safely in New York.

While the British and American armies were marching across New Jersey, the first French forces arrived in America—Vice Admiral the Comte d'Estaing with seventeen ships and four thousand troops. Washington proposed to use them in recovering Newport. But in August, just before the American-French assault was to begin, a storm scattered and damaged the French fleet, and the unsupported land forces withdrew when British reinforcements arrived. D'Estaing took his ships to Boston to refit and, in November 1778, sailed south to protect the French West Indies.

The departure of D'Estaing was a serious disappointment to Washington, for the Americans had no means of their own to combat the British navy. It offered deadly support to British land troops along the coast, and it regularly sent raiding parties to devastate towns far from any army. Though the Americans commissioned hundreds of privateers (probably over two thousand in all), which rendered invaluable service in disrupting the merchant shipping, communications, and supply lines of the enemy, the privateers were no more a navy than the militia were an army; they were simply not up to engaging British warships in a sustained action.

The Congress had tried to create a navy, but it could scrape together the money for only a few ships, which were no match for the Royal Navy. Nevertheless, one of them, commanded by the unpopular but unsinkable John Paul Jones, carried the war to the British Isles, raiding coastal towns and seizing British ships. Unfortunately there were not enough Joneses to divert the British navy from North America, and Clinton kept most of his troops near the coast within reach of naval assistance. Without naval assistance of his own Washington dared not risk an all-out assault on the British army, and after following it from New Jersey to New York he had camped outside the city at White Plains and waited for the French fleet to return or to draw the British ships to other waters. For a year and a half he waited while the fighting was carried on mostly by small forces remote from New York, the strategic center. In the fall of 1779 all prospect of French naval support disappeared when D'Estaing took his fleet from the West Indies back to France.

Meanwhile a British expeditionary force had occupied Georgia, and Clinton prepared to go ahead with the Southern campaign he had been ordered to conduct. Leaving an army equal to Washington's to hold New York, he pulled his troops out of Newport (thus freeing New England of all British troops) and, in December 1779, sailed with an expeditionary force of over eight thousand for Charles Town, South Carolina. He took it on May 12, 1780, along with its defending general, Benjamin Lincoln, and his entire force of fifty-five hundred men. The Carolinas now lay open to a British sweep. On June 8 Clinton sailed for New York, leaving Cornwallis in command with instructions to secure the British hold on South Carolina and then to recover North Carolina. Cornwallis was at first successful. On August 16, 1780, near Camden, he intercepted and routed over three thousand men under General Horatio Gates who were coming to the defense of South Carolina. Washington sent General Nathanael Greene, his ablest commander, to pick up the pieces.

With the assistance of Daniel Morgan, a Virginia rifleman, Greene built a mobile fighting unit, which owed much to the Southern militiamen who appeared whenever a fight was in the offing. A group of these tough campaigners had already demonstrated their worth before Greene arrived by capturing a British force atop King's Mountain in North Carolina (October 7, 1780). Greene and Morgan lured Cornwallis into trap after trap, chewing off a bit of his force here and a bit there (notably at Hannah's Cowpens on the

⑤ **The convergence of troops on Yorktown, 1781**

Broad River, January 17, 1781, and at Guilford Courthouse, March 15).

In April 1781 the two generals turned their backs on each other: Greene headed south to pick off more British outposts in South Carolina and Georgia, while Cornwallis, having failed in the Carolinas, set out to conquer Virginia. By July, after a few inconclusive engagements, he had settled at Portsmouth, from which he later moved to Yorktown. Portsmouth and Yorktown both lay on the seacoast, the only safe place for a British army in America; but the coast would remain safe only so long as the British navy commanded the sea. And Yorktown, at the end of the peninsula between the York and the James rivers, was particularly vulnerable (earlier in the war Washington had warned one of his own generals not to encamp there for fear of being cut off). Without naval support Cornwallis could be isolated from his own forces in Charles Town and Savannah and from Clinton's forces in the North.

In New York Clinton still looked out at Washington's waiting army, and Washington still waited for the French navy. The French had sent five thousand land troops under the Comte de Rochambeau to occupy Newport in July 1780, but the eleven warships that accompanied them under the Comte de Barras had been promptly bottled up inside the harbor by a superior British fleet.

In August 1781 Washington's patience was finally rewarded by news that Admiral de Grasse with twenty warships was heading for the Chesapeake but would be able to stay only a short time. Washington immediately decided to dash south for a try at Cornwallis. Leaving behind a part of his New York troops to fool Clinton, he marched the rest to the head of Chesapeake Bay and placed them aboard transports for the last leg of the journey. Additional forces under An-

④ **Southern campaigns, 1778–81**

thony Wayne and the French volunteer, the Marquis de Lafayette, were already within marching distance of the target. Barras meanwhile had managed to slip out of Newport and was sailing south loaded with siege guns. When the British naval squadrons discovered what was going on, they hurried to the Chesapeake to drive off Barras and de Grasse but found themselves outnumbered and outgunned. French naval power was at last decisive. Back went the British fleet to New York for repairs and reinforcements, and Washington with fifty-seven hundred Continentals, thirty-one hundred militia, and seven thousand French began to close in on Yorktown. On October 19, when a relief expedition was already under way from New York, Cornwallis gave up. With the bands playing "The World Turned Upside Down," seven thousand British troops marched out of Yorktown and stacked their arms in surrender.

Peace. Yorktown was as much a French as an American victory. And because the war, too, was a French war, it could not end at Yorktown. France was ready for peace but encumbered by a commitment to Spain. Vergennes, upon concluding the treaty of alliance with the United States on February 6, 1778, had continued his efforts to bring Spain into the war; he finally succeeded after agreeing not to stop fighting until Spain had won Gibraltar from England. Since the United States had agreed not to make peace without French consent, Americans were indirectly bound to await the capture of Gibraltar also. Spain, on the other hand, refused to recognize the independence of the United States, and after entering the war on June 21, 1779, accorded only a devious and frosty tolerance to the American cause. Once Spain had seized the thinly held territory of West Florida (a former Spanish possession) from the British, it confined itself mainly to blockading Gibraltar.

After the defeat at Yorktown, most Englishmen were ready to give up the struggle for the colonies even though George III was bent on continuing it. On March 20, 1782, Lord North was forced from office, and the king was obliged to accept a ministry favorable to peace, which immediately sent agents to get in touch with the American commissioners in France.

Congress had first formulated American war aims in August 1779, when it optimistically sent John Adams to France as minister plenipotentiary. Adams was then forbidden to enter into any peace negotiations with Great Britain unless it first recognized the "liberty, sovereignty, and independence, absolute and unlimited, of these United States." After that recognition had been granted, he was to insist on certain boundaries for the new nation: the Mississippi on the west, the thirty-first parallel and the Flint and St. Mary's rivers on the south, and roughly the present boundary on the north.

In June 1781 the French minister to the United States, the Chevalier de la Luzerne, persuaded Congress to revise its arrangements for making peace. John Adams was replaced as sole negotiator by a five-man commission consisting of himself, John Jay (minister to Spain), Franklin (minister to France), Henry Laurens (designated as minister to the Netherlands but captured by the British en route and held in the Tower of London), and Thomas Jefferson (who was unable to go and was dropped from the commission). The commissioners' instructions were weak: they were still to insist on British recognition of American independence before undertaking peace negotiations, but they were free to accept any settlement "as circumstances may direct and as the state of the belligerent and the disposition of the mediating powers may direct." What was worse, they must do nothing without the knowledge and concurrence of the French and, indeed, must be governed by their advice and opinion.

Yorktown, 1781

These instructions put the commissioners under the direction of Vergennes, a position none of them relished. When secret information reached them that he would not support the American demand for prior recognition of independence, and that his secretary, Rayneval, had secretly encouraged the British to think of a boundary well to the east of the Mississippi, with Spain and England dividing up the territory between, they decided they would do better to negotiate with the British separately rather than to sit down at the peace table under French direction. Violating their instructions, they negotiated with British representatives without insisting on advance recognition of independence, and they did not keep Vergennes informed of what they were doing.

By playing on British desires to destroy the American alliance with France, the commissioners were able to secure both recognition of independence and the boundaries prescribed in John Adams' original instructions. In preliminary articles signed on November 30, 1782, they presented this diplomatic triumph to Vergennes as an accomplished fact. Actually there had been no violation of the alliance, for the treaty based on the articles was not to go into effect until France and England had concluded a treaty of their own. The commissioners' coup enabled Vergennes to exert pressure on Spain to give up the fight for Gibraltar, and in the end Spain settled for East and West Florida and Minorca. The final treaties were signed at Paris on September 3, 1783, and the last British troops left New York on November 25. The Declaration of Independence was at last a statement of fact, not a wish.

The Experimental Period

At Lexington, Concord, and Bunker Hill Americans had fought against Parliamentary taxation. After July 2, 1776, they had fought for independence, though in the beginning probably few of them had any clear idea of what independence would mean besides the end of British tyranny. Between 1776 and 1789 they explored the possibilities of their new freedom. These thirteen years may be considered the Experimental Period in American history, the time when Americans were trying their wings, discovering their nationality. They formulated ideas and ideals that had been only half articulate before, and they found ways and means to put their ideas and ideals into practice. During this period the Americanisms discussed earlier (see Chapter 3) underwent further development, and some of them were transformed from characteristic attitudes into national principles.

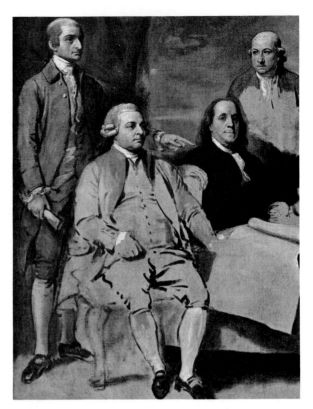

The Peace Commissioners: John Jay, John Adams, Benjamin Franklin, and Henry Laurens

The fruition of Americanisms. American ideas about the separation of church and state and about education advanced less rapidly during the Experimental Period than did political and social concepts. But the assumption that widespread education was desirable did show itself in a revival of schooling, which had lapsed during the war, and in the proliferation of new educational institutions, most of them private. Many academies were founded (especially in New England) to furnish instruction at the secondary level, and sometimes beyond, to both boys and girls. And the number of colleges in the United States doubled: in 1776 there were nine; by 1789 as many more had been opened or chartered; and every state but Delaware had at least one in operation or being organized. Writers in newspapers and pamphlets argued about what kind of education was best suited to Americans. Many demanded that it be made more practical, and new textbooks reoriented traditional subjects like arithmetic and grammar in this direction.

The colonists' wariness of allowing their clergy a hand in government gave rise to a greater separation of church and state. Though most states continued to levy taxes in support of the Protestant religion, the Anglican Church lost the exclusive claims to that support which it had enjoyed in the Southern colonies. Under all the state constitutions people could at least specify which Protestant church their taxes should support. And in Virginia the principle of complete separation of church and state received its finest expression in an act drafted by Thomas Jefferson and adopted by the Virginia legislature in 1786. Beginning with the assertion that "Almighty God hath created the mind free," the act provided that "no man shall be compelled to frequent or support any religious worship, place, or ministry whatsoever."

Jefferson was also author of the phrase that translated social mobility into an American principle. By declaring on July 4, 1776, that "all men are created equal," the United States committed itself to a doctrine that was to prove the world's most powerful lever for social and political change. The declaration was intended simply to justify the colonists' withdrawal from the mother country, which had refused to treat them as the equals of Englishmen. But no great imagination was needed to see wider implications in Jefferson's axiomatic statement of human equality.

Its relevance to black slavery was inescapable. As soon as Americans complained that British taxation would reduce them to slavery, they began to feel uneasy about their own enslavement of Africans; they even forswore the slave trade in their nonimportation agreements. In the Experimental Period most of the states, Southern as well as Northern, forbade the further importation of slaves, and the Northern states provided for the eventual liberation of those already within their borders. Many Southerners also freed their slaves voluntarily at this time. But Americans were not yet ready to face up to the racial meaning of their egalitarian creed. No Southern state provided for the legal abolition of slavery; Jefferson himself continued to hold slaves throughout his lifetime; and Southern slaves continued to do the work that accounted for the major exports of the whole United States. Eventually Americans would have to pay for their failure. Meanwhile the contradiction between the creed of equality and the practice of slavery was heightened as white Americans gradually turned their written commitment into an active force to better their own lives.

The principle of equality was as hostile to aristocracy as to slavery. Having got along without a titled nobility for a century and a half, Americans were determined to continue without one and looked suspiciously at anything that smacked of special privilege. States forbade their citizens to accept titles from foreign nations. And when officers of the Continental Army formed the Society of the Cincinnati in 1783, they met with a storm of protest from critics who feared that the association might become the nucleus of an aristocracy. In Connecticut even a medical society, seeking to raise the standards of the profession by licensing practitioners, was at first denied a charter because its members were to be chosen for life and might thus become a privileged order.

The Revolutionary War itself had an equalizing effect on property: wealthy merchants had lost heavily from the British blockade of commerce, while many a poor farmer had prospered in selling produce to the armies. Wartime finance, with its reliance on steadily inflating paper currency, favored debtors (who were most often farmers) at the expense of creditors. The confiscation and sale of loyalists' lands and the abolition of primogeniture (the inheritance of a man's entire estate by his eldest son) by the state governments likewise contributed to a more equal distribution of property by breaking up some of the larger concentrations of wealth. Although in many cases the initial purchasers of loyalist lands were large-scale speculators, the overall effect of the confiscations was probably to increase the number of landowners, because speculators sold the confiscated lands in small lots. By the time the war ended many Americans regarded equality of property as a goal in itself. When economic depression struck in the 1780s, legislators in some states sponsored bills favoring debtors, on the grounds that republican government required a general equality of property.

The emerging doctrine of equality can also be detected in the reform of voting laws. Property qualifications had disfranchised only a small minority of adult males in most colonies (because most owned property) and there had been few complaints. But every state except Massachusetts reduced the amount of property required for voting. There remained, nevertheless, a strong belief that political rights should be confined to property-holders. Only two states, Georgia and Pennsylvania, opened the franchise to all taxpayers. And in most states there were higher property qualifications for holding office than for voting. In the eighteenth century it was assumed that a man without property had no reason to participate in govern-

Negroes for Sale.

A Cargo of very fine ſtout Men and Women, in good order and fit for immediate ſervice, juſt imported from the Windward Coaſt of Africa, in the Ship Two Brothers.—
Conditions are one half Caſh or Produce, the other half payable the firſt of January next, giving Bond and Security if required.
The Sale to be opened at 10 o'Clock each Day, in Mr. Bourdeaux's Yard, at No, 48, on the Bay.
May 19, 1784.   JOHN MITCHELL.

UNEXPLORED

Hudson Bay

NEWFOUNDLAND

PACIFIC OCEAN

Fr.

Claimed by U.S. and Gr. Britain

Claimed by Russia, Spain, and Gr. Britain

UNITED STATES

Mississippi R.

ATLANTIC OCEAN

LOUISIANA

Claimed by U.S. and Spain

Florida

PUERTO RICO

Gulf of Mexico

Fr.

CUBA

HISPANIOLA

☐ British
☐ United States
▨ Spanish
▧ Russian

North America in 1783

ment either by voting or by holding office. The major purpose of government was to protect property, so a man without any was thought to have little stake in society. Moreover, only property could free a man from the control of employers or landlords. Without property that would support him, a man was not a free agent and could not be trusted with authority or even with a voice in the selection of those who were to wield it. Hence the concern already noted for the maintenance of a wide distribution of property. If America were to become like Europe, with a mass of propertyless workers and peasants, liberty would fall with equality; and authority, concentrated in the hands of a few, would turn into tyranny.

Authority in the hands of the many, of the people, was the essential characteristic of a republic; and with independence colonial insistence on responsible representative government turned into a conscious pursuit of republicanism. Although nothing in the Declaration of Independence had precluded the possibility of monarchy, Americans took it for granted that the new states would be republics. After severing their ties with England, Connecticut and Rhode Island, which in effect were republics already, simply continued the governments defined by their old charters. In other colonies the provincial congress, which replaced the representative assembly (but usually with a larger membership), acted without formal authority until independence was declared. Then, sooner or later, it drafted a written constitution establishing and defining a new government, usually similar in structure to the old one but more responsible to the people.

Since the colonial representative assembly (or lower house) had always been the branch of govern-

ment most directly dependent on the people, the state constitutions enlarged both the size and the powers of the lower houses in the new legislatures. In some states the lower house chose both the upper house and the governor. Two states, Pennsylvania and Georgia, did without an upper house during the 1780s. And in other states there was a marked change in the composition of this body: the members were not as "upper" in wealth or social position as their colonial counterparts. Many were former members of a colonial lower house. They sat, not as the favorites of a governor, but as representatives of the whole people, indistinguishable in this respect from the lower house.

Determination that the government should be the servant of the people and not their master also prompted the inclusion of bills of rights in most of the state constitutions. The Virginia Bill of Rights began by asserting that "all men are by nature equally free and independent, and have certain inherent rights, of which, when they enter into a state of society, they cannot by any compact deprive or divest their posterity." It then enumerated the rights that lay beyond the reach of government, such as freedom of religion and of the press and the right to trial by jury.

In most states, after the provincial congress had drafted and approved a constitution, it went into effect without being submitted to a popular vote. But Massachusetts (the last state to adopt a constitution) elected a special convention to draft one and submitted its work to direct vote by the people. Once it had been ratified in 1780, it could be changed only by another popularly elected convention called for that specific purpose. This was a step that other states had groped for but never quite reached. The purpose of writing out a constitution was to set limits to government by a fundamental law embodying the will of the people. British jurists had often maintained that the unwritten British constitution, consisting of traditions and customs, was superior to government, but custom and tradition had failed to protect the colonists from what they regarded as tyranny by the British government. They wanted something in black and white by which to measure any departure by their own governments from the proper limits of authority. They began to get what they wanted when their provincial congresses wrote and adopted state constitutions. But keen minds soon noted a flaw in this procedure: as the town of Concord pointed out in 1776, a constitution adopted by a legislative body could be altered or abolished by the same body and thus would constitute no protection against legislative tyranny. The device of a special convention and popular ratification elevated the constitution above the legislature and made it easier for the other branches of government to nullify unconstitutional legislation. The courts, for example, could and would refuse to enforce any law that violated the constitution. The Massachusetts invention of the constitutional convention was so widely admired by other Americans that subsequent constitution-making in America followed the Massachusetts method.

Building a national government. The same passion for responsible government that resulted in written constitutions and constitutional conventions prevented for a long time the creation of an effective national government. Americans, like other people of the eighteenth century, believed that republican government was not adaptable to large areas. In a large republic the central legislature must inevitably sit so remote from most of its constituents that it would eventually escape their control and thus cease to be republican. On the other hand, a small republic could never survive in a world of aggressive large nations. There was only one way, it was thought, to overcome these difficulties: a number of small republics might join in a federation and exert their united power for specific purposes.

Americans had formed such a federation in 1774 in the Continental Congress, and after independence the Congress had continued to exercise governmental powers for the whole nation. It was composed of delegates (usually several from each state) appointed annually by the state legislatures. Each state had one vote, which was determined by the majority of its delegates (if they were evenly divided the state's vote was lost).

In the absence of a more effective central organization, Congress served a useful purpose. But it existed only by common consent, and from the beginning the members felt the need for a more binding union. As Americans joined against a common enemy and became aware of their shared principles and beliefs, their feeling of nationality grew stronger. Something more than an unstable succession of congresses was necessary to embody this sentiment and to demonstrate to other nations that the United States too was a nation and not merely a diplomatic alliance of thirteen small republics. Congress accordingly, in the intervals between dealing with the everyday problems of the war, often discussed the formation of a permanent national government. As early as July 12, 1776, a committee had brought in the draft of a constitution, but acceptance had foundered on how expenses and voting power should be apportioned among the states and on the old question of Western policy.

On November 17, 1777, Congress finally agreed on a constitution to be presented to the state legislatures for approval or rejection. The Articles of Confederation provided for a congress like the existing one. Each state, whatever its size, was still to have only one vote, to be cast, as before, by delegates appointed by the state legislatures; each state (by taxing itself) was to contribute to the common expenses according to the value of its lands; none was to be

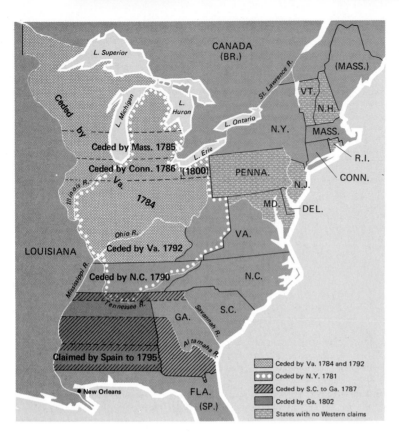

Ceded by Va. 1784 and 1792
Ceded by N.Y. 1781
Ceded by S.C. to Ga. 1787
Ceded by Ga. 1802
States with no Western claims

deprived of its Western lands for the benefit of the United States; and each was to retain its "sovereignty, freedom and independence, and every power, jurisdiction, and right" not expressly delegated to Congress. Congress was permitted to decide on war or peace, appoint military and naval officers, requisition the states for men and money, send and receive ambassadors, enter into treaties and alliances, establish a post office, coin money, borrow money or issue paper money on the credit of the United States, fix weights and measures, regulate Indian affairs, and settle disputes between states.

Although the states found much to object to in the Articles of Confederation, the need to give permanent form to the union moved all but Maryland to accept them by 1779. Maryland's refusal, though probably prompted by narrow, partisan, and pecuniary motives, forced the settlement of a problem that might have wrecked the union—the problem of Western lands.

The West had always been a divisive force, as Bacon's Rebellion, the failure of the Albany Congress, and the Regulator movement all testified. Even more serious trouble lay ahead. Colonial assemblies from Pennsylvania southward had failed to extend full representation to their Western regions as population increased there. Pennsylvania remedied the inequality in its state constitution, but Virginia and the Caro-

linas did not, and the result was Western resentment against the Eastern-dominated state governments.

Concurrent with these internal disputes, the state governments quarreled with one another about the West. The Revolution had dissolved their ties to England but not their territorial boundaries, which had been fixed by royal charters. By their charters, Georgia, the Carolinas, Virginia, Connecticut, and Massachusetts extended to the Pacific Ocean, while Maryland, Delaware, Pennsylvania, New Jersey, and Rhode Island were limited to a few hundred miles on the seacoast. The "landless" states wanted Congress to take control of unoccupied Western lands and restrict the western boundaries of the "landed" states. The landed states resisted any such proposal and squabbled with one another over their conflicting charters. Virginia, whose charter was the oldest, could claim most of the West all to itself. The people of every state, when they looked west, found reason for jealousy or distrust of their neighbors.

The problem was aggravated by land speculation. Before the war, speculators from Pennsylvania, Maryland, and New Jersey (all landless states) had purchased land from the Indians and sought authorization from the king to establish a new colony (Vandalia) in the Ohio Valley. Though bitterly opposed by Virginia's Ohio Company, they had been on the verge of success when the Revolution upset their plans. Now they argued that Congress had inherited the king's authority over all unoccupied lands; and, supported by their state governments, they pressed Congress to recognize their claims. The landed states had fought them off by including in the Articles of Confederation a guarantee that no state should be deprived of territory for the benefit of the United States. But Maryland stubbornly refused to approve the Articles as long as the proposed union lacked control over Western lands. Without Maryland the union was stalled, for it was not to go into effect until unanimously approved.

Maryland could produce better arguments than the mere greed of its land-speculators. The landed states would be able to command such an abundant source of revenue by selling their Western lands that their citizens would pay few or no taxes. People from the landless states would consequently move to the landed ones. Maryland, next door to the leviathan Virginia, would be depopulated.

In Virginia the sentiment for union was strong, and some patriots wanted to give up the state's Western territory, which they thought was too large for a single republican government anyhow. Rather than jeopardize republicanism in Virginia, they preferred to see new states formed in the West and joined to the old ones by the Articles of Confederation. Thomas Jefferson accordingly led Virginia (on January 2, 1781) to offer Congress its claims to all lands north of the Ohio. The transfer was contingent on a number of conditions that in effect canceled speculative claims to the region and required that the land be divided into "distinct republican States," which should ultimately be admitted to the union on equal terms with the old ones. When Virginia's cession was made known, Maryland capitulated (though the speculators still tried to block the way) and approved the Articles of Confederation in February 1781. New York had already ceded its shadowy Western claims, and the other landed states eventually followed suit (Georgia held out until 1802).

Congress under the Confederation. In the Articles of Confederation the American people got what most of them at that time wanted. Having just suffered from the power of a distant British government, they were wary of allowing much authority to their own central government. They charged Congress with the responsibility for making decisions about a multitude of their common concerns, but they neglected to give it the powers to carry its decisions into effect. It could pass resolutions, make recommendations, enact ordinances; but it had no courts, no way of enforcing its orders either on individuals or on states. It could not even levy taxes to pay its own expenses but had to rely on the several states to furnish its funds. In fact,

Congress was allowed less authority than the colonists had once acknowledged in Parliament: Congress did not even have the right to regulate trade. The disadvantages of such a powerless central government soon became apparent.

After the coming of peace diminished the urgency of united action, the states became increasingly enamored of their own power and increasingly casual, even contemptuous, in their relations with Congress, ignoring its resolutions, refusing to fill its requisitions for funds, sending inferior men to represent them or sometimes none at all. Congress was unable to cope with the situation because the Articles of Confederation had provided it with no means to enforce obedience. The weakness of the national government made the years from 1783 to 1789, in the phrase of one historian, the "Critical Period" of American history.

A man elected to Congress during these years might arrive at the meeting place on the appointed day and find a dozen or more delegates like himself eager to proceed to business. But the Articles of Confederation required that each state be represented by at least two delegates and that the representatives of at least seven states be present to make a quorum. Unless more than seven states were represented, every decision had to be unanimous; and the assent of nine states was necessary in most matters having to do with war and peace (including treaties) and with appropriating money. Because the states were often slow about appointing delegates and the delegates themselves slow in taking up their duties, the first arrivals at a session sometimes had to wait several weeks before enough members were present to transact business. Even after a session was organized, it led a precarious existence; for if one or two delegates fell sick, the rest might have to twiddle their thumbs until more arrived or the sick got well.

Each delegate was elected for a one-year term and was prohibited from serving for more than three years in six. As a result, the membership of Congress was constantly shifting. The government was further handicapped by the failure of the Articles of Confederation to provide a regular executive department. Congress exercised executive powers through special commissions and committees and won some continuity by appointing three secretaries to manage crucial executive matters (Benjamin Lincoln, followed by Henry Knox, as Secretary of War; Robert Morris as Superintendent of Finance; and Robert Livingston, followed by John Jay, as Secretary for Foreign Affairs).

These officers struggled to give the United States the appearance of a government. But Congress, pursuing its intermittent existence, belied the appearance. Even when it could scrape together a quorum it had no permanent headquarters or capital. A mutiny in the Philadelphia barracks frightened it out of that city in 1783, and thereafter the delegates wandered from Princeton to Annapolis to Trenton to New York— talking endlessly about where they should settle permanently. Shortly after they began their travels, Oliver Ellsworth, a congressman from Connecticut, observed dryly, "It will soon be of very little consequence where Congress go, if they are not made respectable as well as responsible, which can never be done without giving them a power to perform engagements as well as make them." Congress, in short, had responsibility without power. It could recommend endlessly but no one inside or outside the country paid much attention to what it recommended.

The impotence of Congress made the United States a beggar in the eyes of the world. During the Revolution, Congress had boldly capitalized on popular enthusiasm for the cause of independence by printing paper money, but the money had become worthless before the war's end. Congress had also begged money and supplies from France, but after the peace France preferred to keep its ally poor and humble. Dutch bankers, with more vision than many Americans, did continue to lend. But when Congress turned to the states for funds or for the power to levy a 5 percent tariff on imports, the states turned the beggar down. The power to levy tariffs needed the unanimous approval of the states, and each time it was proposed (in 1781 and again in 1783) at least one state refused; and the others insisted on conditions that would have made the power meaningless anyhow.

The one area in which the United States enjoyed at least the appearance of power was the wilderness north of the Ohio River, a region thinly populated by squatters, Indians, and French. When Virginia offered to cede the area in 1781, Congress had been prevented from taking any formal action to accept it because of pressure from speculators who objected to the terms attached to the cession. Early in 1784, when Virginia renewed the offer, Congress was stalled for lack of a quorum. But by March 1 enough members were present to act favorably, and the United States gained formal authority over the Northwest.

Now Congress might begin to raise the funds it needed by selling land in the newly acquired territory. On April 23 the delegates passed an ordinance, drafted by Thomas Jefferson, that embodied the results of much previous discussion in Congress. It divided the territory into states, each of which was to be admitted into the Union on equal terms with the existing states as soon as its free population equaled any of theirs. Until then the inhabitants could govern themselves according to the constitution and laws of any of the existing states.

To prepare for the sale of lands to individuals, Congress passed an ordinance in 1785 providing that the Northwest be surveyed into townships six miles square along lines running east-west and north-south. Each township was divided into thirty-six lots one mile square (640 acres). A lot (later called a section) was the smallest unit that could be purchased, and neither a township nor a lot was to be sold for less than a dollar an acre in specie. To speed up the transformation of the national domain into hard cash, land offices were to be established in all the states.

Surveying and the settlement of Indian claims proceeded slowly. Before the lands were ready for public sale, a group of ambitious and not very scrupulous speculators from New England came to Congress with a proposition. Calling themselves, like an earlier group, the Ohio Company, they offered to buy a million and a half acres, for which they would pay in currency so badly depreciated that the price amounted to less than 10 cents an acre in specie. Presumptuous as the offer was, the United States needed the money desperately, and Congress decided to accept it. The Ohio Company also agreed to take an option on 5 million additional acres, to be turned over to a subsidiary company known as the Scioto Company. By no coincidence, this company included several congressmen.

To oblige the Ohio Company, Congress passed a new ordinance for governing the Northwest. Jefferson's ordinance of 1784 had never gone into operation, because the area as yet contained no authorized settlers. It did, however, contain many squatters who had helped themselves to public lands and stoutly resisted eviction. Because of the difficulty anticipated in establishing property rights against squatters, and because of the frontier's reputation for violence and disorder, many Easterners believed that congressional rule would be more appropriate than self-government

Continental currency

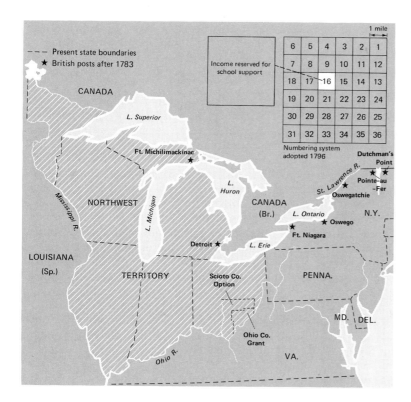

The Old Northwest

- - - Present state boundaries
★ British posts after 1783

Income reserved for school support

6	5	4	3	2	1
7	8	9	10	11	12
18	17	16	15	14	13
19	20	21	22	23	24
30	29	28	27	26	25
31	32	33	34	35	36

Numbering system adopted 1796

1 mile

CANADA

L. Superior

Ft. Michilimackinac ★

NORTHWEST

L. Michigan

L. Huron

CANADA (Br.)

Mississippi R.

Detroit ★

L. Erie

St. Lawrence R.

Oswegatchie ★

Dutchman's Point ★★

Pointe-au -Fer ★

L. Ontario

Oswego ★

Ft. Niagara ★

N.Y.

LOUISIANA (Sp.)

TERRITORY

Scioto Co. Option

PENNA.

MD. DEL.

Ohio Co. Grant

Ohio R.

VA.

during the initial years of settlement. Accordingly, the Northwest Ordinance of 1787 provided for a period during which a governor, a secretary, and a court of three judges, all appointed by Congress, would hold full powers. Once the population had reached five thousand free adult males, a representative legislature would be established, but none of its actions would be valid without the approval of the governor, who would still be appointed by Congress. The legislature could send a representative to Congress, but he would have no vote. The whole area was to be divided into not fewer than three or more than five territories, each of which would be admitted to the Union on equal terms with the existing states when it attained a population of sixty thousand. Slavery was forbidden throughout the area; no person was to be "molested" for his religious beliefs or mode of worship; and "schools and the means of education" were to be encouraged. Though the ordinance did not say how the encouragement was to be effected, the Land Ordinance of 1785 had already reserved one lot in each township "for the maintenance of public schools."

The Northwest Ordinance established for the United States a Western policy that embodied the most cherished American principles. Though the ordinance applied to only a part of the West, it set a precedent that guided the territorial expansion of the nation until the end of the nineteenth century.

National humiliation. One serious obstacle stood in the way of Congress' noble aspirations for the American West: the United States held only a tenuous grip on the area. England had never completely evacuated the Northwest, nor had Spain recognized American possession of any territory south of the Ohio. As the weakness and poverty of the new nation grew more apparent, European statesmen intrigued to push its western boundary back to the Appalachians.

When England made peace in 1783, it was not fully persuaded—nor was the rest of Europe—that the United States would last. While the king officially proclaimed the treaty and commanded his subjects to comply with it, his ministers sent secret orders to the governor-general of Canada to retain Britain's trading posts and military garrisons in the Northwest. The United States, with its own armies disbanded and the French forces gone, was in no position to compel the British to withdraw. To excuse their continued occupation of the posts, the British charged that the Americans had violated the treaty.

Again the weakness of the national government was to blame. The treaty required that neither side make laws impeding the collection of private debts contracted before the war, and it required that Congress "earnestly recommend" to the states the restoration of confiscated loyalist property. Congress did recommend the restitution, and the fact that the states did not follow the recommendation was not technically a violation of the treaty. But when some states passed laws impeding the collection of British debts, they violated the treaty as surely as England did in keeping troops on American territory. Congress was as helpless to prevent one violation as the other. It sent John Adams to England as American minister; and he protested the British garrisons with characteristic Adams vigor, but in vain, for England knew that no American troops stood behind him.

England showed its contempt for the government of its former colonies by failing to establish a legation in the United States to match the American legation in London. More ominously it dickered with the influential Allen brothers, Ethan and Levi, for help in acquiring Vermont. Claimed by both New Hampshire and New York, Vermont had asserted its independence of both and applied for statehood. Congress was reluctant to antagonize either claimant by admitting Vermont into the Union, and there was danger that the Vermonters might attach themselves to Canada (Vermont was not admitted until 1791).

In the Southwest, Spain was grasping for the area that later became the states of Kentucky and Tennessee. Americans were moving into it at such a rate that by 1790 it contained more than a hundred thousand of them, but their presence was hardly a guarantee of permanent American possession. Barred by the mountains from trade with the East, the settlers relied on the Mississippi River to float their produce to market at New Orleans. New Orleans belonged to Spain, and so did the lower Mississippi. The Spanish had gained Louisiana in 1763, the Floridas in 1783; and they maintained forts on the west bank of the Mississippi as far north as St. Louis, on the east bank as far as the present site of Memphis. Anyone who wanted to use the river had to do business with Spain.

Although commercial exports from the Southwest were still meager, everyone in the region was expecting future prosperity through the Mississippi trade. Spain was well aware of that expectation. In 1784 it closed the river to navigation by Americans and waited for the settlers to abandon their feeble Congress for the solid commercial advantage of Spanish citizenship. For a time it seemed that the settlers might do just that, for they were far from pleased with the way Eastern Americans were treating them. In 1772, by the Watauga Compact, pioneers in the Tennessee area had formed a government of their own, which lasted until 1776, when North Carolina organized them into Washington County. In 1784, after its land-speculators had established claims to the most valuable land, North Carolina ceded the region to Congress in order to avoid the expense of protecting it from the Indians. When the state changed its mind the next year and tried to regain possession, many settlers grew disgusted and began to look favorably toward Spain. In Kentucky, the Western region of Virginia, a similar secessionist movement and a similar flirtation with Spain threatened to disrupt the Union.

As the Southwest began to draw away from the United States, Spain in 1785 sent Don Diego de Gardoqui to wring from Congress a formal recognition of Spain's exclusive control over the Mississippi. Congress instructed its Secretary of Foreign Affairs, John Jay, to insist in his negotiations with Gardoqui on the right of Americans to navigate the Mississippi through Spanish territory to its mouth. This was a subject about which the two men had tilted inconclusively once before, during the Revolution, when Jay had gone to Spain in search of assistance in the war against England. Jay now found Gardoqui as adamant as ever about refusing to recognize an American right of navigation but willing to make other concessions. The Spanish would agree to recognize American territorial rights as far south as the old border of British West Florida and as far west as the Mississippi and to give American merchants new trading privileges in Spain. In return, he asked only that the United States agree to give up navigation of the Mississippi for twenty-five years. The offer was attractive to New Englanders and to the Middle states, whose merchants badly needed new markets. But it offered nothing to Southerners that they did not, in their own view at least, already have. And it was anathema to the settlers on the Ohio River, most of whom had come from the South. In Congress the Northern delegates now pushed through a vote that allowed Jay to accept the offer. Thus, even before he presented his treaty for ratification, his negotiations had polarized Congress on North-South lines.

But the Northern majority consisted of only seven states, and nine were required for ratification. As Northerners began talking of a separate confederation, and Westerners talked of betrayal, Gardoqui's shrewdness became apparent. Though he did not get his treaty, he had brought on a sectional confrontation that threatened the Union's very existence.

While Gardoqui led Jay into alienating the Westerners, the Spanish governor of Louisiana, Esteban Rodriguez Miro, was wooing them with bribes and privileges. General James Wilkinson, a veteran of the Revolutionary War and a consummate double-dealer, took a trip to New Orleans in 1787. While there, he took a secret oath of allegiance to Spain in return for trading concessions. The following year he accepted a Spanish pension, with the understanding that he would lead his neighbors in the Tennessee region to repudiate the United States. Wilkinson was not the only Southwestern traitor. Daniel Boone, James Robertson, and John Sevier all accepted Spanish gold.

Instead of doing what they were paid to do, however, they cheerfully deceived both sides while they waited to see what was going to happen. If, as seemed likely, the United States should break up, they were ready to learn Spanish.

The United States had troubles even in the Mediterranean. For years European countries had been protecting their Mediterranean shipping from pirates by paying an annual tribute to the rulers of Morocco, Algiers, Tripoli, and Tunis. As long as American ships carried the British flag, they were safe; but after 1776, when they began to fly the Stars and Stripes, pirates swarmed out upon them. The captured American captains and crews were put on the auction block and sold as slaves. Congress bought protection from Morocco in 1787 but had neither money nor guns to stop the other North African pirates.

Nor were pirates the only difficulty to beset American trade. The whole American economy was in a precarious position. With the coming of peace, American merchants had sensed a huge demand for the British dry goods and hardware to which American consumers had been accustomed before the war. The merchants placed their orders, and warehouses and stores were soon bulging, with the British extending liberal credits. The American merchants in turn extended credit to retailers and consumers, and the country indulged itself in a buying spree. Only when it came time to pay the bills did the Americans discover their situation.

The colonial economy had been a complex one, in which Americans paid for British imports by carrying their own and other people's goods to market in various ports throughout the world, but mostly within the empire. Now they were no longer a part of the empire, and Britain closed its West Indian ports to American vessels. Prices of American produce dropped, merchants found themselves cut off from usual channels of trade, and depression settled over the land—while British merchants called for payment.

Americans blamed themselves and their merchants. Having won their political independence, they had promptly mortgaged it by extravagant purchases from their old masters. It seemed that the British, by craftily extending liberal credits and closing their ports to Americans, had rewon economically the position of dominance that they had lost politically. Congress instructed John Adams to ask England for a commercial treaty, but he was no more successful in this than in pressing for the evacuation of British garrisons in the Northwest.

There were loud demands for retaliation against the British restrictions on American trade, and some states passed laws to discourage imports. But such partial legislation by single states, each imposing different restrictions, only added to the difficulties by injuring the economies of sister states. What was needed was an overall national regulation of commerce, not simply to discourage unnecessary imports, but to create a balanced economy in which manufacturing, agriculture, and commerce would all find their place. Only in this way could the United States become economically as well as politically independent and insure itself against domination by Britain or any other nation. But the American Congress, with no power to regulate commerce, could not even begin to direct the economy toward such a goal.

The Crisis of American Nationality

Many Americans found the impotence of the national government intolerable. The Revolution had widened their vision beyond the affairs of town or county or colony and had taught them to think, as Alexander Hamilton put it, "continentally." They knew that the only way to solve the difficulties of the United States was to strengthen the national government—they had known it before the ink was dry on the Articles of Confederation. Now, as the weakness of the government became more and more embarrassing, they spoke out ever more loudly.

Thinking continentally. The Americans had had plenty of practice in making and breaking governments. Their usual method had been to call an extralegal convention—like the Stamp Act Congress or the Continental Congress or the provincial congresses that replaced the royal governments. Conventions were also summoned whenever the people of a state or region wanted to achieve a public purpose for which their regular government had proved inadequate. Several interstate conventions had met during the war in an effort to regulate prices. Connecticut held a convention in 1783 to protest the founding of the Society of the Cincinnati and the granting of extra pay to army officers. And, as we have seen, Massachusetts called a convention to draft a state constitution.

It was only natural, then, for people who had begun to think "continentally" to turn to a convention for the purpose of strengthening the continental government. As early as 1784 they had talked of it, but at that time public sentiment was overwhelmingly against it. The opposition did not arise from a deficiency of national patriotism or from too much local patriotism. Nationalism, which has proved the most lively—and deadly—force in the modern world, attached itself in America to the Union rather than to the states. As Thomas Paine, in his first publication after the peace, wrote: "Our citizenship in the United

Thinking locally

It is the opinion of the ablest writers on the subject, that no extensive empire can be governed upon republican principles, and that such a government will degenerate to a despotism, unless it be made up of a confederacy of smaller states, each having the full powers of internal regulation. This is precisely the principle which has hitherto preserved our freedom. No instance can be found of any free government of considerable extent which has been supported upon any other plan. Large and consolidated empires may indeed dazzle the eyes of a distant spectator with their splendour, but if examined more nearly are always found to be full of misery. The reason is obvious. In large states the same principles of legislation will not apply to all the parts. The inhabitants of warmer climates are more dissolute in their manners, and less industrious, than in colder countries. A degree of severity is, therefore, necessary with one which would cramp the spirit of the other. We accordingly find that the very great empires have always been despotick.... It is under such tyranny that the Spanish provinces languish, and such would be our misfortune and degradation, if we should submit to have the concerns of the whole empire managed by one legislature.... The attempt made by Great Britain to introduce such a system, struck us with horrour, and when it was proposed by some theorist that we should be represented in parliament, we uniformly declared that one legislature could not represent so many different purposes of legislation and taxation. This was the leading principle of the revolution, and makes an essential article in our creed.

From The Letters of Agrippa, 1787, attributed to James Winthrop.

States is our national character. Our citizenship in any particular state is only our local distinction."

This sentiment was echoed by statesmen, poets, painters, and schoolmasters. George Washington, the nation's hero, was a great Virginian but a greater American. "We are known by no other character among nations," he declared in 1783, "than as the United States." Connecticut during the 1780s produced a host of brilliant young men who celebrated in literature and art not their own state but America. John Trumbull depicted the great events of the American Revolution in a series of historical paintings. Joel Barlow attempted an American epic in *The Vision of Columbus*. Noah Webster wrote schoolbooks designed to teach American English. Jedidiah Morse published an *American Geography*. And Ezra Stiles, the president of Yale, preached of *The United States Elevated to Glory and Honor*. Some authors, to be sure, wrote the history of their own states (Jefferson, for example, published his *Notes on the State of Virginia* in 1785), but the local pride they exhibited was different in kind from the national pride that was evident throughout the Union.

Yet, however proud of their country's past and confident of its future, Americans needed leadership and a government capable of elevating the United States to the glory and honor they wanted for it. National policy was drifting, and continental-minded men warned that the nation faced collapse or conquest if its government was not strengthened. But their appeals met resistance from people who feared that a stronger government might become aristocratic or tyrannical; it might threaten the principles that had brought the Union into being—the principles of equality and of responsible, republican government. In 1785, for example, when the legislature of Massachusetts proposed a general convention to strengthen the national government, its delegates in Congress objected. Would-be aristocrats, they argued, would use such a convention to establish a government based on special privilege, loaded with lucrative positions for themselves, and bolstered by a standing army.

Because of such sentiments on the part of honest and patriotic citizens, a national constitutional convention, though often talked of, had failed to materialize. By 1786, however, Americans had become so impatient with British trade restrictions, conflicting state commercial laws, and national economic helplessness that they arranged for an interstate meeting at Annapolis, Maryland, to consider the extension of national authority to the regulation of commerce. Probably from the beginning, one of the delegates, James Madison, had hoped for something more than an increase in congressional power. It was Madison who had originated Virginia's call for the meeting. By

Thinking continentally: George Washington

September 1786, when the delegates began to assemble, he and other continental-minded patriots were alarmed by the sectional antagonisms that Jay's proposed treaty had aroused. The accumulating threats to the Union were too great to be dealt with by a convention called to consider regulation of trade. When representatives from five states had convened, though more were on the way, they drew up a proposal to Congress and the several states and dissolved the convention. What they proposed was another convention the next year at Philadelphia for the larger purpose of making "the constitution of the Federal Government adequate to the exigencies of the Union."

The message reached the states along with some disturbing news from Massachusetts. In the summer of 1786 the citizens in the economically depressed western part of the state, laboring under a heavy burden of debt, had called a number of local conventions to demand changes in the state government: they objected to the state senate (the upper house of the legislature) as a needless expense and an aristocratic influence; they objected to the heavy taxation of land; and they objected to the high fees charged by lawyers and county courts. After the conventions had voiced their protests and adjourned, mobs prevented the county courts from sitting and thus put an end to the collection of debts. Then, during the winter of 1786-87, some two thousand Western farmers rose in armed rebellion under the leadership of Daniel Shays, a veteran of the Revolutionary War.

Though Shays' Rebellion was easily quelled by the loyal militia of Massachusetts, it alarmed Americans in every part of the United States. By threatening law and order, the rebellion threatened property: the closing of the courts in western Massachusetts had halted mortgage foreclosures and deprived creditors of property owed to them. Other states, too, had depressed areas and discontented debtors who, it was feared, might imitate the Shaysites. Property was also endangered from other directions. In several states, the coming of peace had brought no end to the flood of paper money that inflated values and defrauded creditors. Rhode Island made it illegal to refuse the state's worthless paper money as payment for debts.

Even before Shays' Rebellion, people had realized that something must be done about this undermining of property rights. To many, Madison included, it seemed that the principles of the Revolution were threatened more by the vicious actions of state governments than they could be by the supposed aristocratic danger from a stronger national government. Such a government was needed not only to answer the needs of the union but to curb the irresponsibility of the states toward their own citizens. As Madison saw it, the very existence of republican government was at stake. Others agreed. After the shock of Shays' Rebellion, every state but Rhode Island agreed to send delegates to Philadelphia to revise the Articles of Confederation.

The great convention. The United States in the Revolutionary period produced six men of indisputable greatness: Franklin, Washington, Jefferson, Madison, Hamilton, and John Adams. Four of them—Franklin, Washington, Madison, and Hamilton—were among the fifty-five delegates sent by the state governments to the convention that met in Philadelphia from May 25 to September 17, 1787. Jefferson and Adams would doubtless have been there too if they had not been representing the United States in Europe, for the convention was an extraordinary assem-

I find also the pride of independance taking deep and dangerous hold on the hearts of individual states. I know no danger so dreadful and so probable as that of internal contests. And I know no remedy so likely to prevent it as the strengthening the band that connects us. We have substituted a Congress of deputies from every state to perform this task: but we have done nothing which would enable them to enforce their decisions. What will be the case? They will not be enforced. The states will go to war with each other in defiance of Congress; one will call in France to her assistance; another Great Britain, and so we shall have all the wars of Europe brought to our own doors.... I feel great comfort on the prospect of getting yourself and two or three others into the legislature. My humble and earnest prayer to Almighty god will be that you may bring into fashion principles suited to the form of government we have adopted, and not of that we have rejected, that you will first lay your shoulders to strengthening the band of our confederacy and averting those cruel evils to which it's present weakness will expose us, and that you will see the necessity of doing this instantly before we forget the advantages of union, or acquire a degree of ill-temper against each other which will daily increase the obstacles to that good work.

From Thomas Jefferson, Letter to Edmund Randolph, February 15, 1783.

blage of talent. The delegates had a wealth of experience and tradition to draw upon: the heritage of British political and constitutional ideas stretching back to Magna Carta and beyond; the experience of five generations of colonists in representative assemblies, town meetings, and county courts; the searching debates about authority that preceded the Declaration of Independence; the drafting of state constitutions; the running of state governments and of a rudimentary national government. In no period of American history could a group have been gathered with more sophistication in political thought or with more practical experience in the construction and reconstruction of governments.

Almost without exception the delegates were men who thought continentally; and they were eager for a central government that would preserve and embody the national feeling that had grown out of the Revolution, a government that would be respected at home and abroad. The only way to achieve that end, they believed, was to give the central government more authority than Congress had been allowed. It had to be able to levy taxes so that it could support itself and not be starved into impotence, so that it could raise the armies and build the navy that might one day be needed to defend the independence so dearly won. It had to be able to regulate commerce so as to bargain effectively with foreign nations. It had to offer better protection to private property than the existing national or state governments did. And it had to have coercive powers to enforce its decrees.

The delegates, while agreeing on these objectives,

realized that two obstacles stood in the way of attaining them. The first was the fear of the American people that a national government, if given enough power to do its job, would quickly seize more than enough, that it would fall into the hands of a select group of the wealthy and clever who would use it to their own advantage and to the disadvantage of ordinary men. The American people would not accept an effective central government unless they could be sure of controlling it.

The second obstacle was rivalry among the states. Each state feared that a strong national government might give unfair advantage to the others. For example, it might levy taxes that would injure one state and benefit another. Fortunately, quarrels over the West were momentarily at a minimum because of Virginia's renunciation of claims to the Northwest and because the status of future states in the territory was determined by Congress (in the Northwest Ordinance) while the convention was sitting. The convention itself, after preliminary debates, skirted the knotty question of whether new states should be equal to old and decided simply that "New States may be admitted by the Congress into this Union."

But another form of state rivalry could not be bypassed and threatened to deadlock the convention: in a national government composed of states, how was representation to be apportioned? Under the Articles of Confederation, each state, no matter what its size, had one vote in Congress (this manner of voting was also followed in the convention). Such an arrangement gave undue advantage to the citizens of small states: 68,000 Rhode Islanders had the same influence on decisions as 747,000 Virginians. The large states would not be satisfied with any national government in which their influence was not at least approximately commensurate with their size. But the small states believed that unless they retained an equal vote the large states would be able to advance their own interests at the expense of the small states.

The rivalry between small and large states masked a more serious rivalry between North and South, which had already appeared in voting alignments in the Continental Congress. The Southern states, where slave labor produced crops for export, were wary of subjecting their labor or its produce to a government dominated by the more numerous Northern states, where free labor, diversified farming, and large commercial interests prevailed.

When the convention opened, Edmund Randolph of Virginia presented a plan, drafted by his colleague James Madison, that was designed to overcome both the fears of the people and the fears of the states. Madison, who at thirty-six was the most astute political thinker of his day, proposed to rest the government of the United States on the people rather than on the state governments and to apportion representation not by states but by population. The population of the Southern states (including slaves) equaled that of the Northern states and was expected to grow more rapidly in the future. In a government where representation was proportioned according to population, the South would be safe.

Nor would small states be endangered by large ones. Their fears, Madison perceived, were partly an illusion: the people of a small state did not necessarily have different interests from the people of a large state. The people of Delaware, for example, probably had more in common with their neighbors in Pennsylvania than with distant Rhode Islanders.

To keep the government from seizing more power than it was assigned, Madison proposed to divide it into different branches that would check and balance one another: a two-house legislature, an independent executive, and an independent judiciary. Each would have specific functions and would see to it that the others did not overstep their bounds. The Americans had already endorsed the principle of separation of powers in their state governments, but their discussions of national government had usually revolved around the granting of further powers to the existing unicameral Congress. Only a few, like Jefferson and John Jay, had seen the need for separation of powers in the national government itself; but as soon as Madison made the proposal, its advantages were obvious, and many of the fears about the government's escaping control were dispelled. Pierce Butler, a delegate for South Carolina, said that "he had opposed the grant of powers to Congress heretofore, because the whole power was vested in one body. The proposed distribution of the powers into different bodies changed the case, and would induce him to go great lengths."

The delegates spent two weeks revising Madison's plan and working out its details, without altering its basic structure. Then on June 15 William Paterson of New Jersey suddenly came up with a new plan calling for a continuation of the existing unicameral Congress with increased powers, but with each state retaining its equal vote. Paterson and his supporters would allow Congress the power to tax, to regulate trade, and to enforce its own decrees, but they wanted the national government to remain what it had been, an assembly of the states, not of the people, its members chosen by the state governments, not by popular election. Paterson's plan was rejected, but the small-state delegations had rallied to it and finally threatened to bolt the convention unless each state was given an equal vote in at least one house of the national legislature. To pacify them, the other members of the convention agreed on July 16 that all the states would have equal representation in the upper house; but to this concession they attached several provisions, designed mainly to protect the interests of the South: representation in the lower house and direct taxation would be apportioned according to population, with five slaves to be considered the equivalent of three free persons; all bills for raising or spending money would originate in the lower house; a census would be taken every ten years.

These conditions in effect gave the voters of slaveholding states a larger representation in the lower house than the voters of nonslaveholding states. And if Southern population grew as rapidly as expected, the representation would be increased. On the other hand, the voters of small states (mostly Northern) would have a far larger share of power in the upper house than their numbers would entitle them to.

Once they had made this Great Compromise there was no longer any serious danger that the delegates would fail in their attempt to strengthen the national government. They had started out in substantial agreement about what needed to be done, and they had overcome, in large measure at least, both the rivalry of the states and the fear of tyranny. They still argued about details; but within three and a half months of assembling, they had finished their job.

Their proposed Constitution provided for a national government with authority to collect taxes, make treaties with foreign countries, maintain an army and a navy, coin and borrow money, regulate commerce among the states and with foreign nations, and make any laws necessary to carry its powers into execution. The United States Constitution and all the treaties and laws made under it were to be the supreme law of the land, superior to state laws and binding on state courts. Moreover, the federal government would have its own executive and its own courts to enforce its treaties, Constitution, and laws, and to settle disputes between states. As a last resort it could call on the militia for help.

The national legislature, or Congress, was to consist of an upper house, or Senate, and a House of Representatives. Each state was to have two senators, both appointed by the state legislature for six-year terms, and one representative for every thirty thousand persons, to be popularly elected for a two-year term by the same persons who were qualified to vote for members of "the most numerous Branch of the State Legislature." The executive, known as the President, was to be elected every four years by an electoral "college" to which each state might appoint (in any way its legislature prescribed) as many members as the total of its representatives and senators in Congress. It was intended, of course, that the members of this body should exercise their own discretion in selecting the best man in the country. The man with the second largest number of votes became the Vice President, who was to preside over the Senate.

The Constitution hedged both the federal and the state governments with specific prohibitions. To protect private property, it forbade the state governments to pass laws impairing the obligation of contracts, or to coin money, issue paper money, or make anything but gold and silver legal tender in payment of debts. To prevent the states from encroaching on the sphere of the federal government, it forbade them to make treaties, levy import or export duties, or engage in war unless actually invaded. Conversely the states were protected by clauses prohibiting the federal government from levying direct taxes except in proportion to population, from levying export taxes at all (a protection for the tobacco- and rice-exporters of the South), and from restricting immigration "or Importation of such Persons as any of the States now existing shall think proper to admit" before the year 1808 (a protection for the slave trade until that time). Republicanism and individual rights were protected by clauses forbidding either the states or the federal government to grant titles of nobility, or to pass bills of attainder or ex post facto laws. The federal courts were confined to trial by jury in criminal cases, and the federal government could not make any religious test a qualification for public office or suspend the writ of habeas corpus "unless when in Cases of Rebellion or Invasion the public Safety may require it."

Apart from these prohibitions, the Constitution did not contain any guarantee of individual rights such as freedom of speech or religion. In the last days of the convention, Elbridge Gerry of Massachusetts and George Mason of Virginia proposed that this omission be corrected, but their colleagues rejected the suggestion as unnecessary on the grounds that the Constitution defined and limited the powers of the national government to specified actions and that the state constitutions already contained bills of rights. But in case experience should prove this or any other of their decisions to be unwise, the convention provided a means of correction: once the Constitution was adopted, amendments to it could be proposed by a two-thirds vote of both houses of Congress or by a new constitutional convention, to be called if two-thirds of the state legislatures requested it. The proposed amendments would become part of the Constitution if ratified by three-fourths of the states. The convention adjourned on September 17, after sending a copy of its work to Congress for transmission to the states.

Ratification. The constitution drafted at Philadelphia was the greatest creative triumph of the Experimental Period, and it showed how much its authors had learned during those experimental years. After the war the initial reaction against monarchy and aristocracy had led Americans to create state governments with feeble executives and ineffective upper houses; the new Constitution proposed a powerful executive and a Senate equal in power to the House of Representatives. The Articles of Confederation had created a national government controlled by the state governments and having no direct relation to the individual citizen; the new Constitution proposed a national government independent of the state governments, with a House of Representatives elected directly by the people of the United States and with federal courts acting directly on them. The Articles of Confederation had placed the national government in the hands of a single congress of delegates and had provided it with little authority; the new Constitution split up the national government to prevent abuses and gave it real authority.

The members of the Philadelphia Convention had been empowered only to revise the Articles of Confederation. Actually, they had drawn up a completely new government to take the place of the debating society that Congress had become. Knowing that their ambitious plan would meet opposition, and unwilling to have it defeated by the stubbornness of a few states, the delegates boldly proposed that as soon as nine states had accepted the new Constitution it should go into effect among those nine (revisions of the Articles of Confederation required unanimous approval). The convention also proposed the revolutionary technique of bypassing the state legislatures, where power-hungry state politicians and pressure groups might exert an influence as pernicious as the speculators had exerted against ratification of the Articles of Confederation. In each state the voters would elect a special convention to judge the new constitution. The state government would issue the call for the ratifying convention but would have no part in accepting or rejecting the Constitution. The new national government, if adopted, would thus be authorized directly by the people; its power would derive from them.

The prestige of its authors, especially Washington and Franklin, as well as its intrinsic merits assured the Constitution a hearing. But its adoption was not at all certain. Several members of the convention, including the influential Edmund Randolph, had refused to sign the completed document. When it reached Congress, Richard Henry Lee took an immediate dislike to it. Why, he asked, should Congress approve its own dissolution? Why should nine states be allowed to withdraw from the Confederation to form a new and dangerously powerful government? Before transmitting the document to the states, Lee proposed at least the insertion of a bill of rights.

Lee's proposal was defeated by what he termed "a coalition of monarchy men, military men, aristocrats and drones whose noise, impudence and zeal exceeds all belief." When the Constitution reached the American people, many reacted as Lee had. But in every state the legislature eventually, if sometimes reluctantly, issued the necessary call for a popular ratifying convention.

The opponents of the Constitution were moved less by a desire to perpetuate the superiority of the state governments than by the old fear that a strong national government would escape from popular control and become oppressive. The system of checks and balances, they felt, was not adequate insurance against tyranny. The House of Representatives was too small to represent so many people and would be filled with the rich and well-born. The failure to include a bill of rights seemed an ominous indication of the direction the national government would take. Madison had argued at the convention, and now wrote in the newspapers, to persuade people that there were no grounds for the long-accepted notion that a large republic would fall into tyranny. In a large republic there would be so many different groups with such varied and opposing interests that they would be unable to submerge their differences and combine into a tyrannical majority. The danger of a tyrannical coalition was far greater in a small republic, Madison pointed out, because of the fewer divergent interests and the greater ease of communication.

The supporters of the Constitution were generally more aggressive than their opponents, and sometimes their tactics were unworthy of their cause. In Pennsylvania they pushed through the call for a convention after the legislature had voted to adjourn; they rounded up a quorum only by forcibly detaining two members. Everywhere they campaigned with a vigor and invective born of urgency. This, they felt, was the crisis of American nationality. If the Constitution failed to be adopted, the Union might be doomed.

Opposition to the Constitution was generally weakest in the small states, which would have more than their share of power in the new government. But the Federalists, as the supporters of the Constitution called themselves, knew that it was imperative to win over the four largest states: Massachusetts, Pennsylvania, New York, and Virginia. For any one of them to abstain would imperil the success of the new government. Pennsylvania, in spite of determined opposition, fell in line first, on December 12, 1787. Massachusetts ratified on February 6, 1788, by a narrow majority, which included several anti-Federalist delegates. They had been persuaded after John Hancock proposed that a recommendation for a bill of rights accompany ratification.

In Virginia the opposition, led by Patrick Henry,

was weakened when Edmund Randolph swung back in favor of adoption. The state accepted the Constitution by a vote of eighty-nine to seventy-nine on June 26. Meanwhile every other state but New York, North Carolina, and Rhode Island had voted for ratification. Several had, like Massachusetts, included recommendations for amendments. In New York Alexander Hamilton, John Jay, and James Madison had campaigned for the Constitution in an impressive series of newspaper articles, known as *The Federalist*. Though these were perhaps the most searching discussion of the Constitution ever written, they did not prevent the election of a hostile ratifying convention. Only after news of Virginia's decision reached New York did the state fall into line, on July 26. North Carolina did not ratify until November 21, 1789; and Rhode Island withheld its approval until May 29, 1790. But the rest of the country did not wait for them. As soon as the four big states had given their assent, Congress arranged for its own demise by ordering national elections to be held in January 1789.

The United States was at last to have a government that would embody on a national scale the American principle of responsible representative government. The world had said that republican government was impossible for a country the size of the United States, that only a federation of republics or a powerful monarchy or aristocracy could extend so wide. But here was a new kind of republic, a federation that would be more than a federation, a government that would remain responsible to the people though its territory and population expanded tenfold, a union in which the people would be joined not as citizens of rival states but as a nation of equals.

Suggestions for Reading

A good brief survey of the military history of the Revolution is Howard Peckham, *The War for Independence** (1958). Christopher Ward, *The War of the Revolution*, 2 vols. (1952), is more comprehensive. Don Higginbotham, *The War of American Independence** (1971), emphasizes the political and social aspects of military policies. Piers Mackesy, *The War for America* (1964), views the conflict from the British perspective. The standard account of naval operations is G. W. Allen, *Naval History of the American Revolution*, 2 vols. (1913), but for the exploits of John Paul Jones see S. E. Morison, *John Paul Jones: A Sailor's Biography** (1959). T. G. Frothingham, *Washington, Commander in Chief* (1930), is still a good assessment of the general's military genius, but more thorough accounts will be found in the two major biographies of Washington: D. S. Freeman, *George Washington*, 7 vols. (1948–57), and J. T. Flexner, *George Washington in the American Revolution* (1968). John Shy, *A People Numerous and Armed** (1976), probes the social implications of the war, and Charles Royster, *A Revolutionary People at War* (1979), examines the interaction of republican ideals and military service.

The classic account of the diplomacy of the Revolution is S. F. Bemis, *The Diplomacy of the American Revolution** (1935). R. B. Morris gives a lively and detailed narrative of the peace negotiations in *The Peacemakers** (1965). Clarence Ver Steeg, *Robert Morris* (1954), deals largely with financing of the Revolution. A more extensive study is E. J. Ferguson, *The Power of the Purse: A History of American Public Finance, 1776–1790** (1961).

Since 1909, when Carl Becker offered his opinion that the Revolution, in New York at least, was a contest about who should rule at home, many historians have addressed themselves to the effect of the Revolution on social conflicts within the participating states. J. F. Jameson, *The American Revolution Considered as a Social Movement* (1926), argued that the Revolution acted as a leveling movement in the direction of greater democracy and accelerated social change. Not all of the studies of individual states in the period from 1776 to 1789 bear out this contention. For example, Richard McCormick, *Experiment in Independence: New Jersey in the Critical Period, 1781–1789* (1950), finds little evidence of class conflict, but E. W. Spaulding, *New York in the Critical Period, 1783–1789* (1932), and Edward Countryman, *A People in Revolution* (1981), find a good deal, as do Staughton Lynd, *Class Conflict, Slavery and the United States Constitution* (1968), and Merrill Jensen, *The American Revolution within America* (1974). Robert Brown, *Middle-Class Democracy and the Revolution in Massachusetts, 1691–1780* (1955), argues that there was little democratizing of Massachusetts during the Revolution, because Massachusetts already had democratic government, with the vast majority of adult males enjoying the right to vote. Chilton Williamson, *American Suffrage from Property to Democracy, 1760–1860* (1960), finds that the majority of males in most colonies had the right to vote but that the majority became larger during the Revolution as a result of reductions in property qualifications. E. S. Morgan, *The Birth of the Republic** (1956), emphasizes the growth of common principles rather than conflicts among Americans of the period 1763–89. J. T. Main, *The Social Structure of Revolutionary America** (1965), and A. H. Jones, *The Wealth of a Nation To Be* (1980), contain valuable statistical information about the distribution of property, and Main's *Upper House in Revolutionary America, 1763–1788* (1967), shows the democratizing effect of the Revolution on this legislative branch. J. K. Martin, *Men in Rebellion: Higher Governmental Leaders and the Coming of the American Revolution** (1973), similarly shows how the Revolution opened up opportunities for political leadership to a wider spectrum of the population. And see again, on internal social conflicts, Alfred Young, ed., *The American Revolution** (1976). L. K. Kerber, *Women of the Republic** (1980), and M. B. Norton, *Liberty's Daughters** (1980), show how the Revolution expanded the role of women in American society.

The first general study of the loyalists, C. H. Van Tyne, *The Loyalists in the American Revolution* (1902), saw them as exemplars of the colonial upper class. More recent studies, particularly Wallace Brown, *The King's Friends* (1965), show that they came from all classes. The most comprehensive account of them is R. M. Calhoon, *The Loyalists in Revolutionary America, 1760–1781* (1973). Their point of view is analyzed in L. W. Labaree, *Conservatism in Early American History** (1948); W. H. Nelson, *The American Tory** (1962); and M. B. Norton, *The British Americans: The Loyalist Exiles in England, 1774–1789* (1972). Two good biographies of prominent loyalists are L. H. Gipson, *Jared Ingersoll* (1920), and Bernard Bailyn, *The Ordeal of Thomas Hutchinson* (1974).

John Fiske, *The Critical Period of American History, 1783–1789* (1883), painted a black picture of the United States under the Articles of Confederation and told of the nation's rescue by the Constitution of 1787. Merrill Jensen, *The Articles of Confederation** (1940, 2nd ed., 1959), and *The New Nation** (1950), sought to redeem the reputation of the Articles, which he saw as a true embodiment of the principles of the Declaration of Independence. J. N. Rakove, *The Beginnings of National Politics* (1979), challenges Jensen's interpretation. Irving Brant, *James Madison the Nationalist, 1780–1787* (1948), gives a view of the period through the eyes of one of America's most perceptive statesmen. Gordon Wood, *The Creation of the American Republic, 1776–1787** (1969), traces the development of popular influences in government during the period. W. P. Adams analyzes the state constitutions in *The First American Constitutions* (1980). Two studies analyze political factionalism and voting blocs: J. T. Main, *Political Parties before the Constitution** (1973), on the state level, and H. J. Henderson, *Party Politics in the Continental Congress* (1974), on the national level.

Most modern accounts of the Constitutional Convention take their point of departure from Charles Beard, whose *Economic Interpretation of the Constitution of the United States** (1913) exercised a powerful influence. Beard maintained that the authors of the Constitution had invested heavily in public securities and sought to bolster the national government in order to gain protection for the economic interests of their own class. Beard's thesis has been attacked and all but demolished by Robert Brown, *Charles Beard and the Constitution** (1956), and Forrest McDonald, *We the People: The Economic Origins of the Constitution** (1958). In *E Pluribus Unum** (1965), McDonald gives his own view of the economic and political maneuvering that brought about the Philadelphia convention, while J. T. Main, in *The Antifederalists** (1961), examines the forces of opposition. Max Farrand, *The Framing of the Constitution of the United States** (1913), is still a good account of the convention itself, but there is no substitute for the records of the convention and the debates in it, which are published in Max Farrand, ed., *Records of the Federal Convention of 1787*, 4 vols.* (1911–37), and C. C. Tansill, ed., *Documents Illustrative of the Formation of the Union of the United States* (1927). J. E. Cooke, ed., *The Federalist* (1961), is the definitive edition of these papers, which are also available in a reliable paperback edition by Clinton Rossiter (1961).

For the reader who wishes to approach this period through the original sources, a wealth of material, besides *The Federalist* and the *Records* of the convention, is readily available in complete modern editions, now in process of publication, of the *Papers* of the period's great men. These editions, besides printing everything that a man wrote, include letters and communications written to him. Among the men whose *Papers* are thus being published are Thomas Jefferson (J. P. Boyd, ed.), John Adams (Lyman Butterfield and R. J. Taylor, eds.), Benjamin Franklin (L. W. Labaree and W. B. Willcox, eds.), Alexander Hamilton (H. C. Syrett and J. E. Cooke, eds.), and James Madison (W. T. Hutchinson, W. M. E. Rachal, and R. A. Rutland, eds.).

*Available in a paperback edition.

1789–1861

THE NATIONAL EXPERIENCE

The preamble to the federal Constitution set ambitious goals: "to form a more perfect Union;" to "provide for the common defence;" to "promote the general Welfare;" and to secure for the American people justice, liberty, and domestic tranquility. To achieve those ends the Constitution enlarged the powers of the federal government and curtailed those of the states. But the definition of federal powers was vague, and the division of authority between nation and states imprecise. These ambiguities have never been fully and conclusively resolved, but the early Presidents and Congresses made numerous crucial decisions about policies and procedures that ultimately hardened into enduring precedents. Early in the nineteenth century a vigorous Supreme Court made it clear that the federal judiciary would be a coordinate branch of the government, using its jurisdiction over cases arising under the Constitution to interpret that document and to rule on the constitutionality of both federal and state legislative acts.

One of the most dangerous ambiguities of the Constitution was whether the phrase "a more perfect Union" was intended to mean a perpetual Union. Though opposition to the new Constitution evaporated soon after ratification, state loyalties remained strong, and the federal government, remote from the average citizen, easily aroused the suspicions of those who disliked its policies. For many years after 1789 most Americans thought of the federal Union as an experiment, a possible means to certain desirable ends, seldom as an end in itself. Not until well into the nineteenth century did a substantial body of citizens develop a sense of national identity, a love for the Union as an absolute good, and a determination to preserve it at any cost. Meanwhile, disaffected groups everywhere applied the principle of state sovereignty to justify challenges to federal authority and even, as a last resort, secession from the Union. Ultimately the fate of the Union had to be settled "at the cannon's mouth."

Uncertainty about the future of the Union did not impede steady progression from a deferential political society, in which the common people accepted upper-class gentlemen from established families as their natural leaders, to a modern democracy, in which adult white males of all classes participated in the political process. By the time of Andrew Jackson's presidency, political leaders had accepted parties as essential and constructive adjuncts of politics in a republic. At the same time the base of political democracy had broadened as property restrictions on voting were abolished, the national nominating convention replaced the secret party caucus in the selection of presidential candidates, and presidential electors were chosen by popular vote rather than by state legislatures. Politicians learned how to appeal to a mass electorate, and in the closely contested party battles a growing proportion of the voters turned out on election day. Political democracy advanced in all sections of the country.

American society in the young republic was notable for its fluidity, for "the general equality of condition among the people." The emphasis was on equality of opportunity—on the principle that there must be no special privileges for the few, no artificial barriers in the way of those bent on improving their social or economic status. Indeed, to achieve material success became almost a moral duty, for Americans believed that individual improvement contributed to the improvement of the nation.

Americans differed on how government should enhance the nation's economic well-being. But government, especially at the state and local level, played a significant role in the improvement of transportation and thus in the development of interregional trade and a national market economy. The federal policy of territorial expansion provided what seemed at the time limitless lands for farmers and an inexhaustible treasure of natural resources. Federal land policy was designed to stimulate western settlement rather than to create government revenue.

By the middle of the nineteenth century the country had entered a period of accelerated economic growth, characterized by agricultural expansion in the South and West and by the rise of the factory system and urbanization in the Northeast. The relatively high cost of labor prompted American manufacturers to invest in labor-saving devices and to adopt the methods of modern mass production, including the assembly line and interchangeable parts. By 1860 the corporate form of business enterprise was making rapid progress, especially in transportation and the textile industry.

Industrialization and the growth of cities brought economic and social dislocations, giving rise to the fear that Americans were losing their souls in the quest for material gain. The Protestant clergy often pointed to signs of moral decay and a loss of national purpose, while the Evangelicals among them offered redemption through religious revivals. Another reaction to the social malaise was a massive and sometimes violent anti-Catholic nativist movement directed against the growing tide of German and Irish immigrants. Still another response produced a crusade for moral reform. With a perfectionist view of mankind's potential and a conviction that the millennium was imminent, the reformers organized to advance causes such as temperance, women's rights, and world peace.

Yet it was Southern slavery, which was expanding westward, that many Northern reformers identified as America's greatest social evil. During the 1830s they launched a radical movement for the abolition of an institution in which Southerners had an enormous capital investment and which played a crucial role in both the regional and national economy. In the 1850s the antislavery movement broadened its appeal by focusing on opposition to the further expansion of slavery and to the admission of additional slave states. That issue contributed to the disruption of the existing party system and to the birth of the Republican party, which in 1860 elected Abraham Lincoln President. Southern panic over the implications of this political revolution culminated in a secession movement and the formation of the Confederate States of America. The inability of statesmen to find a peaceful solution to the problem of slavery represented the greatest failure of the American political system. Because of that failure, for the next four years the country's resources and manpower were consumed in a tragic civil war.

6
ESTABLISHING NATIONAL INSTITUTIONS

In adopting the Constitution, Americans gave the United States an effective government with powers that would enable it to shape the future of the nation. But the men who drafted the Constitution were well aware that they had left many details undecided and that the first officers of the new government would have a greater opportunity than their successors to determine what the United States should be and become.

Launching the New Government

Fortunately many of the leaders of the Philadelphia convention were eager to finish the job they had begun. Franklin was too old now to do more than give his blessing, but most of the nation's other great men repaired to New York in 1789 to launch the new government and help shape its institutions. There had never been any question about the candidate for President: Washington's election was unanimous and unopposed. His progress from Mount Vernon to New York was marked by a succession of triumphal arches, cheering spectators, and pretty girls strewing his path with flowers and offering him crowns of laurel. He bore it all with his usual dignity. Though he would rather have stayed at home, he was excited by the

opportunity to give stature to the nation he had done so much to create.

The Vice President, John Adams, who had just returned from England, was a more complicated man, vain enough to invite laughter, but so quick, so keen, so talented in every way that hardly anyone dared laugh. Benjamin Franklin had once said of him that he was "always an honest man, often a wise one, but sometimes, and in some things, absolutely out of his senses." Adams soon found that the Vice Presidency carried little prestige or power, and an Adams could not be comfortable without a good deal of both. During Washington's Administration the Vice President set the pattern for future holders of the office by keeping himself in the background.

More influential in the first years of the new government was James Madison, the young Virginian who had played so large a role at Philadelphia. Madison's old political opponent, Patrick Henry—a powerful figure in the Virginia legislature—had succeeded in preventing Madison's election to the Senate, but his neighbors had elected him to the House of Representatives. There, in spite of his lack of humor, his small frame and unimposing appearance, Madison quickly became the dominant figure. In the early months he was also Washington's principal adviser.

Madison, like many Americans who had lived through the Revolution, was passionately interested in the art of government. So were his two friends,

142

George Washington, 1790, by Trumbull

Thomas Jefferson and Alexander Hamilton, both of whom Washington also called on for advice and assistance. Hamilton, the younger of the two, had a brilliant analytical mind and great talents as an administrator. He also had large ambitions, both for the United States and for himself. Thomas Jefferson was as intensely devoted to the new nation as Hamilton but had a greater range of interests and loyalties. Jefferson was interested in government because he was interested in human beings, of whom he thought well. The new government, he believed, was going to be a good thing for them, but he remained less committed to it than to them.

A strong executive.

In this galaxy of leaders, Washington was the most limited and at the same time the strongest. His strength came, not only from the fact that he had earned the unbounded confidence of the people, but from his simplicity of mind. As commanding general of the Revolutionary armies, he had devoted himself wholly to winning the war. As President of the United States he devoted himself with equal singleness of purpose, equal detachment, and equal success to making the new government respected at home and abroad.

The biggest part of the job, Washington felt, was to establish respect for his own office. In the first flush of republican revulsion from England, Americans had identified executive power with hereditary, irresponsible monarchy, and they had accordingly neglected or suppressed it in their new governments. Most of the state constitutions, while affirming the need for a separation of powers, had actually made the executive the creature of the legislature; the Articles of Confederation had provided for no real executive. The Constitutional Convention had rectified that error by creating the office of President and assigning extensive powers to it: command of the army and navy, responsibility for foreign negotiations, and authority to appoint other governmental officers. Some of the powers were to be shared with the Senate, but the line of demarcation between the executive and legislative branches was not clear. It was up to him, Washington believed, to establish the extent of executive power and to organize the office so that future Presidents would be able to keep it strong.

Simply by taking office Washington went a long way toward achieving that end, for his own immense prestige could not fail to lend weight to any position he accepted. But he took pains to surround himself with more of the trappings of honor than he allowed himself at Mount Vernon. When he rode abroad it was on a white horse, with a leopard-skin saddlecloth edged in gold, or in an elegant coach pulled by six cream-colored horses. He rented one of the most sumptuous mansions in New York and stationed powdered lackeys at the door. He held "levees" in the manner of European monarchs, passing among the dignitaries to give each a moment of the presidential presence.

Some of Washington's associates thought this was going too far; others could not get enough of it. After the President's inauguration on April 30, 1789, his admirers in Congress had brought on a heated debate by proposing to address a formal congratulatory message to "His Highness the President of the United States and Protector of their Liberties." John Adams and Richard Henry Lee argued strenuously that some such title was needed to testify to the President's eminence, especially for the edification of the foreigners for whom he would personify the United States. The idea horrified ardent republicans, and James Madison carried the majority with him by proposing that the message be addressed simply to "George Washington, President of the United States."

By eliminating ostentatious titles Madison had no intention of minimizing the executive office. He had written most of the President's inaugural address as well as the congressional reply to it. In the first crucial months of the new government his was the hand that guided President and Congress alike in the legislation that organized the executive office and gave it the strength the President sought.

Though the Constitutional Convention had not directly provided for any executive departments except the Treasury, it clearly envisaged them in stating that the President should have power to call for the opinions of the principal officer in each such department. One of the first acts of the new government was to pass laws establishing the departments of the Treasury, State, and War, which, together with the offices of Attorney General and Postmaster General, were the only executive departments under Washington.

Had Washington and Madison been less insistent on executive independence, these departments might have formed the nucleus of a "cabinet" responsible to the legislative branch, as in the emerging British system. Such a development was prevented when Madison persuaded the House of Representatives, against considerable opposition, that the heads of departments, though appointed by the President with the consent of the Senate, should be subject to removal by the President alone.

Washington's first appointments to the new offices included Jefferson at State and Hamilton at the Treasury. His other choices were less distinguished: Henry Knox as Secretary of War and Edmund Randolph as Attorney General. Washington did not regard his secretaries as a team or cabinet that must act collectively. Rather, he thought of them as assistants, and in the first years they held no regular meetings. The President might refer decisions to them when he was absent from the seat of government, and he expected them to take the initiative in developing plans within their own fields of responsibility. But he kept the reins in his own hands. Executive decisions were his decisions.

Legislative decisions were not. Washington made only very general suggestions for legislation and scrupulously refrained from disclosing his views on specific measures being considered by Congress. He was extremely reluctant to use his veto power and did so only twice during his Presidency. It was his business, he believed, to administer the laws, not to make them. Consequently, while he established the authority and independence of executive action within the range allowed by the Constitution, he took no active part in the formation of public policy by legislation.

In the absence of presidential initiative three men guided Congress: Madison, Hamilton, and Jefferson. For the first five months Madison had the job to himself, for no other member of Congress combined the requisite political talents with the imagination that the new situation demanded. Hamilton acquired a position of leadership by his appointment to the Treasury on September 11, 1789, because in creating that department Congress had provided for a close connection between the Secretary and the legislature. At Madison's insistence, Congress had authorized the Secretary to prepare plans for collecting revenue and sustaining public credit and to present them to the House of Representatives, which under the Constitution had the sole right to initiate money bills. Washington approved Hamilton's active participation in the affairs of the House for, though he refrained from legislative matters himself, he did not think it necessary or desirable that his department heads should do so.

Jefferson did not accept the Secretaryship of State until January 1790 and did not arrive in New York until two months later. His office was less closely connected with legislative affairs than Hamilton's. Moreover, while Hamilton ran the Treasury pretty much by himself, Washington took an active part in the management of foreign affairs and frequently overruled his Secretary of State. Nevertheless, Jefferson's close friendship and alliance with Madison gave him considerable influence in Congress.

The Bill of Rights. In ratifying the Constitution, six states had suggested amendments to specify the popular rights that the government must never invade. Many of the legislators who had been elected to the first Congress under the new Constitution arrived in New York prepared to carry out the suggestions. Although Madison had opposed a bill of rights both before and during ratification, when it became clear

Washington and his Cabinet: Henry Knox, Alexander Hamilton, Thomas Jefferson, and Edmund Randolph

to him that the people of the United States were determined to have one he decided to draft it himself.

Madison had initially opposed a bill of rights, for two reasons. First, he thought that declarations of popular rights, while useful against a monarch, would be ineffective against a republican government, in which the people themselves were ultimately the lawgivers. Second, he feared that any explicit statement of rights would prove too narrow and might be used to limit freedom instead of limiting authority: a wayward government might construe the specified rights as the only rights of the people. The debates over ratification had introduced another ground for fear: many advocates of amendment, including some members of Congress, wanted to reduce the authority of the federal government in relation to that of the state governments. In order to forestall amendments that might weaken the new government or that might undermine American freedom, Madison wanted to frame the bill of rights himself.

From the proposals he first presented to Congress in June 1789 there emerged the first ten amendments to the Constitution, which were ratified by the necessary number of states in December 1791. Known as the Bill of Rights, the amendments protected freedom of religion, of speech, and of the press, and the rights to assemble, to petition the government, to bear arms, to be tried by a jury, and to enjoy other procedural safeguards of the law (see Appendix). They forbade general warrants, excessive bail, cruel or unusual punishments, and the quartering of troops in private houses.

To prevent the government from ever claiming that the people had no rights except those specifically listed, the Ninth Amendment provided that "The enumeration in the Constitution of certain rights shall not be construed to deny or disparage others retained by the people." The Tenth Amendment reassured the state governments about their relationship to the federal government by affirming, "The powers not delegated to the United States by the Constitution, nor prohibited by it to the States, are reserved to the States respectively, or to the people."

Madison fought hard for his amendments, because in preparing them he had convinced himself that a bill of rights might be more effective than he had originally supposed. If a republican legislature proved hard to control, specific prohibitions would at least form a rallying point around which popular resistance could gather. The amendments would also assist the executive and judiciary branches in checking the legislature, for the amendments would be part of the Constitution, which every officer of government must swear to uphold. Even the state governments might be brought into action to resist encroachments, a thought that recurred some years later to Madison and Jefferson alike (see p. 162).

While Madison guided the Bill of Rights through Congress, the Senate passed a judiciary bill establishing the Supreme Court and thirteen inferior district courts. When the bill came to the House of Representatives, some members wanted to eliminate the provision for district courts and leave the everyday enforcement of federal laws to the state courts. But Madison persuaded the majority that the states could not be trusted in the matter. The Judiciary Act of 1789, as finally passed, established thirteen district courts and three circuit courts with both concurrent and appellate jurisdiction. It also explicitly provided that the Supreme Court should review decisions of state courts and nullify state laws that violated the United States Constitution or the laws and treaties made under it.

The Shaping of Domestic Policy

By adopting the Bill of Rights and by establishing federal courts to uphold the Constitution, Americans completed the work of the Constitutional Convention and made the legacy of the Revolution secure. The next pressing problem was to recover the nation's economic credit.

National credit and national debt. At the Constitutional Convention it had been understood that the new government would levy taxes to pay not only its own expenses but the debts of the old government. The debts were the debts of the nation, regardless of which government contracted them. On July 4, 1789, Congress established customs duties on all imports and two weeks later placed a tonnage duty on all shipping, with high rates for foreign vessels, low ones for American. When Alexander Hamilton took office at the Treasury, it became his task to apply the income from these duties to the national debt.

Hamilton found that the United States owed $54,124,464.56, including interest. It was widely assumed that the amount would be scaled down, at least the amount owed to creditors who were themselves citizens of the United States. Much of the domestic debt was in the form of certificates that had been either issued as pay to soldiers during the Revolution or bought by patriotic citizens to further the war effort. But by now most of the certificates were held by speculators or merchants who had bought them at much less than face value when the credit of the government fell and hard times forced the owners to sell. The restoration of national credit, it seemed to many Americans, did not require payment at face value to those who had themselves discounted that value. Hamilton thought otherwise. In his Report on Public Credit, presented to Congress on January 14, 1790, he proposed to fund—that is, to pay—the entire national debt, both foreign and domestic, at its face value. Existing certificates of indebtedness would be redeemed by interest-bearing government bonds worth the original value plus the unpaid interest, calculated at 4 percent.

The very boldness of the proposal won acclaim, and there was no real opposition to the full payment of the nation's obligations. The only question—and a large one—was who should be paid. On this question Madison and Hamilton came to a parting of the ways.

Hamilton insisted that payments be made to whoever held the certificates. Many of his associates had known that his report would contain such a recommendation and had begun buying up certificates wherever they could be found. Madison, shocked by the scramble, rose in the House of Representatives to offer an alternative to Hamilton's scheme. Madison proposed to pay the face value of the certificates only to original holders who still possessed them. To subsequent purchasers he would have paid the highest market value that the certificates had formerly commanded (fifty cents on the dollar). He would have paid the difference between this amount and the face value to the soldiers and citizens who had supported the Revolution and who had then been obliged to part with their certificates at less than face value because of the government's inability to maintain its credit.

Madison's plan would not have reduced the amount paid by the government. It would simply have prevented speculators from making large profits at the expense of the government's original creditors. Unhappily for Madison, and not by accident, the speculators included many members of Congress, who did not hesitate to wrap their own shady transactions in the national honor. Men who had agents combing the country for certificates stood on the floors of Congress and denounced Madison's proposal as an attempt to make the government evade its just obligations. Madison, hitherto the master of Congress, now saw his motion defeated in the House of Representatives by a vote of thirteen to thirty-six.

Madison's proposal was defeated not by greed alone. If accepted, it would have jeopardized the basic purpose of funding the debt: to restore national credit. The credit of the government had to be sustained without regard to the motives or merits of its creditors, because when the government had need for more money than it could obtain by current taxation (and every government has such a need in national emergencies), it would have to rely on bankers and speculators, men with money to lend. Their confidence had to be purchased in advance.

Before bringing Hamilton's funding scheme to a vote, Congress took up an even more controversial matter, which Hamilton had also recommended in his report—the assumption by the national government of debts owed by the state governments. Such a move was not necessary to sustain national credit, and many supporters of the funding measure failed to see the point of it. Gouverneur Morris, a staunch conservative, was in London when he heard of the scheme and wrote back in puzzlement: "To assume the payment of what the States owe, merely because they owe it, seems to my capacity not more rational, than to assume the debts of corporations, or of individuals." Senator Robert Morris of Pennsylvania, to whom the letter was written, had other views. "By God," he said, "it must be done."

The crucial difference between Gouverneur Morris and Robert Morris was that one was in England and the other in America. Robert, like other speculators in America, had an opportunity to take advantage of assumption before it became a fact. During the Revolutionary War the states, like the national government, had borrowed money by issuing securities. Many of these state securities had since depreciated even more than national ones. Speculators, including congressmen, now rushed to buy them. And with the prospect of making fortunes they lined up behind the assumption of state debts as they did behind the funding of the national debt.

But there was more opposition to assumption than to funding because Hamilton's proposition contained no allowance for states that had already paid a large proportion of their debt. These states included Virginia, Maryland, North Carolina, and Georgia. The largest debts were owed by Massachusetts and South Carolina. As a result, Virginians, for instance, having been taxed by the state government to pay its debt, would be taxed again by the federal government to help pay the debts of Massachusetts and South Carolina.

The inequity of the scheme enabled Madison to muster a small majority against it on a test vote in the House. But he did not dare to push his advantage, because the speculative interests threatened to vote against funding unless they got assumption as well. Much as he disliked Hamilton's funding plan, Madison knew that the rejection of funding altogether would mean the total destruction of national credit and possibly of the national government itself.

In July 1790, after Hamilton and his friends agreed to a partial allowance for states that had already paid a large part of their debts, Madison and his friends agreed to a bill providing for both funding and assumption. The fact that the two sides had been able to reach a compromise was heartening, but the line of division was ominous: Hamilton spoke for the merchants and creditors of the North, who would benefit enormously from funding and assumption, because they had accumulated most of the government's certificates of indebtedness; Madison and Jefferson spoke for the planters and farmers of the South, whose taxes would flow steadily north to pay the debt. The same division was evident in a simultaneous dispute about the location of the national capital, settled by a thirteen-to-twelve vote in the Senate that moved the government for the next ten years to Philadelphia and thereafter to a new federal district (Washington, D.C.) on the Potomac River. The differing interests of North and South, which Madison had already perceived in 1787, were beginning to affect national politics.

The Hamiltonian program. Hamilton's victory, for it amounted to that, was not simply a successful swindle. The speculative frenzy set off by his measures was a calculated part of one of the boldest programs ever envisaged for the development of the nation and the nation's economy. Hamilton believed that the future of the United States depended on a large-scale expansion of industry and commerce. The suspension of imports from England during the war had forced the growth of manufacturing in America, and the production of hardware and textiles had continued in some measure afterward. To effect the kind of growth that Hamilton wanted the primary need was capital, capital in large quantities concentrated in the hands of people willing to risk investing it. By means of funding and assumption Hamilton created

It is now proper ... to enumerate the principal circumstances from which it may be inferred that manufacturing establishments not only occasion a positive augmentation of the produce and revenue of the society, but that they contribute essentially to rendering them greater than they could possibly be without such establishments. These circumstances are:

1. The division of labor.
2. An extension of the use of machinery.
3. Additional employment to classes of the community not ordinarily engaged in the business.
4. The promoting of emigration from foreign countries.
5. The furnishing greater scope for the diversity of talents and dispositions, which discriminate men from each other.
6. The affording a more ample and various field for enterprise.
7. The creating, in some instances, a new, and securing, in all, a more certain and steady demand for the surplus produce of the soil.

Each of these circumstances has a considerable influence upon the total mass of industrious effort in a community; together, they add to it a degree of energy and effect which are not easily conceived.

From Alexander Hamilton, Report on Manufactures, 1791.

just such a group of wealthy investors, or, to use a less attractive word, profiteers. Hamilton was no profiteer himself—he was too interested in power to give much attention to his own finances. But he was well satisfied with the huge speculative profits that others reaped from his measures, for those profits meant capital for business investment. Moreover, funding and assumption, by restoring national credit, would make investment in American enterprises more attractive to foreign capital.

Hamilton's measures were prompted not merely by economic considerations but by his consistent determination to strengthen the national government and to overcome the centrifugal force of the state governments. He anticipated that all the capitalists created by funding and assumption would be eager to maintain the national credit and the national government, if only to protect their investments. By the same token, the assumption of state debts would deprive the state governments of such support. The national government, working hand in glove with powerful investors, would grow strong as industry and commerce grew.

Hamilton's scheme generated its own support. The opportunity to get rich easily and by methods not strictly illegal was more than congressmen could resist. Washington was disturbed by the rumor that "the funding of the debt has furnished effectual means of corrupting such a portion of the Legislature as turns the balance between the honest voters whichever way it is directed." Hamilton, who was doing the direct-

ing, assured the President that "there is not a member of the Legislature who can properly be called a stock-jobber or a paper-dealer. . . . As to improper speculations on measures depending before Congress, I believe never was any body of men freer from them." Washington believed him.

Hamilton's next objective was a national bank with capital supplied partly by the government and partly by private investors. But since the investors would be permitted to pay in government bonds for three-fourths of the bank stock they purchased, the bank's notes would rest very largely on the national debt. With the government furnishing most of the capital and assuming most of the risk, the bank could offer an irresistible invitation to wealthy citizens to invest their money. Furthermore, the national debt, if utilized for a bank, could be a national advantage. In arguing for funding and assumption, Hamilton had emphasized the fact that where a national debt "is properly funded, and an object of established confidence, it answers most of the purposes of money." He intended to make it serve this purpose through the bank: notes issued by the bank would serve as a much needed medium of exchange (specie being scarce) and would greatly facilitate business and the financing of new commercial and industrial enterprise. Besides acting as a central exchange, the bank would handle government finances; and it would expedite borrowing both by the government and by individuals. Through this government-sponsored expansion of credit, the bond between private capital and the na-

Those who labour in the earth are the chosen people of God, if ever he had a chosen people, whose breasts he has made his peculiar deposit for substantial and genuine virtue. It is the focus in which he keeps alive that sacred fire, which otherwise might escape from the face of the earth. Corruption of morals in the mass of cultivators is a phenomenon of which no age nor nation has furnished an example. It is the mark set on those, who not looking up to heaven, to their own soil and industry, as does the husbandman, for their subsistance, depend for it on the casualties and caprice of customers. Dependance begets subservience and venality, suffocates the germ of virtue, and prepares fit tools for the designs of ambition. This, the natural progress and consequence of the arts, has sometimes perhaps been retarded by accidental circumstances: but, generally speaking, the proportion which the aggregate of the other classes of citizens bears in any state to that of its husbandmen, is the proportion of its unsound to its healthy parts.... While we have land to labour then, let us never wish to see our citizens occupied at a workbench, or twirling a distaff ... for the general operations of manufacture, let our workshops remain in Europe.

Jefferson's view of the good society

From Thomas Jefferson, *Notes on the State of Virginia,* **1787.**

tional government would be tightened.

When the bill to charter the bank came before the House early in February 1791, Madison attacked it with arguments he would not have used two years earlier. Before the adoption of the Constitution, he had argued strenuously that Congress should assume all the powers it needed to do its job. Under the new government he had hitherto taken a generous view of the extent of congressional authority. By now, however, he was thoroughly worried over the emerging shape of Hamilton's program and intent on stopping it. He argued that because the Constitution did not specifically empower Congress to issue charters of incorporation it had no right to do so. Hamilton answered that the Constitution empowered the government to do anything "necessary and proper" to carry out its assigned functions.

This was the first great debate over strict, as opposed to loose, interpretation of the Constitution. Congress readily accepted Hamilton's loose construction and passed the bill. Washington weighed the question more seriously, listening carefully to Madison and Jefferson as well as to Hamilton. Though he remained doubtful to the end, at the last minute, on February 25, 1791, he signed the bill. Hamilton's program moved ahead another step.

Having provided capital and credit, Hamilton was now ready to direct the expansion of manufacturing. In December he presented to Congress his Report on Manufactures, a scheme to make investment in industry attractive by means of protective tariffs and bounties. It was Hamilton's aim to direct the nation toward a balanced economy that would include manufacturing as well as agriculture and commerce. Only through such a balance could the United States make the most of its resources, reduce its foreign debt and its reliance on foreign nations, and attain true independence. But Hamilton was not allowed to add this capstone to his economic edifice. Farmers and merchants, fearing that protective tariffs would prompt retaliatory action by other countries against American agricultural exports, preferred free competition to keep down the price of manufactures. And almost everyone wondered whether the United States could afford a measure that would discourage importation, since the government's principal income came from import duties. To raise them to protective levels might reduce the volume of imports so drastically as to endanger the national credit. Moved by these considerations, Congress dealt Hamilton his first defeat by shelving his report.

Madison and Jefferson, who engineered the defeat, were both alarmed by the apparent intent of Hamilton's program. No one had done more than Madison to resuscitate and strengthen the central government a few years earlier at the Constitutional Convention, but in the Hamiltonian system he saw the beginnings of a national government so strong that it would endanger the individual liberties he had been trying to protect in the Bill of Rights. Jefferson, even more than Madison, was wary of governmental power.

The Shaping of Domestic Policy **149**

To this distrust of government, Jefferson joined a dislike of cities and of the merchants and manufacturers who thrived in them. Farmers, he believed, enjoyed a greater virtue and a closer contact with their Maker than did the inhabitants of cities. From Paris he had written to Madison in 1787, "I think our governments will remain virtuous for many centuries; as long as they are chiefly agricultural. . . . When they get piled upon one another in large cities, as in Europe, they shall become corrupt as in Europe." Jefferson and Madison were both convinced that the federal government would have all the strength it needed and would be less likely to exceed its authority if it depended not on an alliance with powerful creditors but on the support of the producing classes, especially the farmers, who formed the bulk of the population. Opponents of the Constitution had feared that a strong central government would be manipulated to bring power and wealth to a few. Hamilton seemed bent on justifying their fears, which he and Madison had earlier joined to combat in *The Federalist*. Moreover, Hamilton's program was driving a wedge between the North, where capital and credit were accumulating, and the South, whose farmers and planters feared that the accumulation was at their expense. Almost all the stock in Hamilton's United States Bank was purchased by Northern and European creditors; and Hamilton made it plain that the bank was intended to assist the expansion of commerce and industry, not agriculture, which in his view needed no encouragement. He dismissed out of hand a proposal that the bank lend money to Southern planters on the security of tobacco warehouse receipts.

Thus, within three years of the inauguration of the national government, its leaders had reached a fundamental disagreement over its scope and policy. The disagreement was perhaps less dangerous than it seemed at the time, because both sides were still determined to make the new government work and because slavery, the issue in which Southerners most feared interference, had gone unchallenged. In 1793 when they introduced a bill in Congress requiring all courts, state and federal, to assist slave owners in recovering fugitive slaves, Northern congressmen readily supplied the votes to pass it, in spite of the fact that its terms were so vague as to imperil the rights of every free black.

Nevertheless, the gap between the views of Hamilton on the one hand and of Jefferson and Madison on the other was about as wide as constitutional government could stand. Each now aimed more at defeating and suppressing the other than at bargaining. Fortunately, Washington stood above the quarrel, and both sides could still join in persuading him to accept another term when the national elections were held in 1792. But during his second term the dissension spread from domestic to foreign affairs, increasingly open, increasingly bitter, and accompanied by a public rhetoric that grew increasingly violent, as each side became convinced that the other was betraying the republican ideals of the Revolution.

Foreign Affairs Under Washington

The Constitution assigned to the President the conduct of relations with Europeans and Indians, and Washington undertook the task himself. While he gave Hamilton a free hand in developing financial policy and refused to meddle in congressional enactments of that policy, he gave Jefferson no such freedom as Secretary of State. He turned to Jefferson for advice, but he sought advice from other department heads as well. As foreign affairs assumed greater and greater complexity, he began the practice of calling together the Attorney General and the Secretaries of State, War, and the Treasury to discuss policy. During these meetings, from which grew the Cabinet as an institution, Jefferson and Hamilton again revealed their differing conceptions of the national welfare.

Jeffersonian neutrality. The discord in foreign affairs first showed itself in 1790, when a threatened war between Spain and England offered the United States an opportunity to press American claims against both countries. Spain had seized three British vessels trading in Nootka Sound, Vancouver Island, which had been Spanish territory ever since its discovery. England demanded the return of the ships, reparation for damages, and recognition of British trading rights in the area. It seemed likely that Spain would fight rather than submit.

Washington's advisers all agreed that the United States should remain neutral in case of war, but they did not agree on what the United States should do if England decided to march troops through American territory in the Mississippi Valley in order to attack the Spanish in Florida and Louisiana. Since Hamilton had just tied his funding program to duties on British trade, he was reluctant to do anything that might offend England and was ready to declare American neutrality at once. Jefferson, on the other hand, had just come from five years as the United States Ambassador to France, where he had seized every opportunity to bargain for national advantages. He wanted to bargain now, to keep both Spain and England guessing about America's intentions and to make them bid high for assurance of American neutrality. In particular, he hoped to make England open its West Indian ports to American ships.

As it happened, Spain gave in to the British ultimatum. No war occurred, and the ports remained closed, with Hamilton giving the British secret assurances against retaliatory regulations by the United States. But another European war was clearly in the making, and mounting tensions in Europe generated a notable increase in the cordiality of European countries toward the United States. In 1791 England sent a minister plenipotentiary, George Hammond, to reside in Philadelphia; the United States in turn sent Thomas Pinckney to London. Full diplomatic relations had thus been established between England and the United States when war finally did break out in 1793 between England and France—and something close to war between Hamilton and Jefferson.

Thomas Jefferson, as American minister to France during the 1780s, had learned to admire French civilization and French people. Just before returning to the United States late in 1789, he had witnessed the beginnings of their revolution. He was skeptical that a people who had lived so long under absolute monarchy could successfully undertake republican government. But he heartily approved their efforts to curb their king. When he took up his post as Washington's Secretary of State, he brought with him a warm sympathy for the French and their cause, a sympathy that was not destroyed by the execution of Louis XVI in 1793 or by the reign of terror that followed.

Hamilton, by contrast, watched with horror as the French Revolution overturned the foundations of society, destroying monarchy and aristocracy, exalting democracy and demagogues. His horror mounted when the French Revolutionists launched the "war of all peoples against all kings," with England and Spain as primary targets. England, even under King George III, seemed to Hamilton a safer friend for Americans than mob-wracked republican France. Hamilton was moved not simply by his repugnance for the French Revolution but by the belief that, if the United States had to choose sides, England was more to be feared than France, because England had the stronger navy. American commerce was more vulnerable to English sailors than to French soldiers.

Hamilton agreed with Washington's other advisers that the United States should stay out of the war, but he wanted to use the crisis as an opportunity to scrap the French alliance. The treaties of 1778, he argued, had been made with the French monarchy and were no longer binding now that the monarchy had been overthrown. The United States should therefore declare its neutrality and refuse to receive the minister, Edmond Genêt, sent by the new French republic early in 1793.

Jefferson argued that the treaties had been made with the French nation and were still binding. He was as certain as Hamilton that the United States should stay out of the war but wanted the country to do so without publicly announcing its intention. A declaration of neutrality would affront the French and would destroy the possibility of bargaining with the British, who still had troops stationed in the American Northwest and still withheld trading privileges in the empire. Washington decided the matter on April 22, 1793, by issuing a proclamation of neutrality addressed to American citizens only and not actually mentioning the word "neutrality." The treaties with France were not repudiated, and Citizen Genêt was accorded formal recognition. But the bargaining power that Jefferson valued was gone. Shortly afterward he announced that he would retire at the end of the year.

Genêt was a fool. From the moment of his arrival he assumed powers that no independent country could permit a foreign envoy: he commissioned American ships to sail as privateers under the French flag; he set up courts to condemn the ships they captured; he arranged an expedition of Western frontiersmen to attack Spanish New Orleans. Jefferson tried hard to like him but gave up in disgust. Finally Washington demanded Genêt's recall.

While Genêt was losing friends for France, the British government was losing them for England. Under the slogan "free ships make free goods," Americans claimed the right as neutrals to carry noncontraband goods (including naval stores) to and from the ports of belligerents. France had lifted some of its mercantilist restrictions regulating trade with its West Indian islands, and American ships were swarming there to take advantage of the new opportunity. But England adhered to its rule of 1756 that trade closed in peacetime could not be opened to neutrals in wartime. In December 1793, without warning, British naval vessels began seizing American ships trading with the French West Indies.

The seizures combined with an Indian episode in the Northwest to bring the United States, in spite of Hamilton, to the brink of war with England. The record of Washington's government in dealing with hostile Indians had not been good. He had arranged a treaty with Alexander McGillivray, the half-breed chieftain of the Creeks, but the Creeks had broken it as soon as it was made. He had sent General Josiah Harmar to crush the Miamis in Ohio, but they had crushed him. He had sent Arthur St. Clair with a larger force in 1791, but St. Clair, like Braddock in 1755, had been surprised just short of his objective and completely routed. In February 1794, as General Anthony Wayne gathered a force to try again, the governor-general of Canada, Lord Dorchester, made a speech to the Indians in which he in effect exhorted them to do their worst. Reports of the speech reached

Congress along with news of the Caribbean seizures.

The House of Representatives was then debating whether restrictions against British commerce (suggested by Jefferson shortly before his resignation) might lead England to reduce its own restrictions against American commerce. News of the seizures precipitated an overwhelming demand for much stronger anti-British measures, to which Hamilton felt sure England would react by declaring war on the United States—if indeed the United States did not declare war first. The country was swept by war hysteria; volunteer defense companies sprang up. Mobs mistreated English seamen and tarred and feathered pro-British Americans. To prevent a plunge into actual warfare, Hamilton urged Washington to send a special mission to England. Hamilton seems to have thought of heading it himself, but Washington gave the job to Hamilton's alter ego, John Jay.

A Hamiltonian treaty. Although Jay had had abundant experience as a diplomat, in the eyes of most Americans much of it had been unsuccessful experience. As envoy to Spain during the Revolution, he had failed to gain either alliance or recognition of American independence. As Secretary for Foreign Affairs under the Articles of Confederation, he had conducted the nearly disastrous negotiations with Gardoqui. In both cases failure arose less from lack of skill on his part than from the fact that the other side held all the cards. This time, with England engaged in a major European war, Jay was in a strong position to play the game that Jefferson had recommended all along: namely, to convince the English that unless they made concessions they could not count on continued American neutrality. Edmund Randolph, the new Secretary of State, agreed with the Jeffersonian strategy. He instructed Jay to consult with Russia, Sweden, and Denmark about the possibility of an armed-neutrality agreement in order to bring pressure on England to stop seizures of neutral shipping.

Once again, however, Jay found himself on the losing side through no fault of his own. Denmark and Sweden, which shared the American view of the rights of neutral ships, took the initiative, and just after Jay's departure for Europe the United States received an invitation from them to join in forming an alliance of neutrals. Randolph wanted to accept, for he felt that such backing would strengthen Jay's hand. But Hamilton persuaded Washington to decline, on the grounds that the alliance would jeopardize Jay's mission by antagonizing the British. Not content with rejecting the assistance of other neutrals, and eager to create a friendly climate of opinion in England, Hamilton weakened Jay's position still further by informing George Hammond, the British minister in America, of Washington's decision.

With this information to guide him, Lord Grenville, the British foreign minister, felt safe in conceding little. He promised again to surrender the Northwest posts—provided the United States permitted the continuation of the English fur trade with the Indians in the area; he promised recompense for the American ships that had been seized without warning in December 1793 in the Caribbean—provided the United States compensated British creditors for pre-revolutionary debts whose collection had been impeded by state governments. He refused to compensate American slave owners for slaves kidnaped or liberated by the British during the Revolution, and he refused to give any guarantee against the British navy's practice of stopping American vessels to impress alleged British subjects as seamen. Instead of stopping the seizure of neutral ships, he required the United States to give up its own view of neutral shipping rights for the duration of England's war with France and for two years thereafter. He consented to reciprocal trading rights between England and America but restricted American trade with the British West Indies to vessels of no more than seventy tons, and even these he allowed only in return for an American promise to ship no molasses, sugar, coffee, cocoa, or cotton from the islands or from the United States to any other part of the world. The only generosity he showed was at the expense of the Spanish: it was agreed that both British subjects and Americans should have the right to navigate the Mississippi through Spanish territory to the sea.

When the treaty containing these terms reached Washington on March 7, 1795, Hamilton was no longer at the Treasury. He had resigned at the end of January, a little more than a year after Jefferson, but he retained as much influence over the President out of office as in. His replacement, Oliver Wolcott, Jr., had been his assistant and continued to consult him on every important matter. Hamilton thought that the treaty was satisfactory and that failure to ratify it would mean war. Washington reluctantly agreed, but he could see that other Americans might not. To avoid a premature hardening of opposition, he tried to keep the terms secret until he could present the treaty for ratification at a special session of the Senate called for June 8. It was impossible. By the time the Senate met, rumors of the contents had produced wide public hostility, which increased as the details became known. Nevertheless, the senators, after striking out the clause regarding trade with the West Indies, accepted the treaty by the exact two-thirds majority required.

As the treaty came before Washington for his signature, the press was denouncing Jay, the treaty, the Senate, and even the President. Popular meetings in Boston, Philadelphia, New York, and other cities

The Treaty of Greenville, 1795

General Wayne had defeated the Indians of the Northwest at the Battle of Fallen Timbers (August 20, 1794) and had gone on to devastate their settlements. In the Treaty of Greenville (August 3, 1795) they gave up most of the territory that was to become the state of Ohio. In the next year the British at last honored their agreement to evacuate their posts in the Northwest.

Meanwhile, Spain had become fearful that the United States would throw its small weight on the British side in the precarious European balance. The clause about the Mississippi in Jay's Treaty suggested that England and the United States might be contemplating joint action against Louisiana. Taking advantage of this fear, Thomas Pinckney, who was sent to negotiate a treaty, won for the United States everything it had been seeking from Spain: free navigation of the Mississippi, permission for American traders to deposit goods for shipment at the mouth of the river, acknowledgment of the American southern boundary at the thirty-first parallel and the western boundary at the Mississippi, and an agreement by each country to prevent Indians within its territory from making incursions into the territory of the other.

The Senate accepted Pinckney's Treaty unanimously on March 3, 1796. With it the danger of secession in Kentucky and Tennessee (admitted to the Union in 1792 and 1796) disappeared; with the Mississippi open to trade, any attachment to Spain lost its charm for the Americans of the Southwest. Although Washington's foreign policy had produced some vastly unpopular concessions to Britain, it must be credited with the restoration of reciprocal trading rights and with achieving, at last, recognition by both Spain and Britain of United States sovereignty over the area first won from Britain in 1783.

urged Washington to reject it. In the Cabinet everyone but Randolph urged him to sign. Dismayed by the public antagonism, Washington hesitated. In the meantime, the British minister handed to Oliver Wolcott some intercepted dispatches written by the French minister, Jean Fauchet. In them Fauchet, referring to some transactions with Randolph, seemed to imply that Randolph had turned over state secrets to him for money. Although the dispatches had nothing to do with the treaty, they discredited the only Cabinet member who opposed it. Washington signed the treaty, and, after confronting Randolph with the dispatches, refused his explanations and accepted his resignation.

The winning of the West. Jay's Treaty was the low-water mark of foreign affairs under Washington.

Negotiating the Treaty of Greenville

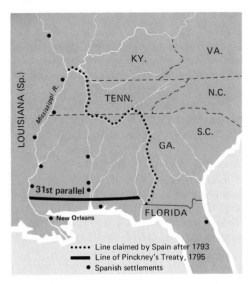

Pinckney's Treaty, 1795

Map legend:
- Line claimed by Spain after 1793
- Line of Pinckney's Treaty, 1795
- Spanish settlements

Federalists Versus Republicans

Alexander Hamilton, by dictating domestic policy to Congress and foreign policy to the President, gave the national government its initial direction. Although Madison and Jefferson managed to modify some of his measures, in all essentials Hamilton prevailed. But in their efforts to defeat him, Madison and Jefferson set a pattern of political action that in ten years' time gave them control of the government and thereafter became the only way of gaining or keeping control. They started a political party.

The Republican challenge. The framers of the Constitution, Madison included, had not thought well of parties. "Faction" was the word generally used for party in the eighteenth century, and a faction meant, by Madison's own definition, a group orga-

New states, 1791-96

nized to procure selfish advantages at the expense of the community. Denunciation of factions or parties was a standard ingredient in every discussion of politics in the eighteenth century, as safe and as platitudinous as denunciation of corruption and praise of honesty.

The parties of the time deserved denunciation. In the British House of Commons, and to some degree in the colonial assemblies, politicians had joined forces from time to time in order to make legal raids on the public purse. Because neither Madison nor Jefferson had any such end in view, they did not at first think of their opposition to Hamilton as constituting a party. Madison, to be sure, had a following in the House of Representatives and was an old hand at collecting votes in support of his measures. But in lining up opposition to indiscriminate funding and wholesale assumption, neither Jefferson nor Madison anticipated a continuing, organized opposition.

It was only as the full dimensions of Hamilton's program revealed themselves that the two men deliberately set out to gather and consolidate their strength against him inside the government and out. Jefferson was aware that Washington consulted Hamilton on every kind of measure, including matters that seemed to belong properly in the Department of State; in response, he tried to extend his own influence within the executive departments. Washington liked Jefferson, as did most of the other members of the presidential entourage. And yet Jefferson made little headway in his campaign. Though he succeeded in having the Mint established under the State Department instead of the Treasury, his attempts to get the Post Office transferred to the State Department failed, and so did his efforts to get his friend Tench Coxe appointed as Comptroller and Thomas Paine as Postmaster General.

Madison was more successful. In the House of Representatives he was often defeated, but every defeat strengthened the loyalty of his followers. Though he lacked Jefferson's personal charm and was not eloquent in debate, he knew how to work in the corridors; and on the floor his colleague from Virginia, William Branch Giles, was an able spokesman of his views. John Beckley, the perennial Clerk of the House, who seemed to know everybody's secrets, turned over valuable information to him. As the Madison forces hardened around a nucleus of Southern congressmen, they began to call themselves the "republican interest," and by 1792 they even dared to say the "republican party"—a phrase that gradually acquired capital letters.

Their opponents, not considering themselves a party, appropriated the name of Federalists, which had been used earlier by the advocates of the Constitution of 1787. This maneuver identified the Republicans with the Antifederalists of that period. Actually, though many former Antifederalists joined the Republicans, the identification was not warranted. The national leaders of the Republican party had supported the Constitution in 1787 and still did; the Federalists of the early 1790s were distinguished, not by any special reverence for that document, but by a conception of the national welfare that included a permanent national debt, a national bank, and dependence on England.

Madison and Jefferson believed that the source of Federalist strength, apart from Washington's support of Hamilton, was typical of faction or party in the traditional sense: it lay in the corruption of congressmen through the speculative opportunities that accompanied funding and assumption. Their own strength, they believed, lay with the people at large. Perhaps because they assumed that the people were on their side, they did not at first organize their party except within the government itself; they did, however, take steps to let the people know, through the press, what their side was.

Before 1791 the *Gazette of the United States* was the only newspaper that gave full coverage to national politics, and its editor, John Fenno, was an ardent Hamiltonian. Madison and Jefferson persuaded the poet Philip Freneau, whom they knew to be Republican in sentiment, to establish a newspaper that would report national issues from their point of view. On October 31, 1791, the first issue of the *National Gazette* was published, and the Republicans gained a medium for spreading attacks on the Hamiltonian program (some of them written by Madison) throughout the country.

At the same time spontaneous popular societies that might have furnished the basis for Republican party organization at the local level began to form. Admiration for the French Revolution and discontent with the government's evident bias in favor of England prompted the formation of these "Democratic Clubs," first in Pennsylvania and then all over the country. The clubs, which were imitations of the Jacobin societies in France, felt that they were continuing the tradition of the Sons of Liberty of the 1760s and 1770s. They sympathized with the French Revolution and passed resolutions against the government's pro-British foreign policy; they supported the Republicans in Congress and in elections for Congress. But before Madison and his friends could capitalize on their support, the Federalists found an opportunity to discredit the clubs and capture a wide popular following for themselves.

The Federalist response. The Federalist opportunity arose from a tax on whiskey passed by Congress in 1791 to help pay the expenses of funding and assumption. Excise taxes, especially on alcoholic beverages, were unpopular in the eighteenth century. A cider tax nearly caused rebellion in England in 1763, and so did a rum tax in Massachusetts in 1754. By 1794 the federal excise tax on liquor did cause rebellion, or what looked like it, in Pennsylvania. Farmers in the western part of the state generally turned their surplus grain into whiskey. This could be transported over the mountains more easily than wheat or corn, and it brought a better price in the Eastern markets. But the profit was small even without the excise, and hence there was much evasion of the tax. In July 1794 the United States marshal, summoning offenders to court, met with mass resistance.

The governor of the state, Thomas Mifflin, thought that the courts could handle the situation, but Hamilton wanted an immediate show of force. Washington weighed the situation, delayed until the rebels' rejection of every overture had turned public opinion against them, and then marched fifteen thousand militiamen to western Pennsylvania. No rebel fired a shot against him, and Washington returned to Philadelphia, leaving Hamilton to complete the arrest of the ringleaders.

When Congress assembled shortly after his return, Washington delivered an address that made clear how he felt about all organized opposition to the policies of the national government, whether from whiskey rebels, Democratic Clubs, or Republicans. Although there is no evidence that the clubs had anything to do with the rebellion, Washington had somehow got the notion that they had. In spite of the fact that the Constitution guaranteed the right to assemble, he rebuked the clubs as "self-created societies." Dismayed by his disapproval, many of them dissolved at once, and the rest expired within a year or two.

Washington's personal popularity was thus revealed as the strongest weapon in the Federalist arsenal. The Republicans were not fully aware of how strong it was or of how it could be used against them. Nor was Washington aware. He continued to regard himself as standing above party and seems never to have realized that as he came more and more to rely on Hamilton he was choosing sides in a party conflict. Hamilton did realize it and used Washington's prestige to turn popular opinion against the Republicans.

When the President signed Jay's Treaty, in spite of popular meetings that urged him not to, the Republicans, instead of conceding defeat, carried the battle to the House of Representatives. Although the Constitution gave only the Senate the authority to approve or reject treaties, the House, under Madison's leadership, asserted its right to examine treaties before appropriating funds to implement them. On this basis, the House demanded copies of the papers that had

Political buttons: supporting the President, 1782-93

passed to and from Jay during the negotiations. Washington, defending the integrity of the executive department, indignantly refused; Hamilton, by decrying the demand of the House as an insult to the President and a step toward war, soon had Congress flooded with petitions supporting the President. Republican efforts to secure counterpetitions were less successful, and Madison saw his majority dwindle to a minority. The House in the end supported the treaty.

The election of 1796. When the Republicans attacked the treaty in the House of Representatives, they had an eye on the presidential election that was to take place later in the year. In the elections of 1788 and 1792 there had been no serious contest for the Presidency. In 1796 it was probable, though not certain, that Washington would retire. If he did, the Republicans would have a chance to challenge Hamilton at the polls. But the Republican hope of unseating the Federalists received a strong setback when Madison's attack on the treaty foundered against Washington's popularity.

As the election approached, Washington gave the Federalists another advantage by delaying his decision to withdraw. The Republicans were wary of advancing any candidate of their own unless the still insuperable national hero was out of the race. It was understood that if Washington chose not to run, Adams would be the Federalist candidate; for Hamilton, though influential among politicians, did not have a wide enough popular following to assure election. For the same reason the Republicans had settled on Jefferson rather than Madison. In September Washington finally announced his retirement and published a farewell address drafted by Hamilton. The address contained a strong warning against partiality for foreign countries (meaning France) and against political parties (meaning Republicans). Washington still refused to think of the Federalists as a party.

Having secured Washington's support for a Federalist successor, Hamilton set about substituting a more pliable candidate for the prickly, independent Adams. Because of Adams' popular following, Hamilton could not renounce him publicly, but he hoped to

achieve his purpose by manipulating the electoral vote.

The maneuver was made possible by the peculiar constitutional provisions for electing the President. Each state could select its members for the Electoral College in any manner it saw fit. Six did it by popular vote, nine by vote of the state legislature, and one, Massachusetts, by a combination of the two. Most candidates for the college announced beforehand for whom they would vote; but this practice was not universal, and the college as an institution retained some small measure of choice. Each elector cast two ballots, without specifying which man he preferred for President; the candidate who received the largest vote became President, and the candidate with the second largest vote became Vice President. Since this was a system designed for a partyless government, complications arose when political parties appeared. If all the electors who favored the strongest party voted for both its candidates, a tie vote would result. In order to elect the party's preferred presidential candidate some electors had to divert their second vote from the party's vice-presidential candidate to some other candidate. This could be dangerous: if too many votes were diverted from the party's vice-presidential candidate he might be left with fewer than the presidential candidate of the opposing party, who would then become Vice President instead. There was also the possibility that if both parties wanted the same man for Vice President, he might receive more votes than either presidential candidate and thus become President.

It was this latter possibility that led Hamilton to arrange for Adams' running mate on the Federalist ticket to be Thomas Pinckney of South Carolina. Pinckney, who had just returned in triumph from his Spanish mission, enjoyed great popularity in the South, where the Republicans were strongest. Southerners would certainly give most of their votes to Jefferson, but they might be persuaded to designate Pinckney as second choice. If a substantial number of electors did so, the combined Federalist-Republican vote might be large enough to put Pinckney into the Presidency.

But Hamilton was not the only one who knew how to play with the electoral system. When the votes of the Electoral College were cast, it appeared that his advocacy of Pinckney had failed. Adams' friends in Connecticut and New Hampshire, refusing to endanger his success, had scattered their second votes, and the Southern Republicans had given Pinckney nothing. Even so, he had fifty-nine votes; but Adams with seventy-one became President and Jefferson with sixty-eight became Vice President. Jefferson's running mate, Aaron Burr of New York, had only thirty.

Had the Federalist electors of Connecticut and

New Hampshire given Pinckney their second votes, Hamilton's strategy could have succeeded. Pinckney would have tied Adams' vote, and tied presidential elections, according to the Constitution, were to be decided in the House of Representatives. There, with Jefferson out of the contest, Southern Republicans might have joined with Hamilton's forces to make Pinckney President. For Adams it was a bitter thing to have come so close to losing and to know that Hamilton was to blame.

The Presidency of John Adams

The new President was a man of conflicting emotions, ideas, and loyalties. Round of face and frame, he looked like an English country squire and often behaved like one, lashing out at those who crossed him as though he were lord of the manor. Yet he was sometimes remarkably patient when there was real cause for anger. Like Washington and Jefferson and George III, he loved the land and found high office uncongenial and inconvenient. Yet no man wanted the Presidency more or would have found defeat more humiliating.

Adams had had a distinguished career during the Revolution, both in the Continental Congress and in negotiating the peace treaty. His political experience and his study of history had given him strong ideas about the proper form of government: liberty, he believed, could be preserved only where a strong executive presided over a legislature divided into two houses, the upper representing the wealthy and well-born, the lower representing the people at large. This idea, expounded at length in his *Defence of the Constitutions of the United States* (1787), had influenced the Philadelphia convention and had helped produce the strong executive office that Adams inherited from Washington. As President, Adams continued to think that the executive must stand above the other branches of government and mediate differences between them.

The President and the politicians. Adams, like his contemporaries, spoke of political parties only to condemn them. Though he had been elected in a contest between parties, the circumstances were not such as to endear either side to him. The Republicans had branded him a monarchist because of his openly avowed advocacy of a strong executive, while the Federalists had almost betrayed him for Thomas Pinckney.

In his inaugural address Adams did his best to minimize party differences. Answering for the first time the accusations that had been made against him

during the campaign, he assured the Republicans that he did not want a monarchical or aristocratic or, indeed, any but a republican government. Lest anyone think him an enemy of the French alliance, so dear to Jefferson, he affirmed his personal esteem for the French nation, "formed in a residence of seven years, chiefly among them" and his "sincere desire to preserve the friendship which has been so much for the honor and interest of both nations."

The Republicans were delighted. Newspaper editors who had been warning of the approach of tyranny suddenly discovered the President's "incorruptible integrity," his intelligence, his patriotism. Jefferson had always liked Adams. The two had become estranged in 1791 when one of Jefferson's friends published a private letter from him criticizing Adams' political writings. Before the inauguration they made it up and took rooms in the same Philadelphia boardinghouse. In assuming office as Vice President, Jefferson hailed the man "whose talents and integrity have been known and revered by me through a long course of years."

The political backers of both men were suspicious of the new harmony and uneasy about the effect it might have on the party organizations they had been building. Before coming to Philadelphia, Jefferson had drafted an open and generous letter to Adams, declaring his pleasure in the outcome of the election. He had always served as a junior to Adams and would be glad to continue doing so. He sent the letter to Madison to deliver at his discretion. Madison thought it best not to: if made public, it might alienate Jefferson's supporters and embarrass him in a future contest. Jefferson himself avoided getting too close to the Administration: the separation of powers, he decided, should prevent his sitting in the President's Cabinet.

Federalist leaders, equally cautious, were worried about Adams' charity toward the Republicans and blocked him when he proposed appointing Madison as special envoy to France. Adams, who had already told Jefferson of his intention, with some embarrassment withdrew the nomination when Oliver Wolcott, Jr., the Secretary of the Treasury, threatened to resign in protest. Thereafter relations between the President and the Vice President deteriorated, for Adams' behavior seemed to indicate that in spite of his good beginning he would not stand very far above party.

It might, in the end, have been better for Adams if he had used his famous temper on Wolcott. Since there was as yet no tradition requiring Cabinet officers to submit their resignations when a new President took office, Adams inherited the Cabinet that Washington left behind. And a sorry lot they were. Besides Wolcott at the Treasury, there was James McHenry in the War Department and Timothy Pickering at State. Hamilton, in suggesting McHenry's appointment to Washington, had said that "he would give no strength to the administration, but he would not disgrace the office." Three years later, Hamilton had to admit that "my friend McHenry is wholly insufficient for his place." Timothy Pickering had originally served as Postmaster, a position that strained his talents to their limits. After Randolph's resignation Washington had given Pickering the State Department temporarily but was unable to persuade a more competent man to take the job.

Apart from their palpable mediocrity, the only thing that Wolcott, McHenry, and Pickering had in common was that they all took orders from Hamilton. Adams was too keen a man not to perceive the quality of their minds, but he did not realize that the advice they gave him came by mail from the man who had nearly blocked him from the presidency. Even had he known, he might have hesitated to drop them. They had been appointed by the great Washington, and it would have been brash for a president who had barely won the office to cashier the advisers whom the national hero had thought adequate. Even if Adams had

let them go, he might have had difficulty replacing them. Cabinet officers received a salary of only $3,000 a year, and a man of talent who could earn much more in private business might be reluctant or unable to make the financial sacrifice, especially since there was as yet little prestige in any appointive office. Washington had kept second-rate men simply because he could not get first-rate ones.

Surrounded by incompetent advisers who remained loyal to a politician who had betrayed him, Adams could have preserved the strength of the executive department only by showing a resolute determination to make his own decisions. Instead, he spent much of his time at home in Quincy, Massachusetts, leaving the members of his Cabinet to deliberate by themselves. Consequently his Administration drifted into policies with which he did not fully agree and from which he finally extricated it only at the expense of his political career.

The end of the French alliance. In the opening months of his Administration Adams' cordiality for France, and for Jefferson, cooled rapidly. During Washington's Presidency the French government had become increasingly angered by the apparent partiality of its American ally for England. Although the commercial treaty of 1778 stated that the United States would give no nation greater trading privileges than it gave to France, Congress had never given France anything more than equality with other nations—and that only on paper. In operation, the laws that Congress passed consistently favored England. Jay's Treaty had outraged France, and the French minister to America, Pierre Adet, had warned that his country would henceforth treat American ships "in the same manner as they suffer the English to treat them." Actually the French had already intercepted several American vessels bound for England and had impounded them in French harbors. Now France announced that it would no longer recognize the treaty principle that free ships made free goods and that it would treat American sailors serving on British ships as pirates. France went even further: it refused to have anything to do with the American minister, Charles Cotesworth Pinckney (brother of Thomas).

President Adams proposed to meet the crisis diplomatically by sending a three-man mission to France, the mission for which he had considered Madison. The members of his Cabinet were at first opposed not only to Madison but to any mission. Only after Hamilton cautioned them not to get too far ahead of public opinion did they fall in with Adams' plan. The commissioners appointed were the Virginia Federalist lawyer, John Marshall; the rejected minister to

John Adams **by C. W. Peale**

France, C. C. Pinckney; and an astute but unpredictable Massachusetts politican, Elbridge Gerry. To announce the mission the President called a special session of Congress in May and delivered a message that he and the Cabinet alike had thought the proper accompaniment to negotiations. It called for strengthening coastal defenses, arming merchant vessels, completing three frigates begun in 1794, and establishing a provisional army.

Jefferson, the former advocate of bargaining from strength, now thought that the recommended belligerence would be offensive to France and would make the mission's task impossible. As it turned out, French corruption as much as American and French belligerence prevented the mission's success. The French minister of foreign affairs, Talleyrand, in messages conveyed only by go-betweens, informed the envoys that the price of official negotiations would be a bribe of $250,000 for himself and a loan of several million dollars for France. After weeks of fruitless exchanges, Pinckney and Marshall departed in disgust, leaving Gerry to continue the futile mission until he was ordered home.

When Adams reported the affair to Congress incredulous Republicans demanded to see the commission's papers. Adams did not follow Washington's example in the case of the Jay's Treaty papers, probably because he knew that the record would fully sustain him. He turned the papers over, concealing only the names of Talleyrand's go-betweens as W, X, Y, and Z. The American press was soon full of the XYZ Affair, and Congress supported the President in retaliating against France by actions just short of war. The treaties of 1778 were repudiated. Commercial intercourse was suspended. American ships were authorized to seize French armed vessels, and for the next two years French and American ships fought an undeclared war on the seas.

It would have been foolhardy to go to such lengths without preparing for full-scale war. But the President and his advisers could not agree on the kind of preparation to make. The most ardent Federalists saw in the crisis an opportunity to strengthen themselves as well as the government at the expense of the Republicans. They wanted a large standing army, not merely to repel a French invasion but to overawe and if necessary to suppress their political opponents. Hamilton also dreamed of leading an army of conquest into Florida and Louisiana. Adams, while denouncing the French and their American friends, had a more realistic and more comprehensive view of the national interest. He thought it wise to keep a small army in readiness, but he discounted the possibility of a French invasion, and he had no ambition to rule by military force or to conquer territories peopled by the French and the Spanish. What the country really needed, he believed, was a navy to defend its commercial interests in the shifting tides of European conflict. To concentrate on an army would leave the United States no choice but to side always with the country whose navy dominated the seas, in other words, with England. Though Adams' own sympathies lay with England, he thought it was bad policy to let the safety of American commerce depend on the good will of any foreign country. Accordingly, in May 1798 he persuaded Congress to establish a Department of the Navy, with Benjamin Stoddert, a Maryland merchant, as Secretary. In Stoddert, Adams gained his first loyal adviser in the Cabinet.

While Adams and Stoddert proceeded with the construction and commissioning of warships, the High Federalists, as the more extreme branch of the party came to be called, continued their buildup of the army, dragging the reluctant President with them, and levying heavy taxes to pay for it. Washington was persuaded to accept command again, and Hamilton was eager to join him. Adams agreed to make Hamilton a general but refused at first to rank him above Henry Knox, Daniel Morgan, and Benjamin Lincoln, Hamilton's seniors in the Revolutionary army. Hamilton, perhaps with more than military ends in view, declined to play second fiddle to anyone but Washington and made his refusal a test of strength. When Washington, still willing to play Hamilton's game, joined with the Cabinet in demanding that Hamilton be his second in command, Adams was forced to back down.

After this victory, the High Federalists pressed hard for a declaration of war against France. The harder they pressed, the more apparent it became that their aims were domestic rather than foreign. England's depredations against American shipping had continued unabated, while France, according to re-

ports from Elbridge Gerry, had become far more conciliatory in response to the violent American reaction to the XYZ Affair. Gerry was denounced by the Federalists upon his return in 1798, but he was courted by the Republicans and heeded by the President. George Logan, an ex-Quaker from Philadelphia who had conducted an unauthorized peace mission of his own, confirmed Gerry's view of the shift in France's attitude. Adams objected to private citizens meddling in the country's foreign relations and got the Logan Act passed to prevent it in the future, but he was impressed by what Logan told him. Similar reports were arriving from the President's son, John Quincy Adams, also in Europe, and from Rufus King, the American minister in London, and from William Vans Murray at The Hague. In January the President received from Murray a letter sent by Talleyrand to the French chargé at The Hague, specifically stating that an American envoy to France would "undoubtedly be received with the respect due to the representative of a free, independent and powerful nation."

Adams did not assume that Talleyrand's character had improved, but he suspected that American firmness had worked a change in French policy. To declare war now would be to lose all the advantages of neutrality, to sacrifice the national interest to party politics. To make a gesture toward peace, on the other hand, would still leave the United States a free hand and would reduce party tensions at home. Such a reduction would not please the High Federalists, who had visions of a Republican rebellion that the new army commanded by old heroes would crush. That way, Adams believed, lay disaster for the Union, and he decided for once to be President. In February 1799, without consulting his Cabinet further, he sent to the Senate the nomination of William Vans Murray as minister to negotiate a new agreement with France.

The XYZ Affair: political cartoon, 1798

160

Having done so, Adams went off to Quincy, leaving the High Federalists furious and frustrated and the Republicans delighted. With party tensions eased, Adams was not in any hurry to get his mission under way. He was by no means sure that it would succeed, and he wanted to have his new naval vessels ready in case it should fail. By October, three squadrons were fit for duty, and Adams gave orders for Murray to proceed to Paris, where he would be joined by Oliver Ellsworth (Chief Justice of the United States) and William R. Davie (former governor of North Carolina). When the three-man commission arrived, they found Napoleon Bonaparte in control. He was eager to line up a coalition of neutral nations against England and ready to renew Franco-American relations on friendly terms. Although the American commissioners were unable to secure compensation for former French seizures, they did obtain a "convention" that recognized the principle of "free-ships free-goods" and thereby put an end to French spoliation of American commerce. The President's declaration of independence from party pressures had thus saved his country from a needless war and gained it greater freedom on the seas.

The Alien and Sedition laws. In sending the mission to France, John Adams had risen above party, as he believed a President should. But he never fully admitted, even to himself, how much he had been and still remained a member of the Federalist party. After his initial *rapprochement* with Jefferson had faded, his very devotion to the national interest and to the dignity of his office betrayed him, as it had Washington, into regarding himself and his supporters as impartial patriots and the Republican opposition as a criminal conspiracy.

After the disclosure of the XYZ Affair, Adams had been deluged by addresses from groups of patriotic citizens declaring their readiness to fight the French. In his public replies he commended his correspondents and deplored the "few degraded or . . . deluded characters" who viewed the crisis differently. "These lovers of themselves," he announced, "who withdraw their confidence from their own Legislative Government, and place it on a foreign nation, or Domestic Faction, or both in alliance, deserve all our contempt and abhorrence." The references to Republicans were oblique but unmistakable. Even Hamilton thought the President might be pushing anti-Republican sentiment a little too far. But other Federalist leaders (without specific encouragement from either Adams or Hamilton) persuaded Congress to pass legislation designed to harass, if not destroy, the Republican opposition.

The Alien Acts, three in number, were passed in June and July 1798. One, the Alien Enemies Act, was a nonpartisan measure that simply provided for the restraint of enemy aliens in time of war. Since war was never declared against France, the act did not operate during Adams' Presidency. The other two were partisan measures aimed against immigrants, who were widely suspected of being Republican in politics. The Naturalization Act required that an alien seeking citizenship must have resided for fourteen years in the United States, five of them in the state where naturalization was sought. The Alien Friends Act, which was to run for two years only, gave the President power to deport any alien whom he considered dangerous to the welfare of the country.

The Sedition Act, which was passed in July 1798, was one of the most repressive measures ever directed against political activity in the United States. It provided fines and imprisonment for persons unlawfully combining or conspiring "with intent to oppose any measure or measures of the government of the United States," or counseling or advising such opposition, or writing, printing, uttering, or publishing "any false, scandalous, and malicious writing or writings against the government of the United States, or the President of the United States, with intent to defame . . . or to bring them or either of them, into contempt or disrepute." The blatant political purpose of the act was admitted in the date it was to expire: March 3, 1801, when the next President would be inaugurated. The act would last long enough to gag Republican criticism of the Administration until the next election was safely over; it would expire soon enough to permit Federalist criticism in case the election brought in a Republican administration.

The first victim of the Sedition Act was Matthew Lyon, Republican representative from Vermont. On the floor of the House, Lyon and the Connecticut Federalist Roger Griswold had already engaged each other with canes, fire tongs, and spit. In the autumn following the passage of the Sedition Act, Lyon, who was up for reelection, directed his campaign against the Federalist party's conduct of the government. Although his attacks were returned measure for measure by his opponent, Lyon was indicted, convicted, and sentenced (by a Federalist judge) to four months in jail and a $1,000 fine. He was reelected while serving his jail sentence.

The Republicans were alarmed—and rightly so. The Alien and Sedition Acts demonstrated that the Federalists were prepared to abandon the principles of the Enlightenment, of the Revolution, and of the Constitution. When Madison sponsored the first amendments to the Constitution, he had recognized that they might one day have to be defended against an ambitious executive or legislature. He had suggested that the federal courts might protect them, but

The fate of Frenchmen will be the fate of Americans. The French boasted that they were the most civilized and humane people in the world. We can say no more of ourselves. Their Jacobins were wicked, cruel, profligate, atheistical— ours are the same. Their pretence ever was, to consult the good of the people—ours make the same. The people in that country have been robbed, enslaved, and butchered—we shall be served in the same manner, unless we arouse instantly, and rescue our government from the fangs of those who are tearing it in pieces. The struggle will be great, but, if successful on our part, it will also be glorious. Look at your houses, your parents, your wives, and your children. Are you prepared to see your dwellings in flames, hoary hairs bathed in blood, female chastity violated, or children writhing on the pike and the halberd? If not, prepare for the task of protecting your Government. Look at every leading Jacobin as at a ravening wolf, preparing to enter your peaceful fold, and glut his deadly appetite on the vitals of your country. Already do their hearts leap at the prospect. Having long brooded over these scenes of death and despair, they now wake as from a Trance, and in imagination seizing the dagger and the musket, prepare for the work of slaughter. GREAT GOD OF COMPASSION AND JUSTICE, SHEILD MY COUNTRY FROM DESTRUCTION.

From *The Connecticut Courant*, September 29, 1800. Signed "Burleigh."

thus far the courts had shown a disposition to restrain the states more than the national government. They had declared a few state laws unconstitutional, and in the case of *Chisholm* v. *Georgia* (1793) the Supreme Court had awarded judgment against the state of Georgia in a suit brought by citizens of South Carolina. This affront to state sovereignty caused so many protests that an eleventh amendment to the Constitution had been adopted to deny federal jurisdiction in suits brought against a state by foreigners or by citizens of another state.

The Eleventh Amendment, which had been ratified in January 1795, was a direct blow at the federal courts, whose prestige was already at a low ebb. Men of high talents refused to serve on them. John Jay had resigned as Chief Justice of the United States in 1795 in order to run for the governorship of New York. The judges who remained and who presided at sedition trials had no more scruples about the constitutionality of the Alien and Sedition Acts than John Adams had had when he signed them.

Since there seemed to be no other way of protecting the Constitution from the Federalists, Madison and Jefferson turned to the state governments. With the election of Adams, Madison had retired temporarily from Congress and returned to Virginia. In the Virginia legislature, he now secured passage (December 24, 1798) of a series of resolutions affirming the authority of the states to judge the constitutionality of federal legislation and declaring the Alien and Sedition Acts unconstitutional.

Madison's resolutions did not go beyond the statement of unconstitutionality. But Vice President Jefferson had framed another set, for the state of Kentucky (November 16, 1798), which declared the acts to be "void and of no force." When the other states declined to support Virginia and Kentucky, Kentucky reaffirmed in another set of resolutions (November 22, 1799) that "nullification" by the states was the proper remedy for unconstitutional actions by the federal government. But the other states still refused to follow suit and allowed the Alien and Sedition Acts to expire under their own terms. Though the resolutions of Kentucky and Virginia failed in their immediate object, they posed a question that would trouble the nation for many years to come. The Philadelphia convention had not decided which was sovereign, state governments or national government, and the resolutions were a reminder that the question was still open.

The election of 1800. The steadily declining fortunes of the Republicans convinced them that in order to survive they would have to build a national organization. As a result of the XYZ Affair they had lost congressional seats in the elections of 1798; even Virginia, the Republican stronghold, had returned five "certain Federalists" and three moderates who leaned toward Federalism. With Jefferson directing party strategy, the Republicans resolved to do better in the next election. Following regional patterns of local government, they appointed county committees in the South and township committees in the North to instruct the voters about the vices of Federalists and the virtues of Republicans. The local committees were supervised by state committees, which in turn took their direction from a caucus of Republican congressmen in Philadelphia. By now there were Republican newspapers scattered throughout the country, the most prominent of which was Philadelphia's *Aurora*. The editors, defying the Sedition Act, charged the government with aristocratic and monarchical pretensions and with levying heavy taxes to support an expensive navy, a standing army, and a corrupt funding system.

The charges struck home, for they were substantially correct. Armies and navies are always expensive, and in 1798 the Adams Administration had levied an extremely unpopular direct tax on houses, lands, and slaves to pay the rising costs. What was worse, in 1799 the army had been ordered into action to enforce collection of the tax, after a mob led by one John Fries released two tax-evaders from prison in Northampton County, Pennsylvania. Although the army, as in the case of the Whiskey Rebellion, could find no one to fight, the use of it lent support to Republican accusations of tyranny.

Federalist newspapers replied by calling Republicans the tools of the godless French. Federalist attorneys and judges made full use of the Sedition Act to silence Republican editors, but the wheels of the law did not turn rapidly enough to make more than a few martyrs. The Federalists also caucused at Philadelphia and tried to organize support at the local level. But their efforts were hampered by their own divisions. The rank and file of the party approved John Adams' peace mission to France and would have been outraged by a proposal to support any other candidate for the Presidency. The High Federalists, however, considered Adams a traitor. Pickering thought that the

mission to France would "subvert the present administration and with them the government itself." Hamilton declared he would never again support Adams and even wrote a pamphlet attacking him.

In spite of the defection in his own camp, Adams made a strong bid for reelection. By the spring of 1800 it had become probable that he would take New England and New Jersey, that Jefferson (the natural Republican candidate) would win most of the South, and that a deadlock would neutralize Pennsylvania. New York and South Carolina, both uncertain, held the balance. In New York the legislature chose the presidential electors, and the state was so divided that the thirteen representatives from New York City held the balance of power in the legislature. In 1800 Aaron Burr, perhaps the Republican's best working politician on the local level, was able to offer the city a slate of thirteen extremely influential and popular candidates for representative. They took the city by five hundred votes, thus assuring Republican control of the state legislature and of New York's electoral votes in the coming national contest.

New York City had hitherto been the private preserve of Alexander Hamilton, and the significance of his defeat was not lost on John Adams. The President knew that he had been right about the peace mission, regardless of party considerations; but he knew now that he was also right politically and that the High Federalists were wrong. After putting up with their insolence for three years, he had had enough. On May 6 he asked for and received McHenry's resignation from the War Department. On May 10 he asked for Pickering's; when Pickering refused, Adams simply discharged him.

While Adams was cutting loose from the High Federalists, the Republicans had decided that Aaron

ELECTORAL VOTE

Jefferson (Dem.–Rep.) 73
Burr (Dem.–Rep.) 73
Adams (Fed.) 65
Pinckney (Fed.) 64*

*One R.I. elector cast one of his ballots for Jay.

Tie resolved by House of Representatives. Jefferson elected.

VT. 4
N.H. 6
MASS. 16
N.Y 12
R.I. 4
CONN. 9
PENNA. 8 ... 7
N.J. 7
DEL. 3
VA 21
MD. 5 votes to each party
KY 4
N.C 8 ... 4
TENN. 3
S.C 8
GA. 4

Note: For all election maps in this book, the electoral vote will be given within each state. When a state's electoral vote is split, as were the votes of Pennsylvania, Maryland, and North Carolina in this election, the split will be shown with the number of electoral votes going to each candidate. The graphic presentation in such cases is not intended to indicate the geographic distribution of votes within the state.

The election of 1800

Burr would again make the best running mate for Jefferson. The Federalists' vice-presidential candidate was Charles Cotesworth Pinckney. Hamilton, who had been responsible for the choice, used the same strategy as in 1796: to throw support to a vice-presidential candidate in the hope that he would overtake both presidential candidates.

The outcome of the election was in doubt for some time, for electors were still chosen at different times and in different ways; but when the ballots were finally counted, Adams had sixty-five electoral votes, and Pinckney sixty-four. The Republican machine, working a little too well, had given Jefferson and Burr each seventy-three. It had been understood that Burr was the vice-presidential candidate, but no Republican elector had diverted one of his two ballots to preclude a tie. To prevent this situation from recurring, the Twelfth Amendment to the Constitution, adopted in 1804, required the Electoral College to vote separately for President and for Vice President. But in February 1801, as directed by the Constitution, the choice between Jefferson and Burr was thrown into the House of Representatives, where each state was to

have only one vote. With Federalist representatives supporting Burr, voting went on for a week through thirty-five ballots without the necessary nine-state majority being reached. The deadlock was finally broken when James Bayard, the single Congressman from Delaware, withdrew his support from Burr and, with other Federalists from South Carolina, cast a blank ballot. Jefferson was declared elected.

Since Republican candidates for Congress were also victorious, the election of 1800 brought to an end Federalist control of the national government. Nevertheless, the Federalists could look forward to a continuing influence: the United States judiciary, manned by Federalist appointees, enjoyed a lifetime tenure. The last acts of the Adams Administration made the most of this fact. A new judiciary act of February 27, 1801, created six circuit courts with sixteen new judgeships, and Adams, instead of leaving the appointment of the new judges to his successor, filled the offices with loyal Federalists. Even more significantly, Adams in January 1801 appointed as Chief Justice of the United States John Marshall of Virginia, an ardent Federalist. Under Marshall the Court was to rise to new heights of prestige and power, to the considerable annoyance of Marshall's fellow Virginian in the White House.

Jefferson liked to think of his election as the "Revolution of 1800." But the election had been no landslide. John Adams had only eight votes fewer than the winners. If he had taken either New York or South Carolina, he would have won; and he might have taken them had he parted sooner from the High Federalists. Actually John Adams' capture of the Federalist party marked as great a political change as Jefferson's triumph at the polls, a change possibly more crucial to the preservation of national unity. Hamiltonian policies, tied to urban business interests at home and to Great Britain abroad, had repeatedly threatened to divide the nation. By sending the mission to France and by repudiating Hamilton, Adams reduced the gap between Federalist and Republican views of the national interest. His action came too late to win an electoral majority for himself or his party, but it did ensure peace, not only between the United States and France, but between two groups of Americans who had drifted dangerously far apart.

Suggestions for Reading The period covered by this chapter is surveyed by J. C. Miller, *The Federalist Era** (1960). L. D. White, *The Federalists** (1948), assesses the achievements of the Washington and Adams Administrations in establishing the bureaucratic machinery of national government. The political foundations of Federalist power are analyzed in Manning Dauer, *The Adams Federalists** (1953). In *The Economic Origins of Jeffersonian Democracy** (1915), Charles Beard saw the rise of the Republican party as a continuation of the small-farmer hostility to the Constitution, which he had described in his *Economic*

*Interpretation of the Constitution of the United States** (1913). Joseph Charles, *The Origins of the American Party System** (1956), denies that there was any such continuity.

Norman Risjord finds elements of continuity in voting patterns in Maryland, Virginia, and North Carolina in *Chesapeake Politics, 1781–1800* (1978), and A. F. Young, *The Democratic Republicans of New York: The Origins, 1763–1797* (1967), finds some elements of continuity in that state. But Paul Goodman finds none in *The Democratic-Republicans of Massachusetts* (1964). In *The Partisan Spirit* (1972), Patricia Watlington discloses a complex relationship between state and national politics in Kentucky. Noble Cunningham, *The Jeffersonian Republicans** (1957), describes the political organizing activities of the Republicans and is particularly good on the election of 1800. A good general account of the first parties is W. N. Chambers, *Political Parties in a New Nation** (1963). Richard Hofstadter, *The Idea of a Party System** (1969), stresses the absence of such a system in the 1790s. Richard Buel, *Securing the Revolution: Ideology in American Politics, 1789–1815** (1972), emphasizes the role of public opinion. Lance Banning, *The Jeffersonian Persuasion* (1978), argues for an ideological continuity in the Republicans and the Revolutionary opposition to England. Richard H. Kohn, *Eagle and Sword* (1975), gives valuable insights into the politics of the late 1790s.

Two aspects of political discontent during the 1790s are treated in E. P. Link, *Democratic-Republican Societies, 1790–1800* (1942), and L. D. Baldwin, *The Whiskey Rebels** (1939). R. A. Rutland, *The Birth of the Bill of Rights, 1776–1791** (1955), discusses the origins of the first ten amendments. Irving Brant, *The Bill of Rights** (1965), is more comprehensive and deals with the later interpretations of the amendments. L. W. Levy, *Legacy of Suppression** (1960), shows that the First Amendment offered less firm protection for freedom of speech and the press than has generally been supposed. J. M. Smith, *Freedom's Fetters** (1956), is the most complete account of the Alien and Sedition Acts. J. M. Banner, *To the Hartford Convention* (1970), emphasizes the Federalists' adherence to republican principles of government.

S. F. Bemis, *Jay's Treaty** (1923, rev. ed., 1962) and *Pinckney's Treaty** (1926, rev. ed., 1960), definitively treat two important episodes in foreign relations in the Federalist decade. Felix Gilbert, *To the Farewell Address** (1961), discusses the origins of attitudes classically expressed in Washington's warning against alliances. Alexander De Conde, *Entangling Alliance* (1958) and *The Quasi-War** (1966); L. M. Sears, *George Washington and the French Revolution* (1960); Charles Hazen, *Contemporary American Opinion of the French Revolution* (1897, reprinted 1964); L. S. Kaplan, *Jefferson and France* (1967); and A. H. Bowman, *The Struggle for Neutrality* (1974), discuss relations with France. In *Number 7* (1964), Julian Boyd gives evidence of Hamilton's efforts in the Nootka Sound crisis to turn American policy in favor of the British. Harry Ammon, *The Genet Mission** (1973), is a good account of that episode. J. A. Combs, *The Jay Treaty* (1970), analyzes the differing views of Republicans and Federalists on foreign policy.

So many men of large stature shared in the making of public policy during the 1790s that much of the history of the period has been written in the form of biography. D. S. Freeman, *George Washington*, 7 vols. (1948–57), is the most complete account; Vol. VII was written after Freeman's death by J. A. Carroll and M. W. Ashworth. J. T. Flexner, *George Washington and the New Nation* (1970) and *George Washington: Anguish and Farewell* (1972), conclude a perceptive four-volume study. E. S. Morgan, *The Genius of George Washington* (1980), briefly assesses his understanding of military and political power. J. C. Miller, *Alexander Hamilton: Portrait in Paradox* (1959), is the best biography of Hamilton. Hamilton's great reports are conveniently gathered in J. E. Cooke, ed., *The Reports of Alexander Hamilton** (1964). Irving Brant, *James Madison: Father of the Constitution, 1787–1800* (1950), the third volume of a six-volume study of Madison, contains a wealth of information about the formation of the Republican party. Gilbert Chinard, *Honest John Adams** (1933), is good, but C. P. Smith, *John Adams* (1962), is more thorough. J. R. Howe, *The Changing Political Thought of John Adams** (1966), is a sensitive interpretation. Stephen Kurtz, *The Presidency of John Adams** (1957), is very good on the election of 1796; Zoltan Haraszti, *John Adams and the Prophets of Progress** (1952), is a charming account of Adams' notes in the margins of his books. Dumas Malone, *Jefferson and His Time*, 6 vols. (1948–81), is authoritative. A stimulating interpretation of Jefferson's thought is D. J. Boorstin, *The Lost World of Thomas Jefferson** (1948). Merrill Peterson, *Thomas Jefferson and the New Nation** (1970), is an excellent one-volume biography.

*Available in a paperback edition.

7

JEFFERSONIAN
REPUBLICANISM

The peaceful inauguration of Thomas Jefferson as President, on March 4, 1801, was an event of uncommon significance, for it marked the first occasion under the new Constitution when executive power passed quietly from one political party to another. Only a short time before, Federalist partisans had attacked "mad Tom" Jefferson as a "Jacobin" and an atheist, and many of them had regarded the Republican party as a treasonable organization against whose activities the Sedition Act was a justifiable defense. The Jeffersonians, in turn, had denounced the Federalists as a "faction" of monarchists with "aristocratical tendencies," ready even to conspire "with the enemies of their country." Each party had suspected the other of plotting to subvert the Constitution.

Moreover, as we have seen, few Republican or Federalist leaders viewed political parties as either legitimate or essential to a republican electoral process. To most, parties were intrinsically evil and corrupt; they promoted selfish interests, appealed to the passions of the populace, and distracted public leaders from calm deliberation and pursuit of the common good. Jefferson never acknowledged the legitimacy of the Federalists, and he viewed his own party as a temporary expedient for uniting the people against a threat to republican institutions. The Federalists, on their side, had questioned Republican legitimacy by accusing the Jeffersonian "faction" of seeking to usurp functions that belonged to the government itself.

Yet, though deeply troubled, the Federalists accepted their loss of control of both Congress and the executive department. Since they still controlled the New England states, a powerful base for future political activity, and since they believed the Republicans incompetent, they comforted themselves with hopes of an early return to power. Besides, Jefferson may have reassured certain Federalist leaders privately that no Jacobin reign of terror would follow the "Revolution of 1800." Hamilton found solace in his jaundiced view of Jefferson as a man inclined "to temporize; to calculate what will be likely to promote his own reputation and advantage." This trait, he thought, would cause Jefferson to accept financial policies "which being once established, could not be overturned without danger to the person who did it." For these reasons the heated rhetoric of the campaign was to have no violent aftermath; and the two-party system, whatever theoretical objections Americans may have had to it, won a more secure footing and a practical legitimacy it had never enjoyed before.

After a decade of protest against Federalist policies, Jefferson was now obliged to spell out policies of his own. This, in broad outline, he did in a brilliant inaugural address (the first to be delivered in the new capital on the banks of the Potomac) that affirmed his liberal democratic philosophy and his faith in the wisdom of the people. He soothed the Federalists by inviting them to join Republicans "in common efforts for the common good." He cautioned Republicans

The unfinished Capitol

that though the will of the majority must prevail, "the minority possess their equal rights, which equal law must protect." He reminded members of both parties that in spite of the acrimonious campaign just past

> every difference of opinion is not a difference of principle. We have called by different names brethren of the same principle. We are all Republicans, we are all Federalists. If there be any among us who would wish to dissolve this Union or to change its Republican form, let them stand undisturbed as monuments of the safety with which error of opinion may be tolerated where reason is left free to combat it.

These conciliatory words reveal Jefferson's basic strategy in dealing with the Federalists. Though still opposed to parties and convinced that good citizens would spurn them, his method was not harsh repression but gentle absorption. He would undermine the party system by winning the support of all reasonable Federalists ("the honest part"), leaving the irreconcilables a small and harmless faction. "Nothing shall be spared on my part," he wrote privately, "to obliterate the traces of party and consolidate the nation, if it can be done without the abandonment of principle." It is ironic that a party leader as skilled as Jefferson never understood how indispensable and inevitable the party system was and that he failed to esteem the role he played so well.

Economy and Simplicity

The new regime. The rustic simplicity and democratic manners that Jefferson thought proper for the leaders of an agricultural republic seemed appropriate in the crude, half-built capital city of Washington,

D.C. Though he was a learned and cultivated gentleman to the manner born, his informality was natural. Unlike his predecessors, he sent his annual messages to Congress to be read by a clerk, lest reading them in person should suggest that he was imitating the British monarch speaking from the throne. Jefferson abandoned the elegant weekly presidential levees that had so delighted the aristocracy of Philadelphia, the former capital. At his infrequent state dinners and receptions and in his dealings with the diplomatic corps he avoided anything that smacked of the pomp of European courts. In the White House he lived simply and made himself accessible to citizens who claimed to have business with him.

Although Jefferson believed in the sovereignty of the people and tended to romanticize the independent farmer, he did not assume that untrained men could handle the responsibilities of important administrative posts. He rejected the notion that society should be governed by a political élite based on wealth or birth, believing instead that it should be governed by the "natural aristocracy" of virtue and talent. The men in the key posts of his Administration were able, educated, and experienced upper-class Republicans of as high a caliber as their Federalist predecessors. James Madison, Jefferson's close friend and political collaborator, a Virginia aristocrat who had led the fight against the Federalists, joined the new Administration as Secretary of State. Albert Gallatin of Pennsylvania, a gifted and devoted Jeffersonian, accepted the crucial office of Secretary of the Treasury and served with such distinction that he won the respect of many Federalists.

In spite of his doubts about the value of political parties, Jefferson, far more than his predecessors, played the dual role of President and party-leader. As party-leader he was concerned about the weakness of the Republicans in the Northern states, where Federalists had identified Republicans with the interests of the South. To strengthen his party in the bastion of Federalism, Jefferson appointed three New Englanders to major offices: Levi Lincoln of Massachusetts as Attorney General, Henry Dearborn of Massachusetts as Secretary of War, and Gideon Granger of Connecticut as Postmaster General. Jefferson also made skillful use of the patronage. Though permitting many Federalists to remain in minor or non-policy-making offices, he was determined that Republicans should have their fair share—two-thirds or three-fourths, he once suggested. He removed Federalists whom Adams had appointed after the election of the preceding year who were guilty of "malversation" (misconduct in public office) and who had shown "open, active and virulent" partisanship. As a wise politician he showed some restraint, but party advantage—his desire to undermine the Federalists—clearly governed his policy; nearly all his appointees were Republicans.

Republican policies. Jefferson disliked Hamilton's mercantilist theories and favored a more passive federal policy. The success of his Administration, therefore, cannot be measured in terms of positive legislation or innovative action. His ideal was "a wise and frugal Government, which shall restrain men from injuring one another . . . [and] leave them otherwise free to regulate their own pursuits of industry and improvement." The principal responsibilities of such a government, Jefferson explained, would be to honor the Bill of Rights, seek equal justice for all men, respect the rights of the states ("the surest bulwarks against antirepublican tendencies"), and practice strict economy, "that labor may be lightly burthened."

But the Jefferson Administration soon discovered—as would future administrations when power passed from one party to another—that it could reverse the actions and repudiate the commitments of its predecessor only at the risk of confusion. "Some things," wrote the cautious Jefferson, "may perhaps be left undone from motives of compromise for a time, and not to alarm by too sudden a reformation." He and his fellow Republicans, therefore, thought it best not to tamper with some of Hamilton's economic measures. The Bank of the United States, for example, continued its operations undisturbed until 1811, when its charter expired. By then many Republicans, including Madison and Gallatin, favored granting the Bank a new charter, a proposal that failed in each house of Congress by a single vote. Nor did the Republicans reverse Federalist measures for funding the national debt, or for federal assumption of the Revolutionary debts of the states, or for encouraging American shipping. "What is practicable," Jefferson confessed, "must often control what is pure theory."

Indeed, in his quest for national unity Jefferson even sought to win greater political support from the banking, commercial, and manufacturing interests, and in this he had much success. In Providence, Rhode Island, he ordered federal funds to be transferred from a Federalist-controlled to a Republican-controlled state bank. "I am decidedly in favor of making all the banks Republican," he wrote, "by sharing deposits among them in proportion to the disposition they show." To justify such fiscal politics, he explained that it was important "to detach the mercantile interest" from the enemies of republicanism "and incorporate them into the body of its friends."

Though still committed to the primacy of agriculture, Jefferson developed a greater respect for other economic pursuits. In his first message to Congress he referred to manufacturing, commerce, and navigation, along with agriculture, as "the four pillars of our prosperity"; and he even suggested, though somewhat vaguely, that "within the limits of our constitutional powers" measures to protect them from "casual embarrassments" might be "seasonably interposed."

The "Revolution of 1800," however, did not lack substance, for the Republicans lost no time in disposing of some of the Federalists' pet measures. They refused, of course, to renew the Alien Act when it expired in 1801. They reduced the residence requirement for naturalization from fourteen years to five; once again, Jefferson hoped, America would become an "asylum" for "oppressed humanity." The Sedition Act also expired in 1801, and Jefferson saw to it that those who had been imprisoned for violating it were freed and urged that all fines be refunded.

The Judiciary Act of 1801, which had enabled Adams to appoint sixteen staunch Federalists to circuit-court judgeships, together with the partisan behavior of Federalist judges in cases brought to trial under the Sedition Act, intensified Jefferson's general distrust of judges and of the federal judiciary. With his encouragement the Republican Congress repealed the Judiciary Act of 1801 and abolished, as a needless extravagance, the circuit judgeships that act had created. Thus, defeated ("lame duck") Federalists, to whom Adams had given "midnight appointments," lost their jobs; and the courts, as one Republican explained, ceased to be a "hospital for decayed politicians." Still not satisfied, Jefferson urged Congress to initiate impeachment proceedings against some of the more indiscreet Federalist judges. The House of Representatives did impeach District Judge John Pickering, whose heavy drinking and mental instability had rendered him incompetent, and the Senate voted his removal. The House then turned on the Supreme Court and, in 1804, impeached Associate Justice Samuel Chase, an arch-Federalist who had used the bench as a political stump. However, in this case the Senate did not interpret Chase's offenses as misdemeanors within the meaning of the Constitution and refused to convict him. Thereafter, Jefferson had to rely on new appointments, when vacancies occurred, to reduce Federalist influence in the courts.

The most crucial aspect of the Jeffersonian revolution was the significant change it attempted in fiscal policy. According to the new President, government tends "to multiply offices . . . and to increase expense"—to leave to labor only a small portion of its earnings and to "consume the whole residue of what [government] was instituted to guard." Unlike Hamilton, Jefferson believed that a public debt and the accompanying interest charges benefited only a small class of investors while acting as a "mortal canker" on the rest of the community. With the able support of Secretary of the Treasury Gallatin, he strove to retire the whole public debt, which had grown to $83 million, at the earliest possible date—in sixteen years, according to the original plan. Since the excise tax along with other internal taxes was to be repealed, the only way to retire the debt was through revenues from import duties and the sale of public lands and through the most rigid government economy. To cut costs in the executive department Jefferson reduced the number of officers in the diplomatic corps and revenue service. He urged Congress to abolish other public offices, to replace wasteful general appropriations with grants of "specific sums to every specific purpose," and to hold the Treasury Department responsible for all funds spent.

Jefferson was convinced, too, that military and naval expenditures could be cut without jeopardizing national defense. America, he said, was fortunately "separated by nature and a wide ocean from the exterminating havoc" of the Old World and consequently needed no large standing army. For defense against invasion, the country should rely on "the body of neighboring citizens as formed into a militia." Accordingly, the regular army was reduced from four thousand to twenty-five hundred officers and men. Jefferson realized, however, that the state militia systems needed to be improved, and in 1808 the federal government began to take a hand in reorganizing them and in defraying part of the cost of arms and equipment. Moreover, in 1802 Jefferson was instrumental in establishing the U.S. Military Academy at West Point.

Turning to the navy, the new Administration proceeded to sell some ocean-going vessels, lay up others, and halt construction on still others; it discharged many Navy Department employees, reduced the number of officers and enlisted men, and abandoned the improvement of navy yards and dry docks. Shore defense was to be maintained by coastal fortifications and by a fleet of small, inexpensive gunboats

serving as a kind of naval militia. This policy was designed, Jefferson explained, "merely for defensive operations," not to protect commerce or to establish the United States as a sea power. The quarreling European states would thus be kept "at a distance" and at little cost.

Here, in short, was Jefferson's formula for a republican utopia: simplicity, frugality, and "a government founded not on the fears and follies of man, but on his reason"—a government whose authority the ordinary citizen would scarcely feel. For a time all worked according to plan, and in his second annual message Jefferson congratulated Congress for the "pleasing circumstances . . . under which we meet." The United States had become a nation of peaceful, prosperous citizens "managing their own affairs in their own way and for their own use, unembarrassed by too much regulation, unoppressed by fiscal exactions."

Jefferson's cheerful view of the state of the Union was valid enough for most white Americans, but not for those Americans (approximately 19 percent of the population) who were Negroes or of mixed white and Negro ancestry. In 1800 nearly 90 percent of those people (894,000) were still slaves, and the rest were everywhere more or less the victims of a deep and pervasive racial prejudice. Though the federal government had no constitutional power to interfere with slavery in the states, slavery had already provoked several sharp congressional debates during the decade

Population 1800

Population per square mile

☐ Under 2
▨ 2 to 5.9
▨ 6 to 17.9
▨ 18 to 44.9
▨ 45 to 89.9
■ 90 and over

226.5 million

Urban 6%

Rural 94%

5.3 million

1800   1980

of Federalist ascendancy. In earlier years Jefferson, though himself a large slaveholder, had professed, usually privately, antislavery sentiments; but during the eight years of his Presidency, like every other chief executive before the Civil War, he carefully avoided the subject. The "Revolution of 1800" brought no change in the condition of black Americans, and Jefferson seems always to have assessed the state of the Union without giving them a thought.

However, in his annual message of December 2, 1806, Jefferson did remind Congress that the time was approaching when it could constitutionally stop citizens of the United States from participating in the African slave trade—a trade that every state except South Carolina had already made illegal. Congress responded with a law prohibiting the trade after January 1, 1808, and punishing violators with fines and imprisonment. But it was a poor law with no machinery for enforcement, and many thousands of African slaves were imported after it was passed. In 1820 Congress passed another law defining participation in the African slave trade as piracy; but, significantly, not until 1862 was anyone convicted under its terms.

Ferment in the West

The westward movement. In his vision of America as the ideal republic, Jefferson's model was a rather romanticized version of the stable, mellow society of Virginia's rural gentry. However, this model did not fit much of the rest of the country—not even the trans-Appalachian West in whose future Jefferson placed such hope. In 1800 nearly a million settlers were living in the vast area between the Appalachians and the Mississippi River. A new land act that year encouraged others to come by offering land for sale in individual tracts of 320 acres and by permitting four-year credits with a down payment of 25 percent. A revision of this law in 1804 reduced the minimum tract to 160 acres; thus, with public land selling at a minimum price of $2 an acre, a buyer could obtain a farm for an initial payment of $80. This generous federal policy brought a steady tide of immigrants into the West, whose rich lands Jefferson thought would afford "room enough for our descendants to the thousandth and thousandth generation." As the forests were cleared and farms and villages began to dot the land, new states were created from time to time—Kentucky in 1792, Tennessee in 1796, and Ohio in 1803.

Most Westerners liked Jefferson's politics and his philosophy, but they had mixed feelings about his economics. Jefferson's ideal of a stable, self-sufficient

yeomanry free of the corrupting influences of commercialism—far from a reality even in Virginia—was hardly the ideal of the traders and speculators who invaded the West—or, for that matter, of many of the farmers. Soon after they arrived, most Westerners began to dream not of self-sufficiency but of cash crops, of outlets to markets, and of the comforts and luxuries of the East.

Between them and their ambitions, however, stood the Indian tribes that still possessed much of the land coveted by white settlers. The American frontier did not advance in a slow, orderly manner, with contiguous tracts of the public domain successively opened for sale and then compactly settled. Rather, farmers and speculators rushed into new areas, often before Indian claims were cleared and surveys completed, seeking the most fertile parcels. With such an abundance of good land, few buyers were interested in less than the best land. The government was constantly pressured to open additional tracts even before those already open had been fully settled.

The government seldom raised a restraining hand. Even Jefferson, in spite of a professed concern for the welfare of the Indians and a promise that "not a foot of land" would ever be taken from them "without their consent," was more often a party to the land grabs than a protector of Indian rights. "Our system," he told William Henry Harrison, governor of Indiana Territory, "is to live in perpetual peace with the Indians," to protect them from injustice, to introduce among them "the implements and the practice of husbandry and of the household arts," and to persuade them to "incorporate with us as citizens of the U.S." When they became farmers, Jefferson thought, they would no longer need their extensive forests and would trade land "for necessaries for their farms and families." He also suggested means of speeding the process of land acquisition: at the government trading houses "the good and influential" Indians might be encouraged to run into debt, thus forcing them eventually to make a settlement "by a cession of land." If any tribe should be "foolhardy enough to take up the hatchet . . . the seizing [of] the whole country of that tribe and driving them across the Mississippi" would be justified. Jefferson further advised Governor Harrison on ways to cajole the various tribes to make land cessions.

The result of both the planless expansion and the cajolery was that Western Indians were repeatedly induced to make treaties with terms they rarely comprehended, treaties by which they surrendered more and more of their hunting grounds. During the first decade of the nineteenth century in the Ohio Valley alone, the Indians were obliged to cede more than a hundred million acres of land. In 1809, in Indiana Territory, Governor Harrison negotiated the last of a se-

New Orleans, 1803: "a noble bargain"

ries of cessions under particularly dubious circumstances, bargaining with the demoralized remnants of several tribes for nearly three million acres in the lower Wabash Valley. Clearly, Jefferson's desire to satisfy the land hunger of white settlers outweighed his concern for the rights of Indians.

The problem of transportation.

Two other problems confronted Westerners: the mountains that cut them off from the East, and the French, who were preparing to take over from Spain possession of New Orleans and the mouth of the Mississippi. Before Jefferson left office, he found solutions to both these problems. In 1806 Congress authorized the building of a road from Cumberland, Maryland, across the mountains to Wheeling, Virginia, as a government-financed "internal improvement." Jefferson approved the measure, even though, lacking the constitutional amendment he had urged Congress to adopt, it required a stretching of federal power to do so. Construction on the National Road, as it was called, began in 1811 and was completed in 1818. In subsequent years the road was extended westward to Vandalia, Illinois.

The second problem—navigation of the Mississippi River—forced Jefferson to take vigorous action that compromised not only his constitutional scruples but his fiscal policy, his foreign policy, and perhaps even his principles of public ethics. Since 1763 the

mouth of the Mississippi and the immense territory of Louisiana, stretching westward to the Rockies, had been held by a declining and enfeebled Spain; and Spain, in Pinckney's Treaty of 1795, had opened the Mississippi to American navigation and granted Western flatboatmen the right to deposit their cargoes at New Orleans for shipment abroad. This arrangement satisfied the Westerners, who saw in Spain no serious threat to their interests. But they were bound to react violently if Louisiana were to fall into the hands of a stronger power or if their river outlet were closed. As Madison explained: "The Mississippi is to them every thing. It is the Hudson, the Delaware, the Potomac, and all the navigable rivers of the Atlantic states, formed into one stream."

The Louisiana Purchase.

Soon after Jefferson became President two events shocked and angered the Western settlers. The first was the revelation that Napoleon Bonaparte, in the secret Treaty of San Ildefonso (1800), had negotiated the transfer of Louisiana from Spain to France (though formal possession by France was long delayed). The second was a proclamation by the Spanish intendant at New Orleans, on October 16, 1802, that the right of deposit was to be suspended. Taking this as a foretaste of Bonaparte's future policy, indignant Westerners looked to Jefferson for support.

Alarmed, Jefferson feared for a time that Bonaparte might force him to reconsider his basic foreign policy, perhaps even to abandon temporarily his opposition to "entangling alliances." The United States, he told Robert R. Livingston, the American minister in Paris; has always looked upon France as its "natural friend"; but there was

> on the globe one single spot, the possessor of which is our natural and habitual enemy. It is New Orleans, through which the produce of three-eighths of our territory must pass to market. . . . France placing herself in that door, assumes to us the attitude of defiance. The day that France takes possession of New Orleans . . . [we will be forced to] marry ourselves to the British fleet and nation.

To Congress he spoke of "the danger to which our peace would be perpetually exposed whilst so important a key to the commerce of the Western country remained under foreign power."

But before considering more vigorous action, Jefferson tried to negotiate peacefully with France. He instructed Livingston to offer to purchase New Orleans and West and East Florida; he obtained from Congress an appropriation of $2 million for vaguely defined expenses; and he sent James Monroe, who had the confidence of Westerners, as a special envoy

Thomas Jefferson on the Louisiana Purchase and the Constitution

From Thomas Jefferson, Letter to John Breckenridge, August 12, 1803.

to assist Livingston. Monroe arrived in Paris on April 12, 1803, two days after Talleyrand, negotiating for France, had startled Livingston by asking whether the United States would like to buy the whole of Louisiana! The two American diplomats, whose instructions were essentially to buy a city, hesitated, though only momentarily, before agreeing to buy an empire that would double the size of their country.

There were several reasons for Bonaparte's sudden decision to abandon his imperial ambitions in America and to concentrate on Europe. First, he had suffered a major disaster when his troops failed to crush a slave insurrection, led by Toussaint L'Ouverture, in the French colony of San Domingo. Second, the Peace of Amiens of 1802 had really settled nothing, and a renewal of war between France and Great Britain seemed all but inevitable. Third, Bonaparte needed money, and it was obviously wise to sell a province that the British navy could prevent France from occupying in any case. Finally, selling Louisiana to the United States would remove a source of friction and avoid an Anglo-American *rapprochement*. Accordingly, on April 11 Bonaparte told one of his ministers: "I renounce Louisiana. It is not only New Orleans that I will cede, it is the whole colony without any reservation."

Livingston and Monroe soon decided that this was a poor time to quibble over the letter of their instructions. On April 30, 1803, after some higgling over price, they made the purchase for $15 million and a promise (written into the purchase treaty) to give citizenship and religious freedom to Catholics residing in Louisiana. The boundaries of Louisiana

were then only vaguely defined, and the treaty merely stated that they were to be the same as they had been when Spain possessed it. "You have made a noble bargain for yourselves," said the realistic Talleyrand, "and I suppose you will make the most of it." In later years the United States did precisely that.

Westerners were delighted with the terms of the treaty, and their devotion to Jefferson and confidence in the federal government grew correspondingly stronger. But New England Federalists, viewing the West as enemy territory, criticized Jefferson severely for accepting a treaty that was tainted with duplicity. In making the sale, they pointed out, Bonaparte had violated the French constitution and a promise to Spain not to cede Louisiana to another power. Yet Jefferson approved the transaction knowing this to be the case—knowing, too, that the Constitution did not explicitly authorize the acquisition of new territory. Federalists also complained that the purchase of lands they regarded as worthless was a wasteful expenditure and meant a staggering addition to the public debt.

Jefferson was sensitive to such criticism, especially to the charge that he was exceeding the limits set by the Constitution strictly construed. His first impulse was to urge an amendment expressly granting the power to acquire territory from which new states might be created; but the amending process was painfully slow, and Livingston warned that Bonaparte might have a change of heart. Some Republicans argued that the power to acquire territory might be *implied* from the power to make treaties—an argument that could hardly have satisfied Jefferson. Nevertheless, trusting that "the good sense of our country will

Map labels:
BRITISH
OREGON COUNTRY
Lewis 1806
Columbia R.
Lewis and Clark 1805
Snake R.
Yellowstone R.
Clark 1806
Missouri R.
Lewis and Clark 1804-05
Missouri R.
Pike 1805-06
L. Superior
L. Michigan
SPANISH
ROCKY MOUNTAINS
Colorado R.
Pike's Peak
Pike 1806-07
Arkansas R.
UNITED STATES
St. Louis
Mississippi R.
Red R.
Rio Grande
Pike 1806-07
Nachitoches
FLA. (Sp.)
New Orleans
PACIFIC OCEAN
Gulf of Mexico

Legend:
— Louisiana Purchase 1803
--- Present boundaries of the United States

correct the evil of [constitutional] construction when it shall produce evil effects," Jefferson submitted the treaty to the Senate.

During the debate Federalists and Republicans reversed their former positions on questions of constitutional interpretation—a few extreme Federalists even spoke of dissolving the Union. The treaty was finally ratified by a vote of twenty-four to seven, and the House appropriated the money required to fulfill its terms. Thus the United States acquired the whole of the Mississippi River and its western tributaries, some 828,000 square miles of territory, millions of acres of rich farm land, and a vast store of natural resources. The purchase of Louisiana removed a major source of American concern about the internal politics of Europe and, in the long run, produced a basic shift in the national balance of political power. After the treaty was ratified, Jefferson seemed to forget quickly his anxieties about it—except to regret that Spanish West Florida had not been part of the bargain. Though for the present neither threats nor money— he tried both—could pry the Floridas loose from Spain, Jefferson was confident that it was America's destiny to obtain them, too, "and all in good time."

Western exploration. On December 20, 1803, just a few weeks after France had taken formal possession of Louisiana from Spain, the French prefect at New Orleans turned the lower part of the territory over to the United States. The transfer of the upper part was delayed until the spring of 1804, when, at St. Louis, Meriwether Lewis, Jefferson's private secretary, accepted it in behalf of the United States. But Lewis was not there for that specific purpose; in fact, he was there as the result of presidential plans that antedated the Louisiana Purchase.

In January 1803 Congress had secretly appropriated money for an expedition to explore the upper reaches of the Missouri River and from there westward to the Pacific—though none of this territory at the time belonged to the United States. The expedition, which Jefferson had been trying to promote for many years, had several purposes. The President assured the Spanish minister that it would "have no other view than the advancement of geography"; and, to be sure, his scientific curiosity about the great unexplored interior was genuine. Lewis and his fellow explorer, William Clark (a brother of George Rogers Clark), were instructed to make astronomical observations, to study the flora and fauna, and to compile the fullest possible records. But they were to be alert to more practical matters, too, especially trading opportunities and mineral deposits. Moreover, Jefferson was fully aware that explorations had diplomatic value when nations laid claim to unsettled lands.

The Lewis and Clark expedition, which took more than two years to complete, was a remarkable success. The party of forty-five men ascended the Missouri River to the Great Falls, crossed the Rockies, and descended the Snake and Columbia rivers to the Pacific. They brought back with them an enormously expanded factual knowledge of Western North America (first made available to the public when their journals were published in 1814), a large botanical collection, information of value to American fur-traders, and a strengthened foundation for an American claim to the Oregon country. This was only one of several Western explorations that Jefferson promoted. Two others were led by Zebulon Pike: one in 1805 up the Mississippi River in search of its source, and a second in 1806 up the Arkansas River to the Rockies in what is now Colorado. All of them combined the scientific and practical interests that Jefferson himself personified.

Political Complications

Even though Jefferson accommodated his political and economic principles to some of the realities of American life, and though he converted many rank-and-file Federalists to Republicanism, he never managed to appease his more ardent opponents or to bring party politics to an end. Groups of disgruntled old Federalists, such as the so-called Essex Junto around Boston, deplored what they viewed as the growth of democratic "licentiousness" and the decline of public virtue. The new Administration, said Hamilton, seems "to imagine that to govern well, is to amuse the wondering multitude with sagacious aphorisms and oracular sayings." Senator Timothy Pickering of Massachusetts described Jefferson as a "cowardly wretch," a "Parisian revolutionary monster," who debased the public morals by his "corrupt and corrupting system. . . . Men are tempted to become apostates, not to Federalism merely, but to virtue and to religion, and to good government." As the Republicans grew stronger even in New England, Pickering and a handful of Northern Federalists in Congress privately urged that the Union be dissolved before it was too late; but their radical schemes won little support.

Not this old guard, however, but a younger generation of Federalists, more flexible and less embit-

tered, kept the party alive and a significant force in national politics. Aware of the failures that had caused their defeat, they worked to build party organizations, to imitate Republican electioneering techniques, to alter their pro-British, antidemocratic image, and to find popular issues that would broaden their appeal. "We must court popular favor," advised Fisher Ames of Massachusetts. "We must study popular opinion and accommodate measures to what it is." The young Federalists never won a national election, for the intransigence of the old guard and the élitist image that the Jeffersonians had fixed on them were more than they could overcome. Yet they made an important contribution to the development of two-party politics, were partly responsible for a dramatic increase in voting, and helped reconcile to the politics of a new age men who had once scorned popular electioneering.

In addition to the Federalist threat, Jefferson was troubled with factionalism in his own party. Personal rivalries and patronage disputes in New York and Pennsylvania produced for a time local third-party movements, some of whose leaders assumed the label "Tertium Quids." More distressing to Jefferson was the criticism he received from the uncompromising state righters of Virginia, who felt that he had moved too far toward Federalism. His good friend John Taylor observed with dismay that "Federalism . . . has gained a new footing, by being taken into partnership with republicanism." Jefferson's most persistent Virginia critic was the brilliant but erratic Congressman John Randolph of Roanoke, who would tolerate not the slightest deviation from the principles of the Kentucky Resolutions of 1798 (see p. 162). "Asking one of the states to surrender part of her sovereignty," he said, "is like asking a lady to surrender part of her chastity."

Randolph grumbled about several Administration-sponsored measures, even more about Jefferson's successful efforts to exert executive leadership and intervene in the affairs of Congress. He bitterly opposed a proposal to use federal funds to settle the claims of investors who had purchased land from the so-called Yazoo Land Companies. In 1795 these companies had corruptly obtained from the Georgia legislature large grants of the state's Western lands; they sold much of the land to various individuals before a subsequent legislature rescinded the grants and before the state, in 1802, ceded its Western lands to the federal government. Jefferson's desire to settle the matter by compensating the Yazoo claimants caused Randolph to accuse the Administration, quite unjustly, of becoming a party to the fraud. Soon Randolph and a small faction of Republicans were in open rebellion. Randolph completed his break with Jefferson in 1806, when he announced his willingness to

Aaron Burr: he courted disaster

support "*quidism*," that is, a third-party movement. He and his Virginia friends blocked the settlement of the Yazoo claims for many years and tormented Jefferson with accusations of apostasy. However, neither the Quid movements in New York and Pennsylvania nor the Randolph defection in Virginia ever reached the proportions of a national third party; eventually Randolph himself simply lost his influence in Congress.

Meanwhile, Vice President Aaron Burr, whom Jefferson had deprived of patronage and excluded from party councils after the disputed election of 1800 (see p. 164), seemed ready for almost any reckless maneuver that might improve his political fortunes. By 1804 he was willing to accept support from Federalists and dissident Republicans in a campaign for the governorship of New York. A handful of Federalists who had been toying with a scheme to unite New York and New England in an independent Northern Confederacy now hoped to enlist Burr's services. But Hamilton exposed and denounced the plot and played a major role in Burr's defeat. The enraged Burr then challenged his old New York rival to a duel, in which Hamilton, on July 11, 1804, was mortally wounded. In the presidential election later that year, Jefferson replaced Burr with George Clinton of New York as his running mate; together they crushed the discredited Federalists. Charles Cotesworth Pinckney, the Federalist candidate, carried only Connecticut and Delaware.

The talented Burr had wrecked a promising political career by overreaching himself; having been indicted for murder in both New York and New Jersey, he now courted final disaster by entering into a quixotic intrigue whose exact nature was obscured in a maze of conflicting reports. The British minister had heard that for a half-million dollars Burr would separate the Western part of the United States from the East; the Spanish minister had heard that Burr planned to establish a buffer state between Louisiana and Mexico; others had heard that he planned to conquer Mexico and establish an empire. Whatever his scheme was, Burr won the support of two important confederates: General James Wilkinson, who commanded the American troops in Louisiana and had as great a taste for conspiracy as Burr; and Harman Blennerhassett, a wealthy Irish exile who lived on an island in the upper Ohio River. In the summer of 1806 Burr and some sixty men on thirteen flatboats departed from Blennerhassett's Island and floated down the Ohio and Mississippi for some unknown purpose to some nameless glory.

The enterprise collapsed when General Wilkinson shifted sides and sent Jefferson a report that Burr was plotting treason. On Jefferson's orders the fleeing Burr was caught and taken to Richmond, where, in 1807, he was indicted for treason and conspiracy. In the curious trial that followed, Jefferson seemed determined to get a conviction whether or not the evidence warranted it; and the presiding judge, John Marshall, a Federalist, seemed as interested in discrediting Jefferson as in giving Burr justice. In the end Burr was acquitted, for the case against him did not fulfill the terms of the Constitution's definition of treason. According to the Constitution, treason consists in "levying war" against the United States or in "adhering to their enemies, giving them aid and comfort." A conviction for treason requires "the testimony of two witnesses to the same overt act." In his charge to the jury, Marshall insisted that the witnesses must have directly implicated Burr in a specific "overt act" of treason, not merely in planning treason or just loosely in organizing "a military assemblage." Since the witnesses had failed to fulfill this constitutional requirement, Marshall's charge prepared the way for Burr's acquittal. It also set a precedent that made convictions for treason extremely difficult and indictments rare.

Trouble on the High Seas

War and American trade. When Jefferson became President in 1801, he was determined that the United States pursue its destiny free from "entangling alliances" and from the wars and diplomatic duplicity of the Old World. Yet he found himself entangled in world affairs throughout most of his second Administration, and he left office with the country fast approaching total involvement. The abrogation of the French alliance in 1800, it appeared, did not mean that America had closed the door on Europe. Since the United States exported foodstuffs and raw materials, imported manufactured goods, and sent merchant ships to distant ports, it was bound to be affected by the course of international politics and by the state of the world economy.

Even during Jefferson's first Administration, pirates operating from bases on the Barbary coast of North Africa had provoked the President into vigorous action. For many years these corsairs had been harrying American vessels and forcing the federal government, like the governments of Europe, to buy immunity by paying tribute to the rulers of Morocco, Algiers, Tunis, and Tripoli. Jefferson found this costly and humiliating practice intolerable, and in 1801 he dispatched a naval squadron to the Mediterranean. For several years the United States was engaged in virtual war with Tripoli, until the Pasha, in 1805, was obliged to make a satisfactory peace. However, tribute payments to other Barbary states did not cease altogether until 1816.

The Tripolitan War, though a minor affair, had forced Jefferson to modify his naval policy. But the resumption of hostilities between Great Britain and France in 1803—a conflict that raged without interruption for the next eleven years—provided a far more strenuous test of the President's desire to remain at peace with the world. In a larger sense, it was a test of how much the American people were ready to endure and sacrifice for the sake of peace, for peace has its price as well as war. As Jefferson warned Congress, with "the flames of war lighted up again in Europe . . . the nations pursuing peace will not be exempt from all evil." To him the price was not too great, and he thanked "that kind Providence which . . . guarded us from hastily entering into the sanguinary contest and left us only to look on and to pity its ravages." Of the belligerent nations he would ask only respect for the rights to which American vessels and citizens were entitled as neutrals under international law. Since American friendship and trade were useful to them, Jefferson was certain that "it can not be the interest of any to assail us, nor ours to disturb them."

While Jefferson professed confidence in his country's capacity to bring "collisions of interest to the umpirage of reason rather than force," the European belligerents were locked in a conflict whose stakes seemed to justify any means that promised victory. In 1805 Napoleon's smashing victory over the armies of Austria and Russia at Austerlitz made him for the time master of much of the European continent, while Lord Nelson's decisive defeat of the French and Spanish fleets at the Battle of Trafalgar gave Britain control of the high seas. Thereafter, in a savage war of attrition, neither antagonist showed

The bombardment of Tripoli, 1804

much concern for the rights of neutrals or the punctilios of international law. Both rained blows on American shipping interests and insults on sensitive patriots.

Trouble began in 1805, when a British court ruled that goods from the French West Indies bound for Europe on American vessels, even though shipped by way of the United States, were subject to seizure. When the commercial provisions of Jay's Treaty of 1794 expired in 1807 and American diplomats were unable to negotiate a new agreement satisfactory to Jefferson, British interference with American shipping increased. Meanwhile Napoleon had developed a program of economic warfare; his so-called Continental System, elaborated in his Berlin Decree of 1806 and Milan Decree of 1807, closed the European ports under his control to British goods and stated that neutral ships complying with British trade regulations would be confiscated. The British government retaliated with a series of Orders in Council, the most important of which proclaimed a blockade of the ports of France and of the nations under its control. Thereafter American ships bound for western Europe risked seizure by one or the other of the belligerents, depending on whose rules they flouted. In the three years prior to 1807 the British seized at least a thousand American merchantmen and the French half that many.

To Americans the most grievous British wrong was the revival and vigorous application of the centuries-old system of impressment, by which the Royal Navy procured its manpower. In times of crisis British law permitted the commander of a warship, when he needed men, to draft able-bodied subjects of the king wherever they could be found. In applying the system British warships stopped American merchantmen on the high seas to search for deserters; they took off British-born sailors who had become Americans by naturalization; and in the process they heedlessly

Thomas Jefferson: to the manner born

impressed an unknown number of native-born Americans as well. The issue reached a crisis in June 1807, when the British frigate *Leopard* overhauled the United States frigate *Chesapeake* within sight of the Virginia coast and demanded the right to search her for deserters. When the commander of the unprepared *Chesapeake* refused, the *Leopard* fired three broadsides that killed three Americans and wounded eighteen others. The crippled *Chesapeake* submitted to the seizure of four deserters and then returned to Norfolk. This humiliation of an American frigate infuriated both Federalists and Republicans. "Never, since the battle of Lexington," wrote Jefferson, "have I seen this country in such a state of exasperation as at present." Judging from the tone of the press and the speeches of politicians, the country seemed ready to unite behind a war policy. But Jefferson asked for less: he ordered British warships out of American waters and demanded reparations, an apology, and assurance that such an outrage would not be repeated.

The embargo. Jefferson asked something of Americans, too. He called for a supreme effort, not to win a war, but to achieve what he considered the nobler goal of keeping the country at peace. To avoid further provocative incidents, Jefferson proposed a policy that he had long cherished as an alternative to war, a policy he described as "peaceable coercion." On December 22, 1807, in response to his urgent plea, Congress passed an Embargo Act that stopped the export of American goods and prohibited all United States ships from clearing American ports for foreign ports. This act, in effect, required shipowners to abandon their risky but extremely profitable wartime trade and obliged planters and farmers to give up their rich European export market.

Jefferson asked for a greater sacrifice than most Americans seemed ready to make. Angry New England merchants, preferring risks and insults to commercial stagnation, denounced the embargo as a ruthless attempt to transform the federal government's constitutional power to regulate foreign commerce into an unconstitutional power to prohibit it altogether. Many of them defiantly engaged in an illicit trade that severe enforcement measures, some of dubious legality, could not entirely suppress. The Federalists, having at last found a popular issue, enjoyed a modest revival. Some again hinted at secession. The agricultural interest was equally distressed when farm commodities began to accumulate at the ports and prices declined. John Randolph's assaults on the Administration matched those of the Federalists. The embargo, he complained, had furnished "rogues with an opportunity of getting rich at the expense of honest men." Eventually Congress yielded to overwhelming pressure and passed an act repealing the embargo. On March 1, 1809, a disappointed Jefferson, his prestige somewhat diminished, signed it.

"Nature intended me for the more tranquil pursuits of science by rendering them my supreme delight," wrote the weary Jefferson at the close of his second Administration. Retirement was a welcome relief not only from the vicissitudes of domestic politics, in which he counted more successes than failures, but from the trials of international affairs, in which he suffered his greatest defeat.

The Decision for War

By declining to run for reelection in 1808, Jefferson helped to establish the two-term tradition. His favorite, Secretary of State James Madison, easily won the nomination of the Republican caucus over James Monroe, the candidate of the Randolph faction. Though the Federalists, who again nominated Charles Cotesworth Pinckney, regained control of New England and increased their strength in the new Congress, Madison won the Presidency by a decisive majority of 122 to 47 in the Electoral College. His inaugural address reflected the changing conditions of the preceding eight years, especially in its concern for the promotion of commerce and industry. However, in spirit

James Madison: political philosopher

it was still a thoroughly Jeffersonian document that endorsed the domestic and foreign policies of his predecessor. Few Presidents have brought to the White House such rich experience in public life as did Madison; none, save John Adams, was so profound a student of political philosophy. Yet, though Madison had contributed much to the formulation of Republican doctrine and had never been Jefferson's mere pliant tool, he lacked Jefferson's political acumen and force as a party leader and chief executive.

The failure of diplomacy.

The overshadowing problem confronting the new President and Congress was the continuing European holocaust, which still created difficulties for neutrals. Although the embargo had been repealed, the policy of "peaceable coercion" persisted in less drastic forms. However, the Madison Administration blundered badly in applying it. The first substitute for the embargo was a Nonintercourse Act, passed in 1809, which reestablished trade with all nations except Great Britain and France so long as the latter two continued to enforce their obnoxious orders and decrees. This act encouraged the British government to try negotiation. David Erskine, the friendly and sympathetic British minister, concluded an agreement that was highly satisfactory to the United States, though he violated his instructions in doing so. On June 10, 1809, the delighted President renewed trade with Great Britain without waiting for the agreement to be approved in London, and hundreds of American ships cleared their home ports for the first time in many months. Unfortunately the British government repudiated the Erskine "treaty" as soon as it arrived and recalled its too-generous minister. Madison, embarrassed and humiliated, then proclaimed the restoration of nonintercourse, and Anglo-American relations worsened.

On May 1, 1810, nonintercourse gave way to a new policy incorporated in a curious measure called Macon's Bill Number 2. This bill restored trade with both Great Britain and France but threatened to resume nonintercourse with either of them whenever the other agreed to respect America's neutral rights. Now it was Napoleon's turn to try some shifty diplomacy. Proclaiming his love for Americans and his concern for their prosperity, he announced that on November 1, 1810, the French commercial restrictions would be repealed—but he attached conditions that made his promise almost meaningless. Nevertheless, on February 2, 1811, Madison reestablished nonintercourse with Britain, though, in fact, the French continued to seize American ships. Unable to get Britain to repeal its Orders in Council, Madison recalled the American minister, William Pinkney, and thus virtually severed diplomatic relations.

Ironically, a few months later the policy of "peaceable coercion" won a striking victory. On June 23, 1812, beset by an economic crisis at home, the British foreign secretary announced the immediate suspension of the Orders in Council (but not impressment). The announcement came too late. On June 1, Madison had asked for a declaration of war against Great Britain, and Congress soon complied: the House on June 4 by a vote of seventy-nine to forty-nine, the Senate on June 18 by a vote of nineteen to thirteen. The division in both houses was largely political, for all Federalists voted against war, while the Republicans voted for it ninety-eight to twenty-two.

Though the Federalist commercial interests were most directly affected by British impressment and interference with American shipping on the high seas, they considered war with Great Britain the ultimate folly. War would be more devastating to their trade than the Orders in Council had been—and the blow would be dealt by their own government. Moreover, to them, Britain was not only a profitable market but the defender of conservatism, stability, and order against the obscenities of Napoleonic France. Sharing these views with the Federalists were a handful of Republican Congressmen representing Southern coastal districts and about a third of the Republicans representing the Northeast. John Randolph, a severe critic of the war policy, urged Republicans to live up to their principles of economy and retrenchment and not to become "infatuated with standing armies, loans, taxes, navies, and war."

The aims of the prowar Republicans.

An able and highly articulate group opposed the declaration of war, but the majority seemed to support it. Although this majority did not include the New England merchants and shipowners, neutral rights and impressment were nevertheless issues of major importance in the decision to go to war. The grievances Madison stressed in his war message were "the injuries and indignities which have been heaped upon our country"—the British actions "hostile to the United States as an independent and neutral nation." Most Americans felt those insults keenly and resented the implicit unwillingness of the British to concede the reality of American independence. According to one Kentuckian, "we must now oppose the farther encroachments of Great Britain by war, or formally annul the Declaration of Independence, and acknowledge ourselves her devoted colonies." The vindication of national honor, many Republicans believed, would also be a vindication of republican institutions against their foreign and domestic enemies. This notion of an American mission to defend republicanism was widespread; according to Jefferson, "The last hope of human liberty in this world rests on us."

Neutral rights involved economic interests, too; as Madison explained, British policy struck not only at commerce but at agriculture as well. By closing European markets to American staples, the British threatened the prosperity of farmers and planters, many of whom lived hundreds of miles from the sea and might never have seen an ocean-going vessel. "The interests of agriculture and commerce are inseparable," said Representative Langdon Cheves of South Carolina.

The Congress that voted for war contained a remarkable little band of youthful Republicans from the Southern and Western states. Some of them had taken their seats for the first time in November 1811 and had at once begun to badger the President and harangue their colleagues with truculent anti-British speeches. They managed to elect the thirty-four-year-old Henry Clay of Kentucky Speaker of the House; Clay in turn gave important committee assignments to aggressive young Republicans such as Richard M. Johnson of Kentucky, Felix Grundy of Tennessee, and John C. Calhoun of South Carolina. These second-generation Republicans—the Federalists called them "War Hawks"—were critical of the nonbelligerent measures of Jefferson and Madison, indifferent to the state-rights political tradition embodied in the Resolutions of 1798, more nationalistic than the Federalists in their prime, and eager for geographic expansion and economic growth, with none of the anxieties that Jefferson sometimes seemed to feel. To them, after diplomacy had failed, only war could demonstrate America's power and redress intolerable wrongs too long endured: impressment, violations of America's neutral rights, disregard for its dignity as a sovereign power.

Eventually these so-called War Hawks tried to use the war as justification for the acquisition of additional territory. The insatiable Southern and Western demand for land was an indirect and perhaps secondary source of the crisis that culminated in war. Still another source was the growth of formidable resistance among Indians of the Northwest and Southwest to the ceaseless incursions of white settlers on their lands. By the time of Madison's first administration, the Indians evidently had decided that if they were ever to make a stand east of the Mississippi, it would have to be now.

At this crucial time two Shawnees of uncommon ability, Tecumseh and his brother Tenskwatawa ("the Prophet"), managed to unite many of the tribes to defend their lands against further white encroachments. Tecumseh supplied political leadership, while the Prophet provided spiritual inspiration and a call for moral regeneration. Together they organized an efficient Indian confederation supported by braves determined to preserve their lands and uncorrupted

Tecumseh: Shawnee chief

by the white man's proffered gifts of liquor. Terror spread along the frontier. In the summer of 1811, when Tecumseh went south to bid for the support of the Creeks, Governor Harrison decided to take advantage of his absence. He advanced with a force of a thousand men to the outskirts of Prophetstown, the chief Indian settlement, on the Wabash River near the mouth of Tippecanoe Creek. There, on November 7, after repelling an Indian attack, his men destroyed the town. The Battle of Tippecanoe marked the beginning of a long and savage Indian war.

In asking for a declaration of war against Great Britain Madison expressed an opinion held by the majority of Westerners: that the Indians had been receiving arms and encouragement from the British in Canada. Some of the young militants, though lacking evidence, were certain of it. "I can have no doubt of the influence of British agents in keeping up Indian hostility" and of encouraging them "to murder our citizens," cried Richard M. Johnson of Kentucky. Felix Grundy of Tennessee agreed, adding that there would be no peace on the frontier until the British were driven out of Canada. To Westerners, once war was declared, the conquest of the rich lands of Upper Canada was one of the anticipated fruits of victory. To Southerners the conquest of East and West Florida, still in the possession of Spain, Great Britain's ally, might well be another. As early as 1810 Madison, in collusion with American settlers, had seized a portion of West Florida; but nothing short of the whole of the Floridas would now satisfy the expansionists. This "agrarian cupidity," as John Randolph called it, was not a cause of the war with Great Britain, but the war evoked the expansionism that was latent in many of those who voted for it.

In a letter summarizing the causes of the war, Andrew Jackson of Tennessee mentioned neutral rights, impressment, national vindication, Indian pacification, and the desire for territorial conquest. He then condensed all these motives into two phrases: "to seek some indemnity for past injuries, some security against future aggression." Jackson seems to have reflected the sentiment of the majority in the Southern and Western states, and in the presidential election of 1812 they, along with Pennsylvania and Vermont, endorsed the war policy by giving their electoral votes to Madison. De Witt Clinton of New York, the candidate of the Federalists and Peace Republicans, carried the rest of the New England and Middle Atlantic states.

Madison's rather narrow margin in the Electoral College (128 to 89—the shift of one state, Pennsylvania, could have changed the result), together with the bitter resentment of the commercial centers, meant that the country went to war dangerously divided. No patriot, wrote a Boston editor, "conceives it his duty to shed his blood for Bonaparte, for Madison or Jefferson, and that Host of Ruffians in Congress." The revitalized New England Federalists wanted no part of "Mr. Madison's war."

The War of 1812

National unpreparedness. The prowar Republicans were convinced that the war could be won with little effort and a minimum of sacrifice. Henry Clay announced that "the militia of Kentucky alone are competent to place Montreal and Upper Canada at your feet." His friends in Congress must have believed him, for they led into war a country that was not only internally divided but hopelessly unprepared. As war approached, the Madison Administration loyally adhered to Jefferson's policy of relying on small gunboats rather than ocean-going frigates; even in his message to Congress of November 1811 Madison made no recommendation for naval expansion. The following January two-thirds of the representatives who were to vote for war five months later helped to defeat a modest proposal to add ten frigates to the navy. During the debate on this measure, Richard M. Johnson of Kentucky, one of the young militants, vowed that he would not vote a penny for a naval force "destined to entail upon this happy Government perpetual taxes and a perpetually increasing public debt."

Congress made no effort to increase American naval power until months after the outbreak of war, and the new forty-four-gun frigates and seventy-four-gun ships of the line then provided for were not ready for action until the war had ended. Indeed, the United States had an ocean-going navy of only sixteen vessels fit for service with which to challenge the world's foremost sea power, whose warships numbered in the hundreds. The American navy had the advantage of a talented, well-trained group of officers but had only a limited supply of experienced seamen. It had no real fleet organization, each ship operating more or less as an independent unit. Moreover, since most of the ships were expected to function as commerce-raiders, the question of naval strategy seemed superfluous.

But the Republican majority, after all, was thinking primarily of a land war, not of challenging Britain's naval supremacy. With Florida weakly defended, with fewer than five thousand British troops in Canada, and with war raging in Europe, the odds seemed to favor the Americans. Had the United States trained, equipped, and put in the field an army of only fifty thousand men—no serious strain on the country's resources—it might have conquered Canada and Florida with relative ease. Congress seemed to act boldly enough: it authorized an expansion of the small regular army by the recruitment of twenty-five thousand five-year volunteers; provided for the raising of an additional fifty thousand one-year volunteers; and made repeated calls on the state militias, which numbered, on paper, some seven hundred thousand men.

However, even in the regions most enthusiastic for war, Americans were reluctant to abandon their civilian pursuits; neither coercion nor persuasion, such as offers of cash bounties and land grants, had much effect. Never during the war did the army number more than thirty-five thousand men, and even this small force was poorly trained and unimaginatively commanded by over-age veterans of the Revolution and incompetent militia officers. Moreover, militiamen, especially in the Federalist states, generally felt that their duty was limited to state defense, and some refused to leave their states for operations across the frontier.

The members of Congress, including those who had voted for war, hesitated to adopt the fiscal measures demanded by a war policy. Eventually Congress doubled tariff rates and levied a new excise tax, a stamp tax, and a direct tax on the states, but those unpopular measures brought the government little revenue until near the end of the war. It authorized loans, but the Treasury Department managed to market the bulk of about $80 million in securities only at a discount and at high interest rates. Since most New England capitalists opposed the war, and since the Bank of the United States had been abolished in 1811, Secretary of the Treasury Gallatin had to rely on state banks, which were poorly equipped to handle business of this sort. In short, Republican policy over the past decade had been designed for a simple agricultural nation at peace with the world; now Republi-

The war was declared, because Great Britain arrogated to herself the pretension of regulating our foreign trade, under the delusive name of retaliatory orders in council—a pretension by which she undertook to proclaim to American enterprise, "thus far shalt thou go, and no further"...; because she persisted in the practice of impressing American seamen; because she had instigated the Indians to commit hostilities against us; and because she refused indemnity for her past injuries upon our commerce.... The war in fact was announced, on our part, to meet the war which she was waging on her part.... We are told that England is a proud and lofty nation, which, disdaining to wait for danger, meets it half way. Haughty as she is, we once triumphed over her, and, if we do not listen to the councils of timidity and despair, we shall again prevail. In such a cause, with the aid of Providence, we must come out crowned with success; but if we fail, let us fail like men, lash ourselves to our gallant tars, and expire together in one common struggle for FREE TRADE AND SEAMEN'S RIGHTS.

From Henry Clay of Kentucky, Speech in the House of Representatives, January 8, 1813.

cans, in effect, attempted to apply Jeffersonian means to a non-Jeffersonian end. In so doing, they barely escaped national disaster.

The military campaigns. Plans for the invasion and occupation of Canada ended in a fiasco. Effective strategy called for a concentration of forces in an attack on Montreal, whose fall would have cut British communications along the St. Lawrence and the Great Lakes and made the British position in Upper Canada untenable. But, in response to the Western demand for protection from Tecumseh's Indian confederation, the nation's forces were diffused. As a result, the military campaign of 1812 was a feeble, poorly planned, uncoordinated attempt to invade Canada at three separate points. General William Hull marched an army from Detroit toward the British garrison at Malden. But, doubting the wisdom of an invasion before winning control of Lake Erie, and hearing that Tecumseh and his warriors had joined the British, Hull soon lost his nerve and returned to Detroit. There, on August 16, a brilliant British commander, General Isaac Brock, surrounded Hull's army and forced him to surrender without firing a shot. A second invasion across the Niagara River culminated in defeat and surrender when New York militiamen refused to enter Canada to reinforce their countrymen. Finally, General Henry Dearborn led an advance along Lake Champlain toward Montreal. When he reached the Canadian border he found that his militiamen would not cross it and was obliged to march back to Plattsburg. So ended the land campaigns of 1812. If they had made no conquests and won no glory, at least they had cost few lives.

Things went little better the next year. Canadians astonished their would-be "liberators" by vigorously supporting British efforts to drive the invaders out. Two events, however, enabled the Americans to recover lost ground on the Northwest frontier and all but eliminate the danger of another British offensive there. The first was Captain Oliver Hazard Perry's notable victory at Put-in-Bay on Lake Erie, September 10, 1813. When Perry reported, "We have met the enemy and they are ours," he gave the Americans control of the Great Lakes and made the British position at Detroit hopeless. The second event was General Harrison's victory over the retreating British at the Battle of the Thames, October 5, 1813. Here the great Indian leader Tecumseh was killed; with his death the Indian confederacy collapsed, and the Northwest frontier was secure. But the conquest of Canada was as remote as ever.

By 1814 the Americans were striving desperately to prevent the British from invading their land and, perhaps, taking a slice of it. With the defeat of Napoleon and his exile to Elba, the British were able for the first time to give their undivided attention to the American war and to send some of their best troops across the Atlantic. Their plan was to harass the cities on the Atlantic coast with amphibious operations while launching invasions at three points: Niagara, Lake Champlain, and New Orleans.

The most ambitious coastal attack was a thrust up Chesapeake Bay culminating in the capture of Washington on August 24. As the President and other Administration officials fled, the British burned the Capitol, the White House, and other public buildings. Having avenged an earlier American raid on York (Toronto) with this crowning humiliation, and failing

Washington, 1814: a crowning humiliation

in an attempt to capture Baltimore, the British withdrew. The military significance of the raid was negligible, but it underscored the utter failure of the Administration's war policy.

The British invasion plans, however, seriously miscarried, for by 1814 the Americans had found some vigorous young officers and no longer had to rely on untrained, undisciplined militia units. The projected British offensive at Niagara was thwarted by the aggressive operations of General Jacob Brown and his able young subordinate, Winfield Scott. The Battle of Lundy's Lane, near Niagara Falls, on July 25, was itself indecisive, but it ended the British invasion threat from that position. In August a powerful force

of British veterans commanded by Sir George Prevost advanced toward Lake Champlain with the apparent purpose of cutting off the New England states from the rest of the Union. Early in September Prevost paused before the strong American fortifications at Plattsburg to await the outcome of a bitter duel between British and American flotillas on Lake Champlain. On September 11 Captain Thomas Macdonough's American fleet won a decisive victory, forcing Prevost to abandon his campaign and retire to Canada. Clearly, the war on the Canadian frontier had reached a stalemate.

The final campaign took place in the Southwest. Here Andrew Jackson of Tennessee, an authentic

The War of 1812: Northern campaigns, 1812–14

self-trained military genius, somehow managed to make soldiers out of militiamen and to furnish them with supplies. Jackson had already broken the military power of the Southwestern Indians by defeating the Creeks at the Battle of Horseshoe Bend, on March 27, 1814, and had also forced them to cede some of their richest lands in Mississippi Territory. Next he captured and destroyed Pensacola in Spanish Florida to prevent the British from using it as a base and then marched his army to New Orleans to meet the invaders. Placing his men behind earthworks and bales of cotton, he awaited the attack of eight thousand seasoned British troops commanded by Sir Edward Pakenham. Contemptuous of Jackson's motley army of militiamen, sailors, and pirates, Pakenham, on January 8, 1815, led his men in tight formation in a rash frontal assault. American rifles and artillery raked the British columns with a deadly fire. Before the British withdrew, the Americans had killed the British commander and inflicted more than two thousand casualties, while suffering little more than a dozen of their own. The Battle of New Orleans was the last engagement of the war—in fact, it was fought two weeks after a treaty of peace had been signed. But it helped sweeten the bitter taste of the defeats and disappointments of the previous two and a half years, and it launched Andrew Jackson, the Hero of New Orleans, on his dazzling career.

On the high seas in the early months of the war the tiny American navy won a series of stunning victories in single-ship engagements, bolstering public

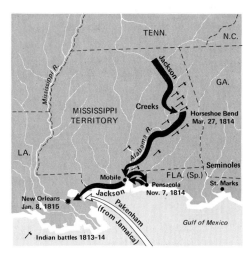

**The War of 1812:
Southwestern campaigns, 1813–15**

morale during the disasters on the Canadian frontier. The most spectacular of these victories were those of the American frigate *Constitution* (Old Ironsides) over the British frigates *Guerrière* and *Java*, and of the *United States* over the *Macedonian*. These successes shocked the British public, which had heard the American navy described as a "few fir-built frigates, manned by a handful of bastards and outlaws"; but they constituted no real challenge to British naval supremacy, nor did they have any great strategic significance.

By 1813 most of the American men-of-war were bottled up in their home ports by a British blockade,

**A spectacular victory:
the *Constitution* and
the *Guerrière*, 1812**

Daniel Webster on conscription and federal tyranny

I would ask, sir, whether the supporters of these measures have well weighed the difficulties of their undertaking. Have they considered whether it will be found easy to execute laws which bear such marks of despotism on their front, and which will be so productive of every sort and degree of misery in their execution? For one, sir, I hesitate not to say that they cannot be executed....

The operation of measures thus unconstitutional and illegal ought to be prevented by a resort to other measures which are both constitutional and legal. It will be the solemn duty of the State Governments to protect their own authority over their own militia, and to interpose between their citizens and arbitrary power. These are among the objects for which the State Governments exist; and their highest obligations bind them to the preservation of their own rights and the liberties of their people....

In my opinion, sir, the sentiments of the free population of this country are greatly mistaken here. The nation is not yet in a temper to submit to conscription. The people have too fresh and strong a feeling of the blessings of civil liberty to be willing thus to surrender it. You may talk to them as much as you please, of the victory and glory to be obtained in the enemy's provinces; they will hold those objects in light estimation if the means be a forced military service.

From Daniel Webster, Speech in the House of Representatives, December 9, 1814.

and by the end of the war only the *Constitution* and a few smaller vessels were still at sea. American cruisers and privateers continued to prey on British commerce and altogether captured more than a thousand merchantmen. These commerce-raiders were a costly annoyance to the British but fell far short of seriously crippling her overseas trade or disrupting her economy. The decisive fact of the naval war was the British blockade of the American coast, which dealt an almost mortal blow to the American carrying trade. In 1814 exports and imports fell to less than 10 percent of what they had been in the peak year of 1807. Flour exports declined from 1,443,000 barrels in 1812 to 193,000 barrels in 1814. The blockade was equally disastrous to American interstate commerce, most of which still moved along coastal waterways. Francis Wayland described the devastating impact of the blockade on the whole economy: "Our harbors were blockaded; communications coastwise between our ports were cut off; our ships were rotting in every creek and cove where they could find a place of security; our immense annual products were mouldering in our warehouses; the sources of profitable labor were dried up." Though the land war was a stalemate, the war on the high seas culminated in a British victory that was well-nigh complete. Floating in the wreckage was Jefferson's gunboat policy.

Disaffection in New England. These disasters were what antiwar Federalists in the Northeast had anticipated—what Josiah Quincy of Massachusetts

had in mind when he said, "This war, the measures which preceded it, and the mode of carrying it on, are all undeniably southern and western policy, not the policy of the commercial states." Feeling betrayed by their own government, convinced that the Madison Administration had deliberately set about to destroy their political and economic power, New England Federalists throughout the war regarded the Republican politicians in Washington, not the British, as their mortal enemies. And, having regained political control of all the New England states, they were in a position to translate their angry polemics into defiant deeds.

Federalist governors contested federal calls on the state militias, insisting that their proper function was to repel invasion, not to invade foreign territory. Federalists discouraged voluntary enlistments; and when Congress debated a militia draft they defended state sovereignty against national tyranny. "Where is it written in the Constitution," asked Daniel Webster, a young Federalist congressman from New Hampshire, "that you may take children from their parents, and parents from their children, and compel them to fight the battles of any war in which the folly or the wickedness of government may engage it?" Federalists resisted tax measures and boycotted government loans. According to a Boston editor, "any man who lends money to the government at the present time will forfeit all claim to common honesty." Meanwhile, defiant New Englanders continued to trade with Canada and even furnished supplies to the British fleet.

The more extreme dissenters, especially the ardent Federalists of the Connecticut River Valley, favored either a separate peace and the withdrawal of New England from the war or else secession from the Union.

In 1814 British depredations along the New England coast and the belief that the federal government would do nothing to check them precipitated a serious political crisis. In October the Massachusetts legislature called for a convention of the New England states to prepare an adequate defense against invasion and to consider amendments to the federal Constitution. The call asserted that in the existing Union the "Eastern sections" had not obtained "those equal rights and benefits which are the greatest objects of its formation." Twenty-six delegates—twelve from Massachusetts, seven from Connecticut, four from Rhode Island, and three from Vermont—assembled in Hartford on December 15 and deliberated secretly for nearly three weeks. Federalist extremists, such as Timothy Pickering, were not among the delegates; the moderates, led by Harrison Gray Otis of Massachusetts, gained control and adopted a final report that was relatively mild.

The report, much of which dealt with the problem of defending the New England coast, began with a gloomy account of the evils the country had endured under the "withering influence" of the Republicans. The Jeffersonians, it claimed, had debauched the civil service; destroyed "the balance of power which existed among the original states" by creating new Western states; and entertained a "visionary and superficial theory in regard to commerce, accompanied by a real hatred but a feigned regard to its interests." As a remedy for these grievances the Hartford report demanded a series of constitutional amendments that would abolish the three-fifths compromise, require a two-thirds vote of both houses of Congress to declare war and to admit new states, prohibit embargoes lasting for more than sixty days, exclude the foreign-born from federal offices, limit the President to one term, and prohibit the election of two successive Presidents from the same state. If these demands were ignored and the war continued, the report recommended that another convention be called and given "such powers and instructions as the exigency of a crisis so momentous may require."

When representatives from the Hartford Convention arrived in Washington with their ultimatum, they found the capital rejoicing over Jackson's victory at New Orleans and over the signing of a treaty of peace. Now their complaints seemed pointless, and their demands were ignored. But the Hartford Convention was remembered; to nationalists it symbolized the disloyalty, the narrow, selfish provincialism, of the Federalists. Consequently, the Federalist party, though for a time it remained strong in several New England states, was itself one of the casualties of the War of 1812.

Oddly enough, New England, in spite of its political disaffection, was the only region that profited materially from the war. Since the British blockade was not enforced along its coast until 1814, it received the bulk of foreign imports. Gold from the rest of the country flowed to its banks, which were thus able to maintain specie payments while other banks were forced to suspend payments. Above all, the war gave a strong impetus to New England manufacturing; between 1810 and 1814 the number of cotton spindles in the area increased sixfold. A war that many had hoped would result in the acquisition of more land for the farmers and planters of the Northwest and South ended without an acre of new territory but with many thousands of spindles whirling in New England factories.

Peace Negotiations

The Treaty of Ghent. Almost from the start of this curious conflict there had been talk of peace. As early as September 1812 the tsar of Russia, anxious that the British give their full attention to Napoleon, offered to act as mediator. President Madison responded favorably and, early in 1813, sent Albert Gallatin and James A. Bayard to work with John Quincy Adams, the American minister in St. Petersburg. The British declined the Russian offer—Russia could not be trusted to support the British position on neutral rights—but soon indicated a willingness to negotiate directly with the Americans. This, too, was acceptable to Madison, though he did not hear of the suggestion until January 1814. He then appointed Henry Clay and Jonathan Russell to join the three commissioners already in Europe, and in August negotiations began in the city of Ghent.

The British diplomats, an unimpressive group, were under the strict control of the Foreign Office in London. The Americans, superior in talent, had received from their government broader powers and greater freedom to negotiate. But they sometimes disagreed among themselves on matters of policy, and during the tedious months of negotiation their personal relations occasionally became tense. Adams' colleagues found him an irritating companion, and Adams, in turn, took a dim view of them, especially of Clay with his taste for cards and late hours. "They sit after dinner and drink bad wine and smoke cigars, which neither suits my habits nor my health, and absorbs time which I cannot spare," wrote the austere

New Englander. Gallatin and Bayard turned out to be the chief peacemakers in dealings not only with the British but with their own colleagues.

Had the two delegations adhered to their initial instructions, the negotiations would have been brief and the result complete failure. The Americans were to insist that the British abandon impressment, agree to respect international law in setting up blockades, and pay indemnity for their illegal seizure of American ships. The British, anticipating decisive military victories in the campaigns of 1814, presented a list of terms that would have jeopardized the sovereignty and future growth of the United States. They demanded territorial cessions in northern New York and Maine, the surrender of American control of the Great Lakes, the creation of an autonomous Indian buffer state south of the Great Lakes, the right to navigate the Mississippi River, and the relinquishment of American fishing rights off the coasts of Newfoundland and Labrador. The Americans made it clear that if the British insisted on these terms the war would continue. "Our negotiations may be considered at an end," wrote Gallatin to his government.

But the British did not insist. News of Macdonough's victory on Lake Champlain and Prevost's retreat from Plattsburg drastically changed the military picture, and the Duke of Wellington, when consulted by the British ministry, argued that failure to gain control of the Great Lakes made the British demands unreasonable. "I confess," he said, "that I think you have no right, from the state of the war, to demand any concession of territory from America." British merchants and manufacturers, eager to resume trade with the United States, favored an end to hostilities. The tax-burdened British public, too, had had enough of war.

As negotiations proceeded, the diplomats dropped one demand after another and eventually agreed to a peace treaty that settled nothing but simply restored conditions as they were before the war. The Treaty of Ghent, signed on December 24, 1814, was silent on impressment and neutral rights, boundaries and fisheries, trade and indemnities—although it referred some of those questions to joint commissions for future settlement. In submitting the treaty to the Senate for ratification, Madison claimed no victory. "The late war," he said with more than a little ambiguity, "has been waged with a success which is the natural result of the wisdom of the legislative councils, of the patriotism of the people, of the public spirit of the militia, and of the valor of the military and naval forces of the country." As Adams described the document, "Nothing was adjusted, nothing was settled—nothing in substance but an indefinite suspension of hostilities was agreed to." Clay, though he signed it, described it as a "damned bad treaty."

Nevertheless, Americans looked back on the war with pride and satisfaction. They ignored the fact that the British had yielded nothing on neutral rights or impressment, because these issues lost their significance when the war ended in Europe. In the selective memories of patriots the military defeats, the bungling of the Canadian campaigns, and British supremacy on the high seas faded into insignificance; the early exploits of American frigates and privateers, Perry's victory on Lake Erie, and, best of all, Jackson's victory at New Orleans were remembered vividly as the crucial events of the war. The very fact that no territory had been lost—that the British had abandoned their extreme demands—contributed to this myth of military success. Moreover, the death of Tecumseh, the collapse of the Indian confederation, and the destruction of Indian military power east of the Mississippi meant that at least one purpose of the war had been fully achieved. Finally, the rise of manufacturing made the country more self-sufficient, and the preservation of their threatened independence gave Americans a greater feeling of national identity than ever before. As Gallatin observed: "The war has renewed and reinstated the national feelings and character which the Revolution had given. . . . The people now have more general objects of attachment. . . . They are more Americans; they feel and act more as a nation."

Postwar settlements. Though memories of the war were to keep alive an undercurrent of Anglo-American hostility for many years, several specific issues that might have caused trouble were resolved soon after the stalemate at Ghent. In 1815 a commercial treaty removed most of the restrictions on Anglo-American trade (except with the British West Indies). An agreement of 1817, signed by Richard Rush, the acting Secretary of State, and Charles Bagot, the British minister, provided for almost complete naval disarmament on the Great Lakes. Though either side could terminate it on six months' notice, the Rush-Bagot Agreement became a permanent policy. Eventually, this agreement led to the demilitarization of the entire American-Canadian border. Another agreement the following year reopened the coasts of Newfoundland and Labrador to American fishermen, established the forty-ninth parallel as the northern boundary of the Louisiana Purchase from the Lake of the Woods to the Rocky Mountains, and provided for a joint occupation of Oregon for the next ten years. Neither the British nor the Americans could have guessed it then, but these postwar negotiations, rather than the War of 1812, were to set the pattern for subsequent Anglo-American relations.

Another long-standing source of diplomatic friction was removed when Spain finally agreed to give up

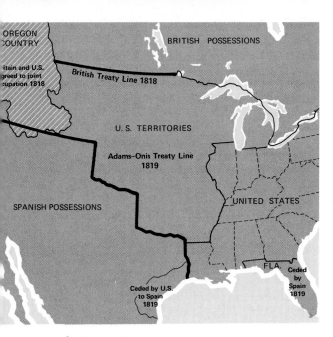

Boundary treaties, 1818–19

the Floridas. Internally weak and rapidly losing its once great empire in South and Central America, Spain maintained only a tenuous hold on the Floridas. Spain's feeble garrison was unable to control the Seminole Indians or to prevent white outlaws and runaway slaves from using the region as a sanctuary. In 1818 Andrew Jackson, giving the broadest possible interpretation to vague instructions from his government, led a military force into the Floridas to punish the Seminoles for depredations along the American frontier. In the process he seized St. Marks and Pensacola, deposed the Spanish governor, and raised the American flag; he also arrested two British subjects for inciting the Indians, tried them by court-martial, and executed them. At home Jackson's highhanded con-

duct added to his popularity, but it immensely complicated matters for Secretary of State John Quincy Adams, who had been negotiating with the Spanish minister, Luis de Onís.

Making the best of a bad situation, Adams brazened his way through. He not only refused to apologize for Jackson's behavior but threw responsibility on the Spanish for failing to preserve order in the Floridas. Spain, he insisted, must either govern the provinces efficiently or cede them to the United States, for they had become "a derelict, open to the occupancy of every enemy, civilized or savage, of the United States, and serving no other earthly purpose than as a post of annoyance to them." This was a challenge that the Spanish were in no position to accept, and in 1819 the Adams-Onís Treaty arranged for the transfer of the Floridas to the United States. In exchange, the American government agreed to assume payment of $5 million worth of claims that American citizens held against the Spanish government. The treaty also drew a boundary between the Louisiana Territory and Spanish possessions in the Southwest. The line followed the Sabine, Red, and Arkansas rivers to the Rocky Mountains, then the forty-second parallel west to the Pacific. Thus the United States gave up its claim to Texas (as part of the Louisiana Purchase) and Spain its claim to territory in the Pacific Northwest. Ratification of the treaty was delayed for two years, but in 1821 Jackson triumphantly reentered the Florida Territory as the first American governor.

Those who had moral sensibilities about the rough tactics of Jackson and Adams soothed their conscience with the argument that since the Floridas were contiguous to American territory, Providence intended that America should have them. A later generation would call this argument "Manifest Destiny." Even so, the age of the Jeffersonians, who believed in man's reason and disliked the cynicism of the Old World, was closing on a slightly sour note.

Suggestions for Reading

JEFFERSON IN POWER
Jefferson's political philosophy has had an enduring influence on American thought; it is analyzed sympathetically in Adrienne Koch, *The Philosophy of Thomas Jefferson* (1943). Dumas Malone, *Jefferson the President: First Term, 1801–1805* (1970), and *Jefferson the President: Second Term, 1805–1809* (1974), are parts of a masterful six-volume biography. Two excellent biographies, written on a smaller scale, are Nathan Schachner, *Thomas Jefferson: A Biography*, 2 vols. (1951), and Merrill Peterson, *Thomas Jefferson and the New Nation: A Biography* (1970). F. M. Brodie, *Thomas Jefferson: An Intimate History* (1974), attempts, with mixed results, a psychoanalytic approach to reveal Jefferson's personal life. R. M. Johnstone, Jr., *Jefferson and the Presidency* (1978), emphasizes Jefferson's strong executive leadership. The contributions of Jefferson's two ablest lieutenants can be stud-

ied in Irving Brant, *James Madison: Secretary of State* (1953); Ralph Ketcham, *James Madison* (1971); and Raymond Walters, Jr., *Albert Gallitan: Jeffersonian Financier and Diplomat** (1957).

The best and most comprehensive survey of the Republican era is Marshall Smelser, *The Democratic Republic, 1801–1815** (1968). Three brief, well-written surveys are also useful: Marcus Cunliffe, *The Nation Takes Shape, 1789–1837** (1959); C. M. Wiltse, *The New Nation, 1800–1845** (1961); and Morton Borden, *Parties and Politics in the Early Republic, 1789–1815** (1967). An older analysis that is a classic, in spite of its hostility to Jefferson and Madison, is Henry Adams, *History of the United States of America During the Administrations of Jefferson and Madison*, 9 vols.* (1889–91). Forrest McDonald, *The Presidency of Thomas Jefferson* (1976), is also highly critical. Two excellent accounts of the party battles and Republican party organization are W. N. Chambers, *Political Parties in a New Nation, 1776–1809** (1963), and Noble Cunningham, *The Jeffersonian Republicans in Power: Party Operations, 1801–1809* (1963). Richard Hofstadter, *The Idea of a Party System** (1969), is a lucid essay on the beginnings of two-party politics in America. Richard Buel, Jr., *Securing the Revolution: Ideology in American Politics, 1789–1815** (1972), focuses on both issues and ideology. The role of the Federalists is traced in D. H. Fischer, *The Revolution of American Conservatism: The Federalist Party in the Era of Jeffersonian Democracy** (1965). L. K. Kerber, *Federalists in Dissent: Imagery and Ideology in Jeffersonian America* (1970), is a study of Federalist political and social thought. L. D. White, *The Jeffersonians: A Study in Administrative History, 1801–1829** (1951), and Noble Cunningham, *The Process of Government under Jefferson* (1978), are expert analyses of Republican administrative organization. J. S. Young, *The Washington Community, 1800–1828** (1966), stresses the failure of the Jeffersonians, because of certain negative attitudes, to develop an effective federal government. Alexander Balinky, *Albert Gallatin: Fiscal Theories and Policy* (1958), is a sharply critical evaluation of Jeffersonian finance.

John Randolph and other conservative Republicans are studied in N. K. Risjord, *The Old Republicans: Southern Conservatism in the Age of Jefferson* (1965), and R. E. Shalhope, *John Taylor of Caroline: Pastoral Republican* (1980). The case for Aaron Burr is presented in Milton Lomask, *Aaron Burr: The Conspiracy and Years of Exile, 1805–1836* (1982), the case against him in T. P. Abernethy, *The Burr Conspiracy* (1954).

FOREIGN POLICY AND THE WAR OF 1812
Two useful works on the Louisiana Purchase are Alexander DeConde, *This Affair of Louisiana** (1976), and A. P. Whitaker, *The Mississippi Question* (1934). The Lewis and Clark expedition and other western exploration in the Republican era are treated fully in Donald Jackson, *Thomas Jefferson and the Stony Mountains: Exploring the West from Monticello* (1981), and Henry Savage, Jr., *Discovering America, 1700–1875* (1979). The best account of the conflict with the Barbary pirates is R. W. Irwin, *Diplomatic Relations of the United States and the Barbary Powers* (1931).

Several excellent works are available on the problems of American neutrality. A good place to begin is with Irving Brant's study of Madison as Secretary of State, mentioned above, and with the same author's *James Madison: The President, 1809–1812* (1956). Brant's multivolume biography of Madison is available in a one-volume abridged edition, *The Fourth President: A Life of James Madison* (1970). Outstanding monographs include J. F. Zimmerman, *Impressment of American Seamen* (1925); L. M. Sears, *Jefferson and the Embargo* (1927); Harry Bernstein, *Origins of Inter-American Interest, 1700–1812* (1945); and Bradford Perkins, *First Rapprochement: England and the United States, 1795–1805* (1955).

B. W. Sheehan, *Seeds of Extinction: Jeffersonian Philanthropy and the American Indians** (1973), stresses the assault on Indian culture by even the best-intentioned whites. Reginald Horsman, *Expansion and American Indian Policy, 1783–1812* (1967), is a fair account of a sordid chapter of American history. The same author's *The Frontier in the Formative Years, 1783–1815** (1970), an excellent work of synthesis, is especially valuable for conditions on the frontier in the years before the War of 1812.

The view that impressment and neutral rights were the fundamental causes of the War of 1812 is presented, with varying emphases, in A. L. Burt, *The United States, Great Britain, and British North*

America from the Revolution to the Peace after the War of 1812 (1940); Bradford Perkins, *Prologue to War: England and the United States, 1805–1812** (1961); and Reginald Horsman, *The Causes of the War of 1812** (1962). R. H. Brown, *The Republic in Peril: 1812** (1964), stresses the desire of Jeffersonians to defend Republican institutions as a force leading to war. R. A. Rutland, *Madison's Alternatives: The Jeffersonian Republicans and the Coming of War, 1805–1812* (1975), is a brief review of the background and causes. J. C. A. Stagg, *Mr. Madison's War: Politics, Diplomacy, and Warfare in the Early American Republic, 1783–1830* (1983), is an excellent synthesis of both the causes and conduct of the war.

Irving Brant, *James Madison: Commander in Chief, 1812–1836* (1961), strongly defends Madison's wartime leadership. The best general account of the war is F. F. Beirne, *The War of 1812* (1949). Two good brief surveys are H. L. Coles, *The War of 1812** (1965), and Reginald Horsman, *The War of 1812* (1969). Military history is treated at length in J. K. Mahon, *The War of 1812* (1972), and briefly in Alan Lloyd, *The Scorching of Washington: The War of 1812* (1975). Marquis James, *Andrew Jackson*, Vol. I: *The Border Captain** (1933), gives an absorbing account of the campaigns in the Southwest. R. V. Remini, *Andrew Jackson and the Course of American Empire, 1767–1821* (1977), is more scholarly and, except for its defensive tone concerning Jackson's attitude toward Indians, is excellent on his role in the war. Federalist disaffection is treated perceptively in George Dangerfield, *The Era of Good Feelings** (1952); J. M. Banner, *To the Hartford Convention* (1970); and S. E. Morison, *Harrison Gray Otis, 1765–1848: The Urbane Federalist* (1969). Excellent analyses of the peace negotiations and postwar diplomacy are in S. F. Bemis, *John Quincy Adams and the Foundations of American Foreign Policy** (1949), and Bradford Perkins, *Castlereagh and Adams* (1964).

*Available in a paperback edition.

8
NATIONALISM AND ECONOMIC EXPANSION

One might have expected the prowar Republicans to be discredited by their mishandling of military affairs. But when peace came the Republican party was still firmly in power. Though the record of Madison's wartime Administration was less than brilliant, the country was still intact, and for several years the economy flourished. Southern cotton-planters were regaining their European markets, and a growing number of Western farmers were taking advantage of cheaper transportation to send their agricultural surpluses to markets in the South, the Northeast, and overseas. Farm-commodity prices were good, and land values were rising. Settlers were swarming into the West, and within a few years after the Treaty of Ghent five new states—Indiana (1816), Mississippi (1817), Illinois (1818), Alabama (1819), and Missouri (1821)—entered the Union. A new economic interest, manufacturing, was growing in importance because of the impetus given to it when the embargo and war cut off the supply of British goods. Shipping, though it would never regain the prominence it once had in the Northeastern maritime states, was recovering from blows the embargo and the war had dealt.

This vast land, with its burgeoning economy and its optimistic, increasingly nationalistic people (9½ million of them by 1820), was no longer the plain, uncomplicated republic that Jefferson had once so admired. Jefferson's party was changing with the country and now counted manufacturers, factory

workers, and other urban groups, as well as farmers and planters, among those it had to serve. Henry Clay, John C. Calhoun, and John Quincy Adams were impatient with the old-fashioned Virginia Republicans' emphasis on constitutionalism, state rights, and laissez faire. They had a vision of national growth, economic expansion, and social progress that required a more dynamic federal government pursuing more positive and imaginative policies. In fighting their political battles, postwar Republicans still used Jeffersonian rhetoric, but the old creed had lost much of its substance. In 1801 Jefferson's remark that "We are all Republicans, we are all Federalists" was only a loose figure of speech; in 1816 it was almost a fact.

The Triumph of Neo-Federalism

The American System. Circumstances had forced Madison, like Jefferson, time after time to compromise traditional Republicanism. In his seventh annual message to Congress, December 5, 1815, Madison's surrender to the nationalists was well-nigh complete; Hamilton himself could hardly have composed a message that embraced orthodox Federalist doctrine more fully. In the name of national defense, Madison urged an expansion of the navy, a reorganization of the

Lockport on the Erie Canal

militia, and an enlargement of the Military Academy at West Point. To establish a stable money and credit supply, he suggested that "a national bank will merit consideration." Because of the resumed flow of cheaper British manufactures, he proposed a federal tariff to provide industry with the protection that "is due to the enterprising citizens whose interests are now at stake." Finally, Madison urged Congress to finance such internal improvements as required "a national jurisdiction and national means," thus "binding more closely together the various parts of our extended confederacy."

Congressional leaders had few qualms about this program of neo-Federalism, and Henry Clay soon labeled it the "American System." The prewar economy, Clay and his supporters thought, had depended too much on the exchange of American raw materials for European manufactured goods, a dependence that exposed it to the whims of other powers and made it the victim of every international crisis. Hence the foundation of Clay's American System was a protective tariff to stimulate domestic manufacturing and thereby to create an enlarged domestic market for the surplus agricultural products of the South and West. Internal improvements, financed with tariff revenues, would encourage interstate commerce; and a national bank would provide banknote currency of uniform value to facilitate an expanding volume of business transactions, as well as the short-term credits required for economic growth. This nationalistic program, Clay believed, would bring to all interests and sections of the country both prosperity and independence from the outside world.

New states, 1812–21

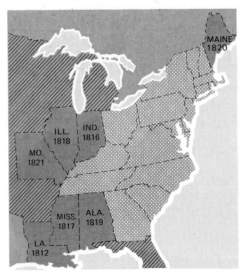

The Tariff of 1816.

The first postwar Congress, one of the most fruitful of the nineteenth century, took long strides toward Clay's goal of an American System. By 1816 the Republican party numbered in its ranks a large cluster of interest groups, both urban and rural, clamoring for protective duties on certain foreign goods entering the American market. Leading the protectionists were those who had invested in New England textile mills and Pennsylvania iron-smelters when the embargo and war had choked off European supplies. Seconding them were the hemp-growers of Kentucky, the wool-growers of Ohio and Vermont, and an assortment of Southerners and Westerners who hoped either to promote industry or to expand their domestic market behind a tariff wall.

The cries of the protectionists grew louder when British exporters, seeking to dispose of surpluses accumulated during the war and to drive competing American manufacturers out of business, flooded the American market with relatively low-priced goods. In the critical years immediately following the war, this British competition forced many small, less efficient American manufacturers to close their doors. Protectionists claimed that the British were plotting to wreck the American economy and asserted that a higher tariff was essential for national economic survival. America's "infant industries" were fragile things, they said, requiring the tender care of the federal government while they matured.

Congress responded with the Tariff of 1816, an act that raised duties to an average of 20 percent to meet both the need for increased revenues and the demand for greater protection. In the House the Western and Middle Atlantic states gave the bill overwhelming support; New England divided seventeen to ten for it, the South twenty-three to thirty-four against. Webster and other Federalists, speaking for the shipping interests, opposed higher duties as an obstacle to foreign trade; John Randolph, like most Southerners, vowed that he would not "agree to lay a duty on the cultivator of the soil to encourage exotic manufactures." On the other hand, Calhoun, the South Carolina nationalist, hoped that the manufacturing interest would "at all times, and under every policy . . . be protected with due care." In 1816 a substantial minority in the South shared Calhoun's point of view; in subsequent years, as conditions and expectations changed, Southern support for the tariff—and for the American System in general—eroded rapidly.

The second Bank of the United States.

Republican leaders, chastened by their fiscal experiences during the war, made their most dramatic surrender to Federalism when they revived both Hamilton's plan and his arguments for a national bank. When the first

Bank of the United States perished in 1811, its business had fallen to the state-chartered banks; within five years the number of those banks had increased from 88 to 246, their issues of bank notes from $28 million to $68 million. Since many state-chartered banks did not maintain adequate specie reserves (gold and silver), their notes often circulated at a discount. The bewildering variety of notes, their fluctuating values, and a rash of counterfeiting soon brought the country to the edge of fiscal chaos. The final blow came when the state banks, except those in New England, suspended specie payments altogether during the war—and showed no disposition to resume specie payments with the restoration of peace.

Meanwhile, the federal government lacked a safe depository for its funds, a reliable agency to transfer them from place to place, and adequate machinery to market securities when it needed to borrow. The absence of a uniform paper currency was a handicap to businessmen engaged in interstate commerce. Even some of the old state-rights Republicans, though they opposed all banks that issued paper currency, favored chartering a new national bank as the lesser of two evils. Madison discarded his constitutional doubts and decided that the question had been settled by "a concurrence of the general will of the nation." Changed circumstances, he concluded, required measures "which may be as proper now as they were premature and suspicious when urged by the champions of federalism." Calhoun, taking a thoroughly nationalistic position, attacked the state banks for usurping the federal government's exclusive power to issue and regulate the country's currency. Clay, who had opposed rechartering the first Bank, confessed that he had not anticipated the evils its demise had caused.

In 1816 a bill to grant a twenty-year charter to a second Bank of the United States, with headquarters in Philadelphia, passed both houses of Congress over the opposition of state banking interests, Federalist partisans, and Virginia conservatives. The functions and structure of the second Bank were essentially the same as those of the first, except that its capital was increased from $10 million to $35 million; and, under the power given it to distribute its facilities over the nation as needed, the number of its branches eventually increased from eight to twenty-five. The federal government again held one-fifth of the stock, and the President appointed five of the twenty-five directors. Its liabilities were not to exceed its capital, one-fifth of which had to be in specie; and it was to report annually to the Treasury Department and open its books to that department for periodic inspections.

This powerful banking corporation served a number of useful purposes: it assisted the government in its fiscal business by helping to market federal securities and by providing a depository for federal funds; it regulated the banknote currency (and thus the credit policies) of the state banks; and it encouraged business enterprise by providing a sound paper currency in national-bank notes and by making available short-term credits, principally to merchants. But as the largest capitalistic institution in the country, exercising immense power over the supply of money and credit, depending as it did upon the government for special favors, it was essential that the Bank be responsibly directed and that its operations be subjected to adequate federal control. In the absence of such control, it was bound to find itself in political trouble, for it would then loom as a potential instrument of economic tyranny, perhaps even a threat to political democracy. Indeed, under the best of circumstances, the Bank, because of its size and strength, was always a tempting political target.

Internal improvements. The War of 1812, by disrupting coastal shipping, had demonstrated the inadequacy of the country's internal transportation system for both interstate commerce and national defense. The Northwest, where high transportation costs still deprived many farmers of outside markets and tied them to an economy of pioneer self-sufficiency, was the most persistent solicitor of federal funds for internal improvements. New England, suffering a loss of population and a decline of political strength, was the center of opposition. President Madison, stretching his constitutional scruples to support projects that were national in scope, approved appropriations for the continued building of the National Road, which had been started during Jefferson's Administration. But he doubted that Congress had the power to subsidize local roads and canals without an appropriate amendment to the Constitution. In 1817 Congress ignored his doubts and passed a bill to distribute among the states for local internal improvements a $1,500,000 bonus that the Bank of the United States had paid the government for its charter. To Madison this was going too far, and in one of his last presidential acts he vetoed the so-called Bonus Bill. Calhoun, disgusted with this narrow view of federal power, grumbled that the Constitution "was not intended as a thesis for the logician to exercise his ingenuity on . . . it ought to be construed with plain good sense." But Madison's veto stalled one crucial part of the American System. Local internal improvements remained, for the time being, the responsibility of the individual states, communities, and private enterprise.

The Era of Good Feelings. In 1816, nearing the end of his second term, Madison supported another Virginian, his Secretary of State, James Monroe, to suc-

Conestoga Wagons, by Thomas Birch, 1816

ceed him to the Presidency. The Randolph Republicans preferred William H. Crawford of Georgia, and some Northern Republicans fretted about the long domination of their party by the "Virginia Dynasty." But Madison had his way, and Monroe won an easy victory over his Federalist opponent, Rufus King of New York. Four years later, with the Federalists too feeble even to run a candidate, Monroe was reelected without opposition.* After a few more years of activity in scattered localities, the Federalist party ceased to exist. The party's war record, the failure of its older leaders to adjust to new conditions, its narrow particularism, and the Republican pirating of its program all contributed to its death. Thus the eighteenth-century ideal of a republic without political "factions" seemed to have been achieved at last. "Surely our government may go on and prosper without the existence of parties," wrote Monroe, who shared Jefferson's views of both the Federalists and the party system. "I have always considered their existence the curse of the country." In his first inaugural address, Monroe told his countrymen that they could rejoice when they reflected "how close our Government has approached to perfection; that in respect to it we have no essential improvement to make."

*One elector from New Hampshire voted for John Quincy Adams.

James Monroe, a representative of the small-planter class of the Virginia piedmont, reached the Presidency at the age of sixty-one after many years of devoted, though not brilliant, public service. Once the favorite of John Randolph and other Virginia state righters, Monroe continued to interpret the Constitution more narrowly than the nationalists in his party. He accepted the tariff and the banking legislation passed during Madison's last year in office as well as the use of federal funds for internal improvements national in scope, but while he was President the American System made only limited progress. Though Monroe was less talented than his distinguished predecessors, his contemporaries found something solid and reassuring in this surviving member of the Revolutionary generation. In Monroe, with his wig, his cocked hat, and his knee-length pantaloons, the postwar generation had a last nostalgic look at the eighteenth century.

The year of Monroe's inauguration, 1817, found the country in a complaisant mood. On a good-will tour that ultimately carried him into once-hostile New England, the new President saw everywhere abundant signs of national unity. His warm reception in Boston caused the *Columbian Centinel*, a Federalist paper, to speak of an "Era of Good Feelings," thus giving a popular label to Monroe's Administrations.

Political factionalism was at a low ebb, and there was relative harmony among the sections. Above all, as Monroe observed in his first message to Congress, the country was in a "prosperous and happy condition. . . . The abundant fruits of the earth have filled it with plenty," However, the "Era of Good Feelings" in fact lasted only about two years—until the middle of Monroe's first Administration—when political strife and sectional bitterness suddenly revived, and the national prosperity came to an abrupt and shocking end.

John Marshall and the Supreme Court

Marshall's role. In these postwar years still another Virginian played a key role in the shaping of public policy and in the molding of the American political and constitutional structure. This was John Marshall, Chief Justice of the United States from 1801 to 1835, who first established the power of the judicial branch of the government and gave it the prestige it had previously lacked. Unlike most of his fellow Virginians, Marshall was from the start an ardent and consistent nationalist, supporting a relatively broad interpretation of federal power. Born in 1755, he saw military service during the revolution and then went home to become one of the most successful lawyers before the

James Monroe: solid and reassuring

Richmond bar. After a term in Congress and brief service as John Adams' Secretary of State, Marshall received his appointment as Chief Justice shortly before the last Federalist President left office. The Supreme Court, at least, would remain in Federalist hands!

In personal appearance and social intercourse Marshall impressed one as a plain, homespun democrat, for he was the most unpretentious of men, an amiable lover of sports and other simple pleasures. But underneath he was a resolute Federalist, suspicious of popular government and contemptuous of what he considered Jefferson's sentimental trust in the people. Marshall was in no sense a scholar or philosopher of the law, but he had a keen intelligence and a tough mind that readily discovered the logic of a case and swiftly drove to its core. According to Joseph Story, whom Madison made an Associate Justice in 1811, Marshall "examines the intricacies of a subject with calm and persevering circumspection and unravels its mysteries with irresistible acuteness." His personal magnetism and intellectual powers gave him enormous influence over his colleagues on the bench, including those appointed by Republicans. During his thirty-four years as Chief Justice he wrote almost half the decisions and dissented from the majority opinion only eight times. Caring little for precedents, avoiding legal jargon, using crisp prose and careful reasoning, Marshall delivered a series of the most momentous decisions in American judicial history.

Judicial review. Soon after assuming his new office, Marshall pronounced a vigorous and, in the long run, decisive opinion on a matter of prime importance to a federal system based on a written constitution. While the Federalists were in power there had been a persistent but inconclusive debate over who was to decide when Congress had exceeded its delegated powers or encroached upon the rights of the states. Since the Constitution is not explicit on this point, the answer had to be found by inference rather than from the plain language of the document. Probably the majority of delegates to the Constitutional Convention had expected the Supreme Court to pass on the constitutionality of the acts of Congress, and Hamilton, in one of his contributions to *The Federalist*, had upheld the principle of judicial review. Jeffersonian Republicans, however, were later to reject this nationalist doctrine and to argue that the federal government was the agent of the sovereign states and that those who had created it must define its powers. The individual states, said Jefferson in the Kentucky Resolutions of 1798, would decide when the Constitution had been violated, as well as "the mode and measure of redress."

That is where things stood when, in 1803, Mar-

John Marshall's liberal construction of the Constitution

[The Constitution] contains an enumeration of powers expressly granted by the people to their government. It has been said that these powers ought to be construed strictly. But why ought they to be so construed? Is there one sentence in the constitution which gives countenance to this rule? In the last of the enumerated powers, that which grants, expressly, the means for carrying all others into execution, congress is authorized "to make all laws which shall be necessary and proper" for the purpose.... What do gentlemen mean by a strict construction? If they contend only against that enlarged construction which would extend words beyond their natural and obvious import, we ... should not controvert the principle. If they contend for that narrow construction which, in support of some theory not to be found in the constitution, would deny to the government those powers which the words of the grant, as usually understood, import, and which are consistent with the general views and objects of the instrument; for that narrow construction, which would cripple the government, and render it unequal to the objects for which it is declared to be instituted, and to which the powers given, as fairly understood, render it competent; then we cannot perceive the propriety of this strict construction, nor adopt it as the rule by which the constitution is to be expounded.

From Gibbons v. Ogden, 9 Wheat. 1, 1824.

shall wrote the Court's decision in the case of *Marbury* v. *Madison*. Of minor importance in itself, this case related to a section of the Judiciary Act of 1789, which, according to Marshall, expanded the Court's original jurisdiction beyond what the Constitution intended it to be. "The question whether an act repugnant to the constitution can become the law of the land, is a question deeply interesting to the United States," Marshall asserted. His answer to the question was clear: The wording of the Constitution establishes the principle "that a law repugnant to the constitution is void; and that courts, as well as other departments, are bound by that instrument." Moreover, "It is emphatically the province and duty of the judicial department to say what the law is. Those who apply the rule to particular cases must of necessity expound and interpret that rule."

Marbury v. *Madison* thus established a precedent for the Supreme Court to rule on the constitutionality of congressional legislation and to act as the final authority on the meaning of the Constitution. This doctrine of judicial review, though denounced by Jefferson and other state-rights Virginians and challenged many times thereafter, has weathered all the storms and survives to this day. Having established the precedent, Marshall and his colleagues never again disallowed an act of Congress—more than a half-century passed before the Supreme Court exercised that power again. But the Marshall Court sometimes applied the positive side of judicial review—that is, it reviewed congressional legislation and ruled it to be constitutional.

National supremacy. As a nationalist Marshall was inclined to interpret the powers of Congress broadly and to assert the federal government's supremacy in the exercise of its constitutional authority. For example, in two important cases, *Martin* v. *Hunter's Lessee* (1816) and *Cohens* v. *Virginia* (1821), the Marshall Court affirmed its right to review and reverse decisions of state courts when they concerned issues arising under the federal Constitution. On thirteen occasions it voided state laws as violations of "the supreme law of the land." One of the most significant of these cases, *Gibbons* v. *Ogden* (1824), involved a New York law giving a steamboat company a monopoly of the business of carrying passengers on the Hudson River to New York City. In rejecting the law Marshall gave the term "commerce" an extremely broad definition and came close to saying that the power of Congress over interstate commerce is absolute. This power, he ruled, "is complete in itself, may be exercised to its utmost extent, and acknowledges no limitations other than are prescribed in the constitution."

The Chief Justice expounded the nationalist doctrine most fully in the case of *McCulloch* v. *Maryland* (1819), which tested the constitutionality of the second Bank of the United States. Conceding that the Constitution does not explicitly grant Congress authority to charter a bank, Marshall insisted that Congress must have some discretion in exercising the powers clearly delegated to it. Surely the authority could be implied from the "necessary and proper" clause. Then Marshall made a classic statement of the doctrine of "loose construction": "Let the end be legitimate, let it be within the scope of the Constitution, and all means which are appropriate, which are plainly adapted to that end, which are not prohibited, but consist with the letter and spirit of the constitution, are constitutional." After this decision the nationalist advocates of the American System had no reason to anticipate any judicial obstacles to their program.

Sanctity of contracts. As a defender of property rights, Marshall also sought to use federal authority through the courts to protect the propertied classes whenever they were harassed by unfriendly state legislatures. He sympathized with creditors and entrepreneurs who considered contracts sacred and inviolable, and he made vigorous use of the clause in the Constitution that prohibited states from "impairing the obligation of contracts." In the case of *Fletcher* v. *Peck* (1810), Marshall gave evidence of the extremes to which he would go to defend this principle. As we have seen (p. 175), the Georgia legislature, in 1795, had granted a large tract of Western land to the Yazoo Land Companies. The following year a new legislature, discovering bribery and fraud, repudiated the grant and thus provoked litigation that ultimately reached the Supreme Court. To Marshall the case was perfectly clear: the grant of land was a binding contract, and the circumstances under which it was negotiated did not concern the Court. The withdrawal of the grant, therefore, was an unconstitutional violation of the obligation of contract.

Another case, *Dartmouth College* v. *Woodward* (1819), enabled the Marshall Court to make an equally extreme application of the contract clause. The case originated in an attempt of the New Hampshire legislature to revise Dartmouth's charter, which dated back to colonial days, and to transform the college into a state institution. The trustees went to court and employed Daniel Webster, a Dartmouth alumnus, to represent them. Webster's sentimental plea in behalf of his alma mater brought tears to the eyes of the unsentimental Chief Justice, who ruled that a charter was a contract and could not be violated. Thereafter, to escape this restriction, the states usually wrote reserve clauses into corporation charters permitting subsequent amendment of the charters' terms.

Marshall's decisions established a body of property rights that provided a constitutional foundation for the subsequent economic growth of the United States. However, some old-line Republicans believed that Marshall had dealt "a deadly blow to the sovereignty of the states." Judge Spencer Roane of Virginia sent angry dissenting opinions to the newspapers, and John Taylor waged a pamphlet war against the Supreme Court. To Jefferson the federal justices were a "corps of sappers and miners" steadily undercutting the powers of the states. "The Constitution," he wrote, "is a mere thing of wax in the hands of the judiciary, which they may twist and shape into any form they please." Yet, except for Marshall's interpretation of the contract clause (which later courts have modified), there was little in these decisions that the dominant element in the postwar Republican party really cared to criticize. Giving his blessing to the nationalistic trend of Republican legislation, Marshall used the Constitution as a flexible instrument adaptable to conditions that the Founding Fathers could never have anticipated. If judicial review was a usurpation, no majority in Congress ever agreed on a practical alternative to it. Rather, it has become an integral part of the federal government's system of checks and balances.

The Monroe Doctrine

Revolutions in Latin America. One of the most striking expressions of postwar American nationalism occurred in the area of foreign policy. While Spain was preoccupied with France during the Napoleonic wars, its South and Central American colonies had had a pleasant taste of freedom from its strict political and commercial control. Their appetite whetted, the colonies revolted and soon expelled the Portuguese from Brazil and the Spanish from all their American possessions save Cuba and Puerto Rico. When, in 1820, revolutions broke out in Spain and Portugal, all hope of recovering the lost colonies perished—unless other European powers could be induced to intervene.

To the people of the United States this was 1776 all over again. Henry Clay, an admirer of the Latin American patriots, rejoiced at "the glorious spectacle of eighteen millions of people, struggling to burst their chains and to be free." When a modest commerce developed with South America, Clay, optimistic about its further expansion, incorporated Pan-American trade into his American System. Both justice and self-interest, thought Clay, required quick recognition of the revolutionary governments.

After 1815 the State Department had pursued a policy of neutrality that recognized the revolutionists as belligerents and permitted them to purchase supplies in the United States; but a Neutrality Act of 1818 prohibited American citizens from serving in the rebel armies. Full diplomatic recognition came in 1822, after negotiations for the purchase of Florida had been completed and after the new governments in South America had shown themselves capable of maintaining their independence. To Clay this recognition was disgracefully late, but the United States was still the first nation to grant it.

The fear of foreign intervention. Granting recognition at that time was in fact a bold step. Thus far the British had refrained from establishing diplomatic relations with Latin America and had even indicated a willingness to see Spain reestablish its authority there. Moreover, the reactionary governments of Russia, Prussia, Austria, and France had formed an alliance pledged not only to preserve the status quo and to suppress liberalism but to intervene in the internal

affairs of any country that threatened the peace and security of Europe. Under this mandate Austria had invaded the Italian states of Naples and Piedmont, and France had invaded Spain to liquidate revolutionary movements for which many Americans felt a deep sympathy. Perhaps the alliance would now apply its policy to the New World and assist Spain in the reconquest of its colonies. France, it was rumored, had an eye on Cuba as a reward for intervening in Spain; and Russia seemed intent on spreading its influence southward from Alaska along the Pacific coast. Actually there was not much danger that any European power would intervene in Latin America without British support, and, when Adams warned Russia that the Western Hemisphere was closed to further colonization, the two countries soon negotiated a satisfactory agreement. Nevertheless, the time seemed appropriate for formulating some kind of policy that would cover all contingencies.

By 1823 Great Britain, too, was ready to take a stronger stand. British liberals resented the reactionary schemes of the continental alliance, and British merchants and manufacturers were determined to maintain the profitable markets they had established in Latin America. Accordingly, the British foreign minister, George Canning, approached the American minister in London, Richard Rush, with a proposal that their governments make a joint statement of policy. Canning told Rush that his government was now convinced that Spain could not recover its colonies and that recognition of their independence was only a matter of time. Great Britain had no designs on any of them, nor would it permit any portion of them to be transferred to another power. If the American government shared these feelings, Canning asked, "why should we hesitate mutually to confide them to each other; and to declare them in the face of the world?"

In October 1823 President Monroe had the British proposal before him and turned to the Republican elder statesmen for advice. Jefferson and Madison both supported his own inclination to accept it. Oddly enough, it was a statesman from New England, the traditional center of pro-British sentiment, who objected most strenuously to accepting British leadership in the Western Hemisphere. Secretary of State Adams opposed any agreement by which the United States would, in effect, commit itself not to annex additional territory. With an eye on Texas and Cuba, Adams argued that "we should at least keep ourselves free to act as emergencies may arise." Moreover, he disliked a joint statement that would make the United States appear "to come in as a cockboat in the wake of the British man-of-war." After long discussion in the Cabinet, Adams noted with satisfaction that his position "was acquiesced in on all sides." The President, it was agreed, would make a statement of *American* policy emphasizing the separateness of the Old World and the New.

The American response. Monroe incorporated his famous doctrine rather unsystematically in his annual message to Congress on December 2, 1823, a message that dealt with many other topics as well. With some rearranging, the relevant passages run substantially as follows: First, wherever American sympathies may lie, it does not comport with American policy to intervene in the "internal concerns" of European powers, or in their wars when they involve matters only "relating to themselves." Second, the United States will not interfere with "existing colonies or dependencies" in the Western Hemisphere. Third, with the Latin American governments "whose independence we have . . . acknowledged, we could not view any interposition for the purpose of oppressing them, or controlling in any other manner their destiny, by any European power in any other light than as the manifestation of an unfriendly disposition toward the United States." Fourth, "the American continents, by the free and independent condition which they have assumed and maintain, are henceforth not to be considered as subjects for future colonization by any European powers." Finally, Monroe warned the autocrats of Europe that "we should consider any attempt on their part to extend their [political] system to any portion of this hemisphere as dangerous to our peace and safety." In brief, the essence of this nationalistic pronouncement was the concept of two worlds, each of which was to refrain from intervening in the internal affairs of the other.

Monroe and Adams, of course, were responsible for the precise phrasing of these principles, but they owed much to earlier Presidents and Secretaries of State. They had brought together the elements of a coherent policy that had been gradually evolving since the Revolution. To European diplomats, the promulgation of a policy that the young republic lacked the power to enforce was a piece of presumptuous impertinence. Canning, who knew that British diplomacy and the British navy had been decisive in preventing continental powers from meddling in America, was particularly annoyed. He was aware that Monroe's unilateral statement could be invoked against Great Britain as well as against other nations. Yet, though the response of the American people was overwhelmingly favorable, within a few years the President's dramatic message had been nearly forgotten. A generation later it would be rediscovered and identified as the Monroe Doctrine; and for many years thereafter it would be accepted as the authoritative and almost definitive statement of American foreign policy.

The Westward Movement

These displays of nationalism in domestic politics and foreign policy reflected the underlying optimism of the American people—their confidence in the destiny a kind Providence had planned for them. To be sure, their nationalistic creed also embraced an awareness of their past: they had their nostalgic and sentimental side; they gloried in their traditions each Fourth of July; and they were deeply stirred when a Webster waxed eloquent upon the Constitution and the Founding Fathers. But most Americans would have agreed with Jefferson's affirmation that he liked "the dreams of the future better than the history of the past," for there existed among them a widespread feeling of emancipation from history. According to one editor, "Our national birth was the beginning of a new history . . . which separates us from the past and connects us with the future only." America was still primarily a promise: as Ralph Waldo Emerson rejoiced, it was "a country of beginnings, of projects, of designs, of expectations."

The general confidence and optimism of the American people were rooted both in a popular belief that the potentialities of men and women are great when they are free to develop them and in the practical social and economic realities of nineteenth-century America. One of the most important of these realities was the virgin land—the seemingly unlimited space and inexhaustible resources that promised a life of greater dignity and abundance than Europe's common people had ever dreamed of. The West—the untapped wealth of the great interior stretching from the Appalachians to the Rockies—helped to give the future its rosy hue; and the West became one of the central interests of the American people in the decades after the Treaty of Ghent.

Advance of the agricultural frontier. Between 1800 and 1840 the gross value of American agricultural production grew at a substantial average annual rate of 3.1 percent. To a limited extent, this growth was due to increased farm productivity resulting from technological innovations, improved methods of cultivation, and the introduction of better crop varieties and livestock strains—all encouraged by cheaper transportation and widening markets. Far more important, however, was a threefold increase in the agricultural population from approximately 5 million to 15 million, which in turn caused a vast amount of new land to be brought under cultivation and produced a significant increase of farm capital in the form of livestock, implements, and buildings.

The growth of agricultural production was closely linked to the westward movement of population and

Flatboats at New Orleans, 1828

the development of new areas for the raising of live-stock and the cultivation of wheat, corn, tobacco, and cotton. After 1815 improved transportation enabled more and more Western farmers to escape a self-sufficient way of life and enter a national market economy. Farmers who engaged in this kind of commercial agriculture specialized in a "money crop"—a crop produced chiefly for sale in nearby and distant markets—and used the proceeds to buy consumer goods manufactured in the Northeast or in Europe. During periods when commodity prices were high, the rate of westward migration, the sale of public lands, and eventually the supply of Western staples increased spectacularly.

"Old America seems to be breaking up and moving westward," observed an English visitor in 1817, during the first great wave of postwar migration. After falling off for a few years during the depression following the Panic of 1819 (see p. 217), the number of emigrants increased again and reached a peak in the 1830s. Whereas in 1810 only a seventh of the American people lived west of the Appalachians, by 1840 more than a third lived there. The table below shows population growth in the new Western states between 1810 and 1840.

	1810	1840
Ohio (1803)	230,760	1,519,467
Louisiana (1812)	76,556	352,411
Indiana (1816)	24,520	685,866
Mississippi (1817)	40,352	375,651
Illinois (1818)	12,282	476,183
Alabama (1819)		590,756
Missouri (1821)	20,845	383,702
Arkansas (1836)	1,062	97,574
Michigan (1837)	4,762	212,267

Some of the people who settled the great Mississippi Valley were recent immigrants from Europe, but most of them came from the older states, whose agricultural populations were also growing rapidly. Kentuckians and Tennesseeans moved to the new cotton lands of the Southwest or crossed the Ohio River into the Northwest; migrants from New England and the Middle Atlantic states generally settled in the Great Lakes region; and people from the South Atlantic states (the largest group of all) invaded not only the Southwest but southern Ohio, Indiana, and Illinois as well. By and large those who moved west came from the lower middle classes and traveled with their few worldly possessions loaded on wagons or flatboats—or even on pack horses or pushcarts.

Factors encouraging migration. Why were these hundreds of thousands of settlers—most of them farmers, some of them artisans—drawn away from the cleared fields and established cities and villages of the East? Apart from the fact that the West happened to be an inviting land of opportunity, certain characteristics of American society help to explain this remarkable migration. The European ancestors of the American people had lived century after century rooted to the same village or the same piece of land until some religious or political or economic crisis uprooted them and drove them across the Atlantic. Many of those who experienced this sharp and devastating break thereafter lacked the ties that had bound them and their ancestors to a single place. Moreover, in the relatively stratified European society men usually inherited the occupations and social status of their fathers, but in American society there was a less rigid class structure. Men changed occupations easily and believed that it was not only possible but almost a moral duty to improve their social and economic

Transportation to the West, about 1840

position. As a result, Americans were, as many European visitors observed, an inveterately restless, rootless, and ambitious people.

The Frenchman Alexis de Tocqueville, who published a remarkably penetrating study of American society after a tour in the early 1830s, observed these traits:

> In the United States, a man builds a house in which to spend his old age, and he sells it before the roof is on . . . he brings a field into tillage and leaves other men to gather the crops . . . he settles in a place, which he soon afterwards leaves to carry his changeable longings elsewhere . . . the tie that unites one generation to another is relaxed or broken . . . every man there loses all trace of the ideas of his forefathers or takes no heed of them.

The reasons for this "strange unrest," Tocqueville believed, were, first, the American "taste for physical gratifications"; second, a social condition "in which neither laws nor customs retain any person in his place"; and, third, a pervasive belief that "all professions are open to all, and a man's own energies may place him at the top of any one of them." These social traits helped to produce the nomadic and daring frontiersmen who kept pushing westward beyond the fringes of settlement, as well as the less adventurous immigrants who followed them across the mountains in search of new homes, material success, and a better life for themselves and their children.

The West had plenty of attractions for a people conditioned to appreciate them. The alluvial river bottoms, the fecund soils of the rolling forest lands,

and, after they adjusted to the lack of trees, the black loams of the prairies were tempting to New England farmers working their rocky, sterile acres and to Southeastern farmers plagued with soil depletion and erosion. The Indian menace east of the Mississippi was now substantially reduced; after 1815 the helpless tribes made a succession of treaties ceding lands, which the government surveyed and put up for sale. In 1820 a new land law ended the credit system but reduced the minimum tract for individual sales to eighty acres and the minimum price to $1.25.* Now it was possible to buy a farm for $100, and the continued proliferation of state banks made it easier for those without cash to negotiate loans in paper money. Western farmers borrowed with the confident expectation that the expanding economy would keep farm prices high, thus making it easy to repay loans when they fell due.

Transportation was becoming less of a problem for those who wished to move west and for those who had farm surpluses to send to market. Prior to 1815 Western farmers who did not live on navigable waterways were connected to them only by dirt roads and mountain trails. Livestock could be driven across the mountains, and high-value products, such as whiskey and furs, might be carried profitably on pack horses or by wagon, but the cost of transporting bulky grains in this fashion was several times greater than their value in Eastern markets. Goods could be shipped across the Atlantic for less than the cost of transportation from western New York or western Pennsylvania to cities along the seaboard.

*New lands, however, were first put up at auction, and the best often sold for a good deal more than the minimum price.

The first step toward an improvement of Western transportation was the construction of graded and planked or macadamized turnpikes. Built by private corporations that charged tolls, most of the turnpikes were designed to connect Eastern cities, but a few served the tramontane West. By the 1820s migrants could follow the Baltimore Turnpike to Cumberland, Maryland, and then the National Road to Wheeling (ultimately, to Vandalia, Illinois); the Lancaster Turnpike and Forbes Road to Pittsburgh; or the Mohawk and Genesee Turnpike to Lake Erie. By reducing transportation costs, these roads stimulated the commercialization of agriculture along their routes.

Two other developments, however, presaged the end of the era of turnpikes and started a transportation revolution that resulted in increased regional specialization and the growth of a national market economy. First came the steamboat. In 1811, four years after Robert Fulton's *Clermont* made its celebrated voyage up the Hudson River, Nicholas J. Roosevelt launched the steam-powered *New Orleans* at Pittsburgh and sent it on a successful voyage down the Ohio and Mississippi. Within twenty years some two hundred shallow-draft sternwheelers were plying the Western waters, and by 1840 the number had increased to 536. Before 1860 the volume of goods

shipped downstream nearly doubled every decade. Steamboats were not only faster but transported up-river freight for about one-tenth of what it previously had cost on hand-propelled keelboats. The indirect results of this decline in transportation costs were a rise in the income of farmers and a further inducement to Western settlement and commercial agriculture.

Next came the Erie Canal, an enormous project in its day, spanning the three hundred fifty miles between Buffalo on Lake Erie and Albany on the Hudson River. With the support of Governor De Witt Clinton and funds from the New York legislature, construction began in 1817 and was completed in 1825. After the Erie Canal went into operation, the cost per mile of transporting a ton of freight between Buffalo and New York City declined from nearly 20 cents to less than 2 cents. Until the 1840s the canal was used primarily by the shippers of farm products and lumber from western New York, but eventually the Western states diverted much of their produce from the rivers to this shorter route to Eastern markets. Meanwhile, the canal boats carried increasing quantities of manufactured goods to the West.

The Erie Canal's immediate success (tolls enabled the state to recover the cost within seven years)

Building the Erie Canal

launched the country into the Canal Age. New York's rivals, especially Philadelphia and Baltimore, strove to tap the West with their own canal systems, but with less success. Ohio and Indiana built canals to connect the Ohio River with the Great Lakes. Between 1815 and 1840 (after which construction declined), various states invested about $125 million in three thousand miles of canals. By the 1830s the country had a complete water route from New York City to New Orleans. By then, however, many were looking to a new marvel, the railroad, for an even more dazzling answer to the West's transportation needs (see p. 316).

In all phases of this transportation revolution government provided a large proportion of the needed funds. State and local governments sometimes helped finance the turnpike companies with land grants or by subscribing to their stocks; the states built most of the important canals; federal and state governments paid for all river and harbor improvements; and in later years federal, state, and local governments aided the Western railroads with various forms of subsidies. Thus even in the years of alleged laissez faire the states had begun to play a more important role in the nation's economic life. In transportation until the 1850s state and local governments were more active than the federal government.

Life on the frontier. Only the hope of a better future could make bearable the hardships of a farm family getting its start on the Western frontier. The propaganda literature of the land-speculators abounds in descriptions of the salubrious climate, the health-giving waters, the ease with which one could make the land bloom, and the increasing comforts of civilization. The realities, for some years at least, were quite different. Clearing a piece of land for cultivation meant backbreaking labor for pioneer families. Disease and death hung over the Western settlements; trained doctors were scarce, and the only resort was to home remedies or the patent-medicine panaceas of itinerant quacks. Malaria, dysentery, pneumonia, smallpox, yellow fever, cholera, and dietary deficiencies took a heavy toll; travelers often commented on the pale and sickly appearance of Westerners. Living in primitive lean-tos or floorless cabins, surviving on a diet mainly of corn and salt pork, making their own clothing from homespun and deerskin, enduring the almost unmitigated bleakness of frontier life, these pioneers would have been hard put to discover the Arcadian quality that some romanticists see in their isolated, self-sufficient agrarian society. A prospective migrant to Illinois warned his family: "What awaits you in this region, which, as of now, is not much better than a wilderness, is a life full of hardships, want and toil. By this choice we shall close ourselves off from the rest of the world for many years."

But the settlers looked beyond the ordeal of these early years, and eventually better times did come. Life softened for them as schools and churches were built, as neighbors became less remote, as transportation improved and Eastern manufactured goods became cheaper and more plentiful, and as the growing villages and county seats acquired printing presses and newspapers, developed small local industries, and offered social diversions to the surrounding country-folk. These cultural amenities, the modest comforts earned from operating a family-size farm, and the feeling of independence derived from landownership, were the ultimate rewards of many who made their homes in the Western wilderness.

For many others, however, this was not enough. The more ambitious Westerners, if they came to farm, thought of agriculture as a business enterprise and of themselves as small capitalists producing for the market. Moreover, to those who invaded the West in search of wealth, farming was only one way—and perhaps the slowest—to gain their end. Along with the yeomen came the frontier boomers, the speculators in real estate to whom land was simply a commodity to be bought and sold for a profit. Indeed, many of the yeomen themselves were as much interested in land speculation as in agriculture. The largest profits in the West were seldom earned by industrious and thrifty farmers; they were often won by shrewd operators who knew how to exploit the vagaries of federal land policy or to buy favors at the local land offices. A long chapter in the history of the West belongs to the land companies—one of the earliest forms of large-scale American business enterprise— whose agents spied out the best tracts, bought them at public auction, and then sold them at higher prices to authentic settlers.

Other Westerners engaged in the fascinating business of promoting towns at strategic trading sites. Many of these proposed wilderness metropolises never materialized, and often the giddy purchasers of unseen town plots wound up with a "business block" knee-deep in swamp water. But important urban centers, such as Cincinnati, Cleveland, Detroit, Indianapolis, St. Louis, Milwaukee, and Chicago, did grow with amazing speed. To them came not only promoters and speculators but men with capital to invest in banking, commerce, and manufacturing. Surprisingly early these cities became the centers of Western political and economic power and of Western culture when it pushed out its first tender shoots.

The significance of the frontier. Near the end of the nineteenth century, in a famous essay, the Midwestern historian Frederick Jackson Turner called his Eastern colleagues' attention to the significance of the

Cincinnati, 1848

frontier in American history. Among other things, Turner claimed that the West had provided a refuge and its rich lands new opportunities for those suffering from economic adversity in the East—a safety valve of natural abundance; that the frontier had been a nationalizing force and the prime influence in the development of a unique American character; above all, that the frontier had provided the most powerful impulse for the growth of democracy in both America and Europe.

Turner doubtless claimed too much, as recent critics have shown. The New West seemed to have contributed little in the way of political innovation, for the new state and local governments were for the most part modeled after those in the East. Apparently the forces generating the trend toward increased political democracy in these years were as much Eastern as they were Western. Socially and culturally the West was dependent upon the East and again showed a greater tendency to copy than to innovate. This was natural enough, for those who moved west were less often critical of the fundamental structure of Eastern society than dissatisfied with their position in it.

But the impact of the New West was not insignificant. Because of its lack of local traditions, its interior position, and its need for military protection and improved transportation, the West was usually the most nationalistic section of the country. The unfamiliar problems confronting settlers on a raw frontier did encourage those who would survive to develop to a high degree qualities such as individualism and resourcefulness. Though the West did not produce a society of social and economic equals, it did foster a

belief that all artificial barriers to advancement must be removed—that all must have an equal chance to make their way in the world. Moreover, Westerners showed great respect for those who, starting with little, achieved success in the competitive struggle.

Finally, the New West was America's treasure house of unused lands and untapped resources. It was a major, though not exclusive, factor in producing the economic growth and rising standard of living from which most white Americans profited more or less. There is some truth in Turner's assertion that "this expansion westward with its new opportunities" accounted for the "fluidity of American life." These Western wilds, he wrote, "constituted the richest free gift that was ever spread out before civilized man."

Slavery and the Cotton Kingdom

Southern expansion. The migration into Alabama, Mississippi, and Louisiana was, as we have seen, a part of the westward movement; and the great majority of the early settlers were pioneer farmers, mostly from Virginia and the Carolinas, who endured the same hardships and cherished the same ambitions as those who settled north of the Ohio River. They engaged in subsistence farming or grazing to begin with, and many of them never managed to produce more than occasional small surpluses for the market. But enterprising farmers in the Southwest knew that many cotton-planters in the South Carolina and Georgia piedmonts had been making fortunes ever since Eli

Whitney, in 1793, invented a gin that efficiently separated seeds from the lint of "uplands," or short-staple, cotton. Before Whitney solved this technological problem, most of the cotton used in European textile mills had come from Brazil, Egypt, and Asia. Southerners had grown small amounts of high-quality "sea-island" cotton on the coast of South Carolina and Georgia, but this variety could not be grown inland. In 1793 the South produced only about ten thousand bales of cotton; but by the 1820s, with the Cotton Kingdom spreading westward and responding to a rapidly growing demand in Europe, the South's annual production rose to a half-million bales.

Cotton prices before 1825 seldom fell below 15 cents a pound and sometimes rose much higher, thus making it an exceedingly profitable crop, especially for those who kept their production costs low by obtaining the most suitable fresh lands and exploiting the labor of black slaves. A fortunate few—some beginning as small farmers, others bringing slaves with them from the Southeast—established large plantations on the rich, silt-loamed prairies of the Alabama-Mississippi Black Belt, or on the alluvial bottom lands of the Mississippi and Yazoo delta. These great cotton-planters, together with the rice-planters of coastal South Carolina and Georgia and the sugar-planters of Louisiana, developed agriculture to the highest levels of efficiency, complexity, and commercialization to be found anywhere in America before the Civil War.

After 1815 the economy of the Deep South was tied to the cultivation of cotton, for investments in new cotton lands and slaves brought higher returns than any of the possible alternatives. Indeed, during the next few decades cotton was a crucial factor in the developing national market economy and in the economic growth of all regions. It accounted for more than half the country's exports and thus paid for a large part of its imports. The cotton plantations provided a substantial market for farm products from the Northwest and for manufactured goods from the Northeast, and the marketing of Southern cotton gave the Northeastern commercial interests a highly profitable trade.

Soon after the War of 1812 the booming Gulf states were ceasing to be part of the New West and were becoming increasingly identified with the Old South, even though they differed socially from Virginia and the Carolinas in many significant ways. Their identification with the South Atlantic states came at a time when Southerners were becoming more, rather than less, conscious of their special sectional problems and interests.

Planting South Carolina cotton

Nat has survived all his followers, and the gallows will speedily close his career. His own account of the conspiracy ... reads an awful, and it is hoped, a useful lesson, as to the operations of a mind like his, endeavoring to grapple with things beyond his reach.... [The conspiracy] was not instigated by motives of revenge or sudden anger, but the result of long deliberation, and a settled purpose of mind....

... It has been said he was ignorant and cowardly ... [but] for natural intelligence and quickness of apprehension, [he] is surpassed by few men I have ever seen.... He is a complete fanatic, or plays his part most admirably. On other subjects he possesses an uncommon share of intelligence, with a mind capable of attaining any thing; but warped and perverted by the influence of early impressions.... I shall not attempt to describe the effect of his narrative, as told and commented on by himself, in the condemned hole of the prison. The calm, deliberate composure with which he spoke of his late deeds and intentions, the expression of his fiend-like face when excited by enthusiasm, still bearing the blood of helpless innocence about him; clothed with rags and covered with chains; yet daring to raise his manacled hands to heaven, with a spirit soaring above the attributes of man; I looked on him and my blood curdled in my veins.

From Thomas R. Gray, *The Confessions of Nat Turner*, 1831.

The survival of slavery. What was it that gave the Old South its special identity? Not physical isolation, for it lacked natural barriers separating it from the rest of the country; nor geographic and climatic uniformity, for it had great diversity of soils, topography, mean temperatures, growing seasons, and average rainfalls. Not a difference in the origins of the white population, for the South, like the North, was originally settled mostly by middle- and lower-class people from northern and western Europe; nor contrasts in cultures or ideologies, for here, too, the similarities outweighed the differences. Not even the economies of North and South were altogether dissimilar, for, although there were important differences, the majority of the white people of both sections were independent yeoman farmers who worked their own lands. However, fewer Southern farmers than Northern farmers benefited from improved transportation and became part of the national market economy. Wealth was less evenly distributed in the South than in the West; less money was invested in education; and the rate of illiteracy was higher. Fewer towns and less local industry developed. In short, the Old South remained more rural and economically less diversified than the North, and a larger proportion of its small farmers lived a life of pioneer self-sufficiency and isolation.

But these differences between North and South were of secondary importance. By far the most significant difference was the presence and survival in the South of Negro slavery, which Southerners themselves called their "peculiar institution." More than anything else, it was slavery, with all its ramifications, that eventually gave the Old South its identity and white Southerners their feeling of separateness from the rest of the Union.

In the eighteenth century, of course, Southern slavery had not been a peculiar institution, for it existed in the Northern colonies and throughout the Western Hemisphere. During or soon after the Revolution, however, the Northern states abolished it, and in the first half of the nineteenth century slaves gained their freedom in most of Central and South America. Some Southerners of Washington's and Jefferson's generation, moved by anxieties about social dangers as well as by the ideals of the American Revolution, were cautiously and rather abstractly critical of slavery. As late as the 1820s a scattering of emancipation societies in the Upper South, supported mostly by Quakers, carried on a discreet campaign for gradual emancipation and the colonization of free blacks outside the boundaries of the United States.

In Virginia, in the late eighteenth and early nineteenth centuries, a prolonged agricultural depression resulting from low tobacco prices and soil depletion led some to believe, or hope, that slavery would soon die. In August 1831, Southampton County, Virginia, was the scene of the South's bloodiest slave insurrection, led by a bondsman named Nat Turner, in which sixty whites and scores of blacks lost their lives. (Turner himself was captured, brought to trial, and executed.) The Turner rebellion, which caused profound alarm throughout the South, precipitated an earnest debate in the Virginia legislature the following January, during which various legislators denounced slavery as a social canker and an economic blight. The antislavery legislators, showing clearly that their concern was less for blacks than for the safety and welfare of whites, demanded a program of gradual emancipation and colonization. But the Virginia emancipationists, like those in other states of the Upper South, were defeated; and soon after 1832 Southern critics were either silenced or driven into exile.

Southern slavery, then, did not die of natural causes; it did not even decline. Instead, with the rise of the Cotton Kingdom and the eventual improvement of agriculture in the seaboard states, it flourished and seemed to have the vitality to survive indefinitely. Since the federal Constitution recognized slavery as a local institution within the jurisdiction of individual states, Southerners saw nothing to prevent them from introducing it into the Southwest. Some moved there with their slaves, while others stayed behind and operated new plantations as absentee owners. Still others took advantage of high slave prices resulting from the labor shortage in the Southwest and sold a portion of their slaves to professional traders who took them to the busy markets in New Orleans and Natchez. There at the slave auctions the self-made men of the Cotton Kingdom, some of whom had started with no slaves at all, purchased "prime field hands" to work their growing estates.

Negro slaves thus became an important element in the migration to the Southwest and played a major role in clearing the land for cultivation. By 1840 almost half the population of Alabama and Louisiana and more than half the population of Mississippi (by then the leading cotton-producing state) consisted of Negro slaves. Yet at all times nearly three-fourths of the white families in the South as a whole held no slaves and depended on their own labor alone. Moreover, the great majority of slaveholders owned just a few slaves; as late as 1860 only ten thousand Southern families belonged to the planter aristocracy operating large estates with slave gangs numbering more than fifty.

Why did Southern slavery survive far into the nineteenth century? Not because Negroes were innately suited to be slaves; nor because white labor could not adjust to the Southern climate and successfully cultivate the Southern crops; nor because the Negroes' health was not adversely affected by living in the malarial swamps, where the sugar and rice plantations and many of the cotton plantations were located. The reasons the South clung so tenaciously to slavery are to be found in the fears, ambitions, and aspirations of white Southerners.

By the nineteenth century the South's peculiar institution was two hundred years old, and to abolish it would have brought painful changes in long-established habits and attitudes. Those who would destroy slavery, warned a Georgian, "would have to wade knee-deep in blood"; indeed, slavery is "so intimately . . . mingled with our social conditions that it would be impossible to eradicate it." Most white Southerners—indeed, most white Americans—believed that blacks were by nature shiftless, untrustworthy, and sexually promiscuous. Slavery, therefore, was a means of controlling an inferior race, of preventing it from becoming a burden on society, and of maintaining the purity and supremacy of the white race. To nonslaveholders slavery symbolized their link with the privileged caste of free whites and the blacks' social and legal subordination. "Now suppose they was free," explained a poor Southern farmer to a Northern visitor, "you see they'd all think themselves as good as we." To the master class the possession of slaves brought great prestige, for in the South the ownership of a plantation worked by slave labor was the sign of success and high social position.

But, above all, slavery survived because it was a viable and profitable labor system representing an enormous investment of Southern capital. Slavery, of course, did not make every master a rich man, nor did every master strive to wring the last ounce of profit from his toiling bondsmen. Nevertheless, in the long run most slaveholders earned good returns on their investments—and this accounts for the generally heavy demand for slaves and for their high price in the market. The system, moreover, was highly adaptable. Slaves were employed not only in agriculture and as domestics but as skilled artisans, as laborers in construction gangs, and as workers in mines, iron foundries, textile mills, and tobacco factories. In short, the master class had no compelling economic reason for wanting to abolish slavery; as late as 1860 it was still a vigorous and remunerative economic institution.

The nature of slavery. In governing their bondsmen most masters were neither inordinately cruel nor remarkably indulgent; they usually dealt with their human property with a measure of compassion but in the manner they deemed necessary to make the system work. They bought and sold slaves, used them as security for loans, and divided them among heirs. As a result of these transactions husbands could be separated from their wives and children from their mothers, for state laws gave slave marriages no legal protection. Except for the deliberate killing or maiming of a slave, the master's power to administer physical punishment was virtually unlimited, and planters could delegate this power to white overseers employed to manage their estates. Most slaveholders used the whip for "moderate correction" only when they believed it essential to maintain discipline; many devised positive incentives for efficient labor; but an element of cruelty was inseparable from slavery, as even many of its defenders recognized. Some slaves fell into the hands of brutal masters, or of men who were corrupted by the power the institution conferred upon them. Since blacks were unable to give testimony against whites, the justice they received in court was, at best, very eccentric.

The standard of living of most slaves was near the subsistence level. They lived on a diet mainly of corn and pork (seasonally supplemented with other foods), adequate in bulk but often unbalanced and monotonous; they wore coarse, skimpy clothing made from some variety of cheap "Negro cloth"; and they lived in cabins that varied in size and comfort but were too often drafty, cramped, and scantily furnished. Their labor routine kept them at work from dawn to dusk. By nineteenth-century standards, they were not often worked excessively, but a long day of hard toil was usually exacted from them. The slaves were most in danger of being overworked to the detriment of their health on the large cotton and sugar plantations of absentee owners managed by overseers, and on the estates of ambitious new planters "on the make."

One cannot pretend to know all that being a slave meant to the Negroes, for slaves were seldom able to express their feelings and most of the evidence comes from white sources. Though organized rebellions were rare, there is no reason to assume that they accepted slavery as their natural lot and cheerfully submitted to their white masters. No doubt they made certain psychological adaptations to their condition; no doubt they enjoyed the occasional holidays and simple pleasures that most masters permitted them; no doubt their untrained intellects seldom dwelt on freedom as a philosophical abstraction. But to conclude from this that they had no idea of the meaning of freedom, no comprehension of its practical advantages, no desire to obtain it, would be quite unwarranted. The evidence of their submission and obeisance suggests not so much contentment as the superior power of the white caste and the effectiveness of its elaborate techniques of control. Moreover, there is some direct and much circumstantial evidence indicating that most plantation slaves consciously played the role of a docile, cheerful Sambo as a protective device in their relationships with whites. Consequently, slaveholders often knew less about the true character of their slaves than they thought. "The most general defect in the character of the Negro," complained one planter, "is hypocrisy . . . and if the master treats him as a fool, he will be sure to act the fool's part." The swift and ruthless suppression of Nat Turner's followers drove home to the slaves the futility of any large-scale insurrection. But it did not deter some of the bolder ones from less spectacular forms of protest. Of these protests, running away was one of

Identification tags for Southern blacks

the most common—and certainly the most irksome to the master class.

White Southerners paid a high price for slavery: artisans and yeoman farmers suffered from the competition of cheap slave labor; most slaveholders were more or less distressed by the obvious paradox of slavery in a republic whose moral commitment was to individual freedom and natural rights; and all were bedeviled by a nagging fear of slave rebellions, a fear that occasionally reached the proportions of mass hysteria. But the blacks, not the whites, were the chief victims of the system. Slavery exposed them not only to its cruelties and meager rewards but to its strong dehumanizing tendencies and its powerful pressures toward emasculated personalities. It destroyed much of the rich and varied cultural tradition that Negroes had brought with them from Africa; it sometimes disrupted slave families and exposed black women to the lust of white men; and it put a premium on docility. Above all, slavery deprived its victims of the opportunity to develop their potentialities and of the freedom that white Americans treasured so much.

Yet, in spite of the damage done to them, Southern slaves found ways to maintain a degree of psychic balance and to avoid total dehumanization. Though slave marriages had no legal support and slave fathers could not be the authority figures traditional in nineteenth-century families, slaves nevertheless customarily lived in family groups. In the plantation slave quarters they were not under the constant scrutiny of their masters; and there, in their relationships with each other, they could play roles other than Sambo and develop a community life of their own. They found opportunities for self-expression in their religious services, in their music and folklore, and in other social activities. In due time these experiences of slave community life, which blended a modified white culture with fragments of African cultural survivals, would provide the ingredients from which a semiautonomous Afro-American subculture would grow.

Missouri and the issue of slavery expansion. Eventually the South's peculiar institution was to have a tragic impact upon the whole nation—indeed, a few intimations of the ultimate tragedy were evident even in the early years. Slavery was a topic of debate at the Constitutional Convention of 1787, and its future under the new Constitution was a subject of inquiry at Southern ratifying conventions. The compromise by which Southerners obtained congressional representation for three-fifths of their slaves (see p. 134) provoked repeated Northern complaints. Antislavery Northerners frequently resisted enforcement of the Fugitive Slave Act of 1793, which enabled Southern masters to recover runaways in the free states. In the Deep South some doubted the wisdom of the federal law closing the African slave trade, and, as we have seen, the law was not very effectively enforced.

But these were minor irritants compared to the succession of national political crises generated by the acquisition of new Western territory and by the ensuing steady march of slavery into the Southwest. Before 1820 five additional slave states (Kentucky, Tennessee, Louisiana, Mississippi, and Alabama) had been admitted to the Union; these increased the total number to eleven, which, as it happened, were balanced by eleven free states. The resulting political equilibrium in the Senate was threatened, however, when the territory of Missouri, settled mostly by Kentuckians and Tennesseeans, petitioned for admission as a slave state. In February 1819, a House committee reported an act authorizing Missouri to frame a state constitution; but Representative James Tallmadge, Jr., a Republican from New York, proposed an amendment to prohibit the introduction of additional slaves into Missouri and to provide gradual emancipation for those already there. The Tallmadge Amendment passed the House on a sectional vote but was defeated in the Senate. When neither chamber would yield, slavery's critics and defenders plunged into an ill-tempered debate that revealed a deep sectional cleavage.

Much of the Missouri debate revolved around constitutional issues. Southerners, especially Virginians, insisting that new states had the same sovereign rights as the old, denied that Congress could make the abolition of slavery a condition of admission. Northerners claimed that the Founding Fathers had thought of slavery as a temporary institution and had not intended that it should spread into the Western territories. In the heat of the debate angry Southerners accused Federalists of deliberately fomenting a crisis in order to win popular support in the North and revive their dying party. Jefferson, who strongly opposed the Tallmadge Amendment, was convinced that the Federalist leader Rufus King was "ready to risk the Union for any chance of restoring his party to power and wriggling himself to the head of it." Northern opposition to slavery expansion, wrote Charles Pinckney of South Carolina, "sprang from the love of power, and the never ceasing wish to regain the honors and offices of the government."

The Missouri Compromise, 1820

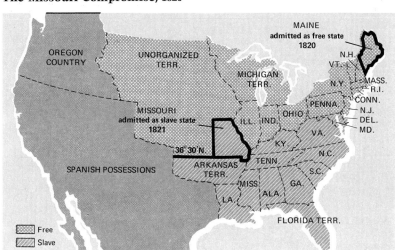

John Quincy Adams on the Missouri crisis

I have favored this Missouri compromise, believing it to be all that could be effected under the present Constitution, and from extreme unwillingness to put the Union at hazard. But perhaps it would have been a wiser as well as a bolder course to have persisted in the restriction upon Missouri.... If the Union must be dissolved, slavery is precisely the question upon which it ought to break....

... If slavery be the destined sword in the hand of the destroying angel which is to sever the ties of this Union, the same sword will cut in sunder the bonds of slavery itself. A dissolution of the Union for the cause of slavery would be followed by a servile war in the slave-holding States, combined with a war between the two severed portions of the Union. It seems to me that its result must be the extirpation of slavery from this whole continent; and, calamitous and desolating as this course of events in its progress must be, so glorious would be its final issue, that, as God shall judge me, I dare not say that it is not to be desired.

From Charles Francis Adams, ed., *Memoirs of J. Q. Adams*, March 3, Nov. 29, 1820.

No doubt political advantage and sectional power—the North already had a substantial majority in the House—were basic ingredients of the Missouri controversy. But the crisis might have looked less portentous had this been all there was to it. Tallmadge himself appeared to have no crass political motive; rather, he seems to have acted from a conviction that slavery was a moral evil that should not be permitted to spread. So did many others whose humanitarian impulses were aroused by the obvious vitality of Southern slavery. In urging his colleagues to prevent its further spread, Representative Arthur Livermore, of New Hampshire, stressed the importance of the decision they were about to make:

An opportunity is now presented, if not to diminish, at least to prevent the growth of a sin which sits heavy on the soul of every one of us. By embracing this opportunity, we may retrieve the national character and, in some degree, our own. But if we suffer it to pass unimproved, let us at least be consistent, and declare that our Constitution was made to impose slavery, and not to establish liberty.

Never before had the peculiar institution been so severely attacked—and so vigorously defended—on moral grounds as it was during the Missouri debate.

The basic issue was not resolved on this occasion; it was simply postponed by a compromise that passed largely through Henry Clay's efforts. In 1820 Congress finally agreed to admit Missouri as a slave state, but it preserved the balance by admitting Maine as a free state. It divided the remaining territory acquired in the Louisiana Purchase along the line 36° 30′ north latitude. North of that line, except for Missouri, slavery was "forever prohibited."

The Missouri crisis made some Americans apprehensive about the future of the federal Union. John Quincy Adams foresaw the possibility of a realignment of political parties along sectional lines, hastening the "emancipation of all . . . [Southern] slaves, threatening in its immediate effect that Southern domination which has swayed the Union for the last twenty years." Tallmadge, said a Georgia congressman, had "kindled a fire which all the waters of the ocean can not put out, which seas of blood can only extinguish." And Jefferson, showing hardly a glimmer of his earlier antislavery sentiments, poured his indignation on Northerners for opening this sensitive issue. "All, I fear, do not see the speck on our horizon which is to burst on us as a tornado, sooner or later. The line of division lately marked out between different portions of our confederacy is such as will never, I fear, be obliterated." Writing thus in 1821, Jefferson had, in effect, formulated the doctrine of an "irrepressible conflict" between North and South.

Another Frontier: Industry and Technology

Beginnings of the factory system. The western edge of settlement was not the only frontier that attracted Americans and promised a future of increased abundance. Since the War of 1812 growing numbers had been drawn to the thriving towns and cities of the New England and Middle Atlantic states. Here lived the pioneers of the American Industrial Revolution—people who devoted their lives to the

Albert Gallatin on American economic progress

promotion of business enterprises and to the application of science and technology to the goals of increasing productivity and profits, lightening the burdens of labor, and multiplying the comforts of human life. Their efforts gradually rendered obsolete the system of household manufacturing that had been almost universal in colonial days. Under this system farm families outside the market economy had made their own clothes and household necessities, while village artisans had produced such items as cloth, shoes, hats, and tools for sale to consumers in local markets. The independent artisan survived longer in some crafts than in others, and household manufacturing was always a part of life on the isolated agricultural frontier; but after 1830 both were clearly doomed by the factory and the spreading market economy.

In a sense the Industrial Revolution, in America as in Europe, was merely an acceleration of technological changes that had no clear beginning and as yet have no foreseeable end. It involved the development and increasing use of power-driven machines in industrial production; the location of those machines in factories that tended to grow in size and complexity; and, with the decline of transportation costs, the distribution of their products in ever widening mass markets. As the domestic market expanded, manufacturing enterprises became increasingly specialized. The early textile mills, for example, marketed their own products and constructed their own machinery; but eventually they concentrated on spinning and weaving, selling their products to wholesalers, and buying their machinery from independent machine shops. The essential features of the Industrial Revolu-

tion, then, were mechanization, specialization, and a trend from local to regional and national distribution.

American industrial technology was in part copied from Europe, especially England, and was in part an outgrowth of the genius of American inventors, skilled mechanics, and entrepreneurs. Manufacturers found an impelling incentive for mechanization in the relative scarcity and high cost of domestic labor. The dearness of labor was the direct result of the high productivity of American agriculture, which forced industry to pay wages comparable to what could be earned on the land. Another incentive was the presence of cheap waterpower to which machinery could easily be harnessed. Moreover, the optimistic American entrepreneurs, anticipating continued technological advances, usually built cheaper machines that wore out quickly, thus making it relatively inexpensive to retool. Nowhere in Europe did environmental conditions provide so many inducements for mechanical innovation; nowhere was there a society so free from the sort of deep-rooted traditions that impede technological change. "Everything new is quickly introduced here," wrote a European visitor in the 1820s. "There is no clinging to old ways; the moment an American hears the word 'invention' he pricks up his ears."

The Northeastern states, for a variety of reasons, were the first to industrialize to a significant degree. In the years before the embargo and War of 1812, their profitable foreign trade had enabled them to accumulate the necessary capital and to build the banks and other commercial facilities that were now useful to industry. Their substantial urban centers provided large local markets, coastal waterways opened regional markets, and turnpikes gave them early access to the hinterland. In addition, the Northeast had superior entrepreneurial talent, a well-educated labor supply, easy access to Southern cotton, and rich resources in the waterpower of New England and the iron and coal of Pennsylvania. In the years after 1815 manufacturing gradually superseded commerce as this region's primary economic concern.

What the pioneers in technology accomplished lacks the romance and drama of the Western frontiersman's elemental struggle for survival. Yet their work was equally vital to national growth and expansion, and its long-run social and economic consequences were much greater. In the field of transportation, for example, the builders of turnpikes experimented with various kinds of road-surfacing and with truss-type and suspension bridges; engineers on the Erie Canal designed new excavating equipment and developed a special cement for use in its eighty-eight locks; and Henry M. Shreve, among others, built flat-hulled steamboats of shallow draft especially adapted to service on the Western rivers. Meanwhile, a patent act adopted by Congress in 1790 (revised in 1793) encouraged numerous people to pursue fame and fortune through the improvement or invention of devices useful to humanity.

The factory system in the United States had its beginnings during the Presidency of Washington. In 1790 Samuel Slater, an English immigrant who knew the secrets of English textile machinery, built a cotton-spinning mill at Pawtucket, Rhode Island, for the merchant Moses Brown. This first successful American factory contained seventy-two spindles tended by nine children, and its machinery was soon harnessed to waterpower. After years of slow and faltering growth, Jefferson's embargo and the War of 1812 gave the American cotton-textile industry a chance to become a significant part of the national economy. By the end of the war cotton factories were counted in the hundreds, most of them in New England, and the number of spindles in operation approximated 130,000. Immediately after the war many of these mills failed because of renewed British competition; but others survived, and by 1840 the number of spindles exceeded 2 million.

In the years of expansion constant improvements were made in the machinery for carding the raw cotton and for spinning it into yarn and thread. But the weaving long continued to be done in the homes of small craftsmen, who sold the cloth in their own shops or who worked for wages for merchant capitalists. After 1814, however, the introduction of the power loom soon brought weaving as well as spinning into the factory. Many American mills specialized in the manufacture of a coarse white cloth called "sheet-

ing," which was in wide demand and could be mass produced. American manufacturers of sheeting could compete successfully with the British in the domestic market, and by the 1830s they were even selling in foreign markets. By 1840 domestic manufacturers were consuming some 270,000 bales of cotton annually, which amounted to about 20 percent of Southern production.

From cotton textiles the factory spread to other industries. In 1793, at Byfield, Massachusetts, John and Arthur Schofield, who came to the United States from Yorkshire, England, built the first factory to manufacture woolens. War in Europe, a series of improvements in carding, napping, and shearing machines, and the introduction of waterpower soon placed the American woolens industry on a secure foundation. Meanwhile, merchant capitalists were taking the manufacture of shoes out of the cobblers' shops and into the homes of semiskilled workers who specialized in making a single part of the finished product. By mid-century, when the shoe industry was being mechanized, the workers were brought into factories where their role changed from that of craftsmen to that of tenders of machines. Similarly, in the iron industry Pennsylvania's furnaces and rolling mills were fast supplanting small local forges.

In 1804 Oliver Evans of Philadelphia, one of the most remarkable pioneers of American technology, developed a high-pressure steam engine that was adaptable to a great variety of industrial purposes. Within a few years it was being used not only in steam navigation but to run sawmills, flour mills, and printing presses—and, in 1828, steam power replaced waterpower at the Slater cotton mills. Earlier, Evans had experimented with the techniques of mass production and built the first completely mechanized flour mill. Eli Whitney and Simeon North, a Connecticut clockmaker, applied those techniques to the manufacture of guns and developed the system of interchangeable parts. Whitney taught his workers to make identical parts from metal molds, or "gigs"; after the perfection of this system, guns could be assembled or repaired in a fraction of the time required by a skilled gunsmith. North then introduced his system in the clock industry, and Connecticut manufacturers were soon mass-producing inexpensive clocks for a national market.

To build a factory equipped with expensive machinery run by steam or waterpower required more capital than the average individual entrepreneur or even partnership could obtain. While these older forms of business organization predominated as late as the 1850s, the ultimate answer to this financial problem was the corporation. Chartered under state laws, corporations could accumulate capital from numerous small investors; and the stockholders enjoyed "limited liability"—that is, they were financially responsible for the corporation's debts only in proportion to their share of ownership. Used first by bankers and the builders of turnpikes, bridges, and other internal improvements, the corporate form slowly spread to manufacturing, especially textiles, after the War of 1812. In 1813 a group of wealthy merchants known as the Boston Associates, including Francis Cabot Lowell, Nathan Appleton, and Patrick Tracy Jackson, formed the Boston Manufacturing Company in Waltham, Massachusetts. With capital exceeding a half-million dollars and with an efficient managerial staff, these men built the first integrated textile factory that performed every operation from the carding of raw cotton to the weaving of cloth with power looms. A decade later the Boston Associates shifted the center of their activities to Lowell, "the Manchester of America," where they chartered the Merrimack Manufacturing Company. During the 1820s and 1830s they chartered additional companies in Massachusetts and New Hampshire, until, by the 1850s, they and their imitators had made the manufacturing corporation an entrenched economic institution.

In other areas, too, the American economy began to show the effects of advancing technology. Eastern merchants used improved transportation and marketing techniques to compete for the trade of the hinterland, with New York merchants rapidly outstripping their rivals. The New York group siphoned much of the Western trade through the Great Lakes and the Erie Canal and captured a large share of the cotton trade between the South and Europe. The skill of Yankee shipbuilders and the initiative of New York merchants combined to improve transatlantic service for passengers and cargo. The New York packet lines, beginning with the Black Ball Line in 1818, were the first to post sailing dates and observe them, whether or not a full cargo was on board. The sleek vessels in this service were built for speed and maximum cargo; they

were, said an English reporter, "probably the finest and fastest sailing vessels in the world . . . beautifully modeled and of the best workmanship." The whaling industry, concentrated at New Bedford and Nantucket Island, Massachusetts, was also more highly organized after the War of 1812 than before, because the depletion of the Atlantic supply necessitated long, expensive voyages to the Pacific. Still another sign of the new era was John Jacob Astor's American Fur Company, a million-dollar corporation chartered in New York in 1808. Until the 1830s, when the fur supply of the Northwest began to near exhaustion, Astor used efficient organization and ruthless methods to destroy his weaker competitors and lay the foundation for the first great American fortune. Eventually he transferred his capital from the fur trade to real-estate operations in New York City.

As mechanical devices played an increasingly important part in the lives of the American people, the study of applied science began to invade the precincts of American education. A network of mechanics' institutes, beginning with one in Boston in 1795, spread through American cities to train men in the mechanical arts. When President Madison, like his predecessors, urged the founding of a national university, he stressed its potential value as a "temple of science" to diffuse "useful knowledge." Nothing came of this, but several private colleges soon added applied science to their curricula. At Harvard, in 1814, Dr. Jacob Bigelow began to lecture on "The Elements of Technology" and tried to awaken his students to the possibilities of this exciting frontier. At Yale, Benjamin Silliman brought a similar message not only to his students but to a wider audience through his *American Journal of Science*, founded in 1818, and through his enormously popular public lectures. In 1825 Rensselaer Polytechnic Institute, the first of its genre, opened its doors at Troy, New York, "for the purpose of instructing persons who may choose to apply themselves in the application of science to the common purposes of life."

If newspapers and periodicals accurately reflected public opinion, the American people were proud of their technological achievements and fascinated by the many useful products of applied science. Looking back at the half-century of economic growth following independence, Tocqueville concluded that "no people in the world had made such rapid progress in trade and manufactures as the Americans; they constitute at the present day the second maritime nation in the world"; their manufacturing makes "great and daily advances"; "the greatest undertakings and speculations are executed without difficulty. . . . The Americans arrived but as yesterday on the territory which they inhabit, and they have already changed the whole order of nature for their own advantage."

Capital and labor. Yet, while they found the promises of the Industrial Revolution irresistible, many Americans were at the same time a little uneasy about what had been happening to their society since industry got a foothold. Carrying with them into the new age the assumptions of a simple agricultural society, they watched apprehensively the growth of cities, the "paper-money speculations" of urban businessmen, and the movement of young people from the land to the factory. They wondered whether the craving for material success was undermining their morals and compromising their virtue. To be sure, those fears were still rather vague and sporadic, for in the 1820s and 1830s the factories (except in textiles) were not very large, and the urban population was a small fraction of the whole—only 10.8 percent as late as 1840. But the trend was clear.

One consequence of the factories and machines was the gradual emergence of two new social classes. The first were the industrial capitalists, whom the rural gentry regarded as vulgarly ambitious and dangerously powerful. With their wealth they gained considerable political power and, as James Fenimore Cooper complained, substituted their "fluctuating expedients for the high principles of natural justice." The second new social class consisted of factory workers, the hirelings who tended machines for a weekly wage and, in the larger establishments, had no personal contact with either owners or ultimate consumers. They were recruited from the farms and, increasingly by the 1830s, from among newly arrived immigrants.

Thanks to a chronic labor shortage, workers' living conditions were, on the average, better in America than in Europe. Visitors to Lowell often commented on the attention that the Boston Associates gave to the welfare of the young women who worked in their mills. The "Lowell girls" lived in comfortable boardinghouses built by the company; their morals were strictly supervised; and they were provided with recreational facilities, educational opportunities, and religious instruction. They published their own monthly magazine, the *Lowell Offering*, "as a repository of original articles, written by females employed in the mills." After a visit to Lowell, Charles Dickens reported that he had seen "no face that bore an unhealthy or an unhappy look." According to Anthony Trollope, Lowell was "the realization of a commercial utopia," where the women were "taken in, as it were, to a philanthropical manufacturing college."

But industrial paternalism soon declined in the Lowell mills as professional managers fought competitors by cutting costs and making increased use of immigrant labor. Even in the 1830s the working day at Lowell was thirteen hours in summer and from sun-

Dispiriting regimen

rise to sunset in winter. Another visitor had a less happy report about conditions among the women employees: "The great mass wear out their health, spirits, and morals without becoming one whit better off than when they commenced labor." Children under sixteen, who constituted two-fifths of the labor force in New England textile mills, worked twelve or more hours a day. Real wages declined; in 1830 it was estimated that some twenty thousand of the lowest-paid women in Eastern cities worked sixteen hours a day for $1.25 a week. The callousness of the factory system in a laissez-faire economy began to be reflected, too, in the crowded dwellings of drab factory towns.

Such conditions ultimately produced disturbing social fissures and a greater awareness of class interests and class identity than had been the case before the rise of industry. When workingmen tried to improve their status through united action, severe tensions developed in the relations between labor and capital. In the 1790s carpenters, printers, and cordwainers had begun to organize in several cities; in the early nineteenth century other skilled trades followed their example. The next step was the formation of city federations of craft unions, six of which united, in 1834, to form the short-lived National Trades' Union. Strikes for higher wages usually failed, first, because labor organizations were still weak and inexperienced and, second, because state courts usually treated them as criminal conspiracies under common law.* Turning briefly to political action in the 1820s, workingmen's parties, especially in New York and Philadelphia, agitated for free public education, shorter working days, and other social reforms to aid the laboring class. Distressed by such novel phenomena as trade unions and workingmen's parties, some conservatives might well have recalled Jefferson's pessimistic predictions about the evil consequences of industrialization.

Economic crisis. The Panic of 1819 introduced the United States to still another hazard of a commercial-industrial economy: the depression phase of the modern business cycle. When Americans first began to experience the rhythmic rotation of booms, panics, and depressions, they were so mystified that many of them turned to the supernatural for an explanation. An angry deity, they said, periodically brought hard times to punish men and women for their moral delinquencies—extravagance, speculation, and greed. This first modern panic followed several years of postwar prosperity. In the boom years, when cotton sold for more than 30 cents a pound and wheat for $2 a bushel, land speculation financed by the state banks became a national disease. Soon the Bank of the United States caught the spirit of the times; rather than acting as a stabilizing force, it extended credit generously to speculators and business-promoters in both the East and the West. Public land sales rose sharply; and between 1814 and 1819, under the impetus of high prices, cotton production doubled.

At length an accumulation of adverse economic forces brought these flush times to a sudden end. First came a decline in the European demand for American agricultural products, especially wheat, flour, and cotton, then a shrinking of the market for textiles. Early in 1819 the Bank of the United States, now under new and more conservative management, began to call in its loans and to exert pressure on the state banks to redeem their notes with specie. The Bank's attempt to save itself from its own recent follies was the immediate cause of a financial panic that forced many state banks to close their doors. In the subsequent depression prices fell disastrously—in 1823, because of the decline in foreign demand, cotton sold for less than 10 cents a pound—and public land sales nearly ceased. Thousands of farmers and planters saw their lands sold at public auction to satisfy the claims of creditors; numerous speculators and business-promoters forfeited property to the Bank of the United States for failing to repay their loans. In the Eastern cities a half-million workers lost their jobs when factories, offices, and shops closed down or curtailed their operations.

Those suffering from economic distress turned to government for relief. Manufacturers demanded higher tariff protection, and after a long battle Congress came to their aid with the Tariff of 1824. To help Western farmers who had bought public land on credit, Congress permitted them to delay payments or to keep as much of the land as they had paid for. Several Southern and Western states passed "stay laws" postponing the time when creditors could foreclose on the property of debtors. The demand for "stay laws" and other measures of debtor relief became bitter issues in the politics of various states, especially Kentucky and Tennessee.

By the mid-twenties prosperity had returned, but not before the panic and depression had created angry feelings that were reflected in national politics. Many accused the Bank of the United States of coldly sacrificing thousands of innocent victims to protect the interests of its stockholders. Thereafter much of the anxiety about the new economic order was focused on the monopolistic Bank, the most powerful of the "soulless" corporations. Senator Thomas Hart Benton of Missouri pictured the Bank as a ruthless "money power" to which the Western cities were enslaved: "They may be devoured by it at any moment. They are in the jaws of the monster! A lump of butter in the mouth of a dog! One gulp, one swallow, and all is gone!"

The ground had been prepared for the growth of the Jacksonian movement, which, in a strange way, benefited from both the acquisitive impulses that the new order had aroused in the American people and the lingering doubts they felt about its results.

---

*The common law, introduced to America from England in colonial days, consists of a body of judicial decisions based on custom and precedent. It became the basis of the legal system in all the states except Louisiana. In the early nineteenth century, state courts repeatedly used common-law precedents to find guilty of criminal conspiracies the combinations of workers attempting to force employers to bargain with them over wages and working conditions.

Suggestions for Reading

POSTWAR NATIONALISM

George Dangerfield has written two superb books on the period from the War of 1812 to the election of Andrew Jackson as President: *The Era of Good Feelings** (1952) and *The Awakening of American Nationalism, 1815–1828** (1965). P. C. Nagel, *One Nation Indivisible: The Union in American Thought, 1776–1861* (1964), is a study of the intellectual roots of American nationalism. An excellent work on the postwar decline of the Federalists is Shaw Livermore, Jr., *The Twilight of Federalism* (1962). The period may also be studied through several good biographies of Republican leaders: Harry Ammon, *James Monroe: The Quest for National Identity* (1971); C. M. Wiltse, *John C. Calhoun: Nationalist, 1782–1828* (1944); and G. G. Van Deusen, *The Life of Henry Clay** (1937). Bray Hammond, *Banks and Politics in America from the Revolution to the Civil War** (1957), provides a sympathetic account of the chartering of the second Bank of the United States and its role in the American economy.

The role of the Supreme Court in the Marshall era is treated fully in A. J. Beveridge's distinguished biography of the great Chief Justice, *The Life of John Marshall*, 4 vols. (1916–19). Leonard Baker, *John Marshall: A Life in Law* (1974) is warmly sympathetic. F. N. Stites, *John Marshall: Defender of the Constitution** (1981), is a good brief biography. Valuable special studies include D. O. Dewey, *Marshall Versus Jefferson: The Political Background of Marbury v. Madison* (1970); R. E. Ellis, *The Jeffersonian Crisis: Courts and Politics in the Young Republic** (1971); and R. K. Faulkner, *The Jurisprudence of John Marshall* (1968). A. M. Bickel, *Justice Joseph Story and the Rise of the Supreme Court* (1971), is a satisfactory biography of one of Marshall's most brilliant contemporaries.

Several excellent monographs on the Monroe Doctrine are available: Dexter Perkins, *The Monroe Doctrine*, Vol. I, *1823–1826* (1927); A. P. Whitaker, *The United States and the Independence of Latin America 1800–1830* (1941); and E. R. May, *The Making of the Monroe Doctrine* (1975). Two fine biographies should also be consulted: J. H. Powell, *Richard Rush: Republican Diplomat, 1780–1859* (1942); and S. F. Bemis, *John Quincy Adams and the Foundations of American Foreign Policy* (1949).

THE WESTWARD MOVEMENT

Two good syntheses of the westward movement in this period are Dale Van Every, *The Final Challenge: The American Frontier, 1804–1845* (1964); and F. S. Philbrick, *The Rise of the West, 1754–1830* (1965). The classic statement of the importance of the West to the whole of American society is F. J. Turner, *The Frontier in American History** (1920). Frederick Merk, *History of the Westward Movement* (1978) is a traditional Turnerian survey. R. A. Billington, *America's Frontier Heritage** (1967), is a sympathetic appraisal of the Turner thesis in the light of modern scholarship. M. J. Rohrbough, *The Land Office Business: The Settlement and Administration of American Public Lands, 1789–1837** (1968), is an excellent study of public land policy in the early national period. P. W. Gates, *The Farmer's Age: Agriculture, 1815–1860* (1960), is a comprehensive study of Southern and Western agricultural development. J. T. Schlebecker, *Whereby We Thrive: A History of American Farming, 1607–1972* (1975), traces changes in technology and marketing. The importance of urban development in the West, long neglected, is stressed in R. C. Wade, *The Urban Frontier** (1959). M. J. Rohrbough, *The Trans-Appalachian Frontier: People, Societies, and Institutions, 1775–1850* (1978), is a good study of social conditions in the West.

G. R. Taylor, *The Transportation Revolution, 1815–1860* (1951), a general study, has much detail on internal improvements in the West. L. C. Hunter, *Steamboats on the Western Rivers* (1949), is a classic. Other valuable studies are P. D. Jordan, *The National Road* (1948); L. D. Baldwin, *The Keelboat Age on Western Waters* (1941); Carter Goodrich et al., *Canals and American Economic Development* (1961); R. E. Shaw, *Erie Water West: A History of the Erie Canal, 1792–1854* (1966); H. N. Scheiber, *Ohio Canal Era: A Case Study of Government and the Economy, 1820–1861* (1969); and E. F. Haites, J. Mak, and G. M. Walton, *Western River Transportation: The Era of Early Internal Development, 1810–1860* (1975).

THE OLD SOUTH AND SLAVERY

The best surveys of the Old South are Clement Eaton, *A History of the Old South*, 3rd ed. (1975); and Monroe Billington, *The American South* (1971). Clement Eaton, *The Growth of Southern Civiliza-*

tion* (1961), and Bertram Wyatt-Brown, *Southern Honor: Ethics and Behavior in the Old South*
(1982), are studies of Southern social and cultural life. U. B. Phillips, *Life and Labor in the Old South*
(1929), is a somewhat sentimental description of life on the plantations. Catherine Clinton, *The
Plantation Mistress: Woman's World in the Old South* (1983), is a valuable study. F. L. Owsley, *Plain
Folk of the Old South* (1949), deals almost as sentimentally with the life of nonslaveholders. E. D.
Genovese, *The World the Slaveholders Made* (1969), attempts to apply a Marxian class interpretation
to the social structure of the Old South. James Oakes, *The Ruling Race* (1982), emphasizes the
restless, acquisitive, entrepreneurial characteristics of the slaveholders. An indispensable book, based
on extensive travels in the South in the 1850s, is F. L. Olmsted, *The Cotton Kingdom* (1861). A new
edition, edited by A. M. Schlesinger, was published in 1953. Gavin Wright, *The Political Economy of
the Cotton South* (1978), is a modern economic analysis.

Slavery may be studied from several perspectives in U. B. Phillips, *American Negro Slavery** (1919);
K. M. Stampp, *The Peculiar Institution** (1956); J. W. Blassingame, *The Slave Community** (1972);
E. D. Genovese, *Roll, Jordan, Roll** (1974); L. H. Owens, *This Species of Property** (1976); and N. J.
Huggins, *Black Odyssey** (1977). Among the best books on special aspects of slavery are Frederic
Bancroft, *Slave Trading in the Old South* (1931); R. C. Wade, *Slavery in the Cities** (1964); R. S.
Starobin, *Industrial Slavery in the Old South* (1970); L. W. Levine, *Black Culture and Black Con-
sciousness** (1977); and A. J. Raboteau, *Slave Religion** (1978). C. N. Degler, *Neither Black Nor
White: Slavery and Race Relations in Brazil and the United States** (1971), is an excellent compara-
tive study. D. L. Robinson, *Slavery in the Structure of American Politics, 1765–1820** (1971), traces the
issue through a series of national debates. The best study of the Missouri Compromise is Glover
Moore, *The Missouri Controversy** (1953).

INDUSTRY AND TECHNOLOGY
Three excellent short introductions to American economic growth are W. E. Brownlee, *Dynamics of
Ascent: A History of the American Economy* (1974); Stuart Bruchey, *Growth of the Modern Ameri-
can Economy* (1975); and T. C. Cochran, *Frontiers of Change: Early Industrialism in America* (1981).
E. P. Douglass, *The Coming of Age of American Business* (1971); and Sidney Ratner, J. H. Soltow, and
Richard Sylla, *The Evolution of the American Economy* (1979), cover all fields of economic enter-
prise. L. C. Hunter, *A History of Industrial Power in the United States, 1780–1930*, Vol. I, *Waterpower
in the Century of the Steam Engine* (1979), is a major study. Books especially valuable for their
interpretations are T. C. Cochran and William Miller, *The Age of Enterprise* (1942); D. C. North, *The
Economic Growth of the United States, 1790–1860** (1961); Stuart Bruchey, *The Roots of American
Economic Growth* (1965); T. C. Cochran, *Business in American Life: A History* (1972); and R. D.
Brown, *Modernization: The Transformation of American Life, 1600–1865** (1976). H. J. Habakkuk,
*American and British Technology in the Nineteenth Century** (1962), is a penetrating analysis of the
relationship between high labor costs and mechanization. Brooke Hindle, *Emulation and Invention**
(1981) focuses on technological creativity in the development of the steamboat and the magnetic
telegraph. Nathan Rosenberg, *Technology and American Economic Growth** (1972), is an excellent
brief synthesis.

The best studies of the early textile industry are A. H. Cole, *The American Wool Manufacture*, 2 vols.
(1926); C. F. Ware, *The Early New England Cotton Manufacture* (1931); P. F. McGouldrick, *New
England Textiles in the Nineteenth Century: Profits and Investment* (1968); and D. J. Jeremy, *The
Diffusion of Textile Technologies between Britain and America, 1790–1830s* (1981). Thomas Dublin,
*Women at Work: The Transformation of Work and Community in Lowell, Massachusetts, 1826–1860**
(1979), examines the changing conditions and status of women workers. The best treatments of the
early labor movement are in J. R. Commons et al., Vol. I of *History of Labour in the United States*,
4 vols. (1918–35); and Edward Pessen, *Most Uncommon Jacksonians: The Radical Leaders of the
Early Labor Movement** (1967). The best work available on the Panic of 1819 is M. N. Rothbard, *The
Panic of 1819: Reactions and Policies* (1962).

*Available in a paperback edition.

9
POLITICS FOR THE COMMON MAN

The rapid economic growth and social change that followed the War of 1812 had a profound effect on the nation's political life. During the 1820s the death of the Federalists (see p. 196) and the subsequent fragmentation of the Republicans brought the first American party system to an end. But in the sixteen years between the presidential elections of 1824 and 1840 a new party system took shape—one that differed from the first in many crucial ways, most notably in the willingness of its leaders to abandon the eighteenth-century ideal of social harmony and to accept parties and political conflict as both inevitable and constructive. As vigorous two-party politics developed in all sections of the country—it had never before existed in the South and West—a growing number of voters turned out in national elections, and control of public affairs became less exclusively the business of prudent gentlemen from old and distinguished families. The Democratic party, under the leadership of Andrew Jackson and Martin Van Buren, made skillful and dramatic appeals to the fears, ideals, and aspirations of the common man; but the National Republicans (replaced by the Whigs in the 1830s), under the leadership of Clay and Webster, also made an effective bid for mass support and became equally adept in the use of the new political tactics. The politics of the Jacksonian era was enlivened by bitterly fought presidential contests—they were the lifeblood of the second American party system—by disputes over who were the friends and the enemies of the people, by ill-tempered conflicts between nationalists and state righters, and at times by a heightened sectionalism. Party battles were waged with intense fervor and with an unprecedented amount of demagoguery and political flimflam, each party predicting that the victory of its rival would bring disaster to the nation. Yet, though the heated rhetoric of political partisans should not be taken at face value, though party leaders were far more pragmatic and less ideological than they sometimes sounded, and though the parties tried to mute divisive sectional issues, these political wars often did involve important questions of public policy.

The New Democracy

The celebration of the Common Man. The Jacksonian era, it was once claimed, marked the "rise of the common man," a vague generalization at best and a doubtful one as well. It is true that in the 1820s and 1830s some ambitious and energetic young white men (most blacks, of course, remained in slavery) found opportunities in their thriving and still relatively fluid society to achieve material success. With economic affluence they or their children could expect soon to gain both political influence and social prestige. This was the road followed by a limited number of men

Andrew Jackson's inauguration

Village mechanic: little social mobility

who began with modest means—in effect, they emerged from the ranks of common men and pushed their way into the ranks of the élite, as Jackson himself did.

However, this evidence of social fluidity did not in any respect mark the Jacksonian era as unique. For in this sense some common men had been rising ever since the colonial period. In the years of prosperity and expansion after the War of 1812, other common men flourished and rose by engaging in manufacturing in New England and the Middle Atlantic states, or by speculating in Western lands, or by growing cotton with slave labor in Alabama and Mississippi. And long after the Jackson era had closed, a portion of the American élite continued to be recruited from the ranks of common men.

But the great majority of common men, in this era as in those that preceded and followed it, neither grew rich nor rose to high social position. Instead they managed only to make a more or less comfortable living and continued to be common men—small farmers, village mechanics, city laborers. The social mobility of Jackson's America was not remarkably great—it

may even have been less than in earlier years—and the existence of social classes was as evident at the end of the era as at the start. To be sure, a major goal stated by the Jacksonians was to remove obstacles to success and to provide equal opportunities for all to prosper materially. Nevertheless, the striking feature of the period was not social fluidity; it was the emergence of a new party system combined with certain changes in political procedures that broadened the base of American democracy and increased the influence of the common man while he *remained* a common man. More than ever before politicians were obliged to square their platforms with the desires and adapt their tactics to the tastes of a mass of ordinary voters. In consequence, the Jacksonian era was notable less for the rise than for the celebration of the Common Man—for its rhetorical equalitarianism, which honored the average voter's moral virtue and common-sense wisdom. "Never for a moment believe," said Jackson, "that the great body of the citizens . . . can deliberately intend to do wrong."

Democratic reforms. This was not the beginning of American democracy, only its expansion; nor was the expansion initiated by President Jackson, for the trend had been evident long before. Armed with the Declaration of Independence and the doctrine of natural rights, political reformers argued that they were seeking no radical innovations but merely harmonizing political practices with the principles on which the nation was founded. They claimed America was safe for political democracy because there was no sharp conflict between classes, no mass poverty, and no need for ambitious men to remake society before they could hope to improve their lot. Indeed, conservative property-holders could yield, if sometimes grudgingly, to the democratic upsurge and to the new form of mass politics without fearing that they were paving the way to their own destruction.

When, for example, political reformers urged the removal of property restrictions on the suffrage, they invariably argued that no one would be hurt. A delegate to the New York constitutional convention of 1821 agreed that if manhood suffrage would in fact impair the rights of property "this would be a fatal objection." But this was not the case: "Will not our laws continue the same? Will not the administration of justice continue the same? And if so, how is private property to suffer?" Unlike Europeans, said another delegate, "We have no different estates, having different interests, necessary to be guarded from encroachments. . . . We are all of the same estate—all commoners."

The best-remembered protest against manhood suffrage was that of Chancellor James Kent, a New York Federalist. Though Kent warned of the "tendency in the poor to covet and to share the plunder of the rich," he did not advocate the rule of a small aristocracy of large property-holders. Rather, he accepted the election of the governor and the lower house of the state legislature by manhood suffrage and asked only that the upper house be chosen by owners of freehold estates worth at least $250. In defending his position he sounded more like a Jeffersonian than a champion of a capitalist plutocracy, for he spoke of the "freeholders of moderate possessions" as the "safest guardians of property and the laws." Like Jefferson, Kent feared the propertyless "crowds of dependents connected with great manufacturing and commercial establishments, and the motley and undefinable population of crowded ports." Another New York conservative, professing "great veneration for the opinions of Mr. Jefferson," quoted his view that cities are "ulcers on the body politic," and expressed fear that manhood suffrage "would occasion political demoralization, and ultimately overthrow our government." But these conservatives frightened few and went down to overwhelming defeat.

Indeed, it is remarkable how easily the reformers carried the day—how feeble the resistance of the conservatives proved to be. The constitutions of the new Western states provided for white manhood suffrage—or at least enfranchised all taxpayers, which was almost the same thing. The Eastern states had originally restricted the suffrage to property-holders, but one by one they gave way, until, in the 1850s, the last of them, Virginia and North Carolina, adopted manhood suffrage. Only in Rhode Island did the movement for reform result in violence—in the so-called Dorr Rebellion—but even there, by 1843, the conservatives had surrendered.

Manhood suffrage alone, however, had only a minor impact on American politics until the mass of qualified voters began to take a personal interest in it. Since the Revolution, a large proportion of the voters had been apathetic; save for an occasional state election, they turned out in limited numbers and seemed willing to accept the leadership of a small political élite. To the mass of village artisans and self-sufficient farmers, both federal and state governments seemed remote, and in an age of laissez faire neither visibly affected their daily lives. Politics was the business of wealthy men who had things at stake and had the experience necessary for the management of public affairs. State and local governments, therefore, were often controlled by a few great families, who ruled through factional alliances and only occasionally faced the challenge of an aroused electorate.

But when ordinary voters became involved in the money economy as small entrepreneurs, industrial wage-earners, or farmers producing for the market, they developed a greater personal interest in questions of public policy such as the tariff, internal improvements, and banking. The shock of the Panic of 1819 and the depression that followed intensified their political concerns and shook their confidence in the old political leadership. The Virginia Dynasty came to an end in 1825; and the subsequent growth of a second American party system, which began at the state level, soon gave politics an unprecedented vitality. Eventually the new system brought two-party politics to every state, and the close political contests that occurred in most of them caused public interest to increase dramatically. Inexpensive party newspapers appeared in every town to arouse and educate the people; and the new breed of politician, skilled in the art of popular appeal, developed the business of electioneering into a unique cultural phenomenon, second only to religious revivalism in its emotional charge. These new, pragmatic political leaders came less often from the well-established American élite; they viewed politics as a profession and loyalty to party as a supreme virtue. Focusing as they did on efficient organization for the presidential campaigns, the parties were like corporations that made bids every four years for the job of administering the federal government.

It was in this new political environment that attendance at the polls began to rise. When Jackson was elected President in 1828, 56 percent of the adult white males voted, which was more than double the percentage of 1824; and in 1840, 78 percent of them voted. Since no state yet had the secret ballot, ordinary voters might still be influenced by their powerful neighbors. Nevertheless, an increasing number paid less deference to the gentry and became more independent in exercising their political rights. To be sure, voting behavior in the new party system was significantly affected by religious and ethnic affiliations and by irrational influences such as family and local traditions, appeals to party loyalty, spectacular electioneering tactics, and pure demagoguery, but local and national issues were seldom irrelevant to the decisions voters made.

Another democratic reform supposedly gave the common man a more direct role in the selection of presidential candidates. From the time of Jefferson, Federalists and Republicans had named their candidates in secret congressional caucuses. This system was used for the last time in 1824; by 1832 "King Caucus" had given way to the national nominating convention, which in theory gave the party rank and file a voice in the nominations. Meanwhile, one state after another transferred the election of presidential electors from the legislature to the voters, and by 1832 only South Carolina adhered to the old system. The states also made an increasing number of state offices elective rather than appointive.

Finally, the idea of a trained—and therefore, presumably, aristocratic—civil service was repudiated so that common men could aspire to state and federal offices as a reward for faithful party service. Party leaders "claim as a matter of right, the advantages of success," said William L. Marcy, a leader of the New York Jacksonians. "They see nothing wrong in the rule, that to the victor belong the spoils of the enemy." In its day the "spoils system" appeared to be another step toward the democratization of American politics. The anti-Jacksonians were critical of this debasing of the civil service, but when they came to power they found the system irresistible and used it with equal enthusiasm.

John Quincy Adams and National Republicanism

The election of 1824. As the end of Monroe's second term approached, a sparsely attended congressional caucus nominated Secretary of the Treasury William H. Crawford as the official Republican candidate for President. Crawford, a Virginian by birth though a resident of Georgia, was a state-rights representative of the planter class. This time, however, there were other ambitious politicians in the field—all professed Republicans—whose supporters repudiated the caucus system as undemocratic and won endorsements for their candidates from state legislatures and mass meetings. Crawford's competitors included John

Quincy Adams, the talented Secretary of State, a nationalist, and the favorite of New England; Henry Clay, Speaker of the House, champion of the American System, and a man of captivating charm; and Andrew Jackson, a military hero with wide popular appeal but, at the time, rather vague political views. With four competing candidates, each attracting somewhat different sections and interests, the Republican party quickly disintegrated as a national political organization. At the start of the campaign Crawford seemed the likely winner, but he suffered a paralytic stroke and consequently lost much of his support.

In the election Jackson won a plurality of the popular vote and ninety-nine electoral votes; he had substantial support everywhere except in New England. Adams' eighty-four electoral votes came chiefly from New York and New England, Crawford's forty-one from the Southeast, and Clay's thirty-seven from the Northwest.* Since none of the four polled a majority in the Electoral College, the choice had to be made by the House of Representatives from among the three leading candidates, with the congressional delegation from each state casting one vote. Clay, who had come in fourth, was thus eliminated from the competition, and Crawford's illness had put him out of the running. The choice was between Adams and Jackson.

Clay, because of his power in the House and his control over the three states he had carried, could swing the election either way. Jackson's friends approached Clay and argued that their man had the stronger claim, because he had polled the largest popular vote; and the Kentucky legislature instructed Clay to support the Hero of New Orleans. But Clay not only feared Jackson as a formidable competitor in Western politics but doubted that he was qualified to be President—doubted, too, that he would support the American System. Adams, meanwhile, was tortured by a conflict between his ambition to be President and his distaste for the political higgling that was required to win the prize. Eventually his ambition triumphed: he made the necessary promises and had an interview with Clay that seemed to satisfy the President-maker and win his support. Adams and Clay were as different as two men could be, and their personal relations had been far from cordial; but Adams was still the logical man for Clay to favor, because he shared Clay's views on public policy. Accordingly, when the House voted on February 9, 1825, Adams, with Clay's backing, won a clear majority on the first ballot (Adams thirteen votes, Jackson seven, Crawford four).

When President Adams subsequently appointed Clay Secretary of State, the disappointed Jacksonians immediately detected a shocking case of political

*Calhoun easily won election as Vice President.

The election of 1824

	Electoral	Popular
Adams	84	108,740
Jackson	99	153,544
Crawford	41	46,618
Clay	37	47,136

No candidate received a majority of electoral votes, and House of Representatives elected Adams.

jobbery. Adams, they claimed, had purchased Clay's support by giving him the post from which he could best hope to succeed to the Presidency. The nation's political virtue, wrote an angry Jacksonian editor, had died "of poison administered by the assassin hands of John Quincy Adams, the usurper, and Henry Clay." For the next three years the enemies of the Adams Administration charged that "bargain and corruption" had betrayed the will of the people. Though Adams doubtless had reached a political understanding with Clay, he had in fact made no corrupt bargain. But neither man ever successfully refuted the accusation. Jackson resigned his seat in the Senate, the Tennessee legislature again nominated him for the Presidency, and the political campaign of 1828 was under way almost as soon as Adams was settled in the White House.

The Adams Administration. Adams' term as President was a tragic episode in an otherwise brilliant public career, which included service as a diplomat, as Secretary of State, and in later years as a congressman from Massachusetts. Unfortunately the superb talents of this son of John Adams did not include a sensitivity to trends in public opinion or the adroitness, tact, and personal warmth essential to presidential leadership. As a result he suffered a series of political disasters. This was all the more unfortunate because Adams represented a point of view on the federal government's role in the national economy, and on its responsibilities to the states and the people, that deserved to be considered on its own merits.

The new President was a champion of national economic growth, especially of commercial and manufacturing expansion, and he looked benevolently upon the new capitalistic enterprises that were spawned by the Industrial Revolution. He was, moreover, as he made clear in his first annual message, a nationalist who believed that the Constitution gave the federal government ample power to direct and encourage this growth and to undertake numerous projects "for the common good." Adams spoke in support of the American System with as much fervor as Clay, especially when he urged the use of federal funds for internal improvements. Citing the National Road as a precedent, he asked: "To how many thousands of our countrymen has it proved a benefit? To what single individual has it ever proved an injury?" After the retirement of the public debt he urged that the proceeds from the sale of public lands be used for roads and canals to facilitate communication "between distant regions and multitudes of men." More, he proposed the building of a great national university at Washington for "moral, political, and intellectual improvement," support for explorations of the interior and of the Northwest coast, and the establishment

John Quincy Adams: scrupulous nationalist

of an astronomical observatory. Adams believed that Congress might even pass laws designed to promote "the elegant arts, the advancement of literature, and the progress of the sciences." Congress would, in fact, betray a sacred trust by not doing so. In an unfortunate phrase, often used against him, he urged Congress not to justify inaction with the excuse "that we are palsied by the will of our constituents." The time was ripe for action, said Adams confidently, for "the spirit of improvement is abroad upon this earth."

But these very sentiments prompted his critics to assail him as a tyrant and an aristocrat. Crawford found them "replete with doctrines which I hold to be unconstitutional." Jefferson accused Adams of seeking to establish "a single and splendid government of an aristocracy . . . riding and ruling over the plundered ploughman and beggared yeomanry." Congress responded to the President's proposals with little enthusiasm—even his friends thought he had gone too far—and after the congressional election of 1826 his enemies had full control of the Senate and the

House. Appropriations for internal improvements far surpassed those provided during previous administrations but fell short by a great deal of Adams' grand design. A new tariff, enacted in 1828, sponsored by both Administration and anti-Administration congressmen from the Middle and Western states, was not the judicious measure he had called for. The bill was poorly drawn, and because of its concessions to the extreme protectionists the Southern cotton interest called it the "tariff of abominations." Yet Adams signed it.

Somehow his good intentions always seemed to lead him to personal disaster. He conscientiously repudiated a fraudulent Indian treaty by which the Creeks were to be shorn of all their lands in Georgia and ordered the negotiation of a new one. But his scrupulous concern for the rights of Indians irritated both Southerners and Westerners. Worse, when the governor of Georgia defied the federal government and threatened to take jurisdiction over the disputed lands, Adams flouted the principle of state rights: he warned that it was the President's duty to vindicate federal authority "by all the force committed for that purpose to his charge." Even in foreign affairs, in spite of Adams' rich experience, the Administration failed to achieve its goals. In 1826, chiefly for partisan reasons, Congress obstructed Clay's attempt to strengthen ties with Latin America by sending delegates to a conference at Panama. Adams also failed to persuade the British to open their West Indian islands to American trade.

At home, while his foes continued their savage attack, Adams further weakened his position by spurning the role of party leader and refusing to use the patronage weapon in his own defense. Many hostile politicians continued to hold office in his Administration—among them Postmaster General John McLean, whose appointment policy seemed to be to reward the President's enemies and punish his friends. Adams was, in fact, the last of the Presidents to look upon parties as an evil and to cling to the eighteenth-century ideal of a national consensus with himself as its spokesman.

The triumph of the Jacksonians. Adams realized that his chances for reelection in 1828 were slim; "the base and profligate combination" of his critics, he wrote bitterly, would probably succeed in defeating him. During the preceding three years the anti-Administration forces had rallied around the charismatic figure of Andrew Jackson. Joining the original Jacksonians was a heterogeneous group that included most of the previous supporters of Crawford and Calhoun and others who disliked the nationalistic American System or had been alienated by the President's inept handling of public affairs and public relations.

Jackson bandanna

Though political divisions did not follow class or occupational lines, the Jacksonians seemed to win a majority of the planters and farmers in the South and West, many small entrepreneurs in all parts of the country, and a substantial number of artisans and factory workers in the towns and cities. What strength remained to Adams and the National Republicans was concentrated in the Northeast, mostly in New England.

Thinking it proper to remain aloof from electioneering, the President gave little help to those who ran his campaign. He would not "exhibit himself" to the public or in any other way actively seek a second presidential term. "If my country wants my services, she must ask for them," was his naive but altogether sincere response to those who urged more vigorous action. But his lieutenants were no match, in any case, for the Jackson organization and its able, hard-hitting leaders, the most important of whom were Senators Martin Van Buren of New York, Thomas Hart Benton of Missouri, and John H. Eaton of Tennessee; and three newspapermen: Amos Kendall and Francis Preston Blair of Kentucky and Isaac Hill of New Hampshire. These men and their associates skillfully exploited the fears and prejudices as well as the ideals of the mass electorate.

In the background of the campaign were a number of specific issues: the tariff, internal improvements, banking, land policy, and at the local level the question of bankruptcy laws and debtor-relief laws. But the politicians and party editors were usually vague on these issues, first, because they feared to divide their friends and hoped to win over the doubtful and, second, because they found other appeals that seemed better calculated to win votes. In a campaign that revolved largely around personalities, few political leaders showed much respect for the intelligence of the American electorate.

Jacksonians described the election as a contest between democracy and aristocracy. Their candidate, they said, was a man of the people who had their interests at heart. Adams was a monarchist, an enemy of the people, a parasite who had lived off the taxpayers all his life, the head of a band of rascally officeholders, an extravagant waster of public funds for his own pleasure, and the darling of the old Federalists. (Actually, many one-time Federalists supported Jackson.) Voters were also reminded of the "corrupt bargain" of 1825 and of the need to vindicate the will of the people. Friends of Adams retaliated by describing Jackson as a crude and hot-tempered frontier brawler, an inexperienced incompetent, a demagogue having no program, and totally unfitted for the responsibilities of the Presidency. At a still lower level, campaign leaders, resorting to mudslinging and character assassination, exchanged charges of pandering, adultery, and murder.

The outcome of such a campaign cannot be explained apart from its element of irrationality. Moreover, sectional feelings doubtless accounted for much of Jackson's Southern and Western support. Even so, many of those who voted for Jackson evidently had come to the conclusion that he would better protect the interests of the people against government corruption and special privilege. Though scarcely more than half the adult males went to the polls, they gave Jackson a substantial popular majority: 647,286 to 508,064. The electoral vote was 178 to 83, with Adams carrying only New England, New Jersey, Maryland, and Delaware. Observing the wild celebration in Washington on the day of Jackson's inauguration, culminating in a boisterous reception at the White House, some observers saw the start of the reign of King Mob, others the triumph of the common man. Webster remarked dryly, "People have come five hundred miles to see General Jackson, and they really seem to think that the country has been rescued from some dreadful danger."

Jacksonian Democracy

The new President. Andrew Jackson was a controversial figure in his day and has been a source of controversy among historians ever since. This may be explained in part by his own complexity, in part by the complexity of the age in which he lived, in part by the divergent expectations of those who supported him. Jackson's original appeal was not as an experienced statesman with a clear-cut program but as an enormously popular and much-loved national hero. To his admirers, Old Hickory, the Hero of New Orleans, was the embodiment of numerous American virtues and towered above the ranks of "mere" politicians. To some, his election represented a victory for the nationalistic West; to others, a victory for the state-rights South; and to still others a victory for those everywhere who would dislodge entrenched privilege from positions of power.

Above all, Jackson's supporters interpreted his victory as a vindication of the common man. Born in poverty to Scotch-Irish immigrant parents in the Carolina back country, lacking formal schooling, he had moved to Tennessee and made his own way as a lawyer, land-speculator, soldier, politician, and planter. He was the first President not to come from a well-established American family in comfortable circumstances—indeed, the first President who, by rising from a log cabin to the White House, embodied the American success story in its most romantic form. However, this does not mean that Jackson was at the time of his election still a crude and simple frontiersman, as his political enemies described him. For he had already held several public offices; he had accumulated lands and more than a hundred slaves and lived in a mansion, "The Hermitage," near Nashville; and he had been allied with affluent speculators and creditors in Tennessee politics. In fact, Jackson had entered the ranks of the gentry of the Southwest and with advancing years had become increasingly mellow and perhaps a little pompous. A visitor who met him after his inauguration reported that he had seen dukes and princes and kings, "but none of such elegance and courtliness of manners, and of so commanding presence, as were possessed by General Jackson."

The election of 1828

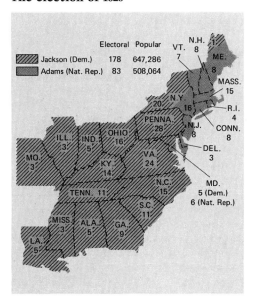

	Electoral	Popular
Jackson (Dem.)	178	647,286
Adams (Nat. Rep.)	83	508,064

N.H. 8
VT. 7
ME. 8
MASS. 15
N.Y. 20
16
R.I. 4
PENNA. 28
N.J. 8
CONN. 8
DEL. 3
ILL. 3
IND. 5
OHIO 16
VA. 24
MO. 3
KY. 14
N.C. 15
MD. 5 (Dem.) 6 (Nat. Rep.)
TENN. 11
S.C. 11
MISS. 3
ALA. 5
GA. 9
LA. 5

Nevertheless, in both background and temperament, Jackson was closer to the people than any of his predecessors had been, and his view of himself as their special defender was not a mere demagogic pose. As the one officer of the federal government chosen in a truly national election, he felt that he was in a position of peculiar responsibility. He was not intimidated by congressmen, whose acts, he felt, were too often controlled by small, selfish groups of powerful constituents, and he used his veto power more frequently than had all previous Presidents combined. Nor would Jackson agree that the Supreme Court had the final word on matters of constitutional interpretation, for he believed that the President's oath bound him to support the Constitution "as he understands it, and not as it is understood by others." Beyond being governed by the dictates of his own judgment, Jackson professed to know of no tribunal to which a public man "can appeal with greater advantage or more propriety than the judgment of the people."

In his dual role as party leader and guardian of the people's interests, Jackson promised to use his appointive power to "reform" the civil service and to make it more responsive to the public will. He would discharge all corrupt or incompetent officeholders who had acquired a "habit of looking with indifference upon the public interest" or who had come to regard their offices "as a species of property" and "a means of promoting individual interests." Long tenure in the civil service, he said, was corrupting; a rotation of civil servants every four years would force them to "go back to making a living as other people do." Jackson saw little to be gained by the experience derived from long incumbency, for in general the duties were "so plain and simple that men of intelligence may readily qualify themselves for their performance."

Jackson thus elevated the spoils system to a democratic principle, though its practical purpose was to reward loyal party workers with public offices. His rejection of an experienced civil service was not a major disaster in an age when the functions of government were relatively few and uncomplicated; but it did nothing to encourage efficiency or to increase the devotion of officeholders to the public interest. One Democrat observed with dismay that "office-seeking and office-getting was becoming a regular business, where impudence triumphed over worth." Clay indignantly described the "lank, lean, famished" Jacksonians who descended on Washington in 1829 with the cry: "Give us bread! Give us treasury pap! Give us our reward!" But Clay and other critics exaggerated the thoroughness with which Jackson applied his principle. In practice he left 80 percent of the officeholders undisturbed during his eight years as President, and at least a few of the removals were not for political reasons but for dereliction of duty.

Andrew Jackson: controversial Democrat

Though Jackson used the spoils system more freely than his predecessors, subsequent administrations, as the new party system developed, used it with far less restraint than he.

In selecting heads of departments Jackson recognized the regions and factions that had elected him. But save for Van Buren, who became Secretary of State, the men he appointed were an undistinguished lot, and he did not depend on them alone for advice. Frequently he counseled informally with a shifting group of men in whom he had confidence, among them the shrewd, talented, ambitious Van Buren; the Second Auditor of the Treasury, Major William B. Lewis of Tennessee, who lived with Jackson in the White House; Francis Preston Blair of Kentucky, who came to Washington to edit the Washington *Globe* as an Administration organ; Isaac Hill, editor of the New Hampshire *Patriot*; Roger B. Taney of Maryland, who later became Attorney General, Secretary of the Treasury, and Chief Justice of the United States; and the Fourth Auditor of the Treasury and later Postmaster General, Amos Kendall, a man of great influence, who helped Jackson prepare many of his state papers. This "kitchen cabinet," as critics called it, played an important role in the development of Administration policies and ideas.

The Jacksonian philosophy. To speak of a Jacksonian philosophy may be to dignify too much the ideas of its pragmatic leaders. The Jacksonians, of course, were never of one mind; nor were their differences with the Whigs always sharp and clear, for the two parties were not ideological opposites. In fact, they were often divided more over means than ends. Nevertheless, there was a Jacksonian way of looking at things, and much of its ideology can be found scattered unsystematically in the President's inaugural addresses, annual messages to Congress, and veto messages.

The Jacksonians lived in a more complex society than had Jefferson, and they generally favored the advances in political democracy that individual states had recently achieved. Yet, at the federal level, they were strikingly traditional and conservative on most questions of public policy. In a sense, John Quincy Adams, who had called for vigorous federal action, had endorsed a more radical program for national economic growth and social progress than they. In contrast, Jackson believed in minimal federal action and warned: "To suppose that because our government has been instituted for the benefit of the people it must therefore have the power to do whatever may seem to conduce to the public good is an error into which even honest minds are too apt to fall." Jackson repeatedly emphasized that the federal government was one of limited powers and cautioned against "overstrained constructions" of the Constitution. He would guard against "all encroachments upon the legitimate sphere of State sovereignty."

Federal intervention in the affairs of the people, Jackson believed, usually came in the form of special favors to influential minorities or of encouragement to monopolistic corporations. There would always be distinctions in society, he conceded, as a result of "superior industry, economy, and virtue . . . but when the laws undertake to add to these natural and just advantages artificial distinctions . . . and exclusive privileges, to make the rich richer and the potent more powerful, the humble members of society—the farmers, mechanics, the laborers—who have neither the time nor the means of securing like favors to themselves, have a right to complain of the injustice of their Government."

As an exponent of federal laissez faire, Jackson promised to reduce the government "to that simple machine which the Constitution created." Experience had vindicated the Founding Fathers in their decision to withhold "the power to regulate the great mass of the business and concerns of the people" and to leave them to "free enterprise . . . aided by the State sovereignties." The people would find happiness not in a "splendid government . . . but in a plain system, void of pomp, protecting all and granting favors to none."

Some Jacksonians favored this formula of state sovereignty, strict construction, and federal laissez faire because they hoped for a return to old-fashioned Jeffersonianism. On numerous occasions Jackson, unlike Adams with his enthusiasm for economic and social progress, looked back wistfully to the simpler, and presumably purer, young republic of Jefferson's day. He praised "the examples of public virtue left by my illustrious predecessors"; and, disillusioned by his own earlier speculations and resulting bankruptcy, he expressed a desire "to revive and perpetuate those habits of economy and simplicity which are so congenial to the character of republicans." Like Jefferson, Jackson described the agricultural interest as "superior in importance" to all others and the cultivators of the soil as the "best part" of the population. "Independent farmers are everywhere the basis of society and true friends of liberty."

But traditional Jeffersonian principles were already hopelessly out of date. Reducing the government's role in the economy made it harder for favored groups to win special privileges, but it also gave free rein to irresponsible entrepreneurs in a period of frantic economic activity. At best, Jackson's followers had mixed feelings about his conception of the ideal society. Many of them doubtless shared his nostalgia, but few could resist the temptations of their age. Indeed, more often than not they liked Jackson because, in one way or another, they expected him to help them get ahead in the world—and it was not Jefferson's world that interested them.

Internal Improvements and Public Lands

After his inauguration in 1829, Jackson faced a problem that every American President has faced: the problem of holding together the disparate groups that had elected him. Typical of the second American party system, the national Democratic party of Jackson's day was essentially a federation of state parties—an unstable coalition of men from many regions with differing needs and interests. Insofar as voters had favored Jackson over Adams for rational reasons, they preferred what they believed would be his stand on most, but seldom all, of the issues that concerned them. Moreover, since the Democrats were loosely organized at the national level, party discipline tended to be lax. Not even the Democratic majority in Congress shared Jackson's view on every issue, and it seldom voted as a unit. Those who differed with the President on questions of secondary importance might rebel momentarily but still remain in the party and continue their general support of the Administration. But those who differed with him on a crucial issue might break away entirely and join the opposition party. This is what actually happened to many of the men who had supported Jackson in 1828, while some of his original opponents turned to him because of his stand on one or another major issue.

The Maysville veto.   On one issue, internal improvements, Jackson was bound to antagonize either his friends in the West who favored federal support or his friends in the South and in New York and Pennsylvania who opposed it. He gave a full statement of his position in 1830 when he vetoed a bill to subsidize the construction of a sixty-mile road from Maysville on the Ohio River to Lexington, Kentucky. In this veto message, as well as in other state papers, apparently in part because of Van Buren's influence, he opposed in principle federal spending for any internal improvements. But, like Madison and Monroe, Jackson insisted that if such appropriations were to be made without a constitutional amendment, they must be for projects that were national and not local in character. The Maysville Road, he protested, had "no connection with any established system of improvements; is exclusively within the limits of a State . . . and even as far as the State is interested . . . [it gives] partial instead of general advantage." The road happened also to be in the home state of his political rival, Henry Clay.

Federal appropriations for such purposes, Jackson feared, would bring logrolling, wasteful spending, and corruption; they would lead to a consolidated government with powers so vast as to endanger the liberties of the people. It would be far better for the government, after the public debt was retired, to distribute its surplus revenues among the states and permit them to manage their own internal improvements. (At the state level the Jacksonians were anything but consistent proponents of laissez faire.) Yet, in spite of these views, Jackson did not veto all the internal-improvement bills that Congress passed, not even all that were for local projects. At most it can be said that his Maysville veto checked the acceleration of such appropriations and diminished the role of the federal government relative to that of the states. Jackson even saw to it that the completed portions of the National Road were turned over to the four states that contained them, thus enabling the federal government to escape the burden of maintenance costs. This policy gave the National Republicans an issue that they exploited in those parts of the West where the need for improved transportation influenced the political affiliations of many voters.

Land policy.   On the question of public land policy Jackson redeemed himself somewhat in the West. In general, Westerners wanted the government to encourage the rapid settlement of unoccupied lands by offering generous terms rather than to seek maximum revenue for the federal treasury. With this in mind, Senator Thomas Hart Benton of Missouri advocated a gradual reduction of the minimum price of public lands of inferior quality from $1.25 (the starting price when land was put up for auction) to 50 cents an acre, after which any lands still unsold might be given free to actual settlers. Another favorite scheme of Westerners was to permit "squatters"—that is, people who had settled on the public domain before the land was surveyed and offered for sale—to purchase at the minimum price the land they had improved. Neither the first of these schemes (called "graduation") nor the second (called "preemption") was enacted into law during Jackson's Administration, but the President clearly shared the Western point of view. In his message to Congress in 1832 he urged that "the public lands shall cease as soon as practicable to be a source of revenue." To give everyone a chance to obtain a freehold, land should be sold to settlers in small tracts at a price barely sufficient to cover the cost of surveys and clearing Indian titles. More, Jackson recommended that each new state be given that portion of the public domain that lay within its boundaries.

Easterners, especially manufacturers, hoped to slow down the westward movement and the resulting depletion of the labor supply. They strongly opposed both graduation and preemption and even looked with favor on a proposal to stop temporarily the survey and sale of new Western lands. Henry Clay, seeking a plan that would satisfy all sections, suggested that rather than giving public lands to individual Western states the proceeds from the sale of the lands should be distributed among all the states, to be used as each saw fit. In 1833 Congress passed such a bill, but the President vetoed it. Land policy thus remained an unsettled issue when Jackson left office.

Religious and Ethnic Minorities

Although President Jackson repeatedly professed his devotion to and trust in "the people" and claimed to speak for them, he never really had in mind all the people who lived within the boundaries of the United States. The idea of equality or of political rights for women interested neither him nor his political opponents. Of the country's three largest racial and religious minorities—Negroes, Indians, and Irish Catholics (the last of whom came in increasing numbers during the 1830s and 1840s)—most Jacksonian leaders showed concern only for the Irish. Because anti-foreign, especially anti-Catholic, sentiment was centered in the Whig party, recent immigrants in general and

A civilized people: Cherokee newspaper and constitution

Irish Catholics in particular voted overwhelmingly Democratic. Their votes were vital to the Jacksonian organizations in the cities of the Northeast.

In the case of the American Negroes, however, whether they were slaves or free persons held down by discriminatory state laws and a rigid caste system, Democratic leaders were at best indifferent to their condition. Jackson was not only one of the largest slaveholders in the Southwest; he was a good deal less troubled about the morality of the institution than Jefferson had been. The Jackson Administration tried to keep the divisive issue of slavery out of national politics, but the President and Postmaster General Amos Kendall showed their hostility to antislavery organizations by refusing to protect their right to use the mails to distribute their literature in the Southern states. Though race prejudice was rampant in all sections and among members of both political parties, it is still true that in the Northern states the Democrats were more aggressively anti-Negro and more prone to make demagogic, racist appeals than the Whigs. In New York State the small Negro vote was almost solidly anti-Democratic.

Indian removals.   Since Indians could not vote, neither party cared very much about them, and Indian policy caused President Jackson relatively little political trouble. Criticism of his policy was limited to a handful of humanitarians concentrated in the Northeast, most of them already affiliated with the anti-Jackson party. Jackson, to the delight of land-hungry Southerners and Westerners, vigorously enforced a plan, initiated by Jefferson and favored by both Monroe and Adams and approved by Congress, to remove all the Eastern Indian tribes to lands west of the Mississippi. Lewis Cass, a Jacksonian politician from Michigan, was certain "that the Creator intended the earth should be reclaimed from a state of nature and cultivated; . . . a wandering tribe of hunters . . . have a very imperfect possession of the country over which they roam." Removal would be better for the Indians themselves, said Jackson, because they were not only unhappy living among the whites but threatened with extinction. "Doubtless it will be painful to leave the graves of their fathers," he conceded, but we need only "open the eyes of those children of the forest to their true condition" to make them appreciate the "humanity and justice" of removal. "Rightly considered," Jackson concluded, "the policy of the General Government toward the red man is not only liberal, but generous." Federal Indian policy, President Van Buren told Congress a few years later, had been "just and friendly throughout . . . its watchfulness in protecting them from individual frauds unremitting."

These unctuous words covered a policy that was callous in its conception and often brutal in its execution. Though the President told Congress that the emigration should be voluntary, most of the tribes were more or less coerced into signing removal treaties. Usually the lands they received in the West were inferior to those they gave up; the migrations

It gives me pleasure to announce to Congress that the benevolent policy of the Government ... in relation to the removal of the Indians beyond the white settlements is approaching to a happy consummation.... Toward the aborigines of the country no one can indulge a more friendly feeling than myself, or would go further in attempting to reclaim them from their wandering habits and make them a happy, prosperous people....

Humanity has often wept over the fate of the aborigines of this country, and Philanthropy has been long busily employed in devising means to avert it, but its progress has never for a moment been arrested, and one by one have many powerful tribes disappeared from the earth. To follow to the tomb the last of his race and to tread on the graves of extinct nations excites melancholy reflections. But true philanthropy reconciles the mind to these vicissitudes as it does to the extinction of one generation to make room for another.... Nor is there anything in this which, upon a comprehensive view of the general interests of the human race, is to be regretted. Philanthropy could not wish to see this continent restored to the condition in which it was found by our forefathers. What good man would prefer a country covered with forests and ranged by a few thousand savages to our extensive Republic, studded with cities, towns, and prosperous farms...?

From Andrew Jackson, second annual message to Congress, December 6, 1830.

themselves were poorly planned and caused much suffering; and in some cases the Indians were literally driven from their old homes by military force. In 1838 a federal officer complained bitterly about the manner in which the Creek Indians in their trans-Mississippi settlements were being cheated by government contractors, noting that more than half of them were "entirely destitute." He was appalled at "the misery and wretchedness that presents itself to our view in going among these people. The fell destroyer Death last year visited nearly every house, and . . . I have witnessed entire families prostrated with sickness— not one able to give help to the other."

Only a few tribes put up organized resistance. In 1832 about a thousand Sac and Fox Indians, led by Chief Black Hawk, defiantly returned to Illinois, but militiamen and army regulars easily drove them back across the Mississippi. This so-called Black Hawk War was hardly more than a skirmish, but the resistance of the Seminoles in Florida was a good deal more formidable. In 1835 many of them, led by Chief Osceola and supported by scores of runaway slaves, rose in rebellion and thus began a costly war that dragged on into the 1840s. The highly civilized Cherokees of Georgia, on the other hand, tried resistance through legal action. When the government of Georgia refused to recognize their autonomy and threatened to seize their lands, the Cherokees took their case to the Supreme Court and won a favorable decision. Marshall's opinion for the Court majority was that Georgia had no jurisdiction over the Cherokees and no claim to

their lands. But Georgia officials, with no objection from the President, simply ignored the decision. At length the Cherokees had to leave, too, and when Jackson retired from office he counted the near-completion of Indian removals as one of his major achievements. "I feel conscious of having done my duty to my red children," he once remarked.

The Tariff and Nullification

Disaffection in South Carolina. Jackson favored a fiscal policy that, in its broad outlines, was consistent with old-fashioned Republican principles: he promised rigid economy and a swift reduction of the public debt in order to "counteract that tendency to public and private profligacy" encouraged by large federal expenditures. But on one critical issue, the tariff, he wavered. Some of his early statements gave encouragement to the protectionists—for example, in his first inaugural address he endorsed protective duties on all products "that may be found essential to our national independence." As Southern opposition increased, however, Jackson's position began to change. By 1832 he advocated a tariff designed primarily to provide the government with revenue, one that would give only "temporary and, generally, incidental protection"; and he warned manufacturers not to expect the people to "continue permanently to pay high taxes for their benefit." This shift in favor of tariff

**The Cherokee
nation on Indian
removals**

From Memorial and Protest of the Cherokee Nation, June 22, 1836.

reduction antagonized the Northern protectionists.
But when South Carolina resorted to direct action to
force a reduction of duties, Jackson denounced the
state and threatened federal action against it, thereby
alienating many Southerners who believed in free
trade and extreme state rights.

Though the tariff was never a clear-cut sectional
issue, protectionist sentiment was centered in the
North and free-trade sentiment in the South. By the
1820s the majority of rural Southerners, especially
those who grew cotton, were convinced that the protective tariff was a discriminatory tax designed, according to a public meeting in Charleston, to elevate
the manufacturing interest and thus to benefit "one
class of citizens at the expense of every other class."
Clay's American System, most Southerners now believed, gave no advantage to the South, because the
South had built few factories and because it exported
two-thirds of its cotton crop to European markets.
Southern exports, they reasoned, paid for most of the
country's imports, and the federal government supported itself chiefly by taxing this exchange—that is,
by levying duties on imports. Hence Southerners complained that they were paying more than their share of
federal taxes; and, to make matters worse, the government spent much of the income from the tariff on
internal improvements, mostly in the North. In short,
the tariff was an unjust tax on Southern farmers and
planters, one that raised the price of the manufactured
goods they consumed and thus the cost of producing
their staple crops. A policy so injurious to them, many

Southerners soon concluded, could not be constitutional. They agreed that the Constitution had empowered Congress to levy moderate duties on imports, but
the purpose was to provide the government with revenue, not to protect industry.

These were the opinions of cotton-growers everywhere, but nowhere were they so strongly held as in
South Carolina. Here a combination of economic
adversity and social anxiety caused a reaction in both
the rice- and cotton-producing districts not only
against the tariff but against nationalism generally.
Looming large in the background was the fear—widespread in this state, whose black population outnumbered the white by a considerable margin—that federal power might somehow be used to weaken or
destroy slavery. The Missouri debate had increased
the concern of white South Carolinians; and in 1822
rumors (which had some basis in fact) of a formidable
slave conspiracy, led by Denmark Vesey, a Charleston
free Negro, created a veritable frenzy. Throughout the
1820s white South Carolinians were inordinately sensitive to the slightest criticism of their peculiar institution from any source. The tariff, many said, was
only the first dangerous manifestation of federal usurpation; the same arguments that justified protection
might subsequently justify congressional emancipation.

More immediately, however, South Carolina was
in the midst of a severe economic crisis. Prior to 1819
the state had flourished, and its proud and aristocratic
planters had lived well on fortunes made from the

Plantation on the Mississippi: competition for South Carolina

Adams, and he faced it even more after the passage of the high Tariff of 1828 while he was seeking reelection with Jackson.

Calhoun and state interposition. By then Calhoun had changed his mind and adopted his state's position that the protective tariff was not only discriminatory but unconstitutional. Now, in 1828, he proposed a remedy in an essay entitled *The South Carolina Exposition and Protest*, which the state legislature published without revealing the name of its author. This document, which indicated that Calhoun had abandoned much of his earlier nationalism, proposed a way for a numerical minority, such as the South, to protect itself from obnoxious legislation adopted by the majority. His solution was nullification, or state "interposition," which he offered as a procedure less drastic than secession from the Union. He hoped that other sections would approve this remedy and thus enable him to protect the interests of the South while continuing his pursuit of the Presidency.

Calhoun was an able student of political theory and a skillful logician. The premises on which he based his doctrine of nullification, however, were not altogether original, for he borrowed much from Madison's and Jefferson's Virginia and Kentucky Resolutions of 1798 (see p. 162). As they had, Calhoun argued that before 1787 the states had been completely sovereign and that in framing and ratifying the new Constitution they had not given up their sovereignty. Rather, the states had merely formed a "compact" among themselves and created the federal government as their "agent" to execute it. This agent had only limited powers, and the sovereign states, not the Supreme Court, were the judges of what powers had been delegated to it.

From these premises Calhoun concluded that if Congress exceeded its delegated powers by enacting, say, a protective tariff, any one of the states might interpose state authority to block enforcement of the law. To accomplish this, the people of a state would elect delegates to a state convention; if the convention decided that the act in question was unconstitutional, it would declare the act null and void within the state's boundaries. Congress might then choose between acquiescing in nullification or proposing a constitutional amendment specifically granting to the government the desired power. Thus whenever a single state challenged the constitutionality of an act of Congress, the cumbersome amending process, requiring ratification by three-fourths of the states, would be the government's only recourse. This system, thought Calhoun, would safeguard sufficiently the interests of the minority South. True democracy, he said, was not the rule of an absolute, or numerical, majority, for such a majority could ride roughshod over the rights

cultivation of rice and cotton. But the Panic of 1819 and the subsequent depression were cruel blows, for they brought a sharp decline in cotton prices—a decline that hit South Carolina planters with exceptional force. Facing the competition of the new cotton states in the Southwest, South Carolinians found production costs on their long-used lands relatively high and their crop yield per acre and profit margin correspondingly low. Charleston's commercial interests were languishing, and the state's population had almost stopped growing as farmers moved west in search of better land. Economic troubles, along with worries about slavery and the security of the white race, caused political unrest and a swing to extreme state rights.

The majority of white South Carolinians had a simple explanation for their plight. Not soil depletion, not the competition of the Southwest, but the high tariff and other discriminatory federal legislation, they said, were to blame. They looked suspiciously at their leading politician, John C. Calhoun, who had supported the Tariff of 1816 (see p. 194) and still in the early 1820s appeared to be a nationalist and protectionist. To have a political future in his state Calhoun had no choice but to revise his views; to advance his ambitions in national politics he had to find some remedy that would satisfy the South without alienating all his friends in the North and West. He faced this challenge while he was still Vice President under of minorities. Instead, he proposed rule by the "concurrent" majority, with the people of each state having a veto over federal legislation. Minority rights would thereby be protected, and only legislation beneficial to all sections would be enacted.

Calhoun's defense of state sovereignty, which could have been used to justify the secession of a state as easily as state nullification of a federal statute, profited both from the ambiguity of the Constitution on the nature of the Union created in 1787 and from the equally ambiguous position of those who supported it in the debates over ratification. His case was further strengthened by numerous assertions of state sovereignty and threats of secession during the previous four decades as well as by the failure of the nationalists to advance a full and systematic counterargument in support of national supremacy and the Union's perpetuity. Indeed, the formulation of an elaborate doctrine of perpetuity had to await the threat to the Union posed by Calhoun's *Exposition and Protest* and by the reckless talk of secession emanating from South Carolina. During the resulting crisis a host of politicians and constitutional scholars—among them, Webster, John Quincy Adams, Associate Justice Joseph Story, and James Madison (who denied that his resolutions of 1798 justified nullification)—formulated the case for a perpetual Union and against the right of a state either to nullify an act of Congress or to secede.

The doctrine of nullification had a full review in the United States Senate early in 1830 during a debate that began over public land policy but soon centered on the nature of the federal Union. Robert Y. Hayne of South Carolina and Webster of Massachusetts, both brilliant orators, were the chief contestants, while Vice President Calhoun listened carefully as presiding officer of the Senate. Hayne explained and defended the doctrine of nullification, enumerated his section's grievances, appealed to the West to join the South in resisting the avarice of the Northeast, and reminded New Englanders that they themselves had toyed with both nullification and secession during the War of 1812. Webster, now an intense nationalist, denied that the Constitution was a mere compact to be interpreted as individual states might please. The people, not the states, had created it, and the Supreme Court was the proper authority to settle disputes over its meaning. Nor was the federal government simply an agent of the states; in exercising its powers it was sovereign and acted directly on the people. "It is," he said, "the people's Constitution, the people's government, made for the people, made by the people, and answerable to the people." The Union was not a voluntary federation of sovereign states; rather, it was older than the states—in fact, had created them—and it was intended to be perpetual. Any attempt to dismember it would be trea-

sonable and would lead to civil war. There may have been flaws in Webster's logic and in his history, but he understood better than Hayne the direction of events and the views of the majority. The South sympathized with Hayne's expression of its grievances, but outside South Carolina few Southerners at that time showed sympathy for the extreme remedy of nullification.

The cold response of Congress to the doctrine of nullification disappointed Calhoun, but the vigorous response of President Jackson produced a major crisis in Calhoun's political career. Jackson had a deep respect for the rights of the states, and he was now convinced that Southerners had reason to complain about the existing tariff; but to talk of nullification or secession, as South Carolinians did, was another matter. Soon after the Webster-Hayne debate, at a public banquet, Jackson rose, looked squarely at Calhoun, and proposed his famous toast: "Our *Federal* Union—*It must be preserved.*" This incident was only one of numerous signs of a growing rift between the President and the Vice President, a rift that Secretary of State Van Buren encouraged in his effort to supersede Calhoun as Jackson's successor to the Presidency. Even a petty social tiff among Administration wives contributed to Calhoun's downfall. Mrs. Calhoun, a South Carolina aristocrat, snubbed the wife of the Secretary of War, Peggy Eaton, the attractive, flirtatious, twice-married daughter of a Washington tavern-keeper. Jackson, still bitter about gossip concerning a previous marriage and divorce of his own recently deceased wife, had no patience for this kind of snobbery, and Van Buren, a widower, made it clear that he shared the irritated President's admiration for Mrs. Eaton. Meanwhile, Calhoun's enemies let Jackson know that back in 1818, Calhoun, as Secretary of War, had denounced Jackson for his high-handed invasion of Florida. Explanations were offered and rejected. In 1831 there was a Cabinet reorganization, and Calhoun's friends were forced out of the Administration. Van Buren was now Jackson's candidate to succeed him, and Calhoun found himself pushed more and more out of his role of national leadership into the position of chief defender of the South.

The nullification crisis. The doctrine of nullification was put to the test in 1832, when Congress passed a new tariff bill that conceded little to the Southern demand for lower duties. After Jackson signed the bill, South Carolina's congressmen sent an address to their constituents stating that "all hope for relief from Congress is irrecoverably gone," and Calhoun now openly announced his support of nullification. The nullifiers won control of the South Carolina legislature, and when it met in October it ordered the election of delegates to a state convention. On November 24, 1832, the convention, by an overwhelming major-

John C. Calhoun: in defense of the minority South

The great and leading principal is, that the General Government emanated from the people of the United States, forming distinct political communities, and acting in their separate and sovereign capacity, and not from all the people forming one aggregate political community; that the Constitution of the United States is, in fact, a compact, to which each State is a party.... Stripped of all its covering, the naked question is, whether ours is a federal or a consolidated government; a constitutional or absolute one; a government resting ultimately on the solid basis of the sovereignty of the States or on the unrestrained will of a majority; a form of government, as in all other unlimited ones, in which injustice, and violence, and force must finally prevail. Let it never be forgotten that, where the majority rules without restriction, the minority is the subject; and that, if we should absurdly attribute to the former the exclusive right of construing the Constitution, there would be, in fact, between the sovereign and subject, under such a government, no Constitution, or, at least, nothing deserving the name, or serving the legitimate object of so sacred an instrument.

From John C. Calhoun, Fort Hill Address, July 26, 1831.

ity, adopted an ordinance that pronounced the tariffs of 1828 and 1832 "unauthorized by the Constitution" and therefore "null, void, and no law, nor binding upon this State, its officers or citizens." The ordinance prohibited state or federal officers from enforcing the tariff laws in South Carolina after February 1, 1833, forbade appeals to federal courts, and warned that any federal attempt to coerce the state would force it to secede from the Union. At this juncture Hayne resigned from the Senate to become governor of South Carolina, and Calhoun resigned as Vice President to take Hayne's place and lead the fight on the Senate floor. The tariff issue had precipitated a serious national crisis.

But South Carolina's position was an uncomfortable one, for no other Southern state was then prepared to approve its radical action. An angry President, vowing that he would "die with the Union," threatened to hang Calhoun; he sent a warship and revenue cutters to Charleston harbor, and he announced his readiness to take the field personally in case of a clash of arms. In a proclamation to the people of South Carolina, Jackson made the strongest possible case for the supremacy of the federal government in the exercise of its constitutional powers and for the perpetuity of the Union, and he warned the nullifiers of the serious consequences of their action. As President he had no choice but to see that the laws of the United States were executed, for his duty was "emphatically pronounced in the Constitution."

Tension increased when the legislature of South Carolina defiantly replied that Jackson's views were "erroneous and dangerous" and that the state would "repel force by force." It increased further when Congress considered a "force bill" authorizing the President, if necessary, to use the army and navy to enforce the laws. Yet Jackson hoped to avoid violence except as a last resort, and South Carolina politicians, feeling their isolation, were eager to find a way to escape from their predicament without losing face. At length Henry Clay came forward with a compromise tariff, the details of which he had worked out in consultation with Calhoun. It provided that tariff schedules would be gradually reduced over a period of nine years, until by 1842 no duty would exceed 20 percent. On March 1, 1833, Congress passed both the compromise tariff and the force bill, and Jackson signed them. On March 15, the South Carolina convention accepted the compromise and withdrew its nullification of the tariff; but, yielding nothing in principle, it solemnly declared the force bill null and void. Since the crisis had passed, Jackson had the good sense to overlook this final petulant gesture.

Though Jackson irritated both the uncompromising protectionists and the state-rights followers of Calhoun, most nationalists praised him for his firm support of the Union; in subsequent sectional crises they remembered him fondly for his bold action against the nullifiers. At the same time, even though most Southerners rejected nullification, the fight over the tariff made them more conscious than ever before of their minority position. Looking back at the tariff crisis, Chancellor Harper of South Carolina was pessimistic about the future:

It is useless and impracticable to disguise the fact that the South is a permanent minority, and that there is a *sectional* majority against it—a major-

Andrew Jackson on nullification

The ordinance is founded ... on the strange position that any one State may not only declare an act of Congress void, but prohibit its execution; that the true construction of that instrument permits a State to retain its place in the Union and yet be bound by no other of its laws than those it may choose to consider as constitutional.... But reasoning on this subject is superfluous when our social compact, in express terms, declares that the laws of the United States, its Constitution, and treaties made under it are the supreme law of the land, and, for greater caution, adds "that the judges in every State shall be bound thereby, anything in the constitution or laws of any State to the contrary notwithstanding." And it may be asserted without fear of refutation that no federative government could exist without a similar provision....

If the doctrine of a State veto upon the laws of the Union carries with it internal evidence of its impractical absurdity, our constitutional history will also afford abundant proof that it would have been repudiated with indignation had it been proposed to form a feature in our Government....

I consider, then, the power to annul a law of the United States, assumed by one State, incompatible with the existence of the Union, contradicted expressly by the letter of the Constitution, unauthorized by its spirit, inconsistent with every principle on which it was founded, and destructive of the great object for which it was formed.

From Andrew Jackson, Proclamation to the People of South Carolina, December 10, 1832.

ity of different views and interests and little common sympathy. . . . We are divided into slave-holding and non-slave-holding states; and . . . this is the broad and marked distinction that must separate us at last.

The Bank War

Criticism of the Bank. Before the controversy over the tariff and nullification had been resolved, Congress and the Administration were engaged in an equally bitter dispute over whether the charter of the Bank of the United States should be renewed when it expired in 1836. Jackson had been hostile to the Bank long before he became President, criticized it repeatedly during his first term in office, made it a major target in his campaign for a second term, and gave it so much attention after his reelection that he seemed almost obsessed with a desire to destroy it. To many Jacksonians the future of the Bank was by far the most crucial national issue, for opposition to it went to the very heart of their philosophy; and Jackson himself doubtless counted his ultimate victory over "the Monster" his greatest single accomplishment. To his critics, however, the destruction of the Bank was a major blunder, a singularly irresponsible exercise of presidential power that did incalculable harm to the country.

After a shaky start this powerful financial institution had settled down to become, in the decade after the Panic of 1819, a conservative, prosperous, and reasonably responsible business enterprise. Since 1823, the president of the Bank had been Nicholas Biddle, an aristocratic, cultivated, and talented Philadelphian, whose acumen as a banker was unfortunately matched by his ineptitude in dealing with politicians. Many of his admiring contemporaries credited him with developing the Bank and its twenty-nine branches into an effective regulator of the expanding American economy. The Bank marketed government bonds and served as a reliable depository for government funds; it was an important source of credit for the business community; its bank notes provided the country with a sound paper currency; it forced the state banks to back their notes with adequate specie reserves and thus helped to create confidence in the entire banking system of the United States. The source of its power was its control of one-fifth of the bank notes and one-third of the bank deposits and specie of the country.

But it was in part the Bank's vast economic power that made it so vulnerable politically, for many Jacksonians believed that democracy was in peril when so much power was concentrated in a single corporation. During the 1820s Biddle ran the Bank with considerable restraint, but he tactlessly admitted to a congressional committee that most state banks might have

Defense of the Bank

The national bank, though not properly a political institution, is one of the most important and valuable instruments that are used in the practical administration of the government.... As the fiscal agent of the executive, it has exhibited a remarkable intelligence, efficiency, energy, and above all, INDEPENDENCE. This ... has been its real crime. As the regulator of the currency, it has furnished the country with a safe, convenient and copious circulating medium, and prevented the mischiefs that would otherwise result from the insecurity of the local banks. As a mere institution for loaning money, it has been ... the Providence of the less wealthy sections of the Union.... Through its dealings in exchange at home and abroad, the bank has materially facilitated the operations of our foreign and domestic trade. The important advantages which have thus been derived from this institution have been unattended by any countervailing evil. As its term advanced, and its officers acquired additional experience, it has been constantly gaining on the public favor.

From the Boston *Daily Advertiser*, September 1832.

been "destroyed by an exertion of the powers of the [United States] Bank." Moreover, its control over the supply of short-term credit was not subjected to sufficient government regulation. Its charter did not assign to it the public responsibilities of a central bank, as did the legislation creating the Federal Reserve System a century later. Instead, this Bank was responsible primarily to its own investors, and its chief function was to earn dividends for them. Many state bankers resented it not only because it forced them to maintain adequate specie reserves but because its federal charter gave it a considerable competitive advantage.

Senator Benton complained that it was to this privileged monopoly that "the Federal Government, the State Governments, and great cities, must, of necessity, apply, for every loan which their exigencies may demand." Biddle's enemies also accused him of corrupting the nation's political life, because many influential politicians and editors were indebted to the Bank for loans. Webster was not only a heavy borrower but was on the Bank's payroll as a legal counsel. "I believe my retainer has not been renewed or *refreshed* as usual," he once wrote to Biddle. "If it be wished that my relation to the Bank should be continued, it may be well to send me the usual retainer."

Thus, by the time Jackson became President the Bank had incurred the hatred of numerous groups for either practical or ideological reasons. Curiously, it antagonized both those who favored "soft money" (more state-bank notes) and those who favored "hard money" (only gold and silver coins). The former included some state banking interests, land-speculators, and small entrepreneurs who felt that their needs were best served by an abundant paper currency. The

latter included Eastern workingmen who resented receiving their wages in paper of uncertain value, and those who, like Senator Benton, considered any currency other than gold and silver dishonest. The hard-money advocates were hostile to banks of any kind, state or national, that issued bank notes; they tended to look upon banking as a parasitic enterprise. Among them was Jackson, who once told Biddle, "I do not dislike your Bank any more than all banks." By using gold and silver in ordinary business transactions, he told Congress, the country would avoid "those fluctuations in the standard of value which render uncertain the reward of labor."

Veto of the Bank bill. Jackson's first message to Congress, in which he questioned "both the constitutionality and the expediency of the law creating this bank," left little doubt that he would veto any bill to recharter it. To be sure, the Supreme Court had already affirmed the constitutionality of the Bank, but to Jackson this was irrelevant. "I have read the opinion of John Marshall," he said, "and could not agree with him."

Biddle, in his campaign to save the Bank, could not avoid getting deeply involved in national politics. He had started as a Jeffersonian Republican and had tried to appease Jackson by appointing some of his supporters to directorships of the branch banks. But Jackson's hostility drove Biddle into the camp of the opposition, and Biddle's loans to congressmen and newspaper editors became increasingly motivated by politics. At length, in 1832, he took the advice of Clay and Webster and applied for a new charter, though the old one would not expire for four more years. Clay assured Biddle that Congress would pass the bill, and he was ready to make a presidential veto an issue in the coming campaign. The bill to recharter the Bank, amended to meet some of Jackson's objections, easily passed both houses of Congress with the support of a substantial minority of the Democrats. Jackson accepted the challenge. "The Bank," he told Van Buren, "is trying to kill me, *but I will kill it.*"

Jackson's veto message, a powerful political document, maintained that the Bank was unconstitutional in spite of the proposed changes in its charter and described the dangers of "such a concentration of power in the hands of a few men irresponsible to the people." Much of the stock was held by foreigners, "and the residue is held by a few hundred of our own citizens, chiefly of the richest class." Their demands for "grants of monopolies and special privileges" had "arrayed section against section, interest against interest, and man against man, in a fearful commotion which threatens to shake the foundations of the Union." Webster bitterly denounced the President for executive usurpation and for demagogically seeking "to inflame the poor against the rich," but the veto stood and became a central issue in the presidential election of 1832. Indeed, Clay, Biddle, and the National Republicans helped to make it so by giving the veto message wide circulation, mistakenly thinking that it would serve to discredit Jackson. Whatever the weaknesses of its reasoning, however it may have exposed Jackson's limitations as a student of money and banking, the election showed that Jackson and his advisers, Kendall and Van Buren, knew how to reach the ordinary voter better than their opponents.

Jackson vindicated. The campaign of 1832 was notable not only for its vindication of Jackson but for two political innovations: the appearance of the first national third party, the Anti-Masonic party, and the holding of the first national nominating conventions. The new party, like so many third parties, at first focused on a single issue: opposition to the Society of Freemasons and to secret societies in general. The party's strength was concentrated in the rural districts of New England and the Middle Atlantic states, especially western New York, where its supporters objected to the secrecy, exclusiveness, and allegedly undemocratic character of these societies. In 1826 William Morgan of Batavia, New York, a former Mason who was about to publish an exposure of the secrets of Freemasonry, suddenly vanished, and a deep and widespread conviction developed that members of the society had murdered him. The resulting popular indignation, intensified by the apparent attempt of influential Masons to block an investigation, eventually took the form of a political movement designed to drive the "grand kings" of Freemasonry out of public office. In September 1831 the Anti-Masonic party held a national convention at Baltimore and nominated William Wirt of Maryland for President, the first candidate to be selected in this fashion. The new party, in spite of its democratic assaults on a presumably privileged group, was essentially anti-Jacksonian—Jackson was himself a Mason—and in a short time most of its leaders joined the National Republicans.

Wirt hoped to win the nomination of the National Republicans, too, but in December 1831 this party held its own convention in Baltimore and nominated Henry Clay for President and John Sargeant of Pennsylvania for Vice President. The Democrats also met in Baltimore, in May 1832, but Jackson had already been renominated by numerous local conventions, and a party platform seemed superfluous. All that remained was to nominate a candidate for Vice President, and Jackson saw to it that his choice, Van Buren, was selected.

National Republicans attacked Jackson for abusing the patronage and the veto power, endorsed Clay's American System, and boldly demanded the rechartering of the Bank, but to no avail. Jackson was then at the peak of his popularity, and with Wirt taking votes away from Clay the outcome of the campaign was never in doubt. Jackson won by a comfortable majority in the popular vote, and in the Electoral College he polled 219 votes to Clay's 49. Wirt carried only Vermont, while the disaffected leaders of South Carolina gave their state to John Floyd of Virginia. To Jackson the significance of the election was clear: he had been given a mandate to press his war against the Bank of the United States until this "Hydra of corruption" had been destroyed.

The Bank destroyed. Nicholas Biddle was not yet ready to surrender. "This worthy President," he said, "thinks that because he has scalped Indians and imprisoned judges, he is to have his way with the Bank. He is mistaken." So the battle went on, and in its final phase the friends and enemies of the Bank fought so recklessly that they impaired the stability of the entire American economy.

Jackson refused to wait for the Bank's charter to expire, for he feared that Biddle might still use the Bank's political and economic power to buy a new charter from Congress. Soon after the election Jackson decided to deprive the Bank of federal support for its financial operations by ceasing to use it as a depository for government funds. He justified his decision by accusing the Bank of "misconduct," charging that it had attempted to influence the outcome of the election by playing on "the distress of some and the fear of others"—a charge that a special congressional committee failed to sustain. Jackson had to remove two uncooperative Secretaries of the Treasury before he found a man in complete sympathy with his scheme: Roger B. Taney, the former Attorney General. Taney accomplished the gradual removal of federal funds from the Bank simply by paying government expenses from existing deposits and by refusing to place current revenues in its vaults. Those revenues were now distributed among numerous state banks—eventually, eighty-nine of them—which critics called "pet banks." The use of state banks of varying degrees of soundness was, as Jackson himself admitted, an unsatisfactory expedient subject to strong political pressures.

Jackson's enemies struck back hard. In a hostile Senate Clay mustered a majority in 1834 to pass a resolution censuring the President for (among other things) removing the deposits and thus assuming power "not conferred by the constitution and the laws." Jackson responded with a message accusing the Senate of usurping the power of impeachment, and privately he vowed one day to "bring that rascal [Clay] to dear account." Not until 1837 were indignant Jacksonian partisans able to get this resolution expunged from the Senate record. Meanwhile, as federal deposits diminished, Biddle began calling in the Bank's loans and contracting credit, in part to protect

himself and in part as a form of economic coercion to force the government to return the deposits and renew the charter. The resulting credit shortage brought delegations of businessmen to Washington to petition for relief. But the angry President told them to "go to Biddle." "I never will restore the deposits," he vowed, "I never will recharter the United States Bank, or sign a charter for any other bank, so long as my name is Andrew Jackson." At length the businessmen turned against Biddle and forced him to relax his credit policy, but not before he had managed to increase his unpopularity and thus to destroy even the faint hope that a drastically revised federal charter could be obtained. In 1836 Biddle received a charter from the state of Pennsylvania, which enabled the Bank to continue in business until 1841, when, because of economic depression and unwise speculations, it was finally forced to close its doors.

The Bank war was over, and Jackson's victory was complete. The anti-Jacksonians fumed at his highhanded tactics; they spoke indignantly of the "reign of King Andrew I"; they renamed themselves the "Whigs" in imitation of the British party that, in the eighteenth century, had sought to reduce the power of the monarch; and they formed a loose coalition of those who opposed the Administration. In 1836, in their extremity, they held no national convention and drew up no platform; still lacking effective national party leadership, they ran not one but three presidential candidates: Webster to appeal to New England, Hugh Lawson White of Tennessee to appeal to the South, and General William Henry Harrison of Ohio to appeal to the West. The Whigs hoped thus to throw the election into the House of Representatives, where they might unite behind a single candidate. The Democrats held a convention at Baltimore, dutifully nominated Van Buren, and presented him on Jackson's record without a formal platform. In the election Van Buren won by a slim majority in the popular vote and by 170 electoral votes to 124 for his several opponents.

Panic and Depression

Economic crisis. Jackson remained in Washington to witness Van Buren's inauguration, and Benton observed that "the rising was eclipsed by the setting sun." It was not easy to follow the dynamic Jackson into the Presidency, not even for Van Buren, whose political adroitness had earned him the title of "the Little Magician." Like Jackson, this New Yorker was a self-made man from a rural family of modest means. After a successful law career that gave him financial independence, Van Buren turned to state politics and,

Plain Sewing: Clay tries to silence Jackson

fully exploiting the state's political patronage, soon became the leader of an efficient Republican machine called the Albany Regency. A career politician who relished the give-and-take of political life, he was a founder of the second American party system and a defender of parties as "inseparable from free governments" and "highly useful to the country." Following the presidential campaign of 1824, when he supported Crawford, Van Buren linked his political fortunes with Jackson's and rose with him, while helping to shape and define Jacksonian principles. But Van Buren was a pale copy of his chief: he lacked Jackson's forcefulness and popular appeal and had to rely on his tact and his skill in the management of men. Unfortunately neither these talents nor the Jacksonian philosophy enabled him to cope with the serious economic problems that beset the nation while he was President. Jackson was fortunate to have left office when he did, for within two months the country plunged into a panic and soon after into a major depression. Van Buren thus had the misfortune of being remembered as a "depression President."

During Jackson's two Administrations, except for the brief "Biddle panic" of 1833–34, the country enjoyed a period of glorious prosperity and unprecedented economic expansion. Southerners found seemingly limitless markets for their cotton at good prices, and planters and slaves poured into the states of the Southwest to open up vast new cotton lands. Between 1831 and 1836, because of rising prices and expanded production, the value of cotton exports trebled. In the West farmers, also finding ample markets and enjoying high prices, continued to be drawn into the spreading money economy. Western cities experienced a phenomenal growth as they developed commercial facilities and manufacturing enterprises to serve local needs. In the Northeast merchants prospered from the flourishing cotton trade, and manufacturers expanded to supply their growing Southern and Western markets. Land prices shot up as speculation once again became a national mania; between 1834 and 1836 the speculators were responsible for a fivefold increase in government land sales. Meanwhile, the states and private entrepreneurs undertook ambitious canal and railroad projects. In the years between 1830 and 1838 state debts increased by nearly $150 million, two-thirds of which were spent for internal improvements.

Funds for this economic activity came from British capitalists, who assumed that investments in state bonds were as safe as investments in federal bonds, and from the multiplying state banks and other domestic investors. Between 1829 and 1837 the number of state banks more than doubled, their note issues trebled, and their loans quadrupled. In an economically "underdeveloped" country with a rapidly growing population, much of this business activity was healthy. But some of it was reckless and speculative—and the economy now lacked even the modest control that the Bank of the United States had once exercised.

Before Van Buren took office, the Jackson Administration, besides trying to divorce the government from business, had adopted fiscal policies that probably intensified the crisis when it came. First, as Jackson himself observed, the deposit of federal funds in numerous "pet banks" tended to multiply state-chartered banks and "had a great agency in producing a spirit of wild speculation." Though most state banks maintained adequate specie reserves, some indulged in "wildcat financiering" by recklessly expanding their note issues and by making loans without demanding adequate collateral. Speculators borrowed paper of dubious value from these institutions and gave it to the government land offices for new lands; the government in turn deposited the paper in the "pet banks," which made the money available again for further speculation. This was a happy situation for those who favored soft money, but it distressed the hard-money advocates who, as Benton said, had not joined "in putting down the paper currency of a national bank in order to put up a paper currency of a thousand local banks." Jackson shared this point of view and, in July 1836, suddenly intervened with his so-called Specie Circular. In the future, he ordered, federal land offices would accept only gold and silver in payment for public lands. This was a severe blow to the speculators, and for a time land sales almost ceased and inflated land prices dropped precipitously.

Next, the Congress, with Jackson's approval, gave an enormous stimulus to costly internal-improvement projects launched by the states. In 1836, with the federal government out of debt and with a treasury surplus of almost $40 million, an act provided that beginning on January 1, 1837, the surplus above $5 million was to be distributed among the states in proportion to population in four quarterly installments. Many states, assuming that they would receive a similar subsidy each year and ignoring the fact that the federal funds were intended to be only a loan, immediately designed ambitious projects that exceeded the limits of their own resources. At the same time, the act deprived the "pet banks" of the bulk of their federal deposits and, in consequence, obliged them to call in their loans from private borrowers.

But the economic crisis had causes more fundamental than federal fiscal policy. For example, most of the inflation that preceded it was caused not by the expansion of state bank notes but by a substantial increase in specie imports, some of it from Great Britain and France but most of it from Mexico; by a decline of specie exports to the Far East; and by Brit-

Martin van Buren: hard-money advocate

ish credits that permitted the purchase of British goods at high prices without the loss of specie. Under these circumstances, in a period of prosperity and free spending, the country sustained a considerable international balance-of-payments deficit. When, eventually, Great Britain suffered from hard times, British investors began to withdraw their support of American economic expansion; and the British demand for American cotton began to decline just as the opening of new Western lands caused a sharp increase in the supply. Business conditions in the United States had been deteriorating for some months, but the real panic began in May 1837, when New York banks, soon followed by banks in the rest of the country, suspended specie payments. It was at this point that the Bank of the United States was missed, for its destruction reduced confidence in the whole banking system, thus stimulating runs on state banks. The state banks in turn were forced to curtail loans in an effort to increase their specie reserves.

The Panic of 1837 was followed by a brief period of economic recovery, but in 1839 the collapse of cotton and other agricultural prices and the decline of foreign investments brought on one of the most severe depressions in American history. Banks and business houses failed by the hundreds, factories closed and unemployment mounted, cotton sold for as low as 6 cents a pound (more than a 50 percent drop from the early 1830s), internal-improvement projects were abandoned, and some states, their credit exhausted, either stopped payments on their debts or repudiated them outright. Recovery did not come until the middle of the 1840s.

The Independent Treasury. Understanding of the causes of business cycles had advanced very little since the depression following the Panic of 1819—President Van Buren attributed the present crisis to "overbanking" and "overtrading." The idea that government might give assistance to distressed farmers, workers, and businessmen was not yet considered. In so far as the government did react to the crisis, it adopted fiscal policies that served to deepen the depression and heighten economic distress. Distribution of funds to the states for internal improvements was stopped, federal spending was curtailed, and the President concentrated on getting the government out of debt. Van Buren also rejected pleas for the withdrawal of the Specie Circular and continued the hard-money policy of his predecessor; he scorned the argument that the crisis justified the chartering of a new national bank. He thus identified himself with the radical, or Locofoco,* wing of his party—the extreme hard-money, antibank, antimonopoly faction that was especially strong among workingmen and reformers in his own state of New York.

One aim of the Locofocos was to divorce the federal government from banking altogether by denying all private banks the use of federal deposits. Van Buren urged such a step repeatedly, and finally, in 1840, Congress passed the Independent Treasury Act. This act authorized the establishment of subtreasuries in various cities where government funds could be placed in vaults for safekeeping. Although this system insured the government from loss, it made economic recovery more difficult, because it deprived the banks of funds that otherwise could have been used for private loans.

Banking was now entirely in the hands of the states. A few, notably New York and the New England states, managed to establish reasonably satisfactory and responsible state banking systems; a couple of Western states adopted the Locofoco philosophy and for a time abolished banking altogether. In many states the Jacksonians established "free banking" systems, which enabled promoters to secure a bank charter without a special act of the legislature. Free banking and so-called general incorporation laws were important aspects of Jacksonian Democracy at the state level. By eliminating the need for small entrepreneurs to have political influence in order to obtain state charters, these laws were expected to provide equal opportunities for all.

---

*"Locofoco" was a popular name for the newly invented friction matches. Radical New York Democrats once carried candles and "locofocos" to a party meeting, because they feared that the conservatives would try to break it up by turning off the gaslights. This incident explains how the Locofocos got the name.

Hard Times: the Panic of 1837

The election of 1840. As the presidential campaign of 1840 approached, the country was still deep in economic depression; the Democrats were bound to lose the support of many voters who would express their discontent by turning against the party in power. The Democratic national convention at Baltimore was a gloomy affair. The delegates renominated Van Buren unanimously, but with restrained enthusiasm, and adopted a platform reaffirming the party position on state rights, banking, internal improvements, and the Independent Treasury. The Democrats were on the defensive throughout the campaign.

The Whigs, however, were in an optimistic mood when their convention assembled at Harrisburg, Pennsylvania. Having been branded the enemies of the common man, a party of aristocrats and monopolists, having endured a succession of humiliating defeats, they now looked forward to giving the Democrats some of their own medicine. They had already attributed the depression to Democratic fiscal measures, charged that the Independent Treasury scheme was a callous attempt of the government to protect itself without regard for the welfare of the country, and accused Van Buren of indifference to the suffering of the people. Now, with a far more efficient party organization, having learned much from the tactics of their enemies and from their own mistakes, they prepared to out-Jackson the Jacksonians in a bid for popular support. The Whigs passed over Clay in favor of a military hero: William Henry Harrison of Ohio, who had defeated the Indians at the Battle of Tippecanoe and the British at the Battle of the Thames. With an eye on the South, they nominated John Tyler of Virginia, a conservative state-rights Whig, for the Vice Presidency. They adopted no platform, for the campaign they planned was to have little relevance to concrete issues.

The campaign was something less than edifying. Though Harrison was descended from an aristocratic Virginia family and lived as an Ohio country gentleman in a sixteen-room mansion, the Whigs transformed "Old Tippecanoe" into a simple frontier farmer and man of the people. When a blundering Democratic editor sneered that Harrison would be satisfied to retire to a log cabin with a barrel of hard cider, the Whigs happily accepted the statement as true. They praised his simple tastes, made log cabins and cider barrels their party symbols, and boasted of their own log-cabin backgrounds. (Webster apologized for not having been born in one.) The Whigs de-

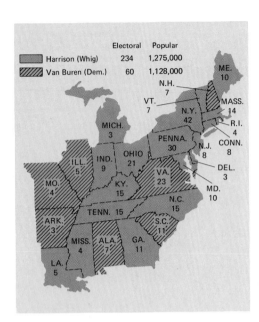

	Electoral	Popular
Harrison (Whig)	234	1,275,000
Van Buren (Dem.)	60	1,128,000

The election of 1840

scribed Van Buren as a squanderer of public funds on lavish entertainment, a man of expensive aristocratic tastes who fancied fine wines, ate from gold plates, and effeminately scented his whiskers with cologne. They dazzled the voters with boisterous mass meetings, barbecues, and torchlight processions; they nicknamed Van Buren "Martin Van Ruin" and "Sweet Sandy Whiskers"; they promised to cleanse the civil service of corruption and to restore prosperity; and they chanted their campaign slogans: "Tippecanoe and Tyler too" and "Van, Van is a used-up man."

The voters responded by turning out in larger numbers than in any previous presidential election—even Jackson had not attracted so large a proportion to the polls. Harrison's popular majority was small, but he won overwhelmingly in the Electoral College: 234 votes to 60 for Van Buren. After twelve years of Democratic supremacy, the Whigs seemed about to have their turn. Equally important, the presidential election of 1840 marked the final emergence of a fully developed American party system, with vigorous two-party politics in every section and in nearly all the states.

The Supreme Court under Taney.

But the Democrats, like the Federalists in 1801, retained a firm hold on the third branch of the federal government: the judiciary. While he was President, Jackson had appointed six new Associate Justices to the Supreme Court, all of them staunch Democrats; and when Chief Justice Marshall died in 1835, Jackson had selected Roger B. Taney, a one-time Federalist but now a state-rights Democrat to replace him. Jacksonians thus controlled seven of the nine positions on the Court, and conservatives such as Webster feared an irresponsible and radical departure from the constitutional doctrines laid down by Marshall. Actually, though the Taney Court modified the Marshall Court's opinions on the rights of corporations and the sanctity of contracts, the main corpus of Marshall's decisions remained almost intact. Even the doctrine of judicial review went unchallenged; in several important cases the Court threw out state and (on one occasion) federal legislation that it found to be unconstitutional.

The chief departure from the extreme nationalism of Marshall was the new Court's tendency to give the states greater power to regulate corporations. This change is best illustrated in the case of *Charles River Bridge* v. *Warren Bridge* (1837). The issue was whether the state of Massachusetts, having earlier given a charter to the Charles River Bridge Company to build and operate a toll bridge, could now grant a charter to a second company to build and operate another and competing bridge. The first company contended that this would constitute a breach of contract, but the Court disagreed and held that the rights of corporations are subordinate to the interests of the community—"that the community also have rights, and that the happiness and well-being of every citizen depends on their faithful preservation." The Court thus provided an admirable statement of two of the basic goals of Jacksonian Democracy: encouragement to new entrepreneurs, and the elimination of special privilege and entrenched "monopoly."

Tyler and Paralysis

The Whig disaster. As the Whigs organized their first administration, they looked forward to a period of progress along the lines of Whig principles. Harrison, who appeared to favor the goals of the American System, seemed ready to accept guidance from Webster and Clay, for he made Webster Secretary of State and gave most of the other Cabinet posts to followers of Clay. Then disaster struck. Only a month after his inauguration the sixty-eight-year-old President died of pneumonia, and for the first time the Vice President succeeded to the Presidency. Unfortunately for the Whigs, their new President, John Tyler, a Virginia aristocrat, sympathized with those Southern planters who opposed nearly everything the Whig majority hoped to accomplish. As a result, within less than a year, the Whigs in Congress were so torn by factionalism that they accomplished little, and the country had to suffer through a period of almost complete political stalemate.

Tyler had once been a Democrat but had broken with Jackson over nullification and the removal of federal deposits from Biddle's Bank. He drifted over to the Whigs because in his state that party was dominated by affluent men of high social status and because he opposed the radical, Locofoco tendencies of the Democrats under Jackson and Van Buren. Tyler was thought to be a political friend of Clay, but he made it clear that the imperious Kentuckian was not going to run his Administration; none of his messages showed any sympathy for Clay's views on banking, tariffs, or internal improvements.

Nevertheless, Clay confidently planned a legislative program that would at last put his American System into full operation. In 1841 he introduced a bill to distribute the proceeds from the sale of public lands among the states to finance internal improvements. In a bid for Western support, this bill also contained a provision for preemption by which squatters on the public domain could purchase 160 acres of land they had improved at the minimum price of $1.25 an acre when the land was put up for sale. To get his bill adopted, Clay had to agree that the distribution of proceeds from land sales would cease if tariff schedules were increased. A year later, in 1842, the Whigs tried to raise the tariff without repealing distribution. But a presidential veto forced them to give up distribution in order to get the increase in duties for which manufacturers were clamoring. Tyler then reluctantly approved the Tariff of 1842 to solve the government's need for more revenue, though it restored the level of duties provided in the Tariff of 1832. The new tariff was virtually the only Whig achievement—Tyler not only forced the abandonment of distribution but vetoed internal-improvement bills with essentially the same arguments Jackson had used.

The final disappointment came when Clay and the majority of Whigs attempted to establish a third Bank of the United States. Tyler approved the repeal of the Independent Treasury Act, but it was well known that he would not accept a new system of national banking in its place. Hence the Whigs tried to disguise their purpose by using other names. First they provided for the creation of a "Fiscal Bank," but Tyler was not deceived and vetoed the bill; then they proposed the chartering of a "Fiscal Corporation," only to be thwarted by another presidential veto. With that, national banking ceased to be a serious issue in national politics for two decades. The angry Whigs in Congress formally read Tyler out of the party, the Cabinet resigned (except Webster, who was involved in diplomatic negotiations with the British), and Clay gave up his seat in the Senate to try again for the Presidency. After making a fiasco of the Whig victory, Tyler and his Southern allies began to drift back to the Democratic party, where in subsequent years they would challenge the Jacksonians for control.

Foreign affairs under Tyler. The political paralysis at home did not prevent the Tyler Administration from solving several problems in the country's foreign relations. Jackson, in spite of his blunt tactics, had already disposed of two issues that had survived the negotiations following the War of 1812: he managed to persuade the British to permit American merchants to trade with their West Indian islands; and, after a rather unnecessary crisis in American-French relations, he made a satisfactory settlement of claims against France for damages inflicted on American shipping during the Napoleonic wars. But new sources of friction in Anglo-American relations had begun to appear during the 1830s and had reached serious proportions by the time Tyler became President. The traditional undercurrent of anti-British feeling, heightened by British travelers who made disparaging comments on American culture and by local politicians bidding for the Irish vote, made it dangerous to permit disagreements to go unsettled.

Trouble began in 1837, when an insurrection broke out in the eastern provinces in Canada. Though many Americans hoped the uprising might ultimately lead to union with the United States, the British suppressed it with relative ease. But while it was in progress Americans along the frontier aided the rebels and afterward gave the defeated rebel leaders refuge. When raids across the border continued from American bases on the Niagara River, Canadian officials one night impetuously crossed the river, killed one American, and burned an American steamer, the *Caroline*, which had been carrying supplies to the rebels. In spite of growing tension, the British government ignored the American demand for reparations and an apology.

Meanwhile, a long-standing controversy over the boundary between Maine and Canada flared up when, in 1838, American and Canadian lumberjacks battled for possession of part of a disputed area along the Aroostook River. Another dispute grew out of a British request that its naval patrols along the west coast of Africa be permitted to stop and search ships flying the American flag to determine whether they were engaging in the slave trade. This request revived memories of British practices during the Napoleonic wars, and the American government would not agree to it. Finally, in 1841, a group of slaves being transported from Virginia to New Orleans on the American brig *Creole* mutinied and sailed to Nassau in the British Bahamas, where government officials freed them. Prodded by angry Southerners, Secretary of State Webster demanded that the slaves be returned, but the British refused.

At this point a new British government decided that the time had come for negotiations and sent Lord Ashburton to Washington as a special envoy. Ashbur-

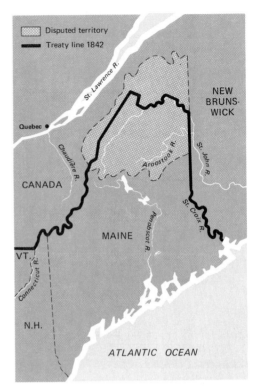

The Webster-Ashburton Treaty, 1842

ton was a happy choice, for he was friendly to the United States and a man of infinite tact; moreover, he had met Webster in England, and the two men liked each other. Neither was an experienced professional diplomat, but both were in a conciliatory mood, and their patient and highly informal negotiations culminated in the important Webster-Ashburton Treaty of 1842.

Except for Oregon, which remained under joint occupation, the treaty settled all border controversies by awarding seven-twelfths of the disputed territory along the Maine boundary to the United States and by making minor adjustments around Lake Champlain and between Lake Superior and the Lake of the Woods. The treaty also included an agreement for the mutual extradition of fugitives accused of any of seven major crimes. As for the slave trade, the United States did not agree to British search of its vessels but did agree to maintain a squadron off the African coast to apprehend slavers flying the American flag. Neither the *Caroline* nor the *Creole* affair was dealt with in the treaty, but Ashburton disposed of them through an exchange of notes that Webster chose to accept as satisfactory. With regard to the *Caroline* affair, Ashburton simply expressed regret "that some explanation and apology for this occurrence was not immediately made." In the case of the *Creole*, the slaves were not to be returned, but he promised that in the future there would be no "officious interference" with American vessels forced to enter British ports by "violence or accident."

Webster, after concluding these negotiations and seeing the treaty ratified by both governments, followed the example of the other Whigs and resigned from Tyler's Cabinet. Thereafter the Tyler Administration, disrupted and lacking congressional support, looked rather futile in the face of increasing sectional conflict.

In the critical years ahead, during a succession of weak administrations, many disheartened patriots would remember the strength and firmness of Andrew Jackson with growing admiration. As the country moved from crisis to crisis, the cry that would be heard more and more frequently was "Oh, for an hour of Old Hickory."

Suggestions for Reading

THE ADVANCE OF DEMOCRACY

The most perceptive contemporary analysis of the workings of American democracy in the Jacksonian era is Alexis de Tocqueville, *Democracy in America*, 2 vols.* (1945). Moisie Ostrogorski, *Democracy and the Organization of Political Parties*, 2 vols.* (1902), though dated, is still a useful general work on the democratization of American politics. Chilton Williamson, *American Suffrage from Property to Democracy, 1760–1860* (1960), supersedes all other works on the extension of the suffrage. The development of the system of nominating presidential candidates and voting for presidential electors is studied in J. S. Chase, *Emergence of the Presidential Nominating Convention, 1789–1832* (1973), and R. P. McCormick, *The Presidential Game: The Origins of American Presidential Politics* (1982). Two important revisionist studies that stress social stratification and a decline in class mobility are D. T. Miller, *Jacksonian Aristocracy: Class and Democracy in New York, 1830–1860* (1967), and Edward Pessen, *Riches, Class, and Power before the Civil War* (1973), the latter a quantitative study of men of wealth in Boston, New York, Brooklyn, and Philadelphia.

The disputed election of 1824, as well as the goals and misfortunes of the Adams Administration, are described in rich detail in George Dangerfield's two books: *The Era of Good Feelings* (1952), and *The Awakening of American Nationalism, 1815–1828**(1965). Three biographies are useful for an understanding of those years: G. G. Van Deusen, *The Life of Henry Clay* (1937); S. F. Bemis, *John Quincy Adams and the Union* (1956); and C. C. Mooney, *William H. Crawford, 1772–1834* (1974). R V. Remini, *The Election of Andrew Jackson** (1963), is the best study of the election of 1828.

THE AGE OF JACKSON

Four recent surveys, based on modern scholarship, deal critically with Jacksonian Democracy: G. G. Van Deusen, *The Jacksonian Era** (1959); C. M. Wiltse, *The New Nation, 1800–1845** (1961); J. C. Curtis, *Andrew Jackson and the Search for Vindication** (1976); and Edward Pessen, *Jacksonian America*, rev. ed. (1978). The latter two are decidedly anti-Jackson. Marquis James, *Andrew Jackson*, Vol. 2: *Portrait of a President* (1937), R. V. Remini, *Andrew Jackson and the Course of American Freedom, 1822–1832* (1981), and R. V. Remini, *Andrew Jackson and the Course of American Democracy, 1833–1845* (1984), are sympathetic and lucid studies of Jackson as President. R. V. Remini, *Andrew Jackson** (1966), brief and breezy, is an admiring portrayal of Jackson as a skilled politician. Two of Jackson's strongest supporters in Congress are the subjects of distinguished biographies: C. G. Sellers, *James K. Polk, Jacksonian, 1795–1843* (1957), and W. N. Chambers, *Old Bullion Benton:*

Senator from the New West (1956). There are also excellent biographies of three key figures in the Jackson Administration: C. B. Swisher, *Roger B. Taney* (1936); W. B. Hatcher, *Edward Livingston: Jeffersonian Republican and Jacksonian Democrat* (1940); and E. B. Smith, *Francis Preston Blair* (1980). An authoritative study of administrative organization is L. D. White, *The Jacksonians: A Study of Administrative History, 1829–1861* (1954). R. B. Latner, *The Presidency of Andrew Jackson: White House Politics, 1829–1837* (1979), examines the workings of the administration. R. P. McCormick, *The Second American Party System: Party Formation in the Jacksonian Era** (1966), is a revisionist study of major importance. W. P. Vaughn, *The Antimasonic Party in the United States, 1826–1843* (1983), is a study of the first American third-party movement.

The meaning of Jacksonian Democracy is still the subject of animated controversy. In addition to the study by Edward Pessen, cited above, the following books, each notable for its distinctive interpretation, provide a sample of the various ways in which Jacksonian Democracy can be viewed: A. M. Schlesinger, Jr., *The Age of Jackson** (1945); J. W. Ward, *Andrew Jackson: Symbol for an Age** (1955); Joseph Dorfman, *The Economic Mind in American Civilization*, 5 vols. (1946–49); Marvin Meyers, *The Jacksonian Persuasion** (1957); Lee Benson, *The Concept of Jacksonian Democracy: New York as a Test Case** (1961); and R. P. Formisano, *The Birth of Mass Political Parties: Michigan, 1827–1861* (1971).

All the above books deal with Jackson's views on banking and are important to a study of the controversy over the second Bank of the United States. But the key work on this topic is Bray Hammond, *Banks and Politics in America from the Revolution to the Civil War* (1957). R. V. Remini, *Andrew Jackson and the Bank War** (1967), is a brief, balanced study stressing the political side of the controversy. Two other works merit consultation: W. B. Smith, *Economic Aspects of the Second Bank of the United States* (1953), and J. M. McFaul, *The Politics of Jacksonian Finance* (1972). The best possible case for Nicholas Biddle is presented in T. P. Govan, *Nicholas Biddle: Nationalist and Public Banker* (1959). J. A. Wilburn, *Biddle's Bank: The Crucial Years* (1967), is a study of sources of public support for the Bank before the election of 1832. J. R. Sharp, *The Jacksonians versus the Banks* (1970), is a study of banking policy at the state level after the Panic of 1837. W. G. Shade, *Banks or No Banks: The Money Issue in Western Politics, 1832–1865* (1972), finds banking to be a durable cause of political divisions.

Angie Debo, *A History of the Indians of the United States** (1970), is an excellent survey. W. E. Washburn, *The Indian in America** (1975), is a cultural study. William Brandon, *The Last Americans: The Indians in American Culture* (1974), emphasizes Indian-white relations. B. W. Dippie, *The Vanishing American: White Attitudes and U.S. Indian Policy* (1982) is a study of white perceptions of the Indian. The tragedy of Indian removals is the subject of Angie Debo, *The Road to Disappearance: A History of the Creek Indians** (1941); M. D. Green, *The Politics of Indian Removal: Creek Government and Society in Crisis* (1982); A. H. DeRosier, Jr., *The Removal of the Choctaw Indians** (1970); and Grant Foreman, *Indian Removal: The Emigration of the Five Civilized Tribes of Indians** (1932). J. K. Mahon, *History of the Second Seminole War, 1835–1842* (1967), is a vivid account of Seminole resistance, F. P. Prucha, *American Indian Policy in the Formative Years** (1962), is a history of federal legislation. R. N. Satz, *American Indian Policy in the Jacksonian Era** (1975), is a balanced account. Land policy in the Jacksonian era is treated fully in R. G. Wellington, *The Political and Sectional Influence of the Public Lands, 1828–1842* (1942), and R. M. Robbins, *Our Landed Heritage: The Public Domain* (1942).

THE NULLIFICATION CONTROVERSY

C. S. Sydnor, *The Development of Southern Sectionalism, 1819–1848** (1948), analyzes the nullification crisis in the broad setting of Southern history. The best study of nullification is W. W. Freehling, *Prelude to Civil War** (1966). M. D. Peterson, *Olive Branch and Sword: The Compromise of 1833* (1982), is a good brief account. Sympathetic analyses of Calhoun's ideas are provided in A. O. Spain, *The Political Theory of John C. Calhoun* (1951); C. M. Wiltse, *John C. Calhoun, Nullifier, 1829–1839* (1949); and M. L. Coit, *John C. Calhoun: American Portrait** (1950). More critical appraisals appear in Richard Hofstadter, *The American Political Tradition** (1948); G. M. Capers, *John C. Calhoun, Opportunist* (1960); and R. N. Current, *John C. Calhoun* (1966).

DEPRESSION AND THE WHIG INTERLUDE

The best biographical studies of Van Buren are John Nivin, *Martin Van Buren: The Romantic Age of American Politics* (1983), and R. V. Remini, *Martin Van Buren and the Making of the Democratic Party* (1959). The Van Buren Administration is analyzed in J. C. Curtis, *The Fox at Bay: Martin Van Buren and the Presidency, 1837–1841* (1970). In a challenging interpretation of the panic and depression, Peter Temin, *The Jacksonian Economy** (1969), absolves the Jacksonians from major responsibility for the inflation and subsequent collapse. Earlier studies of the economic crisis are R. C. McGrane, *The Panic of 1837** (1924), and W. B. Smith and A. H. Cole, *Fluctuations in American Business, 1790–1860* (1935).

R. P. McCormick, *The Second American Party System**, and G. G. Van Deusen, *The Jacksonian Era**, both cited above, are the best introductions to a study of the origin and growth of the Whig party. D. W. Howe, *The Political Culture of the American Whigs** (1979), is the best study of Whig ideology. Four biographies of Whig leaders also need to be consulted: the biography of Clay by Van Deusen, cited above; C. M. Fuess, *Daniel Webster*, 2 vols. (1930, 2nd ed., 1968); R. N. Current, *Daniel Webster and the Rise of National Conservatism** (1955); and I. H. Bartlett, *Daniel Webster** (1978). Sydney Nathans, *Daniel Webster and Jacksonian Democracy* (1973), is an excellent study of Webster's political career during the Jacksonian years. R. G. Gunderson, *The Log-Cabin Campaign* (1957), is a brisk account of the election of 1840. The Tyler Administration is treated competently in O. D. Lambert, *Presidential Politics in the United States, 1841–1844* (1936), and O. P. Chitwood, *John Tyler: Champion of the Old South* (1939). A. B. Corey, *The Crisis of 1830–1842 in Canadian-American Relations* (1941), and J. B. Brebner, *North Atlantic Triangle* (1945), are good monographs on foreign policy under Tyler. Howard Jones, *To the Webster-Ashburton Treaty: A Study in Anglo-American Relations, 1783–1834* (1977), is excellent. R. A. Varg, *United States Foreign Relations, 1820–1860* (1979), is a good general study.

*Available in a paperback edition.

10
AN ERA OF REFORM

Many nineteenth-century Americans, especially but not exclusively those of strong religious convictions, believed that the destiny of their country concerned not only themselves but all humanity. In America's congenial environment men and women could reveal their capacity to govern themselves, to live in harmony with the laws of God's universe, and to eradicate social injustice. They could build an ideal society of righteous men and women whose leaders would be motivated by feelings of unselfish benevolence. In achieving these noble goals America could serve as a model for the rest of the world. To fail would be to betray a sacred trust.

This belief in a divine mission, together with a nagging awareness of their shortcomings, made Americans inordinately sensitive to criticism from European visitors. Tocqueville noted that their "irritable patriotism" caused them to take offense at any comment that was even mildly unfavorable. But if Americans regarded criticism by outsiders as impertinent, many of them periodically displayed an ample capacity for self-criticism. They knew that neither they as individuals nor their society had yet achieved that state of near-perfection toward which they aimed— that social anarchy might yet result from undesirable personal habits, especially excessive drinking, from urban disorders or slave rebellions, or from a general moral decline. Though some cherished an optimistic belief that a benign providence made progress inevitable, others were not satisfied with the pace at which it came, and they sometimes tried to give providence a helping hand. "We could not retard the great forward

movement of Humanity if we would," wrote Horace Greeley, editor of the New York *Tribune*, "but each of us may decide for himself whether to share in the glory of promoting it or incur the shame of having looked coldly and indifferently on."

In the 1820s movements for moral uplift and social reform began to attract people who were unwilling to compromise with evil and were impatient with the slow pace of progress. The causes they championed were by no means peculiarly American—British and American reformers had considerable influence on each other—but there was a millennial quality about the American crusades that was unique. Theodore Parker, a distinguished Boston clergyman, described the aims of the reformers who kept the country in a turmoil for a whole generation: They hoped to create a society

> full of industry and abundance, full of wisdom, virtue, and the poetry of life; a state with unity among all, with freedom for each; a church without tyranny, a society without ignorance, want, or crime, a state without oppression; yes, a world with no war among the nations to consume the work of their hands, and no restrictive policy to hinder the welfare of mankind.

The goals of this perfectionist program, the reformers believed, not only were attainable but could be achieved with relative speed and without violent upheaval. There existed in America, one of them explained, "abundant elements for progress, and a field of action comparatively free from those obstacles

Moral uplift: the road to Hell

which so impede reform elsewhere." Reformers in countries with more rigid class structures and deeply rooted customs might have to resort to violence in order to overthrow injustice, but here "the better course of effecting reform by moral and intellectual means is more trustingly expected." The proper vehicles of reform were the benevolent agencies of the churches and the secular and sometimes more radical reform societies, rather than revolutionary movements or even political parties. To be sure, some clergymen frowned on the crusaders and refused to become involved in secular affairs, but many of them thought it their duty not only to preach the Gospel but to help realize the promise of American life by advancing the cause of reform.

The Religious Background

The decline of orthodox Calvinism. Tocqueville believed that there was "no country in the world where the Christian religion retains a greater influence over the souls of men than in America." Certainly many Americans of the first half of the nineteenth century were still deeply religious, and the church continued to be a powerful force in their lives. But the various Protestant sects, especially those that had been based on Calvinist theology, had gone through some critical times since the eighteenth-century religious revivals and Jonathan Edwards' stout defense of orthodoxy. By the start of the nineteenth century some of the Puritan dogmas—predestination, infant damnation, and the total depravity of man—had already been rejected, or at least qualified, by a more liberal theology that replaced Calvin's God of wrath with a benevolent God of love. The conservatives admonished the faithful to "guard against the insidious encroachments of innovation," but this was no more than a rear-guard action.

Even in the eighteenth century a number of heresies, some of them actually quite old, had begun to trouble the minds of a few New England clergymen—heresies that raised doubts about doctrines such as the Trinity and the divinity of Christ. These early challenges were fortified by the rationalism of the Enlightenment and the more optimistic view of human nature expressed by the philosophers of the American and French revolutions. Respect for the dignity of the individual, confidence in the individual's capacity for self-improvement, and belief in the idea of progress led to a decline in otherworldliness and a growing interest in temporal affairs. Life on earth, according to this new view, was not a mere preparation for the hereafter, at best a kind of winnowing of the saved from the damned; rather, God intended it to have its own beauty and value.

These intellectual trends caused orthodox Calvinism to give way to a theology that was at once more rational and more humanistic. Many leaders of the Revolutionary generation, such as Jefferson and Franklin, withdrew from the established churches and became deists. Deism, which originated in Europe in the early eighteenth century, emphasized the ethics of Christianity but rejected the Trinity, the divinity of Christ, the idea of original sin, and the Bible as divine revelation. It held that God had created the universe and set it in motion to run by natural laws. He did not perform miracles or intervene in the everyday affairs of the world. The humanistic implications of deism were evident in Thomas Paine's *The Age of Reason:* "I believe in the equality of man, and I believe that religious duties consist in doing justice, loving mercy, and endeavoring to make our fellow creatures happy." Though Paine accepted the creed of no church, few intellectuals were prepared to carry rationalism that far, and most church leaders saw no significant difference between deism and atheism.

Unitarianism. In the long run those who worked for a liberalized theology within the churches had a broader influence than the freethinkers who deserted organized Christianity entirely. These liberalizers rebelled especially against the deterministic Calvinist doctrine of salvation only for the elect in favor of the more hopeful doctrine of free will and salvation open to all. The revolt against traditional Calvinism produced several new sects, such as the Universalists, and a division of the Presbyterians into Old and New schools. But the most influential of the organized religious groups produced by eighteenth-century rationalism and humanism was the Unitarian Church. An offshoot of Congregationalism, it never won masses of converts, for it appealed chiefly to the better-educated and more affluent descendants of the New England Puritans. Unitarians, as their name indicates, did not believe in the Trinity—Jesus was mortal, the founder of a great religion but not the son of God. They denied that men and women were conceived in sin or that they were totally depraved; rather, they were capable of goodness and virtue through the development of a Christian character. Moreover, according to this comfortable theology, good Christians received their reward on earth as well as in the hereafter, for they "enjoy the world more than other men [and] find more satisfaction in it." God was a merciful and loving Father, not a vindictive and arbitrary deity who predestined the mass of mankind to damnation. Unitarians were skeptical of finespun theological systems and urged each individual to search the Scriptures for truth. And once found, it must not be perverted into dogma to be imposed on others. Instead, Unitarians preached tolerance of differences among sincerely devout men and women.

William Ellery Channing (1780–1842), pastor of the Federal Street Church in Boston, was the most eminent Unitarian clergyman of the early nineteenth century. Channing stressed the primary responsibility of individuals to their own consciences and helped to link the liberal Unitarian creed with humanitarianism. To him "God is infinitely good, kind, benevolent," and the essence of religion is "the adoration of goodness." Belief in predestination and the God of Calvinism tends "to form a gloomy, forbidding, and servile religion, and to lead men to substitute censoriousness, bitterness, and persecution, for a tender and impartial charity." Channing supported humanitarian reform, "because I have learned the essential equality of men before the common Father . . . because I see in [them] a great nature, the divine image, and vast capacities." In Channing, Unitarianism found its ideal leader, for he balanced its rationalism and tolerance with a humanistic warmth and with an active concern for the welfare of humanity.

The transcendentalists. In the course of time, however, Unitarianism began to crystallize into a new orthodoxy. The Church's well-fed members, though more reasonable and tolerant than their Puritan ancestors, became at least as smug; though given to philanthropy, they were free to pursue individual gain with far less restraint. Unitarianism struck a growing number of New England intellectuals as distressingly cold and formal, its creed as vague and passionless, and its communicants as more concerned with material than with spiritual well-being. "Nothing quieted doubt so completely as the mental calm of the Unitar-

Margaret Fuller

ian clergy," wrote Henry Adams. "For them, difficulties might be ignored; doubts were waste of thought; nothing exacted solution. Boston had solved the universe."

Moreover, eighteenth-century rationalism, the foundation of Unitarianism, was succumbing to a romantic movement that was associated with the German writers Friedrich von Schiller and Johann Wolfgang von Goethe, and with the British men of letters Samuel Coleridge, Thomas Carlyle, and William Wordsworth. The romanticists rejected experience and pure reason as the keys to truth and substituted for them intuition, or spiritual insight, which they believed produced knowledge that could not be derived through the senses. They idealized natural, spontaneous individuals rather than the educated and sophisticated. In a sense, Jacksonian Democracy, with its faith in the intuitive good judgment of common people, was the political manifestation of romanticism in America.

In 1836, a small group of intellectuals living in and around Boston and Concord, Massachusetts, began to meet informally to exchange ideas about philosophy and theology. Though the group had no formal organization or membership list, it was known as the Transcendental Club. The former Unitarian minister Ralph Waldo Emerson was always its moving spirit. In addition to Emerson, this distinguished group included, at one time or another, Unitarian clergymen such as Theodore Parker, George Ripley, and James Freeman Clark; literary figures such as Henry Thoreau, Amos Bronson Alcott, Nathaniel Hawthorne, and Orestes Brownson; and talented women such as Sophia and Elizabeth Peabody, and Margaret Fuller.

The transcendentalists, though as a group comfortable enough, professed to be appalled by the crass materialism of a country preoccupied with economic development and were concerned that spiritual progress was not keeping pace. They were too individualistic and too hostile to institutional restraints to start a church of their own, but the philosophy of transcendentalism was shot through with theological implications. It was clearly an outgrowth of Puritanism and Unitarianism (with a touch of Quakerism and mysticism) as well as romanticism.

The transcendentalists, like the Unitarians, rejected Calvinist dogma and believed in the essential goodness of humanity and in a God of love. But their idealism was warm and affirmative, not the bland concoction of "pale negations" that Emerson found so unsatisfying in Unitarianism. As Theodore Parker explained, transcendentalists held that man has "faculties which give him ideas and intuitions which transcend sensational experience; ideas whose origin is not from sensation, nor their proof from sensation."

The mind of man "is not a smooth tablet on which sensation writes its experience, but is a living principle which of itself originates ideas." Moreover, God dwells in every person, and human nature, therefore, is not simply excellent but divine. Since the transcendentalists discovered no evil in the human mind and had faith in the individual's intuitive knowledge of right and justice, they urged everyone to follow the dictates of conscience even when it led to the defiance of church or state. "To know what is right," said Parker, "I need not ask what is the current practice, what say the Revised Statutes, what said holy men of old, but what says conscience? what, God?" Thoreau, in his famous *Essay on Civil Disobedience*, asked: "Must the citizen ever for a moment, or in the least degree, resign his conscience to the legislator? Why has every man a conscience, then?"

The transcendental belief that God, or the Oversoul, permeated both matter and spirit, and that humanity, blessed with a spark of divinity, enjoyed limitless potentialities, had several consequences. It led to a celebration of individualism and self-reliance and to an admiration of those who had the strength and confidence to strike out on their own—sentiments that abounded in many of Emerson's essays. In this spirit Thoreau, in 1845, built a cabin on Walden Pond near Concord, where he lived for two years to illustrate that individuals can rely on themselves and live a full life without the baubles and trivia of civilized society. Transcendentalism also encouraged a rather naive faith that in the long run everything would turn out well. Emerson wrote: "An eternal beneficent necessity is always bringing things right. . . . The league between virtue and nature engages all things to assume a hostile front to vice."

But although the transcendentalists were optimists, they did not ignore the shortcomings of American society or wait complacently for an inevitable progress to produce the remedies. Instead, they were severe critics of governments, laws, social institutions, and debasing commercialism—whatever prevented humanity from realizing its full potential. "Their quarrel with every man they meet," said Emerson, "is not with his kind, but with his degree." Hence the transcendentalists, though they were not given to organizing or joining reform societies, nonetheless contributed to the country's intellectual climate of reform. Emerson asked,

> What is man born for but to be a Re-former, a Re-maker of what man has made; a renouncer of lies; a restorer of truth and good, imitating that great Nature which embosoms us all, and which sleeps no moment on an old past, but every hour repairs herself, yielding to us every morning a new day, and with every pulsation a new life?

The Protestant sects and revivalism. If Unitarianism was too cold, transcendentalism was too intellectual, perhaps too cheerful, and not sufficiently structured to attract a large following. Most Protestants remained in the Congregational, Presbyterian, Baptist, and Methodist churches or joined one of the numerous evangelical sects that proliferated in the nineteenth century. Even at the popular level, however, the hard tenets of orthodox Calvinism began to soften. Devout Protestants continued to believe in man's sinful condition, but they accepted the doctrine of a benevolent God who offered everyone the chance of salvation through the experience of spiritual conversion and through faith. Moreover, the material opportunities that lay before Americans in a growing and flourishing society discouraged otherworldliness and tempted them to expect virtue to be rewarded on earth as well as in heaven.

Even so, much of orthodoxy still survived in the religion of the common people. In their cosmology, when they thought about such matters, the earth was still the center of the universe; and God continued to be actively and intimately involved in human affairs. Ordinary churchgoers still believed in the Trinity, in the Bible as divine revelation, and in a literal heaven and hell. They might doubt man's total depravity, but they could never accept the transcendentalist's extreme optimism about human nature. For the reality of evil in the world was too manifest, human frailty in the face of temptation too obvious. The continued prevalence of endemic and epidemic diseases, and the resulting short life expectancy and high infant mortality, made most Americans acutely conscious, sometimes almost obsessed, with the imminence of death. This awareness helps explain the persistence of a measure of gloom and pessimism in their outlook on life; it intensified their religious fervor and turned them to the church for strength and solace.

With few exceptions, notably the Quakers, the various Protestant denominations actively proselytized those who were seeking comfort and salvation. Some had greater success than others. After the Revolution the Protestant Episcopal Church, formerly the Anglican Church, was discredited by the fact that much of its clergy had been Loyalist; it grew only slowly, appealing mostly to well-to-do Eastern conservatives. The Congregationalists of New England lost members to the Unitarians. In the newly settled regions of the West they joined with the Presbyterians in 1801 to adopt a Plan of Union, by which they agreed to establish united churches that might select either Congregational or Presbyterian ministers. In the long run the Plan of Union benefited the Presbyterians, because most of the united churches entered their fold. Although the Presbyterians thus experienced a considerable growth, they were far surpassed

Methodist meeting: converts by the thousand

by two other Protestant denominations. One of these, the Baptists, had phenomenal success with their system of autonomous congregations and with an untrained, uneducated clergy that spoke the language of the common people. Their ministers brought a primitive but passionate message of hellfire for sinners and redemption for those who experienced conversion and admitted God into their souls. The second, and most successful of all, were the Methodists, each of whose itinerant ministers rode a circuit of several congregations in the scattered settlements of the West and preached an equally simple Christianity.

After the eighteenth-century religious revivals that historians have called the Great Awakening, revivalism became a periodic phenomenon. During these interludes of religious enthusiasm Presbyterians, Baptists, and Methodists won new converts by the thousands, and church attendance rose significantly. In the course of the Second Awakening, which began around 1800, the religious frenzy spread with increasing intensity from east to west. An innovation of this revival was the camp meeting, which brought crowds together for several days of uninterrupted preaching and prayers. Under the emotional influence of exhorters who called for repentance, many experienced conversion. Since the battle with Satan was often violent, a familiar spectacle was the jumping, shouting, and moaning of tortured souls. When the battle had been won and Satan put to rout, as one witness observed, "hundreds

were prostrate upon the earth before the Lord."

The intensity of religious feeling and the relative autonomy of many individual congregations often led to disputes over questions of doctrine, church organization, and ritual, and these in turn caused schisms and the formation of numerous small fundamentalist denominations. For example, the quest of a group of Methodists in western New York for holiness and perfect love led them ultimately to separate from the Methodist Episcopal Church and to form the Free Methodist Church. The divisions among Baptists produced the Hard-Shells, Soft-Shells, Primitives, and Free Willers, as well as new denominations such as the Campbellites (Disciples of Christ). Among the new sects, one of the most important was the Mormon Church, founded in 1830 by Joseph Smith. The Church of Jesus Christ of Latter-Day Saints, as it was officially called, was based on miraculous revelations that Smith claimed to have received from God and that he incorporated in the Book of Mormon. Still another sect, the Adventists, believed in the imminence of the Bible's prophesied second coming of Christ and of the millennium—the thousand years mentioned in the New Testament book of Revelations during which holiness, peace, and harmony would prevail on earth. Early in the 1840s, William Miller, a Vermont Baptist preacher, after a series of elaborate calculations, predicted the start of the millennium, first in 1843, then in 1844. When Miller's predictions proved incorrect, the disappointment that his Adventist followers experienced led most of them to desert him; but for a few years they numbered into the hundreds of thousands.

During another period of revivalism in the 1820s many of its leaders, for the first time, combined a desire to save souls with an active interest in social reform. Support for reform was especially strong among those who believed that the millennium would precede the second coming of Christ. These so-called postmillennialists felt the urgency of perfectionist reforms as essential steps toward preparing the world for the ultimate reign of God and the final Judgment. The greatest preacher of this new revival was the Reverend Charles G. Finney, who gathered his first harvest of converts from the fertile soil of upstate New York, a land of transplanted New Englanders. Finney preached not only salvation through repentance and faith but the importance of good works and the obligation of the churches to take "right ground . . . on all the subjects of practical morality which come up for decision from time to time." To him original sin was a "deep-seated but voluntary . . . self-interest. . . . All sin consists in selfishness; and all holiness or virtue, in disinterested benevolence." Salvation was not the end but the beginning of life—a life of useful work and benevolent activity. Since Finney's doctrine, as one contemporary observed, encouraged mankind "to *work* as well as to *believe*," Finney became a powerful influence for social reform. In addition to winning the support of many established preachers, he sent out a remarkable group of young converts to advance his work, notably Theodore Dwight Weld, who went into the West to preach and to advance the cause of moral reform.

In 1830 Finney brought his revival to New York City, where he met two remarkable brothers, Arthur and Lewis Tappan, wealthy merchants and pious men who were already devoting most of their energy and fortunes to philanthropy. The Tappans welcomed Finney and organized an Association of Gentlemen to give financial support to both his religious and his reform work. Lewis Tappan, once a Unitarian, had become dissatisfied with that faith and had moved not toward transcendentalism but back to evangelical Protestantism. He had concluded, he explained, that the Unitarians "did not, in an equal degree, consider themselves as stewards, and their property as consecrated to the cause of Christianity; and that they were deficient in a devotional frame of mind."

Religion thus encouraged reform in two different but parallel trends. First, the transcendentalists celebrated the divinity of man and called on everyone to trust their consciences in their quest for right and justice. Thoreau wrote: "It is not desirable to cultivate a respect for the law, so much as for the right. The only obligation which I have a right to assume is to do at any time what I think right." Second, the evangelical Protestant revivalists, believing as most of them did in America's divine mission, made good works a manifestation of holiness and of the experience of conversion, and reform a vital function of the churches. "And what is to reform mankind but the truth?" asked Finney. "And who shall present the truth if not the church and the ministry? Away with the idea that Christians can remain neutral and keep still, and yet enjoy the approbation and blessing of God."

The Movement for Reform

The nature of the movement. William Ellery Channing observed that one of the remarkable circumstances of his age was "the energy with which the principle of combination, or of action by joint forces, by associated numbers, is manifesting itself. It may be said, without much exaggeration, that everything is done now by Societies. . . . You can scarcely name an object for which some institution has not been formed." Though the benevolent societies were numerous, there was a considerable overlapping of both leaders and members. Active reformers tended to be attracted to several causes, and the same names appeared repeatedly among the directors of the various reform organizations.

In its early phase the movement was an inherently conservative effort of clergymen and wealthy philanthropists to fight infidelity and preserve the country's Christian character. It was a battle of the churched against the unchurched, the evangelicals against the secularists, for control of the national spirit. Organizations such as the American Sunday School Union, American Home Missionary Society, and American Bible Society all had as their goal a general moral regeneration. But under the influence of various perfectionist groups the movement, while retaining its religious essence, soon transcended its cramped moralism and grew into a multifaceted crusade for social betterment. The crusade, though millennial in its goals, was a response to a variety of specific social problems—drunkenness, prostitution, crime, ignorance, slums, among others—none of them

William Ellery Channing

new but all of them intensified as industrialization and urbanization increased the complexity of American society and accelerated the pace of life.

The reformers, for a variety of reasons, dismayed their conservative contemporaries and annoyed the uncommitted majority, most of whom were fully occupied with the problems of their own daily lives and wished to be left alone. In the first place, as a leading reformer himself noted, there is a "tendency of every reform to surround itself with a fringe of the unreasonable and half-cracked"; and the reformers had within their ranks a full quota of cranks whose bizarre crusades exposed the whole movement to ridicule. While some worked constructively to improve the public health by, for example, urging women to stop wearing tight corsets or by advocating the eating of whole-wheat bread, others devoted their energies to promoting outlandish food or dress fads. Still others were devotees of the pseudoscience of phrenology and tried to measure character and intelligence by studying the conformation of the skull. A surprising number of them developed an interest in Spiritualism, especially in the ideas of the Swedish philosopher Emanuel Swedenborg, who described a spirit world where all were received and were able to strive for perfection. Reformers were accused, too, of being more concerned with denouncing evil than with advancing constructive remedies. Moreover, as Emerson complained, some of them were "narrow, self-pleasing, conceited men" given to petty bickering and "personal and party heats."

From the perspective of the twentieth century, these reformers seem naive in their optimism about human nature, in their belief that social evils result entirely from the selfish acts of individuals, and in their confidence that social problems can be solved simply by the regeneration of individuals and by appealing to the innate goodness in humanity. In addition, many of them were not very well informed about, or equipped to understand, the problems of urban factory workers, a growing number of whom were recent immigrants. Reform leaders usually came from the old middle-class families of rural and small-town New England; their social backgrounds and economic assumptions caused them to be insensitive to conditions in the industrial centers—or prone to blame the plight of the worker entirely on the use of liquor and tobacco.

Though the shortcomings of the reformers were real enough, the movements they launched were not merely the enterprises of impractical, shortsighted cranks and neurotics. The ranks of reform contained many dedicated men and women who demonstrated a keen understanding of, and sensitivity to, some of the social problems of their day. Their aim in part was to find ways to prevent the unsettling social changes of

The "Tombs": New York City prison

their age from destroying traditional values and thus betraying America's mission to the world. However, the reformers could not transcend the limits of contemporary religious and secular thought, which explains why they were more sensitive to some social evils than to others, why certain organizational methods appealed to them, and why they resorted to the tactics they used in fighting their foes.

The accomplishments of those who made a career of reform, though far short of the goals they had set, were by no means negligible. If they were a trial to their friends, it was in part because their work, by its very nature, forced them to "disregard the peace and proprieties of the social world." Each reformer seemed to bear a burden of personal guilt for the evils in society and felt driven to do something to eliminate them. This sense of individual responsibility, which can easily be lost in a mass society, was in itself a legacy of inestimable value.

Treatment of criminals and the insane. Humane and sensitive men and women who investigated the care of paupers, criminals, and the insane in their own communities found an ample field for reform. These social derelicts, the victims of public ignorance or indifference, were treated almost as they had been in the Middle Ages. In atrocious jails and dungeons young offenders were thrown together with hardened criminals and the violently insane; in neglected almshouses idiots and the destitute were left to the mercy of low-paid, untrained attendants. Humanitarians managed at least to start the painfully slow process of providing prisons with better physical accommoda-

tions. With their more enlightened approach to penology, they urged, with some success, that the community concentrate on reforming, rather than punishing, criminals. Accepting the view that criminals were the products of their environment rather than of some character defect, various states, especially New York and Pennsylvania, experimented with programs designed to change the lives and environments of prisoners. Young offenders were confined in "reform schools" or "houses of refuge," where they could be dealt with in ways thought to be more appropriate for juveniles, and where they could escape the corrupting influence of older criminals. Meanwhile, the states, one by one, responded to the new spirit by abolishing several vestiges of primitive justice: the imprisonment of debtors, public floggings, and public executions.

Since little was known about the causes of insanity, or about therapy, society provided almost no mental hospitals; the insane were either cared for by relatives or committed to jails and almshouses. Among those who took an interest in the treatment of the insane, Dorothea Dix, a Boston schoolmistress, was the most active advocate of state-supported mental hospitals and of experiments in therapy. In 1841 she launched her crusade by investigating the condition of the insane in her own state. Two years later, she presented the legislature with an eloquent but factual memorial that described "the present state of insane persons confined in this Commonwealth, in cages, closets, cellars, stalls, pens! Chained, naked, beaten with rods, and lashed into obedience." Until her death in 1887 she worked with tireless patience to arouse public officials throughout the country, and her sincerity and command of the facts won her considerable success. By the end of the 1850s twenty-eight states were maintaining mental institutions, many of which operated on the assumption that cures could be found for their inmates. However, some of these institutions ultimately became places merely to lodge the unwanted and abandoned.

Temperance. Concern for criminals, paupers, and the insane was intimately related to another goal of the reform movement: temperance. It was commonly believed that excessive drinking was a basic cause of the condition of these unfortunates, as well as of the poverty that plagued city workers. Temperance, therefore, would not merely redeem the individual sinner but would advance the whole program of social reform. Accordingly, the support for this reform was more widespread than for any other. There can be no doubt that drunkenness was a genuine problem, for this was an age of heavy drinking in which the per capita consumption of whiskey, hard cider, and rum was staggering. The temperance movement began with the formation of numerous local societies, which, in 1826, combined to form a national organization, the American Society for the Promotion of Temperance, subsequently the American Temperance Union. Some leaders merely preached moderation in the use of liquor, but others, such as the Presbyterian clergyman Lyman Beecher, sought converts who would pledge total abstinence. Some relied on the voluntary decisions of individuals; others urged the use of the coercive power of state governments. In 1851 Maine, whose temperance forces were led by Neal Dow, a wealthy merchant and reformer, passed the first state law prohibiting the manufacture or sale of intoxicating beverages; within the next decade a dozen other Northern and Western states followed Maine's example, but most of these laws remained in force for only a few years. At its height the temperance movement resembled a religious revival; its flavor is suggested by a stanza from one of its popular songs, "One Glass More":

> Stay, mortal, stay! nor heedless thus
>   Thy sure destruction seal;
> Within that cup there lurks a curse,
>   Which all who drink shall feel.
> Disease and death forever nigh,
>   Stand ready at the door,
> And eager wait to hear the cry—
>   "O give me one glass more!"

If the prohibition laws proved transitory, the temperance crusade itself was by no means a failure, for in the two decades after 1830 the per capita consumption of intoxicants declined significantly.

Dorothea Dix: eloquent reformer

Women's rights. Women took a special interest in temperance, but when they tried to participate actively in this or other reform movements they confronted a wall of prejudice and the rebuff that, except for some limited church and charitable activities, a woman's place was in the home. American men characteristically treated women with deference but would not accept them as equals. Women, according to their male protectors, were physically, intellectually, and emotionally unsuited for participation in public affairs or for the pursuit of professional careers. In the growing cities, where men spent much of their time away from home working in factories or offices, women were expected to devote themselves to child-rearing and homemaking. Accordingly, their lives were almost totally defined by their duties as mothers and wives. To transcend their domestic responsibilities would be to undermine the traits of submissiveness, piety, and purity that were, according to the women's magazines and masculine wisdom, the attributes of True Womanhood.

Except for female seminaries where the daughters of the well-to-do could learn the social graces, schools were closed to girls. Women, though providing much of the labor in textile mills and other industries, were excluded from the professions and from nearly all other rewarding economic activities that might afford attractive alternatives to marriage and homemaking. Their inferior position was reinforced by laws that denied them the right to vote or hold public office, treated unmarried women as minors and made them wards of their nearest male relatives, and recognized the husband as the dominant figure in the family. The husband was even given control over the property his wife brought to the marriage or subsequently inher-

The history of mankind is a history of repeated injuries and usurpations on the part of man toward woman, having in direct object the establishment of an absolute tyranny over her. To prove this, let facts be submitted to a candid world.

He has never permitted her to exercise her inalienable right to the elective franchise.

He has compelled her to submit to laws, in the formation of which she had no voice....

He has made her, if married, in the eyes of the law civilly dead.

He has taken from her all right in property, even to the wages she earns....

He has monopolized nearly all the profitable employments, and from those she is permitted to follow, she receives but a scanty remuneration.

He closes against her all the avenues to wealth and distinction, which he considers most honorable to himself....

He has denied her the facilities for obtaining a thorough education—all colleges being closed against her....

He has created a false public sentiment, by giving to the world a different code of morals for men and women, by which moral delinquencies which exclude women from society, are not only tolerated but deemed of little account in man....

He has endeavored, in every way that he could, to destroy her confidence in her own powers, to lessen her self-respect, and to make her willing to lead a dependent and abject life.

From the Seneca Falls, New York, "Declaration of Sentiments and Resolutions," 1848.

ited. Divorce was rare, but when it occurred the father received custody of the children no matter what the circumstances causing the divorce may have been.

Not only were the boundaries of a woman's life severely confined, she also had to endure a humiliating double standard of morality. Premarital and extramarital sexual activity, though absolutely taboo for respectable women, was at least tolerated, if not condoned, for men. The difference in standards, according to the prevailing belief, resulted from differences in the natures of men and women. Women were not expected to find pleasure in sex; submitting to their husbands' desires was simply another domestic duty. Indeed, in an age when abstinence from intercourse was almost the only way to avoid repeated pregnancies, women had reasons other than social pressures for suppressing their sexuality. The double standard was reinforced by the availability in the cities of lower-class prostitutes, who enabled upper- and middle-class women to remain chastely on their pedestals for men to admire. Men idealized the pure, submissive wife and mother who devoted her life to domestic chores; and, according to one European visitor, they guarded her with "a sevenfold shield of insignificance."

So strict was the prevailing code of respectable female behavior that it was considered unfeminine for women even to speak in public places or to offer prayers in church. When Sarah and Angelina Grimké, members of a South Carolina slaveholding family, came north to join the crusade against slavery, they were denounced for addressing "promiscuous" audiences—that is, audiences of both men and women. In 1838, Sarah wrote bitterly that men had "endeavored to . . . drive women from almost every sphere of moral action." She called on women to think for themselves, "to rise from that degradation and bondage to which we have been consigned by men, and by which the faculties of our minds . . . have been prevented from expanding to their full growth, and are sometimes wholly crushed." In 1840, a group of American women, including Elizabeth Cady Stanton and Lucretia Mott, went as delegates to a World Antislavery Convention in London, but they were denied the right to participate.

This and similar experiences provoked a women's rights movement that became at once an integral part of the general reform crusade and a divisive issue among male reformers, most of whom opposed permitting women to join their organizations. The emergence of the movement, together with the support it received from a segment of male reformers, indicated at least the beginning of a change in attitudes and, especially among middle-class women, a growing confidence that the proscriptions placed on them could be effectively challenged. In 1845, Margaret Fuller published *Woman in the Nineteenth Century*, a book that passionately protested not only against the inferior position assigned to women, but also against their inability to obtain any identity except through their husbands. Mrs. Stanton, one of the most advanced and militant women of her generation, publicly advocated divorce to terminate unsatisfactory marriages, birth control, and recognition that women are "absolutely sovereign" over their own bodies.

In 1848, the first Women's Rights Convention met at Seneca Falls, New York. Here the delegates adopted a statement, drafted by Mrs. Stanton, that paraphrased the Declaration of Independence and proclaimed that "all men and women are created equal." After listing women's specific grievances, the statement demanded that women "have immediate admission to all the rights and privileges which belong to them as citizens of the United States." They had, it concluded, "too long rested satisfied in the circumscribed limits which corrupt customs and a perverted application of the Scriptures" had marked out for them. The Seneca Falls convention was the first of a series that met during the following decade.

In the years before the Civil War, the women of the United States did make some limited gains. A few states gave married women control over their own property, and everywhere two low-status professions, nursing and elementary education, were opened to them. They secured admission to a few high schools and normal schools, and in 1837 Oberlin College became the first coeducational college. Also in 1837 the first women's college, Mount Holyoke, opened its doors. But most important was the example set by a courageous group of women who defied prejudice and played an active and constructive role in public affairs. Dorothea Dix, as we have seen, contributed to improved treatment of the insane; Dr. Elizabeth Blackwell won distinction as a physician; Margaret Fuller for a time edited the transcendentalist journal, *The Dial*, and then served as literary editor of the New York *Tribune*; Emma Willard campaigned for educational reform; Lucy Stone was a popular lecturer as well as a crusader for equal suffrage; and a small host of women, notably Frances Wright, Elizabeth Cady Stanton, Susan B. Anthony, Lucretia Mott, and Sarah and Angelina Grimké, played active roles in the movement to abolish slavery. Indeed, women abolitionists often united antislavery with women's rights to form a double crusade. Angelina Grimké explained, "The investigation of the rights of the slave has led me to a better understanding of my own." Most men (and more than a few women) sneered at these "unsexed" women, citing Mrs. Amelia Bloomer's wearing of pantalettes as evidence of where it would all end. But the feminists had effectively challenged the myth that women were physically and intellectually unfitted for any useful activity outside the home.

However, even in the home the role of women had been undergoing a significant change, one especially evident in Northern middle-class families. As fathers were drawn away from their homes to pursue their careers, families became somewhat less patriarchal; while mothers, no longer mere child-bearers, began to play a more dynamic role in the rearing of children and as decision-makers in family affairs. In the training of children mothers resorted less to physical punishment than to appeals to the consciences of their children—that is, to a form of moral suasion. In evangelical families mothers may thus have played a role as significant as the churches in rearing a generation of men and women driven by their inner consciences and feelings of guilt to launch a crusade for moral reform. These mothers, though lacking any spirit of rebellion against the existing social order, may nevertheless have helped to inspire the movement of which women's rights was so significant a part.

Education. Some reformers revealed their debt to Jacksonian Democracy, as well as their concern for the welfare of the common people, in the crusade for free, tax-supported public education. In the early nineteenth century, except in Massachusetts, the children of the poor obtained their elementary education at home or in church or charity schools, and the children of the rich in private schools or from tutors. The lack of public support, together with the fact that most teaching was done by low-paid, untrained young men who regarded it as a temporary occupation, left a mass of people, both urban and rural, in a state of semi-literacy. In the two decades after 1830 the crucial battle to establish public responsibility for elementary education was fought and won, though in many states it took much longer for the idea to be translated into reality.

Opposition to public schools came from those who considered education a private concern, from taxpayers who objected to paying for the education of other people's children, and from religious groups that maintained their own schools. Support came from practical men who saw the need for them in an increasingly commercial society, where more and more occupations required the ability to read, write, and cipher. It came, too, from those who believed that mass education was essential to a political system based on manhood suffrage. Additional support came from those who viewed public education as a means of providing the common man with better opportunities to advance, thereby achieving a more general diffusion of property ownership and a softening of class lines. In 1848, Horace Mann, secretary of the Massachusetts Board of Education, noted the alarming contrasts of wealth and poverty in his state; he maintained that "nothing but Universal Education can counterwork this tendency to the domination of capital and the servility of labor." Educate the workingman, and he will improve his position and acquire property, for "such a thing never did happen, and never can happen, as that an intelligent and practical body of men should be permanently poor." Education, Mann concluded, "is the great equalizer of the conditions of men—the balance wheel of the social machinery. . . . It does better than to disarm the poor of their hostility toward the rich; it prevents being poor." Urban artisans themselves made state-supported education one of their principal demands. A resolution adopted by the mechanics of Philadelphia in 1830 declared "that there can be no real liberty without a wide diffusion of real intelligence . . . [and] that until means of equal instruction shall be equally secured to all, liberty is but an unmeaning word, and equality an empty shadow."

By the 1850s the states were committed to making tax-supported public education available to all without the stigma of charity. Some of the states had already passed laws requiring local communities to establish elementary schools, and most of the others had at least required that when schools were established they must admit all children, not just those able to pay tuition. As a result, outside the South, where the movement was impeded by rural conditions, by the reluctance of small farmers to lose their children's labor, and by the indifference of the planter class, a steadily growing number of children found free public schools available to them.

But this was only the beginning, for compulsory-attendance laws had not yet been passed, school terms were short, the curriculum was thin, and teaching methods were still based on rote memorization and corporal punishment. Massachusetts led the way in remedying these conditions by establishing, in 1837, a state Board of Education, with Horace Mann as secretary. Mann had devoted many years to teaching and the study of education, and during his eleven years as secretary his annual reports made him the most influential man in the public-school movement. In Massachusetts he worked successfully to improve the curriculum and teaching methods, lengthen the school year, raise teachers' salaries, establish the first state-supported normal school for teacher-training, and organize a state association of teachers. Other states appointed their own boards or superintendents of education, who tried, with varying degrees of success, to achieve similar reforms.

For most American children formal education ceased after a few years in an elementary school. Secondary education was limited to those who could af-

ford to pay the tuition to a private academy, where, in preparation for college, they took courses in mathematics, rhetoric, and the classics. In 1827 Massachusetts passed a law requiring every town of five hundred or more families to set up a public high school, a policy soon adopted by the other New England states. But as late as 1860 only slightly more than three hundred public high schools existed in the United States, with almost a third of them in Massachusetts and only a scattering in the South and West.

In higher education, which was less influenced by reform, the most notable development was the proliferation of private denominational colleges throughout the country. In the two decades between 1830 and 1850 about eighty of these colleges were founded. Most of them had meager endowments, small student bodies, and incompetent faculties; but every village seemed determined to have a college, and every religious sect wanted a network of colleges to train its clergy and indoctrinate its youth. The idea of state-supported institutions of higher learning was an old one, and four states (Vermont, North Carolina, Georgia, and Tennessee) chartered them in the late eighteenth century. The first one actually to win academic distinction, however, was the University of Virginia, founded in 1819. By the 1850s numerous state universities, most of them in the South and West, had been founded, but few were in reality more than small colleges limping along on slender budgets.

Both state and private colleges offered a traditional liberal-arts curriculum, which stressed Latin, Greek, science, mathematics, moral philosophy, and political economy. True universities in the modern sense, with professional schools, graduate teaching, and emphasis on scholarly research, did not emerge until after the Civil War. Too many colleges were founded during these years, and few of them had the libraries and scholars they needed to become centers of creative intellectual life. The idea of academic freedom, moreover, had few defenders, and countless instructors fell victim to the political and sectarian controversies of the age.

Since the colleges served only a tiny fraction of the population, the mass of adults with a thirst for learning searched for other and more accessible avenues to cultural advancement. The "penny press," which began in 1833 when the New York *Sun* went on sale at a penny a copy, put newspapers within the reach of everyone and served up a mixed fare of sensationalism, news, and essays on practical and scientific subjects. Scores of magazines catered to all tastes, but the best of them offered essays, poetry, and fiction by the most distinguished European and American writers. This was an era of organized efforts for self-improvement, and most communities had their debating societies, literary societies, and library associa-

The Emerson School in Boston

tions. The lyceum movement, a nationally organized program of adult education initiated in 1826 by a New Englander, Josiah Holbrook, was the most ambitious of these enterprises. The original plan was to encourage local lyceums to assemble libraries, study scientific subjects, and form discussion groups, but most of them soon concentrated on lecture courses. Though many a fraud and charlatan managed to get on the lyceum lecture circuit, men of letters such as Emerson and Charles Dickens, scientists such as Harvard's Louis Agassiz, and a host of reformers made the program a useful instrument of mass education.

The peace movement. Reformers not content with the piecemeal alleviation of domestic social ills turned to more ambitious projects, such as the cause of world peace. Remembering the dreadful suffering and waste of the Napoleonic wars, some reformers were attracted to the pacifist principles of the Quakers or at least hoped to find nonviolent ways of settling international disputes. Local peace societies, which had begun to appear soon after the War of 1812, united in 1828 to form the American Peace Society. William Ladd, a Maine sea captain, merchant, and farmer, was the founder of the national organization and the editor of its journal, the *Harbinger of Peace*. In a pam-

phlet, *Essay on a Congress of Nations* (1840), Ladd proposed an international congress to interpret international law and a Court of Nations to apply it. Most peace advocates, however, distinguished between the use of force for aggressive and for defensive purposes and condemned only the former. In 1838 the peace movement split when the "ultraists," headed by Henry Clark Wright and William Lloyd Garrison, formed a Non-Resistance Society committed to oppose violence even in self-defense. Their constitution denounced military service, forceful resistance to tyranny, capital punishment, and actions at law for civil damages. This millennial program was designed to put Christian precepts into immediate action—to prepare the way "for the full manifestation of the reign of Christ on earth." It would secure "the reconciliation and salvation of a warring and lost world." During the 1850s all segments of the peace movement weakened as the sectional conflict grew increasingly bitter, and with the outbreak of the Civil War it collapsed.

Communitarianism. Other perfectionists worked for the complete regeneration of society by building model communities that they hoped would form the nuclei of a better social order. Early communitarian projects had been undertaken by several small religious sects, such as the Rappites and the Shakers, with the goal of achieving holiness through a form of Christian communism. In 1825 Robert Owen, a Scottish textile-manufacturer and philanthropist, established the first significant nonreligious communitarian enterprise at New Harmony, Indiana. Owen hoped to abolish poverty and crime through cooperative labor and the collective ownership of property, but within two years New Harmony proved an economic failure. In 1836 the perfectionist John Humphrey Noyes organized a far more successful association of Bible Communists at his home in Putney, Vermont. In 1847, after outraging his neighbors by introducing a system of "complex marriage," involving both polygamy and polyandry, he and his followers moved to central New York, where they formed the Oneida Community. Here, in spite of persistent outside hostility to its sexual practices, the community grew to about three hundred members, established a model educational system, and prospered economically, operating a large farm and several manufacturing enterprises. The Oneida Community survived until 1879, when both internal and external troubles caused Noyes to dissolve it.

Communitarianism reached its peak during the 1840s, when the ideas of the French reformer Charles Fourier were embraced by many transcendentalists and other perfectionists and popularized by his chief American champion, Albert Brisbane. The perfectionists were attracted by Fourier's optimistic view of human nature, his goal of social harmony, and his plan of voluntary associations, or "phalanxes," free of governmental intervention. Association, explained the idealistic Brisbane, offered "the means of effecting peaceably and in the interest of all classes, a complete transformation in the social condition of the world." The successful establishment of only one association, he believed, would inspire men and women to form others. Ultimately the movement would become universal, and there would emerge "a true Social and Political Order in the place of the old and false one." Of the many phalanxes that briefly put Fourier's ideas into practice, the best remembered was Brook Farm near Boston, founded in 1841 by George Ripley. Until its abandonment in 1847 a number of transcendentalists repaired to it, as Ripley explained, "to prepare a society of liberal, intelligent, and cultivated persons" who could lead "a more simple and wholesome life, than can be led amidst the pressures of our competitive institutions."

Young Nathaniel Hawthorne was one of the transcendentalists who went to Brook Farm, but he left with doubts about the divinity of human beings and a conviction that the perfectionist reformers did not understand the true source of evil in the world. "The heart, the heart," he wrote, "there was the little yet boundless sphere wherein existed the original wrong of which the crime and misery of this outward world were merely types." His caution to the perfectionists is perhaps more understandable to our generation than it was to his: "The progress of the world, at every step, leaves some evil or wrong on the path behind it, which the unrest of mankind, or their own set purpose, could never have found the way to rectify."

Children's hour at Oneida

The Crusade Against Slavery

The beginnings of abolitionism. A reform movement with a liberating ideology and perfectionist goals could hardly have ignored the continued existence of human slavery in the Southern states. The evils of slavery had been acknowledged by many leaders of the Revolutionary generation, and organized antislavery activity, especially among the Quakers, dated back to the late eighteenth century. Pressure from antislavery groups had already achieved the abolition of slavery in the Northern states, and in the 1820s a small manumission movement in the Upper South, supported mostly by Quakers, had called for gradual, compensated emancipation with colonization of the free blacks in Africa.

In the early stages of the movement, because of the prevailing prejudice against blacks, both Northern and Southern emancipationists believed that a program of colonization would remove one of the chief obstacles to slavery's demise. In 1817 they helped to organize the American Colonization Society, and in 1822 the first permanent settlement of free blacks from the United States was planted in a territory named Liberia on the coast of West Africa. The American Colonization Society had only limited success in persuading free blacks to migrate, but the colonization movement introduced many future abolitionists to the antislavery cause. Eventually most abolitionists denounced colonization both as a proslavery attempt to strengthen slavery by eliminating a potential danger and as an injustice to the blacks themselves. Nevertheless, the colonization idea persisted among more moderate critics of slavery (including Abraham Lincoln) to the time of the Civil War.

During the 1820s Benjamin Lundy, a New Jersey Quaker, was the most important American emancipationist. Advocating a program of gradual emancipation, compensation to slaveholders, and colonization of the liberated slaves, Lundy helped organize local manumission societies in Tennessee, North Carolina, and Virginia and at the same time edited an antislavery newspaper, *The Genius of Universal Emancipation* in Baltimore. In 1830 young William Lloyd Garrison, a reformer from Boston, got his start as an antislavery crusader writing for Lundy's paper. But Garrison was a man of different temperament and brought a new passion and militancy to the attack. One of his strident editorials led to his arrest and brief imprisonment, after which he left Baltimore and returned to Boston. There, on January 1, 1831, he began the publication of *The Liberator*, a weekly newspaper dedicated to the immediate abolition of Southern slavery without compensation to the masters or colonization of the emancipated blacks. Garrison set the

William Lloyd Garrison: "as harsh as truth"

tone of his crusade in the prospectus printed in the first issue:

> I will be as harsh as truth, and as uncompromising as justice. On this subject, I do not wish to think, or speak, or write with moderation. . . . I am in earnest—I will not equivocate—I will not excuse—I will not retreat a single inch—AND I WILL BE HEARD.

In 1832 Garrison organized the New England Anti-Slavery Society and a year later helped to establish a national organization, the American Anti-Slavery Society. During the next few years abolitionist agents were busy establishing local societies, until by 1840 a network of some two thousand of them with nearly two hundred thousand members stretched across the North. To many, Garrison was the embodiment of abolitionism, and the angry response of the South to his harsh words kept him in the public eye. But he was more an editor and publicist than an effective leader and tactician, and the movement soon grew too large for him to control. Other abolitionists also played significant roles: Wendell Phillips in New England, Gerrit Smith and the Tappans in New York, and Theodore Dwight Weld in the West. Weld, a product of the Finney revival in upstate New York, was perhaps the most successful of the abolitionist organizers. In 1834, at the Lane Theological Seminary in Cincinnati, Weld persuaded the students to engage in a prolonged debate on the subject of slavery. In the course of the debate many students became converts to abolitionism; and when the conservative trustees ordered them to cease discussing slavery, Weld's converts withdrew from Lane in a body and moved to

Pennsylvania Anti-Slavery Society

Oberlin College. In subsequent years the Lane rebels joined Weld as agents and organizers for the American Anti-Slavery Society. Using the techniques of the revivalists, these men won thousands of converts among rural and small-town native-born Protestants in New England, upstate New York, western Pennsylvania, and the Great Lakes region of the Old Northwest.

At length, in 1840, resentment against Garrison, disagreement over his effort to admit women to full participation, and differences over tactics caused a split in abolitionist ranks and led to the withdrawal of the anti-Garrisonians from the American Anti-Slavery Society to form a society of their own. Thereafter abolitionism was only loosely organized at the national level, and the real force of the crusade came from the state and local groups.

Except for communitarianism and perhaps feminism, abolition was the most radical cause of the reformers, for it attacked not only the basic structure of Southern society but an institution whose filaments ran through the whole national economy. To justify their crusade against it, abolitionists described slavery as the greatest social evil in the way of the nation's moral regeneration. Confident of humanity's great potential, they found particularly obnoxious a system that denied individuals control over their own destiny and upheld the right of one human being to hold another as property. To prove its wickedness abolition-

ists dwelt on its corrupting impact on slaveholders and the cruelties inflicted on the slaves, for they were always less interested in presenting a balanced picture than in winning converts. Slavery provided abolitionists with plenty of illustrations of cruelty. In 1839 Weld published a powerful antislavery tract, *Slavery As It Is*, which was simply a documented compilation of atrocities culled from Southern newspapers and court records. The Southern states made themselves especially vulnerable to criticism by refusing to eliminate the system's worst abuses: its physical cruelty, its failure to give legal recognition to slave marriages, the separation of children from their parents, the callous practices of the interstate slave-traders, and the denial to Negroes of opportunities for self-improvement.

Abolitionism also attracted Northern reformers because the Southern manumission societies had failed to accomplish their purpose; slavery, it appeared, would never be destroyed without intervention from the outside. It no longer seemed to be a weak and declining institution that could be left to die a natural death; instead it was flourishing and spreading westward into new territories and states. The reformers were shocked by the Southerners' growing tendency to defend slavery as a desirable and permanent institution and by their increasingly harsh treatment of even native Southern critics. One reformer expressed his dismay at "the sentiments openly expressed in southern newspapers, that slavery is not an evil . . . [and] that it is criminal toward the South . . . to indulge even a hope that the chains of the captive may some day or other, no matter how remote the time, be broken." Moreover, the reformers were acutely conscious of the hypocrisy of America's posing as a model of liberal institutions while remaining one of the last countries in the Western world to tolerate human bondage. Finally, the success of British abolitionists in securing emancipation in the British West Indies (1833) stimulated the reformers to undertake a similar crusade in America.

One small group of Americans, the free blacks, needed no prodding from white reformers to support abolitionism, and in the North they made a significant contribution to the movement. Northern free Negroes always constituted the majority of subscribers to Garrison's *Liberator*, and after the organization of the American Anti-Slavery Society three Negroes always served on its executive committee. Among the most prominent Negro abolitionist agents and orators were Samuel Ringgold Ward, who escaped from slavery in Maryland; Lunsford Lane, who was born a slave in North Carolina and bought his own freedom; Sojourner Truth, who was born a slave in New York and was freed by the state emancipation act; Charles Lenox Remond, a well-educated Massachusetts Negro who lectured in Great Britain as well as in the United States; and Frederick Douglass, who escaped from slavery in Maryland to become editor of an antislavery newspaper, one of the greatest of all antislavery orators, and the preeminent American Negro leader of the nineteenth century. Though most black abolitionists accepted the peaceful tactics of their white comrades, a few helped to build a tradition of militant activism. In Boston, in 1829, David Walker, a free Negro born in North Carolina, published an angry *Appeal to the Colored Citizens of the World*, justifying

violence to destroy slavery and warning white masters of the coming retribution for holding blacks in bondage. In 1843, Henry H. Garnet, in an address before a Negro convention in Buffalo, urged slaves to strike for their liberties: "Let your motto be resistance! . . . No oppressed people have ever secured their liberty without resistance." Many free Negroes guided fugitives to freedom over the so-called underground railroad. Among them was Harriet Tubman, who escaped from slavery in Maryland but returned nineteen times to help several hundred slaves flee from their bondage.

Abolitionist tactics. The tactics of the abolitionists were determined by their optimistic assumptions about human nature, by their faith in the power of truth, by their belief that slavery was essentially a moral issue, and by the restrictive political structure within which they had to operate. They were confronted with the problem that Congress, unlike the British Parliament, had no constitutional power to abolish slavery. At the same time, the pacifism of most abolitionists discouraged the use of force. In its statement of principles, the New England Anti-Slavery Society affirmed that "we will not operate on the existing relations of society by other than peaceful and lawful means, and that we will give no countenance to violence or insurrection." Abolitionists, therefore, relied on "moral suasion." Their first goal was to persuade slaveholders that slavery was a sin requiring repentance, as well as a denial of the "unalienable rights" with which, according to the Declaration of Independence, all men are endowed. Though abolitionists believed in immediate emancipation—slaveholding being a sin, a moral person could not advocate abandoning it gradually—they were practical enough to understand that the actual implementation of emancipation might take a little time. In an era of revivalism they might hope for mass conversions of slaveholders,

Harriet Tubman and fellow escapees

but they could hardly hope that all slaveholders would give up the institution in a single year. Moreover, they understood that there would probably have to be a period of transition while the Negroes were prepared for their new status as freedmen. Hence they usually qualified their "immediatism" by defining it, in one way or another, as a program of emancipation "promptly commenced" but "gradually accomplished." But the theoretical immediatism to which abolitionists were committed strengthened the conviction of indignant Southerners that abolitionists were reckless incendiaries seeking to bring ruin upon the South.

When the abolitionists failed to move the slaveholders to action, when they found it nearly impossible to carry their message into the South, they turned to building up antislavery opinion in the North. Their propaganda hammered relentlessly at their central argument: every person of full age and sane mind has a right to freedom unless convicted of a crime; "mere difference of complexion is no reason why any man should be deprived of any of his natural rights"; "man cannot, consistently with reason, religion, and the eternal and immutable principles of justice, be the property of man"; "whoever retains his fellow-man in bondage is guilty of a grievous wrong." Abolitionists sometimes spoke of the alleged economic waste of slavery, but their indictment was chiefly moral and religious.

Whether moral suasion might be supplemented by some form of political action was a question on which abolitionists differed. Garrison's nonresistance principles turned him against government as an instrument of force and therefore against involvement in politics. Moreover, he viewed the political parties as tools of the slaveholders, the Union as their protector, and the Constitution as a proslavery document

(in his words, "a covenant with death and an agreement with hell"). Most abolitionists, however, though recognizing that Congress could not touch slavery in the states, believed that some things might be accomplished through political action—for example, the abolition of slavery in the District of Columbia, the outlawing of the interstate slave trade, and the exclusion of slavery from federal territories. Hence they took an active part in politics and put pressure on congressional candidates to take antislavery positions. In 1840 a group of political abolitionists organized the Liberty party and nominated James G. Birney for the Presidency, but the small vote the party attracted in this and subsequent elections indicated that most abolitionists preferred to operate through existing parties. With the growth of political abolitionism there was a notable decline in pacifist sentiment, and the sectional conflict of the 1850s prepared many abolitionists to turn from moral suasion to force as the ultimate remedy.

In the early years of the movement most Northerners shared the opinion of Southerners that abolitionists were irresponsible fanatics, and antislavery meetings were frequently broken up by violence. In 1834 a mob invaded Lewis Tappan's house and destroyed the furnishings; in 1835 a Boston mob treated Garrison so roughly that authorities took him to jail for his own protection; and in 1837 a mob in Alton, Illinois, murdered Elijah Lovejoy, an abolitionist editor. After being mobbed on several occasions, Weld warned fellow abolitionists that each would have to decide "whether he can lie upon the rack," or "if cloven down, fall and die a martyr."

Northern businessmen, viewing antislavery agitation as a threat to their profitable trade with the South, more than once joined or encouraged the mobs. Nationalists opposed the abolitionists, because

> *Here are three millions of slaves in a land calling itself free; three millions of human beings robbed of every right, and, by statute and custom, among a people self-styled Christian, held as brutes. Knowledge is forbidden and religious worship, if allowed, is clogged with fetters; the sanctity of marriages is denied; and home and family and all the sacred names of kindred, which form the dialect of domestic love, are made unmeaning words. The soul is crushed, that the body may be safely coined into dollars.*
>
> *What if the black man is inferior to the white? It does not follow that he always must be. Excel him where his chances are equal, before you boast yourself above him. Give him his liberty, and as strong a motive to exertion as you have; a prospect of reward as sure and ample; not only wages for his toil, but respect and honor and social standing according to his worth, and see what he can then become.... His powers have never yet been fairly tried, for he has always had to struggle against difficulties and discouragements which white men do not meet.*

Slavery: an abolitionist's view

From Charles C. Burleigh, "Slavery and the North," 1855.

their crusade endangered the federal Union; conservative churchmen feared that attacks on slavery might divide the churches along sectional lines. However, race prejudice, which was nearly as intense in the North as in the South, was always the fundamental cause of the hostility to abolitionism. The prevailing prejudice exposed Northern free Negroes to many forms of discrimination. They were prohibited from entering most trades and professions and forced into menial occupations; they were excluded from the public schools or sent to segregated schools; they were assigned segregated seats in white churches and on public transportation; they were barred from office-holding and jury duty; they were denied the ballot except in five New England states and in New York (where they had to meet a property qualification not required of whites); and they were prohibited from settling in several Western states. Indeed, it is safe to say that if Southern slaves had been white rather than black, Northerners would have been far less prone to advance practical arguments against antislavery agitation. Even some of the abolitionists were unable to free themselves entirely from the prevailing prejudice and shrank from personal contacts with Negroes, but as a group their racial attitudes were so liberal that their contemporaries often denounced them as "nigger-lovers." There is much evidence that the efforts of abolitionists to eliminate discrimination and segregation in the North, which was a second goal of many of them, greatly intensified Northern hostility toward them.

A broadening appeal. Though abolitionists had only limited success in reducing Northern prejudice

against Negroes, the growing sectional tension of the 1840s and 1850s caused Northerners to listen more sympathetically to what they had to say about the South and the evils of slavery. Eventually abolitionist agitation helped to persuade large numbers of Northerners that even black slavery was morally wrong and therefore could not be accepted as a permanent institution. This agitation also produced an image of slaveholders as unenterprising, undemocratic, arrogant, immoral, and cruel. The slaveholders and their political henchmen, said the abolitionists, formed a sinister "Slave Power" that ruled the South and conspired to rule the entire Union in order to destroy freedom and make slavery a national institution. Theodore Parker described the Slave Power as

> the blight of this nation, the curse of the North and the curse of the South. . . . It confounds your politics. It has silenced your ablest men. It has muzzled the pulpit, and stifled the press. It has robbed three million men of what is dearer than life; it has kept back the welfare of seventeen million more.

Meanwhile, as the abolitionists braved mobs to defend freedom of assembly and of the press, they began to win admiration as champions of civil liberties not only for blacks but for whites. They aroused sympathy when Southern mobs broke into post offices to destroy packages of antislavery pamphlets, for now the right of minority groups to disseminate their ideas through the mails seemed to be at stake. In 1836, when the abolitionists deluged Congress with petitions urging the abolition of slavery in the District of Columbia, Southerners forced through the House a so-called gag rule, which provided that petitions relating to slavery were to be laid on the table without being printed, referred to committee, or debated. Until the repeal of the gag rule in 1844, abolitionists stood as defenders of another sacred liberty: the right of petition.

Most Northerners also sympathized with the more or less systematic efforts of abolitionists to assist fugitive slaves to freedom along the routes of the underground railroad. Few could help feeling compassion for pathetic fugitives seeking their own liberty, and even a Negrophobe might resent the activities of the professional slave-catchers who roamed the free states. In 1842 an important case (*Prigg* v. *Pennsylvania*) involving the constitutionality of the Fugitive Slave Act of 1793 came before the Supreme Court. Though the Court ruled that the act was constitutional, it conceded that a state might prohibit its own officers from helping to enforce it. Thereafter a number of states, under pressure from the abolitionists, adopted "personal-liberty laws" that withheld assistance in the capture of fugitives.

On one issue—whether slavery should be introduced into new territories and states—the abolitionists eventually gained overwhelming Northern support. Northerners continued to agree that the Constitution prevented federal interference with slavery in the Southern states, but by the 1850s they felt strongly that slavery should not be permitted to enlarge its domain. Often this sentiment sprang less from sympathy for the black than from a determination of free white farmers to keep slaveholders out of the territories they coveted. But the abolitionist indictment of slavery proved a handy weapon for them to use against Southern expansionists.

In one fundamental respect the abolitionist crusade was a failure. Since it did not convert the slaveholders, it never achieved its original goal: peaceful abolition through moral suasion. Abolitionists who hoped to eliminate prejudice and discrimination in the Northern states, of course, suffered a second defeat. But in another and unexpected way the crusade was a success. Though it was launched by pacifists, by 1861 abolitionism, which had itself grown increasingly militant, had helped to arm the Northern population morally for the terrible struggle that lay ahead.

The Proslavery Argument

Slavery a positive good. In January 1837 Senator John C. Calhoun boldly took a position toward which many Southern apologists for slavery had been drifting:

> I hold that in the present state of civilization, where two races of different origin, and distin-

Northern caricature of John C. Calhoun

guished by color and other physical differences, as well as intellectual, are brought together, the relation now existing in the slaveholding states between the two is, instead of an evil, a good—a positive good.

There would be no more apologies—no concessions that slavery was at best a necessary evil—as Southern dialecticians spun out the arguments affirming the benign qualities of their peculiar institution. Never before had the justification of human bondage been presented with so much moral fervor and in such elaborate detail as in the antebellum South. Indeed the proslavery argument was one of the most impressive products of its intellectual life. Southern poets, theologians, moral philosophers, social theorists, jurists, and scientists combined their talents to uphold slavery and denounce heresy and radicalism.

This body of proslavery literature is significant not only because it was one of the principal contributions of Southern men of letters but because it was a rare expression in nineteenth-century America of deep pessimism about human nature, of doubt about the liberal tradition, and of skepticism about progress. As one Southerner insisted, "it cannot be denied that we must still look to antiquity for the noblest deeds and grandest thoughts that illustrate the race of men." Romanticism, which found expression in the North in the reform movement and in a remarkable burst of literary productivity, found expression in the South in a cult of chivalry and in an attempt to identify the planter class with traditional aristocratic values.

The nature of the defense. Since the average slaveholder was highly religious, a theological defense of slavery was almost invariably incorporated in the numerous treatises on the subject. Out of the mass of Scriptural arguments, three were of crucial importance. The first identified the Negroes as the descendants of Canaan, the son of Ham, of whom Noah said, "Cursed be Canaan; a servant of servants shall he be unto his brethren." The second pointed to Mosaic law, which authorized the Jews to make bondsmen "of the heathen that are round about you." The third noted that neither the prophets of the Old Testament nor Christ and his apostles ever condemned slavery. Rather, they repeatedly admonished servants to obey their masters and to submit to their earthly lot. The proper role of the church, therefore, was not to attack slavery but to bring spiritual salvation to the slaves and to urge benevolence on their masters.

Turning to history, the defenders argued that slavery had always existed in some form and that it had been the foundation of all the great civilizations of antiquity. Aristotle, whose thought permeates the proslavery argument, taught that in every organized society the men of superior talents would become masters over those of inferior talents. Slavery thus enabled a class to emerge that could devote its genius to art, literature, and other intellectual pursuits. "It is a common remark," wrote George Fitzhugh of Virginia, "that the grand and lasting architectural structures of antiquity were the results of slavery."

Yet, in spite of such generalizations, few Southerners were prepared to defend their own slave system on a class basis—that is, as a desirable condition for certain classes of people of all races. Rather, their defense was essentially a defense of *black* slavery—of the subordination of the black race to the white. Since all Southern slaves had at least some African ancestors, evidence that Africans were innately inferior to whites was crucial to the Southern justification of the peculiar institution. By a curious combination of comparative anatomy and the pseudoscience of phrenology, Southern ethnologists attributed to blacks certain distinct physical and psychic traits that suggested their inferiority to the whites. In the Negro, claimed a Georgia doctor, "the animal parts of the brain preponderate over the moral and intellectual," which explains why he is "deficient in reason, judgment and forecast . . . thoughtless of the future, and contented and happy in the enjoyment of the mere animal pleasures of the present moment." The inevitable conclusion was that "nothing but arbitrary power can restrain the excesses of his animal nature: for he has not the power within himself." These and other alleged racial diversities established the master-slave relationship between whites and blacks as a natural condition, its abolition a profound disaster to both groups.

Belief in the inferiority of Negroes led also to the conclusion that the affirmations of the Declaration of Independence, the provisions of state bills of rights, and the benefits of citizenship did not and were not intended to apply to them. Society must have a class "to perform the drudgery of life," affirmed James H. Hammond of South Carolina, a class "requiring but a low order of intellect," a class that "constitutes the very mud-sill of society." Black slavery provided this class and, by freeing the whites from menial tasks, elevated all members of the privileged caste to a condition of perfect equality.

The South had found in slavery, argued its defenders, a way to avoid the dangers to order and property posed by the laboring classes in free society. Slavery served as a conservative bulwark against all the radical "isms" that threatened the North with revolution. In the South the slaves were "orderly and efficient," and society had within it no element of disharmony. "It is the only condition of society in which labor and capital are associated on a large scale in which their interests are combined and not in conflict. Every plantation is an organized community . . . where *all work*, where *each member gets subsistence and a home*." Slavery, in short, was a practical form of socialism.

In every respect, said Southern apologists, the slaves were better off than so-called free laborers. They were happy and contented, because they were well treated, well fed, well housed, and well clothed; they were cared for in childhood, in old age, and in times of sickness. The free-labor system, which left workers to shift for themselves, was far more cruel and heartless. "I may say with truth," said Calhoun, "that in few countries so much is left to the share of the laborer, and so little exacted from him." Indeed, wrote a Virginian, "a merrier being does not exist on the face of the globe, than the Negro slave of the United States."

The defense of slavery as a positive good in the South at a time when a great reform movement was agitating the North posed a serious threat to the survival of the Union. Slavery was no longer open to discussion in the South, and slaveholders intensely resented its denunciation on moral grounds in the North. Not even the two largest Protestant churches were able to bear the strain, and the slavery issue led to sectional splits—the Methodists in 1844, the Baptists in 1845. Eventually the national political parties would also disintegrate, and thus another major institutional tie would be broken. Abolitionists and proslavery polemicists had raised a moral issue—the right and wrong of slavery—that stubbornly resisted resolution by the best efforts of a generation of able politicians and statesmen.

Suggestions for Reading

RELIGION

All the surveys of American cultural and intellectual history devote much space to religion in the first half of the nineteenth century. The best on this subject are R. H. Gabriel, *The Course of American Democratic Thought*, rev. ed. (1956), and Perry Miller, *The Life of the Mind in America: From the Revolution to the Civil War**, Vol. I (1966). I. H. Bartlett, *The American Mind in the Mid-Nineteenth Century** (1967), is brief and readable. S. E. Ahlstrom, *A Religious History of the American People** (1972), is an outstanding survey that stresses the importance of religious ideas in American culture. Several useful general studies of American religion should also be consulted: E. S. Gaustad, *A Religious History of America** (1966); M. E. Marty, *Righteous Empire: The Protestant Experience in America* (1970); and J. W. Smith and A. L. Jamison, eds., *Religion in American Life*, 4 vols. (1961). H. F. May, *The Enlightenment in America** (1976), is a major study of religious thought in the early years of the Republic.

The revolt against orthodox Calvinism can be traced in H. M. Morais, *Deism in Eighteenth Century America* (1934); Albert Post, *Popular Free Thought in America* (1943); Conrad Wright, *The Beginnings of Unitarianism in America* (1955); R. L. Patterson, *The Philosophy of William Ellery Channing* (1952); D. P. Edgell, *William Ellery Channing* (1955); M. H. Rice, *Federal Street Pastor: The Life of William Ellery Channing* (1961); and Andrew Delbanco, *William Ellery Channing: An Essay on the Liberal Spirit in America* (1981). D. W. Howe, *The Unitarian Conscience: Harvard Moral Philosophy, 1805–1861* (1970), is a lucid, comprehensive analysis of Unitarian thought. Transcendentalism is examined in two distinguished works on American literature in this period: V. W. Brooks, *The Flowering of New England, 1815–1865** (1936), and F. O. Matthiessen, *American Renaissance** (1941). P. F. Boller, Jr., *American Transcendentalism, 1830–1860: An Intellectual Inquiry* (1974), and A. C. Rose, *Transcendentalism as a Social Movement, 1830–1850* (1981), are excellent brief studies. There are good biographies of several transcendentalist leaders: H. S. Commager, *Theodore Parker: Yankee Crusader* (1936); A. M. Schlesinger, Jr., *Orestes A. Brownson: A Pilgrim's Progress* (1939); J. W. Krutch, *Henry David Thoreau* (1948); Richard Lebeaux, *Young Man Thoreau* (1977); R. L. Lusk, *The Life of Ralph Waldo Emerson* (1949); and Paula Blanchard, *Margaret Fuller: From Transcendentalism to Revolution* (1978).

A good survey of Protestant revivalism is W. W. Sweet, *Revivalism in America* (1944). Much valuable detail is added in W. R. Cross, *The Burned-Over District** (1950); C. A. Johnson, *The Frontier Camp Meeting* (1955); B. A. Weisberger, *They Gathered at the River* (1958); W. G. McLoughlin, Jr., *Modern Revivalism* (1959); and D. G. Mathews, *Religion in the Old South** (1977). Two important books tie revivalism to the reform movement: C. C. Cole, Jr., *The Social Ideas of the Northern Evangelists, 1826–1860* (1954), and T. L. Smith, *Revivalism and Social Reform in Mid-Nineteenth Century America** (1957). F. M. Brodie, *No Man Knows My History: The Life of Joseph Smith* (1945), is an outstanding biography of the founder of Mormonism. Sympathetic studies of Mormonism include James Allen and Glen Leonard, *The Story of the Latter-Day Saints* (1976); L. J. Arrington and Davis Bitton, *A History of the Latter-Day Saints** (1979); and K. J. Hansen, *Mormonism and the American Experience** (1981).

REFORM

R. G. Walters, *American Reformers, 1815–1860** (1978), is a good introduction to the reform movement. The most comprehensive general treatment, though dated, is A. F. Tyler, *Freedom's Ferment** (1944). C. S. Griffen, *The Ferment of Reform** (1967), is an excellent brief, interpretive, and historiographical essay. Lewis Perry, *Childhood, Marriage, and Reform* (1980), offers a fresh interpretation. Other useful books are E. D. Branch, *The Sentimental Years, 1836–1860* (1934); and C. S. Griffen, *Their Brothers' Keepers: Moral Stewardship in the United States, 1800–1865* (1960).

In the vast literature on specific reforms, the following are among the best: Blake McKelvey, *American Prisons** (1936); H. E. Marshall, *Dorothea Dix: Forgotten Samaritan* (1937); F. L. Byrne, *Prophet of Prohibition: Neal Dow and His Crusade* (1961); I. R. Tyrrell, *Sobering Up: From Temperance to Prohibition in Antebellum America, 1800–1860* (1979); R. E. Riegel, *American Feminists* (1963); W. L. O'Neill, *Everyone Was Brave: The Rise and Fall of Feminism in America* (1970); Page Smith, *Daughters of the Promised Land** (1970); Gerda Lerner, *The Woman in American History* (1971);

Eleanor Flexnor, *Century of Struggle: The Woman's Rights Movement in the United States**, rev. ed. (1975); M. P. Ryan, *Womanhood in America** (1975); K. E. Melder, *Beginnings of Sisterhood: The American Women's Rights Movement, 1800–1850* (1977); Lois Banner, *Elizabeth Cady Stanton** (1980); C. N. Degler, *At Odds: Women and the Family in America from the Revolution to the Present** (1980); L. H. Tharp, *Until Victory: Horace Mann and Mary Peabody* (1953); Jonathan Messerli, *Horace Mann: A Biography* (1972); F. M. Binder, *The Age of the Common School* (1974); L. A. Cremin, *American Education: The National Experience, 1783–1876** (1980); Lee Soltow and Edward Stevens, *The Rise of Literacy and the Common School in the United States* (1981); and C. F. Carstle, *Pillars of the Republic: Common Schools and American Society, 1780–1860* (1983).

ABOLITION AND PROSLAVERY

The best surveys of the abolitionist movement are Louis Filler, *The Crusade Against Slavery* (1960); Gerald Sorin, *Abolitionism: A New Perspective* (1972); M. L. Dillon, *The Abolitionists: The Growth of a Dissenting Minority** (1974); and J. B. Stewart, *Holy Warriors: The Abolitionists and American Slavery** (1976). G. H. Barnes, *The Antislavery Impulse, 1830–1844* (1933), now dated but a pioneer work, stresses the role of Theodore Dwight Weld at the expense of Garrison. It should be compared with A. S. Kraditor, *Means and Ends in American Abolitionism* (1967). D. G. Mathews, *Slavery and Methodism* (1965), traces the conflict in one of the largest Protestant denominations. Three important facets of abolitionism are examined in R. B. Nye, *Fettered Freedom: Civil Liberties and the Slavery Controversy, 1830–1860*, rev. ed. (1963); Carleton Mabee, *Black Freedom: The Nonviolent Abolitionists from 1830 through the Civil War* (1970); and Lewis Perry, *Radical Abolitionism: Anarchy and the Government of God in Antislavery Thought* (1973). Benjamin Quarles, *Black Abolitionists* (1969), and J. H. and W. H. Pease, *They Who Would Be Free** (1974), describe the role of the Negro in the antislavery movement. Arthur Zilversmit, *The First Emancipation** (1967), traces the abolition of slavery in the Northern states. D. B. Davis, *The Problem of Slavery in the Age of the Revolution, 1770–1823** (1975), is an excellent study of the intellectual origins of the abolition movement. R. G. Walters, *The Antislavery Appeal* (1976), examines its cultural roots. L. J. Friedman, *Gregarious Saints** (1982), is a penetrating psychological study.

Among the best biographies of abolitionist leaders are Benjamin Quarles, *Frederick Douglass** (1948); Robert Abzug, *Passionate Liberator: Theodore Dwight Weld and the Dilemma of Reform** (1980); Betty Fladeland, *James Gillespie Birney: Slaveholder to Abolitionist* (1955); I. H. Bartlett, *Wendell Phillips: Brahmin Radical* (1962); J. L. Thomas, *The Liberator: William Lloyd Garrison* (1963); M. L. Dillon, *Benjamin Lundy and the Struggle for Negro Freedom* (1966); Gerda Lerner, *The Grimké Sisters from South Carolina: Rebels Against Slavery** (1967); T. G. Edelstein, *Strange Enthusiasm: A Life of Thomas Wentworth Higginson** (1968); and Bertram Wyatt-Brown, *Lewis Tappan and the Evangelical War Against Slavery** (1969). J. H. and W. H. Pease, *Bound with Them in Chains* (1972), illustrates the varieties of antislavery thought through the lives of ten abolitionists.

Racism, one of the chief obstacles the abolitionists confronted, is analyzed in William Stanton, *The Leopard's Spots: Scientific Attitudes Toward Race in America, 1815–1859** (1960), and G. M. Fredrickson, *The Black Image in the White Mind* (1971). L. F. Litwack, *North of Slavery** (1961), is an excellent empirical study of race prejudice in the North. Violence against abolitionists is analyzed in Lorman Ratner, *Powder Keg: Northern Opposition to the Antislavery Movement, 1831–1840* (1968), and L. L. Richards, *Gentlemen of Property and Standing: Anti-Abolition Mobs in Jacksonian America** (1970).

W. S. Jenkins, *Pro-Slavery Thought in the Old South* (1935), is a comprehensive analysis of the proslavery argument. Harvey Wish, *George Fitzhugh: Propagandist of the Old South* (1943), and Drew Faust, *A Sacred Circle* (1977), are studies of proslavery thinkers.

*Available in a paperback edition.

11
EXPANSION AND
SECTIONAL CRISIS

The acquisition of Louisiana and Florida in the early nineteenth century quieted for a time the American urge for expansion. Feeling secure from foreign intervention, and satisfied that there was ample space for a growing population, most Americans who moved west in the 1820s and 1830s were content to take up the vacant lands in their already immense country. They occupied the unsettled regions of Mississippi, Missouri, and Illinois and poured into new territories that soon would become states: Arkansas (1836), Michigan (1837), Florida (1845), Iowa (1846), and Wisconsin (1848). Except for the Mexican province of Texas, the vast area beyond Missouri and Arkansas, stretching out to the Rocky Mountains, was then of no interest to the westward-moving settlers. Because explorers reported that the land was too arid for farming, cartographers labeled it the "Great American Desert," and white Americans presented it as a "permanent" gift to the Indians. The donors felt there was room enough and plenty for white men to the east of this "Indian Country."

Or so it seemed until the 1840s, when the impulse to expand suddenly stirred anew. Actually, few Americans had ever assumed that the boundaries of the United States would stand forever unchanged. Though some pressed expansion more aggressively than others, few challenged the idea that providence had destined their country to continued growth. Expansion, however, raised the touchy question of

whether slavery should be permitted to spread into the territories that were acquired. Much of the controversy recently generated by proslavery and anti-slavery propagandists began to center on that problem, and by the end of the 1840s it had precipitated a national crisis. In 1850, after months of bitter debate, a compromise was painfully constructed—a makeshift arrangement that settled nothing yet somehow served to hold the Union together for another decade.

Westward to the Pacific

Manifest Destiny. The reasons for the revived interest in territorial expansion were several. The first and most obvious was that the American people, with their sense of mission, were sorely tempted by the boundless tracts of unsettled or sparsely settled land lying just beyond the borders of their country. During the 1820s and 1830s American fur-trappers, in their search for beaver streams, had been blazing trails, searching out passes through the mountains, and ranging over the fertile valleys of the Far West. The publicity they gave to the region beyond the Great American Desert at once strengthened the myth of the West as a land of romance and adventure and aroused interest in its agricultural possibilities.

274

Dreams of fortunes in gold

Manifest Destiny? *Did this country know itself, or were it disposed to profit by self-knowledge, it would feel the necessity of laying an immediate curb on its passion for extended territory.... We are a restless people, prone to encroachment, impatient of the ordinary laws of progress.... We boast of our rapid growth, forgetting that, throughout nature, noble growths are slow.....*

It is full time that we should lay on ourselves serious, resolute restraint. Possessed of a domain, vast enough for the growth of ages, it is time for us to stop in the career of acquisition and conquest. Already endangered by our greatness, we cannot advance without imminent peril to our institutions, union, prosperity, virtue, and peace....

It is sometimes said, that nations are swayed by laws, as unfailing as those which govern matter; that they have their destinies; that their character and position carry them forward irresistibly to their goal;... that ... the Indians have melted before the white man, and the mixed, degraded race of Mexico must melt before the Anglo-Saxon. Away with this vile sophistry! There is no necessity for crime. There is no fate to justify rapacious nations, any more than to justify gamblers and robbers, in plunder. We boast of the progress of society, and this progress consists in the substitution of reason and moral principle for the sway of brute force.... We talk of accomplishing our destiny. So did the late conquerer of Europe [Napoleon]; and destiny consigned him to a lonely rock in the ocean, the prey of an ambition which destroyed no peace but his own.

From William E. Channing, Letter to Henry Clay, 1837.

A second reason was a growing desire to develop trade with the Far East and the belief, as one expansionist politician expressed it, that along the valley of the Columbia River "lies the North American road to India." Many Eastern businessmen began to look covetously at the three best natural harbors on the Pacific coast, at San Diego, San Francisco, and Puget Sound.

A third reason—and the one that probably explains the rebirth of expansionism at this precise time—was renewed fear that the security of the United States might be impaired by foreign intervention in areas along its borders, especially by British activity in Texas, California, and Oregon. Once again freedom and republican institutions in North America seemed threatened by the aggressive meddling of Europeans.

The expansionist drive was further strengthened by a mystical and romantic concept that, though hardly new, now received an attractive label. In 1845 a New York editor wrote exuberantly that it was America's "manifest destiny to overspread and to possess the whole of the continent which Providence has given us for the development of the great experiment of liberty and federated self-government entrusted to us." This doctrine of Manifest Destiny, quickly taken up by the press and politicians, was in part the kind of rationalization that expansionists everywhere and at all times have used to justify territorial aggrandize-

ment. They invariably proclaim the superiority of their own culture and insist that their conquests merely fulfill a divine mission and are impelled by forces beyond human control. So did Americans when they spoke of their Manifest Destiny. Editors and stump-speakers often advocated expansion in terms so extravagant as to make the United States sound like a nation of swashbucklers. "Make way, I say, for the young American Buffalo," shouted a New Jersey politician, "he has not yet got land enough."

But running through the boasts and the threats was a thread of idealism that tied expansion to America's assumed mission to serve as a model of political democracy. Expansion in these terms was a means of "extending the area of freedom," to quote a popular phrase of the day. America's destiny was not only to teach by precept but to bring more land and more people under its jurisdiction—in short, to spread its democratic institutions over the entire North American continent. Thus, as one politician explained, America would become "a vast theatre on which to work out the grand experiment of Republican government."

Unfortunately, intertwined with the thread of democratic idealism was a thread of racism justifying the conquest of Indians and Latin Americans and their subordination to the authority of the North American republic. The "grand experiment," politi-

Texas has been absorbed into the Union in the inevitable fulfilment of the general law which is rolling our population westward.... It was disintegrated from Mexico in the natural course of events, by a process perfectly legitimate on its own part, blameless on ours.... [Its] incorporation into the Union was not only inevitable, but the most natural, right and proper thing in the world....

California will, probably, next fall away from ... Mexico.... Imbecile and distracted, Mexico never can exert any real governmental authority over such a country.... The Anglo-Saxon foot is already on its borders. Already the advance guard of the irresistible army of Anglo-Saxon emigration has begun to pour down upon it, armed with the plough and the rifle, and marking its trail with schools and colleges, courts and representative halls, mills and meeting houses. A population will soon be in actual occupation of California, over which it will be idle for Mexico to dream of dominion.... All this without agency of our government, without responsibility of our people—in the natural flow of events, the spontaneous working of principles, and the adaptation of the tendencies and wants of the human race to the elemental circumstances in the midst of which they find themselves placed.

From the *Democratic Review*, July 1845.

cians and publicists often noted, was to be carried out "under the auspices of the Anglo-Saxon race." American expansionists, when they spoke of "extending the area of freedom," commonly advanced a racial explanation for the political instability and the weakness of democracy in the countries south of the United States. Thus the same racial attitudes that justified Indian removals, the enslavement of blacks in the South, and discrimination against them in the North helped to make manifest America's "destiny" to expand.

Texas. The first area outside the United States to which settlers moved in substantial numbers was Texas. Mexico, after winning its independence from Spain in 1821, twice rejected American offers to buy this sparsely settled province; but during the 1820s it welcomed Americans who would submit to its jurisdiction and abide by its laws. Among the promoters of settlement in Texas, the most successful was Stephen F. Austin, who obtained a huge land grant from Mexico and planted a flourishing colony on the banks of the Brazos River. Most of the immigrants were Southern speculators, yeoman farmers, and small slaveholders who were attracted by the rich lands suitable for cotton culture and available for a few cents an acre. By 1830 eastern Texas had been occupied by nearly twenty thousand whites and a thousand Negro slaves from the United States.

The Mexican government soon had cause to regret its hospitality, for the American settlers had no intention of giving their allegiance to a nation whose culture was so different from their own. Among numerous sources of friction, one of the most irritating was the fact that Texas did not have its own state government but remained a part of the state of Coahuila, whose legislature the Mexicans controlled. Moreover, the Americans were suspicious of Mexican land titles, which were unlike those they had been accustomed to in the United States. In 1830 the mounting tension had prompted the Mexican government to make a drastic switch in policy: it prohibited further immigration from the United States, stopped the importation of slaves, placed heavy duties on American goods, and dispatched troops to the frontier to see that these laws were enforced. The final blow came when General Santa Anna, who had seized political power in Mexico, not only repudiated his promise to give Texas separate statehood but nearly abolished Mexico's federal system altogether.

To Texans, the parallel between British oppression under George III and Mexican oppression under Santa Anna was clear, and revolution was the obvious and justifiable remedy. For a short time they claimed to be fighting in defense of the old Mexican constitution, but on March 2, 1836, they declared their independence. The struggle was brief. Santa Anna moved into Texas with a large army and won a few minor skirmishes, the most notable being the extermination of a small garrison of Texans at the Alamo mission in San Antonio. But on April 21, 1836, at the Battle of San Jacinto, an army commanded by General Sam Houston decisively defeated the Mexicans and took Santa Anna prisoner. Santa Anna was forced to sign a treaty recognizing Texan independence; and though Mexico later denounced the treaty as having been signed under duress, it made no further attempt to reestablish its authority. The new Republic of Texas then framed a constitution, but in September 1836, when the voters ratified it, they also indicated overwhelming support for annexation to the United States. President Houston forthwith began negotiations with the government at Washington, first for recognition and then for annexation.

American volunteers and supplies had contributed to the Texans' victory over Santa Anna, and proannexation sentiment was strong, especially in the South and West. But opposition to the admission of another slave state began to grow among Whigs and abolitionists in the Northeast. Some practical Whig politicians feared that annexation would lead to war with Mexico; in addition, it would increase the South's power to block legislation favorable to Northern economic interests. Abolitionists and other opponents of Southern expansion charged that the settlement of Texas, the revolution, and the movement for annexation were all parts of a slaveholders' conspiracy to enlarge their empire and open new markets for the vendors of human flesh. Texas thus became an issue in the controversy over slavery.

President Jackson was an ardent annexationist, but he acted cautiously lest he impair Van Buren's chances of winning the presidential election of 1836. Jackson even delayed recognition of Texan independence until the eve of his retirement from office, and Van Buren refused to recommend annexation during his term as President. Rebuffed by the United States, Texas in 1838 turned to Europe for recognition and aid; its leaders began to talk boldly of creating a nation that would expand to the Pacific and rival the United States in size and strength. This was a pleasing prospect to the British, who saw in Texas a buffer to American expansion, a threat to the American cotton monopoly, and a promising new market. Moreover, British abolitionists hoped to persuade the Texans to abolish slavery and prove that cotton could be produced with free labor. As Texan leaders doubtless expected, British interest in their affairs alarmed the United States government, and the talk of abolition frightened the slaveholders of the South.

These developments spurred President Tyler to reopen negotiations with Texas, and he worked vigorously to get a treaty of annexation before his term expired. By April 1844 Tyler's new Secretary of State, John C. Calhoun, had secured the desired treaty, and it was submitted to the Senate for approval. Unfortunately Calhoun also sent a note to the British government concerning its interest in Texas, in which he defended slavery as a positive good and thus strengthened the abolitionist claim that annexation would be the culmination of a proslavery plot. This, along with the continued anxiety about war with Mexico, doomed the treaty; only sixteen senators voted for it, while thirty-five voted against. Annexation was again delayed, and Texas became an issue in the approaching presidential election.

The Santa Fe trade. Meanwhile, a resourceful group of small entrepreneurs had aroused American interest in another of Mexico's remote provinces: New Mexico. Santa Fe and other smaller Spanish outposts on the upper Rio Grande, planted in the seventeenth century, were hundreds of miles from the nearest Mexican settlements, and Spain's rigid trade restrictions had long deprived them of supplies from the United States. In the 1820s, however, the independent Mexican government had opened the Santa Fe trade to Americans. Every spring for the next two decades American merchants assembled their wagons at Independence, Missouri, for the long journey along the Santa Fe Trail. Only a few merchants engaged in the trade—usually not many more than a hundred— but they always found a highly profitable market for their goods. In 1844, to the dismay of the traders, bad feelings generated by the Texas question caused Santa Anna again to exclude Americans from Santa Fe. By then, however, the trade had enlarged the American vision of Manifest Destiny to encompass New Mexico. Though few of the traders had actually settled in Santa Fe, they had opened a route into the Far West, demonstrated that heavily laden wagons could cross the plains, and developed a system of organized caravans for protection against the Indians. Another sparsely settled territory seemed ripe for American plucking.

Oregon. Far to the northwest, in the Oregon country, during the 1830s and early 1840s, merchants, fur-trappers, and missionaries were awakening Americans to the potentialities of still another area, one to which the United States had a solid, though not exclusive, claim. That claim was based on the voyages of Boston merchants to the Oregon coast to buy furs from the Indians in the late eighteenth century; on Captain Robert Gray's discovery of the mouth of the Columbia River in 1792; on the explorations of the Lewis and Clark expedition between 1804 and 1806; and on the founding of Astoria on the Columbia River in 1811 by John Jacob Astor's Pacific Fur Company. In addition, the United States had acquired the French claim to Oregon in the Louisiana Purchase treaty of 1803 and the Spanish claim in the Florida-purchase treaty of 1819. But the British claim was at least as good as the American. Sir Francis Drake, the British insisted, had discovered the Oregon coast in 1579; Captain James Cook and Captain George Van-

Lumber mill, Northwest

couver had visited it again in the eighteenth century; and Alexander Mackenzie had made the first overland trip to Oregon in 1793 as an agent of British fur-trading interests. In short, both the Americans and the British could make strong claims to a huge territory bounded on the south by the forty-second parallel, on the north by the line of 54° 40' (the southern boundary of Russian Alaska), on the east by the Rocky Mountains, and on the west by the Pacific Ocean.

In the early nineteenth century, though neither the British nor the Americans claimed the whole of Oregon, they were unable to agree on a line of division. On several occasions the United States proposed an extension of the forty-ninth parallel to the Pacific, while the British suggested that the line follow the

Fort Laramie, Wyoming

Columbia River from the forty-ninth parallel to its mouth. In 1818 the two countries postponed the settlement of this question and agreed to leave Oregon "free and open" to the citizens of both for a period of ten years. In 1827 they extended the agreement indefinitely, with the proviso that either country could terminate it on a year's notice. There the matter rested until the 1840s.

For many years Americans showed little interest in Oregon, and British fur-traders had the area largely to themselves. After 1821 the Hudson's Bay Company, with its headquarters at Fort Vancouver on the north bank of the Columbia, monopolized the fur trade, and Dr. John McLoughlin, the company's chief factor, gave Oregon the only government it had. McLoughlin was scrupulously fair in dealing with the Indians, and under his efficient direction the company flourished. In the 1830s, however, agents of the Hudson's Bay Company operating in the Rockies began to encounter fierce and ruthless competitors: the intrepid Mountain Men, who hunted beaver skins for the Rocky Mountain Fur Company, directed by Thomas Fitzpatrick, James Bridger, and Milton Sublette. The Mountain Men, along with the agents of Astor's American Fur Company, were the advance guard of American overland penetration of Oregon. One of the most famous of them, Jedediah Smith, a major figure in Western exploration, led expeditions along the Colorado and Gila rivers and through California's interior valleys as well as over much of the Oregon country. Meanwhile, U.S. Army topographical engineers were also exploring the region and preparing maps that subsequently guided emigrant parties on their westward treks.

Efforts by several Eastern promoters to stimulate American migration to Oregon in the 1820s and 1830s ended in failure. But the impulse for settlement soon came from another source. In 1833 an Eastern religious periodical published a report that the Indians of the Oregon country were eager for instruction in the Christian faith. In response to this report (which had little substance to it) the Methodists sent the Reverend Jason Lee, who established a mission in the fertile Willamette Valley; the Presbyterians and Congregationalists sent Dr. Marcus Whitman, who was active farther east, near Fort Walla Walla; and the Catholics sent Father Pierre Jean de Smet, a Jesuit priest from St. Louis, who worked among the Indians in the Rockies. But the Indians showed little interest in the Gospel, and the religious work of the missions proved to be less important than the publicity they gave to Oregon. Scores of missionary letters and reports filled with references to Oregon's fecund soil and salubrious climate found their way into the Eastern press.

As word spread that the Willamette Valley was a new Garden of Eden, the people of the Mississippi Valley began to catch the "Oregon fever." In the late 1830s and early 1840s a trickle of emigrants followed

San Francisco, 1847

the Oregon Trail in quest of free virgin land; in 1843 the first substantial caravans of covered wagons made the two-thousand-mile journey; and soon after the movement to Oregon began to take on the dimensions of a mass migration. The Oregon Trail started at Independence, Missouri, ran northwest to the Platte River, followed the Platte and its north fork into southern Wyoming, made an easy crossing of the Rockies at South Pass, followed the Snake River to a cutoff that led to the Columbia River, and then followed the Columbia to the Willamette Valley. By 1845 at least five thousand Americans had reached Oregon along this route; they had already formed a provisional government and were now demanding that the United States establish exclusive jurisdiction over them. Joint occupation with the British was no longer a satisfactory formula, and a final settlement could not be delayed much longer.

California. South of Oregon lay California, another of Mexico's remote provinces and the fourth area in the Far West where Manifest Destiny seemed to beckon Americans. In the eighteenth century the Spanish, in order to strengthen their control over California and to convert the Indians to Christianity, had encouraged Franciscan friars to build a chain of missions along the coast from San Diego to San Francisco. The missions, at best a mixed blessing to the Indians, were highly successful as large-scale agricultural enterprises; but in 1834 the Mexican government began to deprive them of their lands, and the mission system soon fell apart. Under a succession of weak, inefficient, and often corrupt secular adminis-

trators, California sank into political chaos. But the sparse Mexican population, which in 1846 numbered approximately seven thousand settlers, still managed to live in easygoing comfort, most of them on cattle ranches.

The first American contacts with California were made by whaleboats stopping for supplies. By the 1820s New England merchant ships were putting in along the coast to trade manufactured goods for hides and tallow—a trade vividly depicted in Richard Henry Dana's classic account, *Two Years before the Mast* (1840). Now and then an American sailor deserted his ship and settled down; an occasional party of Mountain Men found its way to California on a trapping expedition; and by the 1830s a few merchants had come to trade with the Indians and Mexicans. Among the merchants was Thomas O. Larkin, who arrived at Monterey in 1832, built a flourishing trade, and worked tirelessly to promote American immigration to California. In the 1840s a few emigrants began to leave the Oregon Trail near the Snake River to follow the California Trail across the Nevada desert and the Sierra Nevada to the Sacramento River Valley. Invariably their goal was Sutter's Fort, the center of a private empire ruled by John A. Sutter, a Swiss immigrant who had acquired Mexican citizenship and was a law unto himself. Sutter welcomed the Americans, furnished them with supplies, and helped them find land. By 1845 California was the home of about seven hundred Americans, almost none of whom expected to give up their American citizenship or to remain beyond the jurisdiction of their government very long.

Sutter's Fort

The "California fever" had become almost as virulent as the "Oregon fever." Emigrants were attracted by the abundance of fertile, unoccupied land and by extravagant descriptions of California as "the richest, the most beautiful, and the healthiest country in the world." Eastern businessmen became increasingly interested in the commercial opportunities, and the American government coveted the harbors at San Diego and San Francisco—the latter was described as "capacious enough to receive the navies of all the world." Reports of British designs on California gave the matter a special urgency. In 1842 Commodore Thomas ap Catesby Jones, commander of the United States Pacific squadron, somehow got the impression that his country had gone to war with Mexico and that British warships were moving toward California. Accordingly, he sailed into Monterey Bay, seized the city, ran up the American flag, and proclaimed the annexation of California to the United States. The embarrassed State Department disavowed Jones' act and made apologies to the Mexican government, but the incident was a clear sign of what the expansionists had in mind.

The Mormon migration. One group of emigrants to the Far West, pursuing a Manifest Destiny of their own, sought to escape the jurisdiction of the United States. These were the Mormons (see p. 255), who in 1847, after many years of persecution, crossed into Mexican territory and established a settlement in the Great Salt Lake basin. From the beginning the Mormon Saints had annoyed the "gentiles" about them with their close-knit communitarian social pattern, their thriving economic life, and their contempt for other religious sects. In their search for a Zion where they could escape this hostility and live in peace, they first moved from New York to Kirtland, Ohio, then to Missouri, then (in 1839) to Nauvoo, Illinois, where their numbers soon grew to fifteen thousand. In 1843,

after five prosperous years, a new crisis developed when Joseph Smith claimed to have received another revelation, this one justifying polygamy. The result was a schism in the Church, a rash of violence, and Smith's arrest and imprisonment. On June 27, 1844, the anti-Mormon mob took him from jail and murdered him. Once more the Mormons were obliged to abandon their homes and renew their wanderings.

Leadership now passed to Brigham Young, a brilliant, strong-willed man, who organized the most remarkable migration and settlement in the annals of the American West. In 1846 Young led almost the whole Mormon community across Iowa to the Council Bluffs on the Missouri River; the next year he sent the first band to the Salt Lake basin, which he had selected for the new Zion. It was, as Young intended, an isolated region, protected on the east by the Wasatch Mountains and on the south and west by a great desert. No place could have appeared less promising; the first to arrive saw only "a broad and barren plain . . . a seemingly interminable waste of sagebrush . . . the paradise of the lizard, the cricket and the rattlesnake." But Young knew from the reports of explorers that fresh water and good soil were available there; and within a decade the Mormons, under his stern leadership and the theocratic control of the Church, had transformed the landscape. Substituting cooperative labor for individual effort of the typical pioneer, they built a thriving city and an efficient irrigation system with which they made the desert bloom. In the critical early years their economy benefited from the sale of supplies to emigrants passing through on their way to California. When their lands were annexed to the United States soon after they arrived, the Mormons tried first to organize their own state of "Deseret." Failing, they acquiesced when Congress created the Territory of Utah. Even then, however, the Mormon Church continued to be the dominant political as well as religious force in the land of the Saints.

Salt Lake City: a new Zion

Polk and the Triumph of Manifest Destiny

The election of Polk. The presidential election of 1844 exposed a variety of tensions that had been growing in American society in recent years. First, the long depression following the Panic of 1837 had kept alive issues of national policy concerning money, banking, and public lands—issues that sometimes divided labor and capital, sometimes farm and city. Second, the entrance of the abolitionist crusade into politics had given sectional differences a moral dimension that made compromise increasingly difficult to achieve. Third, the doctrine of Manifest Destiny was reaching the height of its influence, and the drive for expansion to the Pacific was becoming an irresistible force. Slavery and expansion sorely tried the national party system and ultimately contributed to a fragmentation of the Whig and Democratic organizations.

In 1844 Henry Clay and Martin Van Buren expected to receive the presidential nominations of their respective parties. They found the unsettled Texas question a source of embarrassment, because it had become involved in the slavery controversy. Hence they tried to eliminate it as a campaign issue by mak-

ing separate but very similar statements (apparently after private consultation) opposing the annexation of Texas at that time without the consent of Mexico. The Whig convention unanimously nominated Clay and adopted a platform that avoided taking a stand on Texas or on most other national issues. But the Democratic convention, where expansionist sentiment was stronger, and where a two-thirds majority was required for nomination, rejected Van Buren. On the ninth ballot, after a bitter conflict on the convention floor, the delegates chose James K. Polk of Tennessee, whose commitment to territorial expansion (including the immediate annexation of Texas) was clear and unqualified. To avoid the accusation of sectional favoritism, the Democratic platform cleverly united a demand for the admission of Texas with the dubious assertion that "our title to the whole of the Territory of Oregon is clear and unquestionable; that no portion of the same ought to be ceded to England or any other power." It followed, therefore, "that the re-occupation of Oregon and the re-annexation of Texas at the earliest practicable period are great American measures, which this convention recommends to the cordial support of the Democracy of the Union."

By combining the expansionist desires of South and West, the Democrats had found a winning formula. Throughout the campaign Manifest Destiny transcended all other issues, so much so that Clay began to shift his position on Texas. He would favor annexation after all if it could be accomplished without war and upon "just and fair terms." But this commitment still sounded halfhearted when compared with the spread-eagle oratory and aggressive slogans of the Democrats. Clay converted few of the expansionists but lost some antislavery votes to the Liberty party (see p. 268), especially in New York. In the election Polk won by a small plurality of 38,000 in the popular vote and by a margin of 170 to 105 in the Electoral College.

Though Polk is remembered as the first "darkhorse" presidential candidate, the term is valid only in the sense that he had not been considered for the nomination before the Democratic convention. He was far from a political unknown in 1844. Born in North Carolina, he had moved to Tennessee as a young man and soon became a successful lawyer and planter. He entered politics as a Jacksonian Democrat and served seven terms in the House of Representatives (two as Speaker) and one term as governor of Tennessee. As President, Polk displayed neither extraordinary talent nor a striking personality, but by hard work and stubborn determination he had remarkable success in redeeming the pledges his party had made during the campaign.

Polk's Administration reflected both the continuing influence of Jacksonian principles on the Democratic party and the growing power of the South within the party. As a planter and slaveholder Polk shared the Southern hostility toward abolitionists; if they achieved their goal, he warned, "the dissolution of the Union . . . must speedily follow." He favored a low revenue tariff, and in 1846 his Secretary of the Treasury, Robert J. Walker of Mississippi, helped to frame such a measure, which Congress passed. The Walker Tariff delighted the South, but it angered Northern protectionists and increased their hostility to further strengthening the antiprotectionists by the admission of any more slave states. Polk shared Jackson's views on national banking and persuaded Congress to reestablish the Independent Treasury system, which it had abolished during the Tyler Administration. On two occasions, to the intense annoyance of Westerners in the Great Lakes region, he vetoed internal-improvements bills. In short, Polk blocked every effort to revive the American System of Henry Clay and John Quincy Adams, and in his last message to Congress he devoted much space to attacking that system and celebrating its demise.

The acquisition of Texas and Oregon. Important as these domestic policies were, the Polk Administration's primary concern was with geographic expansion. The Texas question was the first to be disposed

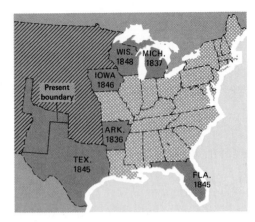

New states, 1836–48

of, for Congress had virtually settled the matter shortly before Polk's inauguration. After the presidential election Tyler assured Congress that the verdict of the voters had been in favor of annexation, and he proposed now that the two houses accomplish it by a joint resolution. Annexation would thus require only a simple majority, rather than the two-thirds majority needed in the Senate to approve a treaty. The introduction of a resolution for this purpose provoked a heated debate between proslavery and antislavery congressmen, but it finally passed the House by a vote of 120 to 98 and the Senate by a vote of 27 to 25. President Tyler signed the joint resolution on March 1, 1845. Polk approved of this action, and within a few months Texas had accepted the terms of annexation. In December 1845 Texas was admitted to statehood.

The problem of Oregon was not so easily resolved, for the Americans and British still had not agreed on a line of division. Indeed, the restless settlers in Oregon and the expansionists in the East were growing increasingly belligerent in their demand that the government make no division at all but, as the Democratic platform of 1844 had insisted, take the whole territory to its northern limits. "Where shall we find room for all our people, unless we have Oregon?" asked Representative Andrew Kennedy of Indiana. America claimed Oregon for a noble purpose, explained John Quincy Adams: "To make the wilderness blossom as the rose, to establish laws, to increase, multiply, and subdue the earth, which we are commanded to do by the first behest of God Almighty." In January 1845 the British government, realizing that continued joint occupation was impossible, proposed arbitration, but the State Department rejected the offer.

In referring to the Oregon question in his inaugural address, Polk seemed to stand firmly on his party's platform; it would be his duty, he said, "to assert and maintain by all constitutional means the

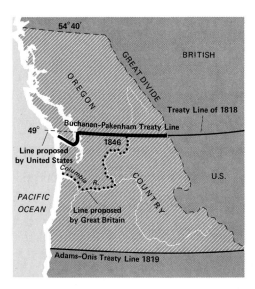

The Oregon controversy, 1818–46

right of the United States to that portion of our territory which lies beyond the Rocky Mountains. Our title to the country of the Oregon is 'clear and unquestionable,' and . . . those rights we are fully prepared to maintain." Meanwhile, there was a good deal of irresponsible saber-rattling on both sides of the Atlantic, and the situation threatened to get out of hand. "We want thirty thousand rifles in the valley of the Oregon," cried Senator Benton of Missouri. "They will make all quiet there . . . and protect the American interests."

But Polk did not want war with England when there was danger of war with Mexico; accordingly, he soon decided to abandon the Democratic platform and try for a compromise. In July 1845 he notified the British minister in Washington, Richard Pakenham, that the United States was willing to renew its offer to divide Oregon along the forty-ninth parallel. Pakenham, without even consulting his government, rejected the offer and held firm to the earlier British demand for a division at the Columbia River. The indignant President then withdrew his offer, concluded that "the only way to treat John Bull was to look him straight in the eye," and decided to pursue "a bold and firm course." In his message to Congress that December, Polk recommended that the British government be given the year's notice required to end joint occupation. He also invoked the almost forgotten Monroe Doctrine to fortify his case: "it should be distinctly announced to the world as our settled policy that no future European colony or dominion shall with our consent be planted or established on any part of the North American continent." Meanwhile, truculent American expansionists, apparently ready for another war with the British, repeated the slogans

"All of Oregon or none," and "Fifty-four forty or fight." Once Congress had approved the termination of joint occupation of Oregon, the only remaining hope for a peaceful settlement seemed to be an offer of concessions by the British.

Fortunately the British Foreign Office disapproved of Pakenham's blunt rejection of Polk's offer to compromise, for it did not believe that the disputed segment of Oregon between the Columbia River and the forty-ninth parallel was worth a war. Indeed, the flood of American settlers and the depletion of the fur resources had already prompted the Hudson's Bay Company to transfer its headquarters from Fort Vancouver on the Columbia northward to Fort Victoria on Vancouver Island. In June 1846 Secretary of State James Buchanan received from Pakenham the draft of a proposal to divide Oregon at the forty-ninth parallel, thus granting to the United States the magnificent harbor at Puget Sound, but to retain for the British all of Vancouver Island and the right to navigate the Columbia River. Polk was at first inclined to reject the proposal, but he decided to submit it to the Senate and let that body assume responsibility for the decision.

After an angry debate the Senate advised acceptance; the treaty was signed on June 15, and the Senate approved it by a vote of forty-one to fourteen. Most of the opposition came from Western Democrats who bitterly criticized Polk for backing down on the demand for the whole of Oregon. But most of the country was satisfied with the settlement, for the British, rather than the Americans, had given up their original claim. Eastern business interests had no taste for a war to secure the area north of the forty-ninth parallel; nor did Southerners, whose interest in Oregon waned once Texas had been safely annexed. Besides, the United States was already at war with Mexico and had a richer prize in view.

War with Mexico

The background. Among the causes of the war with Mexico were the inability of United States citizens to obtain compensation for claims against the Mexican government, the anger of Mexican patriots over American annexation of Texas, a dispute over the southern and western boundaries of Texas, and the instability of the Mexican government, which made negotiation with it difficult and irritating. But even more important was the determination of Polk (and of the expansionists generally) to obtain the provinces of New Mexico and California—with money if possible, by force if necessary. Though Mexico was far from blameless for the war that came—

indeed, welcomed it—the central cause was nevertheless the readiness of the Polk Administration to resort to arms to achieve its expansionist goals.

As soon as the United States annexed Texas, Mexico broke off diplomatic relations, thus closing the normal channels of negotiation. Yet there was need for negotiation, because Texas was not satisfied with its traditional southern boundary, which in Spanish days had been the Nueces River, but claimed instead the Rio Grande. Polk, convinced that the Texas claim was justified, ordered General Zachary Taylor to take fifteen hundred troops into the disputed area. By the summer of 1845, Taylor's small army was encamped at Corpus Christi on the Nueces River; in March of the following year it obeyed Polk's command and advanced to the Rio Grande. To Mexican patriots this act, following soon after what they considered the illegal seizure of Texas, was a further aggressive invasion of their territory, and the war spirit grew among them.

There was now little hope that Polk could persuade Mexico to give up California and New Mexico peacefully, but he decided to try nonetheless. When he learned that Mexico would receive an American commissioner to settle the Texas dispute, he appointed John Slidell of Louisiana as envoy extraordinary and minister plenipotentiary with authority to discuss not only Texas but California and New Mexico as well. Slidell was instructed to offer (1) the assumption by the United States of all claims of its citizens against Mexico if Mexico would accept the Rio Grande boundary; (2) $5 million for the rest of New Mexico west of the Rio Grande; and (3) as much as $25 million for California. Since the Mexican government needed money and since its hold on these distant territories was weak, to Polk it seemed the course of wisdom for Mexico to sell.

When Slidell reached Mexico City on December 6, 1845, news about his purpose had already leaked out, and Mexican nationalists were furious at this brazen attempt to dismember their country. The existing government was collapsing, in part because of its alleged lack of firmness in dealing with the United States, and a new revolutionary government came to power pledged to uphold the national dignity. Neither the old nor the new government would receive Slidell. Mexico, he was reminded, had agreed only to receive a commissioner to negotiate on Texas, and until that question was settled there could be no regular diplomatic relations. The Slidell mission had failed. "Be assured," the angry diplomat wrote Polk, "that nothing is to be done with these people until they shall have been chastised."

Polk apparently agreed. On May 9, 1846, he told his Cabinet that the unpaid claims and the snubbing of Slidell would justify a declaration of war, and he began at once to prepare a war message to Congress. That evening news arrived that on April 25 Mexican troops had crossed the Rio Grande and engaged in a skirmish in which sixteen American soldiers were killed or wounded. Polk hastily revised his war message and sent it to Congress on May 11. After reviewing recent relations between Mexico and the United States, his message concluded: "The cup of forbearance had been exhausted even before the recent information from the frontier. . . . But now, after reiterated menaces, Mexico has passed the boundary of the United States, has invaded our territory and shed American blood on the American soil." Therefore, "war exists, and, notwithstanding all our efforts to avoid it, exists by the act of Mexico herself." Two days later Congress passed a resolution declaring that "by the act of the Republic of Mexico, a state of war exists between that government and the United States," the Senate by a vote of 40 to 2, the House by a vote of 174 to 14. It then appropriated $10 million for war purposes and authorized the recruitment of an army of fifty thousand volunteers.

The country went to war somewhat less united than these votes in Congress suggested. Though most Whig politicians felt they had no choice but to support the military measures, they showed less enthusiasm for the conflict than the Democrats. War sentiment was strong in the Southwest, but it diminished to the east and north. Abolitionists and antislavery Whigs (who called themselves Conscience Whigs) denied that Polk had tried to avoid war and insisted that American blood had been shed not on American soil but on disputed soil that American troops should never have occupied. Senator Tom Corwin of Ohio accused Polk of involving the country in a war of aggression, and added bitterly: "If I were a Mexican, I would tell you, 'Have you not room in your own country to bury your dead men? If you come into mine, we will greet you with bloody hands and welcome you to hospitable graves.'" Another Whig, though seeing no alternative to supporting the war, was distressed to think "that when we pray 'God defend the right' our prayers are not for our own country." In 1847 the Massachusetts legislature resolved that the war was "unconstitutionally commenced by the order of the President" and that it was being waged for "the triple object of extending slavery, of strengthening the slave power, and of obtaining the control of the free states." A new sectional crisis thus began to take shape almost as soon as the war commenced.

The military campaigns. In all probability the Mexicans entered the war with greater unity and enthusiasm than the Americans. They had concluded that war was the only way to check Yankee aggres-

Scott entering Mexico City

sion, and they were confident that their regular army, vastly superior in numbers to the American, could easily defeat the invaders. But the Mexicans were sadly deluded, for they did not take into account their outdated weapons, their limited supplies and inferior resources, and their oversupply of incompetent generals. Though the United States had a regular army of fewer than eight thousand officers and men, it was able quickly to raise a force of sixty thousand volunteers. With this manpower, with superior equipment, and with at least one gifted military commander, General Winfield Scott, the Americans won the war with relative ease.

Polk, who planned the military operations himself, hoped that a few quick victories would persuade Mexico to make the desired territorial cessions. According to Senator Benton, Polk "wanted a small war, just large enough to require a treaty of peace." In the first of three major campaigns, General Taylor crossed the Rio Grande, captured Matamoros, and pushed on to Monterrey. There, in a severe battle (September 21–23, 1846), Taylor defeated the Mexican garrison but permitted it to withdraw rather than surrender. Because of these early victories, Old Rough and Ready, as Taylor's men affectionately called him, became a national hero, but he had betrayed limitations as a tactician and a tendency to be overcautious— serious flaws in a commanding officer. As a result, Polk lost confidence in him, took away half his army for a new offensive at Vera Cruz, and would have been content to let him remain idle for the rest of the war.

But Santa Anna, who had regained power in Mexico, moved north to attack Taylor's weakened forces. At the Battle of Buena Vista (February 22–23, 1847) Taylor added to his national popularity by defeating Santa Anna and forcing him to return to Mexico City. This action ended the war in northern Mexico, but the decisive victories were still to be won elsewhere.

The second offensive was designed to bring the coveted Mexican provinces under American occupation before a peace treaty was negotiated. In the summer of 1846 a force of seventeen hundred men, commanded by Colonel Stephen W. Kearny, marched from Fort Leavenworth to Santa Fe and, on August 18, captured it without firing a shot. After proclaiming the annexation of New Mexico to the United States, Kearny sent part of his troops to join Taylor, left a small garrison at Santa Fe, and took the rest to California. There some of the American settlers, in the "Bear Flag Revolt," had already declared the independence of California; and Captain John C. Frémont, who had arrived earlier at the head of an exploring expedition, was in command of the rebels. Meanwhile, naval forces had landed at Monterey and raised the American flag. Hence, when Kearny arrived late in 1846 the only remaining task was to subdue scattered resistance to American authority in southern California. By January 1847 the United States had virtually undisputed possession of both New Mexico and California.

It took a third American campaign to force Mexico to accept these realities. In March 1847 an army

American advance
Mexican advance
Mexican retreat

commanded by General Scott landed near Vera Cruz, forced that city to surrender after an eighteen-day siege, and then began a slow and difficult advance toward Mexico City. Scott won a decisive victory over Santa Anna at Cerro Gordo (April 17–18, 1847), and by August he was on the high plateau before the Mexican capital. On September 14 American troops forced their way into the city, and soon after Mexico surrendered.

The Treaty of Guadalupe Hidalgo. A new Mexican government was now ready to sign a treaty of peace. Anticipating this outcome, Polk had sent Nicholas P. Trist, chief clerk in the State Department, along with Scott's army "to take advantage of circumstances, as they might arise to negotiate a peace." Trist was instructed to offer essentially the same terms that Slidell had offered. In November 1847, after a long and irritating delay, negotiations were about to begin when Trist received orders from the impatient President to return to Washington. But Trist, convinced that he was on the verge of getting all he had been sent for, decided to ignore his orders and enter into

negotiations. On February 2, 1848, he signed the Treaty of Guadalupe Hidalgo, by which the United States obtained California, New Mexico, and the Rio Grande boundary for $15 million and the assumption of the claims of United States citizens against Mexico. Trist then hurried back to Washington, but he got no thanks from the President. Instead, Polk denounced him as an "impudent and unqualified scoundrel" for disobeying orders and dismissed him from his job.

But Polk could find no fault with the treaty and, notwithstanding "the exceptional conduct of Mr. Trist," decided to submit it to the Senate. By then some of the more rabid expansionists were asking why the United States should settle for only California and New Mexico. Why not take the whole of Mexico? As one partisan of Manifest Destiny asked, why "resign this beautiful country to the custody of the ignorant cowards and profligate ruffians who have ruled it for the last twenty-five years?" But after a volley of bombastic oratory, the Senate, on March 10, 1848, approved the treaty by a vote of thirty-eight to fourteen. Thus the United States gained possession of more than a half-million square miles of territory and became a power on the Pacific with substantial new defense problems and enlarged diplomatic interests.

At the same time, without giving the matter much thought, the United States extended its jurisdiction over additional Indian populations and another ethnic minority, the Mexican-Americans. Unfortunately, the country's dominant Protestant, north-European majority was then ideologically unprepared to accept a multicultural society. The prevailing assumption was that the various peoples who came under American jurisdiction through annexation or immigration would lose their separate identities and become totally assimilated. But the "Anglos" of Texas and California regarded the Mexican-Americans as unassimilable and accordingly made them the victims of cruel stereotypes and ethnic prejudice. Not until the twentieth century did a new concept of cultural pluralism begin to encourage respect for ethnic minorities who maintained their own identities.

Crisis and Compromise

The issue of slavery expansion. On August 8, 1846, three months after the outbreak of the Mexican War, the House of Representatives had under consideration a request from the President for passage of a bill appropriating $2 million to facilitate the purchase of territory from Mexico when a peace treaty was negotiated. The bill immediately provoked several Northern congressmen to announce their opposition to the spread of slavery into whatever territory might be acquired. One of them, David Wilmot, a Pennsylvania Democrat with close ties to the Van Buren wing of the party, finally rose and moved an amendment making it "an express and fundamental condition to the acquisition of any territory" that "neither slavery nor involuntary servitude shall ever exist in any part of said territory." The Wilmot Proviso, as the amendment was called, twice passed the House but each time failed in the Senate, and on several other occasions it was reintroduced and bitterly debated. During the next fifteen years the issue of slavery expansion, which had been a latent source of trouble ever since the Missouri controversy, was to drive a wedge ever deeper between North and South. The stakes seemed to be high, for critics and defenders of slavery alike were convinced that if the institution were not permitted to expand, it would ultimately die.

Support for the proviso came from resentful Northern Whigs who felt that Polk had been less than candid with Congress in explaining the background of the Mexican War. It also came from some Northern Democrats who were discontented with the Walker Tariff, with Polk's veto of internal-improvements bills, with the Oregon compromise, with the rejection of Van Buren in 1844, or, more generally, with what they regarded as the unduly pro-Southern stance of the Administration. What personal motives Wilmot may have had for introducing his proviso are of no great historical importance, because other Northern congressmen were prepared to offer similar proposals had Wilmot not acted first.

More important is the question whether the subsequent long and angry controversy over slavery expansion had substance to it or, as some have claimed, was simply a flight from reality. Polk was the first of many contemporaries to denounce the Wilmot Proviso as "mischievous and foolish" and to accuse "Southern agitators and Northern fanatics" of raising a false issue merely for political advancement. He and other conservatives argued that none of the territory acquired from Mexico was suitable for plantation agriculture with slave labor; hence legislation to exclude slavery from it would be unnecessarily provocative. Such a law would needlessly reenact a "law of nature." From this, presumably, it followed that irresponsible demagogues were creating a great national crisis and endangering the Union over a mere abstraction.

By the end of the 1840s the Southern plantation system may well have reached its natural geographic limits within the existing boundaries of the United States, but it does not necessarily follow that the debate over slavery expansion was therefore meaningless. In the first place, not all Northerners and Southerners were sure that geography alone would keep slavery out of California and New Mexico. Some believed that even if the familiar plantation system could not be developed in these areas, slavery might still be introduced in other forms of agriculture, as well as in industry and mining. Slaves, after all, were employed in many occupations in the South. In the second place, few Americans thought that their country's growth would stop with the territory acquired in the Treaty of Guadalupe Hidalgo. There was a widespread conviction that at least Cuba would one day become part of the United States, and perhaps other Caribbean islands and Central America as well. In these tropical lands slavery would not be merely an abstraction. Indeed, much of the controversy over slavery expansion was waged with an eye on prospective future annexations and with the understanding that laws excluding slavery from existing territories would provide significant precedents.

Finally, and perhaps most important, the issue was decidedly relevant to the moral positions of pro-slavery and antislavery interests in the two sections. When Northerners with antislavery sentiments argued that it would be morally wrong to legalize slavery in New Mexico, they were by implication arguing that it was also morally wrong to tolerate it in Virginia. Constitutional limitations on federal power prevented them from doing anything about slavery in the Southern states; hence their efforts to prohibit it in the territories, where they believed Congress had authority to act, had symbolic as well as practical significance. Southerners understood this perfectly well, which explains in part why they so vigorously opposed all exclusion proposals, such as the Wilmot Proviso, even when applied to territories where slavery was not likely to be introduced. For example, Southern congressmen delayed for two years (until 1848) the passage of a bill creating Oregon Territory, because the bill contained a clause excluding slavery. Representative James R. Seddon of Virginia protested that territorial exclusion was a "direct attack on the institutions" of the Southern states, an "insult and injury, outrage and wrong."

Support for the Wilmot Proviso, however, did not arise exclusively from hostility toward slavery or concern for blacks. Many opponents of slavery expansion, because of sectional tensions over other questions of public policy, seemed to express anti-Southern rather than antislavery feelings. Many more betrayed essentially racist motives—that is, a determination to keep blacks, whether slave or free, out of the Western territories. Wilmot himself assured his colleagues that his purpose was to defend "the rights of white freemen. I would preserve for free white labor a fair country, a rich inheritance, where the sons of toil, of my own race and own color, can live without the disgrace which association with negro slavery brings upon free labor." In short, Northern support for the Wilmot Proviso arose from three sources: from ideological antislavery feelings, from sectional anti-Southern feelings, and from racist antiblack feelings.

Much of the debate over the Wilmot Proviso centered on the question of how much power the Constitution had given Congress to govern the territories. Supporters of Wilmot cited the clause authorizing Congress to "make all needful rules and regulations respecting the Territory or other Property belonging to the United States." Until the 1840s, as Henry Clay observed, this clause had been accepted as giving Congress power over slavery in the territories "by the uniform interpretation and action of every department of our government, legislative, executive, and judicial." Moreover, the power had repeatedly been used. The First Congress had reenacted the Ordinance of 1787, which prohibited slavery in the Northwest Territory; a later Congress had applied the same restriction to the Illinois and Michigan territories when they were created; and overwhelming majorities in the House and Senate had voted in 1820 to prohibit slavery in that portion of the Louisiana Purchase north of the line 36° 30'. After the Mexican

War, when President Polk and many other Southern moderates suggested extending the Missouri compromise line to the Pacific, they were again, in effect, agreeing that Congress did have the authority to regulate slavery in the territories.

Calhoun, however, led proslavery Southerners toward an extreme state-rights position similar to the stand that some Virginians had taken during the Missouri debates. In 1847 he introduced a series of resolutions in the Senate asserting that the territories were the common property of all the states; that Congress had no power to deprive the citizens of any state of their right to migrate to the territories with their property, including slaves; and that only when a territory was ready for statehood could it constitutionally prohibit slavery. Calhoun's position, therefore, was that *all* the territories must be open to slavery—which made even the Missouri Compromise unconstitutional. Some of his supporters went a step further and insisted that it was the duty of Congress to *protect* slavery in the territories if necessary. This being the case, the Wilmot Proviso was, in the words of one Southern congressman, "treason to the Constitution," and its adoption would justify the secession of the South.

Between these uncompromising antislavery and proslavery doctrines, a third doctrine, called "popular sovereignty," began to win the support of moderates in all sections, but especially in the Old Northwest. With two Democratic senators, Lewis Cass of Michigan and Stephen A. Douglas of Illinois, its chief advocates, popular sovereignty was designed in part to remove the explosive territorial question from the halls of Congress. Why not respect the American tradition of local self-government, these moderates asked, and permit the people who actually settled in a territory to decide the question of slavery for themselves? Congress could then organize new territories without reference to slavery. Southerners would escape the humiliation of congressional prohibition, while Northwestern farmers might hope that their numerical superiority over Southern slaveholders would enable them to win the territories for freedom.

The election of 1848. Meanwhile, as the debate over the territorial question dragged on, California and New Mexico were left without government, and the issue was injected into the presidential campaign of 1848. President Polk had failed to unite the Democrats behind his Administration and was not a candidate for reelection. As the election approached the party was torn by factionalism. Calhoun led a group of Southern-rights men unwilling to accept anything less than his extreme position on slavery expansion. Martin Van Buren commanded a faction of disaffected New York Democrats, called the "Barnburners" (presumably because they would burn the barn to get rid of the rats), who had thirsted for revenge ever since Polk defeated Van Buren for the presidential nomination in 1844. Throughout the North, especially in the Northeast, groups of free-soil Democrats endorsed the Wilmot Proviso. When the Democratic convention met in Baltimore, the party leaders, having decided that a Northern candidate was essential, threw the nomination to Lewis Cass of Michigan, a colorless old party wheel horse whose opposition to the Wilmot Proviso and support of popular sovereignty would appease the Southern moderates. The platform praised Polk for his territorial acquisitions and domestic policies but was silent on the slavery question. As a result, the Barnburners and pro-Wilmot delegates left the convention prepared for revolt.

The Whigs, meeting in Philadelphia, again staked their chances on a military hero, General Zachary Taylor. Born in Virginia and now a Louisiana slaveholder, Taylor was expected to reassure Southern Whigs who had grown uneasy about the antislavery sentiments of Northern Whigs. Old Rough and Ready had spent his whole career in the regular army; he had neither political principles nor political experience—and, indeed, had discovered only recently that he was a Whig ("but not an ultra Whig"). After nominating Taylor on the fourth ballot, the convention tried to avoid controversy by writing no platform at all. But this surrender to expediency was more than the Northern Conscience Whigs could bear. Many of them decided that rather than support a slaveholder

Taylor: "Old Rough and Ready"

whose views were unknown and who was uncommitted to a platform they would bolt their party.

Antislavery leaders saw in the disgruntled Van Buren Barnburners, free-soil Democrats, Conscience Whigs, and political abolitionists the elements of a powerful third party, one that would take a firm stand on the territorial question and make a broader appeal than the Liberty party had made in the two preceding elections. In August 1848 delegates representing all these groups met in Buffalo, organized the Free-Soil party, and nominated Van Buren for President and Charles Francis Adams (a Conscience Whig, the son of John Quincy Adams) for Vice President. The platform bluntly demanded that slavery be excluded from the territories and opposed any additional concessions to the Slave Power. It supported federal appropriations for internal improvements and the passage of a homestead act giving actual settlers free farms from the public domain. In a concluding statement the platform summarized the principles of the new party as "Free Soil, Free Speech, Free Labor, and Free Men." Among the Free-Soilers were numerous self-seeking politicians and an abundance of Negrophobes, but the organization also reflected much of the idealism of the antislavery crusade.

In spite of the intensity of feeling about the territorial question, the campaign itself was unexciting, the voters apathetic. Taylor defeated Cass by a small plurality in the popular vote (1,360,967 to 1,222,342) and by a majority of 36 in the Electoral College (163 to 127). The Free-Soil party failed to carry a single state, but its popular vote of 291,263 was impressive for a party organized less than three months before the election. A dozen Free-Soilers were elected to Congress, among them Ohio's new senator, Salmon P. Chase.

Taylor and the crisis. President Taylor was a man of honesty, integrity, and determination; he was capable of quick action, and he had a store of plain common sense. But these virtues were not sufficient to offset his limitations as chief executive in a time of crisis: his lack of training in politics and civil administration, his ignorance of public affairs—above all, his tendency to oversimplify complex problems. In a brief and vacuous inaugural address, he promised to devote his Administration "to the welfare of the whole country, and not to the support of any particular section or merely local interest." This pledge he tried conscientiously to fulfill; though a Southerner, he was a nationalist with no strong sectional loyalties.

When Taylor came into office, California and New Mexico, still lacking civil government, were being ruled by army officers directly responsible to the President. The settlers found this situation annoying under the best of circumstances, but it became intol-

Forty-Niner: months of discomfort

erable soon after the discovery of gold in California. James Marshall had made the discovery in January 1848, along the American River about forty miles from Sutter's Fort; within six months San Francisco and other coastal towns were all but deserted as men rushed headlong into the "diggings" in the Sierra. By the end of 1848 the news had spread to the East, and during the next year some eighty thousand "forty-niners" came to California from the Mississippi Valley, from the Atlantic coast, and from Europe, Asia, and Australia. Most of those from the Eastern states followed the overland trails across the continent, others took the easier but more expensive route by ship around Cape Horn, and still others risked death by taking a shortcut through the jungles of Panama. The miners dreamed of fortunes in gold as they worked the stream beds with picks, shovels, and wash-pans; a few struck it rich, but most of them gained only modest returns from their backbreaking labor and months of discomfort in primitive mining camps. Much of the gold ultimately found its way into the pockets of merchants in San Francisco and Sacramento, who in effect mined the miners by selling them supplies at exorbitant prices.

By the end of 1849 California's population had grown to one hundred thousand, and in the absence of civil government crime and violence were rampant in the cities and mining camps. With military authorities unable to restore law and order, with Congress seemingly paralyzed by the slavery issue, President Taylor decided to take matters into his own hands. As he saw it, there was a simple solution to the problem that had bedeviled Congress ever since the introduction of the Wilmot Proviso. He proposed to avoid the territorial issue by encouraging the people of California and New Mexico to frame constitutions and apply for immediate admission to the Union as states. Californians wasted no time in taking Taylor's advice; by October 1849 a convention had drafted a constitution prohibiting slavery, and in November the voters ratified it and elected state officers to whom the military gladly yielded political authority. The people of New

Mexico took more time, but by May 1850 they too had adopted a free-state constitution. Hence, when Congress met in December 1849, Taylor congratulated the country on the fact that the problem had been solved. All that remained was for Congress to admit California as a free state at once, and New Mexico as soon as it was ready.

The Compromise of 1850. Taylor had miscalculated. Rather than settling the matter, he helped precipitate one of the bitterest sectional debates in American history, one that carried the country dangerously close to disunion and civil war. Southerners denounced Taylor as an apostate and a tool of the abolitionists, while the followers of Calhoun vowed that they would break up the Union rather than see slavery excluded from California and New Mexico. Several other issues intensified the crisis: Texans and New Mexicans were on the verge of a private war over their common boundary; abolitionists were gaining Northern support for their demand that slavery be abolished in the District of Columbia; and Southerners were clamoring for a more effective fugitive-slave law. Legislatures and mass meetings in both the North and the South adopted fiery resolutions, and violence threatened to break out in the halls of Congress. A Massachusetts convention of Democrats and Free-Soilers resolved that "we are opposed to slavery in every form and color, and in favor of freedom and free soil wherever man lives." Mississippi contributed to the atmosphere of crisis by issuing a call for a convention of the Southern states to meet at Nashville in June 1850. Many feared that the friends of Calhoun would use the convention to expedite Southern secession.

Moderates in both sections were convinced that nothing short of a comprehensive settlement of all outstanding issues could save the Union. And it was to Henry Clay, then in his seventy-third year and near the end of his long career, that lovers of the Union looked almost instinctively for a just and durable compromise. On January 29, 1850, Clay offered the Senate a series of resolutions proposing (1) that California be admitted as a free state; (2) that territorial governments be provided for the rest of the Mexican cession without any restriction on slavery; (3) that Texas abandon its claim to the eastern portion of New Mexico; (4) that the federal government compensate Texas by assuming the public debt Texas had contracted before annexation; (5) that the use of the District of Columbia as a depot in the interstate slave trade be prohibited; (6) that slavery in the District of Columbia be abolished only with the consent of its residents and of the state of Maryland and with compensation to the slaveholders; (7) that a new and more rigorous Fugitive Slave Act be adopted; and (8) that Congress declare that it had no power to interfere

Henry Clay: Unionist

with the interstate slave trade. Among the many moderates who labored to secure the adoption of these compromise proposals, Stephen A. Douglas of Illinois was second only to Clay.

Congress debated the proposals for more than seven months, with the moderates under constant attack from both proslavery and antislavery opponents of compromise. Clay opened the memorable debate in February. For two days he spoke in defense of his measures and urged mutual concessions for the sake of the Union. He asked Northerners why they insisted on the Wilmot Proviso when they had a stronger force working for them: "You have got nature itself on your side." He warned Southerners that they would gain nothing and lose a great deal by secession—that secession was certain to lead to civil war, "furious, bloody, implacable, exterminating." On March 4, John C. Calhoun, ill and close to death, listened to a colleague read his last address to the Senate. The present crisis, Calhoun insisted, was due to a breakdown of the old sectional equilibrium, to Northern aggression against the South, and to the destruction of the rights of the states and the creation of a consolidated government. Nothing could save the Union but an end of antislavery agitation, a faithful enforcement of the Fugitive Slave Act, equal rights for the South in the territories, and a constitutional amendment restoring

The Union cannot ... be saved by eulogies on the Union, however splendid or numerous. The cry of "Union, Union, the glorious Union!" can no more prevent disunion than the cry of "Health, health, glorious health!" on the part of the physician, can save a patient lying dangerously ill....

How can the Union be saved? There is but one way by which it can with any certainty; and that is, by a full and final settlement, on the principle of justice of all the questions at issue between the two sections....

But can this be done? Yes, easily; not by the weaker party, for it can of itself do nothing—not even protect itself—but by the stronger. The North has only to will it to accomplish it—to do justice by conceding to the South an equal right in the acquired territory, and to do her duty by causing the stipulations relative to fugitive slaves to be faithfully fulfilled—to cease the agitation of the slave question, and to provide for the insertion of a provision in the Constitution, by an amendment, which will restore to the South, in substance, the power she possessed of protecting herself before the equilibrium between the sections was destroyed by the action of this Government....

If you, who represent the stronger portion, cannot agree to settle them on the broad principle of justice and duty, say so; and let the States we both represent agree to separate and part in peace. If you are unwilling we should part in peace, tell us so; and we shall know what to do, when you reduce the question to submission or resistance.

From John C. Calhoun, Speech in the Senate, March 4, 1850.

the balance between the two sections. If these points were not conceded, if the South were forced to choose between "submission or resistance," it would know how to act.

On March 7, three days after Calhoun had sounded his grim protest against Clay's compromise, Daniel Webster delivered the last great oration of his career. To the dismay of his antislavery constituents, he repudiated his free-soil sentiments and announced that he would speak "not as a Massachusetts man, nor as a northern man, but as an American." Though Webster refuted Calhoun's charges against the North, his speech was clearly an attempt to make the compromise palatable to his own section. He denounced antislavery agitation, urged Northerners not to insist on the Wilmot Proviso when slavery would not expand into the new territories in any case, called for an end to resistance to the Fugitive Slave Act, and concluded with a tearful plea for the Union. Webster's speech immensely strengthened the forces of compromise, but for the remaining two years of his life antislavery men vilified him for his apostasy.

Most of the Northern Conscience Whigs stood firm. Senator William H. Seward of New York spoke for them when he denounced compromise as "radically wrong and essentially vicious." There was only one way to end antislavery agitation, he said, and that was by "yielding to the progress of emancipation." In reply to Calhoun's constitutional defense of the right to carry slaves into the territories, Seward appealed to "a higher law than the Constitution," a divine law that intended these rich lands to be enjoyed by free men.

As the debate wore on and the House and Senate considered numerous variations of Clay's proposals, it

Daniel Webster: courageous orator

Gentlemen of the South not only argue the question of right and of honor; they go further, and they tell us what they will proceed to do if we do not yield to their demands. A large majority of the Southern legislators have solemnly "resolved" that if Congress prohibits slavery in the new territories, they will resist the law "at any and at every hazard."...

And do the gentlemen who make these threats soberly consider how deeply they are pledging themselves and their constituents by them? Threats of dissolution, if executed, become rebellion and treason.... Such forcible opposition to the government would be treason. Its agents and abettors would be traitors. Wherever this rebellion rears its crest, martial law will be proclaimed; and those found with hostile arms in their hands must prepare for the felon's doom....

I have only to add that such is my solemn and abiding conviction of the character of slavery that under a full sense of my responsibility to my country and my God, I deliberately say, better disunion—better a civil or a servile war—better anything that God in His Providence shall send, than an extension of the bounds of slavery.

From Horace Mann, Speech in the House of Representatives, February 15, 1850.

became increasingly evident that opinion in favor of a compromise of some kind was steadily building up in both North and South. Northern businessmen, frightened by the talk of secession, favored a compromise in order to protect their Southern trade and investments. The country had recovered from the depression of the 1840s, and practical men longed for political peace so that they could make the most of a new era of prosperity and economic growth. Those who were indifferent to the moral issue of slavery saw no point in permitting continued antislavery agitation to endanger the Union. The compromisers were further strengthened when the moderates won control of the Southern convention at Nashville and indicated that they were ready to accept a fair settlement. Now the most formidable obstacle to compromise was President Taylor, who bitterly resented Clay's rejection of the Administration's recommendations on New Mexico and California in favor of proposals of his own. The possibility of a presidential veto loomed until Taylor's sudden death on July 9 after an attack of gastroenteritis. His successor, Vice President Millard Fillmore, though a New York Whig of free-soil proclivities, immediately allied himself with Webster and Clay and used his influence in favor of compromise.

Even then, the adoption of a compromise was not easy. When Clay's major proposals had been combined in an "omnibus bill," they were threatened with defeat by a combination of Free-Soilers, antislavery Whigs, and Southern-rights men. But the moderates discovered that each of the measures might be enacted separately, for the moderates could then combine with those who opposed the compromise as

a whole but favored individual parts of it. In the final weeks of the battle, Senator Douglas replaced the exhausted Clay as leader of the compromisers, and by September 1850 all the measures had been passed and signed by President Fillmore.

The Compromise of 1850 as it was finally adopted was essentially like the one Clay had proposed the previous January: California was admitted as a free state; the territories of New Mexico and Utah were created from the rest of the Mexican cession, with no

Millard Fillmore: influence for compromise

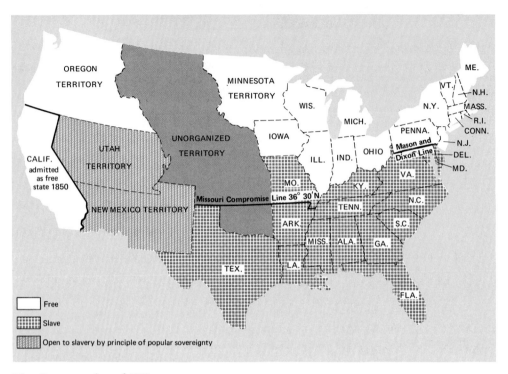

The Compromise of 1850

Legend:
- Free
- Slave
- Open to slavery by principle of popular sovereignty

restriction on slavery; the Texas boundary was fixed as it exists today; Texas was paid $10 million from the federal treasury as compensation for yielding to New Mexico in their boundary dispute; the District of Columbia ceased to be a depot for the interstate slave trade; and what was expected to be a more effective Fugitive Slave Act replaced the old one of 1793.

The Aftermath

Public reaction to the compromise. Few Northerners or Southerners were altogether satisfied with the Compromise of 1850, and some in each section spurned it as an unclean thing. Abolitionists and Free-Soilers refused to be bound by its terms and denounced as unprincipled tools of the Slave Power the Northern congressmen who had voted for it. In 1851 the Massachusetts legislature delivered a stern rebuke to Webster (who had joined Fillmore's Cabinet as Secretary of State) by electing Charles Sumner, a radical Free-Soiler and enemy of the compromise, to the United States Senate.

In the South, "fire-eaters" like Robert Barnwell Rhett of South Carolina and William L. Yancey of Alabama termed the compromise a fatal defeat for their section and called for drastic action. In South

Carolina the secessionists were defeated with the greatest difficulty, and then only because the "moderates" insisted that action be delayed until other Southern states were ready for independence. A state convention in Georgia adopted a series of resolutions, known as the Georgia Platform, that were probably an accurate expression of public opinion in the Deep South. These resolutions accepted the Compromise of 1850 but warned that Georgia would resist, "even (as a last resort) to a disruption of every tie which binds her to the Union," any congressional act abolishing slavery in the District of Columbia, refusing to admit a slave state, excluding slavery from the territories, or repealing the Fugitive Slave Act.

But most Americans in both sections, though doubting the wisdom of some provisions of the compromise, accepted it with great relief and hoped for a respite from sectional agitation. Mass meetings throughout the country celebrated its passage, and the merchants of New York City formed a Union Safety Committee to mobilize public opinion in its defense. Stephen A. Douglas announced that he had resolved "never to make another speech on the slavery question." In his annual message of December 1850 President Fillmore told Congress that he regarded the compromise measures as "a final settlement of the dangerous and exciting subjects which they embraced." And forty-four congressmen of both parties signed a pledge to respect the terms of the compromise and never to support a candidate for public office who threatened to disturb it.

Franklin Pierce. The presidential election of 1852 gave further evidence of the widespread hope that the Compromise of 1850 would in fact be a "final settlement." The Democrats adopted a platform that endorsed the compromise without qualification and promised to resist "agitation of the slavery question, under whatever shape or color the attempt may be made." After many futile ballots the convention dropped the leading candidates—Douglas, Cass, and James Buchanan of Pennsylvania—and nominated another "dark horse," Franklin Pierce of New Hampshire. The Whig party, with its Northern and Southern wings now almost hopelessly divided, wrangled over a platform that unenthusiastically "acquiesced in" the compromise and therefore pleased almost no one. The convention rejected Fillmore and turned to another military hero, General Winfield Scott of Virginia, whose friendship with Seward and whose failure to endorse the compromise made him suspect in the South. In the election, though Pierce's popular majority was not overwhelming, he carried twenty-

seven states with 254 electoral votes, while Scott carried only four states with 42 electoral votes. The Barnburners had returned to the Democratic fold, and the Free-Soil party, with John P. Hale of New Hampshire as its candidate, polled only about half as many votes as it had four years earlier.

Pierce was a Jacksonian Democrat of amiable disposition, modest talent, and almost no capacity for executive leadership. His close ties with Southern Democrats, especially with his Secretary of War, Jefferson Davis, and his sympathy for their views on questions of public policy caused antislavery leaders to damn him as a "doughface"—"a northern man with southern principles." But his promise in his inaugural address that the provisions of the Compromise of 1850 would be "unhesitatingly carried into effect" suited the popular mood. In his first message to Congress, in December 1853, Pierce rejoiced that the recent compromise had "given renewed vigor to our institutions and restored a sense of repose and security to the public mind." With the country prospering, with the hope that sectional issues had been disposed of, some optimists went so far as to predict a new era of good feelings.

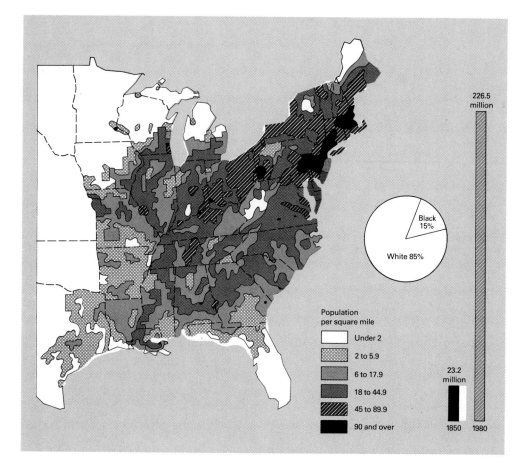

Population 1850

226.5 million

Black 15%

White 85%

Population per square mile

Under 2
2 to 5.9
6 to 17.9
18 to 44.9
45 to 89.9
90 and over

23.2 million

1850   1980

**Harriet Beecher Stowe:
"I will write something"**

Surviving sources of friction. Soon, however, there were abundant signs that the sectional truce would be brief. The disintegration of the Whig party after its defeat in 1852 eliminated another of the institutional ties holding the Union together. The admission of California had upset the sectional balance in the Senate—prior to 1850 there had been fifteen slave and fifteen free states—and the admission of several more free states could not be long delayed. The immigrants who poured into the United States during the 1840s and 1850s (see p. 310) shunned the South and thus further increased the North's numerical majority. Railroad-building and industrial expansion gave the free states an accelerating economic supremacy. Now secessionists could argue that the rights and interests of the minority South were at the mercy of a hostile and overbearing North.

Southern-rights advocates used the controversy that soon began over the enforcement of the new Fugitive Slave Act to prove their point. This provision of the Compromise of 1850 was the one Southerners regarded as their principal gain and the one Northerners found most difficult to accept. It was a harsh measure that subjected alleged fugitives to summary hearings before federal commissioners without trial by jury or the right to testify in their own behalf. Since a commissioner received a fee of $10 if he ruled that a black prisoner was a slave but only $5 if he ruled that the black was free, abolitionists charged that he was being bribed to collaborate with kidnapers who sought to sell free blacks into slavery. Many Northerners were outraged that the new law required them, on the demand of a federal marshal, to assist in the capture of runaways, and thus to become unwilling supporters of slavery. Emerson publicly declared that no man could obey that law "without loss of self-respect and forfeiture of the name of a gentleman." Though in most cases the law was effectively enforced, abolitionists executed a series of dramatic rescues of fugitives and sent them on to Canada and freedom. Moreover, various Northern states passed personal-liberty laws that sought to nullify the Fugitive Slave Act or at least to interfere with its enforcement. This was an assertion of state rights and a form of nullification that Southerners failed to appreciate.

Above all, the Compromise of 1850 could not stop the pens or quiet the voices of the abolitionists. Less than two years after the compromise was passed, the most eloquent and influential appeal in behalf of slaves ever to be written appeared in Harriet Beecher

Stowe's justly celebrated novel, *Uncle Tom's Cabin.* Mrs. Stowe was the daughter of a New England clergyman, sister of seven others, and wife of still another. Her anger over the Fugitive Slave Act prompted her to declare: "I will write something. I will if I live." First published serially in an antislavery weekly, her novel appeared in book form in March 1852. By the end of the year, three hundred thousand copies had been sold. Thereafter the novel, together with its various adaptations for the stage, won thousands of converts to the antislavery cause. *Uncle Tom's Cabin* has more than a few flaws as literature: its situations are contrived; its dialogue is unreal; its slaves are romanticized. Some recent critics also discern in it a kind of patronizing air toward blacks, even a kind of benevolent racism. Yet, although Mrs. Stowe knew almost nothing of slavery firsthand, she understood clearly its tragic aspects; moreover, she had the wisdom to direct her moral indictment against the institution itself rather than against the Southern men and women who were caught in its toils. Indeed, the chief villain of her plot, the cruel overseer Simon Legree, was Northern-born. But these subtleties made the book no more attractive to Southern slaveholders than the cruder forms of abolitionist propaganda.

Slavery, then, still threatened the nation's peace and unity. On the eve of the Civil War Abraham Lincoln wrote to Alexander H. Stephens of Georgia: "You think slavery is right and ought to be extended, while we think it is *wrong* and ought to be restricted. That I suppose is the rub."

Suggestions for Reading

WESTWARD TO THE PACIFIC

Among the surveys of the westward movement, R. A. Billington, *Westward Expansion* (4th ed., 1974), and Frederick Merk, *History of the Westward Movement* (1978), are especially good on American penetration of the Far West. The best books dealing comprehensively with expansion in this period are R. A. Billington, *The Far Western Frontier, 1830–1860** (1956), and J. D. Unruh, Jr., *The Plains Across: The Overland Emigrants and the Trans-Mississippi West, 1840–60** (1975). The impact of the frontier on the lives of women is the subject of S. L. Myres, *Westering Women and the Frontier Experience, 1800–1915** (1982). N. A. Graebner, *Empire on the Pacific* (1955), stresses the desire for Pacific ports as a motive for expansion. A. K. Weinberg, *Manifest Destiny* (1935), is an excellent analysis of the ideology of expansionism. Reginald Horsman, *Race and Manifest Destiny: The Origins of American Racial Anglo-Saxonism* (1981), stresses the racialist dimension. Frederick Merk has written two important books on the motivation and rationalization of expansionism: *Manifest Destiny and Mission in American History: A Reinterpretation** (1963), and *The Monroe Doctrine and American Expansionism, 1843–1849* (1966). H. N. Smith, *Virgin Land** (1950), analyzes the place of the West in American literature and thought. David Pletcher, *The Diplomacy of Annexation* (1973), and P. A. Varg, *United States Foreign Relations, 1820–1860* (1979), deal with the diplomatic aspects of expansion.

The two basic works on the American occupation of Texas are E. C. Barker, *Mexico and Texas, 1821–1835* (1928), and W. C. Binkley, *The Texas Revolution** (1952). A good popular account of the Santa Fe trade is R. L. Duffus, *The Santa Fe Trail** (1930). The best introductions to the fur trade of the Far West are R. G. Cleland, *This Reckless Breed of Men: The Trappers and Fur Traders of the Southwest** (1950); D. L. Morgan, *Jedediah Smith and the Opening of the West** (1953); P. C. Phillips, *The Fur Trade*, 2 vols. (1961); G. G. Cline, *Exploring the Great Basin* (1963); and D. J. Wishart, *The Fur Trade of the American West, 1807–1840* (1979). Two books on the overland trails, reliable and well written, are W. J. Ghent, *The Road to Oregon* (1929), and Jay Monaghan, *The Overland Trail* (1937).

W. H. Goetzmann, *Army Exploration in the American West** (1959), and *Exploration and Empire: The Role of the Explorer and Scientist in the Exploration and Development of the American West** (1966), are valuable studies. The American occupation of Oregon is treated adequately in O. O. Winther, *The Great Northwest* (2nd ed., 1950), and D. O. Johansen and C. M. Gates, *Empire on the Columbia* (2nd ed., 1967). Malcolm Clark, Jr., *Eden Seekers: The Settlement of Oregon, 1812–1862* (1981), is comprehensive, colorful, and well written. Early American interest in California is covered in two general histories: A. F. Rolle, *California: A History* (1963, rev. ed., 1969), and W. E. Bean, *California: An Interpretive History* (1968). Wallace Stegner, *The Gathering of Zion: The Story of the Mormon Trail** (1964), is an excellent account of the Mormon migration. The Mormon settlement in the Salt Lake basin is viewed from several perspectives in Nels Anderson, *Desert Saints: The Mormon Frontier in Utah* (1942); R. B. West, Jr., *Kingdom of the Saints* (1957); T. F. O'Dea, *The Mormons** (1957); and L. J. Arrington, *Great Basic Kingdom** (1958). Preston Nibley, *Brigham Young: The Man and His Works* (1936), is warmly sympathetic. S. P. Hirshon, *The Lion of the Lord: A Biography of Brigham Young* (1969), is more critical.

POLK AND THE TRIUMPH OF MANIFEST DESTINY

The authoritative study of the election of 1844 and the first two years of the Polk Administration is Charles Sellers, *James K. Polk; Continentalist, 1843–1846* (1966). W. R. Brock, *Parties and Political Conscience: American Dilemmas, 1840–1850* (1979), is a valuable interpretive study. A lively and readable introduction to the expansionism of the Polk era is Bernard De Voto, *The Year of Decision, 1846* (1943). Two books deal with negotiations for the annexation of Texas: J. H. Smith, *The Annexation of Texas* (1911), and J. W. Schmitz, *Texan Statecraft, 1836–1845* (1945). F. W. Merk, *Slavery and the Annexation of Texas* (1972), is critical of the proslavery propagandists and their fear of British intervention. M. C. Jacobs, *Winning Oregon* (1938), is a good summary of the Oregon dispute and its settlement. F. W. Merk, *The Oregon Question* (1967), is a collection of excellent interpretive essays. The standard works on the background of the Mexican War are J. S. Reeves, *American Diplomacy under Tyler and Polk* (1907), and G. L. Rives, *The United States and Mexico: 1821–1848*, 2 vols. (1913). D. M. Pletcher, *The Diplomacy of Annexation: Texas, Oregon, and the Mexican War* (1973), is detailed and comprehensive. G. M. Brack, *Mexico Views Manifest Destiny, 1821–1846* (1975), examines the reaction of the Mexican press to American expansion.

Though dated and marred by its biases, the fullest and most authoritative work on the Mexican War is J. H. Smith, *The War with Mexico*, 2 vols. (1919). S. V. Conner and O. B. Faulk, *North America Divided: The Mexican War, 1846–1848* (1971), attributes responsibility to both belligerents but is mostly a defense of the United States. Three other books contribute few fresh interpretations but are brief and readable: A. H. Bill, *Rehearsal for Conflict: The War with Mexico, 1846–1848* (1947); R. S. Henry, *The Story of the Mexican War* (1950); and O. A. Singletary, *The Mexican War** (1960). California from conquest to statehood is treated in Neal Harlow, *California Conquered: War and Peace on the Pacific, 1846–1850* (1982). The military campaigns are traced in K. J. Bauer, *The Mexican War, 1846–1848* (1974), and in two excellent biographies: C. W. Elliott, *Winfield Scott* (1937), and Holman Hamilton, *Zachary Taylor: Soldier of the Republic* (1941). J. H. Schroeder, *Mr. Polk's War: American Opposition and Dissent, 1846–1848* (1973), explores the sources of antiwar sentiment. R. H. Peterson, *Manifest Destiny in the Mines: A Cultural Interpretation of Anti-Mexican Nativism in California, 1848–1853* (1975), is a study of early ethnic prejudice against the country's newly acquired Chicano population.

CRISIS AND COMPROMISE

Allan Nevins, *Ordeal of the Union*, 2 vols. (1947), contains a full, incisive, and well-written account of the issue of slavery expansion and of the Compromise of 1850. D. M. Potter, *The Impending Crisis, 1848–1861** (1976), is a superb synthesis of modern scholarship. Among the most useful books for the politics of slavery expansion are A. O. Craven, *The Growth of Southern Nationalism, 1848–1861* (1953); K. J. Brauer, *Cotton Versus Conscience: Massachusetts Whig Politics and Southern Expansion, 1843–1848* (1967); C. W. Morrison, *Democratic Politics and Sectionalism: The Wilmot Proviso Controversy* (1967); F. J. Blue, *The Free Soilers: Third Party Politics, 1848–1854* (1973); R. H. Sewell, *Ballots for Freedom: Antislavery Politics in the United States, 1837–1860** (1976); W. J. Cooper, *The South and the Politics of Slavery, 1828–1856* (1978); and John Mayfield, *Rehearsal for Republicanism: Free Soil and the Politics of Antislavery* (1980). M. L. Wilson, *Space, Time, and Freedom: The Quest* for *Nationality and the Irrepressible Conflict, 1815–1861* (1974), relates the slavery expansion issue to the ideology of nationalism. Negrophobia as a motive for opposition to slavery expansion is stressed in E. H. Berwanger, *The Frontier Against Slavery: Western Anti-Negro Prejudice and the Slavery Extension Controversy* (1967). J. G. Rayback, *Free Soil: The Election of 1848* (1970), is both scholarly and readable. The Taylor Administration is treated thoroughly in two good biographies: Brainerd Dyer, *Zachary Taylor* (1946), and Holman Hamilton, *Zachary Taylor: Soldier in the White House* (1951).

Of the many books on the California gold rush, the following are among the best: R. W. Paul, *California Gold: The Beginning of Mining in the Far West** (1947); J. W. Caughey, *Gold Is the Cornerstone** (1949); O. C. Coy, *The Great Trek* (1931); A. B. Hulbert, *Forty-Niners* (1931); J. H. Jackson, *Anybody's Gold: The Story of California's Mining Towns** (1941); and James Holliday, *The World Rushed In* (1981).

The best study of the Compromise of 1850 is Holman Hamilton, *Prologue to Conflict: The Crisis and Compromise of 1850* (1964). The role of South Carolina is examined in John Barnwell, *Love of Order: South Carolina's First Secession Crisis* (1982). The crisis and compromise can also be studied through the numerous biographies of national political leaders. Among the most useful are: C. B. Going, *David Wilmot, Free-Soiler* (1924); W. Y. Thompson, *Robert Toombs of Georgia* (1966); G. G. Van Deusen, *William Henry Seward* (1967); F. B. Woodward, *Lewis Cass: The Last Jeffersonian* (1950); R. W. Johannsen, *Stephen A. Douglas* (1973); G. M. Capers, *Stephen A. Douglas: Defender of the Union** (1959); I. H. Bartlett, *Daniel Webster** (1978); R. N. Current, *Daniel Webster and the Rise of National Conservatism** (1955); G. G. Van Deusen, *The Life of Henry Clay* (1937); G. G. Van Deusen, *Thurlow Weed: Wizard of the Lobby* (1947); J. H. Parks, *John Bell of Tennessee* (1950); Rudolph Von Abele, *Alexander H. Stephens: A Biography* (1946); and C. M. Wiltse, *John C. Calhoun: Sectionalist, 1840–1850* (1951).

*Available in a paperback edition.

12
AMERICA AT MID-CENTURY

From the Mexican War to the Civil War the major themes of American political history were a growing sectionalism interacting with a vigorous nationalism, the gradual disintegration of the second American party system, and the formation of a new party system. Outside the realm of politics, however, this period was notable for its positive achievements—its industrial growth, railroad construction, agricultural expansion, and technological innovations. In spite of the mounting political crisis, Americans were concerned most of the time with other affairs. They were occupied with ships and railroads and machines and farm implements, with the settlement and development of the West, and with geographic expansion and Manifest Destiny. Stephen A. Douglas, energetic and tough-minded, idol of a bumptious element in the Democratic party that called itself Young America, cared little for the moral issue of slavery and was impatient with those who did. In the early 1850s Douglas struck a popular note when he urged Americans to forget the sectional quarrel and turn to the main business of building a prosperous and powerful nation. Young America was, to be sure, concerned about its soul, but it was concerned even more about getting things done.

The Emergence of an American Literature

The 1850s were one of the most distinguished and productive periods in the history of American literature. The decade was preceded, however, by many years of literary dependence on Europe. As late as the 1820s American readers were buying more than twice as many books by British as by American authors.

The first writers to win more than local recognition—Washington Irving (1783–1859) and James Fenimore Cooper (1789–1851)—had exploited American themes, but they had spent much of their lives abroad and had observed the conventions of Europe's men of letters. Irving, after writing an amusing and popular *History of New York* (1809) and *The Sketch Book* (1819–20), which depicts village life in rural New York through characters such as Ichabod Crane and Rip Van Winkle, went off to Europe hoping to exchange "the commonplace realities of the present" for "the shadowy grandeur of the past." Cooper used the American frontier as the setting for his five *Leatherstocking Tales* (1823–41), but it is a romantic, unrealistic frontier where the hero, Natty Bumppo,

New York docks

The genius of the United States is not best or most in its executives or legislatures, nor in its ambassadors or authors or colleges or churches or parlors, nor even in its newspapers or inventors ... but always most in the common people. Their manners, speech, dress, friendships—the freshness and candor of their physiognomy—the picturesque looseness of their carriage ... their deathless attachment to freedom—their aversion to anything indecorous or soft or mean—the practical acknowledgment of the citizens of one state by the citizens of all other states—the fierceness of their roused resentment—their curiosity and welcome of novelty—their self-esteem and wonderful sympathy—their susceptibility to a slight—the air they have of persons who never knew how it felt to stand in the presence of superiors—the fluency of their speech—their delight in music, the sure symptom of manly tenderness and native elegance of soul ... their good temper and openhandedness—the terrible significance of their elections—the President's taking off his hat to them not they to him—these too are unrhymed poetry. It awaits the gigantic and generous treatment worthy of it.

From Walt Whitman, Preface to *Leaves of Grass*, 1855.

embodies the courage, nobility, innocence, and naturalness supposedly characteristic of those who live in the wilderness. Though defending American democracy to Europeans, Cooper had little confidence in the future of literature in his native land. "There is scarcely an ore which contributes to the wealth of the author, that is found, here, in veins as rich as in Europe," he complained. A third writer of extraordinary talent, Edgar Allan Poe (1809–49), born in Boston but a Virginian by adoption, was too exotic a figure, too much lost in a weird world of his own creation, too alienated from his optimistic, democratic compatriots, to be the founder or precursor of an American literature.

Yet the call for a national literature as an essential part of a genuine American independence was heard soon after the Revolution and grew stronger with the passing years. In 1815 a group of Boston intellectuals began publishing a literary magazine, the *North American Review*, but rather than breaking new ground it soon came to speak chiefly for a conservative, European-oriented, genteel literary tradition. It often spoke in terms of a cultural nationalism, but it did little in these early years to disturb the local literary establishment. In 1830 William Ellery Channing, in his "Remarks on National Literature," criticized these traditionalists, many of them his Unitarian coreligionists. The true rulers of a country, he said, "are those who determine its mind, its tastes, its principles, and we cannot consent to lodge this sovereignty in the hands of strangers." A decade later a New York editor again asked when an American literature would "breathe the spirit of our republican institutions? . . .

When will it assert *its* national independence, and speak the soul—the heart of the American people? . . . Why do our authors aim at no higher degree of merit, than a successful imitation of English writers of celebrity?"

Eventually several transcendentalist writers made the first successful break with the traditionalists. One of the milestones in this revolt was Emerson's Phi Beta Kappa address at Harvard in 1837, titled "The American Scholar." Calling for a literature of democracy, Emerson advised American writers to stop imitating the "courtly muses of Europe" and to produce a distinctive literature of their own. "Our day of dependence, our long apprenticeship to the learning of other lands draws to a close," he exulted. "The millions that around us are rushing into life cannot always be fed on the sere remains of foreign harvests. Events, actions arise, that must be sung, that will sing themselves." The writer should look to the lives of the common people, who, Emerson believed, were the finest products of this new nation. Writers should turn away from "the great, the remote, the romantic" and "sit at the feet of the familiar, the low. . . . What would we really know the meaning of? The meal in the firkin; the milk in the pan; the ballad in the street; the news of the boat; the glance of the eye; the form and gait of the body."

In the 1840s and 1850s American writers began to heed Emerson's advice. Emerson's own essays, as well as those of Thoreau, marked a turning away from Europe, a trend still more apparent in the novels of Nathaniel Hawthorne (1804–64) and Herman Melville (1819–91) and in the poetry of Walt Whitman

(1819–92). Their masterpieces—Hawthorne's *The Scarlet Letter* (1850), Melville's *Moby Dick* (1851), which many critics call the greatest American novel, Thoreau's *Walden* (1854), and the first edition of Whitman's *Leaves of Grass* (1855)—attracted a limited but appreciative audience of educated men and women. Both Hawthorne, fascinated with the Puritan tradition and with New England's history and legends, and Melville, drawing on his adventures on the high seas, were tormented by deep philosophical questions: the nature of man and the source of evil, which they saw as a powerful and enduring force in the world.

Whitman, far more a buoyant transcendentalist then either Hawthorne or Melville, responded most heartily to Emerson's call. His poetry—sensuous, exuberant, unorthodox, unconcerned about rhyme or meter—was denounced by some as crude, vulgar, even immoral. When *Leaves of Grass* first appeared, Emerson found it a little shocking, because some of the poems dwelt on "the form and gait of the body" somewhat more than he had bargained for; nevertheless, he greeted Whitman "at the beginning of a great career." Drawing his themes from nature and the common people, Whitman called *Leaves of Grass* "the great psalm of the republic." In his preface he expressed the humane, democratic idealism that underlies his poetry: "Love the earth and sun and the animals, despise riches, give alms to everyone that asks . . . hate tyrants, argue not concerning God, have patience and indulgence toward the people, take off your hat to nothing known or to any man or number of men." In effect, Whitman took the ideas of the transcendentalists out of the study and gave them joyous, uninhibited life.

Herman Melville: a fascination with evil

Intimations of Imperialism

During the 1850s America's politicians doubtless understood the spirit of the people at least as well as America's poets did, and the politicians were listened to more attentively. As in the 1840s, they found widespread support for proposals for national geographic expansion. In his inaugural address President Pierce served notice that the acquisition of Oregon, California, and New Mexico was not the complete fulfillment of his country's Manifest Destiny. There were other areas that circumstances might force the United States to acquire, and Pierce announced that his Administration would not shrink from further expansion because of "any timid forebodings of evil." In part he was expressing the continuing belief that eventually all or part of Canada and the rest of Mexico would be annexed to share the blessings of American democracy. But by mid-century some expansionists were looking beyond these adjacent territories to Cuba, Central America, and Hawaii, where commercial and strategic considerations outweighed the hunger for land. This was a sign that Manifest Destiny might very easily be converted into a modern doctrine of imperialism.

Cuba. The Spanish colony of Cuba, a land of slaves and sugar plantations, interested Southerners who hoped to acquire it in order to increase their political and economic power. Cuba also attracted certain Northern commercial interests, especially a small but active group of business-speculators in New York. Moreover, its proximity to Florida and its commanding position at the mouth of the Caribbean Sea and the Gulf of Mexico gave it great strategic importance. The United States had always been apprehensive about the possibility that Cuba might pass from Spain to a stronger power. As early as 1810 President Madison had warned that his country "could not be a satisfied spectator" if Cuba were to fall to some European government "which might make a fulcrum of that position against the security and commerce of the United States."

Until the 1840s the chief aim of American diplomacy had been merely to keep Cuba out of the hands of Britain and France. After the Mexican War, however, proannexation sentiment became so strong that the government changed its policy. In 1848 James Buchanan, Polk's Secretary of State, instructed the American minister at Madrid to offer as much as $100 million for Cuba. The Spanish government responded with a cold refusal.

Unable to gain Cuba by diplomacy, some expansionists (mostly Southerners) were ready to try force. In 1848 General Narciso López, a Venezuelan adventurer, appeared in New Orleans to find arms and recruits for a filibustering expedition against Cuba. The next year, in spite of federal attempts to stop him, López invaded the island with two hundred fifty volunteers, mostly Mexican War veterans, but Spanish troops quickly repulsed them. In 1851 López tried again with a force of four hundred men, but once more he was defeated; this time Spanish authorities

executed him and fifty other captives as pirates. Disappointed sympathizers in New Orleans retaliated by destroying the Spanish consulate, and the American and Spanish governments exchanged angry notes. Eventually the United States paid an indemnity for the damage committed by the New Orleans mob, and Spain pardoned the rest of the captured filibusters. But the government did not disavow its interest in Cuba; indeed, it rejected a British and French proposal for a tripartite agreement designed to assure the island's continued possession by Spain.

The Pierce Administration made the acquisition of Cuba one of its chief goals. It sent Pierre Soulé of Louisiana, a flamboyant French exile and ardent expansionist, as minister to Spain, and it gave him cause to believe that his mission was to acquire the island regardless of methods. Secretary of State William L. Marcy authorized Soulé to renew the attempt to purchase Cuba, this time for $130 million; failing in this, he might try to "detach" it from Spain by intrigue. Lacking the most elementary qualifications of a diplomat, the impetuous minister soon was embroiled in a bitter dispute with the Spanish government. In February 1854 an American merchant vessel, the *Black Warrior*, was seized at Havana for a technical violation of Spanish customs laws. Soulé promptly demanded a disavowal of the act and an indemnity; when he received no immediate reply, he renewed his demands in the form of a virtual ultimatum. The Spanish foreign minister simply ignored Soulé and negotiated a settlement directly with Washington and with the owners of the *Black Warrior.*

At this point Soulé might well have been replaced by a more skillful minister. Instead, Marcy showed no outward sign of disapproval and gave him an even more delicate assignment. Soulé was to confer with John Y. Mason, minister to France, and James Buchanan, minister to Great Britain, about methods of acquiring Cuba and of dealing with possible British and French opposition. In October 1854 the three ministers met for a few days at Ostend and then for a week at Aix-la-Chapelle. They sent their recommendations to the Secretary of State in a confidential memorandum, but its contents were soon known to the public—and the document itself was quite inaccurately labeled the Ostend Manifesto. Largely the work of Soulé, the memorandum declared that the United States would benefit from the possession of Cuba, while Spain would be better off without it. Accordingly, it proposed that another effort be made to purchase the island. If Spain again refused to sell, the United States would have to consider whether Cuba was a threat to its internal peace. If it was, "then by every law human and divine, we shall be justified in wresting it from Spain, if we possess the power."

The Ostend Manifesto delighted Southern expansionists and the Young America element in the Democratic party, and it played no small part in Buchanan's presidential nomination two years later. But the criticism from abroad and the indignation of antislavery Northerners forced the Pierce Administration to repudiate it. Marcy sent a strong rebuke to Soulé, and the shocked and humiliated minister resigned. But Cuba was not forgotten; the Democratic platform of 1856 favored annexation, and in three of his annual messages to Congress President Buchanan urged another attempt to purchase it. Cuba, however, had become a sectional issue, and any further action was impossible.

Central America. For centuries men had dreamed of joining the Atlantic and Pacific by cutting a canal through Panama or Nicaragua, but the United States did not become seriously interested in the idea until after the Mexican War and the acquisition of California. In 1848 the need for faster communication between the East and the Far West led to the signing of a treaty with New Granada (Colombia), which gave the United States transit rights through Panama in exchange for a guarantee of New Granada's sovereignty over this isthmian province. By 1855 a group of American promoters had built a railroad across Panama; until the completion of the first transcontinental railroad in 1869, this was the easiest route to the Pacific coast.

Meanwhile, American diplomats, speculators, and adventurers had become deeply involved in the affairs of the small and politically unstable Republic of Nicaragua, which seemed as promising a site for a canal as Panama. Here, however, the Americans met a formidable competitor in Great Britain, whose worldwide trade, large navy, and extensive colonial possessions gave it a keen interest in an isthmian canal. Indeed, because of the enormous cost of such a project, many assumed that when a canal was built, British capitalists would finance and control it. The British government, watching American movements suspiciously, established a foothold at the mouth of the San Juan River (the probable eastern terminus of a Nicaraguan canal) and claimed a protectorate over the Mosquito Indians on the eastern coast of Nicaragua. This action alarmed the American government, and in the resulting diplomatic exchanges each country warned that it would not permit the other to have exclusive control over an isthmian canal. In 1850 the dispute was settled when Sir Henry Lytton Bulwer, the British minister to the United States, and John M. Clayton, President Taylor's Secretary of State, agreed to the terms of a treaty. It provided, first, that any canal built through Panama or Nicaragua was to be unfortified, neutral in time of war, and open to the ships of all countries on equal terms; second, that

neither country was to colonize or establish dominion over any part of Central America.

The Clayton-Bulwer Treaty was approved by the Senate and remained in force for the next half-century, but it was unpopular from the start. Expansionists disliked the commitment not to acquire territory in Central America, which meant, they said, that the United States had voluntarily applied the Monroe Doctrine against itself. This concession, together with the implicit recognition that Britain had equal interests in Central America, provoked critics to accuse Clayton of having been outwitted by Bulwer— Buchanan suggested that Clayton ought to be rewarded with elevation to the British peerage. Resentment increased when the British government maintained that the treaty applied only to the future and was not an obligation to abandon its existing protectorate over the eastern coast of Nicaragua. Impulsive Southern expansionists applauded when, in 1855, William Walker, a Tennesseean by birth, led a filibustering expedition into Nicaragua and seized control of its government. Walker was soon driven out, and when he tried to return in 1860 he was captured and executed.

In spite of the criticism, the Clayton-Bulwer Treaty was not a bad bargain for the United States, given the circumstances of the time. The British government removed one cause of complaint when in 1859 it voluntarily gave up its protectorate over the Mosquito Indians. Then and later the treaty avoided a race between the two countries for possessions in Central America. Above all, it assured the United States equal access to an isthmian canal at a time when the nation was in no position to ask for more.

Hawaii. Even before the acquisition of Oregon and California made the United States a Pacific power, some Americans had developed an interest in Hawaii. Merchantmen engaged in trade with the Far East, and whaling ships, had stopped there for supplies; by the 1830s missionaries had begun to arrive; other Americans had come in search of land or commercial opportunities. In those early years there was little talk of annexation, but the government was uneasy about the intentions of the British and the French. In 1849, when France seemed ready to seize the islands, Secretary of State Clayton, though denying that the United States desired to establish its sovereignty over them, warned that it "could never with indifference allow them to pass under the dominion or exclusive control of any other power." The Pierce Administration, however, pursued a more aggressive policy; in 1854 Secretary of State Marcy negotiated a treaty of annexation with the Hawaiian government. But British protests and Senate opposition caused Pierce to drop the matter. Thereafter, until the 1880s, the United States seemed content merely to keep Hawaii free from foreign control.

The Gadsden Purchase. The only tangible result of the various expansionist schemes of the 1850s was the purchase from Mexico of another slice of land in the Southwest. In 1853 the War Department surveyed possible routes for a transcontinental railroad. The survey revealed that if a line were built westward from a Southern city it would probably have to enter Mexican territory south of the Gila River. Realizing that this would be an effective argument for a Northern route, Secretary of War Jefferson Davis persuaded President Pierce to send James Gadsden, a Southern railroad-promoter, to negotiate with Mexico. When Gadsden arrived in Mexico City, he found Santa Anna back in power and in need of money. In 1853 they signed a treaty giving the United States a forty-five-thousand-square-mile strip of desert land below the Gila for $10 million. Except for Alaska, the Gadsden Purchase established the present-day continental boundaries of the United States.

International Trade

Europe. After American merchants and shipowners recovered from the disasters they had suffered during the War of 1812, they were severely hurt again by the long depression following the Panic of 1837. By the mid-1840s, however, economic recovery and several other favorable developments combined to encourage a revival of foreign trade, and commerce and shipping once more became a vital source of income for the economy of the Northeast. Mercantile prosperity was stimulated, first, by the fact that the South continued to be the principal supplier of raw cotton for the expanding British textile industry; second, by the repeal of the British Corn Laws in 1846, which opened a large market for American wheat; third, by the passage of the low Walker Tariff the same year (followed by a still lower tariff in 1857), which encouraged the flow of European manufactured goods to the United States; and, last, by a spectacular rise in immigration, which kept American ships filled to capacity on the homeward voyage. As a result, the combined value of American exports and imports increased from $222 million in 1840 to $318 million in 1850, and then more than doubled in the next decade—reaching $687 million in 1860.

More than two-thirds of this commerce was with Europe, and the most valuable part of it was the exchange of American cotton, wheat, and flour for the products of British factories. Until the Civil War, cotton continued to provide more than half the value of the country's exports. As late as 1860 finished manufactured goods constituted only 10 percent of United States exports but nearly half of its imports. As is typical of a still undeveloped country, the value of imported goods and services usually exceeded the value of exports—by $44 million in 1850. This unfavorable trade balance was offset in part by European credits and investments and in part by the export to Europe of much of the gold mined in California. Nevertheless, foreign trade was vital to the national economy. Though Americans still concentrated on their own internal development, they were bound to the outside world by important commercial ties.

China. Before 1860 scarcely more than 5 percent of American trade was with Asia. Ever since the late eighteenth century, however, many New York and New England merchants had been dazzled by the profits they anticipated, and often made, from the penetration of Far Eastern markets. As we have seen, their hope of developing this trade was related to the desire for ports on the Pacific coast. By the early nineteenth century, American merchant ships were stopping in the Philippines, Java, and India, and in 1833 the United States signed a trade treaty with Siam. But the center of activity was at Canton, the one Chinese port open to foreigners, where furs were traded for tea, spices, and nankeens.

Though the United States government never took the initiative in wringing commercial concessions from China, it always capitalized on opportunities afforded by the encroachments of others. When Britain, after the Opium War of 1839–42, forced open several additional Chinese ports and gained various other advantages, American merchants demanded that their government intervene in their behalf. President Tyler responded by sending Caleb Cushing of Massachusetts, a man of rare diplomatic talent, to negotiate with China. In the Treaty of Wanghia (1844) Cushing won access to the ports that had been opened to the British; he established the right of extraterritoriality, which enabled resident Americans accused of crimes to be tried in American rather than Chinese courts; and he obtained a promise of "most favored nation" treatment, whereby privileges granted to other powers would also be granted to the United States. In subsequent years, as the British and French forced China to make further concessions, American merchants were thus able to claim similar rights. However, since the United States merely asked to be given what others had seized by force, relations with China remained friendly.

Japan. From the sixteenth century to the middle of the nineteenth century Japan's only contact with the outside world had been a limited trade with the

Dutch East India Company through the port of Naga-saki. The military shoguns, who dominated the weak emperors, had excluded foreign merchants, mission-aries, and diplomats in order to preserve a feudal society. But during the 1840s some Americans began to take an interest in Japan. The Pacific whaling industry needed a treaty to assure proper treatment of shipwrecked sailors cast up on Japanese shores; merchants engaged in the China trade hoped to make Japan a port of call; and textile-manufacturers were eager for a chance to exploit the Japanese market.

In 1852 pressure from these groups caused President Fillmore to send Commodore Matthew C. Perry to Japan with an imposing fleet of steam warships. Perry bore a letter and gifts to the emperor and an array of gadgets illustrating the wonders of Western civilization. In July 1853 he arrived at Yedo Bay, insisted that his letter be delivered to the emperor, and promised to return in the spring. Perry made his second visit early in 1854 and found Japanese officials conciliatory and ready to negotiate. By combining vague threats of war with skillful diplomacy, he secured a treaty of friendship that opened two small ports to American trade, permitted the establishment of a consulate at one of them, guaranteed the safety of shipwrecked sailors, and gave the United States "most favored nation" treatment. Other Western powers soon negotiated their own treaties and forced Japan to open other ports and make additional concessions.

First Japanese Mission to the United States

The State Department sent Townsend Harris, a brilliant diplomat, to Japan as the first American consul. Pointing to the fate of China under foreign domination, Harris assured Japan that the United States had no territorial ambitions and urged it to protect itself by modernizing and Westernizing under American guidance. "If you accept my proposals," he predicted, "Japan will become the England of the Orient." His case was persuasive, and in 1858 he signed another treaty greatly enlarging the concessions that Perry had won. Ministers were now to be exchanged; American consuls could reside at the six ports then open to foreigners; American citizens could buy property and enjoy freedom of religion at the so-called treaty ports; and Japan could buy warships and merchantmen from the United States. In 1860 the first Japanese diplomatic delegation visited Washington, and soon thereafter Japan began to make rapid strides toward catching up with the modern world.

The clipper ships. The recovery of American foreign trade was immensely aided by a series of dramatic changes in the design of the old three-masted packet ships (see p. 215), changes that produced a fleet of the swiftest and most beautiful sailing vessels ever to engage in ocean commerce. In 1845 the *Rainbow*, a seven-hundred-fifty-ton ship designed by John Griffith, a naval architect, was completed; it had a long, sleek hull with a concave bow, convex sides, and a rounded stern, and tall masts with an enormous spread of canvas. The launching of the *Rainbow*, a ship that incorporated the advances of several decades, marked the beginning of the era of the famed clipper ships.

Among the builders of clippers, Donald McKay, of Newburyport, Massachusetts, was the most successful; his yards produced scores of vessels, including the 1,783-ton *Flying Cloud*, the 2,421-ton *Sovereign of the Seas*, and the 4,000-ton *Great Republic*. Commanded by daring, hard-driving captains, these ships broke all records for speed. In 1851, on its maiden voyage, the *Flying Cloud* covered 374 miles in a day; then, on a voyage from New York to San Francisco, it made a run of 433 miles in a day to break its own record. The *Sovereign of the Seas* soon surpassed that with 495 miles in a day's run. Another clipper, the *Lightning*, set a record of thirteen and a half days for a voyage from New York to Liverpool; still another, the *Oriental*, set a record of eighty-one days for a voyage from New York to Hong Kong.

From the mid-1840s to the mid-1850s the clippers gave the United States a larger share of the world's peacetime carrying trade than ever before, a share that briefly promised to surpass the British, especially in the long-distance trades. The new ships and their masters took a commanding position in the com-

Lightning

Immigration

The role of the immigrant. Between 1830 and 1860 the population of the United States increased from 12,866,000 to 31,443,000. But in spite of this remarkable growth the country was still sparsely settled and short of manpower. The factories needed more and more hands to tend the machines. Revived programs of internal improvements following the depression of the early 1840s created another heavy demand for workers. Above all, the supply of arable land still seemed to be inexhaustible, and the Western states and territories eagerly welcomed new settlers. Depression created temporary unemployment in the Eastern industrial centers, but most of the time before the Civil War there were not enough men and women to meet the labor requirements of cities and farms.

The manpower problem would have been even more acute had it not been for a sharp increase in European immigration to the United States, for industrialization and urban growth had caused a decline in the birthrate among the native-born population. Until the mid-1840s immigrants had been arriving at a slowly accelerating annual rate—8,385 in 1820; 23,322 in 1830; and 84,066 in 1840—but in the decade before 1840 fewer than 600,000 had crossed the Atlantic. In the following decade, however, immigration increased to 1,713,000, and during the 1850s to 2,598,000. Each year between 1850 and 1854 the number of immigrants exceeded 300,000, reaching a peak of 428,000 in 1854—a figure that would not be surpassed until the 1870s.

The overwhelming majority of immigrants still came from northern and western Europe. During the 1850s slightly more than three hundred thousand migrated from Great Britain, about twenty-five thousand from the Scandinavian countries. But Germany and southern Ireland had now become the two principal sources. In addition to the usual incentives—technological unemployment in Europe, the lure of cheap land in America, and the vision of the United States as a country of opportunity, freedom, and social equality—several special conditions helped to bring in a tide of Irish and Germans. In Ireland the failure of the potato crop of 1845 began a succession of famine years that caused widespread misery and actual starvation. As a result, in the fifteen years after 1845 approximately a million and a half Irish, most of them unskilled, illiterate, and in extreme poverty, crossed the Atlantic. In Germany the suppression of the liberal Revolution of 1848 brought many political refugees along with the majority who came in search of improved economic conditions. Between 1850 and 1860 nearly a million Germans arrived.

In the main these immigrants were not systematically recruited, and they were seldom subsidized by

merce of both Europe and the Far East. But the most spectacular role of the clippers came in the early 1850s in the growing trade between the Atlantic coast and California. The older sailing vessels had taken more than five months to make the voyage around the Horn, whereas the clippers made it in three.

The era of the clipper ships, however, soon ended, for by the mid-1850s advances in technology were making them obsolete. The opening of the Panama Railroad in 1855 deprived them of California passengers, who could reach San Francisco along the shorter route in five weeks. Meanwhile, the clippers were losing out in the competition with British ironclad sailing ships, and then ironclad steam vessels, which were less beautiful in design but superior in speed and cargo space. American steamship companies had only indifferent success in their rivalry with the British, who now recaptured much of the ocean commerce they had lost to the clippers. Not until the First World War would the United States again hold the position in the carrying trade that it enjoyed for a decade in the mid-nineteenth century.

Arriving immigrants

organized groups. The Mormon Church helped its converts, and an Irish Pioneer Emigration Fund, supported by British, Irish, and American leaders, paid the passage of a few. In addition, some immigrants helped friends or relatives to join them. But most came on their own. A minority of them were fairly well-to-do middle-class people whose motive for coming, according to one report, was "not want or oppression, but . . . a rage for speculation, or a desire to acquire wealth more rapidly." Usually, however, the immigrants were poor people who could afford to pay their way only because competing merchant ships, needing return cargoes, reduced fares to as low as $30. Immigrants were crowded into steerage quarters, where they suffered from poor food, inadequate sanitary facilities, and the ravages of smallpox, dysentery, and "ship fever."

Much of this immigrant stream poured into the country through New York, some of it through Boston, Philadelphia, Baltimore, and New Orleans. Since there was no public program to help these strangers find homes and jobs or to ease the difficult adjustment to a new environment, many of them at first had unhappy experiences. Although the state of New York, in 1855, gave immigrants some limited protection by establishing Castle Garden as a controlled landing place, they often fell victim to swindlers who cheated them with exorbitant charges for lodgings or transportation or with false promises of employment.

Because the Irish seldom had the means to become farmers, they congregated in the slums of New York and Boston and in the factory towns of New England. A much larger proportion of the Germans arrived with enough money to move to the Middle West, where they acquired farms, became artisans, or established business enterprises in cities such as Cincinnati, St. Louis, Chicago, and Milwaukee. Fewer immigrants settled in the South. Most of them debarked at Northern ports, but even many of those who arrived at New Orleans took steamboats up the Mississippi to the free states. They were drawn north by their preference for the cooler climate, by superior economic opportunities and their unwillingness to compete with slave labor, and, in the case of many Germans, by their opposition to slavery itself.

Though few immigrants found it easy to settle in a new land, though far too many lived in abject poverty in the cities of the East, in the long run most of them did manage to improve their lot, and their cultural, social, and economic contributions were incalculable. From the ranks of the immigrants in subsequent years came many of the country's distinguished leaders in politics, the professions, journalism, the fine arts, banking, industry, and transportation. The English and Germans augmented the short supply of skilled craftsmen; the Welsh and Cornish worked the coal mines of Pennsylvania and the lead mines of Missouri and Wisconsin; the Irish tended the machines in New England factories, built railroads, and dug canals; men and women from all the immigrant groups brought millions of acres of Western land under cultivation. Not the least of the immigrants' contributions was the richness and variety they gave to American society through the customs and amenities they brought with them from their old homes.

Nativism. Notwithstanding the value of the immigrants to a thinly settled country, their growing numbers began to alarm some Americans whose ancestors had arrived in earlier years. By the 1850s aliens constituted half the population of New York City and outnumbered the native-born Americans in Chicago, Milwaukee, and St. Louis. Such conditions helped to produce the first significant nativist, or antiforeign, movement in American history, a movement that briefly became a major force in both state and national politics.

Nativism resulted not only from concern about the numbers of immigrants but from other anxieties as well. A few racists feared that the Celts from southern Ireland would pollute the old American stock, and that the United States would cease to be predominantly an Anglo-Saxon nation. Some criticized the Irish and Germans for being clannish and for preserving Old World customs and habits of dress. Others were distressed by the prevalence of crime and pauperism in the immigrant slums, resented the burden that alien indigents put on public funds and private charity, and accused European governments of deliberately exporting their "undesirables" to the United States. Native workers disliked the immigrants as economic competitors whose low standard of living threatened to depress wages. In New England, for example, Irish workers, recruited in Boston, soon replaced the native-born young women who had been the original source of the labor supply in the textile mills. The mill owners found the newcomers more docile and willing to work for wages lower than the women had received. Conservatives were concerned about the immigrants' growing political power, for many states permitted them to vote before they became naturalized citizens. Most immigrants supported the Democratic party as the party of the common people, and in Eastern cities, such as New York and Boston, Democratic bosses, to the dismay of their political enemies, used them to build party machines.

Though all these anxieties contributed to the nativist movement, the strongest force behind it was anti-Catholicism. In the early nineteenth century Roman Catholics were a small fraction of the population, but in the 1840s and 1850s nearly all of the Irish and approximately half of the German immigrants were adherents of this faith. The long experience of persecution and exploitation by English Protestants in their homeland caused the Irish to cling to their Church with intense loyalty; the fact that they were a minority in the United States, confronted with a hostile Protestant majority, reinforced these feelings and made the Church a central influence in their lives.

Anti-Catholic sentiment among American Protestants was old and deep-rooted, having grown from a combination of bigotry, fear of the temporal power of the Catholic Church, and genuine disagreement over Christian doctrine. With the growth of the Catholic population, there was a corresponding increase in the number of priests and bishops, convents and monasteries, parochial schools and colleges. Frightened nativists viewed every Catholic immigrant as an agent of the pope sent to seize the government and destroy Protestantism. They believed the Church to be the ally of tyranny and reaction in Europe, the enemy of freedom and democracy in America. And their prejudices were confirmed by lurid accounts of immorality in the convents and among the priesthood.

Nativist agitation started in the 1830s. In New York the Reverend George Bourne edited an anti-Catholic weekly, *The Protestant*, while other clergymen organized a Protestant Association "to promote the principles of the Reformation" and to "unfold the true character of Popery." In 1834 Samuel F. B. Morse, portrait-painter and promoter of the telegraph, published an influential anti-Catholic book, *A Foreign Conspiracy Against the Liberties of the United States*, that went through numerous editions. Urging Protestants to unite against the Catholic menace, Morse advocated stricter immigration laws to "stop this leak in the ship through which the muddy waters from without threaten to sink us." Nativists incited anti-Catholic riots, stoned Catholic institutions, and, in 1834, burned the Ursuline Convent School in Charlestown, Massachusetts.

During the 1840s, when Catholic immigrants began to arrive in large numbers, a bewildering array of secret nativist societies sprang up—among them, the Sons of '76, the Sons of America, the Druids, and the Order of United Americans. One of them, the American Protestant Society, was organized for the purpose of combating the "spiritual darkness" of popery and converting Catholics to Protestantism. The Society's missionary efforts were a failure, but it won the support of many churchgoers and gave the nativist movement the aura of a Protestant crusade. Early in the 1850s most of these societies united to form a powerful national organization, the Order of the Star Spangled Banner. Because members were sworn to secrecy and refused to answer questions about their aims and activities, they were usually called the Know-Nothings. However, it soon became evident that their purposes were to defend Protestant-

Popery is a system of mere human policy; altogether of Foreign origin; Foreign in its support; importing Foreign vassals and paupers by multiplied thousands; and sending into every State and Territory in this Union, a most baneful Foreign and anti-Republican influence. Its ... Pope, his Bishops and Priests, are politicians.... Associated with them for the purpose ... of securing the Catholic vote, are the worst class of American politicians, designing demagogues, selfish office-seekers, and bad men.... These politicians know that Popery, as a system, is in the hands of a Foreign despotism.... But corrupt and ambitious politicians in this country, are willing to act the part of traitors to our laws and Constitution, for the sake of profitable offices; and they are willing to sacrifice the Protestant Religion, on the ancient and profligate altar of Rome, if they may but rise to distinction on its ruins!...

Every Roman Catholic in the known world is under the absolute control of the Catholic Priesthood.... And it is this faculty of concentration, this political influence, this power of the Priesthood to control the Catholic community, and cause a vast multitude of ignorant foreigners to vote as a unit, and thus control the will of the American people, that has engendered this opposition to the Catholic Church. It is this aggressive policy and corrupting tendency of the Romish Church; this organized and concentrated political power of a distinct class of men; foreign by birth; inferior in intelligence and virtue to the American people ... which have called forth the opposition ... to the Catholic Church.

From William G. Brownlow, *Americanism Contrasted with Foreignism, Romanism, and Bogus Democracy,* 1856.

ism against Catholicism, to make immigration laws more restrictive, to increase the number of years required for naturalization, and to deprive aliens of the ballot.

Meanwhile nativism had become a political force and, posing as a movement to reform politics and make government more responsive to the popular will, had begun to score successes in local elections. After the presidential election of 1852, many former Whigs joined as their own party disintegrated. However, the movement cut across party lines, for some Democrats joined as well. In addition, a scattering of political abolitionists and other social reformers, viewing the Irish Catholics as enemies of their causes, were temporarily attracted to the nativist crusade. Political nativism reached its peak in 1854 and 1855, when the Know-Nothings captured several state legislatures, elected numerous governors, and claimed the allegiance of at least seventy-five congressmen. Their most spectacular victory came in Massachusetts, where they controlled every state office and had an overwhelming majority in the legislature. In 1856 the nativists formed the American party, nominated Millard Fillmore for President, and polled 22 percent of the popular vote.

Thereafter, nativism rapidly declined. At neither the federal nor the state level were the Know-Nothings successful in implementing their program. In Congress they proposed to extend the time required for naturalization to twenty-one years, but they never managed even to bring their proposal to a vote. In Massachusetts, where nativist legislators were notable chiefly for incompetence, their sole anti-Catholic victory was a requirement that "the common English version" of the Bible be read in the public schools; their only enduring measure directed at the immigrants was a literacy test for the franchise. Elsewhere—in Indiana, for example—the Know-Nothing record was one of complete failure. Nativism, Horace Greeley observed, was "as devoid of the elements of permanence as an anti-Cholera or anti-Potato-rot party would be." Nationally the nativists soon lost their appeal as the country became increasingly absorbed in the slavery controversy—indeed, the American party itself divided when most of the Northern leaders demanded that it take a stand against the expansion of slavery.

Moreover, the Know-Nothings were discredited by charges that their secrecy cloaked a conspiracy against democratic institutions, by the ridicule poured on them following the exposure of their rituals, and by antiforeign riots and election disorders for which they were held responsible. Their religious bigotry and xenophobia failed to destroy traditional

Know-Nothing campaign ribbons

American attitudes that soon began to reassert themselves: a belief in religious toleration, the idea of America as a refuge for the oppressed of the Old World, and a confidence that the United States could in time assimilate as many immigrants as came to its shores. Finally, nativist racism was refuted by a popular argument that held that the mixing of various nationalities was producing a new and unique individual, the American, superior to the old by the very fact of the mixing. As Herman Melville observed, "We are the heirs of all time, and with all nations we divide our inheritance."

Economic Growth

In the two decades before the Civil War, for reasons that are not altogether clear to economic historians, there was an acceleration in the rate of growth and structural change in the American economy. No doubt one major cause for this was the doubling of the labor force as a result of immigration and the natural increase of the population. Most immigrants came as young adults ready to work; some of them contributed not only their labor but special knowledge of production methods useful in agriculture or industry. In addition, this period witnessed a substantial decline in the proportion of the labor force engaged in agriculture from 63.4 to 53.2 percent, and an increase in the proportion working in factories and construction from 13.9 to 18.5 percent. This change was significant, because industrial labor is relatively more productive than agricultural labor. Still another stimulus to economic growth was the abundance and cheapness of raw materials resulting from the abundance and cheapness of land, a condition that partially offset the scarcity and high costs of labor and capital compared to the costs to foreign manufacturers. Finally, the rapid spread of the factory system, the rising productivity of labor resulting from the replacement of manual methods by machines, and the emergence of a class of efficient professional business managers contributed measurably to accelerating economic growth. By 1860 both the agricultural and the manufacturing sectors of the American economy had taken decisive steps in the direction of "modernization"—that is, they welcomed technological innovations that cut labor costs and increased productivity, they readily abandoned traditional methods, and they accepted change rather than stability as in the natural order of things.

Domestic commerce. The flourishing American foreign trade of the mid-nineteenth century required the movement of huge quantities of bulky raw materials and foodstuffs to the seaports on the Atlantic and Gulf coasts as well as the distribution of finished European goods to the markets of the interior. At the same time, internal trade expanded as the population grew and as the economies of the various regions became increasingly interdependent and somewhat more specialized. Much of this commerce continued to move along the country's excellent waterways. Coastal vessels carried cotton, tobacco, and sugar from Southern ports to New York and New England, while the glamorous Mississippi River steamboats, in spite of railroad competition, carried more freight and passengers in the 1850s than ever before.

The paths of inland water transportation were rapidly changing, however, for the canals were diverting a growing amount of business from the rivers to the Great Lakes. The Miami and Erie Canal through Ohio, and the Wabash and Erie Canal through Indiana both connected the Ohio River with Lake Erie at Toledo, while the Illinois and Michigan Canal united the Mississippi and Illinois rivers with Lake Michigan at Chicago. As trade shifted to the Great Lakes and the Erie Canal, New York replaced New Orleans as the chief outlet for Western commodities destined for Northeastern and European markets, and young cities on the lakes outgrew the older cities on the rivers. In the 1830s Chicago had been a small village; by 1860 it had a population of 109,000.

Meanwhile, all forms of water transportation

"Americans took to . . . the railroad"

were beginning to face serious competition from the railroads, with the result that transportation costs for both farmers and manufacturers steadily declined. The principle of running cars on wooden or iron rails had long been in use in the British mining districts for hauling coal, but until the early nineteenth century men or animals had always provided the power. Experiments with steam engines began soon after 1800, and in 1820 John Stevens of New Jersey demonstrated a steam locomotive that successfully pulled a train of cars over a short piece of track. Five years later a small British line, the Stockton and Darlington, became the first commercial railroad to utilize steam power.

This development was enough to stimulate feverish activity in the cities of the Eastern United States, where merchants had been seeking a way to compete with New York for the trade of the interior. In 1828 construction began on the Baltimore and Ohio, and by 1830 a thirteen-mile segment was open for business. A year later the Mohawk and Hudson established service over sixteen miles of track between Albany and Schenectady. In 1833 South Carolina's 136-mile Charleston and Hamburg line was completed and became for a time the longest railroad in the world. Philadelphia soon had a rail connection with the coal fields of eastern Pennsylvania, Boston with Worcester and other interior New England cities. By 1840 these and other lines had a combined trackage of 2,818 miles; by 1850 the trackage had grown to 9,021 miles and by 1860 to 30,627 miles.

Emerson once observed that "the Americans take to this little contrivance, the railroad, as if it were the cradle in which they were born." They took to it (after first showing considerable hostility) in spite of such early inconveniences as irregular schedules, frequent breakdowns, and the likelihood of being showered with sparks from the wood-burning locomotives. A major annoyance was the lack of a standard-gauge track—as late as 1860 there were still a dozen gauges in use—which made it impossible for the rolling stock of one railroad to use the tracks of another. Worse than the inconveniences were the disastrous wrecks resulting from soft roadbeds, broken rails, and collapsed bridges.

Construction engineers gradually increased the safety and efficiency of the railroads. They built solid roadbeds using crushed rock for ballast, substituted cast-iron "T" rails for the old wooden rails covered with iron straps, learned how to make curves and negotiate grades, erected sturdier bridges, and improved the design of locomotives and cars. By the 1850s, though accidents still occurred with painful frequency, technological advances had reduced the risks of travel by railroad to a point where they were not much greater than by steamboat. The speed of the railroads (twenty to thirty miles an hour by 1860),

their ability to get through rough terrain and to tap remote markets, their serviceability in winter when the canals froze or in droughts when rivers were low, made them the ideal solution to the country's transportation needs.

Most of the early small railroad lines were designed to tap the hinterlands of various towns or to give interior areas access to water transportation. However, during the 1850s, in addition to an enormous expansion of railroad mileage, considerable progress was made toward the consolidation of small, independent lines to form trunk lines. In the South, although both Norfolk and Charleston had established rail connections with the Mississippi River at Memphis, most lines continued to be short and to serve merely as feeders for river transportation. The railroad network that had emerged by 1860 was largely a system that united the Northwest with the Northeast. The Baltimore and Ohio had then reached the Ohio River at Wheeling, the Pennsylvania Railroad had connected Philadelphia and Pittsburgh, and several lines had given Boston access to the Erie Canal and the Great Lakes. Meanwhile, the Hudson River Railroad from New York to Albany, together with the New York Central, formed by the consolidation of seven lines between Albany and Buffalo, had given New York a through route to the West. A second railroad, the Erie, had been built across southern New York State from Jersey City to Buffalo. Powerful corporations, controlled by railroad capitalists like Erastus Corning of Albany and John Murray Forbes of Boston, directed the construction and consolidation that produced the trunk lines. Most of the funds came from American and British investors, a little from state and local government subsidies.

In the West, where most of the railroad construction of the 1850s took place, various lines in Ohio, Indiana, and Illinois linked the Ohio and Mississippi rivers with the Great Lakes. The most important of these north-south lines was the Illinois Central, which by 1858 had given Chicago a connection with the rivers at Cairo. Other railroads ran eastward from Chicago, now the transportation hub of the West, to meet the Eastern trunk lines. By 1860 both the Erie and the New York Central either controlled or had agreements with a series of lines that gave them access to Chicago. Railroad bridges now spanned the Mississippi River, and new lines had penetrated as far west as Burlington, Iowa, and St. Joseph, Missouri.

Railroad-builders in the West, where traffic was initially lighter, depended on public support more than those in the East. State and local governments aided them with loans, subsidies, and stock subscriptions, and in 1850 Congress passed a momentous bill providing the first of many railroad land grants. This act, whose chief sponsor was Senator Stephen A.

Railroads in 1850

Railroads in 1860

Douglas, was for the benefit of the Illinois Central; it gave the state of Illinois three square miles of land in alternate sections on both sides of the proposed line (six square miles for each mile of track), with the understanding that the land would be turned over to the company as the railroad was built. Southern support was obtained by making a similar grant for a line from the Ohio River to Mobile. By 1860 approximately 28 million acres from the public domain had been granted to various states for railroad construction.

After 1850 there was much talk of a transcontinental railroad to be built with a federal subsidy, but sectional disagreement over the location of the route delayed action until after the start of the Civil War. Meanwhile, in 1855 the firm of Russell, Majors & Waddell, aided by a government subsidy, established regular overland freight service by wagon train between Kansas and California. Three years later the Butterfield Overland Mail Company began to run subsidized semiweekly stagecoaches between St. Louis and San Francisco. In the spring of 1860 Russell, Majors & Waddell introduced the pony express, which carried mail from St. Joseph, Missouri, to Sacramento in ten days. But in less than a year and a half the pony express was put out of business by a device that was revolutionizing communication: the electric telegraph. In 1844 Samuel F. B. Morse had demonstrated its practicality, and by 1860 the country had been tied together with fifty thousand miles of telegraph wire. In October 1861, when the Pacific Telegraph Company completed its line to San Francisco, communication between the Atlantic and Pacific coasts became a matter of minutes.

Agriculture. The revolution in transportation, the rapid growth of industry, and advances in agricultural technology profoundly affected the life of the American farmer. In New England the rural population declined as many families, or at least the younger members, moved west in search of better land, or to the cities to find employment in factories. Farmland sold to sheep raisers made commercial wool production more feasible. In the 1850s a large proportion of the country's raw wool came from New England, while much wheat and corn were grown in New York and Pennsylvania. But farmers in the Northeast were rapidly turning from these crops to the production of fruits and vegetables, and to dairying for the growing cities nearby. Railroads enabled the owners of orchards, truck gardens, and dairy herds to make daily shipments to city markets, and in this highly specialized and commercialized form Eastern agriculture found new life and became a rewarding enterprise.

In the South the 1850s were generally prosperous years for the producers of the great staples (tobacco, rice, sugar, and cotton) with slave labor. By then the heart of the Cotton Kingdom had shifted from the Southeast to the Alabama-Mississippi Black Belt, the Mississippi Delta, the valleys of the Arkansas and Red rivers, and the prairies of eastern Texas. With cotton selling for 10 to 12 cents a pound, production rose from 2,469,000 bales in 1849 to 5,387,000 bales in 1859, and the South came near to monopolizing world markets. Able-bodied young slaves sold for $1,500 in the New Orleans market. In eastern Virginia, where a generation earlier soil depletion had produced agricultural stagnation, conditions had greatly improved. The slave-plantation system gained new vitality from the introduction of fertilizers, improved methods of cultivation, and systems of crop rotation; but the sale of surplus slaves in the markets of the Southwest continued to be vital to the economy of the older plantation districts. Throughout the South the plantations, though highly commercialized agricultural enterprises, were less affected by technological changes than the farms of the Northeast and Northwest. Planters continued to cultivate the staples with gangs of slaves using simple hoes and plows. As for the mass of nonslaveholding farmers, they often planted a few acres in cotton or tobacco, but in the main they raised corn and hogs for their own subsistence and generally remained outside the market economy.

By 1860 the Old Northwest had become the center of commercial wheat, corn, beef, and pork production. Responding to the growing demands of the East and of Europe, native-born farmers and German and Scandinavian immigrants had opened up the virgin lands of northern Illinois and Indiana, southern Michigan and Wisconsin, and eastern Iowa and Minnesota. With their help the corn crop had increased from 592 million bushels in 1849 to 839 million bushels in 1859, the wheat crop from 100 million bushels to 173 million bushels. Illinois and Indiana now led in hog production, Illinois in corn production, and Illinois, Indiana, and Wisconsin in wheat production.

Widening markets, the high cost of labor, and the abandonment of self-sufficient agriculture for specialized crops stimulated the improvement of farm implements and mechanization. To cut through the tough prairie sod, Western farmers needed plows that were more efficient than the old ones made of wood or cast iron. In 1847 John Deere began to supply this need when he opened a factory at Moline, Illinois, to manufacture steel plows that cut deeper furrows. The fifties also saw the substitution of grain drills for hand planting and the introduction of mowers to harvest the hay crop. Most important for the wheat farmers was the invention of mechanical reapers to replace hand sickles and cradles. In 1831 Cyrus Hall McCormick, a Virginian, built a successful reaper, and in 1847 he moved to Chicago to begin manufacturing reapers on a large scale. The use of the reaper overcame the constraints of a short harvest period, reduced the risks of loss of a year's crop, and enlarged the production potential on a single-family farm. With a reaper a farmer was able to cut as much wheat in a day as had been possible with a sickle in two weeks. Mechanization advanced another step when threshing machines outmoded the old method of flailing wheat by hand.

Having entered the market economy, a growing number of Western farmers thought of agriculture as a business enterprise rather than, in Jefferson's terms, as a way of life. Technological advances enabled them to cultivate more acres but also forced them to make heavier investments in implements and machinery. The railroads opened new markets to them but increased their dependence on the middlemen who financed, transported, stored, and marketed their crops. Specialization made them more efficient but

McCORMICK'S
PATENT
VIRGINIA REAPER.

increased their dependence on Eastern manufacturers for things they had once made for themselves. In short, the farmers were being caught up in the capitalist world of merchants, manufacturers, bankers, and railroad-operators, and by 1860 some of them were showing signs of dissatisfaction with their place in this world. Out of their discontent would grow the farmers' movements of the post-Civil War years.

Industry. In 1851, at London's Crystal Palace Exhibition, the products of American industry and technology were shown to the world. More than a hundred of them won prize medals, including the McCormick reaper, which attracted by far the greatest admiration. The success of the American exhibits was an indication of the rapid progress the country had made in manufacturing since the founding of the first textile mills in the early nineteenth century.

The industrial growth of the 1850s far surpassed that of any earlier decade. The capital investment of a half-billion dollars in 1849 had nearly doubled by 1859, the number of manufacturing establishments had increased from 123,000 to 140,000, and the annual value of their products had grown from $1,019 million to $1,886 million. Manufacturing was concentrated in the New England and Middle Atlantic states, but some industries, such as meat packing and farm equipment, were growing in the Northwest as well. The market was almost entirely a domestic one, with the Northeast exchanging its industrial surpluses for the foodstuffs and raw materials of the agricultural South and West.

Yet industry in the 1850s had certain characteristics indicating that the United States was still in the early stages of the Industrial Revolution. First, most of the manufacturing involved the processing of the products of American farms and forests. In 1860 the leading industry was the milling of flour and meal, whose value was about one-eighth of the total value of manufactures. Other important industries included lumber-milling, distilling, brewing, leather-tanning, and meatpacking. A second indication of industrial immaturity was the smallness of the typical manufacturing enterprises; on the average they employed fewer than ten workers and had a capital value of less than $7,500. Finally, as we have seen, the United States was still a large consumer of foreign manufactured goods and primarily an exporter of agricultural products.

Nevertheless, by 1860 the direction of American economic development was clear. Textile-manufacturing had already become the core of New England's economy: the investment in mills and machinery was more than $100 million, and the number of cotton spindles in operation had grown to 5,236,000—a 100 percent increase since 1840. In 1844 Charles Goodyear

First Singer sewing machine, 1851

had patented a method of "vulcanizing" raw rubber to make it resist heat and cold, and a new rubber-goods industry was soon manufacturing hundreds of products. In 1846 Elias Howe had patented a sewing machine, and five years later Isaac Singer had begun to manufacture and market an improved model. By the 1850s these machines were being used in factories making shoes and ready-made clothing. The iron industry had expanded to supply the needs of the producers of farm machinery and at least some of the needs of the railroads. Between 1840 and 1860 pig-iron production rose from 321,000 tons to 920,000 tons a year. Originally the locomotives for American railroads had to be imported, but by the 1840s Pennsylvania iron-manufacturers were able to meet the domestic demand. Their rolling mills were still unable to turn out heavy rails, however, and the railroads continued to import them from Great Britain.

During the years of rapid industrial growth in the 1840s and 1850s, the chronic shortage of skilled workers and the relatively high cost of labor kept alive the American manufacturer's keen interest in increased efficiency and technological advances. As a result, by

Just as sure as there is a sun at noonday, capital, under its present hostile and unnatural state, is fast reducing labor to utter dependence and slavish beggary.... This talk about the continued prosperity, happy condition, and future independence of the producing class of this country ... is all fiction, moonshine. There is at this very moment a great strife between capital and labor, and capital is fast gaining the mastery—the gradual abasement of the workingmen and women abundantly sustain this position—the various "strikes" among the operatives and workingmen in New England and other sections of the country, which have almost invariably proved abortive and ineffectual, evidently show that combined, incorporated, and protected capital can "starve out" and dismay the disorganized, competing, and dependent laborers, whose daily toil provides the scanty portions to satisfy the pinching necessities of those dependent upon them....

Let the American laborers recollect that the same grasping system which has driven thousands from the Old World in utter destitution to this country for refuge, is here being nourished; and should they suffer it to go on, their children will look in vain for an asylum for their ills and oppressions; and perchance ... curse the day that gave them existence and the beautiful heavens and earth that mock and aggravate their misery.

From Fitchburg, Mass., Voice of Industry, 1845.

the 1850s the United States had outstripped all other industrial countries in turning out products whose manufacture involved the use of precision instruments. A few industries began to apply the methods of modern mass production. The manufacturers of guns, clocks, sewing machines, and farm implements introduced assembly lines on which unskilled workers, performing standardized tasks, made the finished product from interchangeable parts. During the 1850s, two British commissions visited the United States to study manufacturing techniques, especially the remarkable progress of American technology. The British visitors were struck by the inventiveness of American artisans and by the fact that they seemed to be as fascinated by mechanical improvements as their employers.

Meanwhile, in America's growing industries the corporate form of business organization spread rapidly—during the 1850s the number of manufacturing corporations nearly doubled. Their securities were traded on Wall Street and in other financial markets along with those of federal and state governments and transportation corporations. Industry and the building and organizing of railroads were rivaling commerce as the road to wealth and economic power. Thus Amos and Abbot Lawrence of Boston, Phelps, Dodge & Company of New York, and many others got their start in mercantile enterprises but transferred their capital to manufacturing, railroads, and mining. The industrial entrepreneur had already become an important figure in the country's economic life.

By 1860 American factories employed 1,311,000 workers, the mines and transportation a half-million more. Although skilled labor was still in great demand, each craft felt severely threatened by the steady encroachments of the machines and of mass production. Already the factories had made nearly obsolete several old and honorable crafts, notably those of the cordwainers, coopers, and ironsmiths. As the factories grew in size and the ranks of the unskilled were filled with recent immigrants, the relations of labor and capital became increasingly impersonal. Employers began to think of their workers less as human beings than as commodities to be bought at the lowest price. They paid their employees $6 a week or less for a working day of twelve to fifteen hours. They often ignored feeble state laws fixing maximum hours or regulating the labor of children. And they viewed with indifference the poor sanitary conditions and the high rate of industrial accidents in their factories. Conditions such as these touched the lives of only a small fraction of the population, but by the 1850s there had emerged in the factory slums of Eastern cities an unskilled, propertyless proletariat. The Industrial Revolution thus raised to prominence the problem of poverty in an affluent society.

Middle-class reformers who took an interest in the plight of the laboring population usually urged low-paid workers to form their own cooperative workshops or to go west and become farmers. They seldom approved of direct economic action through trade unions. This, however, was how factory workers eventually improved their condition. The promising labor movement of the 1830s (see p. 216) had been destroyed by the depression following the Panic of 1837, and it took many years for another movement to get started. A formidable legal barrier was partially removed when the Massachusetts Supreme Court, in the case of *Commonwealth* v. *Hunt* (1842), ruled that trade unions were not in themselves conspiracies in restraint of trade, a rule that courts in other states soon accepted. But when workers resorted to strikes or boycotts they still ran into trouble with the courts, which continued to interpret such activities as violations of the old common-law doctrine of conspiracy. Trade unions were also handicapped by a hostile press, by generally unfavorable public opinion, and by the ability of employers to recruit strikebreakers.

In the 1850s, though conditions showed little improvement, only a few American workingmen belonged to trade unions. In 1852 the International Typographical Union was formed; by the end of the decade the stonecutters, hat-finishers, iron-molders, and machinists had also established national organizations. The other skilled crafts were organized only locally, while the mass of unskilled workers had no unions at all. Strikes for higher wages or shorter hours occurred in the shoe and textile industries and on the railroads, but they usually failed. Though trade unionism had made a new beginning, a powerful labor movement would not emerge until after the Civil War.

Economic Discontent in the South

The colonial South. On the surface the economic conditions of the 1850s would seem to give no cause for sectional conflict. Because of the growing demand for raw cotton in world markets, the South was prospering, and its economy appeared to be neatly complementary to that of the North—each section needed the products of the other. And yet, throughout the decade, there was in the South an undercurrent of economic discontent.

After the Panic of 1837 Southern cotton played a less dynamic role in the economic development of the country than it had before. Industry now played the role that cotton once played; and, with the growth of the West, Northeastern business interests were relatively less dependent on the Southern market. In short, the South, though still flourishing and enjoying substantial economic growth, saw its economic power diminishing within the Union.

Far more than that of the Northeast, even more than that of the Northwest, the economy of the South

Cotton: the basis for agricultural prosperity in the South

was based on agriculture. In 1860 the eleven states that were to form the Southern Confederacy produced less than one-tenth of the country's manufactured goods; they contained about half as many manufacturing establishments as the Western states. Moreover, Northern ships carried Southern staples to European markets, and most Southern imports came indirectly via New York City. An Alabama editor complained,

> With us every branch and pursuit of life, every trade, profession, and occupation, is dependent upon the North. . . . In Northern vessels [the Southerner's] products are carried to market, his cotton is ginned with Northern gins, his sugar is crushed and preserved by Northern machinery; his rivers are navigated by Northern steamboats . . . his land is cleared with a Northern axe, and a Yankee clock sits upon his mantel-piece; his floor is swept by a Northern broom, and is covered with a Northern carpet; and his wife dresses herself in a Northern looking-glass.

Southerners resented this dependency and searched for ways to strengthen their economy. As early as 1837 a group of Georgians had sponsored a convention at Augusta "to attempt a new organization of our commercial relations with Europe." During the 1840s and 1850s a series of commercial conventions urged the establishment of direct trade between Southern and European ports. While some Southerners planned steamship lines, others favored the building of railroads to divert Western trade to Southern cities. Neither goal was achieved.

For a time there seemed to be a better prospect of improving the South's industrial position. During the depression years of the 1840s, when the price of raw cotton was low, interest in manufacturing increased in the older states of the Southeast, and a number of factories were built. William Gregg of South Carolina, a vigorous propagandist for industrialization, demonstrated its profitability at his highly successful cotton factory in Graniteville. In the 1850s, however, the revival of agricultural prosperity once again made it clear that the South's comparative economic advantage was in the production of staples, and Southern industry therefore found it difficult to compete for capital. Moreover, Northern manufacturers were usually able to undersell their Southern competitors and to provide superior products. As a result, the South's economy remained overwhelmingly agricultural.

Rumors of a Northern conspiracy. Agriculture, Jefferson had taught and Southerners believed, was the most productive pursuit of man. Yet the North had surpassed the South in wealth and population and, according to this widely held though highly inaccurate analysis, had reduced the region to a colonial status. Many Southerners seemed to think they were the victims of a sinister conspiracy planned by a close-knit body of Northern bankers, merchants, manufacturers, and their political agents. The chief haunts of the conspirators were New York and Washington; their distinguishing characteristics were their essential unproductiveness and their skill in amassing wealth from the labor of others. They were accused of exacting exorbitant middlemen's charges, of rigging prices, of manipulating the money market, thus causing much of the wealth produced in the South to flow steadily into their coffers. The price of Southern property, wrote an indignant Virginian, "is dependent upon the speculative pleasure of the Merchants, Bankers, and Brokers of New York. And why? Because Wall Street can depress the money market when it pleases." The South, said a Mississippian, had permitted itself to fall into a condition of "serfdom" and to become

Mid-century America: "The Follies of the Age"

"the sport and laughing stock of Wall Street." A Southern editor described New York as "a mighty queen of commerce . . . waving an undisputed commercial scepter over the South." With an "avidity rarely equalled," she "grasps our gains and transfers them to herself."

But, according to this sectional indictment, Northern capitalists did not make their profits solely from their adroit maneuvers in a free economy. Rather, in advancing their conspiracy they had enlisted the support of the federal government. According to Senator Robert Toombs of Georgia, no sooner had the government been organized than "the Northern States evinced a general desire and purpose to use it for their own benefit, and to pervert its powers for sectional advantage, and they have steadily pursued that policy to this day." They demanded, and received, a monopoly of the shipbuilding business; they demanded, and received, a monopoly of the trade between American ports. The New England fishing industry obtained an annual bounty from the public treasury; manufacturers obtained a protective tariff. Thus, according to Toombs, through its policy of subsidizing "every interest and every pursuit in the North," the federal treasury had become "a perpetual fertilizing stream to them and their industry, and a suction-pump to drain away our substance and parch up our lands."

By the 1850s the notion that Northern profits were largely a form of expropriation of Southern wealth, that the South was "the very best colony to the North any people ever possessed," was having a powerful effect on Southern opinion. Much of this analysis of the antebellum economic relationship between North and South has been effectively challenged by modern economic historians. But what is important historically is not the inaccuracy of this economic analysis but the fact that most Southerners apparently believed it to be true. The attitudes they shared were characteristic of those held by nineteenth-century farmers and planters concerning the "middlemen" who financed, transported, and marketed agricultural commodities. Since they regarded the activities of middlemen as nonproductive and parasitic, they were bound to consider marketing costs exorbitant. Southerners had convinced themselves, remarked a Northerner, "that in some way or other, either through the fiscal regulations of the Government, or through the legerdemain of trade, the North has been built up at the expense of the South." Not even agricultural prosperity could banish this thought from the Southern mind.

Suggestions for Reading

AMERICAN LITERATURE
The surveys of American intellectual history listed at the end of Chapter 10 all deal with American writers of the pre-Civil War years. The best special studies are F. O. Matthiessen, *American Renaissance** (1941); Harold Kaplan, *Democratic Humanism and American Literature* (1972); and Larzer Ziff, *Literary Democracy: The Declaration of Cultural Independence in America** (1981). The biographies of individual writers should also be consulted: J. W. Krutch, *Henry David Thoreau** (1948); R. L. Rusk, *The Life of Ralph Waldo Emerson* (1949); G. W. Allen, *Waldo Emerson: A Biography* (1981); Mark Van Doren, *Nathaniel Hawthorne* (1949); J. R. Mellow, *Nathaniel Hawthorne in His Time** (1980); Arlin Turner, *Nathaniel Hawthorne: A Biography* (1980); Newton Arvin, *Herman Melville* (1950); and G. W. Allen, *The Solitary Singer: A Critical Biography of Walt Whitman** (1955).

EXPANSIONISM AND FOREIGN TRADE
Several excellent monographs on American interests in Cuba and Central America are available: M. W. Williams, *Anglo-American Isthmian Diplomacy, 1815–1915* (1916); Dexter Perkins, *The Monroe Doctrine, 1826–1867* (1933); Basil Rauch, *American Interests in Cuba, 1848–1855* (1948); and R. E. May, *The Southern Dream of a Caribbean Empire, 1854–1861* (1973). E. S. Wallace, *Destiny and Glory* (1957), is a vivid account of filibustering.

The most useful special studies of American-Far Eastern relations that deal with this period are: Tyler Dennett, *Americans in Eastern Asia* (1941); A. W. Griswold, *The Far Eastern Policy of the United States** (1938); P. J. Treat, *Diplomatic Relations Between the United States and Japan, 1853–1905*, 3 vols. (1932–38); F. R. Dulles, *China and America: The Story of Their Relations Since 1784* (1946); and L. H. Battistini, *The Rise of American Influence in Asia and the Pacific* (1960). Arthur Walworth, *Black Ships off Japan* (1946), is a readable account of the Perry mission to Japan. H. W. Bradley, *The American Frontier in Hawaii: The Pioneers, 1789–1843* (1942), is the best study of early American interest in Hawaii.

The standard works on the growth of American foreign trade are E. R. Johnson et al., *History of Domestic and Foreign Commerce of the United States*, 2 vols. (1915), and J. H. Frederick, *The Development of American Commerce* (1932). The commerce of New England and New York City are the subjects of two distinguished books: S. E. Morison, *Maritime History of Massachusetts: 1783–1860** (1921), and R. G. Albion, *The Rise of New York Port, 1815–1860* (1939). The best books on the clipper ships are A. H. Clark, *The Clipper Ship Era* (1910); C. C. Cutler, *Greyhounds of the Sea* (1930); and Robert Carse, *The Moonrakers* (1961).

IMMIGRATION AND NATIVISM

Three surveys of immigration to the United States are valuable for this period: Carl Wittke, *We Who Built America* (1939, rev. ed., 1964); M. L. Hansen, *The Atlantic Migration, 1607–1860* (1940); and M. A. Jones, *American Immigration** (1960). Oscar Handlin, *The Uprooted** (1951, 2nd ed., 1973), and Philip Taylor, *The Distant Magnet: European Emigration to the U.S.A.* (1971), focus on the immigrants and their problems. Four specific immigrant groups are the subjects of individual volumes: T. C. Blegen, *Norwegian Migration to America*, 2 vols. (1931–40); R. T. Berthoff, *British Immigrants in Industrial America, 1790–1950* (1953); Carl Wittke, *Refugees of Revolution: The German Forty-Eighters in America* (1952) and *The Irish in America* (1956). The immigrant populations of two Eastern cities are studied in Oscar Handlin, *Boston's Immigrants** (1941), and Robert Ernst, *Immigrant Life in New York City, 1825–1863* (1949). J. P. Dolan, *The Immigrant Church: New York's Irish and German Catholics, 1815–1865** (1975), considers the Church's social role.

A perceptive account of mid-century nativism is in Allan Nevins, *Ordeal of the Union*, 2 vols. (1947). R. A. Billington, *The Protestant Crusade, 1800–1860** (1938), emphasizes the anti-Catholic aspect of the movement. I. M. Leonard and R. D. Parmet, *American Nativism, 1830–1860** (1971), is a study of the origins and political significance of nativism. T. J. Curran, *Xenophobia and Immigration, 1820–1930* (1975), is a brief survey. Two special studies are also useful: Sister M. E. Thomas, *Nativism in the Old Northwest, 1850–1860* (1936), and W. D. Overdyke, *The Know-Nothing Party in the South* (1950).

ECONOMIC DEVELOPMENT

All of the books on agriculture, industry, transportation, and technology listed in the suggested readings for Chapter 8 are useful for this period. There are also several good chapters on the American economy at mid-century in Nevins, *Ordeal of the Union*, cited above. Allan Pred, *Urban Growth and City Systems in the United States, 1840–1860* (1980), is a major study of a related topic.

A good introduction to the history of the railroads is J. F. Stover, *The Life and Decline of the American Railroad* (1970) and *Iron Road to the West: American Railroads in the 1850s* (1978). Problems of railroad promotion and finance can be studied in F. A. Cleveland and F. W. Powell, *Railroad Promotion and Capitalization in the United States* (1909); A. M. Johnson and B. E. Supple, *Boston Capitalists and Western Railroads: A Study in the Nineteenth Century Railroad Investment Process* (1967); L. H. Haney, *A Congressional History of Railways in the United States to 1850* (1908) and *A Congressional History of Railways in the United States, 1850–1877* (1910). An outstanding history of the New England railroads is E. C. Kirkland, *Men, Cities and Transportation*, 2 vols. (1948). Railroad promotion in the Southeast is described in U. B. Phillips, *A History of Transportation in the Eastern Cotton Belt to 1860* (1908). T. C. Cochran, *Railroad Leaders, 1845–1890* (1953), contains important material on early railroad promoters and their social attitudes. The following histories of individual railroads are useful: F. W. Stevens, *The Beginnings of the New York Central Railroad*

(1926); J. F. Stover, *History of the Illinois Central Railroad* (1975); Edward Hungerford, *The Story of the Baltimore and Ohio Railroad, 1827–1927*, 2 vols. (1928) and *Men of Erie* (1946); and R. C. Overton, *Burlington West* (1941). Two books deal with the impact of the railroads on the American economy: R. W. Fogel, *Railroads and American Economic Growth** (1964), and Albert Fishlow, *American Railroads and the Transformation of the Ante-Bellum Economy* (1965).

In addition to the listings in the suggested readings for Chapter 8, the following books on industry and technology are worth consulting for this period: G. S. Gibb, *The Saco-Lowell Shops: Textile Machinery Building in New England* (1950); P. G. Faler, *Mechanics and Manufacturers in the Early Industrial Revolution: Lynn, Massachusetts* (1981), for the shoemaking industry: P. E. Paskoff, *Industrial Evolution: Organization, Structure, and Growth of the Pennsylvania Iron Industry, 1750–1860* (1983); J. A. Kouwenhoven, *Made in America** (1948); D. J. Struik, *Yankee Science in the Making* (1948); and Mitchell Wilson, *American Science and Invention: A Pictorial History* (1954). The best book on labor in this period is N. J. Ware, *The Industrial Worker, 1840–1860* (1924). Alice Kessler-Harris, *Out to Work: A History of Wage-Earning Women in the United States** (1982), is a general study of women in the labor force. Hannah Josephson, *The Golden Threads* (1949), is excellent on the women textile-workers of New England. Two good general treatments are J. G. Rayback, *History of American Labor** (1959), and H. M. Pelling, *American Labor** (1960). R. H. Bremner, *From the Depths** (1956), deals with the emergence of the problem of poverty in America.

The causes of economic discontent in the South can be studied in R. R. Russel, *Economic Aspects of Southern Sectionalism, 1840–1861* (1924); J. G. Van Deusen, *The Ante-Bellum Southern Commercial Conventions* (1926); Herbert Wender, *Southern Commercial Conventions, 1837–1860** (1930); and Clement Eaton, *The Growth of Southern Civilization, 1790–1860** (1961).

*Available in a paperback edition.

13
DESTRUCTION OF THE UNION

The men who fashioned the Compromise of 1850 hailed it as the "final settlement" of the slavery question, but in reality it only postponed disunion. Postponements in history have been of great value at times, however. This one gave the nation another decade to try to find a peaceful solution to the quarrels caused not only by the existence of slavery in the society but by the accompanying fact that most Americans of European descent had not made room in their sense of a free society for Americans of African descent. As slaves, the Afro-Americans were accounted for; as free people their own sense of where their freedom might take them was not likely to conform to the picture of the nation held by people who had defined the American free life in a way that excluded them.

Many white Americans of good will saw the Democratic party, with its doctrine of opposition to privilege and advocacy of pragmatic solutions to problems, as the most likely source of the difficult solution. Perhaps tranquility would make one possible. In the election of 1852, Americans seemed to be voting for just such stability when they chose Franklin Pierce, a charming, quiet, well-educated man from New Hampshire. Pierce's lack of a grand plan seemed a good sign that work to reconstruct the national sense of unity could proceed on a day-by-day basis.

No such process took place. Instead, distrust infused every issue and quickly weakened the political means by which continued compromise might have

been affected. The Whig party—which had contained, uneasily, the contending "cotton" Whigs and "conscience" Whigs—gave way totally by 1856. Distrust eroded the effectiveness of the Democratic party as well. Pierce's personality proved unequal to the task of keeping conflict in check and his intellect produced no useful idea around which reunion could be built.

Each of a succession of crises in the 1850s hinged on the question of slavery in the expanding nation. While many antislavery people wanted neither slavery nor the black people who were the slaves in the developing areas of the west, the Southerners saw Northern efforts to contain slavery as likely to result in its extinction. The end of slavery would, they thought, destroy their way of life and make the South a place of undisciplined biracial discord. Many Northerners, for their part, believed the slaveholders would not rest until federal law forever protected their property everywhere in the union.

Those Northern fears proved valid. As soon as the South lost equality in the Senate as a result of the compromise measures, Southern spokesmen insisted on an interpretation of the Constitution that would guarantee the survival of slavery both as an economic basis of society and as the only acceptable solution to the emotional question of race relations in the South. The free farmers of the North and their political representatives were equally determined to reserve the ter-

Federal arsenal, Harper's Ferry

ritories for free white Americans. As the possibilities for accommodating those positions receded, Southerners reasserted their familiar belief that the states retained their sovereignty under the Constitution, while a majority of Northerners held the Union indivisible. Few Northerners believed blacks were equal to whites, but most of them believed slavery was wrong and that it should not be allowed to spread further. The crises of the 1850s successively exposed and hardened those conflicting positions.

The Divisive Issue

The Kansas-Nebraska bill. Early in January 1854 Senator Stephen A. Douglas, chairman of the Committee on the Territories, introduced a bill for the organization of the Nebraska Territory, the region that lay west of Missouri, Iowa, and Minnesota. Douglas was the man for the job. When he resettled in Illinois, he wrote, in 1833, to his family back in New England, "I have become a Western man." For the rest of his life he viewed the region of his new home as the true America and committed his great political talents to its development and political organization. Standing five feet four inches, with a firm, big chest and pugnacious look, Douglas—sometimes volatile and always openly ambitious—hoped to reach the White House as the champion of an America that governed itself with local laws. He came to be distrusted and disliked with equal fervor by proslavery planters who refused to commit the future of slavery to such popular decisions and by black leaders of the antislavery movement like Frederick Douglass. Although his theory was never tested, Douglas claimed that Westerners would exclude slavery from their growing region and thus contain the obsolete institution in the South, where it would eventually be abandoned. Perhaps he was being disingenous with this assertion and, not caring about slavery one way or the other, only wanted to see the West developed prosperously. But certainly Douglas cared far more for the Union than for any questions raised by an abolitionist or secessionist.

In the Senate, Douglas was eager, as he had long been, to extinguish Indian titles on the plains so that the tribes could be driven from their lands on which white people would settle. He sought to establish the basis for a transcontinental railroad with an eastern terminus in Chicago, the potential metropolis of his own state of Illinois. "The tide of immigration and civilization must be permitted to roll onward," Douglas preached. The country needed a "continuous line of settlements, with civil, political and religious institutions all under the protection of the law." He hoped this nationalistic program would win him the Democratic nomination for the Presidency in 1856.

Douglas knew that his Nebraska bill would face large obstacles. Promoters in both New Orleans and in St. Louis, along with their allies in the Congress, were working for rail routes to the Pacific along lines that would originate in their cities and not Chicago. President Pierce's Secretary of War, Jefferson Davis of Mississippi, had begun surveys of three possible routes, of which he clearly favored the most southern. To facilitate its development, Pierce had sent James Gadsden to Mexico with instructions to purchase land south of the Gila River, an objective quickly arranged. The rivalries among the cities cut across the lines of disagreement about slavery, but, as that disagreement grew more virulent, advocates of Western expansion took rigid positions. By 1854, Senator David R. Atchison of Missouri was prepared, as he put it, to see all of Nebraska "sink in hell" before he would permit its organization except on a basis safe for slavery.

Douglas realized from the outset that his bill would fail without Southern support. If it failed, so, too, would his chances for the Presidency. In the text of his bill, he used the exact language used earlier in the Utah and New Mexico acts of 1850: "when admitted as a State . . . , the said Territory . . . shall be received into the Union, with or without slavery, as their constitution may prescribe at the time of their admission." That language expressed Douglas' own point of view. "The Little Giant," always a proponent of popular sovereignty, now reached for phraseology that might skirt the slavery question and still contribute to the "final settlement." Yet as Southerners pointed out, that language did not satisfy them, because the Missouri Compromise of 1820 did not allow slavery north of 36°30′ latitude in the territories, and if the institution was excluded before the transition to statehood, it would not then have support at the time of transition. Douglas tried to adjust the language: "all questions pertaining to slavery in the Territories, and in the new states to be formed therefrom are to be left to the people residing therein, through their appropriate representatives." Still not satisfied, Senator Archibald Dixon of Kentucky proposed the outright repeal of the Missouri Compromise. Douglas conceded. He knew the concession risked the antagonism of antislavery Northerners, but he had confidence in popular sovereignty as a solution to the slavery issue. He expected that the geography of both Kansas and Nebraska would be hostile to a slave economy and therefore make them free states. At the least his concession would get the issues of slavery out of the Congress and into the territories, and permit the building of empire to resume.

In that spirit Douglas failed to assess accurately the extent to which slavery had become a moral issue.

Mr. Haley and Tom jogged onward in their wagon, each, for a time, absorbed in his own reflections. Now, the reflections of two men sitting side by side are a curious thing,—seated on the same seat, having the same eyes, ears, hands and organs of all sorts, and having pass before their eyes the same objects,—it is wonderful what a variety we shall find in these same reflections!

As, for example, Mr. Haley: he thought first of Tom's length, and breadth, and height, and what he would sell for, if he was kept fat and in good case till he got him into market. He thought of how he should make out his gang; he thought of the respective market value of certain supposititious men and women and children who were to compose it, and other kindred topics of the business; then he thought of himself, and how humane he was, that whereas other men chained their "niggers" hand and foot both, he only put fetters on the feet, and left Tom the use of his hands, as long as he behaved well; and he sighed to think how ungrateful human nature was, so that there was even room to doubt whether Tom appreciated his mercies. He had been taken in so by "niggers" whom he had favored; but still he was astonished to consider how good natured he yet remained!

As to Tom, he was thinking over some words of an unfashionable old book, which kept running through his head again and again, as follows: "We have here no continuing city, but we seek one to come; wherefore God himself is not ashamed to be called our God; for he hath prepared for us a city." These words of an ancient volume, got up principally by "ignorant and unlearned men," have, through all time, kept up, somehow, a strange sort of power over the minds of poor, simple fellows, like Tom. They stir up the soul from its depths, and rouse, as with trumpet call, courage, energy, and enthusiasm, where before was only the blackness of despair.

Mrs. Stowe on human property

From Harriet Beecher Stowe, *Uncle Tom's Cabin: or, Life among the Lowly*, 1852.

It was in these years that 300,000 Americans read Uncle Tom's Cabin (see pp. 298–99). The book struck a nerve of guilt in white Southerners, who reacted with defensive anger. Northerners, seeking a brave new start in the West, not only felt compassion for Eliza, crossing treacherous floating ice with her baby in her arms to escape a slave trader who planned to separate them, but did not want to encounter any such scenes of anguish in Kansas. Opponents of slavery in the territories would not be satisfied with the mere probability that slavery would be turned down on the Kansas plains; they would take no chances. Members of the Free Soil party as well as free-soilers in the Democratic party joined antislavery Whigs in attacking the repeal of the Missouri Compromise and in opposing the final version of the Kansas-Nebraska bill.

The bill included the repeal and called for the Platte River country to be divided into two territories, each to be organized immediately on the basis of popular sovereignty. Because the northern territory, Nebraska, was west of Iowa, a free state, few feared the development of slavery there. Kansas, to the south and immediately west of Missouri, a slave state, was another matter. Missourians seemed to think of Kansas as their own backyard, and Southerners in Congress abandoned their initial coolness to the Kansas-Nebraska bill and endorsed it as a measure "reasonable in its operation and effect" and fair to the South.

The Republican party. "The Appeal of the Independent Democrats," a pamphlet written by Salmon P. Chase of Ohio, voiced the outrage of free-soilers, but they could not dissuade President Pierce from endorsing the Kansas-Nebraska bill. On March 3 the Senate passed the controversial measure. After President Pierce then put intense pressure on members of the House and after nearly three months of heated debate, the House passed the bill with a margin of thirteen votes. On May 30, the Kansas-Nebraska bill became law. New England and the Northwest exploded in angry demonstrations as "anti-Nebraska" people came together across party lines to denounce Douglas and his bill. Douglas sardonically noted that he could travel from Washington to Chicago in the light of his own burning effigies. Some of the strongest opponents of the act were Democrats. The Northern wing of the party had divided evenly on the issue in the House of Representatives. The territorial issue, which had already severely damaged the Whigs, now threatened to divide the Democrats as well.

As early as February, 1854, in Ripon, Wisconsin, a gathering of anti-Nebraska Whigs and Democrats united to form a new party and spoke of themselves as "Republicans." Similar meetings took place elsewhere and after President Pierce signed the Kansas-Nebraska bill one of these fusionist groups met at Jackson, Michigan, and adopted the name "Republican Party."

The term "Republican" was employed to suggest both protest and reaffirmation. It implied a criticism of both aristocratic slaveholding and opportunistic land-grabbing and invoked the civic virtue of the less individualistic days of the early republic. The organizers of the new party, deliberately taking the name of Thomas Jefferson's party, sought to establish a connection with the opposition to slavery's expansion that had existed in the earliest days of the republic when the Northwest Ordinance banned slavery in the territory that became the states of the Midwest. As the successors to the Northern Whig party, the Republicans sought to brand the Democratic party as a haven for selfish apologists for slavery.

The new party was made up entirely of voters from one section, the North, and was devoted to the containment of slavery within the states where it was already established. Much as Northern Democrats had done, the Republicans stressed their belief in the dignity of free labor and, in both Pennsylvania and Indiana, members of the new movement called their organizations by the radical name, the "People's Party." Although some enthusiastic new Republicans, like Charles Sumner and George W. Julian, opposed slavery's expansion on purely antislavery grounds, many held that the spread of slavery both endangered the independent way of life of white American farmers and artisans, and decried the movement of black Americans into open lands that should be white as well as free. Ever since the election of 1852, the Whig party had been in disarray. Now the Northern Conscience Whigs, Free-Soilers, political abolitionists, and many Northern Democrats alienated by the Kansas-Nebraska Act joined the new Republican party. The Republicans did a masterful job of associating the entire Democratic party with slavery in the public's mind.

By 1854 the Whig party, badly eroded, maintained its organizations intact in only a few states, but whether the Republicans would become the chief party to oppose the Democrats was still uncertain. The Know-Nothings who organized as the American party also had a strong claim to make. Democrats sustained heavy losses in the congressional elections that year, and it was uncertain which of the components of the alliance opposed to the Kansas-Nebraska Act was stronger, the Republican party or the American party.

The latter, claiming to be a party of reform that would clean up politics by excluding foreigners, was winning votes on the hatred and fear of Catholics and foreign-born citizens that was strong in the cities, the Middle Atlantic states, and the entire border-state region. Because so many of the foreign-born were Catholics, because many had no aversion to the use of alcohol and were thought to be ignorant of ways to avoid political bribes, and because most were Democrats, a voter who chose to oppose the Democrats by voting for the Know-Nothings could be voting against demon rum, corruption, Catholicism, and the "slave power conspiracy" as well. Although some opponents of Pierce's Nebraska policy, like George W. Julian and William H. Seward, were firmly opposed to nativism, there was so much cooperation between the Republican anti-Nebraska forces and the American party that distinguishing the head from the tail of the victorious combination was not easy. But as the Pierce Administration began organizing the Kansas territory, the attention of the country focused on a chaotic contest that worked to the benefit of the Republicans.

The test in Kansas. Critics of "popular sovereignty"—a policy under which decisions were to be made by the majority of adult male settlers—preferred to call it "squatter sovereignty," and the phrase was apt. Nobody expected trouble in Nebraska, and there was none, but in Kansas general and sustained disorder discredited popular sovereignty as a workable solution to the question of slavery in the territories. The customary lawlessness of the frontier was heightened by special causes of dispute. The government had permitted speculators to make claims in Kansas before legal titles had been wrested from the Indians, and early purchasers were making claims where they supposed towns would spring up and along the line of the anticipated transcontinental railroad. The speculators, greedy, not for homesites, but for a rise in values, came from everywhere, but Missourians, on the scene early, regarded Kansas as their rightful territory, their natural place to expand.

Preparing to fight matters out on the basis of popular sovereignty, because that was now the law, free-soil forces determined to make themselves the more numerous party in Kansas. In Massachusetts, Eli Thayer, a wealthy cotton manufacturer, organized the Emigrant Aid Company to give financial help to those willing to undertake the westward trek. To John Greenleaf Whittier, the poet of antislavery, the emigrants were crusaders, rearing "a wall of men . . . on freedom's southern line." All told, only 1,240 settlers came to Kansas under the Emigrant Aid Company's auspices, and efforts to promote Kansas in the Southern states inspired even fewer emigrants. Most of the Kansas settlers came, as they usually did when new

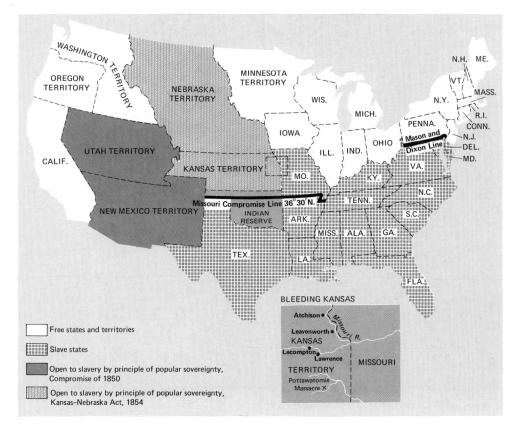

Free states and territories

Slave states

Open to slavery by principle of popular sovereignty, Compromise of 1850

Open to slavery by principle of popular sovereignty, Kansas–Nebraska Act, 1854

BLEEDING KANSAS
Atchison
Leavenworth
KANSAS
Lecompton
Lawrence
TERRITORY
Pottawatomie Massacre ✕
MISSOURI
Missouri R.

The Kansas-Nebraska Act, 1854

territories were opened, from neighboring states. A majority were free-soilers, but many others were from Missouri, and though the slaveholders among them were few, even the nonslaveholders abhorred abolitionism. If abolitionists were unpopular, so too were the black people they sought to free. The number of Afro-Americans in Kansas was miniscule, but the majority of Kansas settlers (including the Emigrant Aid Company settlers) wanted to exclude the free blacks as well as slaves. "Free soil" was for whites only.

When Andrew H. Reeder, the Pennsylvanian chosen by Pierce to be the first territorial governor of Kansas, arrived there in the fall of 1854, he found more than eight thousand settlers ahead of him. The first elections he called set the pattern for many Kansas elections to follow. The proslavery forces won overwhelmingly, electing a territorial delegate to Congress in the fall of 1854 and a proslavery legislature the following spring, but both elections were riddled with fraud. Encouraged by Senator Atchison to believe that their own security depended on establishing a government in Kansas that would protect slave property, Missourians living in the counties adjacent to the border had crossed the state line to cast illegal ballots. Governor Reeder threw out the most blatantly fraudulent returns, but permitted the main result to stand. President Pierce vacillated and did nothing. The new Kan-

sas legislature expelled antislavery members, drew up a territorial slave code so severe that it set the death penalty for anyone aiding a fugitive slave, and, defying freedom of speech, made it a crime to espouse abolitionist sentiments.

The free-soil forces denounced the actions of the "bogus" legislature, as they called it, and organized their own "shadow" government. They drew up the so-called Topeka constitution, which provided for the end of slavery by 1857. It also excluded free blacks from entry into Kansas. The free-soilers announced new elections for a state legislature and established a capital at Topeka. Now two governments, complete with capitals, governors, and legislatures, confronted each other: one was the product of fraud, the other lacked legal foundation.

For three weeks in late November 1855 armed bands of "Border Ruffians" from Missouri roamed the countryside. They claimed to be helping the legal government of Kansas restore order, but their real intent was to terrify the free-soil settlers. The free-state men met the invaders with "Beecher's Bibles," named for Henry Ward Beecher, a popular antislavery preacher who had declared rifles a better force than Bibles for morality in Kansas. Finally the free-state "governor," Charles Robinson, struck a truce with Governor Wilson Shannon, whom Pierce had sent to replace Reeder.

Free-Soilers, Kansas, 1856

Shannon denied that he had sent for the Missourians, and Robinson explained that the free-state men had no intention of disobeying territorial laws.

With the coming of spring 1856, trouble broke out again. In Leavenworth violence at a free-state election resulted in several deaths. Free-staters were justifiably indignant when President Pierce attributed the violence in Kansas to the Emigrant Aid Company and placed no blame on the raiders from Missouri. Pierce, by rejecting the Topeka or free-state constitution as illegal, almost invited an attack on the new free-state capital at Lawrence. In May the attack occurred. A roving band of Missourians broke up the free-state printing press at Lawrence, burned a hotel, and intimidated the inhabitants.

"Bleeding Kansas." One grim free-stater made himself the agent of a savage retribution. The roving survivor of many failed enterprises, John Brown had come to Kansas in the fall of 1855 to settle down with his large tribe of sons and their families and support the antislavery cause. An early advocate of armed resistance, Brown, thinking of himself as God's instrument of revenge, led a small band of his sons and followers in a midnight attack on the sleeping community of Pottawatomie Creek. He ordered them to kill five of the settlers with broadswords he had deliberately sharpened for the purpose and then made off with their horses. Although his victims were asso-

ciated with the proslavery party, not one was a slaveholder, and none had done special services for the Missourians. Within days the whole of southeast Kansas was in arms. John Brown went into hiding with his men, but the Missourians took revenge by burning the free-state town of Osawatomie and killing one of Brown's sons, while seeking Brown himself.

A summer of guerrilla war followed. The death toll for the first year of settlement under popular sovereignty rose to over two hundred, while property losses in barn-burnings, theft, and general destruction reached nearly $2 million. Pierce removed Shannon and sent yet another governor, John W. Geary, to replace him. In September 1856, Governor Geary brought order to the territory with federal troops. Though he persuaded the Missourians to abandon hostilities, nobody believed that the question of slavery in the territories was settled.

Tempers in Congress soon matched those on the frontier. In May 1856, just as the Missourians were burning the hotel in Lawrence, Senator Charles Sumner of Massachusetts, a famous antislavery orator, gave a ringing denunciation of the "Crime Against Kansas." In the course of a two-day speech during which he urged the admission of Kansas as a state under the Topeka constitution, he lashed the Administration for its alleged partiality to the proslavery settlers and defined the "crime" as the "rape of a virgin" territory, comparing it to the "hateful embrace of slavery." Pursuing his sexual metaphors, Sumner insinuated that the aged Senator Andrew P. Butler of South Carolina had taken slavery and, presumably, a slave as his mistress; then he referred to the "loose expectoration" of Butler's speech. That reference to a partial paralysis caused by a stroke prompted the senator's young cousin, Congressman Preston Brooks, to walk into the Senate a few days later and cane Sumner into unconsciousness. Brooks was censured by the House and then resigned only to be triumphantly re-elected, a fact that many Northerners saw as a stinging example of the slaveholders' arrogance. Following the painful attack, Sumner did not return to the Senate for several years, and his empty seat became a focus of antislavery determination. To Northern supporters the senator from Massachusetts was a martyr to Southern barbarism; to Southerners he was an unmanly creature capable of fighting only with words. Southerners saw Brooks as a hero who had defended the honor of his family and the South. No incident showed more clearly how rigid the lines of hatred had become.

The election of 1856. The Pierce Administration had provided the nation with neither tranquility nor stability. Neither South nor North had gained from its domestic or its foreign initiatives and, in terms of morale, the nation had lost severely. Cuba had not been secured (see p. 306) and the effort to get it by sordid negotiations that had a proslavery objective made a mockery of the claim that Americans sought to assist the Cuban people. The Kansas-Nebraska Act had neither strengthened slavery nor impeded it, and, in the process, the concept of popular sovereignty had been degraded into a euphemism for no restriction whatever on slavery. In the gamble to organize Kansas for statehood the Administration had forced the slavery issue into open conflict. Now the country and the Democratic party drifted rudderlessly toward a crucial presidential election.

Only the Republicans faced the future with confidence, for they had made important gains since the congressional elections two years earlier. In New York, where many Whigs had voted for Know-Nothings in 1855, Senator William H. Seward now faced the destruction of his old party and cast his lot with the Republicans. In Ohio, Salmon P. Chase, elected governor in 1855, announced his departure from the Democratic party. He joined the Republicans at the same time as did his old Whig antagonist Benjamin Wade. The two men disliked each other, but they disliked slavery even more. Other important public figures, including the Whig, Abraham Lincoln, were cooperating with the Republicans while still retaining their old party labels. By 1856 most state governments in the North were under the control of political leaders sym-

pathetic to the Republicans. They reflected a growing popular conviction that only the new party could halt the aggressions of the "slave power conspiracy."

Even the Know-Nothing threat to Republican ascendancy disappeared in the February before the presidential elections. At the American party convention one wing withdrew because it was unable to get an antislavery plank included in the platform. Some antislavery Americans later endorsed the Republican candidate, but others, including particularly the Southern wing, supported Millard Fillmore, whom the fading Whigs selected as their presidential candidate.

In February, the Republicans met in Pittsburgh to establish a national organization and, in June, they convened in Philadelphia. The platform, bold and radical, containing quotations from the Declaration of Independence, was, if not abolitionist, nonetheless highly critical of slavery. Strongly free-soil, it denounced the repeal of the Missouri Compromise. The Republicans asserted that Congress had a duty to prohibit slavery—"a relic of barbarism"—in the territories. The platform did not condemn the Kansas territory, or indeed the Midwestern states, for their policy of excluding free blacks, and many Republicans tacitly accepted the view that blacks could not be citizens. They aimed specifically to contain slavery where it already existed and made no effort to attract Southern votes. They condemned the Ostend Manifesto—which asserted that the United States would be justified in taking Cuba by force if Spain refused to sell—as an imperialist design of the Administration to expand slave territory into the Caribbean (see p. 306). Former Whigs in the party applauded the Republican call for internal improvements, particularly for federal aid to the construction of a Pacific railroad.

The Republicans chose John C. Frémont, a popular soldier and explorer as their presidential candidate. Never a nativist, and thoroughly antislavery, the "Pathfinder of the West" had no more political experience than William Henry Harrison and Zachary Taylor had had, but, like them and Washington and Jackson as well, he had a warrior's glamour. Frémont knew how to dramatize himself. Flamboyant and self-assured, he had, as one of his detractors said, every qualification of genius except talent.

The Democrats nominated James Buchanan, one of the architects of the Ostend Manifesto. An amiable but mediocre Pennyslvanian, he enjoyed the inestimable advantage of having been minister to England while troubles in Kansas were ruining the chances of abler men. Recognizing the destructive potential of the slavery question, the Democratic platform denied the authority of Congress to legislate on slavery in the territories and avoided the question of whether the population of a territory could exclude slavery before achieving statehood. The Democrats might well have

Buchanan and his Cabinet

lost to the Republicans had they been more explicit on this latter point, which raised the fine question of just when the people would become sovereign under the Democratic formula of popular sovereignty. Could they constitutionally vote to exclude slavery while still a territory? Or must they wait for statehood? The platform also endorsed the Ostend Manifesto, which voiced a continuing belief that expansion would shore up the declining representation of the slave states in Congress. But more than platform promises, the Democrats offered, once again, the chance to avoid a critical regional confrontation.

Buchanan won the election, becoming the eighth President, consecutively, to serve one term, or less. He received 174 electoral votes against 114 for Frémont. The Whig candidate, Fillmore, won only the 8 votes of Maryland. In the popular vote, however, Buchanan had only 45 percent of the total. Without the South he would have lost the election, for Frémont carried all but five of the free states. Without a single vote from the South, Frémont could have won had he been able to carry Pennsylvania and either New Jersey, Illinois, or Indiana. The Whig voters in those four states had to be won over in the next election. Because the Democrats could neither resolve nor bury the slavery issue, they appeared on the road to extinction like the

Whigs and the Know-Nothings. (They were spared, as it turned out, when the Civil War resolved the problem for them.) The lesson for the Republicans was plain. Next time, with a stronger candidate and, perhaps, a less strong platform, they could win.

The Buchanan cabinet was composed of Democrats who the President hoped could be counted on to hold a safe and steady central position in the intensifying regional struggle. In fact, his advisors had the strongest proslavery bias of any cabinet yet formed. Appointed Secretary of State was Lewis Cass, the presidential candidate in 1848, who had stood against the Wilmot Proviso. He resigned in 1860 when the President refused to promise military support to preserve the Union. Howell Cobb of Georgia was the Secretary of the Treasury. An anti-states-rights Democrat, he had fought moves toward secession as Speaker of the House during the debates over the Compromise of 1850 and had worked resolutely inside Congress and out to silence debate of the inflammatory slavery question. At the head of the War Department was John B. Floyd of Virginia, who resigned in the wake of charges of corruption and of having shipped large supplies of guns from Northern to Southern arsenals in 1860. (During the civil war, Floyd was charged with cowardice as an inept Confederate general.) Jeremiah

Black, first Buchanan's Attorney General and, following Cass' resignation, Secretary of State, was an eccentric lawyer who had taken many anti-abolitionist positions. So, too, had the other members of the Buchanan cabinet. Only as substitutions were made late in the Administration, as Southerners withdrew, were there any members of the cabinet who could be called anti-slavery men. This strong pro-Southern sentiment in the White House was echoed in the Supreme Court, where five of the nine Justices were from slaveholding states.

The House Divided

The Dred Scott decision. During the campaign the Democrats had charged that the Republicans were a sectional party devoted to a single issue: the exclusion of slavery from the territories. Once reelected, the Democrats hoped to deprive their opponents of that issue and save their party. In his inaugural address, James Buchanan referred to a momentous case, then pending before the Justices of the Supreme Court, that would settle the question of slavery in the territories. He urged the public to accept the verdict, whatever it might be, as final. Actually, Buchanan had already been told that Southern Democrats would be pleased with the Supreme Court decision in the case of Dred Scott.

Dred Scott was a black man, once the property of John Emerson, an army doctor who had bought him as a slave in Missouri and had then taken him into Illinois, a free state, and from there into Wisconsin Territory, north of the 36°30' latitude of the Missouri Compromise. Later, he was brought back to Missouri. After Dr. Emerson died, Scott, in 1846, sued in the state courts of Missouri for his freedom, on the grounds that he had lived in free territory. He won his case, but, on appeal to the Missouri Supreme Court, the decision was reversed. Meantime, Mrs. Emerson, who had the use of her first husband's property during her lifetime, remarried, and under Missouri law, the executor of her estate, her brother, John F. A. Sanford, could dispose of her property on behalf of the Emerson's daughter. Sanford was a citizen of New York, which gave Scott's lawyers the right to present his case in the federal courts, because Scott, if free, could claim to be a citizen of a different state than Sanford was.

Thirteen years after Scott's first appeal to the courts, the Supreme Court was ready to rule. The justices faced two central questions. First, did Dred Scott have a right to bring his case into the federal courts? This was another way of asking whether a black per-

Dred Scott: he lost his case

son, either free or slave, could be a citizen of the United States. Free blacks had been denied the right to enter claims to Western lands, and they had often been denied passports to travel abroad. Second, was the Missouri Compromise of 1820 constitutional?

Both questions were politically volatile. The Supreme Court might have avoided them by following the formula already used in the Missouri courts: Scott's residence in free territory had not altered his slave status, based on the contention that he returned

Chief Justice Taney: he rendered the decision

to Missouri voluntarily. Instead, the majority of the justices decided to undertake a broad decision. They did so, in part because they knew that the public had been expecting such a decision since 1850, and in part because three of the justices, two of them antislavery and one proslavery, were determined to get a decision on the Missouri Compromise.

The justices' opinions filled 235 pages, not all of which contributed clarity to an issue of freedom or slavery that had deliberately been allowed to become entangled in complex constitutional questions precisely to avoid a clear resolution of the slavery question. Five concurred in the long, involved, but forceful opinion of Chief Justice Roger B. Taney of Maryland—that became the law of the land—which declared that Scott could not claim the rights of a United States citizen. Black people, Taney pronounced, had been regarded for more than a century before the Constitution was adopted as "beings of an inferior order" with "no rights which any white man was bound to respect." That statement was not good history, as Justice Curtis argued in a brilliant dissent. Curtis pointed out that in four of the original states which ratified the Constitution free blacks had been entitled to vote.

The court might have stopped there and avoided a decision on the constitutionality of the Missouri Compromise, but divisions among the justices forced them to speak on that issue as well. The Fifth Amendment, said Justice Taney, had denied Congress the right to deprive persons of property without due process of law, and therefore the Missouri Compromise prohibiting slavery north of the 36°30' line had violated the Constitution. Slaves were property, and neither Congress nor the territorial governments could deprive citizens of property "without due process of law."

The Supreme Court had only once before declared an act of Congress unconstitutional and had never before interpreted "due process" to involve substantive rights to property. Earlier uses of the phrase had referred to such procedures as the right to trial by jury or the right to examine witnesses. Further, by a slim margin the Court now ruled on a political question, the future of slavery in the territories, which had long divided the parties, the Congress, and the nation. Although the proslavery justices vainly hoped the Dred Scott decision would settle the slavery controversy, their political response to what was, finally, a moral issue of overriding importance only intensified differences about the slavery issue rather than relieving them.

Even mildly antislavery Northerners were outraged by the harshness of Justice Taney's language. Republicans believed that Justice Curtis's powerful dissent had come closer to the truth in pointing out that Congress was given the power to "make all need-

Frederick Douglass

ful rules" for the government of the territories. They observed that most of the Justices were Democrats, four having been appointed by Andrew Jackson, and that the Northern Democrat, Justice Robert C. Grier of Pennsylvania, who sided with the Southern justices, was a political associate of President Buchanan. Many Northerners wondered if the Supreme Court and the President were not conspiring to extend slavery throughout the nation.

Although they had more at stake in all the quarrels than any other group in the country, Afro-Americans had little power with which to effect their outcome. But they were not silent. Black abolitionists in the North, whether freeborn natives of the northern states or former slaves from the South, like Frederick Douglass, spoke powerfully before black, white, and integrated audiences, calling for both the end of slavery in the South and the achievement of the vote and other rights of free citizens in the North. Douglass's newspapers, such as *The North Star*, never faltered either in their excoriation of the slaveholders or their belief that emancipation would one day come. Another black leader and Douglass's one-time editorial collaborator, Martin R. Delany, had grown so disillusioned when his fellow medical students of Harvard had him expelled and when the Fugitive Slave Act became law, that he left the United States for Africa (where he engaged in the scientific surveying of Nigeria) and urged others to do the same. After the Dred Scott decision, many other free black people despaired of their future in America. Delany did not return to this country until the Civil War dramatically reopened the prospect of freedom for his people.

Before that war came, many Democrats had hoped for a Supreme Court decision that would cut the ground from under the Republicans and settle the slavery question for good, but once the decision came it increased tension rather than alleviating it. Buchanan's prior knowledge of Taney's ruling gave credence to Northern fears that the slaveholders were indeed engaged in a conspiracy with men in power. Republicans, having built their party on the proposition that the federal government could block slavery's expansion, were more critical of Buchanan than ever. The decision was an invitation to them to disband, but they responded to it with sharp criticism of both Buchanan and Taney. Many Democrats also found it unsettling. Stephen Douglas quickly saw that the Dred Scott decision had troublesome implications for his proposal of popular sovereignty. The ruling that Congress could not legislate about slavery in the territories reinforced the Kansas-Nebraska Act, which it had sponsored, but the decision also cast doubt on whether a territorial legislature had any more right than Congress to exclude slavery. Many Northerners feared that slavery might be too deeply entrenched by the time a territory got its constitution drawn to be abolished.

Lecompton vs. Topeka. The Supreme Court had cast doubt on the constitutionality of popular sovereignty, while events in Kansas were making popular sovereignty appear ridiculous in practice. Two governments were operating there: the proslavery government, now at Lecompton, which enjoyed legitimacy, and the free-state government at Topeka, which commanded the support of the majority of the settlers. The United States House of Representatives had approved the Topeka constitution, but the Senate would not, claiming that its ratification in Kansas had been irregular.

Soon after his inauguration, President Buchanan sent a fourth governor, Robert J. Walker, to the territory. Buchanan hoped Walker would be able to get a constitution adopted through a fair vote, so that Kansas could be admitted to statehood. A native Pennsylvanian who had moved to Mississippi and had risen in the Democratic party of his adopted state, Walker seemed qualified to bring harmony to the troubled territory. He undoubtedly counted on strong support from Buchanan in his effort.

Walker knew that, although the free-soil settlers were three times more numerous than the proslavery settlers, the real abolitionists among the free-soilers were few. He hoped therefore to get the free-soilers to cooperate with the proslavery faction long enough to establish a legal government. To that end he called a constitutional convention, but when the proslavery legislature planned the election for delegates, the free-soilers refused to participate, claiming that the legislature had divided the voting districts unfairly. Even though they might have won, fraud notwithstanding, the free-soilers would not lend legitimacy to a rigged election. As a result, proslavery delegates dominated the constitutional convention, which met in Lecompton. They drew up a document that attempted to please free-soilers and proslavery voters alike by prohibiting the entry of free blacks into Kansas.

The Lecompton constitution was thoroughly unsatisfactory to the free-soilers. It included a clause confirming the slavery of the three hundred slaves already in Kansas. Voters were given no opportunity to vote for or against that clause in the constitution. Their only option was to vote for or against another clause prohibiting the entry of additional slaves. The people could not vote for or against the general body of the constitution, a limitation that prevented any action to free those slaves already in Kansas. On that account, the free-staters declined to vote, and the Lecompton constitution was overwhelmingly ratified with a clause permitting additional slavery.

Though disappointed, Governor Walker continued his efforts to secure free-soil participation. He persuaded the free-soilers to vote in the elections for the territorial legislature, and they handily won a large majority. The new legislature then called a referendum on the Lecompton constitution for January 4, 1858. This time the proslavery voters refused to participate, and the referendum voters called for the constitution's reform.

Before the referendum, and against Governor Walker's wishes, President Buchanan had already asked Congress to admit Kansas to the Union under the Lecompton constitution. Walker had come east to persuade Buchanan to support him in his efforts to get a constitution acceptable to the majority of Kansas voters. Buchanan, increasingly submissive to the Southerners in his cabinet, refused and Walker resigned. Stephen A. Douglas was as angry with Buchanan as Walker was, for he recognized that the Northern Democrats would not tolerate another capitulation to the Southern wing of the party. Realizing that his own support came from Midwestern Democrats, and that he needed that support for reelection to the Senate, Douglas defied the President and led the opposition in the Senate against the Lecompton constitution. This was a momentous decision for Douglas to take and one that foreshadowed the fundamental division within the Democratic party—and the nation.

Although Douglas lost his struggle in the Senate, the House of Representatives blocked the admission of Kansas under the Lecompton constitution. By a compromise the constitution was then resubmitted to the voters of Kansas. It was again defeated, in August 1858, by a margin of nearly ten to one. The question of admitting Kansas was set aside, but it was clear that once it came into the Union it would be as a free and not a slave state and the South's position would be further eroded. Only after much of the South had seceded did the territory achieve statehood in 1861, with a nonslavery constitution. In the meantime, however, the rupture in the Democratic party had widened.

The Panic of 1857. In retrospect, the slavery issue so dominated the era that it is easy to overlook the major economic crisis begun by the Panic of 1857. Some people who had been rich or comfortable, became poor while a few others, capitalizing on economic shifts, became richer. Many poor people who had had jobs, lost them and were destitute. Many politicians, with no remedies for the situation, chose to discuss the issue in sectional terms. Partisans compared the Northern and Southern economies and thrust blame on the selfishness of the other.

The problem lay not in sectionalism but in the difficulties of financing an underdeveloped country, which the United States was, and supplying unpredictable demands for American agricultural exports which had to be sold on the markets of an internationally capitalist economy. As usual when such a crisis occurred, the weakest link in a chain of overextended credit broke. The failure of the New York branch of the Ohio Life Insurance and Trust Company precipitated the panic, and within months foreclosures, bankruptcies, and unemployment spread through the Northeast. The nation entered a severe depression from which it did not fully recover for over two years. There had been excessive investments in railroads and much real estate speculation. Americans borrowed as never before to cover investments in lands along the lines of railroads yet to be built. Bankruptcies occurred, and the rate of investment turned sharply downward.

International conditions underlay the disaster. Basic to the new economic expansion, and general throughout the industrialized countries of western Europe as well as the United States, was the discovery of rich new deposits of gold in California and Australia. This new wealth facilitated the flow of goods among nations, and America was becoming increasingly tied to international trade. During the 1850s the American West had benefited from the European demand for its agricultural products. The end of the Crimean War in 1856 and the return of Russian exports deflated the wheat market, and Western farmers suffered accordingly. Only the market for cotton held firm.

The South passed through the crisis relatively unscathed, but the commercial and industrialized economy of the Northeast suffered. Aggrieved manufacturers, blaming the lack of protection from cheaper foreign goods for their inability to sell their products, attacked the low tariff supported by Southern politicians. Some, who regarded the revenue-only Tariff of 1857 as the result of a conspiracy, joined the Republican party. Similarly, workers at numerous protest meetings looked past the increasingly capitalistic industrial and commercial economy that was failing to provide them with secure jobs or satisfactory farm income and chose to blame, instead, the slave-holding Southerners. They, too, felt that the "slave-power" had once more sacrificed the nation's well-being to its own sectional interests. Many became Republicans. Responding to those charges Southern leaders boasted that their economy was superior in that it produced cotton, a commodity that Europe had to have, and rested on slavery, a better organization of labor than that of the "wage slaves" of the North, who had no one to provide for their welfare when they were out of work.

Although the panic was relatively brief, it had a large political impact. With Westerners clamoring for homestead legislation to secure financial relief, the Republicans embraced that issue as well as tariff protection, and attracted many laborers, farmers, and manufacturers who were little moved by the question of slavery.

The election of 1858. The Democrats, faced with a congressional election during a depression, tried to dress ranks. It was no use, for President Buchanan and Stephen Douglas had broken irreparably over the Lecompton constitution, and the President had removed Douglas' patronage and purged his followers. Buchanan thought that only stern measures directed at antislavery proponents would convince the South of the devotion of the Democratic party. Though handicapped in his fight to retain his Senate seat, Douglas knew that his constituents in Illinois would tolerate no further surrenders to Southern pressure on the territorial question. In criticizing the handling of the Lecompton constitution as a perversion of popular sovereignty, Douglas believed that he was fighting not only for his own political life but for the survival of the Democratic party, one of the few trans-sectional institutions left in the country. Only on the basis of popular sovereignty could the party survive.

Douglas' challenger for his Senate seat—still filled by vote of the legislature—was Abraham Lincoln, a lawyer from Springfield, who two years before had abandoned a long and loyal attachment to the Whigs to join the Republicans. Lincoln, forty-nine years old, was largely but splendidly self-educated. A man of many moods but great steadiness of character, Lincoln had an air of melancholy that was broken by bursts of rough frontier humor. Though Easterners knew little about him, he was no newcomer to Illinois politics. Lincoln had served a term in Congress during the Mexican War, which he strenuously opposed, and in 1852 he had nearly been elected senator. A superb politician, he could surprise and amuse his audiences with homely analogies drawn from the common experiences of the frontier farmers he knew so well. In a time when politicians sometimes doubled as traveling entertainers, even Lincoln's remarkable appearance, though it amused sophisticates, was an asset. People remembered the tall man—he was 6' 4"— with long, powerful arms, an axe-handler's hands, and a sad, brooding face under a thatch of black hair. He was a singular man and yet one of their own kind, and, most of all, he impressed them with his sincerity and common sense. Abraham Lincoln revered the Declaration of Independence and its principles; he believed in equality of opportunity—"the right to rise"— among whites; and he considered slavery an impediment to that right. He was deeply convinced that slavery should spread no farther. Congress, he believed, had the right and responsibility to prohibit slavery in the territories. Stephen Douglas still spoke for letting the people of each territory decide.

New states, 1858–61

The great debate: Lincoln

I have stated upon former occasions ... what I understand to be the real issue in this controversy between Judge Douglas and myself. On the point of my wanting to make war between the Free and the Slave States, there has been no issue between us. So, too, when he assumes that I am in favor of introducing a perfect social and political equality between the white and black races. These are false issues.... The real issue in this controversy—the one pressing upon every mind—is the sentiment on the part of one class that looks upon the institution of slavery as a wrong, and of another class that does not look upon it as a wrong. The sentiment that contemplates the institution of slavery in this country as a wrong is the sentiment of the Republican party.... They look upon it as being a moral, social, and political wrong; and while they contemplate it as such, they nevertheless have due regard for ... the difficulties of getting rid of it in any satisfactory way and to all the constitutional obligations thrown about it. Yet ... they insist that it should, as far as may be, be treated as a wrong; and one of the methods of treating it as a wrong is to make provision that it shall grow no larger.

From Abraham Lincoln, Speech at Alton, Illinois, October 15, 1858.

The Lincoln-Douglas debates. In 1858, these two politicians, seeking votes in Illinois, conducted a debate that became the nation's most famous seminar on slavery and freedom. At Freeport, Lincoln asked Douglas whether there was any lawful way for the inhabitants of a territory to exclude slavery before achieving statehood. Lincoln was trying to make Douglas state frankly how badly the Dred Scott decision had damaged popular sovereignty. Douglas' answer was not new, but for a presidential aspirant it was hazardous. Douglas pointed out that slavery was by its nature an institution that would dissolve unless protected by a slave code and by local police enforcement. Without these defenses slavery could not, Douglas insisted, last a day or even an hour. Therefore the opponents of slavery in a territory simply had to see to it that every effort to enact a slave code was defeated. This answer satisfied pragmatic Northern Democrats, but it further antagonized the South, already hostile to Douglas because of his stand on the Lecompton constitution. Though he had done no more than state what most thoughtful Southern Democrats knew to be true, especially after the Kansas experience, his stand seemed to render meaningless the South's constitutional triumph in the Dred Scott decision. Even the moral victory the decision represented was sullied. Douglas was saying, after all, that slavery could not be taken anywhere it was not wanted, and his opponents in the South would not forget that he had said it.

In the campaign Lincoln and Douglas outlined their positions on slavery and race with painful frankness. Resorting to racist demagoguery, Douglas attempted to stigmatize Lincoln as an abolitionist in areas where blacks were disliked and distrusted. Denying those charges, Lincoln said he did not believe in social or political equality. He nevertheless held to his belief that slavery was a wrong that should be contained. Throughout their many debates Douglas evinced an insensitivity to the moral issue that slavery had become for an increasing number of Northern voters.

The Republicans won a plurality of the votes in Illinois but the Democrats won a majority in the legislature, which returned Douglas to the Senate. Yet Lincoln had run well, and across the North the Republicans carried enough districts to gain more seats in the House of Representatives than any other party. The election was a rebuke to Buchanan. It left Douglas as the leader of the Northern Democrats, although the Southern Democrats easily retained control of the party caucus in Congress. The depression affected voter attitudes in many areas, especially in Buchanan's home state of Pennsylvania, where only anti-Lecompton Democrats survived. If the Republicans could win the cooperation of a handful of Know-Nothings, they would have a majority in the House.

Most significantly, the contest had established the stature of Abraham Lincoln. He had given the principles of the Republican party their most forceful statement, and he had expressed the people's growing concern over the cost of slavery when he likened the nation to a dwelling and declared: "A house divided against itself cannot stand. I believe this government cannot endure, permanently half *slave* and half *free*." He went on to tell the Republicans at their state convention that he did not "expect the house to *fall*. . . ."

The great debate: Douglas

We ought to extend to the negro race ... all the rights, all the privileges, and all the immunities which they can exercise consistently with the safety of society. Humanity requires that we should give them all these privileges; Christianity commands that we should extend those privileges to them. The question then arises, What are those privileges, and what is the nature and extent of them? My answer is, that that is a question which each State must answer for itself.... If the people of all the States will act on that great principle, and each State mind its own business, attend to its own affairs, take care of its own negroes, and not meddle with its neighbors, then there will be peace between the North and the South, the East and the West, throughout the whole Union.

Why can we not thus have peace?... The moment the North obtained the majority in the House and Senate by the admission of California, and could elect a President without the aid of Southern votes, that moment ambitious Northern men formed a scheme to excite the North against the South, and make the people be governed in their votes by geographical lines, thinking that the North, being the stronger section, would outvote the South, and consequently they, the leaders, would ride into office on a sectional hobby.

From Stephen A. Douglas, Speech at Alton, Illinois, October 15, 1858.

Douglas and Lincoln assumed positions in 1858 from which neither would retreat in 1860 as they faced each other in the contest for the Presidency of the United States.

By that time, severe crises had brought the moral issues raised by slavery into the Northern constituencies and strengthened Lincoln's position that slavery must be contained. Those same crises had made Douglas' position, that slavery concerned only those who had a direct interest in it, seem irrelevant in the South and inadequate in the North.

Personal liberty laws. As the South lost power in Congress, its leaders, as if insisting on a symbolic recompense, demanded the systematic enforcement of the Fugitive Slave Act (see p. 293). When federal law enforcement officials tried to do so in Boston in 1854, members of the black community alerted their white abolitionist allies to the fact that Anthony Burns, a Marylander who had escaped to their city, was in danger. Hearings were underway that were likely to result in Burns being returned to his master. A rally was called and, following passionate speeches by Wendell Phillips and Theodore Parker, a group of men—black and white—moved to the jail and began battering the door with a log, seeking to free Burns. In the struggle a guard was killed and when additional police arrived the would-be rescuers were arrested.

Attempts to buy Burns' freedom were thwarted by the unwillingness of rich (and safe) men to acknowledge the Fugitive Slave Act and to do business with slavery by buying a slave. When Burns was brought to trial, five hundred black Bostonians joined by five hundred black citizens from the strong anti-slavery town of New Bedford patrolled the streets outside the courthouse. Inside, the commission ruled that Burns was still a slave and must be returned to his master. Conducted by state militia and federal infantry troops and marines, Burns was led to a ship and sent back to slavery.

Nothing could have roused Northern antislavery sentiment more effectively than the Anthony Burns case and others like it. Every slave returned under the Fugitive Slave Law aroused more people in the North to the cruelty of slavery. The sight of people being sent back to slavery made visible the evils of the institution which could be ignored when they existed only in a far-off region. Proslavery Southerners and their numerous Northern sympathizers were enraged when citizens helped slaves escape. But even worse in their estimation than these individual actions were the personal liberty laws passed in Northern states to impede the enforcement of the Fugitive Slave Act. By strengthening the rights of alleged slaves to proper legal defense, and by making illegal the use of state and local police and jails to detain them, angry state legislatures made "slave-catching" a difficult business. Ironically, Southern whites, traditional champions of states' rights, charged that the personal liberty laws were unconstitutional. In 1859 the Supreme Court endorsed that view.

Early in 1859 tension mounted higher. A Southern commercial convention meeting in Vicksburg in May called for the reopening of the Atlantic slave trade. If even a handful of Southerners could voice such ideas in the middle of the nineteenth century,

The House Divided **341**

then slavery, many Northerners thought, had driven the South into collective madness.

Heightened Violence

Harper's Ferry. In 1859, John Brown carried his war on slavery into the South. After the Pottawatomie killings and the guerilla fighting in Kansas in the summer of 1856, Brown had escaped authorities and dropped from public view. But he had not been idle. With the help of Gerrit Smith, a wealthy abolitionist from upstate New York, Brown secured the backing of a distinguished group of intellectual and financial leaders in the Boston area who called themselves the "Secret Six." With their help, Brown diverted contributions made for the relief of free-soil Kansas settlers to the purchase of guns and ammunition. On the night of October 16, 1859, he led a band of eighteen men from Maryland into Virginia, where he seized hostages among the citizens and occupied the fire-engine house of the federal arsenal at Harper's Ferry. He held the engine house for two days, in a state of siege, before surrendering to a small force of United States marines sent out from Washington under the command of Colonel Robert E. Lee. With many of his men killed and others wounded, John Brown quietly awaited trial in the Charles Town jail where he resisted all talk of efforts to rescue him and prepared his own defense.

Although Brown explicitly denied the charge at his trial, evidence indicates that he had intended to raise a slave insurrection. Once in Ralph Waldo Emerson's hearing he had stated that he believed in two things, the Bible and the Declaration of Independence and that it would be "better that a whole generation of men, women and children should pass away by a violent death than that a word of either should be violated in this country." Emerson reflected comfortably that the old man must have been speaking "symbolically," but he was wrong. Although Brown was sincere in his friendship for the oppressed slave, his fanaticism best explains his actions from Pottawatomie Creek to Harper's Ferry. Whether or not that fanaticism extended to insanity, as his friends and relatives hoped to show in presenting his defense, their obvious interest in saving Brown from execution cast suspicion on their claim, and Brown himself would have none of that defense.

John Brown knew how to die. From jail in Charles Town his words stirred the souls of many who had previously been impervious to abolitionist arguments. "I am," said Brown in his final appeal to the courts, "yet too young to understand that God is a respecter of persons. I believe that to have interfered

John Brown: martyr

as I have done in behalf of His despised poor, is no wrong, but right." In his captivity Brown was magnanimous and he went to the gallows with dignity. The hangman made him a martyr. The parallels between the crucifixion of Christ and the execution of John Brown were abundant, not least in the conspicuous absence of the Secret Six, who with one exception agreed that Brown could best serve the cause of abolition by dying. In the end John Brown was a better prophet than revolutionary leader. He said on December 2, 1859, the day he died, that "the crimes of this *guilty land: will* never be purged *away;* but with Blood."

Reactions North and South. Although most sober-minded Northerners deplored Brown's actions, white Southerners did not hear their words. Instead, they listened only to the tales of the tolling bells that rang all day as Brown was hanged. Memorial services were held throughout the North as citizens like Henry David Thoreau mourned a man who had tried to free the slaves and who had now become a martyr to the cause of freedom. To most Southerners Brown was worse than a madman who had intended to visit death and destruction upon guilty and innocent alike. He was, they thought, exactly what was to be expected if Republicans came to power. The discovery of maps among his belongings showing likely points of assault deep in the southern Appalachians carried Virginia's fears into the Lower South. Edmund Ruffin, a vociferous Virginia fire-eater, distributed among Southern governors nine hundred captured pikes that Brown had had forged from bowie knives and iron staves. It required no paranoid imaginings to see that those crude but quiet weapons were better designed for midnight assassination than for a frontal assault against firearms. A wave of fear of slave insurrections perhaps greater than that which followed Nat Turner's revolt in 1831 swept the South and it was in this highly charged atmosphere that the election campaign of 1860 was to be conducted. In many communities hysteria vented itself in attacks on persons who held unorthodox opinions on slavery. This outburst of hatred showed that the region deeply distrusted outsiders and that there lurked an abiding fear of what the slaves might do if a realistic possibility of freedom presented itself.

The contest for the Speakership. On the Monday following Brown's execution, Congress convened and set about the routine business of electing a Speaker of the House. This time the task required two months of extravagant recrimination and verbal abuse that was without precedent. By combining with Southern Know-Nothings and Whigs, the Democrats prevented the nomination of the Republican choice, John Sherman of Ohio, but they could not command enough votes to elect a Democrat. The Democrats opposed Sherman because he had endorsed a controversial book about the South and slavery by Hinton Rowan Helper, *Compendium of the Impending Crisis of the South*. Helper was a white man from Northern Carolina who charged that slavery was ruining the nonslaveholders, socially and economically. He likened slaveholding to throwing strychnine into a public well, so dangerous was it to the safety of white people. Though he called for immediate emancipation, Helper was not a friend of the blacks. He feared the Africanization of America and recommended the deportation of the emancipated slaves. His racist book did touch a sensitive Southern problem, the economic impotence of nonslaveholders in a society dominated by the plantation system and by owners of slaves.

Name-calling was not new in Congress, but there was no humor, style, or eloquence in the verbal duels over the Speakership. Radical Southerners, insinuating that people like John Sherman had provoked Harper's Ferry, angrily renewed their threats to secede from the Union. The Republicans sneered at these threats of secession and declared they would no longer be bluffed by such talk. In this charged atmosphere, members of Congress began to carry pistols to the stormy sessions. Never able to garner the votes needed to elect Sherman, the Republicans at last settled for a

man of inferior talents, William Pennington of New Jersey, who had the necessary Know-Nothing support.

In early February 1860, on the day after Pennington became Speaker of the house, Jefferson Davis introduced in the Senate a series of resolutions that defined the position of extreme Southern Democrats. Davis demanded a national slave code for the protection of slave property in the territories and a congressional declaration that personal liberty laws and attacks on slavery were unconstitutional. The Mississippi Senator argued for the resolutions on the floor of the Senate but pressed for their adoption only in the caucus of Democratic senators. His aim was to embarrass Douglas, who opposed the resolutions, and to impose a proslavery orthodoxy on his party as it met to choose a presidential candidate.

The election of 1860. The Democrats who met in Charleston in April were divided even before they arrived. Senator Douglas was the favorite of most of the Northern Democrats. President Buchanan still opposed him, however, and Administration supporters at the convention found allies among the Southern fire-eaters—men like William Lowndes Yancey—who had come to Charleston to find an excuse for secession. For this reason they demanded the impossible: a party platform calling for federal protection of slavery in the territories. Unfortunately for Douglas, the convention took up the platform before nominating a candidate. The majority of the platform committee then brought in a document very like the Davis resolutions that were being debated in the Senate. Since Douglas clearly could not run on such a platform, his supporters had no choice but to fight for the adoption of a minority report. On grounds of principle and politics, they could not recede from the popular sovereignty position. As an Ohio delegate warned, if the majority report was adopted, "you cannot expect one Northern electoral vote, or one sympathizing member of Congress from the free states." Without those the Democrats could not win the Presidency.

After several days of struggle, a compromise was adopted in a vote boycotted by the Southern delegates. After a solemn speech by Yancey in which he detailed Southern grievances, the delegates of the Lower South withdrew. The remaining delegates defeated an effort to nominate Douglas and at last decided to go home and hold another convention in Baltimore in June.

The Republicans, convening in Chicago, seized the opportunity presented by the split among the Democrats. On May 18, to a wild ovation, they nominated Abraham Lincoln, the rail-splitter of Sangamon County. Hannibal Hamlin of Maine was nominated as the vice-presidential candidate. Lincoln held firmly to the basic Republican principle that slavery must be contained. But his nomination rather than that of

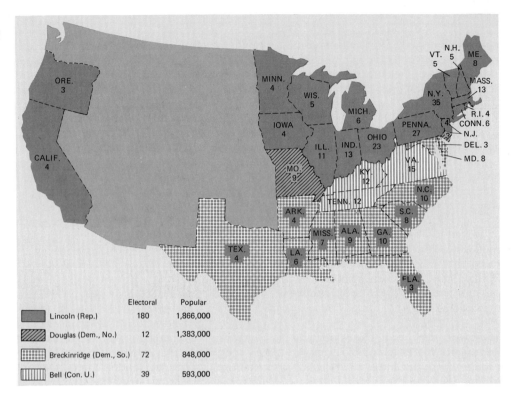

	Electoral	Popular
Lincoln (Rep.)	180	1,866,000
Douglas (Dem., No.)	12	1,383,000
Breckinridge (Dem., So.)	72	848,000
Bell (Con. U.)	39	593,000

William H. Seward represented a victory for the more restrained statement of that principle. As senator, Seward had given wide circulation to his views on the "irrepressible conflict" between slavery and freedom and to his advocacy of a "higher law" than the Constitution. In comparison, Lincoln seemed steadier, safer. He was already popular in the Midwest as well as in Seward's own state of New York. In February Lincoln had come east to speak at Cooper Union in New York City. There he had outlined with powerful simplicity the historical basis for Congress' right to exclude slavery from the territories. "There is a judgment and a feeling against slavery in this nation, which [has] cast at least a million and a half of votes," he said.

To striking workers in New England, he had spoken of the rights of free labor, saying he wished all men could quit work when they wished to quit. Lincoln also had a practical political advantage over Seward. The former governor of New York, who had long fought the Know-Nothings of his state, could not hope to attract members of their American party to the Republicans. Yet their votes were essential to victory, especially in Pennsylvania, a key state lost by the Republicans in 1856.

Lincoln campaigned on a platform broader than Frémont's had been. The platform adhered firmly to the basic Republican policy of containing slavery within the states where it existed, but it affirmed also the belief that it should not be disturbed there. It condemned John Brown's raid. The Republicans also gained by the addition of important economic issues. The Democrats, by frustrating Republican efforts to secure homestead legislation, the Pacific Railroad bill, and an increase in the tariff, had alienated many voters who saw in those measures hope of economic recovery. The Republicans now built those issues into their platform. No longer a "one idea" party, they nevertheless struck Southern Democrats as enemies dangerous to the South and its institutions.

Halfway between the unproductive convention at Charleston and the Republican nomination of Lincoln in Chicago, the Constitutional Union party met in Baltimore. Here was an old party with a new name. Old border-state Whigs, known for their long service to the Union, hoped to head off secession by nominating John Bell of Tennessee, with Edward Everett of Massachusetts as his running mate. The Constitutional Union men declared for "the Constitution of the country, the union of the states, and the enforcement of the laws."

In June, Democrats, also meeting in Baltimore, recognized their peril. They even saw the possibility of Southern secession if the Republicans won. Although Douglas would have withdrawn his candidacy in favor of a compromise, he would not retreat from popular sovereignty as the essential plank in the platform. Most Northern Democrats shared his conviction. The convention fell apart almost immediately over the question of accreditation. Bolters from the Charleston convention came to Baltimore and challenged the credentials of the more moderate delegations their states had sent in their stead. Southern delegates again seceded to a separate convention, and the remaining Democrats nominated Douglas to run with Herschel V. Johnson of Georgia. The Southern Democrats nominated John C. Breckinridge of Kentucky, with Joseph Lane of Oregon as their vice-presidential candidate. They called for federal protection of slavery in the territories.

The stage was set for a fateful four-way contest. Whether the nation would move toward war or peace depended on its outcome. Lincoln did not campaign himself, but the Republicans, capitalizing on their many youthful supporters, organized smart marching bands that demonstrated vigorously throughout the North. The Republicans not only reaffirmed their stand against the extension of slavery into the territories and attacked the vulnerable record of the Democrats for eight years of bickering, corruption, and vacillation, but also placed exceptional emphasis on a series of economic proposals, concentrating in each locality on the issue that would appeal most strongly. Protective tariffs were stressed in manufacturing states; homestead legislation, internal improvements, and a Pacific railroad were advocated farther West, where they were popular. The Republicans also reassured the foreign-born that they were in no danger from a Republican election.

The strongest argument brought against the new party was that a vote for the Republicans was a vote for disunion, that the South would secede if Lincoln was elected. Therefore the Republicans played down the sectional issue, claiming that Southern Democrats were once again crying "wolf" with their threats. Lincoln shared that opinion. Douglas knew better. The only national candidate in the field, he was also the first presidential candidate to undertake a nationwide personal campaign. In the South he urged acceptance of popular sovereignty as the only possible way for the Democrats to save themselves and urged that the South, in spite of its fear of Lincoln, not secede whatever the outcome of the election.

With no support in the South, Republicans were deprived of their claim to be a national party, but their appeal to so broad a spectrum of interest, from capitalist entrepreneur to the rural and industrial working class, established a widely democratic base for the new party. In spite of Douglas' ranging campaign, the election in effect involved two separate contests— Breckinridge against Bell in the South, and Lincoln against Douglas in the North. In the electoral vote that resulted, the Republicans won an overwhelming majority. Concealed by that majority was a profound division of opinion in the country. Taking only 40 percent of the total ballots cast, the Republicans collected 180 electoral votes, as compared with only 12 for

Douglas, 72 for Breckinridge, and 39 for Bell. In the popular vote Douglas had 1,382,713, no disgraceful showing compared with Lincoln's 1,865,593. Southerners knew that those figures rested on the great increase of population the Midwest had experienced since the last census. The election had been decided in the North; the South's electoral votes had been only incidental to the result. With only a third of the total white population in the country, the states of the future Confederacy saw that decisions concerning slavery could now be made without them.

Secession: The Confederate States of America. In retrospect, the formal secession of states from the United States seems almost unavoidable and the process by which it was accomplished orderly rather than revolutionary. The concern for legal form was itself a

CHARLESTON

MERCURY

EXTRA:

Passed unanimously at 1.15 o'clock, P. M., December 20th, 1860.

AN ORDINANCE

To dissolve the Union between the State of South Carolina and other States united with her under the compact entitled "The Constitution of the United States of America."

We, the People of the State of South Carolina, in Convention assembled, do declare and ordain, and it is hereby declared and ordained,

That the Ordinance adopted by us in Convention, on the twenty-third day of May, in the year of our Lord one thousand seven hundred and eighty-eight, whereby the Constitution of the United States of America was ratified, and also, all Acts and parts of Acts of the General Assembly of this State, ratifying amendments of the said Constitution, are hereby repealed; and that the union now subsisting between South Carolina and other States, under the name of "The United States of America," is hereby dissolved.

THE

UNION
IS
DISSOLVED!

tribute to Southern loyalty to the concept that American liberties were guarded by a government of laws rather than of men. Even those Southern leaders most determined to secede did not ride behind a man on horseback. But, when looking at the steps by which the Union was broken, it is essential to be alert to the deep emotion that underlay the process. The South still thought of itself as the heartland of the nation—of the Union. Southerners, persuaded as they were that their enemies in the North not only had sullied that Union but also, with the election of Lincoln, had turned their own country against them, still could view the dissolution of George Washington's United States of America only with great distress. Indeed, the passion they came to feel for the Confederate States of America was in no small measure a transferal of the affection felt for the nation they left behind.

Southern Unionists spoke out eloquently to save that nation, but the electorate in the region as a whole seemed almost to have lost its will to resist the tug toward disunion. When called to the polls to ratify secession, the most important election ever held in the South, fewer men voted than had voted in the recent presidential election. It was as if those who did not vote, did not want to face the consequences of a decision, either way, while those who were more than ready to decide, the advocates of secession, were seasoned politicians. Robert Barnwell Rhett of South Carolina, Robert A. Toombs of Georgia, and William Lowndes Yancey of Alabama seized the initiative and took skillful advantage of the crucial absence of presidential leadership that resulted from the peculiar American system of electing a new president (and repudiating an old one) in November, but not placing him in office until March.

The South Carolina legislature had stayed in session to await the results of the election. Wary of being left out on a limb as they had been when they made gestures of secession in 1832 and 1850, the South Carolinians initially planned their secession convention for January, to allow other states to make the first moves, but extreme voices prevailed. Amid well orchestrated rumors of resignations from the national Congress and references to the spector of Republican rule and John Brown's slave insurrection, the meeting was set for December. On December 20, 1860, South Carolina left the Union and, by February 1, 1861, Mississippi, Florida, Alabama, Georgia, Louisiana, and Texas followed her lead. Delegates of these seceded states soon met at Montgomery, Alabama, and adopted a Constitution, based on that of the United States of America, on February 7, 1861. A new republic, the Confederate States of America, was born.

Failure of compromise. President Buchanan, now a lame duck, refused to recognize secession, but the right of a state to leave the Union seemed sanctioned by political theory that ran back to Jefferson and Madison. Buchanan could not countenance forceable coercion and he urged Congress once again to compromise. Had the nation allowed the lower South to go in peace, the people in the most disadvantaged position—other than the slaves within the seceded states—would have been the slaveholders of the upper South. With the other slaveholding states out of the Union, they would have been in a highly constricted minority position. With the Gulf Coast and Texas gone, there would have been no route for the expansion of slavery into the Caribbean or Mexico and none into the northwest territories either. The slaveholders within the Union would have been exceedingly vulnerable to new efforts by antislavery forces in the North.

Their only hope, short of joining the Confederacy, which in the winter of 1861 a majority did not yet want to do, was to write yet another compromise. Such a document would have to reassure the secessionists that slavery was secure within the Union and allow the departing states to return. Like all the great nineteenth century compromises, this new one could be counted on not to enhance the position of any of the Americans who were black.

The nation had no leader. President Buchanan still had the powers of office with which to assert leadership, but he did not have the temperament for it and his repudiation at the polls limited his moral authority. President-elect Lincoln, had no formal power and he carefully refrained from any public commitments that might suggest an inappropriate anticipation of the responsibility which was to be his only in March. In private, however, he strongly counseled Republicans in Congress, like Representative Charles Francis Adams, to hold firm against further concessions to the slaveholders.

With neither the President nor the President-elect asserting public leadership, the efforts of compromise took place in the Congress. On December 18, two days before South Carolina seceded, John J. Crittenden of Kentucky introduced resolutions in the Senate that would have protected slavery in the territories south of the 36°30' line of the old Missouri Compromise extended westward to the Pacific, and in territory "hereafter acquired." This phrase, hinting strongly of Caribbean acquisitions into which slavery could expand, was the source of many misgivings by men otherwise anxious to compromise. Lincoln objected to it strongly. Also troubling to nonslaveholders in the Senate was the provision for a federal slave code and the repeal of all personal liberty laws. The compromise Crittenden proposed called for a series of constitutional amendments to secure those objects and one other; he asked for an "unamendable" amendment that would guarantee slavery forever. The Republicans stood fast. They were unwilling to return to the Missouri Compromise, which permitted slavery below the line of Missouri's southern border. Although few Republicans really feared that slavery would take root in the arid Southwest, they knew that some Southerners wanted to acquire slave territory in the Caribbean. While maintaining a perilous silence himself, President-elect Lincoln warned his followers privately: "Entertain no proposition for a compromise in regard to the extension of slavery. The instant you do, they have us under again; all our labor is lost, and sooner or later must be done over. . . . Have none of it. The tug has come, and better now than later." In January, from a contrary position, thirty Southern Congressmen, sent a message to the people of their region that "the argument is exhausted." With almost all the members of the deep South delegations leaving their seats and returning to their states, a determined Crittenden, aware that the Congress would not accept his resolutions, proposed as a last resort that they be offered as a referendum to the people of the country. The Republicans prevented that step. The congressional plans to achieve compromise had failed.

In February the Virginia General Assembly took up the effort for compromise by inviting delegates of all the states to Washington to seek a solution. The Peace Conference, at the Willard Hotel, with former President John Tyler in the chair, fared no better than the Congress. Many states boycotted the meeting, including all the Lower South states. In several weeks of discussion the delegates proposed constitutional amendments similar to Crittenden's but they also could not get them adopted by the Congress.

By this time the Confederate government was established in Montgomery, and the Southern states were seizing federal arsenals and forts. In his annual message, President Buchanan had spoken in conciliatory tones of Southern grievances. He denied the right of South Carolina to secede but then disclaimed his own authority to use force to prevent the state from doing so. Though rightly convinced that the secession threats were in earnest, Buchanan erred by delaying to take firm measures. He acted for peaceful ends but inadvertently encouraged the South to believe that secession could be accomplished without war.

Buchanan abruptly changed his course early in the year. When the state-rights Southern members of his Cabinet withdrew, he replaced them with staunch Union men. In his last message to Congress, on January 8, 1861, the President referred to the Union as "a sacred trust" and declared that he would collect federal revenues and protect government property throughout the United States.

One such property was the federal fort at the mouth of the Charleston harbor, Fort Sumter. Its defender, Major Robert Anderson, was already a hero in the North. To the consternation of the South Carolinians, he had moved his small garrison from an undefendable fort to the stronger Fort Sumter and, there, stood in defiance of the Southern fire-eaters, who wanted war. In January, President Buchanan had sent supplies to Anderson on an unarmed merchant ship, but the South Carolinians fired on the "Star of the West" before it entered the harbor, driving it off. Short on provisions, Fort Sumter became a symbol, along with Fort Pickens in Florida, of all that was left of federal authority in the seceded states. What the new President would do was the question uppermost in the North, where anger mounted daily.

Two new Presidents. Jefferson Davis of Mississippi, elected provisional president by the delegates to the Confederate Convention at Montgomery, Alabama, stepped out on the portico of the Alabama capital and was sworn in as President of the Confederate States of America on February 18, 1861. A week later Abraham Lincoln of Illinois arrived in Washington to become the sixteenth President of the United States. The two men, born a year and less than a hundred miles apart in Kentucky, were both products of the frontier experience. Their differences spoke the difference of North from South. Davis's father, taking his family to Mississippi, raised cotton and, when prospering, sent his son to Transylvania University. When financial reverses came, Jefferson transferred to West Point, which was free. Even before becoming a hero in the Mexican War, he had been elected to Congress and in the 1850s was first a Senator, then Secretary of War, and then, again, a Senator.

Tall and handsome, Davis was serious almost to the point of humorlessness, and he would not permit himself any emotional interchange with the men with whom he worked. As did the Lincolns, he and his much younger wife suffered the private anguish of the loss of a child during the public ordeal of the war. The Confederate President was proud of his family, but not sure enough of its aristocratic strength to be able to rely on it easily for self-confidence. Instead he demanded deference from colleagues and took criticism poorly. In his insistence on directing military actions, he provoked quarrels among his generals. He did not grow into greatness as President; instead he grew more and more reserved and remote from people who might have helped him. But in February 1861, the firm, upright Mississippian, well known to his colleagues, had inspired confidence. Introducing him on the Montgomery portico, William Lowndes Yancey said: "The man and the hour have met."

In contrast, Lincoln—having done virtually no campaigning, taken no public positions since the election, and forced to make a secret trip into Washington from Philadelphia to avoid an assassination threat in Baltimore—arrived in his capital an object of newspaper scorn and a man unknown to many people in government. Lincoln's father, poorer than Davis', had not provided for his son, who had to break from his family in order to escape poverty and succeed as a lawyer. Lincoln brought to the White House a confidence few, at first, guessed him to have. A deeply emotional man, he was perfectly in touch with his countrymen, from whom he demanded—and received—great sacrifices. Lincoln did, indeed, grow into greatness as President.

Jefferson Davis's Cabinet was never strong and was subject to constant change. Judah P. Benjamin, Attorney General, Secretary of War, and finally, Secretary of State, was perhaps the most able cabinet mem-

Jefferson Davis

ber, but it is telling that he was but one of six Secretaries of War. Alexander H. Stephens, the Vice President, was soon one of Davis's chief critics. Another weakness was that the states-rights doctrine led Southern governors to be more grudging in their support of the war effort than governors of the Northern states were to be.

Lincoln, in contrast, chose strong men and had far fewer changes in his Cabinet. Those who thought Secretary of State William H. Seward, Secretary of the Treasury Salmon P. Chase, or Secretary of War Simon Cameron—and later Edwin M. Stanton—would dominate the inexperienced President were wrong. Lincoln was soon in command, and he learned at the helm in one of the most difficult crises in American history.

Fort Sumter. On the day after the inauguration, word came from Major Anderson, for the first time, that he had nearly exhausted his supplies and would have to surrender the fort unless supplies reached him within six weeks. Consequently Lincoln found himself with less time for conciliation than he had hoped to have.

The President's new Cabinet gave him advice that reflected the political past of its members. At first only Montgomery Blair, the new Postmaster General, and Secretary of the Treasury Chase favored sending supplies. Former Jacksonian Democrats, they undoubtedly remembered the old General's style of dealing with South Carolina in the nullification crisis (see p. 235). The counselors of caution were headed by Seward, who feared that forceful provisioning of Sumter would push the border states to secession. He had on his own authority promised Confederate commissioners in Washington that the government would not reinforce the garrison. For three weeks Lincoln vacillated. In that time Seward came to stand alone in the Cabinet against the relief of Sumter. He went so far as to suggest that Lincoln put him in charge of managing the crisis, evacuating Sumter, and relieving Fort Pick-

ens—located at Pensacola, Florida—instead, and move toward war with Spain and France to reunite the country in a common cause. Lincoln rejected most of the advice, but he did order additional troops sent to Pickens.

On March 30, Lincoln uneasily made up his mind about Fort Sumter. He allowed word to reach Governor F. W. Pickens of South Carolina that he would try to provision the fort, but that he would send no troops without notice, unless South Carolina attacked first. On April 6, Lincoln sent Pickens an awkward notice that he would supply Sumter "with provisions only." If the shipment was not "resisted," additional arms

The Stars and Bars above Sumter

would not be delivered to the fort. With this message, which the secessionists chose to read as an ultimatum, President Lincoln had shifted the decision to Governor Pickens and, more tellingly, to the President of the Confederacy. In Montgomery, Jefferson Davis met with his Cabinet on April 9 and made up *his* mind. He instructed General P. G. T. Beauregard, in command in Charleston, to ask Major Anderson to state when he would evacuate the fort and, further, to fire if Anderson refused to set a time. Major Anderson replied that he would leave Sumter by noon on April 15, "should I not receive prior to that time controlling instructions from my government or additional supplies." Davis wanted to be sure that Anderson was forced out before federal warships, rumored to be preparing to force their way into the harbor, arrived with supplies—and with their naval guns. At 4:30 on the morning of April 12, the Palmetto Guard of South Carolina opened fire on the fort. Thirty-three hours of bombardment damaged Sumter badly but, oddly, in view of the huge number of casualties in the war that followed, no one was killed during the assault. On April 13, with his ammunition gone, Anderson surrendered. His garrison left Charleston aboard one of the tardy relief ships that arrived in time only to observe the engagement. The Civil War had begun.

Suggestions for Reading

GENERAL

*The Impending Crisis, 1848–1861** (1976) by D. M. Potter is a masterful interpretation of the decade of the 1850s. The notes and excellent (if dated) bibliography in J. G. Randall and D. H. Donald, *The Civil War and Reconstruction* (2nd rev. ed., 1969) will direct readers to specialized studies. Another important and readable study of the period is Allan Nevins, *Ordeal of the Union*, 2 vols. (1947), and its sequel, *The Emergence of Lincoln*, 2 vols. (1950). Also significant for its interpretation of politics is R. F. Nichols, *The Disruption of American Democracy* (1948). Eric Foner has had a penetrating look into Northern ideology in *Free Soil, Free Labor, Free Men** (1970). V. J. Voegeli, *Free But Not Equal: The Midwest and the Negro During the Civil War** (1967), Eugene Berwanger, *The Frontier Against Slavery* (1967), and Saul Sigelschiffer, *The American Conscience* (1973) underscore the antipathy of white people toward black, despite a dislike of slavery. Bertram Wyatt-Brown, *Southern Honor: Ethics and Behavior in the Old South** (1982) is a provocative look at Southern white men whose mastery was coming under increasing pressure in the antebellum period.

On Northern attitudes toward the operation of the Fugitive Slave Act, see S. W. Campbell, *The Slave Catchers** (1970). Eric Foner, cited above, provides the best single analysis of the ideas of the Republican Party, while A. W. Crandall describes its birth and growth in *The Early History of the Republican Party, 1854–1856* (1960). G. G. Van Deusen, *William Henry Seward* (1967), traces the development of Republicanism in New York State; the same is done for Massachusetts in M. B. Duberman, *Charles Francis Adams** (1961), and D. H. Donald, *Charles Sumner and the Coming of the Civil War** (1960). Two important studies of the new party are M. F. Holt, *Forging a Majority: The Formation of the Republican Party in Pittsburgh, 1848–1860* (1969), an area where ethno-cultural factors and local issues appear to have been more important than the slavery issue, and his *The Political Crisis of the 1850's** (1978). J. H. Silbey, *Transformation of American Politics, 1840–1860* (1967), and R. P. Formisano, *The Birth of Mass Political Parties, Michigan, 1827–1861* (1971), emphasize local issues also. For background history of the Republicans in the Free Soil movement, see F. J. Blue, *Free Soilers; Third Party Politics, 1848–54* (1973), and J. G. Rayback, *Free Soil: The Election of 1848* (1970). R. W. Johannsen's excellent biography *Stephen A. Douglas* (1973) supersedes its many predecessors. For a probing treatment of the Lincoln-Douglas debates see D. E. Fehrenbacher, *Prelude to Greatness: Lincoln in the 1850's** (1962). This work, D. H. Donald, *Lincoln Reconsidered** (1956), and the biographies of Lincoln listed at the close of Chapter 14 should be consulted for the election of 1860.

THE KANSAS-NEBRASKA ACT AND THE DRED SCOTT CASE

A major concern of the general works cited above, the Kansas-Nebraska Act, receives special analysis in J. C. Malin, *The Nebraska Question, 1852–1854* (1953), and in a splendid essay, R. F. Nichols, "The Kansas-Nebraska Act: A Century of Historiography," *Mississippi Valley Historical Review*, XLIII, 2 (1956). On the aftermath of the act, P. W. Gates, *Fifty Million Acres: Conflict Over Kansas Land Policy, 1854–1890* (1954), is of major significance, as are two studies of John Brown: J. C. Malin, *John Brown and the Legend of Fifty-Six* (1942), and the essay on that disturbed figure in C. V. Woodward, *The Burden of Southern History** (1960). The best modern biography of Brown is Stephen Oates, *To Purge This Land With Blood** (1970). For the views of black Americans on Brown, see Benjamin Quarles, *Allies for Freedom* (1974). On the *Dred Scott* case see D. E. Fehrenbacher, *The Dred Scott Case* (1978), and Walter Ehrlich, *They Have No Rights: Dred Scott's Struggle for Freedom** (1979).

SECESSION AND THE WAR

Among the many accounts of secession, some of the best are in Potter and in Nevins, cited above; A. O. Craven, *The Growth of Southern Nationalism, 1848–1861* (1953); R. A. Wooster, *The Secession Conventions of the South* (1962); W. L. Barney, *The Road to Secession* (1972); and *The Secessionist Impulse: Alabama and Mississippi in 1860* (1974). Also useful is W. C. Wright, *The Secession Movement in the Middle Atlantic States* (1973). Two older works remain admirable for their scope: D. L. Dumond, *The Secession Movement, 1860–1861* (1931), and U. B. Phillips, *The Course of the South to Secession* (1939). Of special significance is D. M. Potter, *The South and the Sectional Conflict** (1969), the distillation of many years of study by one of the South's great historians. Of equal importance are two volumes of essays by C. V. Woodward, the one cited above, and *American Counterpoint** (1971). Challenging, but important for complete understanding of the political struggle, is T. B. Alexander, *Sectional Stress and Party Strength: A Study of Roll-Call Voting Patterns in the United States House of Representatives 1836–1860* (1967). There are two important and somewhat conflicting analyses of the secession winter of 1860–61 in D. M. Potter, *Lincoln and His Party in the Secession Crisis* (1942), and K. M. Stampp, *And the War Came: The North and the Secession Crisis, 1860–61** (1950). A lively account of Lincoln as President-elect is W. E. Baringer, *A House Dividing* (1945) but, for the Northern side of the story, nothing surpasses J. C. Levenson, ed., *The Letters of Henry Adams, vol. 1, 1858–1868* (1982). On the causes of the Civil War see T. J. Pressly, *Americans Interpret Their Civil War** (1954); K. M. Stampp, ed., *The Causes of the Civil War** (1974); and E. C. Rozwenc, ed., *The Causes of the American Civil War** (1972). On the Fort Sumter confrontation see R. N. Current, *Lincoln and the First Shot** (1963). For a spirited scholarly debate on the secession crisis, G. H. Knoles, ed., *The Crisis of the Union, 1860–1861* (1965), offers good reading.

*Available in paperback edition.

1861-1901

THE NATIONAL EXPERIENCE

Facing the last four decades of the nineteenth century, Americans of 1861 revealed the blindness with which their country moved into the future. Few of them dreamed they were on the brink of one of the bloodiest wars in history. Few expected any war at all. No one had planned it, and neither side had prepared for it. Once it started, both sides assumed it would be over shortly—surely by Christmas. The past was a poor guide to policy, for history suggested that threats of secession were empty bluster and that sectional disputes were always settled by compromise. Until well into the war, efforts at compromise continued along traditional lines, including assurances that slavery would be protected in the South. The abolition of slavery was an afterthought, not an original war aim of the Union. The war itself generated endless innovations, including the ways war was fought.

When the war was over, six hundred thousand men were dead, the 4,000,000 people who had been slaves faced an undefined freedom, and the Union was yet to be reconstructed and a peace made. Again, the future was veiled in obscurity. The Constitution was silent on problems of reconstruction and emancipation, and again history was no guide to policy. Northerners had no experience of wielding the power of victor over vanquished of the the same nationality. Southerners had no experience of defeat and what was required of the defeated. Abject submission struck them as "unAmerican." Slaves had little experience of freedom—of how to assert it, or defend it. Untutored by the past, blind to the future, Yankees, rebels, and freedmen struggled through Reconstruction as they had struggled through the war. Acknowledging the failure of large parts of their program for protecting the ex-slaves' rights, a Republican administration abandoned the enforcement of laws safeguarding citizens and their rights and returned to sectional compromise. This left black Southerners to the care of Southern whites. In the realm of race relations, unfortunately, the past was accepted as a guide. In contrast, in order to industrialize their economy, the dominant whites of the New South looked not to their history but to the example of the North.

After the war Northerners picked up where they had left off. They turned again to such unfinished national business as the expulsion of native Americans from lands white settlers coveted, the industrialization of the economy, and the urbanization of society. In these matters there was little history to guide them, and what there was often proved misleading. The Far West was so little known that even the stupendous Grand Canyon, first sighted by Coronado's men in 1540, had to be rediscovered in 1858 and first explored in 1869. When the pioneers of the New West tried to apply what they had learned in the humid forests of the East, they found that in the arid, treeless new frontier the old frontier tools, weapons, methods, and institutions did not work. What was more, the Indians, who stood in their way, were not prepared to yield.

Like other industrializing societies, America started from an agricultural background. Even the North, where industry had begun to take hold before the war, was still predominantly agricultural and rural. Americans proceeded with frustrating efforts to apply country-bred ideas and institutions to industrial and city-bred problems. The vast numbers of European immigrants who joined them were even more rural in origin and no wiser than the older Americans in the ways of "modernization."

In the politics of the Gilded Age, Americans did turn often to their history for guidance. In some respects they were well served, for their history endowed them with a government of no-longer-questioned legitimacy and with democratic means of changing its leadership and its Constitution. They did change the Constitution to conform in some measure to the results of the war and the ideals that inspired it. But Northerners also changed their politics in reaction against the very crusade they had just fought. Tired of the struggle for a more egalitarian nation, they turned to local loyalties and more material concerns. At the end of the period another generation, believing it was destined to free Cuba, marched into a war that led to the acquisition of overseas colonies on two sides of the world. In approving that policy, Americans consciously departed from tradition.

Historians have sometimes been harsh in judging the late nineteenth century. Yet, as ever, the people of that era did not enjoy the benefits of hindsight when they confronted an uncertain future and embarked on the adventure of shaping it.

14
THE CIVIL WAR

Americans rushed to war. Jubilant Southerners, after years of seething under Northern criticism, heard a signal to act in the cannon fire in the Charleston harbor. Cheering the fall of Fort Sumter, they reached for their guns. All across the region young women serenaded men leaving to join military companies. Far to the north, in Maine, a sober young colonel, facing boisterous farm boys equally eager for excitement, pleaded *"for work in preparation for war, and not a few months of holiday entertainment."* His recruits grew quiet as he told them that the war would be more than a matter of gathering a band of "hurrah boys to frighten and disperse a Southern rabble by bluster; after which to enjoy a quick return to our homes."

The colonel was right. Although he lost an arm, he survived four years of war, but thousands of men who fought with him for the Union and thousands more who fought for the Confederacy did not. As the conflict began, no one knew that more than half a million men would be dead before it was over, nor could anyone foresee its other consequences. The victor emerged as a powerful, modern nation-state, while the vanquished saw their way of life repudiated by the modern world. The war, far in our past now, remains the country's greatest tragedy. It was once common to justify the Civil War by saying that a mature nation was forged in the searing crucible of war, or, to put it

another way, that the United States, having set aside childish things, proved its nationhood and assumed its responsibilities as a world power. More recently, observers have challenged the validity of those images and asked themselves if there had been all that much innocence before the Civil War, or maturity after it.

A claim cannot be accurately made that one side went to war to free slaves held by the other side. But when the war started, one of the most enlightened nations on the globe held four million people in bondage, and when it was over, they were free. Other nations dispensed with anachronistic slave systems without bloodshed on the scale that the United States experienced, but that was a comparison seldom drawn by those who came to measure the Civil War in terms of glory or noble tragedy.

Preparation for War

Two Presidents call for troops. The day after the Fort Sumter surrender, Abraham Lincoln, aware of the inadequacy of the 16,000-man standing army, called up 75,000 militiamen. Men like those in Colonel O. O. Howard's Maine regiment immediately reported for duty from all of the free states as well as from Unionist

Grave at Antietam

areas of the slave states. But if Northerners were enthusiastic about Lincoln's bold action, those controlling Virginia's future were not. Members of a convention that only two weeks earlier had rejected secession, now angrily denounced the call for troops. Virginia seceded, as did Arkansas and North Carolina in May and Tennessee in June. The Union had lost any hope of isolating the Deep South, and the Confederacy had doubled its supply of manpower and more than doubled its manufacturing capacity with the addition of these Upper South states. Soon Jefferson Davis's calls for troops went forth from his new capital, Richmond. Men responded eagerly not only in the eleven states of the Confederacy, but in Maryland, Missouri, Kentucky and the Oklahoma Indian territory.

Opening strategies. The Confederacy counted on the demand for cotton by the flourishing textile industries of Europe to provide the support needed for victory. In 1858 James Henry Hammond of South Carolina had said: "No power on earth dares make war on it. Cotton is King." His Confederate compatriots took his words to heart and built their diplomatic strategy on that commodity. One possibility would have been to sell cotton immediately and aggressively and buy war materiel with the proceeds. Instead, the South withheld cotton from the world market in order to

force textile producers, England, in particular, to respond to a desperate need for the commodity with military assistance for the South. Many thought the war's outcome would depend on the wisdom of this decision.

President Davis had already done more than rely on King Cotton and summon an army to sustain his cause. Immediately after Sumter, he had invited ship captains to sail as privateers to prey on Northern merchant ships. Two days later, President Lincoln ordered a blockade of Southern ports to stop exportation of cotton and importation of war goods. Gideon Welles, his able Secretary of the Navy, directed this attempt to close the South's immense coastline, and his men responded to the challenge. Once the United States Navy recovered from the loss of ten ships scuttled when the federal shipyard at Norfolk, Virginia, was abandoned on April 20, it never faltered. Other ships were built and purchased to produce the beginnings of a modern armor-clad, heavily armed, steam-propelled ocean and river fleet. Despite quarrels among officers and corruption connected with the building and fitting of ships, the Union Navy's quiet confidence stood in sharp contrast to the more flamboyant successes and failures of the Army. Rebel blockade runners succeeded in getting through to some ports, but regular shipments of badly needed supplies from Europe could not be counted on to arrive at Southern ports.

The alignment of states in 1861

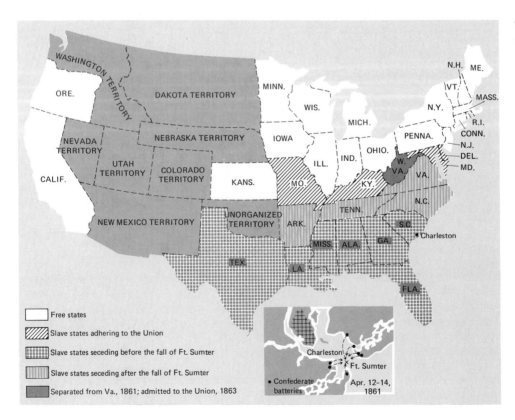

Free states

Slave states adhering to the Union

Slave states seceding before the fall of Ft. Sumter

Slave states seceding after the fall of Ft. Sumter

Separated from Va., 1861; admitted to the Union, 1863

Charleston

Ft. Sumter

Confederate batteries

Apr. 12–14, 1861

The border states. Both Presidents concentrated on gaining the loyalty of the unseceded border states, slaveholding states abutting those that were nonslaveholding. Of these, only Delaware was unequivocally loyal to the Union. Kentucky divided bitterly. Its governor, seeking neutrality, sent troops to neither side, but individual Kentuckians were fiercely partisan. Senator John J. Crittenden, who had tried hard to avoid the war, saw one son go off to the Union forces and another to the Confederate. Maryland was also torn by conflicting loyalties and in the city of Baltimore Union troops reporting to Washington had to pass through taunting, rock-throwing crowds.

The Union could tolerate neither this treatment of volunteers nor the possibility of Maryland's secession, which would make the nation's capital an island within the Confederacy. Lincoln, instituted martial law, sent federal troops to occupy Baltimore, and suspended the writ of habeas corpus, allowing pro-Confederates to be imprisoned without formal charges by a grand jury. In spite of the extreme danger to the

Battle of the Kearsage and Alabama, by Edouard Manet

Major campaigns of the Civil War

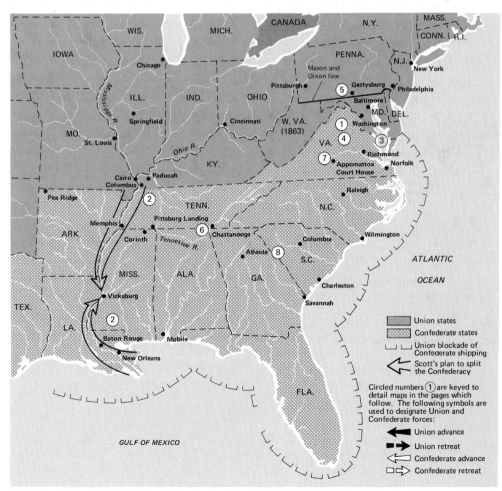

Union, no further authoritarian measures were promulgated. Meeting in Frederick, in the northwest part of the state where Unionism was strong, the Maryland legislature, affirmed its loyalty to the Union and rejected secession.

Unionist sentiment was also strong in the mountain regions of North Carolina, Tennessee, and western Virginia, where there were few slaves. A portion of eastern Tennessee never did acquiesce to that state's secession, and the counties of the western part of Virginia broke with the rest of the state. In 1863, West Virginia was admitted to the Union.

In Missouri, local quarrels exploded into civil war within the state. When Unionist veterans of the struggle in Kansas, called Jayhawkers, attacked people on remote farms whom they believed to be Confederate sympathizers, rebel bands retaliated. Governor Claiborne Jackson tried to lead his state into the Confederacy by seizing the arms in the federal arsenal in St. Louis. But Congressman Francis P. Blair, Jr., and Captain Nathaniel Lyon thwarted this effort by using both regular soldiers and recruited civilians—among them German immigrants—who arrested a contingent of Jackson's militia comprised of men from old Missouri families. Nativism whetted pro-Confederate sentiment as people threw rocks at the soldiers escorting the prisoners. Shooting started and when civilians were killed, many previously neutral Missourians sought formally to take the state into the Confederacy. In June, former Governor Sterling Price, in command of a pro-Confederate army, tried to arrange a truce, but the time for compromise was over. Lyon replied to Price: "This means war."

Bull Run. Soldiers fought in ugly skirmishes in Kentucky and western Virginia as well, but the first major battle was in northern Virginia on July 21, 1861. Union General Irvin McDowell marched twenty-five miles into Virginia to a stream called Bull Run where he met Generals Joseph E. Johnston and P. G. T. Beauregard. Union congressmen arrived with picnic baskets in their carriages to see a fight that they hoped would end the rebellion. Both sides fought hard and, for the first time, Northern soldiers heard the weird wail of the Rebel Yell as determined Southerners successfully counterattacked. Defeated Union soldiers (preceded by the chastened congressmen) hurried back to Washington with the bitter realization that they had been beaten. Confederates celebrated their victory, but Jefferson Davis, also on the battlefield, was disappointed that his generals had not pursued the enemy back into the Union capital.

At Bull Run both sides learned that one short, brisk battle would not end the war. Southern rebels would not yield to a show of force. Their rebellion was conservative. A professional officer corps trained at

① **The first Battle of Bull Run, July 21, 1861**

West Point—men whose loyalties were to their home states and not to the United States—defended an established way of life and fought on their own territory. If the North would not let the seceding states go in peace, it would have to invade, as General McDowell had, terrain familiar to local defenders.

The South's industrial capacity was scarcely 10 percent of the North's, but with such enterprises as Richmond's Tredegar Iron Works (in which slaves labored) it was not insignificant. The product of the new nation's agrarian economy was immense and, with the victory at Bull Run, its confidence was great.

The defeated Union soldiers at Bull Run had been heading for the enemy's capital city when, instead, they were forced to take refuge in their own. Richmond and Washington were close to the boundaries of the regions each sought to rule, but during the balance of 1861, most of the fighting was guerilla warfare in the west, and soon commentators spoke of Eastern and Western theaters of war. A more telling description would show the war to have been one struggle for the capital cities and another for domination over enemy armies and countryside "out west"—which, away from the centers of national politics, was almost anywhere else in the country that men fought in a people's war.

Black civilians. In Missouri, an organized federal army struggled successfully to hold the state in the Union. On August 10, Lyon, attacking Price at Wilson's Bridge, was killed and his men retreated, leaving a large portion of the state in Confederate hands. Union reinforcements were sent to General John C. Frémont, the former presidential candidate who had been summoned from Europe. He established an elaborate headquarters in St. Louis and was soon acting more like the president that he might have been than the army commander that he was.

Frémont was repelled by the spectacle of Union soldiers returning black people who had sought refuge behind Union lines to their masters, and he could think of no more telling way to punish rebels than by depriving them of this valuable property. On August 30, 1861, without consulting Washington, Frémont declared martial law in Missouri and ordered that the property of citizens who took up arms against the United States be confiscated and that "their slaves, if any they have, are hereby declared free men." Reaction was strong among white citizens not only to the prospect of a large number of black people entering a free society but also in response to what seemed a dictatorial attack on the property rights of citizens living in a state that was still in the Union. President Lincoln, fearful of what Frémont's order would do to his support from slaveholding citizens not only in Missouri but also in the other border states, revoked the proclamation. He also began the politically tricky process of easing Frémont out of his command.

Lincoln's repudiation of Frémont's emancipation proclamation was a harsh blow to antislavery advocates, but in the fall of 1861, the Union Navy gave the abolitionists a splendid new opportunity. On November 7, Flag Officer Samuel DuPont seized Port Royal, one of the Sea Islands, a chain of flat, fertile islands lying along the South Carolina and Georgia coasts, which guarded Savannah and Charleston. As Union troops landed, the planters fled to the mainland, abandoning not only the plantations, on which a fine grade of cotton was raised, but also the people who grew it. The slaves who were left behind were apprehensive—with some reason, it turned out—that they might be treated no better by their new Yankee masters than by their old ones. Fortunately, entrepreneurs, who might have sold them back into slavery in Cuba or coerced them into involuntary labor in the cotton fields, were thwarted by a group of "hoe and trowel" abolitionists. These men and women, like the excellent teacher, Laura Towne, taught school and functioned as prototypical social workers, helping the Sea Islanders with the hard work that freedom and self-sufficiency entailed.

Before these promising experiments got underway, the slaves who either had been abandoned or had escaped to Union lines were unclear about their status. In the border states, it was federal policy to return them to their masters, who might or might not be Unionists. But, in May 1861, General Benjamin F. Butler of Massachusetts, in command of the Union enclave at the mouth of Virginia's James River, Fort Monroe, came up with a new approach. Sympathetic to the plight of escaping slaves who were terrified of being returned to their masters and seeing no reason why valuable property should be returned to rebellious slaveholders, Butler declared free slaves in Union custody to be contraband of war. Critics said this new category made black people no different from a bale of cotton or any other seized property, but Butler had

Contraband, 1862

established an intermediate legal status for the former slaves from which, as contrabands, they proceeded to establish themselves as freedmen.

On the Sea Islands, by luck, the general in command, Rufus Saxton, was an enlightened and determined man, also from Massachusetts. He implemented a land policy that enabled the freedmen, working on their own family-size farms, to raise cotton and subsistence crops. When the planters returned after the war, the title to those lands became the center of intense controversy, but while the war continued, so too did the remarkable Port Royal Experiment. The freedmen learned to be independent farmers and Northern observers learned that there was a sensible and unthreatening way for the former slaves to move into a free society.

The Trent Affair. Such domestic readjustments were still remote in 1861 when the United States Navy's aggressiveness precipitated an international crisis that threatened to bring Great Britain into the war on the side of the Confederacy. President Davis had named John Slidell of Louisiana and James Mason of Virginia, commissioners in, respectively, Paris and London. (Lacking diplomatic recognition, Confederate ministers to France and Great Britain would not be received.) The two men had escaped the blockade at Charleston and reached Havana, where Captain Charles Wilkes learned they were to board the British vessel *Trent* for passage to England. When the ship sailed, Wilkes intercepted it and, to the consternation of its captain, removed the two men. Jefferson Davis, initially enraged by Wilkes's action, was delighted to learn that both Prime Minister Lord Palmerston and

Union camp, 1st Connecticut Artillery

Foreign Secretary Lord John Russell, as well as the British press, were incensed. There was talk in London of war against the United States, and troops were sent to Canada.

Many Americans had long thought that Canada should be brought within the United States. Fortunately for the Union, however, neither President Lincoln nor Secretary of War Seward had any appetite for war with Great Britain, even if Canada were to be the prize. With the United States' limited martial resources fully engaged in the war with the South, there was no reason to expect that such a new conflict could have been won. More important for the keeping of the peace, the British, when tempers cooled, did not want war either. Palmerston sent a stiff letter requesting, but not demanding, an apology and providing the Americans with a way out by suggesting that perhaps Wilkes had acted without authority. This fabrication gave Lincoln and Seward the opening they needed. Without formally apologizing, they ordered Mason and Slidell freed and allowed them to continue on their way to Europe.

Battlefields and Emancipation

Strengths South and North. In its first year of existence, the Confederate States of America established a new government and its people elected their provisional president, Jefferson Davis, to an uncontested six-year term as President. The new nation planned an economic and diplomatic strategy for gaining European allies; defeated an invading foe at Bull Run; admitted, although to little practical effect, Missouri and Kentucky into the Confederacy; and organized a determined army. General Beauregard, first at Sumter and then at Bull Run, was aggressive; General Joseph E. Johnston, a seasoned army officer, was in confident command of the army in Virginia, despite ominous quarrels with President Davis; Albert Sidney Johnston, another experienced officer much admired by his President, was in command in the West. There Leonidas Polk, an Episcopalian bishop turned general, was threatening the federally held section of Missouri, as well as southern Illinois and Kentucky, with a thrust northward along the Mississippi River. The Confederacy was on the move even though its most famous soldier, Robert E. Lee, had not yet come to the fore. There was strength south of the Ohio and the Potomac, even though the South's independence was by no means secure.

Polk's bold thrust, so heartening to Confederate morale, was an example of what may have been precisely the wrong strategy for the South to follow. Military experts have suggested that with their limited manpower, the Confederates, rather than putting their immense energy into offensive actions, should have secured their borders and prepared a strong defense. If they had confined themselves exclusively to frustrat-

Confederate camp, Orleans Cadets

ing Northern invasions, they might have broken the Northern will to reunite the Union by force and achieved their independence. The restraint that such a policy would have required was, however, uncongenial to the bold Southern temper.

The North had a strategy too. General Winfield Scott, the able seventy-five-year-old veteran of the War of 1812 and the Mexican War who commanded the Union forces, called for containing the South and dividing it at the Mississippi River. His scheme, soon named the Anaconda Plan, invoked the ugly image of a huge snake choking its prey to suggest that the South should be surrounded and slowly squeezed to death. His successors learned that penetration of the South, rather than encirclement, would be necessary to defeat a determined foe, yet Scott's basic concept proved valid. Unrelenting pressure and not one spectacular battle would accomplish victory for the North, but Scott would not be in command when it was achieved.

Age was held against him, and almost everyone, Lincoln included, hoped a brilliant, aggressive, young general would come forward to put down the rebellion. George B. McClellan seemed to be that man. In the summer of 1861, Lincoln chose the thirty-five year old West Point graduate—turned railroad executive—to train and discipline the large army massed at Washington. McClellan set about his job with great enthusiasm and soon won the affection of his men. In November, partly at his own urging, he was named to replace General Scott, who was sent off to a dignified

retirement at West Point. At the same time, Henry W. Halleck, a West Point scholar of war who also had gone on to a business career, was placed in command at St. Louis, from which Frémont had been removed to a lesser command. Lincoln did not yet know it, but both these able administrators, McClellan and Halleck, were to prove dangerously disappointing as field commanders.

Manpower. The men McClellan was training were part of the largest army in history. From the time of the original call for troops, the overwhelming majority of soldiers in the Union Army, as in the Confederate Army, were volunteers. By the war's end, 2,000,000 men had fought in the North's immense citizens' army; in the South, where statistics were less reliable, somewhere between 600,000 and 1,000,000 men went to war. On both sides, bounties were paid to volunteers. These payments attracted the poor and unemployed and were an added incentive for the thousands of young men who saw in the war a chance for excitement and an escape from the tedium of an often unfulfilling life on the farm or in the factory.

In the Confederacy, men enlisted with even greater eagerness than did their brothers in the North. Eventually, 90 percent of the South's white males of fighting age were at war, while the North never drew on as much as half of all the available men. Despite the many volunteers, both sides were driven to calling up men involuntarily. In the summer of 1862, the

Confederate Congress passed the first conscription act in the nation's history. Initially, white men between eighteen and thirty-five were drafted for three years' service. As the manpower shortage grew acute, all males between seventeen and fifty were subject to the draft. In 1863, the Union Congress also passed conscription legislation. Thousands of men were brought into the war by the draft, but many thousands more, on both sides, volunteered knowing that if they did not, they would be conscripted.

Women at war. Women did not fight the war, but many of them took over the management of families, businesses, and farms. In the South particularly, women bore perhaps the greatest managerial responsibilities they had ever shouldered. In the midst of wartime shortages and a disturbed economy, they ran plantations, disciplined a labor force, met mortgage payments, arranged loans for working-capital, marketed commodities, and secured foodstuffs and supplies for an extensive family of relatives and slaves. Many found the war to be the most compelling experience of their lives. In the North, women were no less fascinated by the awesome excitement of the struggle. "I have always longed to see a war, and now I have my wish," wrote the sometimes more pacific Louisa May Alcott as she went off to work, briefly, in a hospital for wounded men. Julia Ward Howe, determined that the ardor of battle should not cool, wrote the fiercely martial "Battle Hymn of the Republic." Like other intellectuals, she helped move the nation away from its prewar commitment to idealistic, individual betterment toward a more conservative exhaltation of the Union.

Other women found jobs in new occupations. The first "government girls"—447 of them—came to Washington to work as Treasury clerks at respectable wages. The Confederate government also employed women and by the end of the war women were too well established to be dislodged totally from clerical positions in governmental offices. Women also went to work in some one hundred thousand new positions in factories and arsenals. Many new working women were underpaid, particularly seamstresses who received as little as four or five cents for sewing a shirt. Victims of government contractors competing to produce soldiers' clothing at the lowest possible price, they struck in protest. The Working Women's Protective Union, founded in 1864, supported the action and sent a delegation representing ten thousand seam-

Workers at the Watertown Arsenal

New roles for women: in the hospital

stresses to call on Lincoln. The President intervened with the Quartermaster General, but it was too late in the war to produce results.

Clara Barton, the pioneering nurse, claimed the war accelerated women's occupational advances by fifty years. Despite the blood and grime, nursing became a compelling new opportunity for women. Dr. Elizabeth Blackwell, who had already broken a barrier in becoming the first woman in the United States to graduate from medical college, established a training program for women recruits. The South, slower to accept the idea of women nursing men, recognized women nurses officially only in December 1862.

Dr. Blackwell did much important work through the Women's Central Relief Association of New York, an early volunteer organization that helped spur the War Department to organize the United States Sanitary Commission. Men prominent in business and society administered this private agency, which assumed responsibility in the North for the care of the wounded. Working outside the democratic scrutiny

that could have been exercised if the agency had been a public one, the commissioners functioned effectively, but sometimes with greater efficiency than humanity. Another volunteer organization in which women were prominent, the American Freedmen's Aid Commission, helped black refugees from slavery who had been displaced by the war. It sent hundreds of schoolteachers not only to Port Royal, but elsewhere in the South as areas were opened up by the progress of the Union armies. In nearly every walk of life women made strides and were able to maintain certain of their gains after the fighting ceased.

Other women, however, wondered whether the war had any value at all. In the upper South many grieved as husbands, sons, and fathers fought on opposite sides. As men and mules grew scarce, women pulled plows and wrote to their men at the front about broken machinery, poor crops, and shortages of money and food. They were mindful of the price being paid for "the rich man's war."

Fort Donelson and Shiloh. As 1862 began, no battle had yet settled things, but neither had any serious peace-making begun. In February, an invasion of the Confederate heartland by two obscure Union officers, Flag Officer Andrew Hull Foote and General Ulysses S. Grant, broke the stalemate. Foote, a sixty-five year old seasoned naval officer, was a devout New Englander so committed to temperance that he had ended the Navy's grog rations. Grant, thirty-nine, was a West Pointer who after service in the Mexican War had come to detest the peacetime army. Stationed in the remote Pacific northwest away from his family, he grew depressed and drank. Forced to resign from the army, he rejoined his wife in St. Louis and failed as a farmer, woodcutter, and bill collector; at thirty-eight he had to ask his father for a job. He was a clerk in the family's leather business in Galena, Illinois, when the war broke out. All West Point graduates were now in demand to command the hastily raised volunteer regiments, but rumors about Grant's drinking made it difficult for him to get a commission. Finally, when an incompetent colonel was removed, he was given a command and ordered to enter the fighting in Missouri.

Grant took hold immediately. His troops performed willingly for an ordinary man like themselves. Fighting well in the campaign to secure Missouri for the Union, Grant, along with several other colonels, was promoted to the rank of brigadier general and soon given the command at Cairo, Illinois, where the Mississippi and the Ohio rivers join. He and Foote blocked Polk's advance up the Mississippi and, in January 1862, persuaded a reluctant General Halleck to sanction an offensive against two forts built by the Confederates to protect the Kentucky-Tennessee border; Fort Henry on the Tennessee River and Fort Donelson on the Cumberland River.

Foote's gunboats successfully assailed Fort Henry, and Grant's soldiers then marched ten miles to attack Fort Donelson, where Foote's gunboats could not operate effectively. Two of Grant's generals came close to allowing the Confederates to escape, but the Union force rallied and closed in on the rebel defenders. Confederate General Simon Bolivar Buckner, assuming that Grant, an old hiking friend from Mexican War days, would be accommodating, asked for a truce. Grant's reply read simply:

> Sir: Yours of this date proposing armistice and appointment of Commissioners to settle terms of capitulation, is just received. No terms except an unconditional and immediate surrender can be accepted. I propose to move immediately upon your works.

The war had gained a grim new character. Buckner surrendered, and Lincoln was as delighted with the firmness of a general who demanded unconditional surrender as with the first major Union victory.

The victorious momentum was slowed, however, when Halleck, choosing to believe rumors of Grant's drunkenness and jealous of his success, replaced him as commander. Still, General Don Carlos Buell did occupy Nashville in February and a Union government was established in Tennessee. Having been restored to his command in April, Grant moved south along the Tennessee River to continue his penetration of the middle South. As his large advance force made camp, without setting out pickets, in the vicinity of a crossroads church at Shiloh, Generals A. S. Johnston and P. G. T. Beauregard were directing a secret march of Confederate forces from Corinth, Mississippi. On Sunday morning, April 6, 1862, the surprise attack on Grant's front-line commander General William Tecumseh Sherman found soldiers sleeping in their tents.

The grim two-day battle of Shiloh began as two huge armies were soon locked in combat. A snow of peach blossoms fell as gunfire destroyed a ten-acre orchard where resolute Union soldiers, with terrible losses, stemmed the massive Confederate charge long enough to save other fleeing units from destruction.

At day's end the trees were nothing but splinters spiking the sky. The Northerners had experienced the first of many brave but reckless Confederate charges in which men rushed straight into merciless and effective enemy rifle fire. Instead of ballshot, guns were now equipped with cylindrical bullets, called minie balls (after their French inventor), that greatly increased their lethal accuracy. Both officers and men seemed unaware of how much more dangerous frontal assaults now were and Confederate soldiers, letting forth a Rebel Yell, appeared almost eager to make these deadly charges.

On the first day at Shiloh the tactic worked. The Union army had been driven back almost into the river at Pittsburg Landing, but the exhausted Confederate soldiers had lost their commander. General A. S. Johnston, having sent his surgeon to care for Union prisoners, was wounded in the leg and died for want of a tourniquet. Years later Jefferson Davis still mourned him: "I realized our strongest pillar had been broken." Union General Buell arrived that night with reinforcements, and the next day the federal armies counterattacked successfully. Beauregard retreated to Corinth. Grant, whose losses exceeded his foe's, did not pursue. More men—23,741—fell in those two days than had fallen in the Revolutionary War, the War of 1812, and the Mexican War together. Of those, 3,477 were dead. Grant, having seen "an open field . . . so covered with dead that it would have been possible to walk across the clearing, in any direction, without a foot touching the ground," wrote: "At Shiloh I gave up all idea of saving the Union except by complete conquest."

That conquest had to wait, however, despite important Union gains on the Western rivers. In April, Flag Officer David G. Farragut seized the Confederacy's largest port, New Orleans, near the mouth of the Mississippi River. Far upstream, General John Pope captured New Madrid, Missouri, and, midriver, Island 10, permitting the capture of Memphis, Tennessee, in June. On the Tennessee River, gunboats raided as far south and east as Florence in northern Alabama, although the Union mounted no decisive invasion of the central Confederacy. Halleck, taking the field himself, replaced Grant and began a useless grand march on Corinth, an important railroad center. When he reached the town, the Confederates had left and its capture had no result. There was no march on Mobile. Instead, Union attention turned eastward.

The Peninsular Campaign. General McClellan's army, huge and fit, made a splendid appearance as it maneuvered around Washington, but Confederate generals skillfully moved out of its way. Abandoning plans for an assault south toward Richmond, McClellan persuaded President Lincoln to allow him to go down the Potomac and out along the Virginia coast by boat to invade the peninsula formed by the York and James rivers. The object of the Peninsular Campaign was to take Richmond from below.

Once again, gunboats on riverways and in harbors were crucial to the progress of the war. Confederate Secretary of the Navy, Stephen Mallory, alert to the advances in the technology for naval warfare, steampower, rifled ordinance, and shell guns, had the *Merrimack*, one of the warships scuttled at Norfolk, raised,

The *Monitor*
and the *Merrimack*

reconditioned, stripped of its superstructure, armed in four-inch Tredegar iron plate, and renamed the *Virginia*. Nobody had seen anything like this amazing vessel before. She appeared at Hampton Roads on March 8, 1862, and threatened to destroy the Union fleet around Fort Monroe, but the very next day she met her match. The *Monitor*, a Union ironclad designed by a determined and persuasive Swedish-born engineer, John Ericsson, arrived and fought a wearing and indecisive battle with the *Merrimack*. The ships, though not highly maneuverable, pointed the way for naval design. Soon all warships other than ironclads would be obsolete. After the battle, the *Monitor* withdrew and the *Merrimack* remained in the lower James River to assist in the protection of Richmond as McClellan invaded the peninsula below the city. When the Confederates were forced to abandon Norfolk in May, they scuttled the *Merrimack* (as she has continued to be called) to keep her from Northern hands.

McClellan's army had begun its embarkation on March 17. As the troops went ashore at Hampton Roads and slowly started north, Confederate General John B. Magruder, with a far smaller force, maneuvered adroitly in an attempt to frustrate the invasion. The general in command, Joseph E. Johnston, urging Thomas J. "Stonewall" Jackson to keep Union forces busy in the Shenandoah Valley, rushed troops from the Washington area to the peninsula to aid Magruder. Jackson took the hint. The fiery, sternly religious general had moved down into the beautiful Shenandoah Valley to resist invading federal troops. As he drove them back, he turned his valley campaign into an offensive. Learning of an attack on Harper's Ferry, close to Maryland and Pennsylvania, Lincoln ordered General Nathaniel Banks to block Jackson. Fearing a further attack on the capital itself, the President kept General McDowell's troops from leaving to join McClellan.

On the peninsula, the Confederates had been forced from Williamsburg and Yorktown. Union ships, among them the *Monitor*, moved up the James and attacked a Confederate emplacement less than eight miles south of Richmond. Because the strong rebel guns discouraged an invasion of the Confederate capital by water, a land approach seemed both essential and sure of success. During May, Joseph E. Johnston retreated across the Chickahominy—one of the many streams bounded by swamps and thickets that filigree the Virginia tidewater country—to within three miles of Richmond. On May 31, realizing McClellan's force was divided by that same stream, Johnston attacked at Seven Pines (or Fair Oaks), and another confused and murderous battle raged. O. O. Howard, a general now, was wounded in the arm in a fierce encounter; Johnston was also badly wounded.

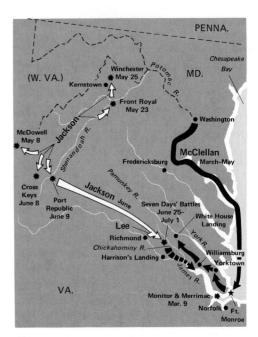

③ **The Peninsular Campaign, 1862**

At the end of the grim day, the two Union corps were intact. During the night reinforcements arrived, and the next day the Confederates were driven back to their original lines.

On June 25 McClellan again started his men toward Richmond, but this time he had to face Robert E. Lee, a handsome fifty-five-year-old aristocrat related by marriage to George Washington. His home was Arlington, the Custis mansion overlooking Washington, D.C., but Lee had left his home state of Virginia to study at West Point and later serve as its superintendent. As a senior officer when the war began, he might well have commanded the Union Army; instead, although tormented by divided loyalties and a prescient awareness of the tragedy that the war would become, he went with Virginia. Initially he held a minor command, but by 1862 he was military advisor to President Davis. With Richmond in grave danger and Johnston wounded, Lee moved onto the field himself. Soon his aggressive, inspiring presence was pacing the Southern defeat of McClellan in the fateful Seven Days' battles.

As McClellan came forward, Lee was ready with his own offensive plan. On June 25, his men crossed the Chickahominy to take Mechanicsville, where a large Union army was poised. Generals A. P. Hill and James Longstreet were to attack in the center, and Jackson, brought east from the valley, was to strike the Union from the left. But Jackson was late, and when Hill attacked without him on June 26, he was repulsed with heavy losses. Undaunted, Lee moved again. The next day, at Gaines Mill, he fought the battle that was decisive in saving the Confederacy and prolonging the

Crossing the Chickahominy, **by Alfred Waud**

war by almost three years. Lee attacked with courage that was matched by recklessness; if he had failed, no sure defense of Richmond would have remained. McClellan's men, under savage fire, held their ground until late in the day when Confederate General John B. Hood—young, tall, blond-bearded, and fearless—led an assault that forced McClellan to retreat. The Confederate assault did not, however, achieve the destruction of the Union army.

On June 28, McClellan's organizational abilities were tested as he strove to move his vast support system—herds of cattle and hundreds of supply wagons—south to the James River, out of Lee's way. He also called, desperately, for help. Although he could scarcely manage the large armies he already had, he complained to Lincoln that it was not his fault he was losing battles but the President's for not sending promised reinforcements. With this plea, he fell into the fatal wartime error of blaming others for his troubles rather than simply facing the realities with which he was confronted. For two more days at Savage's Station and at White Oak Swamp, Lee continued to press McClellan. On July 1, the Union's embattled army turned and fought well, but in the end Lee again rebuffed the attack. McClellan was not the man to take Richmond, but Lee was the man to defend it. Beaten, the Union Army of the Potomac evacuated the peninsula and moved back to Washington.

The wartime economy. Issues other than those of the battlefield commanded attention during even as encompassing a conflict as the Civil War. Before the fighting had started, the Congress in March 1861, as promised in the Republican platform, had returned to protectionism with the Morrill Tariff. In July 1862 and again in June 1864 tariff rates were increased to produce additional income for the war effort and, it was argued, to stimulate production. Economists, however, have found little correlation between tariff rates and goods produced and, surprisingly, the demand for war materiel—for guns and uniforms and rations—did not result in great industrial growth during the 1860s. Many observers since, perhaps in part seeking to justify the Civil War, have assumed that it marked the end of a quiet rural economy and the beginning of a great commercial and industrial expansion. In fact, the opposite proved true. The war interrupted the steady growth in production that the United States experienced throughout the nineteenth century.

The makers of civilian goods converted certain of their factories to the manufacture of war materiel, but only 1 percent of the iron consumed between 1861 and 1865 went into small arms production. From the point of view of economics and tactics, the Civil War can be called the last great pre-industrial war—one fought on foot, or on horseback, with effective rifles, but with artillery that was not sophisticated. But it was also a time of transition into the modern, industrial world. Railroads played a crucial role as tracks torn up by a fleeing army were skillfully reconstructed to supply its pursuers; aerial observations of enemy positions were made from balloons; messages moved along telegraph wires; and photography was employed to inform the public of the war's grim progress. The beginnings of an iron-clad navy also pointed to the future, but with this exception, the war made few technological demands and none that resulted, at the war's end, in major new modes of production. Destruction of many of the South's meager industrial centers did not, as was to happen in Japan and Germany after World War II, pave the way for efficient replacements. Instead, the South was to endure decades of industrial as well as agricultural poverty. In the realm of morale, however, the Civil War anticipated the great wars of the twentieth century by bringing—particularly in the South—not just armies, but the whole of the civilian population into the struggle.

The war had to be paid for, and there was innovation in arranging the necessary financing. In the North, neither tariff levies—the traditional source of federal income—nor increased excise (consumption) taxes, nor even the new income tax—the nation's first—produced sufficient funds. Secretary of the Treasury Salmon P. Chase, a brilliant and flexible politician, found the money the Union needed both by borrowing and by issuing paper currency. To sell government bonds, Chase turned to the private sector; the leading banker in the marketing of the securities was Jay Cooke of Philadelphia. The famous "five-twenties"—bonds paying 6 percent interest and redeemable in not less than five or more than twenty years—accounted for more than 22 percent of the $2,683,000,000 borrowed to pay for the war. In contrast, the income tax yielded only $55,000,000. In addition to the longer term bonds, the government sold short term bonds which, along with newly issued paper currency, comprised 62 percent of its total obligations. Congress declared the new notes, the famous "greenbacks," to be legal tender, which meant that debts—including the government's debts—could be paid with them rather than with gold.

In the North, the demand for goods caused inflation. Wages did not keep pace with prices and money passed from the hands of workers to those of entrepreneurs. Their profits were used for postwar investment, but the result during the war was a drop in real income for workers and people with fixed incomes. The Northern economy was strong enough to keep inflationary excesses in check, but in the South severe shortages of goods drove prices up drastically. The Confederacy issued paper money to keep pace with a demand that could not be met, resulting in uncontrollable inflation. By December 1864, it took more than thirty-four Confederate dollars to buy one dollar in gold. By the war's end the value of money had depreciated so drastically that for decades thereafter there were bitter jokes about worthless Confederate money.

Congressional action. In Washington, congressmen, remembering the Republican promise of free soil, free labor, free men, passed the Homestead Act of May 1862. Citizens or men intending to become citizens who were heads of families could receive 160 acres of undeveloped land. It was expected that these plots would be used for farming and they were not available for attachment for debt. After five years' residence, the farmer was to own his farm at no cost (see p. 444). In July, the Congress passed the Morrill Act, which set apart lands in the states to become the sites or provide the financial base for colleges, many of which stressed agricultural training. Sixty-nine of these land grant colleges were established, many of which later evolved into great universities.

The next winter, with a strong nod to the business community and the need to service the federal debt, Congress passed the National Banking Act of 1863. This legislation created neither a central bank like the old Second Bank of the United States nor one modeled on those of European countries, but it did establish a system of federally chartered banks that increased the role of the Treasury Department in the nation's commerce at the expense of the authority of the state governments.

Emancipation. While these measures of future potential were under consideration, the war was never far from the congressmen's minds. After an embarrassing Union defeat at Ball's Bluff in the fall of 1861, the legislators created the watch-dog Joint Committee on the Conduct of the War. From the start of the conflict the Congress had also concerned itself with the great issue of emancipation. Under the first Confiscation Act of August 1861, designed to punish rebelling Southerners, captured slaves who had been used by their owners actively to support the war effort of the Confederacy were to be set free. In July 1862, after bitter debate, a second Confiscation Act was passed which declared the slaves of all adherents of the rebellion to be free. In practice, these acts achieved little as the United States government had no actual jurisdiction over the rebel slaveholders, but the message for the future was unmistakable. The Southerners who had predicted that the Republicans, urged on by abolitionists, would seek to end slavery were being proven correct.

President Lincoln, committed to winning the war, had avoided the slavery issue. He did not want to lose the support of the war effort that existed among Unionist slaveholders in the border states and anti-black citizens elsewhere in the North. Neither did he want to lose the potential of support for restoration of the Union among slaveholding opponents of secession within the Confederacy itself, but as hope of any such crack in Southern solidarity waned, Lincoln moved

against slavery. When the war was going poorly for the Union in the summer of 1862, the question of emancipation became inescapable. The war's cost in human lives seemed too great to justify as a struggle merely for the political concept of Union. Southerners knew they were fighting to save their unique society, while Northerners could have let the Southern states go without disturbing the pattern of their daily lives. If they were to continue to fight they needed a cause worthy of the sacrifices the President was demanding of them. Frederick Douglass, speaking for other abolitionists, had defined that aim as early as May 1861: "The American people and the Government at Washington may refuse to recognize it for a time; but the 'inexorable logic of events' will force it upon them in the end; that the war as waged in this land is a war for and against slavery."

The inexorable logic was working. Although many Americans, North and South, tried with considerable success not to talk about the issue, most understood that it was the existence of chattel slavery that divided the Union. Many white soldiers, even those prejudiced against black people, thought it inhumane to force slaves to return to their masters and reasoned pragmatically that valuable property was being handed back to the enemy. They had been told they could take the guns, horses, and cotton that came their way; why could they not take the slaves as well. General Butler had been sustained by President Lincoln when he made people desperately seeking freedom "contraband of war." In March 1862, Congress enacted an article of war declaring that no officer could return a runaway slave to his master and passed a bill freeing slaves in the District of Columbia, with compensation awarded former owners. In July, border state politicians, with stunning lack of foresight, rejected Lincoln's offer of compensated emancipation in their region, but by then the President was confident of their loyalty.

Abraham Lincoln, now ready to face the fundamental human questions raised by slavery, told his
cabinet that it was time to declare all slaves within the
rebelling Confederacy to be free. As Union soldiers
captured rebel territory, slavery would end. The cabinet sustained the President in his resolve, but Secretary of State Seward, in light of McClellan's defeat in
the Peninsular Campaign, feared that emancipation
might seem a move of desperation. He urged the President to wait for a victory before making the announcement and Lincoln agreed.

Antietam. This victory, if such it was, came in September. General John Pope, who had been called east
to replace McClellan, had invaded Virginia in August
and lost the second Battle of Bull Run. Now the Confederates took the offensive and invaded Maryland.
By mid-September, Jackson had taken Harper's Ferry,
Virginia, and continued on to Hagerstown, Maryland,
near the Pennsylvania border. Lincoln, fearful not
only for Maryland but for his capital as well, restored
McClellan to command of the Army of the Potomac.
On September 17, McClellan attacked Lee's army
along the Antietam Creek at Sharpsburg. At the close
of a grisly and inconclusive battle, Lee drew back
across the Potomac. The North had its slim victory but
at the cost of more lives than had ever been lost in a
single day. Four thousand men had been killed on the
soil of what Emily Dickinson called "scarlet Maryland."

His confidence restored, Lincoln now moved to
make the purpose of the war match its grim toll. On
September 22, just after Antietam, Lincoln announced
that all slaves held in states or portions of states in
rebellion against the United States would, after January 1, 1863, be "forever free."

The Emancipation Proclamation brought fervor
to the Union's cause at home and did the Confederacy great damage abroad. Members of the strong British antislavery societies were delighted and would
hear no more of any support of the Confederacy. Simi-

larly, European workers applauded and declared the
Union's cause to be a struggle for the release of other
oppressed workers, the slaves. Karl Marx hailed Lincoln, whose lot it was "to lead the country through the
matchless struggle for the rescue of an enchained race
and the reconstruction of a social world." British textile workers, despite economic hardships they were
enduring because of reduced production, were unwilling to press for support of the Confederacy in order to
get the needed cotton. The South's cotton diplomacy
failed in Britain; now with the advent of the Emancipation Proclamation no other European nations could
contemplate an alliance with the Confederacy without flaunting a contempt for recognized standards of
civilized conduct.

Despite this gain of security from European intervention, Lincoln was taking a domestic political risk.
Antietam had blocked one of several Confederate in-

④ **Virginia and Maryland, 1862**

vasion efforts in the fall of 1862, but it was in no way a decisive victory. Many Americans were anxious to have the war over on almost any terms. In exchange for peace, a strong segment of the Democratic Party was ready to return to the status quo that had prevailed before the war, including the existence of slavery.

These Peace Democrats disagreed not only with the War Democrats, who joined the Republicans in the wartime coalition known as the National Union Party, but also with their numerous fellow party members who remained Democrats even as they supported the war. The Peace Democrats, called Copperheads by their opponents, sought in the election of 1862 a repudiation of President Lincoln that would lead to negotiations to end the war. The Democrats made the usual gains of an opposition party in an off-year election, but not enough to dissuade Lincoln from his commitment to emancipation.

One of the hallmarks of Abraham Lincoln's greatness was his capability of growing to meet the imperatives of a moral issue that he had been slow to grasp. The President had once been reluctant to champion the slaves and never was dissuaded from the concept that it would be wise to relocate black Americans in Africa or the Caribbean. He held this view even though these people had been Americans for generations and the United States was their home. Had there been the wherewithal for them to go (and there was not) few would have risked leaving the only security they knew, the sense of home that they had painfully earned as enslaved laborers on plantations. But, despite his insensitive belief in "colonization" of the slaves, Lincoln had come to understand that slavery was a moral wrong that had to be ended. Discouragingly inconclusive news from the battlefields only strengthened his resolve.

In October 1862, Braxton Bragg—a tall, dark-bearded, determined, but quarrelsome Confederate general—invaded Kentucky, only to be halted at Perryville by Buell and a young, new commander, Philip H. Sheridan. Bragg retreated back into eastern Tennessee, but Lincoln had no confidence that another Confederate offensive could not be mounted in the West. This possibility seemed all the more likely when Grant, having invaded northern Mississippi, was, at Christmas, driven back to Memphis.

Meanwhile, in November, Lincoln had again removed McClellan, despite his success at Antietam. Now Ambrose Burnside, another veteran of Antietam, drove south again into Virginia to meet Lee, Jackson, and Longstreet at Fredericksburg. He sent waves of troops up Marye's Heights into certain death, and then sent more—to no avail. Twelve thousand men fell; twelve hundred were known to have been killed, and seventeen hundred were missing and very likely dead. The next day Burnside wanted to attack again, but his commanders dissuaded him. Fredericksburg was as uselessly wasteful of life as any battle in the Republic's history.

Days as tragic as this one drove Abraham Lincoln not into negotiations for peace but into a new determination to make the war worth its terrible costs. He was unflinching in demanding such sacrifices of his people and, as he grieved for the dead, he led his nation into a still greater commitment. On January 1, 1863, he signed the Emancipation Proclamation. The war to save the Union became a war to free the slaves.

The Decisive Campaigns of 1863

Chancellorsville. In the spring of 1863 Lincoln once again exhorted a new general to move south. After Fredericksburg, Burnside had gone the way of Pope and McClellan, and the President turned now to another brash soldier, Joseph Hooker. Leading an immense army through the beautiful Virginia spring to Chancellorsville, the arrogant Massachusetts commander carried with him an extraordinary letter from President Lincoln that read in part:

> I have heard, in such a way as to believe it, of your recently saying that both the Army and Navy and the government needed a dictator. Of course it was not for this, but in spite of it that I have given you the command. Only those generals who gain success can set up dictators. What I now ask of you is military success, and I will risk the dictatorship.

Hooker's aim, skillfully conceived, was to drive Lee back to Richmond. But his immense army of 134,000 did not intimidate Lee, who cooly divided his army of 60,000 men in two parts and attacked. The battle was joined on May 1, 1863, at Chancellorsville, a house at a crossroads in tangled second-growth forest country called the "Wilderness." Hooker had placed his armies well and knew from his observation balloons where Lee's men were. When one Confederate army abandoned the crossroads area, Hooker, instead of attacking, pulled back to build a strong defensive position. Lee had to find a weakness in Hooker's vast line and he did so, but only by boldly risking a further division of his army. He sent Jackson to the left to attack Union General Howard, who was driven back by the assault. Riding back from that action, Jackson was shot by his own men, who presumably mistook him for an enemy scout. He died several days later;

another great Confederate general had been lost on the battlefield.

The only Union attack at Chancellorsville floundered in the almost impenetrable underbrush, and its survivors retreated. Hooker should have driven more of his army forward; instead, Lee attacked with great power. During the fierce assault Hooker seemed unable to control his armies or himself. As he stood irresolutely on the porch of the Chancellorsville house, a shell severely injured him. Unluckily for the Union cause, he did not relinquish command; that night he ordered his armies to fall back along a turnpike north of the crossroads. Two days later, with General George G. Meade's troops conducting a successful rearguard action to prevent Lee from destroying the whole of the Union army, the battered federal troops escaped back across the Rappahannock. President Lincoln had had no need to worry about Hooker earning a dictatorship.

The Battle of Gettysburg. Now Robert E. Lee, who had steadfastly defended the state of Virginia, began a great offensive that might have won the war for the Confederacy. In June, he led his army up the Shenandoah Valley, across Maryland, and into the Cumberland Valley. His men, under Richard S. Ewell, pene-

trated as far as Carlisle and were close to reaching the Pennsylvania capital of Harrisburg. From there Lee could have gone eastward to Philadelphia or made an arc to the southeast which might have encompassed Baltimore and Washington. Hooker, well to Lee's rear, proposed either attacking one of the major components of Lee's army under General A. P. Hill or, more daringly, turning his back on Lee and moving directly on Richmond. Lincoln rejected both proposals and, as Lee neared Harrisburg, he replaced Hooker with General George Gordon Meade, a Philadelphia aristrocrat who was as irascible in his disdain for newspaper reporters as he was able in the management of huge armies. Meade moved north and drew Lee's forces south to meet the threat.

At the town of Gettysburg, on July 1, 1863, Confederate advance forces attacked Union forces under General John F. Reynolds, who was killed. Howard took command and led his men into a strong defensive position on Cemetery Ridge south of the town. Across a narrow valley the Confederates under General Hill brought their artillery onto Seminary Ridge. Late in the afternoon Union General Winfield Scott Hancock arrived to take command and soon a huge Union force had been moved into the area to face Lee's onslaught. On July 2, against the advice of Gen-

⑤ The war in the East, 1863

eral James Longstreet, who urged his commander to force Meade to attack and destroy him as he made an assault, Lee chose to stay on the offensive. He ordered Longstreet to make a flanking attack on the Union forces, while other attacks were made along the federal lines. Longstreet's attack did not begin until four o'clock in the afternoon and a day of fierce fighting ended inconclusively. That evening, Meade held a council of war; after discussing a withdrawal in order to get their badly placed armies in order, his generals elected to remain at Gettysburg and fight.

At one o'clock the next afternoon, under cover of heavy support from Confederate artillery, a division under General George E. Pickett began a frontal assault on the Union position. For a brief moment of intense suspense, observers thought Pickett's Charge would break the Yankee line, but soon the withering Union fire broke the Confederate ranks and desperate survivors fled. Although no one yet knew it, the Confederacy died that afternoon. Lee began a retreat southward back across the Potomac, but to Lincoln's intense disappointment, Meade did not force his exhausted men to pursue him and destroy the Confederate army. Bells rang all across the North on Independence Day to celebrate the grim victory at Gettysburg. The cheers doubled as word came of a second victory at Vicksburg.

The Siege of Vicksburg. While Lee struggled both to protect his capital and to seize his enemy's, Grant had his eye on the seemingly insignificant, pretty little town of Vicksburg on the Mississippi River. A tranquil target for a huge military enterprise, its guns guarded passage of the river, and Union control of that river would split the Confederacy east and west. Such a division—originally General Winfield Scott's plan in 1861—had been Grant's goal since he moved on Forts Henry and Donelson. When he was restored to active command in the fall of 1862, the plan had been for him to move overland toward the town from the east while Sherman went downriver to attack from the south. By the year's end, Confederate troops had frustrated Grant's advance, while, at Chickasaw Bluffs, they also turned Sherman back. All through the winter, Grant and his engineers schemed at ways to get around Vicksburg so they could assault it from the south. Great rains, adroit defensive moves by the Confederates, and the tangled lay of land and water defeated all these efforts.

In April 1863, the final offensive to gain Vicksburg began. The Union Navy had long since secured the Mississippi from the Gulf north to Baton Rouge, and from Louisiana General Nathaniel Banks was ordered to move north to Port Hudson, below Vicksburg. On the night of April 16, Admiral David Porter, in one of the most spectacular actions of the war, took his gunboats south past the blazing Confederate guns on the bluffs of Vicksburg. One vessel was lost and all were damaged, but the flotilla made it through to join Grant's foot soldiers, moving south through the bayou country west of Vicksburg. The Union Army under Grant and Sherman crossed the Mississippi and moved northeast up Big Black River behind the town.

General Joseph E. Johnston, sent to the assistance of Vicksburg's commander, General John C. Pemberton, was poised to attack forty miles due east near Jackson, Mississippi, but a Union force moved on that town and drove Johnston to the north. On May 16, at Champion's Hill, Grant made a major, but unsuccessful, assault on the well-placed Confederate defensive line at the rear of Vicksburg. When other attempts to take the city by assault failed, Grant settled down to starve the townspeople and soldiers into submission. In mid-June, Johnston abandoned hope of rescuing them, and on July 4, 1863, with both civilians and soldiers sick and starving, Pemberton surrendered. Soon the Union Navy patrolled the whole of the Mississippi River. Grant, who caught the public's eye in a way that the austere Meade could not, became the Union's greatest hero.

Draft riots. As the North was celebrating its battlefield victories, ugly riots broke out at the homefront. Under the provisions of the newly enacted draft law, men between twenty and forty-five were subject to conscription, exempting only men in certain occupations and those who were the sole support of dependent families. In addition, one detested feature of the law permitted a man to avoid service by hiring a substitute or by paying a fee of $300 to the government. In July, as the first draft calls went out, poor men and women, many of them immigrants who had hated enforced military duty in Europe, went into the streets of several Northern cities in protest. The target of their anger was not the rich people who could escape going to war, but their black neighbors who were both easily visible scapegoats and emblems of the slavery that had somehow caused the war and hence the draft. In New York an orphanage for black children was burned and at least seventy-four people were killed, some by torture. Hundreds more were beaten before order was restored.

The Gettysburg Address. Abraham Lincoln had the rare quality of being able to lift his countrymen's sights from the ugliest dimensions of the war to the most worthy. In November 1863, he took a train to Gettysburg to dedicate the cemetery where hundreds of soldiers were buried. Travelling there, he wrote on a stray piece of paper the greatest of all American speeches. The brief Gettysburg Address reiterated the fundamental premise of the Declaration of Indepen-

Four score and seven years ago our fathers brought forth on this continent, a new nation, conceived in Liberty, and dedicated to the proposition that all men are created equal.

Now we are engaged in a great civil war, testing whether that nation, or any nation so conceived and so dedicated, can long endure. We are met on a great battle-field of that war. We have come to dedicate a portion of that field, as a final resting place for those who here gave their lives that that nation might live. It is altogether fitting and proper that we should do this.

But, in a larger sense, we can not dedicate—we can not consecrate—we can not hallow—this ground. The brave men, living and dead, who struggled here, have consecrated it, far above our poor power to add or detract. The world will little note, nor long remember what we say here, but it can never forget what they did here. It is for us the living, rather, to be dedicated here to the unfinished work which they who fought here have thus far so nobly advanced. It is rather for us to be here dedicated to the great task remaining before us—that from these honored dead we take increased devotion to that cause for which they gave the last full measure of devotion—that we here highly resolve that these dead shall not have died in vain—that this nation, under God, shall have a new birth of freedom—and that government of the people, by the people, for the people, shall not perish from the earth.

Abraham Lincoln, November 19, 1863.

dence: "All men are created equal," in the context not of a pursuit of happiness, but rather in the course of a tragic war. What was at issue, he claimed, was whether a nation committed to such a proposition could "long endure." "These men shall not have died in vain," he suggested, if a "government of the people, by the people, for the people" were to be sustained.

As Lincoln spoke, it was far from clear that his Republic would endure. In Tennessee, the Confederates seemed to be consolidating their strength so powerfully that the new nation might be able to secure its independence. If the Confederacy could control that state, it could once again drive north into Kentucky and this time, perhaps, reach across the Ohio River. If, on the other hand, the Northerners held Tennessee, they had access to the middle South. But it was not merely a matter of military strategy; the agony of the people of Tennessee was precisely what the war was all about. Cotton planters in the delta and other long-settled families were passionately Confederate, while townsmen from mountainous eastern Tennessee, where there were few slaves, were devoted to the Union. These Unionists, who resented the slave owners and hated the slavery that gave the planters their power, were led by Andrew Johnson. Governor of Tennessee in the 1850s, he was, in 1861, the only senator from a seceding state who did not resign. In March 1862 Lincoln had appointed him military governor of his state.

Chattanooga. Since Shiloh in the spring of 1862, during the Confederates' attempt to invade Kentucky that fall, and on to January 1863 when armies clashed indecisively at Stone's River, the two forces had surged across Tennessee. Time and again, William S. Rosecrans, now the Union's commander in the state, seemed about to defeat the Confederates. But in October, while pursuing Bragg, he himself had been trapped with a large army in Chattanooga, a mountain town in the extreme southeastern corner of the state.

President Lincoln sent Secretary of War Edwin M. Stanton to Louisville to put a man neither had met but both trusted in command in Tennessee. Ulysses S. Grant, arriving from Vicksburg and accepting the new assignment, replaced Rosecrans with stalwart George H. Thomas as commander in Chattanooga and proceeded on to the town. After a painful ride, over a treacherous mountain trail, on horseback—he had injured his leg—Grant arrived on October 23. Without even changing to dry clothes, he listened calmly to the generals' excuses, issued orders regrouping all the armies then in the Western theater of the war, ordered his most trusted lieutenant, General Sherman, to join him, and immediately opened the "cracker line" for desperately needed supplies. On November 23 his well-grouped troops attacked. In the assault, the famous (if militarily unimportant) Battle of Lookout Mountain was waged as Union soldiers, without clear orders but aware of the artillery firing from atop this

(6) Fighting around Chattanooga, 1863

mountain, charged through clouds to take its summit. November 25 brought a successful attack on Missionary Ridge that defeated Bragg and opened the way for the relief of Knoxville to the north and an invasion of Georgia to the southeast.

Chattanooga, even more than Vicksburg or his later Virginia campaign, marked Grant as a man with a comprehensive sense of the surging shifts of a great battle and a vast campaign. Once Chattanooga was won, Lincoln had no doubt about who should direct all of his armies in the final assault on the Confederacy. At his request, the Congress, in March 1864, restored the rank of Lieutenant General, once held by George Washington, and Lincoln appointed Grant to the command of all Union forces.

Fort Pillow. April 12, 1864, was one of the ugliest days of an ugly war. The military importance of the action was small; the reverberations through history immense. A Confederate cavalry division led by General James R. Chalmers, under orders from General Forrest to "attend to" Fort Pillow, attacked that Tennessee post manned by 262 black and 295 white Union soldiers. The Confederates, arriving at dawn, surrounded the fort; during the morning Forrest arrived to take command. The placement of the attackers was skillful and the chances of a successful defense slim.

At midafternoon a surrender ultimatum was issued and, when it was refused, Confederate troops stormed the fort. The survivors surrendered, when, to the cry "Kill the damned niggers!" black prisoners were shot or buried alive and wounded men were burned to death in their tents. Like similar wartime events, from the burning of the Pequot Indians in their village in 1637 to My Lai in 1969, the documented evidence of atrocities at Fort Pillow called forth cries of untruth. But whether in denial of guilt or its acceptance, Fort Pillow has lived with the South ever since.

Black soldiers and sailors. Two-hundred thousand blacks joined the Union Army and Navy. There had been black sailors since the Navy's birth and black Americans had fought in the army in the Revolutionary War and, notably, in the War of 1812, but they had soon been mustered out. Abolitionists who, with some logic, thought that black men should be allowed to participate in a war to end slavery, tried to enroll black soldiers as the Civil War began. Democrats vehemently objected, claiming it would lead to equality of the races. Exactly the point, said some abolitionists of both colors, who pressed harder on Lincoln to allow black men to enlist. One argument for doing so must have struck a sardonic note in the ears of the men most concerned. The abolitionist canon ran that slavery had degraded the enslaved people; if one followed that concept logically, the slaves should have been deprived of the manly virtues required of fighting men. Abolitionists like the self-confident Frederick Douglass urged the army to accept black soldiers who could prove their manhood and their patriotism.

Lincoln initially blocked the enlistment of black troops to appease both Northern conservatives and border-state slaveholders. In the summer of 1862 he permitted limited recruitment. The first two regiments, raised in Massachusetts, were composed of free Northern blacks. At no point was the recruitment effort allowed to look like John Brown's cry to create a slave insurrection and only with the Emancipation Proclamation was the open recruitment of black Americans countenanced. The first regiment recruited from former slaves, the Second South Carolina, with a white abolitionist preacher, Thomas Wentworth Higginson, as its colonel and a handsome, stalwart former slave and future judge, Prince Rivers, as one of its sergeants, was a proud unit. No black officer commanded a regiment, but Martin R. Delany, back in America, (see p. 336) was a major and the senior Afro-American officer in the Union army. There was also discrimination in the matter of compensation; black soldiers were paid $3 a month less than white privates were paid.

Although many black regiments performed menial tasks, some saw combat and those that did acquitted themselves well. The black soldiers comprising the Fifty-fourth Massachusetts attacked Battery Wagner at the entrance to the Charleston harbor in July 1863 in an unsuccessful attempt to take the city. The assault was so fierce that a quarter of the men were killed. One of the dead was the regiment's young white colonel, Robert Gould Shaw. Today these black soldiers, wonderful portraits each, still march into battle at the side of their colonel in the finest artistic expression to derive from the Civil War, Augustus St. Gaudens' great bronze relief on the Boston Common.

The War's End

The Wilderness Campaign. In May 1864 Grant's immense army met Lee's in the same country in which Lee had beaten Hooker a year earlier. In one sense the grisly Battle of the Wilderness scarcely went better than Chancellorsville had. The thicket made madness out of the maneuvers of both armies; friend shot friend, and foes swapped positions at crossroads. The huge numbers of Grant's army proved a liability, not an asset, as the men tried to move along narrow roads and through the dense underbrush. At dusk on May 7 the fighting ceased and wounded men died in anguish in the burning brush. But the next morning, Grant, who had lost 17,666 men, did not hesitate. He moved his battered army not northward in defeat, but forward, to the south.

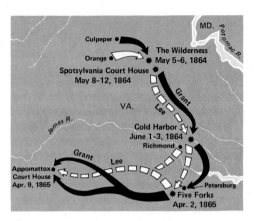

⑦ **Grant's campaign around Richmond, 1864–65**

Reaching Spotsylvania Court House on May 8, the Union troops found Confederates had gotten there first. Although the Southerners later had to yield the town's crossroads, their presence prevented a major breakthrough that might have carried Union soldiers all the way to the Confederate capital. At Spotsylvania, Lee's men hastily erected an excellent defensive line. Time and time again the Union forces fiercely attacked the Confederate defenses only to withdraw when reinforcements were unable to withstand the artillery fire. On May 12, at the terrible Bloody Angle,

Grant and his generals in Virginia

men climbed over the bodies of dead and dying comrades to reach the Confederate emplacement. Still, at no point could Grant break the line sufficiently to get through and defeat Lee.

Grant moved farther south, hoping to force his way through Lee's defensive line at Cold Harbor, but there his efforts were even less successful. Once again wave after wave of troops fell in carnage so terrible that one corps commander refused to make another attack. Those who did walked straight into bullets. Grant now gave up attempting a frontal assault on Lee and moved south of the James River—and Richmond. He skillfully maneuvered the huge army across the river but his assault on Petersburg, a town at a critical rail junction, was not quick enough to be successful. As he entered the Wilderness, Grant had made a famous pledge to "fight it out on this line if it takes all summer." It took all summer—and fall and winter. For ten months the Union army laid siege to Petersburg; for virtually the rest of the war Lee was locked into a defense of his capital.

Grant's command post on the James River, City Point, became the Union's military headquarters. From there he sent Banks on an unsuccessful campaign to take Mobile, Sheridan into the Valley of Virginia to harass Lee from the rear, and Sherman on his March to the Sea. But in the summer of 1864, there were not yet any results to show for these plans. President Lincoln had to face an election campaign with no great prospects of success.

Presidential leadership. The most extraordinary thing about the Union election of 1864 was that it was held. Few governments have risked being overthrown in the midst of a civil war by placing themselves before the electorate. The nation's political habits were strong, however, and the Constitution was essential to the concept of union for which, in part, the war was being fought. The Confederacy had no presidential election campaign, and yet, paradoxically, had a greater need for one than did the Union. Confederate congressional elections in 1863, conducted on a nonpartisan basis, produced a show of unity rather than healthy debate about issues. The new nation, if it were to survive, needed to demonstrate that it could both change and continue. There was reason to ask whether Jefferson Davis was the man to conclude the war successfully and establish a lasting domestic order. No one doubted his unshakable commitment to the cause, but his tireless work in its furtherance produced more confusion than confidence. The "strangely muffled man" retreated from his friends and from the people as the war progressed. He could not find the voice that could define his goals and rally

Union command post, City Point, Virginia

379

the public to him. Depending on his West Point training and experience in both the Mexican War and the War Department, he involved himself in military affairs, where he displayed an almost quixotic obsession with offensive tactics. His efforts led not to single-handed direction of the war but to quarrels with his generals.

Davis's dismissals of Beauregard, Bragg, and Joseph E. Johnston proved more of a discouragement to the war effort than signals of decisive changes of strategy. Robert E. Lee was certainly able, but by deferring to Lee as much as he did, Davis overvalued the Virginia campaigns at the expense of those in northern Mississippi and Tennessee. In the civilian sphere he was even less able to bring forth a strong team to support his leadership. Cabinet members kept coming and going, and he never managed to discredit fully the criticism from his vice president, Alexander H. Stephens. The capital of the Confederacy was in Virginia, but the South's zealously ideological sons had neither the philosophical vision nor the political ability of the founding fathers. These qualities might have emerged, as they had in the Lincoln-Douglas debate, but Davis's six-year single term prevented any similarly searching public discussion of basic issues in the Confederacy.

In the North, Lincoln was subjected to intense criticism. In 1864 he was a controversial incumbent and not yet the immortalized figure that his assassination made him. Legitimate questions were raised about his stewardship in view of not only his deep bouts of depression, but also the long bloody war which he seemed unable to win.

The Democratic party, discredited in some eyes for its inability to preserve the Union, had by no means withered away. It had challenged the Republicans vigorously in the election of 1862, and it remained strongly critical of President Lincoln. The Democrats wanted the war to end, but they differed in their views on how this was to be achieved. One of the Peace Democrats, Clement L. Vallandigham, a congressman from Ohio who had been defeated for reelection in 1862, contended in a speech in 1863 that the war had become a struggle not to free black slaves but to enslave white people. He urged immediate negotiations to achieve peace. Regarding such talk as endangering the war effort, General Burnside, in command of the Department of the Ohio, had Vallandigham courtmartialled. Convicted of aiding the enemy, he was sentenced to close confinement until the war's end, but Lincoln commuted the sentence to banishment. While Vallandingham was in the Confederacy, Peace Democrats, conscious of the issue of infringement of First Amendment rights to free speech, nominated him for governor of Ohio. He was not elected, but when, having made his way to Canada, he reentered the North, he was allowed to move freely. Many Democrats shared his views that a peace should be negotiated while others, including congressmen who had entered the war as generals, urged a more strenuous commitment to winning the war than they saw Lincoln providing.

The President faced criticism of this latter kind even within his own party. In 1863 Secretary of the Treasury Salmon P. Chase, using his considerable charm and the patronage available to him as the seller of government bonds, attempted to win support for the presidential nomination, but he overplayed his hand. His inept supporters soon made Chase appear to be a spoiler who diminished the war effort instead of a desirable alternative to Lincoln. He resigned from the cabinet and was replaced as Secretary of the Treasury by William Pitt Fessenden of Maine. The President's opponents, including abolitionist Wendell Phillips, called a convention of radicals in May 1864 which nominated General Frémont, but his candidacy never achieved recognition by party regulars. At the Republican Convention in Baltimore in June 1864, in the midst of the inconclusive Wilderness Campaign with its appalling casualties, Lincoln's renomination was unanimous, save for the Missouri delegation's protest vote for General Grant.

Lincoln and Andrew Johnson, the War Democrat from Tennessee who was the vice-presidential candidate, ran on a National Union ticket in order to command the votes of both Republicans and Unionists among the Democrats. Their platform committed the party to the indivisibility of the Union, the defeat of the rebellion, the avoidance of any compromise with the Confederacy, and a Constitutional amendment to end slavery. Despite this strong stance, Lincoln still faced opposition within his own party that focused on the issue of Reconstruction.

Lincoln was committed to emancipation, but he had no plan to establish a new social order for the freedmen. He knew of the family-farm experiments at Port Royal and of the various wage-labor schemes of Northern entrepreneurs who were raising cotton in the Mississippi delta. There, Chaplain John Eaton had been placed in charge of refugees who lived in destitution in displaced person camps. With the assistance of the Freedmen's Aid Societies, Eaton tried to ward off those who thought involuntary labor schemes were the only way to discipline the freedmen and make them productive while they earned their subsistence. At some point the President would have to take a stand on these choices facing the freedmen.

Lincoln, the old Whig, was enough of a believer in the "thinking people" to hope that white Unionists in the reconquered states would, in addition to solving the freedmen's problems, also return the Southern states to the Union. In December 1863, he announced a "Proclamation of Amnesty on Reconstruction" and promised full pardon and return of property, save for the return of slaves, to any rebel who would repudiate rebellion by pledging allegiance to the United States. Any state in which as many as 10 percent of the people took such a pledge could establish a government and receive recognition. The document contemplated emancipation, but it did not block a forced-labor substitute for slavery; it would ensure only a government loyal to the nation. Tennessee already had a Union government, and others were established in occupied Louisiana and Arkansas. In Louisiana, the black population immediately began pressing for the right to vote and the new state constitution of 1864 permitted the legislature to grant it.

To ensure that emancipation would be accomplished, the Senate, in April 1864, voted for the Thirteenth Amendment, which would end slavery everywhere in the nation. (Not until after the election did the House act on the measure and send it to states for ratification.) In July, Radicals concerned with the safety and well-being of the freedmen and with what they saw to be treason of the secessionists, successfully advocated the Wade-Davis bill. It called for reentry of states only when 50 percent of the citizens had signed an "iron-clad oath" stating that they had never voluntarily supported the Confederacy. The legislation sought to safeguard the freedmen by making their rights enforceable in federal courts, but it did not call for votes for black men. Lincoln, by not signing the bill as Congress recessed, gave it a veto that could not be overridden by the absent congressmen. The President did not want to disrupt the governments in Tennessee, Arkansas, and Louisiana. He hoped the border states would vote their own emancipation, and in general, he wanted no talk of punishment to discourage Southerners or border-state citizens from regaining a loyal relationship to the Union.

Radicals were furious with Lincoln. With the war going poorly, there was even talk of getting the President to step aside for another candidate. In August, Lincoln was so pessimistic that he alerted his cabinet to the need to work with the as yet unnominated "President-elect to save the Union between the election and the inauguration; as he will have secured his election on such ground that he cannot possibly save it afterwards."

Victories and the election of 1864. Military success saved Lincoln's election—and the Union. William Tecumseh Sherman, spare and restless, with sandy-red hair and a wiry beard, was a brilliant, caustic man. He had entered north Georgia at the start of May 1864 to meet Joseph Johnston, who, after Chattanooga, had replaced Bragg. Grant ordered Sherman to "move against Johnston's army, to break it up and to get into the interior of the enemy's country as far as you can, inflicting all the damage you can against their war resources . . . " In May, Johnston fell back toward Atlanta. The armies skirted each other and fought inconclusive engagements. Some, like Sherman's assault on Kenesaw Mountain, resulted in bloody rebuffs. The rain and mud halted him in June, but on July 8, the first Union soldiers crossed the Chattahoochee River and were at Atlanta's door. On July 17, Jefferson Davis, exasperated by Johnston's retreats, replaced him with General John B. Hood. By July 18, all of Sherman's troops were across the river and ready for battle. At Peachtree Creek, north of town and at the city limits, the Confederacy fought fiercely in Atlanta's defense. Ladies in the city, thinking Hood successful, planned a victory ball, only to see him abandon the town on September 1 when he realized he was in danger of being encircled and trapped. Sherman had not destroyed the Confederate army, but he had taken a great prize.

The Union celebrated the victory at Atlanta less than a week after the Democratic Convention had adopted a platform calling for a negotiated peace. The confused party had, at the same time, nominated a frustrated but still glamorous warrior, George B. McClellan, as its presidential candidate. George H. Pendleton was chosen to run for the vice-presidency. In his acceptance speech, McClellan refused to be bound by the platform calling for an immediate end to hostilities without a guarantee that the Union would be preserved. Instead, as a foe of emancipation, McClellan indicated that he would fight on until the South abandoned independence as a goal. If the South then asked for peace, he would not make emancipation a condition to be met: "The Union is the one condition of peace," he declared. "We ask no more." McClellan campaigned vigorously and, despite Union victories at Atlanta and Mobile, one of the last of the Confederate ports, which had been taken by Farragut in August, might have succeeded if it had not been for General Philip H. Sheridan.

Earlier in the summer of 1864 Confederate cavalry under General Jubal Early rode out of Virginia, through Maryland, and turned toward Washington. The politicians in the capital were frightened; desk soldiers and civilians armed to defend the city and Grant sent a corps from City Point to join them. On July 11 Early entered Silver Springs, just beyond the city, but the arrival of the City Point reinforcements deterred him from entering the capital. No Union commander had been able to deal successfully with the Confederate cavalry troops who ranged threateningly out of the valleys of western Virginia. Now Grant sent one of his ablest soldiers to "make the Shenandoah Valley . . . a barren waste."

Philip Sheridan was young, small, black-eyed, immensely self-confident—and able. His temper had

Lincoln's second inaugural address

... The Almighty has His own purposes. "Woe unto the world because of offences! for it must needs be that offences come; but woe to that man by whom the offence cometh!" If we shall suppose that American Slavery is one of those offences which, in the providence of God, must needs come, but which, having continued through His appointed time, He now wills to remove, and that He gives to both North and South, this terrible war, as the woe due to those by whom the offence came, shall we discern therein any departure from those divine attributes which the believers in a Living God always ascribe to Him? Fondly do we hope—fervently do we pray—that this mighty scourge of war may speedily pass away. Yet, if God wills that it continue, until all the wealth piled by the bond-man's two hundred and fifty years of unrequited toil shall be sunk, and until every drop of blood drawn with the lash, shall be paid by another drawn with the sword, as was said three thousand years ago, so still it must be said "the judgments of the Lord, are true and righteous altogether."

With malice toward none; with charity for all; with firmness in the right, as God gives us to see the right, let us strive on to finish the work we are in; to bind up the nation's wounds; to care for him who shall have borne the battle, and for his widow, and his orphan—to do all which may achieve and cherish a just, and a lasting peace, among ourselves, and with all nations.

From Abraham Lincoln, Inaugural Address, March 4, 1865.

made him unpopular in the regular army, and many doubted the wisdom of giving him this independent command. But his fierce energy was contagious: his men fought for him. With Early as an opponent, they had plenty of fighting to do. Sheridan beat Early at Winchester, although not decisively, and moved south into the beautiful Shenandoah Valley with instructions that "nothing should be left to invite the enemy to return. Take all provisions, forage, and stock wanted for use of your command; such as cannot be consumed, destroy." In just one phase of his campaign, Sheridan's men burned two thousand barns filled with grain desperately needed by Lee's armies and drove off or slaughtered seven thousand animals. Sheridan boasted that when he was through the ninety-mile-long valley would have "little in it for man or beast." War had been taken to the civilians, and Virginians never forgot it. When Sheridan, after a spectacular ride, rallied fleeing men and defeated Early at Cedar Creek, Lincoln had the victory to assure his reelection.

On November 6, 1864, voters in the North, including many soldiers who voted in the field, gave Abraham Lincoln a plurality of 494,567 votes out of more than 4,000,000 cast. McClellan carried only Delaware, Kentucky, and his home state of New Jersey; he almost took New York. When far into the night the returns came in, the President, responding to a serenade, stated that the victory given his administration might be "the very salvation of the country."

Shortly before the election, in October 1864, Chief Justice Roger Taney, the gaunt relic of Jacksonian days and author of the discredited Dred Scott decision, died. To replace him, President Lincoln appointed former Treasury Secretary Salmon P. Chase, his recent rival for the presidential nomination and an early advocate of black enfranchisement and other civil rights. Lincoln had already appointed four justices: Noah Swayne, from Virginia and later Ohio where his wife had freed her slaves; Samuel F. Miller of Iowa; David Davis from Illinois; and Stephen J. Field, the court's first justice from California. With Chase, they comprised a majority and gave the court a new, less Southern cast. In 1864, in *ex parte Vallandigham*, the justices upheld the government's right to arrest civilians if military considerations required it.

The March to the Sea. A week after the election, Sherman burned Atlanta and began his famous March to the Sea. Georgians were in for the treatment the farmers of the Shenandoah Valley had experienced. There was no mass slaughter of civilians, although there were poignant examples of capricious cruelty. The devastation of farms did significant damage to Confederate morale. Other commanders killed more Southerners than Sherman did, yet Southerners hated no Union commander as they hated him.

Two vast armies moved: on one side, the Army of the Tennessee, now under General Howard; on the other, the new Army of Georgia, under General

Ruins of Atlanta roundhouse

Henry W. Slocum, with which Sherman rode. Howard, the "Christian General," tried to stop some of the worst abuses, but his commander, whose concept of total war anticipated those held by twentieth century warriors, declared, "I can make the march, and I can make Georgia howl."

While Sherman moved toward the sea, the Confederacy began one last, desperate offensive led by John Bell Hood. The Confederate general's left arm had been crippled at Gettysburg and only a stump remained of his right leg after an amputation at Chickamauga. But strapped in the saddle, he set off to retake Tennessee and his native Kentucky. At Franklin, Tennessee, on November 30, 1864, Hood's men attacked

⑧ **Sherman's Drive, 1864–65**

with extraordinary bravery, rushing straight into the murderous bullets of the defending Union soldiers. All afternoon and well into the night Hood futilely tried to break the Union's hold. Late that night the Northerners fell back to Nashville.

There, George H. Thomas, in command of the Army of the Cumberland, took direct command of the army facing Hood. So successful were Confederate cavalry raids and so slow was Thomas in counterattacking that the usually calm Grant was alarmed. On December 6 he ordered Thomas to attack Hood at once. When Thomas did not do so, Grant was ready to replace him. Thomas knew this, but he would not order an attack when weather conditions were so bad that he did not think he could win. On December 15, when Grant was in Washington preparing to go to Nashville himself, Thomas finally did move. His force was more than twice the size of Hood's and he planned his attack well. Hood, defeated, led the remnants of his brave army to northern Mississippi and resigned his command. The last great Confederate offensive had been broken.

With Hood in the West, General William J. Hardee, with only 13,000 soldiers, had been left to the hopeless task of stopping Sherman's 57,000 men. Reaching the coast, Sherman ordered siege guns for an assault on Savannah, but Hardee evacuated the city on December 21. After Christmas, Sherman moved out onto the Sea Islands to prepare for an attack on Charleston, which fell on February 18, 1865. Wilmington, North Carolina, was now the only major port open to the Confederacy.

The war had to end. Union soldiers had destroyed two-thirds of the South's industrial assets. Half of the region's farm tools and untold numbers of animals were gone. A quarter of the South's young white male adult population was dead. Anyone in the Confederacy could see that there was no longer any hope, but surprisingly few Southerners would face the fact. They had seceded from the United States to preserve a way of life they cherished as paternal and humane. Sustaining that secession with a hideously painful war had only strengthened their resolve. Somehow, even after Hood had failed, loyal Confederates chose to believe that Robert E. Lee, still gallantly on guard with the stalwart Jefferson Davis in Richmond, would prevail. In January, Davis put Lee in command of all Confederate armies.

As 1865 began, Sherman set out to treat the Carolinas as he had Georgia. In fifty days his 80,000 men marched 425 miles. Columbia, South Carolina, was burned on February 17; in April, Sherman's army, paced by Confederates once again under the command of Joseph E. Johnston, stood outside the North Carolina capital of Raleigh.

Five Forks.   The war's last great battle took place not in North Carolina, but, like the first, in Virginia. On

Robert E. Lee

Lincoln: "with malice toward none"

March 29 Sheridan, the Shenandoah behind him, sought to give Lee the fatal blow. He moved behind Petersburg which, though still under siege, had never been surrounded. Lee and Pickett, with gallant indifference to the fortunes of war, were at a shadbake when the action began on April 1. They rode through infantry fire to lead the futile attempt to hold off Sheridan. Pickett's men, singing "Annie Laurie," were digging in to resist Sheridan's dismounted cavalry, but there were too few of them to stop the furious assault when it came. Sheridan took Five Forks, Petersburg was cut off, and the supply line to Richmond closed. The day after the battle, Grant ordered an assault on Petersburg. One last time the town's defenders fought bravely to hold it, but now the Union soldiers broke through. Lee knew he could no longer defend Richmond. President Davis and his government fled while Lee's troops moved southwest along the Appomattox River.

Appomattox.   Sheridan was soon in pursuit. On April 6, seven thousand Confederates surrendered. Two days later, Union forces captured two trains carrying desperately needed rations. Now Lee knew he could no longer keep the Confederate Army in the field. On April 9 at Appomattox Court House he and Grant met. No political terms were set; Lee simply surrendered his army. Grant, knowing how little forage there was, allowed the officers to keep their horses. He later agreed that any enlisted man who had a horse could take it home "to put in a crop." It was a simple and generous ending of a terrible war.

Five days later, on the Friday evening of April 14, 1865, the Lincolns went to the theater to see a relaxing comedy, "Our American Cousin." During the performance, John Wilkes Booth, an actor with a twisted sense of Southern honor, entered the presidential box and shot Lincoln in the back of the head. He jumped onto the stage allegedly crying Virginia's motto, "Sic Semper Tyrannus," tripped, wrenching his ankle, and fled. Secretary of State Seward was wounded at home by another assailant, but other attacks on high officials were aborted. Pursued, Booth was trapped in a barn and killed; months later his fellow conspirators were hanged. Lincoln, carried to a house across the street from the theater, lived only through the night.

On April 17, Sherman, accepting Joseph E. Johnston's surrender, had told no one of Lincoln's death. When he gave the Confederate General the news, beads of sweat stood out on Johnston's forehead. Both men feared that their men, in desperation, would take the war into the mountains as guerillas. Their fears were misplaced; the soldiers accepted the news of Lincoln's death with numbed silence. By May 26, west of the Mississippi, the last of the Confederate armies surrendered. On May 10, at Irwinville, Georgia, President Davis and his wife were taken into custody. The Confederate States of America ceased to exist. The Civil War was over.

The painfully reunited nation grieved as the funeral train carried Abraham Lincoln's body away from his capital westward, back to Illinois, for burial. The President had known the toll the war took on the men who fought it and he, himself, died believing "those dead shall not have died in vain." The survivors wanted to think so too as, private and general, they slowly made their way homeward.

Suggestions for Reading

GENERAL

The finest account of the war is Shelby Foote, *The Civil War, A Narrative*, 3 vols. (1958–74). For a look from under a blue rather than a grey visor, see Bruce Catton's trilogy, *The Army of the Potomac: Mr. Lincoln's Army* (1951), *Glory Road* (1952), *A Stillness at Appomattox** (1953), and his numerous other works on the war. C. V. Woodward, ed., *Mary Chesnut's Civil War** (1982), is the superb account of the life and death of the Confederacy written by a civilian who had lived at its center. Comparable is R. M. Myers, ed., *Children of Pride* (1972), the letters of a Georgia family caught in a social revolution. George Fredrickson, *The Inner Civil War** (1965), is a fine treatment of the effects of the war on the nation's intellectual life. Daniel Aaron, *The Unwritten War* (1973) examines the failure of our greatest writers to meet fully the challenge presented. The most valuable, critical look at the literature of the war and, perhaps, at the war itself is Edmund Wilson, *Patriotic Gore** (1962).

Two works, valuable not the least for their fine bibliographies, are J. G. Randall and D. H. Donald, *The Civil War and Reconstruction* (1969), and J. M. McPherson, *Ordeal by Fire* (1982). E. B. Long, *Civil War Day by Day* (1971), a daily almanac, and M. M. Boatner, *The Civil War Dictionary* (1959), are useful reference works.

THE CONFEDERACY

The best study of the Confederacy is E. M. Thomas's excellent *The Confederate Nation, 1861–1865* (1979). Clement Eaton, *A History of the Southern Confederacy** (1954) is also valuable; less critical of the cause is E. M. Coulter, *The Confederate States of America, 1861–1865* (1950). Frank Vandiver, *Their Tattered Flags* (1970) is a short, vivid account of the Confederacy and its leaders and so, too, is C. P. Roland, *The Confederacy** (1960). W. B. Yearns, *The Confederate Congress* (1960), and T. B. Alexander and R. E. Beringer, *The Anatomy of the Confederate Congress* (1972), examine the Southern political scene. On Jefferson Davis, the literature is large: the most valuable biography is Hudson Strode, *Jefferson Davis*, 3 vols. (1955–64). P. D. Escott, *After Secession: Jefferson Davis and the Failure of Confederate Nationalism* (1978), is critical of Davis as a civilian leader; Frank Vandiver, *Jefferson Davis and the Confederate State* (1964), is far less so. T. L. Connelly and Archer Jones, *The Politics of Command* (1973), examines critically the related question of Davis's conduct of the war.

Excellent proof that sensible books last are Bell Wiley, *Southern Negroes, 1861–1865** (1938), and *The Plain People of the Confederacy* (1943). For other civilians, see his *Confederate Women** (1975). On the still-argued question of the response of British workers to the Confederate cotton policy, see Frank

Owsley, *King Cotton Diplomacy* (1931), and Mary Ellison, *Support for Secession* (1972). Two excellent works on munitions are Frank Vandiver, *Ploughshares into Swords** (1952) and C. B. Dew, *Ironmaker to the Confederacy* (1966), a study of the Tredegar ironworks in which slave labor was used. E. M. Thomas shows the toll on states' rights in *The Confederacy as a Revolutionary Experience* (1971), and D. H. Donald incisively examines the failure of the Confederacy in *Why the North Won the Civil War* (1960).

THE UNION

Biographies are a good if lengthy way to approach the story of wartime politics. M. B. Duberman, *Charles Francis Adams, 1807–1866** (1961) is excellent on wartime diplomacy. G. G. Van Deusen, *William Henry Seward* (1967), B. P. Thomas and H. M. Hyman, *Stanton* (1962), and John Niven, *Gideon Welles* (1973). focus on the executive branch; see also Howard K. Beale, ed., *The Diary of Gideon Welles*, 3 vols. (1960). On the Senate see the second volume, *Charles Sumner and the Rights of Man* (1970), of D. H. Donald's fine biography. For contrasting views of Lincoln's relations with the Radicals, see T. H. Williams, *Lincoln and the Radicals** (1941), and Hans Trefousse, *The Radical Republicans** (1969).

On the economy of the North, an old study, E. D. Fite, *Social and Industrial Conditions in the North during the Civil War* (1910), is still valuable, as are P. D. Gates, *Agriculture and the Civil War* (1965), and R. P. Sharkey, *Money, Class and Party** (1959). Judicial matters are well treated in H. M. Hyman, *A More Perfect Union* (1973).

LINCOLN

The Lincoln literature is immense. S. B. Oates, *With Malice Toward None** (1977) is a sensible, balanced, readable recent biography. Perhaps the most intriguing and, in some ways, still the most bold is W. H. Herndon, *Herndon's Life of Lincoln** (1983), the ancestor of all subsequent work on the sixteenth President. Notable too are G. R. B. Charnwood, *Abraham Lincoln* (1917); Carl Sandburg, *Abraham Lincoln,** 4 vols. (1939); J. G. Randall, *Lincoln the President*, 4 vols. (1945–55), completed by R. N. Current; and B. P. Thomas, *Abraham Lincoln** (1952). Distinguished collections of essays are R. N. Current, *The Lincoln Nobody Knows** (1958), and D. H. Donald, *Lincoln Reconsidered** (1956). R. P. Basler, ed., *The Collected Works of Abraham Lincoln*, 9 vols. (1953–55), allows interested students to read Lincoln for themselves. W. B. Hesseltine, *Lincoln and the War Governors* (1948), and T. H. Williams, *Lincoln and his Generals** (1952), remain important.

EMANCIPATION

The decision on emancipation is treated in all the biographies of Lincoln (too often with extravagant rhetoric), and its effect on the people most immediately concerned is well presented in a fine documentary history, J. M. McPherson, *The Negro's Civil War** (1965). The same historian's *The Struggle for Equality** (1964), is an excellent study of the abolitionists' wartime efforts to persuade the President to agree to free the slaves. B. I. Wiley's pioneering work, *Southern Negroes, 1861–65** (1939), mentioned above is ably supplemented by W. L. Rose who, in *Rehearsal for Reconstruction** (1964), studies how former slaves became independent farmers when the white planters on the Sea Islands fled Union forces. The unsympathetic attitude of many Northern soldiers toward the freedmen is discussed in Louis Gerteis, *From Contraband to Freedman* (1973). In *The Armies of the Streets* (1974), Adrian Cook examines the draft riot of 1863 in New York City, whose victims were black citizens. R. F. Durden, *The Gray and the Black* (1972), is a fine account of the Confederacy's debate over racial policies. Black members of the Union army and navy are the subject of D. T. Cornish, *The Sable Arm** (1966); see also the fascinating T. W. Higginson, *Army Life in a Black Regiment** (1971), by a Northern clergyman turned colonel. J. W. Blassingame, *Black New Orleans, 1860–1880** (1973), and Peter Kolchin, *First Freedom; The Responses of Alabama's Blacks to Emancipation and Reconstruction* (1972) are studies of the transition from slavery to freedom. Of great value is Ira Berlin, ed., *Freedom: A Documentary History of Emancipation, 1861–1867, Series II, The Black Military Experience* (1982), a remarkable one-volume collection of documents written largely by black soldiers.

Benjamin Quarles in *Lincoln and the Negro* (1962), and LaWanda Cox, in a splendidly argued study, *Lincoln and Black Freedom* (1981), speculate on what Lincoln's hopes for the freedmen were. On

Lincoln's Reconstruction policies, see Herman Belz, *Reconstructing the Union* (1969), and W. B. Hesseltine, *Lincoln's Plan of Reconstruction* (1960).

MILITARY EVENTS

For readers eager to skirt the tawdry celebrations of war that Civil War books can be, Shelby Foote, *The Civil War: A Narrative*, 3 vols. (1958–74) is recommended once again. It is both reliable and well written. There are also many fine accounts of single battles; two of the best are J. L. McDonough, *Shiloh** (1977), and Stephen Sears, *Landscape Turned Red* (1983), a study of Antietam. No one writes better about the rebels at war than T. L. Connelly in *Army of the Heartland: The Army of Tennessee, 1861–1862* (1967), and *Autumn of Glory* (1971).

Memoirs of the generals who fought the war can be considered to comprise a separate genre of American letters. The two most distinguished are both by Northern generals, but an exploration of many others can be fascinating. W. T. Sherman, *Memoirs of General William T. Sherman** (1984), and U. S. Grant, *Personal Memoirs of U. S. Grant** (1982), are stern, powerful accounts of what those warriors wrought. There are also valuable collections of letters of enlisted men and lesser officers; one of the most intriguing is O. W. Holmes, Jr., *Touched with Fire* (1969). The common soldier has had admirable attention in B. I. Wiley, *The Life of Johnny Reb** (1943), and *The Life of Billy Yank** (1952).

Biographies of the generals are legion. Here, the most magisterial work belongs to the Confederacy with D. S. Freeman, *R. E. Lee, A Biography*, 4 vols. (1934–35); there is a one volume abridgement by R. B. Harwell (1961). A work that brings Lee down to human size is badly needed. T. L. Connelly, *Marble Man** (1977), is a study of the myths that have helped hide Lee from us. Lee's Union counterpart is the subject of Hamlin Garland, *Ulysses S. Grant* (1898); a trilogy: Lloyd Lewis, *Captain Sam Grant* (1950); Bruce Catton, *Grant Moves South* (1960); and *Grant Takes Command* (1968); and W. S. McFeely, *Grant: A Biography** (1981).

The reprint, *The Official Atlas of the Civil War* (1958), with an introduction by H. S. Commager, of the beautiful *Atlas to Accompany the Official Records of the Union and Confederate Armies*, and the first volume of V. J. Esposito, ed., *The West Point Atlas of American Wars*, 2 vols. (1959), are excellent. So too are many of the collections of drawings and photographs of the war. One of the most distinguished, which contains the work of Timothy O'Sullivan and other artists that worked with Matthew Brady as well as that of other photographers, is W. C. Davis, ed., *The Image of War, 1861–1865*, 3 vols. (1981).

*Available in paperback edition.

15
RECONSTRUCTION

The American Revolution brought great and, in some cases, uniquely American political changes with the birth of a new nation. The Second American Revolution, as the Civil War has been called, forced a country aged by battle to confront one of the most ancient themes of world history, slavery and emancipation. Slavery had existed for as long as history had been written, and now, the American republic experienced, as older societies had, the dramatic shift of a portion of its population from a rigidly enforced legal servitude into an as yet undefined condition of freedom. Intense argument and dramatic political action characterized the Era of Reconstruction, the period after the Civil War when the nation struggled to restructure itself in order to give meaning to the freedom that the former slaves had achieved.

Proud optimists thought that simply ending slavery was all there was to the job. They did not realize that the freed people would have to struggle to find their next meal in a society that often was anything but welcoming. Despite this uncertain beginning, the former slaves made their way into the economy and achieved a remarkable entry into the body politic as well. But initial optimism yielded to pessimism and shame as these ambitious hopes were cruelly rebuffed. The American people's outraged sense of fairness was unmatched by actions sufficient to end the mistreatment of the black former slaves during Reconstruction and long afterwards.

Yet, if freedmen were slowed in the pursuit of a chance to share equally in the lean rewards of an impoverished South, no one could take away the fact that when the Civil War was over 4,000,000 Americans who had been slaves were slaves no longer. They were a freed people—a free people—and, by their very presence, they said to their country that they had to be taken into account in a new way. The nation would have to reconstruct itself to adjust to their new emancipation.

Andrew Johnson and Reconstruction

"Malice toward none." In March 1865, as the war was ending, Abraham Lincoln, in his second inaugural address, had committed the nation to a peace in which the victors would bear "malice toward none." This magnificent phrase carried a promise of forgiveness of former slaveholders in the South, but implied reliance on their benevolence to provide for the welfare of their former slaves. The President was also mindful of the claims of the freedmen to something more than economic dependence on their former masters. Conferring with highly educated, free-born black leaders from New Orleans, he contemplated the

Richmond, Virginia: the ruins of war

possibility of a suffrage, limited by literacy or property ownership, that would give strength to a leadership group among the black citizens. He was groping towards a Reconstruction policy, and so was the Congress (see p. 395).

On March 3, 1865, the Congress adjourned according to its usual schedule, which meant the legislators were to be out of Washington all through the crucial spring, summer, and fall that followed the war. On their last day in Washington, the law-makers, with the President's approval, established the Freedman's Savings Bank, an interstate federally sponsored private bank in which the freedmen were urged to put their savings as they sold crops or earned wages. The legislators and the President also created the Bureau of Refugees, Freedmen, and Abandoned Lands—a welfare agency, soon known as the Freedmen's Bureau—which was to provide relief supplies and transportation for Union war refugees, black and white. The agents were also directed to divide lands abandoned to the United States Army into forty-acre lots and distribute them to freedmen families. The drafters of the legislation expected that the land would be farmed after the manner of the Port Royal experiment of the Sea Islands (see p. 361). Lincoln, having signed the bills, appointed a well-meaning and devout Christian, General O. O. Howard, to head the Freedmen's Bureau.

With Lincoln's assassination, all eyes turned to the new President, Andrew Johnson, to see what his Reconstruction policies would be. Radicals hoped that his stern wartime attitude toward slaveholding planters in his home state of Tennessee would herald a policy favorable to the freedmen. Shrewder friends of the retention of white supremacy in the South guessed, correctly, that the insecure new President would respond well to the flattering proposition that he could come to be thought of as the great President who reunited the Union. They proposed that he should do so by restoring a social structure not unlike the one that had existed before the war.

Born to poverty in North Carolina, Johnson was apprenticed to a tailor and, at eighteen, moved to Greenville in mountainous eastern Tennessee to practice his skilled trade. His wife, Eliza McCardle, taught him to write and Johnson, a good Jacksonian, joined volunteer associations, including a debating club, and became an active citizen in the small city. He entered politics and, before the war, served not only in the Tennessee legislature and as governor, but also in both houses of Congress. Having risen from being an indentured worker, Johnson was an example of the advancement possible in a society that opened opportunities to even its poorest members. At the Civil War's end, he had a unique opportunity to extend at least some of these possibilities to another group of poor

Americans, the freed slaves, but Johnson could not bring himself to identify his own position with theirs.

Northern advocates of black rights had misunderstood the President's policies as wartime governor of Tennessee. When he had ruled in favor of the former slaves rather than their former masters, he did so not so much to assist improverished freedmen as to punish rich planters, who had long considered themselves superior to men like him. In a pathetic, but moving, drunken inaugural speech when he was sworn in as vice president in March 1865, Johnson exposed not only his awareness of the realities of social and economic injustice but also his lack of confidence. When he became President, powerful members of the very class he had feared and despised, seized the opportunity. With flattery and, even more, with appeals to his

"Taking the oath," 1866

Prisoners from the Front, 1866, by Winslow Homer

staunch support for the Union and to his determination to be thought to be a responsible President, they encouraged him to follow a policy that would sustain black subordination in the South.

On May 29, 1865, Johnson issued two proclamations. The first granted amnesty to former Confederates who would take an oath of loyalty to the Constitution and the federal laws. Their property was to be restored to them, except for slaves and any lands and goods that were already in the process of being confiscated by federal authorities. Fourteen classes of persons were excepted from the general amnesty, including the highest-ranking civil and military officers of the Confederacy, all those who had deserted judicial posts or seats in Congress to serve the Confederacy, and persons whose taxable property was worth more than $20,000. To regain their rights, men in these categories were required to make individual applications for amnesty directly to the President. The former leaders of the South would be applying to him in order to regain the chance to once again be its leaders. With the pardons granted, Johnson would have the most powerful voices in the South indebted to him politically.

The second proclamation, in which Johnson outlined his requirements for the reconstruction of North Carolina, foreshadowed the policy he would follow in future proclamations to other states. He appointed

William W. Holden, an announced Unionist, as provisional governor and directed him to call a convention for the purpose of amending the state constitution "to restore said State to its constitutional relations to the Federal government." Johnson stipulated that only those who had taken the loyalty oath could vote for delegates or serve in that capacity at the convention. Although he did not include a provision that 10 percent of those in the body politic must be loyal, Johnson believed he was following Lincoln's plan of Reconstruction. He also accepted the governments already established in Arkansas, Louisiana, Tennessee, and Virginia which had been brought back into the Union under Lincoln's plan.

In addition to these formal proclamations and programs of political restoration of the South, Andrew Johnson gave informal instructions that not just political rights but lands as well were to be given back to Confederates. A few Freedmen's Bureau agents and a good many black farmers protested this abrogation of the will of Congress expressed in the legislation creating the Freedmen's Bureau. But their protests were of no avail. By the end of the year almost all of the acreage that the freedmen thought would be distributed to them was returned to Confederate planters.

The easy terms that Johnson set for the restoration of Southern states bothered many Northerners. Governor B. F. Perry of South Carolina forwarded every pardon petition he received and President Johnson responded with almost equal generosity. Soon many he pardoned turned up as duly elected congressmen and officers of the restored state governments. Others, knowing Johnson would grant their pardons, did not wait for them before being elected to office. A Confederate general, Benjamin G. Humphreys, was governor of Mississippi and the former vice president of the Confederacy, Alexander H. Stephens, was elected senator from Georgia. The persisting loyalty of the Southern voters to their former leaders alarmed the North.

There were other signs of Southern obstinacy. Some states refused to repudiate the Confederate war debt, and South Carolina merely "repealed" its ordinance of secession, thus refusing to admit that rebelling had been unconstitutional. Mississippi would not ratify the proposed Thirteenth Amendment, formally ending slavery. Southern Unionists and freedmen complained that they were not safe under the Johnson state governments; in late summer of 1865 Governor Holden warned the President that there was "much of a rebellion spirit" left in North Carolina. He feared that Johnson's "leniency" had "emboldened" the enemies of the government. Privately Johnson counseled Southern leaders to avoid antagonizing Congress, but he was too stubborn to modify his plan or even to alter his pardoning policy.

Only after a public outcry against the leniency of his terms did Johnson require the returning states to disavow their ordinances of secession, repudiate the Southern war debt, and ratify the Thirteenth Amendment. That amendment, which would end slavery forever in the United States, had cleared Congress in January 1865, but had required the approval of at least some of the former Confederate states to reach ratification by three-fourths of the states. The agreement that slavery must end seemed only grudgingly forthcoming.

The defeated South. "The country between Washington and Richmond was . . . like a desert," wrote one observer. Another described the path of Sherman's march as "a broad black streak of ruin and desolation." Agriculture, the South's economic bulwark, had been battered wherever armies had clashed and passed. Houses and outbuildings had been burned, crops destroyed, and livestock killed. Seed to plant new crops was often unavailable, and many farmers could not afford to buy it when they found it. Credit was almost unobtainable. Horses and mules to plow the land were even harder to find. Labor was scarce because a quarter of a million soldiers had lost their lives and many freedmen were reluctant to work for their former masters.

Much of Southern industry had been badly damaged, and assets that would have supported desperately needed loans had been wiped out. At one stroke, emancipation had destroyed a credit base made up of billions of dollars invested in slaves. Land values plummeted. The appearance of cities that had stood in the path of the armies was bleak. Charleston, South Carolina, was "a city of ruins, of desolation, of vacant houses, of widowed women, of rotting wharves." Columbia lay in ashes, as did most of Richmond.

Most white Southerners, accepting defeat with fortitude and resignation, set about reworking their land. Many felt considerable relief that slavery was over; with its demise any formal responsibility for the welfare of their slaves also ended. They, like the freed people, were anxious about how the races would now live together. Some whites at first feared that blacks would engage in violent vengeance. Others could not adjust to dealing with a free labor force. They continued to think of themselves as members of a superior group and to believe in the old myths about paternalistic masters and contented slaves. Consequently they were shocked and hurt when their former slaves rejoiced in freedom.

For their part, black Southerners felt an urge to test the meaning of freedom, but few interpreted "Jubilee Day" as a license for perpetual celebration. While some continued to expect support from their former masters, most freedmen responded by cautiously but firmly throwing off the constraints of slavery as a first step toward building a responsible life. They ventured to move about freely from place to place, which slavery had forbidden, and to reunite members of their families—parents, spouses, children—whom slavery had separated. They wanted to leave the regimented conditions of plantation life and live instead in family

Freedmen, Richmond, Virginia

units. They yearned especially for a farm of their own on land they had long worked and thought of as theirs.

In the spring of 1865, both groups of farmers, the former slaves and their former masters, knew that unless vegetable crops were planted, no one would eat the following winter; unless cotton or some other cash crop was raised, there would be no money to buy even so much as a replacement for a broken hoe. The point in contention was the conditions under which fields were to be worked, which, in the end, came down to a quarrel over who was to control the land.

Organizing Southern agriculture. During the war, the Union government had turned over some plantations that had been abandoned, as Unions armies approached, to slaves living on those lands. Southern freedmen hoped for months that this pattern would be followed and that they would receive a portion of their former master's land and some assistance in working it—the famous forty acres and a mule—from the government. The desire for a normal family life and for the privacy and independence of a small farm—normal American expectations in the mid-nineteenth-century—moved Southern blacks to resist signing up to work for their old masters.

The Freedmen's Bureau agents, young Union Army officers who thought a great, progressive change in the Southern economy was in the making, sought both to introduce Northern concepts of wage labor into the region and to honor the need to retain the status quo in sufficient degree to assure survival. The Bureau required both former slaves and former masters to sign contracts, a practice new to both. But the freed people were uncomfortable about signing with an "X" or having their old master sign for them handwritten contracts that called for the planting and harvesting of crops "in the usual way as before the war." Such wording sounded too much like more slavery to them. Not much more reassuring were formally printed contracts in which clauses calling for wages were neatly struck through with a pen-stroke. Those wages that were agreed to were paid not weekly, but only when the crops were harvested and sold—and then only if the planter made a profit sufficient to care for his own family as well as the freedmen living on his land.

The Bureau contracts gave the workers a lien on the crops they had raised to protect the wages due them. But the freed people, scarcely prepared to go into court to enforce the lien, were dependent on appeals to their former master's good will or the intervention of the Bureau agents if their fair share of the crop's value was to be paid to them. Often the agents, finding the white planters easier to understand and identify with, were more sympathetic with them than

with the workers. There is evidence of their using both threats of force and actual physical coercion to make the black freedmen work.

As the Freedmen's Bureau agents, resented by the landlords and distrusted by the freedmen, became less and less active in monitoring Southern labor practices after 1866, the planters and the freedmen began to make their own arrangements. The black workers, hating work in field gangs that had been standard under slavery, found a way to approximate having a farm of their own by striking bargains with their former masters or other landlords. The white planters, short of cash and relieved to be free of the obligation to care for the freedmen's children and elderly dependents, agreed to allow their former slaves to have a plot of land to farm on their own, provided they cared for their own families.

These informal but binding tenancy agreements, similar to those into which impoverished white farmers had begun entering before the war, called for the tenant and the landlord to divide the proceeds from the annual crop into shares that varied according to the condition of the land and the proportion of work, animals, seed, fertilizer, and other necessities each supplied. Merchants put up the money for the goods that had to be bought in return for a lien on the crop. So low was the return on what was raised on sharecroppers' farms that the farmers often found themselves in perpetual debt. The system had many defects. It pushed the poor farmers of the region into a burdensome tenancy, a peonage of a kind, and allowed them only meager return for their labor. But it

Cotton Market in New Orleans, by Edgar Degas

School for black children

Most of my children were very small ... but after some days of positive ... treatment ... I found but little difficulty in managing ... the tiniest and most restless spirits. I never before saw children so eager to learn.... Coming to school is a constant delight ... to them. They come here as other children go to play. The older ones, during the summer, work in the fields from early morning until eleven or twelve o'clock, and then come to school ... as bright and as anxious to learn as ever....

The majority learn with wonderful rapidity. Many of the grown people are desirous of learning to read. It is wonderful how a people who have been so long crushed to the earth ... can have so great a desire for knowledge, and such a capability for attaining it.... One's indignation increases against those who, North as well as South, taunt the colored race with inferiority while they themselves use every means in their power to crush ... them.

From a letter by Charlotte Forten, a Northern black woman teaching in South Carolina.

did permit the resumption of cotton and tobacco culture, and it allowed the freedmen to engage, within the bonds of poverty, in a family life of their own. For all its liabilities, it was better than slavery or gang labor.

Reordering Southern society. In 1865, with the agricultural economy still chaotic, the conflicting expectations of whites and blacks in the South complicated the major problems of restructuring the region. The Freedmen's Bureau agents provided relief from starvation. They distributed medicine, seed, and rations to destitute whites as well as blacks so that farming could begin again. Staffed by army officers, the bureau lacked the personnel, the budget, and the mandate to do more than ease the worst burdens of the Southern people. Even its most generous efforts could not dispel the taste of defeat among white Southerners who despised the Union uniform so visible in their midst. These soldiers, seeking acceptance from fellow white people, often sided with them rather than with the freedmen who counted on their help. Conscientious Bureau agents did protect some freedmen from exploitative planters, provide others with help in locating and reaching their families, formalize marriages, and provide facilities for Northern teachers to begin the education of illiterate blacks. Many of the schools and colleges that have played such a vital part in educating black Southerners were begun with Bureau help. These efforts at restructuring the society did not, however, transform the attitudes of all Southern whites towards blacks, and during 1865 reports reached the North about many incidents of whippings, mutilations, and murders of freedmen.

These private acts of vengance were accompanied, in the public sphere, by the Black Codes passed by the legislatures of the Southern states. These laws looked to many like the old slave codes, but were actually more like the laws governing free blacks in antebellum times. Blacks could now own property, witness, sue and be sued in court, and contract legal marriages; in some states they could even serve on juries. But despite these seemingly liberal provisions, the thrust of the new codes revealed Southern determination to keep blacks in an inferior position. Interracial marriage was forbidden and, in Mississippi, black artisans had to buy a special license in order to engage in certain trades. Everywhere special punishments were prescribed for black vagrants and for those

School for Freedmen

Visit from the Old Mistress, by Winslow Homer, 1876

who broke labor contracts. In some states blacks who could show no means of support could be bound out by the courts to do labor in the fields. The vagrancy laws were used not so much to rid the streets of wanderers as to control a labor force without the consent of the laborers.

In many societies and over many centuries, involuntary servitude of a lesser sort than slavery has followed emancipation. This seemed now to be coming about in the United States. The black codes severely restricted the activities of the freed people. In Mississippi, which had the most restrictive code, black farmers, some of whom had become successful working on rich delta lands abandoned during the war, were denied the right to lease land outside towns. Blatantly, the mobility open to the freedmen who sought to become prosperous independent farmers was to be blocked. The unstated premise of the codes was that the freed people were to continue to be a dependent and dependable source of farm labor, much as they had been when they were slaves.

Congress and Reconstruction. Congressmen, returning to Washington in December 1865, were well-posted on these alarming events in the South. The Republican majority had come to have grave doubts about Johnson's program. The Radicals, a minority within the party, were genuinely concerned for the safety of the freedmen whom they considered to be the most trustworthy Unionists in the South. Most of the black people had supported the Northern cause during the war, and many of them had served in the Union army. The Radicals, therefore, worked for the rapid advancement of the freedmen and the exclusion of the old Southern leaders from politics at all levels. They saw to it that the Congress excluded Southerners

who had been elected to serve as senators and congressmen. The seating of these representatives was to have marked the completion of President Johnson's program of Reconstruction. Instead, the Radicals in Congress set out to devise their own plan for reordering the South.

Thaddeus Stevens, an able congressman from Pennsylvania, with close personal ties to his black housekeeper's family, led the fight. At this early date he opposed black suffrage, because he feared that the Southern planters would use their economic power to control the freedmen's votes and because he was convinced that an economic base was the primary need of the people. Instead of the vote, he proposed to give the

Thaddeus Stevens

Veto of the Radicals' plan

The power ... given to the commanding officer over all the people of each district is that of an absolute monarch. His mere will is to take the place of all law. The law of the States is now the only rule applicable to the subjects placed under his control, and that is completely displaced by the clause which declares all interference of State authority to be null and void....

It is plain that the authority here given to the military officer amounts to absolute despotism. But to make it still more unendurable, the bill provides that it may be delegated to as many subordinates as he chooses to appoint, for it declares that he shall "punish or cause to be punished." Such a power has not been wielded by any monarch in England for more than five hundred years. In all that time no people who speak the English language have borne such servitude. It reduces the whole population of the ten States—all persons, of every color, sex, and condition, and every stranger within their limits—to the most abject and degrading slavery.

From Andrew Johnson, Veto of the Reconstruction Act, 1867.

freedmen land. He would confiscate the holdings of former Confederates and divide it into small freeholds. "Forty acres . . . and a hut," he declared, would "be more valuable . . . than the . . . right to vote." Stevens had in mind the coastal areas of South Carolina and Georgia that extended beyond the Sea Islands, where freedmen were already farming land, under possessory titles, that had been assigned them by the government on estates confiscated during the war. Stevens wanted this policy extended throughout the South, but Johnson had already restored to the former owners the lands that Stevens wanted redistributed.

Senator Charles Sumner of Massachusetts, another Radical, pinned his hopes on suffrage. He called first for votes solely for educated blacks and black veterans but soon advocated general black suffrage. He argued that freedmen required the vote for their own protection. Other Radicals agreed with Sumner and, in New Orleans, the blacks made their own voice heard on the matter. Turning their backs on a limited suffrage proposal that would have formally divided the black community along caste lines, the black citizens of Louisiana demanded "universal suffrage"—for fieldhands as well as free-born literate men—and staged a mock election, complete with a registration system and polls, to prove both the capacity and desire of black citizens to participate in the political process. In New Orleans, to the embarrassment of white supremists, the candidate of the black activists received more votes in the mock election than did the regularly elected governor in the regular election. Alert now to just how ambitious the freedmen were, chagrined moderates in Congress quickly sought to discover a middle road short of suffrage between Johnson's simple restoration and the Radicals' more sweeping plans. The moderates dominated the Joint Committee on Reconstruction, which was created in December 1865 to formulate a plan for the South.

As the Joint Committee began its work, signs of Southern intransigence multiplied. Republican congressmen received countless letters from Southern Unionists, both black and white, complaining that they were being threatened. Both Radicals and more moderate members of the party, agreeing that the safety of the freedmen had to be secured and that the Black Codes should be circumscribed by federal legislation guaranteeing rights to the freedmen, enacted two bills early in 1866. The first, passed in February, extended the life and expanded the powers of the Freedmen's Bureau; the second was a Civil Rights bill. Unabashadly, Moderates, who supported both bills, warned that if the black Southerners were not safeguarded in their own region, they could be expected to leave the South and come North. Congress intended that the Freedmen's Bureau agents would enforce the Civil rights bill; they were authorized to conduct courts not only to adjudicate labor disputes but to hear other complaints of injustice as well.

President Johnson, contending that such provisions would lead to "military jurisdiction"—military rule—considered both bills unconstitutional in time of peace. Accused persons tried in the Bureau courts would be tried and even convicted, he stated, without benefit of jury, rules of evidence, or right of appeal. In a message vetoing the Freedmen's Bureau bill, Johnson rebuked Congress for continuing to exclude the Southern members. Although his observations about the dubious constitutionality of the legislation had some merit, they angered congressmen who knew that freedmen were not getting justice in Southern courts. Four days after the veto, which the Congress narrowly sustained, Johnson harangued a crowd gathered outside the White House to hear him deliver a Washington's Birthday greeting. In a rambling speech he denounced his opponents as traitors, suggested that they wanted to kill him, and compared himself to the crucified Christ. Johnson clearly saw himself as the martyred champion of the Southern states and constitutional liberty.

Furious, Congress turned to the Civil Rights bill, which granted the freedmen the protection of federal citizenship in order to secure for them the same rights and protection as whites, regardless of local statutes. Further, it authorized the use of troops to enforce its privileges and penalties. Again the President resorted to a veto. But this time Congress overrode him and in April the strong Civil Rights Act of 1866 became the law of the land. Unlike so many similar Reconstruction measures, this law has never been overturned. Heartened by this success, congressional leaders put through a mildly amended version of the Freedmen's Bureau bill. Once again Johnson vetoed it, but this time the Congress overrode his veto. Some Republican senators had supported Johnson's veto of the first Freedmen's Bureau bill, but only three of them supported his veto of the amended bill. The broad middle section of the Republican party had joined forces with the Radicals to guarantee civil rights for the freedmen. The President in his obstinacy had consolidated his adopted party into opposition.

The Thirteenth and Fourteenth Amendments. These civil rights measures were designed to enforce the Thirteenth Amendment to the Constitution, which states in part that "neither slavery nor involuntary servitude, except as a punishment for a crime where of the party shall have been duly convicted, shall exist in the United States." Far from being a mere stamp of approval on the Emancipation Proclamation, the amendment, proposed during the war and ratified in December 1865, was necessary to prevent any involuntary servitude measures that might be devised as a substitute for slavery. In Maryland, since long before the war, slavery had been undergoing a transition from a plantation labor system to that of slave-leasing for nonagricultural pursuits. The change had been accompanied by less rigid discipline and the state government had been seeking methods of social control other than that of slavery. One law, which could have set a dangerous precedent, was a nonvoluntary child apprentice system, but, when challenged in a federal court, it was declared unconstitutional under the Thirteenth Amendment. Without the amendment

and the Civil Rights Bill enforcing it, no legal redress would have been possible for the black people who resisted seeing their children forced into a new bondage and other injustices. In Louisiana, when country people had come into New Orleans to sell chickens, local judges were sometimes ready to find them guilty of vagrancy and sentence them to six months labor on a sugar plantation that was short of workers. Now when such injustices occurred, there was a Constitutional principle with respect to involuntary servitude that could be appealed to in the courts.

As valuable as the Thirteenth Amendment was, clearly it was not enough to safeguard the freedmen's uncertain position as citizens. In the Dred Scott case Chief Justice Roger B. Taney had given his opinion that no black, whether free or slave, could be regarded as a United States citizen or was entitled to the privileges that the Constitution granted citizens. Many Republicans, remembering that decision, were afraid to depend on an act of Congress, which would be subject to Supreme Court review, to secure civil rights for the freedmen. They decided that only an amendment to the Constitution would safeguard the freedmen and secure a new electorate in the South loyal to the Union. The Fourteenth Amendment, proposed in April 1866 by the Joint Committee on Reconstruction, was passed by Congress on June 19 and sent to the states for ratification. First it defined American citizenship: "All persons born or naturalized in the United States, and subject to the jurisdiction thereof, are citizens of the United States and of the State wherein they reside." The amendment then prohibited states from passing laws "which shall abridge the privileges or immunities of citizens of the United States," from depriving "any person of life, liberty, or property, without due process of law," and from denying "to any person within its jurisdiction the equal protection of the laws."

The second and third sections of the Fourteenth Amendment attempted to bring about a basic change in the Southern electorate. The second section gave the Southern states a choice of either accepting black voters or losing some of their political power; they could either enfranchise all male citizens or else they would lose seats in the House of Representatives proportionate to the number they excluded. Some Radicals would have prefered a specific guarantee of universal manhood suffrage, but practical politicians realized that such a guarantee might lead to the defeat of the amendment in the North, for only a few Northern states had enfranchised blacks. The third section disqualified from officeholding at the state and federal level all who, before the war, had taken an oath to support the Constitution in order to hold public office and who had subsequently supported the Confederacy. Only Congress could remove this disability.

Other sections of the amendment disavowed the Confederate war debt, validated the United States war debt and disallowed all claims for loss of property, including slaves.

The battle joined. The congressional elections of 1866 caught the voters in a widening rift between President and Congress, with the Fourteenth Amendment as the central issue. As had been true with the Thirteenth Amendment, favorable action by some Southern legislatures was needed to secure ratification by the required three-fourths of the states. President Johnson opposed the Fourteenth Amendment and encouraged Southern legislatures to oppose it too. Of all the former Confederate states only Tennessee ratified the amendment. Vainly hoping to prompt other states to follow suit, Congress seated Tennessee's delegates.

Johnson continued not to implement Republican congressional measures, especially the Civil Rights Act and the Freedmen's Bureau Act. As commander in chief, he replaced military officers serving as agents in the Freedmen's Bureau who showed themselves to be genuinely committed to the freedmen's cause. He interpreted acts of Congress passed over his veto so narrowly that he almost negated their intent and his critics said he was violating his constitutional responsibility to execute the laws of the land. Though Johnson claimed to be working for peace and reconciliation, he was actually trying to unite moderate and conservative Republicans with willing Democrats into a new National Union party, the name Lincoln and he had used in 1864. His purpose was to elect his own supporters to Congress in 1866.

The new party held a convention in Philadelphia in August, but the delegates could do no more than state grand principles. There was little community of interest in the conglomeration of conservative Republicans, Democrats, and former Confederates who attended. Republicans grew skittish, moreover, at the reappearance of their old enemies, the "rebels" and the "Copperheads." At one point Governor Orr of South Carolina, a huge man, walked down the aisle arm-in-arm with Governor Couch of Massachusetts, a slight man. The scene dramatized the Republican fear that the Southerners were about to overpower the Unionists.

Andrew Johnson did his own cause great damage in his personal campaign to win support for conservative congressmen. In a "Swing Around the Circle" throughout the Middle West, he met hecklers on their own terms and sacrificed the dignity of his office at every whistlestop. The President was losing the sympathy of the voters and he had almost entirely lost the confidence of those who had counted on the chief executive to safeguard the lives of the freedmen. In recent outbreaks of racial violence in Memphis and New Orleans scores of black citizens had been killed and hundreds wounded. The President, when warned of impending trouble, had done nothing to prevent those occurrences, even when Union troops were available and could have been used to keep the peace.

Radical Reconstruction. When the results of the election were in, Republicans committed to a Reconstruction program far different from President Johnson's had won a commanding victory. Many Democrats and most of Johnson's Republican supporters were swept out of office and the election was seen as a mandate for the ratification of the Fourteenth Amendment as a basis of Reconstruction. Both the Radicals and the moderates knew that securing sufficient support in the South to ensure the adoption of the amend-

Reconstruction

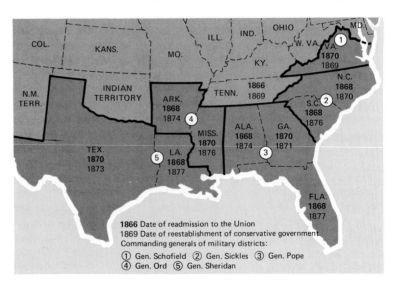

1866 Date of readmission to the Union
1869 Date of reestablishment of conservative government
Commanding generals of military districts:
① Gen. Schofield ② Gen. Sickles ③ Gen. Pope
④ Gen. Ord ⑤ Gen. Sheridan

ment would require forceful measures, which they were prepared to take.

On March 2, 1867, in its final hours and after long debate, the outgoing Thirty-ninth Congress passed a bill "to provide for more efficient Government of the Rebel States." This Reconstruction Act established military rule throughout the South two years after the war was over. The severity of the act was partly owing to the determination of the Radicals—but even more to the unwitting aid of the Democrats who had joined with them—to defeat less harsh proposals offered by moderate Republicans. Johnson's veto, not unexpected, condemned the bill as "utterly destructive" to "principles of liberty," but his veto was promptly overridden.

The new law divided the ten Confederate states into five military districts (Tennessee had already been readmitted to Congress), each under the command of an army general, backed by troops, who was granted full authority over judicial and civil functions. Each of these military governors had police power in his district; each had as his immediate assignment the registration of a new, verifiably loyal electorate. Among the voters who were to be registered were adult males who only two years ago had been slaves. This action, remarkable in the history of emancipation, could have achieved the grant of franchise for over a million black men, and it did result in many thousands of freedmen becoming voters. Excluded from the franchise were former Confederates who had been excluded under the provisions of the proposed Fourteenth Amendment.

In each of the ten states, newly registered voters elected delegates to a state constitutional convention at which a new constitution was adopted that granted universal manhood suffrage. Although the conventions interpreted that grant variously, most new state constitutions excluded former Confederate leaders from voting and officeholding, and some excluded any who had sympathized with the Confederacy. An estimated 150,000 whites were thus disfranchised. The Reconstruction Act further declared that after a state had presented an acceptable constitution to Congress and had ratified the Fourteenth Amendment, Congress would then admit that state's members.

Even with this impressive program of political reform underway, congressional leaders feared that Johnson might use his authority as commander in chief to subvert their intentions and passed two more measures to trim his power. The Army Appropriations Act directed the President and the Secretary of State to issue their orders to the five commanders for the governing of the South through the General of the Army—Ulysses S. Grant's new title—while the Tenure of Office Act provided that any officeholder appointed by the President with the Senate's consent was to serve until the Senate had approved a successor. If the President replaced a Cabinet member while the Senate was out of session, the replacement would serve after the Senate reconvened only with its consent; otherwise, the former incumbent would resume his duties.

The Tenure of Office Act was designed to keep Johnson from using the power of appointment to destroy those who opposed his views on Reconstruction and, in particular, to prevent his replacing Edwin Stanton, Secretary of War. Stanton was the only member left in the Cabinet who was friendly to the Radicals, and many Radicals, including Stanton himself, believed that the safety of the nation depended on his remaining in office. The Tenure of Office Act further provided that, unless the Senate approved a change, Cabinet members were to hold office "during the term of the President by whom they may have been appointed, and for one month thereafter." These two acts, the second of dubious constitutionality, were passed on March 2, the day on which the Reconstruction Act was passed.

A changed South. Freedmen, emboldened both by the results of the 1866 election and the initiatives in Congress, began to move forward on both the economic and political fronts. In the Low Country of South Carolina, black workers, unhappy about low or unpaid wages, struck against the planters who had hired them, counting on newly elected black officials to support them in these actions. During the last half of 1867, black and white delegates to the conventions wrote liberal constitutions, elected legislators and governors, and ratified the Fourteenth Amendment. Black delegates and black legislators were in no instance dominant in the deliberations, but the image of servants insolently seizing the seats of their masters has been so firmly implanted in the minds of so many white observers of Reconstruction that it can be forgotten both how unprecedented and how unremarkable their participation was.

All but three states were readmitted to the Union in 1868. There was much foot-dragging over the disfranchisement of former Confederates, who were often the most popular leaders in their states. Endless discussions of this bitter point delayed the writing of constitutions in Virginia and Texas; in Mississippi ratification of the new constitution was defeated because of it. Not until 1870 did those three states win congressional approval of their constitutions and reenter Congress. Georgia, admitted in 1868 but cast out again when its new legislature dismissed duly elected black members, was also readmitted in 1870, when the dismissal was rescinded.

The new constitutions of the Southern states were in many respects better than the antebellum

... Those Union men who really maintained their integrity and devotion to the Federal Union through the war, and embraced the republican view at its close, were ... mostly of that class who are neither rich nor poor, who were land-owners, but not slave-owners. The few who were of the higher class had been so completely shut out from the intellectual movements of the North during those momentous years, that, as a rule, they were utterly confounded at the result which was before them. They had looked for the nation to come back to them, when its power was re-established, absolutely unchanged and unmodified. It came back, instead, with a new impetus, a new life, born of the stormy years that had intervened, putting under its feet the old issues which had divided parties, scornful of ancient statesmanship, and mocking the gray-beards who had been venerated as sages in "the good old days of the Republic."

But for those Southern men, who, knowing and realizing all these changes, facing all these dangers and discomforts, recognizing the inexorable logic of events, and believing in and desiring to promote the ultimate good which must flow therefrom, in good faith accepted the arbitrament of war, and staked their "lives, fortunes, and sacred honor," in support of this new dispensation of liberty, words enough of praise can not be found! Nor yet words enough of scorn for their associates and affiliates of the North, who not only refused them the meed of due credit for their self-sacrifice and devotion, but also made haste to visit them with coolness, indignity, and discrediting contempt, because they did not perform the impossible task which the Wise men had imposed upon them.

From Albion W. Tourgée, A Fool's Errand; By One of the Fools, 1879.

constitutions. The states now assumed responsibility for many social services that had formerly been left to local officials and private initiative. States without public school systems now established them, along with hospitals and other institutions for the care of the indigent, homeless, and the physically handicapped. Tax systems were made more equitable, penal codes more humane, and the rights of women more comprehensive. For the first time in its history, South Carolina had a divorce law. In states where planters had enjoyed advantages over upcountry farmers, districting for representation in the legislature was made fairer. The new constitutions also empowered state governments to undertake programs in economic recovery, especially for the rebuilding of the ruined railroads. Some of these constitutions, modern for their time, served the Southern states long after Reconstruction had ended.

Southern racial conservatives denounced the new governments, mainly because they detested the political coalition that had created them and that served in the first legislatures. They called resident Northerners who held office in the new governments "carpetbaggers," a name suggesting that as transients they had no stake in Southern society. They denounced Southern whites who cooperated with the new regimes as "scal-

awags"—runty, poorly-bred cattle—suggesting at once both smallness of means and disloyalty. The spectacle of blacks voting and holding public office shocked the conservatives, but pragmatic scalawags found it useful, if awkward, to cooperate with their black colleagues. These latter politicians, using the time-honored "you vote for my bill, I'll vote for yours" procedure, were, in a few instances, able to develop real local political power that workers could appeal to when planters threatened their interests. Robert Smalls, representing the Sea Islands in South Carolina, could intercede when striking freedmen were threatened with violence and succeed in both restoring the peace and protecting his constituents' wages. Although black Southerners never held office in proportion to their numbers, their very presence in government fostered resentment and complaints of "Negro rule."

Behind the criticism of the "Black Republicans" lay the assumption that none of the groups participating in the governing of the South were fit to do so. Actually there was little truth in the stereotypes that conservatives fastened on the Republican coalition. Many scalawags were prominent and affluent leaders who found Republican economic policies not unlike the old Whig program. Others were small farmers, who sensed that their interests would be better protected than they had been before the war. They were willing to cooperate with the Republican party, even with its commitment to black rights, until tax policies were adopted that favored entrepreneurs rather than farmers. The carpetbaggers included all sorts of people who had business in the South after the war. Some were military personnel, some were planters, and some were adventuring businessmen and speculators. Unlike politicians with outside incomes, many carpetbaggers who held office had to depend on their incomes as officeholders for a living. There were fewer carpetbaggers than there were scalawags and blacks, but their undoubted loyalty to the Union and their connections with the federal government gave them considerable influence. Working through local groups called Loyal Leagues or Union Leagues, they organized the black Republican vote in the South.

One great weakness of the Republican coalition was that it had come to power as a result of policy generated in Washington. Members of the once-powerful class of planters, now excluded from public office, would always regard the Republican governments as fraudulent and alien. Indeed, most white Southerners would not recognize the legitimacy of governments which they saw as having been imposed upon them. Yet idealism and high purpose marked the early stages of the Republican effort to rebuild the South.

The impeachment of a President. Congress had been right in suspecting that Johnson would use his control of the army to weaken programs called for in the Reconstruction acts. His behavior was technically correct, but by instructing district commanders not to question the past behavior of those who took an oath of allegiance, he permitted Southerners of doubtful loyalty to the Union and of undoubted hostility to their black fellow citizens to regain the vote and the power that went with it. To the dismay of the advocates of the new Reconstruction policies, Johnson removed three generals who were sympathetic to Rad-

ical policies and, in December 1867 in his message to Congress, he rashly challenged Congress by declaring that he would maintain his rights as President, "regardless of all consequences."

The Radicals in Congress had contemplated impeaching Johnson for some time and held hearings that produced impressive evidence of Johnson's refusal to execute laws designed to safeguard the freedmen and other Unionists, but they could not agree on legal grounds for action. Their opening came when Johnson resolved to test the constitutionality of the Tenure of Office Act. While Congress was in the 1867 summer recess, he dismissed Stanton and appointed Grant as temporary Secretary of War. When Congress reconvened, the Senate refused to consent to Stanton's removal. Grant, spoiling Johnson's plan to hold the office, abandoned an empty room to Stanton and protested that he had never agreed to break the law. Grant's critics suggested that he had done so after a hint from the Radicals that he might himself become a presidential candidate. Johnson, angry with Grant, now embarked on an opera-bouffe search for a more cooperative general. As stand-in, he finally produced General Lorenzo Thomas, but Johnson had no success in installing his protégé in the War Department. Stanton, barricading himself in his office, cooked his own meals and regularly consulted with the Radical leaders. Removing Stanton was bad enough, but trying to replace him with a pliable Secretary of War convinced even moderate Republicans that Johnson now intended to have a free hand in his use of the army to undo what the military Reconstruction Acts were bringing about in the South, and to do so in face of specific laws passed by the Congress. Even moderate Republicans gave up on the President. Aware that in the 1867 fall elections the voters had given the Radicals signs of displeasure over the measures they had taken, the Republican moderates had in December blocked a vote of impeachment, but by February their patience was gone.

Confident that most citizens believed Johnson had broken the law, the Republican majority in the House of Representatives voted, unanimously, on February 24, 1868, to impeach Johnson for "high crimes and misdemeanors in office." The Radicals then drew up a list of specific charges, centering on his alleged violation of the Tenure of Office Act. The most significant was the charge that Johnson had been "unmindful of the high duties of his office . . . and of the harmony and courtesies which ought to exist . . . between the executive and legislative branches." He had attempted to bring Congress into "contempt and reproach." Essentially the House, by this charge, was accusing Johnson of disagreement with congressional policies. A conviction on that charge might have established a precedent for the re-

U. S. SENATE
Impeachment of the President
ADMIT THE BEARER
MARCH 13. 1868
Geo. T. Brown
Sergeant-at-Arms.

To be taken up at MAIN ENTRANCE
U. S. SENATE

Philp & Solomons. Wash. D.C.

moval of any President who could not command a majority in the House of Representatives on an important issue.

To convict the President, two-thirds of the Senate sitting as a court presided over by the Chief Justice would have to agree that Johnson had broken the law (with the implication that he had no right to test the constitutionality of an act of Congress) and that he was not "fit" to hold his office. Johnson's able legal defense successfully disposed of the contention that he had broken the Tenure of Office Act by arguing that Stanton had been appointed by Lincoln and not by Johnson and had served beyond the term of the President who appointed him. On the issue of fitness, cautious senators were troubled by the magnitude of the possible consequences of the removal of a President on the political charge that he had not worked for "harmony" with Congress. By a margin of only one vote, the Senate acquitted Johnson. Chief Justice Chase, who presided at the trial, was in sympathy with the President's arguments, and additional Republican senators would have voted for acquittal had their votes been needed. Many of those who voted to acquit the President did so because they distrusted the radicalism of Benjamin Wade, acting President of the Senate, who would have become President if Johnson had been convicted. Wade's views on public finance, labor, and woman suffrage were fully as radical as his views on civil rights for blacks, and were far more shocking to the moderate Republicans. After Johnson's narrow escape, Stanton resigned and the Senate adjourned. The defeat of the impeachment was an ominous sign for the future of the new Republican governments in the Southern states.

The Supreme Court and Reconstruction.

The Supreme Court was not entirely silent during the prolonged struggle between the President and the Congress over the direction of Reconstruction. The Court had started off boldly late in 1866. In the case, *Ex parte Milligan*, it had ruled unanimously that neither Congress nor the President had the power to create military courts to try civilians in areas remote from war. That noteworthy civil liberties decision freed several men who had been condemned by such courts for military subversion in the North during the war, but, ironically, it was a threat to the newly established civil rights of the freed people. The *Milligan* decision cast doubt on the legality of the courts the Freedmen's Bureau was then conducting in Southern states.

Congress, by passing the Reconstruction Acts in the spring of 1867, delivered an overt challenge to the Court. Unsure of the Court's response, the Radicals began to talk of reducing its size, with some even urging that it be abolished. In 1867, by a five-to-four decision in the twin cases, *Cummings v. Missouri* and *Ex parte Garland*, the Court invalidated the use of loyalty oaths, pronouncing them ex post facto and bills of attainder. In the same year, however, the Court grew more cautious in its rebukes to Radical Reconstruction policies. In the cases *Georgia v. Stanton* and *Mississippi v. Johnson*, the Court was challenged to rule on the constitutionality of the Reconstruction Acts. In both instances it refused jurisdiction on technical grounds.

The Court had been in low repute since the Dred Scot decision, but when Lincoln replaced pro-Southern Justices with staunch Unionists some of its prestige had returned. This change, however, did not ensure that the rights of black citizens would be sustained. In 1873, almost unaware of what the implications of its actions were, the Court robbed the Fourteenth Amendment of its power to protect the freedmen in their precarious postwar position.

In the *Slaughter-House Cases* of 1873, the Court, in a matter unrelated to racial issues, held that the states could define the rules by which its citizens could conduct their lives—in this case, butchers could be required to use a central slaughterhouse—despite an appeal of individual citizens to the new Fourteenth Amendment's guarantee that no person could be deprived of his liberty without due process of law. Shrewd lawyers soon saw that this principle could be used to permit local authorities to establish jurisdiction over the lives of black citizens and make the Fourteenth Amendment impotent as an instrument for their protection. This was precisely what happened once the Radicals were driven from office in the South. Black citizens were deprived of federal protection of many of their basic civil rights for many decades. No longer did the Fourteenth Amendment serve, as Justice Miller in *Slaughter-House* contended that it should, "that race and that emergency."

The Ebullient North

The gilded age.

The Northern economy began to gain strength in the postwar years. Only briefly did it stumble over reconversion to peace. The demobilization of 800,000 Union veterans within six months, and the abrupt cancellation of war contracts, threw a million people out of work. The economy was further restricted in 1867 when Secretary of the Treasury Hugh McCulluch, who considered gold and silver the only sound basis for currency, began to withdraw from circulation nearly $100 million in greenbacks that had been issued during the war. Within a year, however, railroad expansion and other commercial ventures ended the wartime retardation of the economy and spurred a strong recovery.

The South had seceded from a union of states. It returned to a nation hardened by war and vindicated by victory. The new spirit of nationalism in the North had revealed itself clearly in economic legislation enacted during the war years. The absence of traditional Southern opposition in Congress then had made it easy for Republicans to adopt a protective tariff and reduce foreign competition in industry, to create a national banking system, to put through a homestead act, and to start funding a transcontinental railroad. Those measures signaled a new era of expansion in industry, agriculture, and transportation—all under the favoring hand of the national government.

Prosperity fed a mood of confident materialism and Mark Twain, with sardonic aptness, christened the era "The Gilded Age." Seizing the opportunities of wartime economic expansion and inflation, entrepreneurs amassed new wealth that they now sought to invest. They had not far to look. Technological advances opened thousands of new opportunities to put capital to work. Mills in Bethlehem and Pittsburgh, Pennsylvania, made use of the Bessemer Process in which oxygen was forced through molten iron to produce steel, a metal far more adaptable to manufacturing needs than iron (see pp. 458–59). In the new oil industry, the perfection of refining techniques, the opening of the first pipeline, and John D. Rockefeller's mastery of marketing techniques resulted in similarly strong growth. Industrial production in the country increased dramatically and natural resources, seemingly inexhaustible, were ruthlessly and often wastefully exploited.

The iron horse symbolized the new age of energy. The forty thousand miles of railroad track laid in the decade after 1865 stimulated heavy industry and opened the farther West to agriculture. Food for an expanding army of industrial workers rolled eastward. Congress made loans and land grants that sped the construction of the Central Pacific Railroad eastward from California and the Union Pacific westward across the plains. For every mile of track laid, the railway company received 6,400 acres of free land. The government also made generous loans on second-mortgage bonds: $16,000 for each mile of level ground covered $48,000 in the mountains, and $32,000 in the high plains. As the two roads raced for their share of the federal subsidies, they sacrificed quality to speed. Still, their accomplishment was spectacular. The Union Pacific built 1,089 miles of track; the Central Pacific, 689. They met at Promontory Point, west of Ogden, Utah. At ceremonies there on May 10, 1869, the blows of a silver sledge drove in the golden spikes connecting the rails. Now only a week's journey separated the Atlantic Ocean from the Pacific.

Foreign affairs under Johnson. National confidence also marked the able conduct of foreign relations by Secretary of State William H. Seward. During the war the French under Napoleon III had affronted the Monroe Doctrine by setting up a puppet government in Mexico under the pliant and ambitious Austrian Archduke Maximilian. Fully occupied with fighting the Confederacy, Lincoln and Seward had denounced the French action but had been unable to challenge Napoleon's bid to restore French imperial power in the Western Hemisphere. Seward lost no time once the war was over. In 1866 President Johnson sent fifty thousand veteran troops to the Mexican border, and Seward demanded the withdrawal of French forces. This bold action was of assistance to the Mexicans who, bravely asserting their independence, expelled the French.

A vigorous expansionist, Seward believed that trade with other countries would help convince the world of the superiority of American democracy. In 1868 he signed a treaty of friendship and commerce with China. In 1867 he negotiated a treaty to buy the Virgin Islands from Denmark for $7,500,000. The Senate rejected that treaty but at the same time approved one that Seward had arranged with Russia for the purchase of Alaska for $7,200,000. The Tsar's government, with a territory already so vast that Alaska seemed superfluous, was reluctant to commit the naval forces necessary to protect its North American domain, which it did not want to fall into British hands. The Russian minister in Washington, Baron Edoard de Stoeckl, was inordinately fond of intrigue and enjoyed the machinations—including the bribing of some Representatives whose votes for the necessary appropriation were needed—which resulted in the completion of the sale. At the time, many Americans joked about Seward's "icebox," for it seemed more a frozen wasteland than the immensely valuable state that it has become.

The election of 1868. Members of Congress had been bold and imaginative in discussing social programs for the freedmen, but much of this constructive discourse had been deflected into strident criticism of President Johnson during the impeachment crisis. Not one of the senators or congressmen emerged as a strong national leader, and the Republicans, determined to win the White House, turned instead to the greatest of the war heroes, Ulysses S. Grant. At the war's end, both Johnsonian conservatives and congressional radicals had sought Grant as an ally. The general, while disclaiming any political ambition, was concerned about slipping back into the obscurity from which he had rescued himself during the Civil War. He wanted the presidency, the only office comparable to his exhalted position as Commanding General during the war. Grant and his wife skillfully avoided any talk of the White House in 1864 so that President Lincoln had felt no usurping pressure, but they felt no such loyalty to President Johnson. Grant broke with the President in the Tenure of Office struggle and, thereby, persuaded the Radical Republicans that he would be amenable to their policies. He was nominated by the Republican convention with Speaker of the House Schuyler Colfax of Indiana as the vice-presidential candidate.

Johnson's hope of creating a new national party had been dashed by his inability to bring Southern representatives loyal to his policies into the Congress, by his disastrous performance on the Swing Around the Circle in the election of 1866, and by his bitter quarrels with Congress that ended in the impeachment trial. The Democratic Party looked not to him for a bid to retain the White House, but to Horatio Seymour, who had served as governor of New York during the war. For vice president they chose Francis P. Blair, Jr., a member of the famous Jacksonian political family who had been a Union general and could stoutly maintain that the Democrats were not a party of disloyalty. Their platform called for amnesty for former Confederates and restoration of their political rights, which would have resulted in the readmission of Mississippi, Virginia, and Texas, the last three states not represented in the Congress. The Democrats maintained that black suffrage should be left to the states, but the Republicans held the same position on that point, with the large exception of contending that such suffrage was essential in the South.

The Democrats' only hope for victory was to focus public attention on the question of money and the repayment of the war debt, which was under hot debate. During the war the government had issued some $450 million in greenbacks. The value of that currency had fluctuated over the years, but it was always below the value of coins and gold-backed currency. Attacking McCulloch's retirement of greenbacks, the Democrats adopted the "Ohio Idea," sponsored by George H. Pendleton, congressman from that state, who demanded that the notes be reissued to redeem outstanding war bonds not explicitly requiring redemption in gold. This demand for cheap money appealed to debtors, especially farmers with long-term mortgages who stood to benefit from inflation. It appealed also to critics of the war-profiteers who had speculated in the bonds. The Republicans, on the other hand, pledged themselves to the redemption of the national debt in gold. They knew that conservative financiers would approve this adherence to sound money. Grant and his advisors were listening to these hard money men and not to the farmers whose debts would be harder to pay if money increased in value or wage earners who would find jobs harder to

get if there were less money in circulation and, therefore, fewer buyers for the goods they might produce. The Republicans were hoping that both the farmers and the workers would remember the passions of war vividly enough to distrust the Democrats' amnesty proposals for the South. With this strategy, the Republican party turned its back on the working-class people whom some of its founders and many of its more radical members during Reconstruction had vowed to protect.

In the campaign of 1868, the Republicans, with extravagant rhetoric, concentrated on the alleged treason of the Democrats and waved the "bloody shirt" of war to demonstrate their own valor. They knew they could count on the support of the Southern states where black voters, as well as federal officeholders, both local and from the North, were loyal to the party of liberation and Union. The Democrats lost whatever appeal they might have enjoyed from the Ohio Idea when Seymour repudiated that plank in the platform. Even with all their advantages, however, including Grant's great popularity, the Republican victory was not a landslide. Grant carried the Electoral College by 214 votes to 80 but received only 53 percent of the popular vote. Of the former Confederate states, Seymour carried Louisiana and Georgia and showed strength in all the Border States. Mississippi, Virginia, and Texas had not been readmitted to the Congress, and their votes were not counted. The most interesting facet of the election was that black men voted in significant numbers in a national election for the first time. Grant did not owe his victory to them, but without them he would have had only a minority of the popular vote. He owed them a political debt.

The Grant Era

Government under Grant. An immensely popular war hero was in the White House and members of his own party were in the majority in both houses of Congress while Lincoln appointees made up a majority of members of the Supreme Court. Nothing, it seemed, could stand in the way of a Republican triumph for Reconstruction now that the frustrating battles with President Johnson were over. And yet, black Americans, who had the highest hopes as Grant entered the White House, saw their aspirations severely curtailed by the time he moved out. This trend was foreshadowed as early as 1869 when Secretary of War John A. Rawlins, the only true champion of black rights in the original Grant cabinet, died of tuberculosis.

Rawlins had been Grant's chief of staff during the war and, more important, he had been a friend who was not afraid to criticize his commander. With his death in September 1869, Grant lost not only his wisest counselor on public issues, but also an intimate friend who might have helped the President achieve a greater sense of purpose. Rawlins was replaced by William W. Belknap, a weak and, it turned out, corrupt man of little intelligence. Unfortunately, Belknap and not Rawlins was typical of the many men who sat in the Grant Cabinet. One exception was the Secretary of State, Hamilton Fish, an elegant, honest, quiet, and intelligent former Whig from New York. Fish was, however, unsympathetic toward people of a color other than his own and was wary not only of the freedmen in the South, but also of insurgents in Cuba who tried vainly to get support from the United States government. He also was only barely tolerant of President Grant's almost obsessive determination to annex the Dominican Republic, a goal that was frustrated by the Senate, led by the Chairman of the Foreign Relations Committee, Charles Sumner. Grant thought that black Americans, frustrated in their attempts to establish themselves satisfactorily in the South, might move to the island and establish a black state. Both people who wanted the freedmen to succeed within the Union and those who did not were highly dubious of the proposed segregated state. Although his break with the President over this issue was to cost Sumner his chairmanship of the Foreign Relations Committee, the Senator blocked annexation.

Fish proved himself to be a master of diplomacy when conducting American relations with Europe. The greatest problem facing him in that sphere arose from the wartime claims of the United States that the British government had permitted their shipbuilders to supply the Confederacy with warships that had done great damage to Union cargo ships. The most famous of these Confederate raiders was the *Alabama*, and the complaints to Britain about their raids were called the Alabama Claims. Senator Sumner was, as Massachusetts politicians with Irish American constituents are apt to be, an outspoken critic of England, and called not only for reparations equal to the lost cargoes, but for "indirect claims"—vast sums to compensate for losses to the Union caused, indirectly, by the raiders.

Fish, skillfully sidestepping the sensitive and difficult Sumner, conducted gentlemanly negotiations with the British minister to Washington. Under the Treaty of Washington of 1871, the claims were referred to an international board of arbitration. Charles Francis Adams was the leading member of the commission that presented the American case to the board which determined that Britain should apologize and pay the United States $15,500,000 to cover the direct claims. Britain did so and not only was a major crisis in Anglo-American relations resolved but also a much-neglected precedent for the peaceful settlement of international disputes was established.

While these negotiations were under way, the nation was treated to a far less edifying spectacle. During the postwar boom in transcontinental railroad building (see p. 454), the press revealed in the fall of 1872 that prominent members of Congress had accepted bribes, in the form of stock, in return for promises not to investigate Crédit Mobilier, a corporation established to build the Union Pacific Railroad. Crédit Mobilier's purpose was not to get the road built, but to divert profits from building contracts to the Union Pacific's promoters. The fraudulent enterprise was conducted blatantly and exposed. Though many members of Congress, including Vice President Schuyler Colfax and future president James A. Garfield, were tainted by the scandal, only Congressman Oakes Ames was censured by the House for his leading role in the unethical business. Save for the involvement of the Vice President, (Colfax was replaced by Henry Wilson as the Republican candidate for Vice President in 1872) the Congressional scandal did not touch the White House, but the Grant administration could take small comfort in that omission. Evidence of greed had already been revealed within the Executive Mansion itself in a scandal that involved members of the President's own family.

In the fall of 1869, James Fisk, Jr., and Jay Gould, two bold and unscrupulous young speculators, had attempted to corner the gold market on the basis of inside information about the government's handling of the money supply, which they claimed they were receiving from their partner, Abel R. Corbin, President Grant's brother-in-law. The price of gold was bid up to dizzying heights, but when Grant learned that his sister and very possibly his wife were carrying speculative gold accounts, he moved, effectively, to bring the market under control. He and Secretary of the Treasury George Boutwell, one of the honest and able members of his cabinet, sold $4 million in gold at a time that the insiders were claiming the government would not do so. That sale caused the market to recede suddenly. When the crash came on "Black Friday," September 24, 1869, many investors were ruined, but Gould and Fisk were not. The gold market, which fluctuated in part because of the variable value of the greenbacks, was steadied and no general economic collapse occurred.

In their management of the money supply, Grant and Boutwell, ignoring their party's espousal of the gold standard, counted on the continued use of the greenbacks issued during the war. In 1870, however, in *Hepburn v. Griswold* the Supreme Court decided that the wartime act stipulating that contracts could be discharged by greenbacks—which had a shifting value—as well as by the currency originally stipulated, was unconstitutional. The administration wanted the decision reversed and Grant's first two appointments to the Supreme Court (after Edwin M. Stanton had died before being seated and E. R. Hoar had been rejected by the Senate) were men known to favor continued use of the greenbacks. In 1871, with new Justices William Strong and Joseph P. Bradley voting with the majority, the Supreme Court held, in the second *Legal Tender Case*, that the wartime currency could be used to pay debts currently and was not legal simply during the years of military emergency. Although the Strong and Bradley votes were often pointed to as the product of a corrupt conspiracy, some observers have noted that there is nothing unethical about a president's appointment of justices who agreed with administration policy.

Corruption was not confined to Washington and Wall Street. At City Hall in New York, "Boss" William Marcy Tweed relieved the city of an estimated $200 million. That figure included the proceeds from fraudulent bond issues and the sale of franchises as well as graft collected from corrupt contractors and merchants dealing directly with the city government. Since the governor of New York was a Tweed henchman, the "Boss," though a Democrat himself, had little trouble silencing the Republican legislature with bribes. Control of the police, the courts, and the district attorney made Tweed almost invulnerable. At last, when the city was nearly bankrupt, Samuel J. Tilden successfully challenged Tweed for control of the Democratic organization in the city. Tilden gained a national reputation for having "smashed" the ring. Tweed's was only the most notorious of the party machines; others operated in Philadelphia, Chicago, and Washington. In their heyday they had little trouble

Mississippi Senator: Blanche K. Bruce

winning the cooperation of otherwise reputable public figures.

Southern state governments were under particular scrutiny by observers of corruption who hoped to discredit black law makers who differed very little from their white colleagues. Although there were more black citizens than white in three states, no black man was elected governor. Only in South Carolina did blacks make up a majority in one house of the legislature for one session. Two men, Hiram R. Revels, a dignified minister, and Blanche K. Bruce, a skillful politician, were sent to the Senate by Mississippi and fifteen black men entered the House of Representatives. These gains were significant, but they did not represent domination of politics. Many Southern whites condemned what they called "Black Reconstruction" simply because they objected to any black participation in the political life of the South, and they seized upon any incident of corruption to discredit Republican rule.

In the South, as elsewhere, there were such incidents. Bold efforts to rebuild the South's transportation system foundered in the end on the wholesale theft of railroad stock. In South Carolina the Land Commission designed to help blacks buy farms ended up as a device for transferring state funds to the private accounts of unscrupulous assessors and their friends in high places. Florida's bill for printing costs in 1869 was more than the entire cost of running the state government in 1860. "Damn it," expostulated Henry Clay Warmoth, carpetbag governor of Louisiana and one of the worst spoilers, "everybody is demoralized down here. Corruption is the fashion." He had a point. But it took two to make a deal, and many of those who bribed the legislature for favors were native Southerners and Democrats.

Blacks, seldom the beneficiaries of these schemes, were learning to survive in a white world. Nevertheless, the presence of blacks in the legislatures and their loyalty to the carpetbag Republicans enabled disfranchised whites to blame corruption on the experiment in political equality. Even the performance of the honest and efficient Radical government of Mississippi and of remarkable black leaders like South Carolina's Secretary of State Francis Cardozo changed few opinions. Political association with blacks and carpetbaggers became increasingly suspect among Southern whites. Scalawags found themselves ostracized by their neighbors. As one former Whig planter explained when he withdrew from the Republican party, a man with four marriageable daughters could do no less.

If social pressure could block some democratic goals, there were others that were achieved. The Fifteenth Amendment, put forward by the more radical Republicans in February 1869 and supported by President Grant when he was inaugurated, was ratified on March 30, 1870. It forbade the states to deny the right to vote "on account of race, color, or previous condition of servitude." Its sponsors hoped it would prevent unfriendly legislatures from disfranchising freedmen in the future; those hopes were later dashed. The amendment's most immediate effect was to enfranchise Northern black citizens since, in the South, blacks were already voters under the new state constitutions. Proponents of the amendment hoped it would give a strong signal that the ballot box was designed to provide the freed people with sufficient access to those chosen to govern them to protect them from violence.

The Ku Klux Klan. In Pulaski, Tennessee, just after the passage of the Civil Rights Bill of 1866, white men, determined to intimidate their black neighbors and force them into submission, founded the Ku Klux Klan. General Nathan Bedford Forrest was the Grand Wizard of the secret terrorist organization that operated outside the law and soon had Dens, led by Grand Cyclops, across the South. The Klan's strength increased in direct proportion to southern black citizens' assertions of their rights. As the freedmen responded to the opportunities presented by both federal legislation passed to implement the three constitutional Reconstruction amendments and their own state constitutions, the Klan reacted with rides in the night. A tortured corpse was a grim warning to an aspiring citizen who might be considering starting his own farm or running for office.

Shortly after the ratification of the Fifteenth Amendment, Congress created the Justice Department and gave the Attorney General a staff of lawyers with which he could prosecute violaters of the new federal civil rights legislation. Grant's first Attorney General, E. R. Hoar, had not favored aggressive federal

Klansmen with captive

Amos T. Akerman, Georgia Attorney General

action in the civil rights field, but his successor, Amos T. Akerman, appointed with the backing of Southern Republicans, was a native of New Hampshire who had long lived in the South and had been a colonel in the Confederate army. He knew the Klan at first hand in his home country of north Georgia. Congressmen also learned about the Klan through extensive hearings. In the spring of 1871, with the active support of President Grant, Congress enacted the strong Ku Klux Klan Act designed specifically to bring those who attacked black people into the federal courts.

Akerman, assisted by able United States Attorneys located in the South, directed the prosecution of cases that were heard by conscientious federal judges, most notably Hugh L. Bond. In some areas, such as North Carolina, cases were well-enough presented and promptly heard to restrain the Klan. But in South Carolina no jury would convict a white man, and freed Klansmen took terrible reprisals on people who had appeared as witnesses in their trials. Precisely because he was a general, President Grant was reluctant to use the army to maintain civilian order, but in 1871, under the provisions of the Ku Klux Klan Act, he lifted the writ of habeas corpus in nine counties of South Carolina. Akerman worked closely with carefully chosen army officers who arrested violators and held them for trial. Elsewhere across the South federal marshalls also brought Klansmen to court. These vigorous prosecutions and the resulting convictions continued after Akerman, under pressure both from opponents of his civil rights policy and from railroad men who disliked his stern scrutiny of their activities, was forced to resign. The six hundred convictions, and threats of more, did much to break up the Klan as an organized force. Black voters felt free to participate in the election of 1872.

The Liberal Republican movement. As the 1872 election approached, Grant's popularity was still great, but the strongest challenge to his reelection came not from the opposition Democrats, but from dissidents within his own party. Those who led it have been called, in an apt phrase, "the best men"—well-educated gentlemen who deplored disorder and corruption and wanted not so much government by the people as government—good government, they insisted—for the people.

As they looked around, they saw a lack of intellectual force in the government and corruption reaching into city halls, state legislative chambers, the houses of Congress, and even the White House. They also considered the use of military officers to assist in the Ku Klux Klan cases to have been the exercise of military rather than civilian rule. In the increasingly high tariffs that fed the profits of newly rich industrialists and the unrestrained supply of greenbacks, they saw a failure to observe the "laws" of liberal capitalism expounded by Adam Smith and John Stuart Mill.

They proposed cures for all these problems. In commercial matters, they would follow the principles of free trade, redeem the greenbacks, and establish a stable currency, even though this might be painful in credit-starved agricultural areas of the country. In the South, where their disgust with the Klan was matched by their dislike and distrust of blacks, they would restore governing responsibilities to "thinking people," men like themselves who, before the war, had maintained order in the region. In the matter of corruption in government, they put forth their favorite proposal, Civil Service Reform. Only people of merit would be allowed to work for the government; they hoped that both bribery and stupidity would be banished.

Senator Carl Schurz of Missouri, a German immigrant, who was both an intellectual and a war hero, led the revolt. In his state Radical Republicans had all but proscribed the rights of party members who wanted to restore political rights to the many former Confederates in the state. Schurz organized a campaign that placed B. Gratz Brown in the statehouse. By 1872, the Missouri Liberals had been joined by anti-Grant midwestern Republicans, War Democrats (particularly in Ohio), and patricians in the northeast. Two brilliant journalists, E. L. Godkin, the British editor at *The Nation* and Henry Adams, grandson and greatgrandson of Presidents, who edited *The North American Review*, added lustre to the cause. Adams' father, Charles Francis Adams, the patriarch of the movement, hoped for the presidential nomination, which it would be beneath his dignity to seek, but the Liberals' Convention in Cincinnati in 1872 proved more chaotic than reverential and made the quixotic choice of Horace Greeley for President.

Greeley, editor at the influential *New York Tribune*, was a bright and interesting man, but political consistency was not one of his virtues. His advocacy of high tariffs made a mockery of the Liberals' anti-protectionist doctrine, his long-held antislavery positions made him unattractive to potential Liberals in the South, and his formerly staunch Whig and Republican loyalties turned Democrats away. What was more, he was almost the antithesis of the charismatic political candidate. In a most unusual move, the Democratic party ran no campaign in 1872 and instead endorsed Greeley.

Grant and his allies were smart enough politicians not to be complacent. The President took a stance above the battle, from which he could keep his eye on every happening in the campaign, while his loyalists again waved "the bloody shirt" of the regular Republicans' patriotism. On posters, Ulysses Grant and Henry Wilson were pictured as "the tanner and the cobbler." Grant had hated working in his father's tannery and his senatorial running mate, who had once been apprenticed to a shoemaker, had not made many shoes lately, but they did make a strong and successful appeal for the workingclass vote. They got this support despite evidence that Grant had long depended on and favored some of the richest of the nation's capitalists. In appealing to the workingclass, the Republicans stole much of the thunder of the nascent National Labor Reform Party. The voters, somewhat bemused by Greeley and his erudite supporters and still intensely loyal to General Grant, as most people called their President, gave him a strong reelection victory. Greeley's death a few weeks after the election symbolized the demise of the Liberal Republican movement.

The collapse. On September 18, 1873, Jay Cooke & Company failed. The pious banker, who had so successfully sold government bonds to finance the war, overextended his bank in his efforts to sell securities of the Northern Pacific Railway. Once again, such a failure, and the panic that ensued, exposed weakness in the whole of the economy, most notably in railroad speculations and in the European market for agricultural exports. Many of the huge European investments in American western expansions were withdrawn at the time of the Franco Prussian war of 1870–71. The result was a depression which, by some reckonings, lasted six years; other economists link it to the nation's economic difficulties that persisted until the end of the century. One of the immediate results in 1873, when many banks failed, was the collapse of the Freedman's Saving's Bank. Its investments had been managed by Henry D. Cooke, who sold conservative securities to buy his brother's Northern Pacific bonds, which greatly depreciated in value. As the bank's troubles grew fatal, Frederick Douglass, brought in, many said, so that a black man could be blamed when failure came, was made head of the bank by the white trustees to restore depositors confidence. When the bank closed its doors, thousands of poor blacks found that their passbooks, recording hard-earned small deposits, were worthless. Efforts to get the Congress to make compensation for the losses in the bank, which it had sponsored, were to no avail.

The nation's economic problems, coupled with the continuing reports of scandals within the rank of the Grant administration and the Republican party, enabled the Democrats to regain control of the House of Representatives in the election of 1874 for the first time since before the Civil War. As the new majority took its seats in 1875, investigations were launched into each of the cabinet departments. The most serious allegations were made against George M. Robeson, Secretary of the Navy, who had received what amounted to bribes from naval suppliers; Columbus Delano, Secretary of the Interior, whose son sold surveying contracts; and William W. Belknap, who regularly accepted payments from the holders of lucrative Indian trading posts. Robeson rode out the storm, but Delano was forced to resign, and the House voted a bill of impeachment against Belknap. In the summer of 1876, when other Americans were celebrating at the great Centennial Exposition in Philadelphia, which featured the immense and varied manufacturing capacities of the Republic, Washingtonians were treated to a dramatic impeachment trial in the Senate. The evidence against Belknap was indisputable, and he won acquittal only because President Grant had accepted his hasty resignation just hours before the House voted the indictment that led to the Senate's trial. The senators, therefore, were not trying an incumbent official and to save Belknap enough senators concluded that, despite his guilt, they lacked jurisdiction over the case.

As sorry as these scandals were, another struck closer to Grant personally. His private secretary, Orville Babcock, was shown to have been directly involved in widespread and lucrative schemes to defraud the government of taxes on the production of whiskey. Even when Attorney General Benjamin H. Bristow confronted Grant with damning evidence, Grant refused to fire Babcock. Instead, feeling under siege himself, he came to despise Bristow. Knowing of his secretary's guilt, the President nevertheless gave Chief Justice Waite, whom he had appointed following the death in 1873 of Chief Justice Chase, a deposition which, when read in Babcock's trial in St. Louis, won his acquittal. After the trial, when Hamilton Fish found Babcock at work as usual in the White House, he was appalled. The Secretary of State persuaded Grant to send Babcock off to inspect lighthouses, but his demotion, like Belknap's resignation, was not enough to save the moral reputation of the Grant administration.

The still-popular President, often talked about for a third term, was neither put forward as a strong contender for renomination nor permitted to control the choice of his successor. Grant took only slight comfort in the fact that the Republican convention passed up Bristow and gave the nomination to the pious and innocuous Rutherford B. Hayes (see p. 414). When they left the White House, the Grants, once again feeling homeless, set off on a two-and-a-half-year trip around the world.

The end of Reconstruction. The greatest tragedy of the Grant Era was not the corruption on which a frustrated nation fixed its attention, but the failure to complete the basic work of Reconstruction. In the end, the physical safety of the freedmen was bought only at the cost of the deprivation of their economic independence and political equality. White supremacy was reasserted through a combination of political skill and outright physical violence.

A handful of neighbors riding to a family's remote cabin to murder or torment a man unwilling to be quiet about his rights as a worker and voter or an organized band of Ku Klux Klansmen spreading terror across a county—each gave evidence that violence would not be avoided if it were needed to drive black citizens back into a subordinate position in the South. Army officers in the Freedmen's Bureau or under the direction of a Military District commander and the Justice Department had been able to prevent some of this violence. More was stopped when black citizens could count on the support of local black sheriffs or other politicians participating in the integrated administrations that were governing the Southern states. The white supremacists concluded that it would take violence, skillfully directed, to break the power of these administrations and reestablish white domination.

Their method, differently, but effectively, applied in several states, came to be called the "Mississippi Plan." In 1875, Mississippi had a carpetbagger governor, Adelbert Ames, a Union general from Maine; a scalawag senator, James L. Alcorn, a native planter who had been willing, to a degree, to cooperate with his black constituents; and a black Senator, Blanche K. Bruce. One of the state's congressmen, John R. Lynch, was black, as were members of the state legislature, sheriffs, and other local officials. The "white liners" had their work cut out for them. In an off-year election campaign that fall they proved equal to the task. Instead of refusing to engage in politics as long as black citizens held the vote, the white supremacists now reentered politics determined to dominate the black voters. The Democratic party was frank about its aim: its slogan, printed prominently in the *Yazoo City Democrat*, the *Hinds County Gazette*, and the *Aberdeen Examiner*, was "Carry the election peaceably if we can, forcibly if we must."

Adelbert Ames, from Maine to Mississippi

In town after town across the state, the Democrats organized in a disciplined way and not only put forward their "white line" candidates forcefully, but demonstrated what their opponents could expect if they continued to resist. In Macon, as investigating Senators were later told, the Republican candidate for county treasurer was "shot down walking on the pavements, shot by the democrats" because he was running for office and "because he made a speech and said he never did expect to vote a democratic ticket, and also advised the colored citizens to do the same." Such murders were carefully reported in order to frighten voters in neighboring towns. The survivors of a bloody assault on a Republican meeting in Clinton fled to Jackson and begged Governor Ames to protect them. When he asked the President for federal troops to provide that protection, still another of Grant's Attorneys General, Edwards Pierrepont, replied: "The whole public are tired of these autumnal outbursts in the South." He told the governor to first exhaust all local means of keeping order, all of which had already proved insufficient.

When election day came, there was no violence. There was no need for any; the intimidation had worked. Democrats were elected to a majority in both houses of the state legislature and Governor Ames was impeached and removed from office. Neither Senator Bruce nor Senator Alcorn was reelected. Neither was Congressman Lynch, although he regained his seat for a term in the 1880s and long remained a symbol of the reluctance of black citizens to play a docile role in politics.

Conservatives had already regained control in Georgia, Tennessee, North Carolina, and Virginia when first Texas in 1873, and then Arkansas and Alabama in 1874 were "redeemed" by Democratic exponents of white authority. With the recapture of Mississippi in 1875, only Louisiana, Florida, and South Carolina remained in Radical hands. They rejoined the other states of the old Confederacy as a result of the election of 1876 (see p. 414). In South Carolina, a gentleman planter and former Confederate general, Wade Hampton, was elected governor with the help of the Red Shirts, a band that had studied the Mississippi Plan well.

The Redeemers had succeeded in ending Reconstruction, but they had had a potent ally. Poverty was less overtly cruel than violence but no less an effective way of limiting the lives of poor-but-free people. In many cases Southern farmers who had owned many slaves, who had owned none, or who had been slaves were willing to share their corner of the region with each other. But, as each group struggled to scratch out a living, the competition for spare markets led landlords, seeking the cheapest possible labor force, to drive a wedge of hatred between impoverished white and black workers. In the rest of the nation, the white majority gave up trying to define a humane policy favorable to the freed people and turned its attention to other matters. The promises that Reconstruction had held out to black Americans as well as the aspirations they cherished were not forgotten, but their fulfillment was long deferred.

Suggestions for Reading

GENERAL

In the absence of a satisfactory comprehensive study of Reconstruction, it is well to begin with W. L. Rose, *Rehearsal for Reconstruction: The Port Royal Experiment* (1964), a brilliant assessment of both the possibilities and limitations which the freedpeople confronted. Two useful one-volume studies are K. M. Stampp, *The Era of Reconstruction 1865–1877* (1965), and J. H. Franklin, *Reconstruction After the Civil War* (1961). R. W. Patrick, *The Reconstruction of the Nation* (1967), is a more detailed survey. An eloquent and radical account is W. E. B. DuBois, *Black Reconstruction in America* (1969), and the opposite point of view is represented by C. G. Bowers, *The Tragic Era* (1929). Important articles are assembled in K. M. Stampp and Leon Litwack, eds., *Reconstruction: An Anthology of Revisionist Writings* (1969).

THE PRESIDENT AND CONGRESS

The best works on President Johnson's programs are E. L. McKitrick, *Andrew Johnson and Reconstruction* (1960); E. L. McKitrick, ed., *Andrew Johnson: A Profile* (1969); and LaWanda and J. H. Cox, *Politics, Principle, and Prejudice* (1963). An old defense of Johnson is H. K. Beale, *The Critical Year* (1930).

The most interesting and critical study of Congress is M. L. Benedict, *A Compromise of Principle: Congressional Republicans and Reconstruction, 1863–1869* (1974). In *An American Crisis* (1963), W. R. Brock sees the Radicals trying to establish the domination of the legislative branch. For a differing view, consult H. L. Trefousse, *The Radical Republicans** (1969), and D. H. Donald, *The Politics of Reconstruction, 1863–1867** (1965). Biographies of two leaders are Fawn Brodie, *Thaddeus Stevens** (1966), and D. H. Donald, *Charles Sumner and the Rights of Man* (1970). On the contribution of the abolitionists see J. M. McPherson, *The Struggle for Equality** (1964), and on relations with labor David Montgomery, *Beyond Equality** (1967). The best studies of the attempt to remove the President from office are M. L. Benedict, *The Impeachment and Trial of Andrew Johnson** (1973), and H. L. Trefousse, *Impeachment of a President* (1975).

JUDICIAL ISSUES

Constitutional changes of the period are treated in H. M. Hyman, *A More Perfect Union* (1973), and S. I. Kutler, *The Judicial Power and Reconstruction Politics* (1968). The most thorough study of the Supreme Court in this period is Charles Fairman, *Reconstruction and Reunion, 1864–88* (1971). On the most controversial amendment to the Constitution see J. B. James, *The Framing of the Fourteenth Amendment* (1956). A searching, critical examination of the motivation behind the Fifteenth Amendment is William Gillette, *The Right to Vote** (1965). An important study is Herman Belz, *Emancipation and Equal Rights: Politics and Constitutionalism in the Civil War Era** (1978).

POSTWAR SOUTH

E. M. Coulter, *The South During Reconstruction, 1865–1877* (1947), has a conservative bias, but is the most comprehensive treatment in one volume. On individual states some of the best works are V. L. Wharton, *The Negro in Mississippi, 1865–1890* (1947); on South Carolina, W. L. Rose, *Rehearsal for Reconstruction: The Port Royal Experiment** (1964); Joel Williamson, *After Slavery: The Negro in South Carolina During Reconstruction, 1861–1877** (1965); and, on Louisiana, J. G. Taylor, *Louisiana Reconstructed, 1863–1877* (1974), Peyton McCrary, *Abraham Lincoln and Reconstruction* (1978), and John Blassingame, *Black New Orleans, 1860–1880** (1973). Perceptive essays on emancipation are in Eric Foner, *Politics and Ideology in the Age of the Civil War** (1980), and *Nothing but Freedom: Emancipation and its Legacy* (1983).

On federal policies and the Southern response, military aspects are handled by J. E. Sefton, *The United States Army and Reconstruction, 1865–1877* (1967). The Freedmen's Bureau is treated in W. E. B. DuBois, "Of the Dawn of Freedom," *The Souls of Black Folk,** (1903), G. F. Bentley, *A History of the Freedmen's Bureau* (1955), and W. S. McFeely, *Yankee Stepfather: General O. O. Howard and the Freedmen** (1968). Northerners in the postwar South are the subject of L. N. Powell, *New Masters: Northern Planters during the Civil War and Reconstruction** (1980); Otto Olsen, *Carpetbagger's Crusade; The Life of Albion Winegar Tourgee* (1965); and Jacqueline Jones, *Soldiers of Light and Love: Northern Teachers and Georgia Blacks, 1865–1873* (1980). Four studies cast much light on the transition from slavery to freedom: J. L. Roark, *Masters Without Slaves: Southern Planters in the Civil War and Reconstruction** (1977); Robert Higgs, *Competition and Coercion: Blacks in the American Economy, 1865–1914** (1977); L. F. Litwack, *Been in the Storm So Long: The Aftermath of Slavery** (1980); and Vincent Harding, *There is a River: The Black Struggle for Freedom in America** (1981).

Southern resistance to Reconstruction is illuminated in Michael Perman, *Reunion Without Compromise: The South and Reconstruction, 1865–1868** (1973) and his *The Road to Redemption: Southern Politics, 1869–1880* (1984), as well as A. W. Trelease, *White Terror: The Ku Klux Klan Conspiracy and Southern Reconstruction* (1971). Steven Hahn, *The Roots of Southern Populism* (1983), examines the poverty of Southern white farmers and their attempts to find a constructive voice of protest.

GRANT ERA

On the Grant Presidency see W. B. Hesseltine *Ulysses S. Grant, Politician* (1935); Allan Nevins, *Hamilton Fish; The Inner History of the Grant Administration* (2 vols., 1957); and W. S. McFeely, *Grant: A Biography** (1981). For the breakdown of Northern support for Reconstruction, see the scathing, racist view of black legislators by J. S. Pike, an abolitionist who visited South Carolina and wrote *The Prostrate State* (1874), and V. L. Wharton, *The Negro in Mississippi, 1865–1890* (1965). For black farmers who gave up on the South, see N. I. Painter, *Exodusters: Black Migration to Kansas after Reconstruction** (1979).

*Available in paperback edition.

16
THE NEW SOUTH: REUNION AND READJUSTMENT

The first centennial anniversary of American independence made 1876 a time of reckoning as well as a year for celebration. Ceremonies of commemoration, centering at the International Exhibition in Philadelphia, went forward with due pomp and display. But citizens who took thought about just what there was to celebrate in this particular year must have been troubled by their reflections. The safest theme was material progress. Surely the hundred-year-old nation was richer, bigger, stronger, and more populous under General U. S. Grant than it had been in the time of General George Washington. Furthermore, it had survived a terrible Civil War and had emerged from that ordeal with the Union still intact, with a stronger central government, and with slavery abolished. All these were valid reasons for celebration, and patriotic celebrants dwelt on them gratefully, to the exclusion of themes that were less safe and more painful. Yet even the "safe" themes of material and political progress exposed their uglier aspects during the centennial year.

On the material side the national economy slumped toward the bottom of the longest and most severe depression up to that time. In national politics the year 1876 was noted for the exposure of scandals and corrupt deals that completed the disgrace of President Grant's Administration, the most shameful of the century. The same year witnessed a presidential election with the most doubtful and disputed results on record. As seamy and sordid in their politics as the national and state governments, many of the country's cities were also disgraced by gigantic slums filled with disease and human misery. Those who celebrated the rise of the new industrial establishment—a central theme of the Philadelphia Exhibition—had to admit that a great part of its factories and furnaces and work force stood idle throughout the centennial year.

Both those who looked to the West—traditional avenue of escape—and those concerned about the South—perennial source of conflict—had cause for dismay in 1876. Two violent events a few days apart at the peak of the centennial celebration symbolized these troubles in the West and in the South. On June 25 General George A. Custer and 265 of his troops were wiped out in battle with Sioux Indians in Montana; and on July 4 an incident between a black militia company and two white men at Hamburg, South Carolina, provoked a pitched battle between militia and armed white terrorists, followed by the murder of four black prisoners. It was a rough time for a national birthday party.

Sectional Compromise Restored

For the South and its embittered relations with the Union, the national crises of 1876 proved to be a turning point. For sixteen years, ever since Fort Sumter, North and South had settled their differences by

Cotton to market: the South was still rural

armed force—not only during the four years of war but in some measure during the twelve years that followed. And while it is true that a great deal of compromise of principle and conciliation of the white South and Northern racism had gone into Reconstruction, in the last resort military force was still available—and still used. For example, after the bloody outbreak in Hamburg, South Carolina, President Grant reversed his policy of no further military intervention in Southern states and ordered the army into that state to maintain order. More federal soldiers were in the state than at any period since the war by the time of the presidential election. That election, but more particularly the crisis over inaugurating the disputed winner, unexpectedly provided the opportunity to put an end to the policy of force and adherence to principle, and to reinstate the tradition of compromise in sectional disputes on the classic model of 1850. This would mean the end of Reconstruction and the start of a new era.

The electoral crisis of 1876.

It looked like a good year for the Democrats. Republican prospects for 1876 had been clouded by economic depression, political scandals, and growing reaction against Grant's Southern policy. The elections of 1874 had returned the Democrats to control of the House of Representatives for the first time since the Civil War. During the next two years the depression that had started in 1873 deepened, and discontent increased. The Republicans themselves were divided into factions over Reconstruction policy. "We have tried for eight years," wrote Joseph Medill, the influential Republican editor of the Chicago *Tribune*, "to uphold Negro rule in the South officered by carpetbaggers, but without exception it has resulted in failure." Reaction had set in, and devotion to the equalitarian ideals of Reconstruction was in short supply. Reformers, later known as "mugwumps" (p. 502), continued to fill newspapers with exposure of scandals in the Grant Administration. Mounting disgust with corruption in high office helped to block the leading contestant for the Republican nomination, James G. Blaine of Maine, formerly Speaker and currently minority leader in the House of Representatives. Charged with accepting bribes for favors to a railroad company and handicapped by the disfavor of President Grant, Blaine was eliminated from the race for nomination.

The Republicans nominated Rutherford B. Hayes, a comparatively obscure figure from the strategically important state of Ohio. Three times governor of his state, Hayes had a creditable war record, an unblemished reputation, and an association with mild civil-service reform. In short, he was the ideal nominee for a party bedeviled by smirched reputations and beset by scandal. Of Whig antecedents and puritani-

Rutherford B. Hayes: conciliatory conservative

cal conscience, Hayes was conservative in his economic and financial views, and conciliatory toward Southern whites. To balance the ticket, the Republicans chose Congressman William A. Wheeler of New York for Vice President.

Stressing the issue of reform, the Democrats nominated Samuel J. Tilden, governor of New York. Before his election to the governorship in 1874, Tilden had won fame by helping to smash the notorious ring of Boss Tweed, head of Tammany Hall, and by sending Tweed and others to jail; as governor, he had shattered a powerful organization of grafters known as the Canal Ring. Tilden had made a private fortune as a corporation lawyer serving railroads, and his conservative economic views and hard-money doctrines were more pleasing to the business community of the East than they were to the South and the West. Popular enthusiasm for Tilden's candidacy was further limited by his railroad associations, his secretive habits, and his poor health. In order to make up for these drawbacks, the Democrats named for Vice President Thomas A. Hendricks of Indiana, who had served his state as senator and governor and held soft-money views.

The campaign of 1876 was a struggle of exceptional bitterness and trickery. For the first time in twenty years the Democrats had a reasonable hope of winning a presidential election, and they bore down hard on Republican corruption in high places and alleged misrule in the South. Their opponents countered with bloody-shirt oratory, charging that the Democrats were sympathetic to the rebels and attacking Tilden's personal integrity. When the returns came in, the Democrats seemed to have carried the day, for the majority of popular ballots were cast for Tilden with nearly a quarter of a million to spare. And, while Tilden was conceded 184 electoral votes, only one vote short of the 185 required for election, Hayes was conceded only 165. But nineteen of the twenty contested electoral votes lay in the three Southern states that were still under Republican government—South Carolina, Louisiana, and Florida. The twentieth vote, from the Republican state of Oregon, was claimed by the Democrats on a technicality. Tilden needed only one of the twenty votes to assure his election, while Hayes had to have them all to win a bare majority of one vote. Republican managers promptly claimed all the votes and announced a Hayes victory. Charging that the Democrats had used intimidation and fraud against black voters, Republican returning boards in the three Southern states threw out enough Democratic popular votes to give those states to Hayes. Both parties had resorted to chicanery in the election, but modern scholars hold that Tilden deserved more than enough of the con-

tested votes to win. On December 6 Republican electors met and cast the votes of the three states for Hayes, but on the same day a rival set of Democratic electors cast the votes of the same states solidly for Tilden.

Congress, with a Democratic House and a Republican Senate, now faced the problem of deciding which returns were authentic and which candidate had won. The Constitution was not explicit on who should count the electoral votes, and the law was silent. As the weeks passed an ominous deadlock ensued. To break the deadlock a compromise was worked out between the political parties—but not between the sections. That came later.

The solution proposed by moderate congressmen was to refer the disputed returns to an electoral commission created for the purpose, consisting of fifteen members drawn in equal numbers from the Senate, the House, and the Supreme Court. Seven were to be Republicans, seven Democrats, and one was expected to be Justice David Davis, an independent. Counting on Justice Davis to break the tie in their favor, Democrats supported the measure in greater numbers and with more enthusiasm than the Republicans. At the last moment, however, Davis was elected United States Senator by the Illinois legislature, and his place on the commission was filled by a Republican Justice of the Supreme Court. The commission then decided

The election of 1876

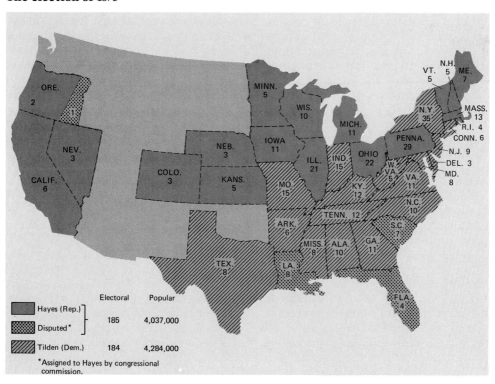

	Electoral	Popular
Hayes (Rep.)	185	4,037,000
Disputed*		
Tilden (Dem.)	184	4,284,000

*Assigned to Hayes by congressional commission.

by strictly partisan votes of eight to seven to accept the Republican returns for all twenty contested electoral votes. This in effect removed Tilden from the race and authorized the election of his opponent; but to seat Hayes required formal action of the House, and there it met resistance from the Democratic majority. Enraged by what they denounced as a "conspiracy" to defraud them of their victory, many Democrats refused to abide by the vote of the commission and staged a filibuster that threatened to prevent any election whatever and bring on anarchy. It was during this anxious interval of three weeks before inauguration day that the sectional compromise was worked out.

The Compromise of 1877. There could be no doubt that the majority of Southern whites wanted Tilden, the man they voted for, elected President. That would have guaranteed what they called "home rule" and other favors for the South. When it began to appear that Tilden was destined to be the loser, however, Southern leaders determined to salvage what they could out of defeat. Southern conservatives, some of Whig background, approached like-minded friends of Hayes, himself a former Whig, with offers of help in the electoral crisis and the possibility of future political support in exchange for a firm Republican commitment to "home rule" in the Southern states. In the short run that meant withdrawal of the federal troops that sustained the Republican governments of South Carolina and Louisiana in power, governments with as strong a claim to legitimacy as Hayes' claim to the electoral votes of those states. More important, "home rule" meant Republican abandonment of freedmen, carpetbaggers, scalawags, and Radicals, and the virtual nullification of the Fourteenth and Fifteenth Amendments and the Civil Rights Act. In short, it meant forfeiting many of the fruits of the Civil War and Reconstruction and, some thought, the honor of the Republican party. Had such a commitment been made by Tilden, a Democrat, it would have lacked the authority and permanence it gained by Republican endorsement.

Hayes nevertheless readily fell in with this policy. Not only was he looking for help in being inaugurated but he was looking ahead for conservative white allies to support a reconstituted Republican party in the South along old Whig lines. While he knew that "home rule" was always the main objective of the ex-Confederates, Hayes and his friends found other means of attracting Southern Conservatives. The depression had dried up sources of Northern investment, and carpetbaggers had exhausted the credit of the states. The only major source of capital left was the federal Treasury, and Southern congressmen were knocking at its doors with literally hundreds of bills

for internal improvements—for building levees and controlling floods along the Mississippi, for clearing harbors, rivers, and canals, for constructing bridges, public buildings, and railroads. The largest appropriation sought was a subsidy of more than $200 million for the construction of the transcontinental Texas & Pacific Railroad with southern terminals. Persuaded by intermediaries that Hayes would be friendly toward his bill, Thomas A. Scott, president of the Pennsylvania Railroad as well as the Texas· & Pacific, brought his lobby to the aid of Hayes. Southern seekers of appropriations had already discovered that Republicans were consistently more sympathetic to their internal-improvement bills than were their fellow Democrats of the North.

Meanwhile the filibuster tactics of the Democrats continued in the House, and as the deadline approached without a settlement Republicans grew more alarmed and intensified their efforts to win over Southern Democrats, thus enabling the latter to demand a higher price for their support. Southern strategists knew more was expected of them than they could deliver and that, as one of them candidly admitted later, they were playing "a bluff game." But they played it for all it was worth and with great skill. Hayes was not only committed to withdraw the troops and turn over two states to Conservative control but also to appoint a Southern Democrat to his Cabinet and permit him to hand out federal offices to his friends. The Republican candidate and his spokesmen emphasized that the new Administration would take a conciliatory policy toward the needs and wishes of Southern whites generally and particularly toward bills for internal improvements. All this was very gratifying and essential to the sectional compromise, but without the votes of Northern Democrats the Southerners could not have brought off a peaceful solution to the crisis. Other motives were at work here, and certainly among them was a rational fear of anarchy and a yearning for peace. At last Hayes' cause prevailed, and he was declared elected only two days before he took office.

The politics of reconciliation. Faithful to his promises of conciliating the Conservative South, President Hayes appointed a Southern Democrat to his Cabinet, an ex-Confederate general from Tennessee. After a few weeks of hesitation and some vigorous prodding by Southern parties to the compromise, the President ordered the troops out of the capitals of Louisiana and South Carolina, and the last two carpetbagger governments promptly collapsed. All the Southern states and the border states as well were now under Conservative control. Within a year Louisiana received more federal appropriations for internal improvements than any other state in the Union. The

The "strong" government, 1869–77   The "weak" government, 1877–81

Texas & Pacific did not get its subsidy, but the South got its road to the Pacific by way of Hayes' support of Collis P. Huntington rather than through the support he gave Tom Scott. In his courtship of the South's ex-Whig Democrats, Hayes appointed many of them to federal offices, rejecting Republican applicants to do so. Admirers cheered the President with the rebel yell during his three visits to the South. It was the first of many experiments to come in the alliance of Southern Democrats with conservative Northern Republicans.

Conciliation pleased Southern whites and eased somewhat the old tensions between North and South. But certain results of that policy disappointed the President. For one thing the ex-Whig Democrats of the South did not rally in numbers to the Republican standard as he had hoped they would. A ground swell of agrarian discontent and radicalism below the Potomac made it difficult for conservative Democratic leaders there to continue their cooperation with business-minded Republicans. Finally, congressmen of Hayes' own party resisted his policy of appeasing the South and appointing Democrats to office. And so the Republicans returned to the practice of bloody-shirt oratory and to charges of Southern disloyalty. Only a few Republicans, mainly of the abolitionist tradition, seemed disturbed by their party's desertion of the carpetbaggers and the freedmen and by its repudiation of the goals of Reconstruction policy.

The most durable aspect of conciliation was "home rule," for never between 1877 and the Little Rock crisis of 1957 were federal troops used in the South for purposes precluded by the Compromise of 1877. Eighty years is a long period as sectional compromises go—longer than any previous one lasted.

Subordination of the Freedmen

The abandonment of equality. By constitutional amendment and statutes, the United States was presumably committed to the principle of equal civil and political rights for the freedmen and to the use of federal power to guarantee them. Yet after Reconstruction the country quickly broke this commitment and virtually forgot about it for more than two generations. That the North was also remiss was indicated by racial discrimination in employment, the policies of labor unions, and the discriminatory laws of Northern cities and states. Furthermore, the Radical promise of equality was an embarrassment to Hayes' effort to reconcile the estranged South and to put aside bitter war memories.

In short, the white people of the North and South were reconciled at the expense of black people. When Hayes visited Atlanta in the fall of 1877, he told the freedmen that their "rights and interests would be safer" if Southern whites were "let alone by the general government." This sentiment was greeted with "immense enthusiasm"—by the whites. "Let alone" became the watchword of government policy in race relations as well as in industrial and business affairs. Many of the former champions of the freedmen in the North took up the new slogan and dropped their concern for the rights of the black. The *Nation* declared that the federal government should have "nothing more to do with him" and doubted that he could ever "be worked into a system of government for which you and I would have much respect."

The plea for reconciliation, the let-alone philosophy, and the prevailing disillusionment with high ideals and promises also had their effect on the Supreme Court. In a long series of decisions the Court favored white supremacy, state rights, and laissez faire and virtually nullified the Fourteenth and Fifteenth Amendments insofar as they applied to the rights of freedmen. In 1876 Chief Justice Morrison R. Waite, in *United States* v. *Cruikshank*, decided that the Fourteenth Amendment "adds nothing to the rights of one citizen as against another" and does not extend federal protection to other rights except when they are infringed by a state. Applying the same interpretation in the *Civil Rights Cases* of 1883, the Court pronounced the Civil Rights Act of 1875 void. This act had provided that all persons, regardless of race, were entitled to "the full and equal enjoyment" of all public facilities such as inns and railroads, as well as theaters and other places of amusement. In holding that the Fourteenth Amendment was a prohibition against states only, the Court said in effect that the federal government could not lawfully protect blacks against discrimination by private individuals. The court joined the President in adhering to laissez faire.

Now, with the official approval of the federal courts, the acquiescence of many Northern liberals and Radicals, and the cooperation of the Republicans, the white South completed the relegation of blacks. Their formal freedom was not seriously challenged, but their equality most certainly was.

Racism and oppression. Part of the Compromise of 1877 had been a public pledge on the part of the Southern Conservatives to protect the rights of the freedmen abandoned to their care. The pledge soon proved to be of little value. The Conservative idea of protection was the old one of paternalistic responsibility for inferiors with few rights to protect. Blacks continued to vote in many parts of the South for two decades or more, and Conservatives sought the vote of black citizens, assuring them that Southern whites were their "best friends." They tolerated elected black officials and appointed some to local, state, and federal jobs. Black state legislators and a few black congressmen continued in office until the end of the century. When these tactics failed, they coerced, bribed, and defrauded black voters or resorted to piecemeal disfranchisement. Nevertheless, competition for black votes continued through the eighties and into the nineties with a fluidity and freedom unknown after wholesale disfranchisement.

Conservatives left no doubt about their intention to "keep the Negro in his place" and to preserve white dominance in social, economic, and public relations.

The enforced intimacy of slavery had left its traces in Southern residential patterns, and the "distant intimacy" of paternalism separated the races so widely by social distance that formal segregation was often unneeded. Status was defined by race. But in public or private institutions such as schools, hospitals, asylums, orphanages, poorhouses, institutions for the blind, deaf, or dumb, and even many prisons, the prevailing practice, often unsupported by law, was segregation of the races—with as little equality for blacks as later under the law. Even so, this was an advance over the antebellum rule of exclusion, a change initiated by the Radicals, continued by the Conservatives, and often supported by the blacks. It was an advance in the sense that it was better to get separate and inferior services than none at all. In public accommodations—in trains, streetcars, and public parks, for example—race relations were more fluid and variable than elsewhere. Exclusion and erratic segregation were combined with a degree of racial integration that would later—after the turn of the century—be unthinkable.

In the 1890s, whatever fluidity, moderation, or variety remained in race relations was swept away by a new wave of Southern racism that imposed segregation by law. "Jim Crow law" made the system universal, rigid, and thorough. It was law rather than custom that reached into every corner of society and put the authority of the state and city in the voice of the railway conductor, the theater usher, or the hoodlum of street and playground. The Southern movement was supported by a rising mood of racism in other parts of the nation and met little resistance from Northern opinion or federal courts. In 1896 the Supreme Court in *Plessy* v. *Ferguson* explicitly sanctioned Jim Crow law by declaring "separate but equal" facilities constitutional.

Another reason for Southern whites to replace custom with law to control the black population was the arrival of a new generation of blacks. Unlike their parents, the younger generation was not born in slavery, was less bound by habit to bow to white demands, and was more prone to resistance. And when the law did not humble young blacks sufficiently to satisfy the mob, the mob was ready to take the law in its hands and resort to lynching—a crime that reached its peak between 1889 and 1899, when an average of some 187 lynchings a year occurred in the United States. About four-fifths of the lynchings took place in the South, and the great majority of the victims of the lynch were black.

So long as blacks voted in large numbers and cast their votes for an opposition party, as they did into the nineties, Conservative Democratic control was insecure—especially in the black belt. Failing to coopt the black vote and dissatisfied with chicanery, ballot-box stuffing, and other fraudulent controls, Conservatives turned increasingly to outright disfranchisement by law. Throughout the eighties they had experimented with restrictive measures of several kinds to reduce the black electorate. This disfranchisement movement, like that for the Jim Crow laws, received encouragement from Northern opinion and the federal courts. Elitist Northern advocates of "good government" had turned against democratic ideals of universal suffrage and blamed recent immigrants and minority races for lowering standards. In 1898 the Supreme Court in *Williams* v. *Mississippi* threw open the legal road to disfranchisement by approving the Mississippi plan, written into the state constitution, for depriving

Lynch mob, 1893

black citizens of the franchise by means of a literacy test.

The reactionary reforms of Southern politics came in waves, with two high tides eventually sweeping all states of the region, one in the early 1890s, the other in the years 1898 to 1902. The chief advocates of disfranchisement were upper-class Democrats of the black belt, who had most to gain from it; the main opponents were Republicans, Populists, a radical third party, and blacks, who had most to lose. The main devices of disfranchisement were the poll tax, registration laws, and literacy and property qualifications, some with the "understanding clause" or the "grandfather clause" as loopholes to admit desirable poor whites and illiterates.* Disfranchisement was a disastrous blow to the democratic process. Both voter participation and party opposition had been rising before the blow and fell sharply thereafter among whites as well as blacks. Black voter turnout dropped an average of 62 percent, white 26 percent, and overall turnout 37 percent. While an average of 73 percent of adult males voted in the nineties before disfranchisement, the Southern turnout in the next decade averaged only 30 percent. Opposition parties virtually collapsed, and Southern politics became a one-party system. It had

changed from a democracy to a more or less broadly based white oligarchy and was to remain so for nearly a half century.

The Atlanta Compromise. After the Civil War, the great majority of the black population remained on the land owned by whites, where many were locked into debt peonage (see p. 425). The black exodus to the Northern cities was not to begin till a later generation, but large numbers did move to the cities and towns of the South. There they entered trades and crafts, and for some years after the war greatly outnumbered white workers. Employers, however, increasingly discriminated against black labor, often at the demand of white workers, who brought pressure to drive blacks out of the better-paid, more attractive work and confine them to "Negro jobs." Gradually, blacks disappeared from some of the skilled trades they had traditionally monopolized and were excluded almost entirely from certain of the newer industries such as cotton textiles. Generally barred from emerging labor unions, they were occasionally used as strikebreakers, thereby earning additional ill will from the unions.

By the 1880s a new middle class, consisting largely of business and professional people, had grown up among the freedmen. Proportionately smaller and much poorer and weaker than the corresponding class

*That is, they might qualify by "understanding" a passage read to them or claiming a grandfather who could vote before 1867.

Students at Tuskegee Institute

of whites, the minority middle class nevertheless shared some of the attitudes and aspirations of its white counterpart. A member of that class, Booker T. Washington, became head of an industrial school for blacks at Tuskegee, Alabama, in 1881. There he preached the doctrine of work, thrift, self-help, and sobriety, conformed humbly to segregation in the South, condoned disfranchisement, and said little about lynching. Washington's attitude of humility contrasted strikingly with the influence he came to wield in dispensing Republican patronage and in shaping philanthropic and educational policies. He believed that education for blacks should stress industrial training rather than intellectual development, and his views attracted support from people of wealth and power in the North.

Booker Washington's reputation as a leader also owed much to the favor he won in the eyes of dominant whites of the South. They greeted with enthusiasm a famous speech he gave in Atlanta in 1895 at their invitation, setting forth what later came to be

**Booker T. Washington:
preacher of patience**

known as the Atlanta Compromise. In it he made sweeping concessions to the white desire for segregation, abandoned the Reconstruction demand for black equality, emphasized economic opportunity rather than political and civil rights, and identified himself and his people with the industrial and social order established by the Conservatives. To his own race he preached patience, conservatism, and the primacy of material progress as a means of attaining independence and self-respect. To those who accepted this program there appeared to be no viable alternative under white supremacy, but to the blacks who rejected Washington's Atlanta doctrine it looked more like a capitulation than a compromise.

Politics in the New South

The new regime. The new rulers of the South, claiming they had "redeemed" their states from the carpetbaggers, earned the name Redeemers. Predominantly Democrats, they often called their party the Conservative or Democratic-Conservative party out of regard for the ex-Whigs they had attracted as members. In the top ranks of the reconstituted party, along with numerous old Whigs, were to be found many businessmen and industrialists or lawyers who served their interests. High in the councils of the party and political offices of such states as Georgia, Alabama, Tennessee, and Virginia sat representatives of railroad, mining, manufacturing, and banking interests—often the foremost officials of those industries. They shared power and exchanged favors with planters in most states, but the combination did not represent a restoration of the old order. It represented instead a new phase of the revolution that had been touched off by the overthrow of the Confederacy, and in that revolution the new order played a more important and

lasting role than did Reconstruction—enduring longer, in fact, than had the antebellum Cotton Kingdom of slavery and planters.

The new state constitutions framed by the Redeemers embodied a strong reaction against the Reconstruction regimes. They revealed suspicion and distrust of legislatures and placed such hampering restrictions upon government that positive action of any sort became difficult. The new Southern Redeemer governments also reacted against Reconstruction through their policy of "retrenchment," which meant cutting taxes and starving or eliminating tax-supported public services. The chief beneficiaries of the tax policy were the railroads, the utilities, and the factories, whose burdens were lightened; and the chief victims were the public schools. The schools, which bore the stigma of carpetbagger support, were gravely crippled by Redeemer retrenchment as well as by general poverty and depression. The Redeemers also cut appropriations for other public institutions, but none so severely as those for prisons. The state governments actually turned prisoners, largely black, into a source of revenue by leasing them as cheap labor to industrialists with the right political connections. The convict-lease system, often marked by brutal exploitation, became an ugly blot on the reputation of the new regime.

This was not an era free of corrupt government and lax public morals across the country, and it would be unfair to single out the Redeemers for special censure. They invited such censure, however, by the attack they made on graft and corruption in their campaigns to overthrow the carpetbaggers. Faced with no effective party of opposition, protected by long tenure of office, and consequently immune from criticism and exposure, the Redeemers acquired habits of laxity that eventually covered several of the state governments with disgrace. In the eighties one scandal after another came to light. Some were exposed only by the

The New South through a glass darkly

absconding of state treasurers, nine of whom were guilty of defalcation or embezzlement, and one of whom defrauded Louisiana of more than a million dollars. Such losses, as an Alabamian said, made a mockery of "niggardly economy in public expenditure."

Stirrings of revolt. The "Solid South" won its name prematurely. Hardly had "home rule" been restored when revolt began to stir against the Redeemer regime. Once the pressure of occupation troops was removed, ancient class, party, and sectional antagonisms within the South began to reassert themselves. Local state parties calling themselves Independents, Greenbackers, or Readjusters organized for action. They were often cheated at elections and won only limited success, but they provide a clue to what was seething beneath the surface solidarity of Southern politics. Before the Redeemers put through their disfranchisement "reforms" described earlier, the opposition parties threatened the stability of their regime.

The most disruptive issue of all was the "readjustment," or repudiation, of state debts. So disruptive was it, in fact, that it unseated the Redeemers in some states and threatened the security of the whole regime. By the end of Reconstruction, the Southern states had incurred a total debt of about $275 million, and in nine states there was talk of scaling the debts down or partially repudiating them. In one way or another these nine states contrived to reduce their total liabilities by $150 million. Naturally the states' creditors and bondholders protested bitterly, and in each state a faction of Redeemers fought the debt-readjusters. In Tennessee the fight brought the Republicans back to power, and in Virginia it led to the triumph of a third party calling itself the Readjusters. The advocates of repudiation argued that much of the debt was a heritage from carpetbagger looting, that the

states themselves had derived little benefit from the sale of Reconstruction bonds, and that in any event the section was too impoverished and ravaged to carry the burden of Reconstruction debts.

Encouraged by the revolt against the Conservative Democrats, the Republicans began to dream of returning to power in the South through an alliance with local third parties. Even though the Republicans had little in common with these parties save their opposition to Democrats, they put aside President Hayes' commitment to the Southern Conservatives and threw their support to the reformers and debt-repudiators. "Anything to beat the Bourbons" was the Republican policy. The Conservatives responded by reviving the tactics of fraud and intimidation once used against the carpetbaggers, employing them so effectively that by 1883 they had beaten all but the last spark out of the Independent revolt and had shattered Republican hopes of exploiting it. Not for a decade was there to be further talk of insurgency in the South. This period of political torpor was not to be broken until the agrarian revolt of the 1890s.

The doctrine of the New South. There had been antebellum advocates of industrialism in the South, but they had looked on factories as a means of buttressing the old social order. Propagandists of the New South, by contrast, sought to replace the old order with an economy like that of the North, a business civilization of cities, factories, and trade, with new values and new aims. This was what the "New South" meant to its champions in the 1880s. "As for Charleston," declared an editor from that city in 1882, "the importation of about five hundred Yankees of the right stripe would put a new face on affairs, and make the whole place throb with life and vivid force."

Propaganda for the New South point of view found full voice during the 1880s and 1890s in such journals as the Atlanta *Constitution*, edited by orator

Henry W. Grady: spokesman for "the New South"

Henry W. Grady. Full of the bustle and salesmanship of business enterprise, Grady exuded optimism and good will. In an address on "The New South" delivered in 1886 to the New England Society of New York he proclaimed: "We have sowed towns and cities in the place of theories and put business above politics. We have challenged your spinners in Massachusetts and your iron-makers in Pennsylvania. . . . We have fallen in love with work." As models for young Southerners, Grady held up the businessman, especially the self-made man, the millionaire. What Grady and his friends were preaching was laissez-faire capitalism freed of restraints, a new industrial way of life, and a businessman's scale of values.

One sign of the popularity of the New South doctrine was the Southerner's eagerness for Northern approval. "Beyond all question," declared a Richmond journal, "we have been on the wrong track and should take a new departure." And Henry Watterson, a Louisville editor and orator, thought that "the ambition of the South is to out-Yankee the Yankee." But the appeal of the New South doctrine would have been less compelling had it not been embellished by sentimental tribute to the past: a heritage "never to be equalled in its chivalric strength and grace," as Grady put it. The invention of a legendary Old South and the cult of the "lost cause" revealed the curiously divided mind and the conflicting impulses of the Southern people in the new era. They marched hopefully in one direction and looked back longingly in the other.

A literary revival of the 1880s brought to national attention Southern fiction writers of the "local color" school, including Joel Chandler Harris, Thomas Nelson Pare, Kate Chopin, and George W. Cable. They sought out the picturesque, the quaint, and the exotic and wrote in colorful dialects of the region. Expressing the florid romanticism of the New South spirit, they combined a celebration of the lost cause with support of the new order. An exception was Cable, who published *The Silent South* (1885), a strong indictment of Southern racial policy, and moved to Massachusetts in 1885.

The inner tensions of the Southern mind were reflected in the career of the Georgia writer Joel Chandler Harris, author of *Uncle Remus* (1881). A gentle, rather wistful man of humble origins, Harris portrayed the old slave in quaint dialect with humor and affection, casting a spell of charm over memories of the antebellum plantation. But while he was writing his nostalgic stories about the Old South, Harris was also chief editorial-writer for Grady's Atlanta *Constitution*, doing his daily best to encourage the growth of the New South of business and industry. Both the admirers of the old order and the propagandists of the new advocated sectional "reconciliation," urging that the North abandon its reformist aims and accept the new order in the South. In political terms reconciliation was simply an alliance between conservatives of both regions built on foundations of white supremacy.

The Colonial Economy

The agrarian pattern. The dream and design of the new leaders of the South was to build an urbanized, industrialized society like that of the Yankees. But the habits and economic realities of the Old South were slow to change and hard to shake off. Despite all the factories that were constructed and the proliferation of small agricultural market towns in the interior, 96.1 percent of the North Carolinians and 94.1 percent of the Alabamians were still not classified "urban" by the census of 1890. Only 8.5 percent of the population of the South Atlantic states below Maryland was urban in 1890, as compared with 51.7 percent of the population of the North Atlantic states from Pennsylvania up. By 1900 the urban population of those Northern states had further increased by nearly 7 percent, that of the Southern states by only 1 percent. The New South was still the most rural and agrarian section in the settled portions of the country.

On the surface it would seem that deep changes had occurred in the distribution of land ownership in the South. The census of 1880 reported an amazing increase in the number of farms since 1860, and the average farm turned out to be less than half its former size. Optimists concluded that the Civil War had broken up the concentration of land in the hands of planters and had brought about "economic democracy." The truth was, however, that the old plantation lands had been parceled out in small plots among

Sharecroppers: trapped in the system

sharecroppers, each plot counting as a new "farm," and that large tracts of new land had been brought under cultivation. The sharecropper had replaced the slave, and his share of the crop depended largely on the tools, work animals, and feed the landlord furnished.

Ownership of the land tended to shift from the old planters into the hands of merchants or other

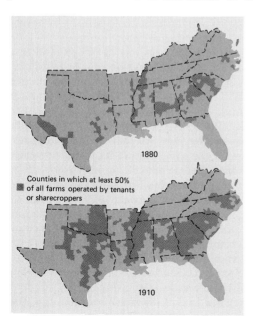

1880

Counties in which at least 50% of all farms operated by tenants or sharecroppers

1910

The increase of farm tenancy in the South

townsmen. Moreover, whatever efficiency and planning, whatever virtues of proprietorship, had resided in the old plantation system were largely missing from the sharecropper system. The old evils of land monopoly, absentee ownership, soil-mining, and the one-crop system were not only retained but intensified. From a strictly economic point of view, cropping was probably worse for the agriculture of the region than slavery had been.

The most desperate need of the Southern farmer after the war was credit. With little or no cash in hand, with few banks and no longer any factors from whom to borrow, the farmer was at the mercy of the country merchants, who enjoyed a local monopoly over credit and exploited their customers by charging outrageous prices. Merchants advanced supplies for the year with a mortgage, or "lien," on the future crop. The farmer pledged an unplanted crop for a loan of an unstipulated amount at an undesignated but enormous rate of interest averaging about 60 percent a year. Trapped by the system, a farmer might continue year after year as a sort of peon, under debt to the same merchant and under constant oversight. The lien system imposed the one-crop system, for the merchant would advance credit only against cash crops such as cotton or tobacco. The one-crop system was more characteristic of the new agricultural order than the old, and the South became more and more dependent on other sections for products it might have grown itself. The system not only impoverished farmers but stifled their hopes and depleted their incentive.

*Blacks who had lived on plantation as slaves

During the last quarter of the nineteenth century, farmers the country over were plagued by low crop prices and depression. Southern farmers shared these ills with farmers elsewhere, but they also suffered from a combination of burdens peculiar to the South. Among these was the heritage of military defeat, pillage, and occupation that had cost the section every third horse or mule. On top of these burdens were heaped the ills of sharecropping peonage and the lien system. By the 1890s a spirit of grim desperation had settled on the farmers of the South, a spirit that long manifested itself in a suspicion of city folk and their ways and a resentment of wealth and its display. This spirit was to enter into the soul of the Populist movement in the years ahead (see p. 514).

Industrial stirrings. Toward the end of the 1870s the depression that had settled over the nation in 1873 started to lift. Once again Northern investors began to show interest in opportunities below the Potomac and freed the springs of capital. The propagandists of the New South boasted that the South, like the West, was an empire ripe for exploiting. "The way to clear and large profits is open," announced a Philadelphia editor in 1877. A book appeared in 1888 on *How to Get Rich in the South* and another in 1894 describing the South as *The Road to Wealth*. The Redeemers welcomed investors with open arms, tax exemptions, and promises of cheap and docile labor.

With the willing cooperation of Southern legislatures, speculators rounded up huge grants of public lands and mineral resources. Florida attempted to grant several million more acres than were in its public domain, and Texas surrendered an area larger than the state of Indiana. In 1877 the law reserving federal lands in five Southern states for homesteaders was scrapped, and the rich Southern empire of timber, coal, and iron was thrown open to unrestricted exploitation. In the next decade nearly 6 million acres of federal lands were sold, most of them to Northern speculators, who indulged in a reckless destruction of forests and a rifling of other resources.

Exploitation of this sort, as well as more laudable schemes of industrial development, would have been impossible without dramatic improvements in transportation. Between 1880 and 1890 railroad mileage in the South, starting from a low base, increased from 16,605 miles to 39,108, a growth of 135.5 percent, 50 percent greater than the national rate of growth in mileage in the same period. Railroads opened to development the landlocked mineral resources of the South, particularly the iron mines of Tennessee, Virginia, and Alabama. Between 1876 and 1901 pig-iron production increased seventeen times in the South, as compared with an eightfold increase in the country at large. Alabama, with its unrivaled deposits of iron ore, coal, and limestone in unique proximity, quickly outstripped its Southern competitors, and by 1898 Birmingham was the largest shipping point for pig iron in the country and the third largest in the world.

So long as the Southern economy stuck to its traditional role of supplying raw materials of mine,

The growth of the railroad network in the South

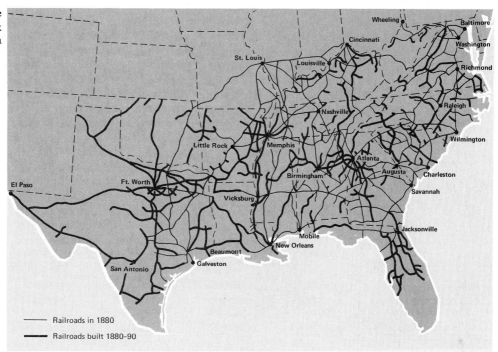

Railroads in 1880
Railroads built 1880–90

forest, and farm, it met with encouragement from Northern bankers and investors. Production of lumber and forestry products soared sensationally, as did the output of such fuels as coal and oil, and such ores as iron, sulfur, bauxite, phosphate rock, and manganese. Eastern capital entered each of these enterprises, and Eastern control followed. The same pattern was followed in the modern era of oil production, which opened with an unprecedented gusher at Spindletop, near Beaumont, Texas, in January 1901.

The tobacco industry, the oldest in the region, discovered new markets and developed new techniques of manufacture during the new era. The genius of concentrated control was a tall, rugged, red-headed North Carolinian named James Buchanan Duke, called "Buck," whose rise paralleled that of the industry. He started out in 1865 with two blind mules and a load of tobacco, all the war had left on his father's small farm. "Tobacco is the poor man's luxury," he observed, and on that insight he founded a fortune. By 1889 his industry was thoroughly mechanized, his firm was producing half the country's cigarettes, and the following year he absorbed his main competitors into the American Tobacco Company.

Linn Iron Works: Birmingham's first industry

Tobacco: new techniques of manufacture

The true symbol of the New South, however, was the cotton mill, and the zeal of its promoters stirred up a veritable "cotton mill crusade." Actually, the industry was confined largely to the Carolinas, Georgia, and Alabama. Cotton-manufacturing began in the Old South and continued to grow through the Civil War and Reconstruction, but between 1880 and 1900 the amount of capital invested in the Southern mills increased sevenfold. Much of the growth came at the expense of New England, which was unable to compete with the Southern supply of nonunion workers accustomed to long hours and low pay. The chief textile products of the South were unfinished goods that were sent north for final processing, and in this, as in the use of cheap labor, the cotton mills were typical of the South's new industries.

The colonial status. For all its boasts of industrial progress, the New South lagged far behind the rest of the country. The region remained poor, its economy undeveloped, technologically backward, and stagnant. By the end of the century the South had a smaller percentage of the nation's factories and a slightly smaller percentage of the nation's capital than it had in 1860. With few exceptions, the industries that did take root in the South were low-wage industries that gave the first rough processing to the agricultural, forestry, and mining products of the region. Transportation costs made it more economical to do this processing near the source of raw material, and large supplies of cheap, unskilled labor were an even stronger attraction to such industries. Cotton yarn, cottonseed oil, cane sugar, polished rice, fertilizers, liquors, and tobacco, and such forestry products as turpentine, resin, and lumber constituted the bulk of the South's industrial output. The final processing of these products was usually done in the North, and from the final processing came the greatest profits.

There was no law relegating the South to a raw-material economy, no plot to exclude Southerners from the better-paying jobs and the more profitable industries. What, then, were the reasons for the persistent economic backwardness of the section? A lost war, a late start, and a lack of capital were some of the reasons. More important and enduring reasons were the kind of economic system Southerners erected in place of the old one and the institutions and attitudes to which they clung. Among these was a credit system that entrapped great numbers of blacks and whites in debt peonage, stifled their initiative, bound them to a stagnant one-crop agriculture, and immobilized them as a labor force. Racism crippled the economy further by depriving blacks of education, skills, and the means of self-advancement.

Industrialization was seen as a way out, but the development of manufactures was handicapped by some special barriers. One of these barriers was the system of regional freight-rate differentials adopted in the seventies and eighties by private railway associa-

"Poor whites" in Kentucky

Wharf in Virginia: a tributary economy

tions and later given legal sanction by the Interstate Commerce Commission. These differentials meant that shippers of manufactured goods in the South and West were charged far higher rates than shippers in the privileged "Official Territory," north of the Ohio and Potomac and east of the Mississippi. The system discouraged the Southern producer from competing in the richest market area, the Northeast, but enabled the Northeastern producer to penetrate the Southern market. At the same time, favorable "commodity rates" were provided for Southern raw materials. Taken together, these rate differentials discouraged the South from developing manufactures of its own and encouraged it to concentrate on raw materials. A price differential imposed on Birmingham steel by the Pittsburgh steel-masters and their allied railroads had a similar effect. "Pittsburgh Plus" meant that buyers of Birmingham steel had to pay the Pittsburgh price *plus* the freight charge from Pittsburgh. Later, the "Birmingham Differential" replaced the freight charge with a straight additional charge of $3 a ton.

During these years the Northeast assumed something like an imperial power over the other sections, and the national economy fell into a neomercantilism reminiscent of colonial days. The Northeast discouraged the rise of competing manufactures by the combination of regionalized freight rates, steel-price dif-

ferentials, and patent control, and reduced foreign competition in its domestic markets by the protective tariff. It also monopolized the carrying trade and promoted ample supplies of raw material for its factories. In brief, the Northeast became for a long time the workshop of the nation, reserving for its own coffers the profits of processing, transporting, and distributing goods. The South was left to produce the raw materials for the new economic order, to serve as a tributary of industrial power.

Division of labor was, of course, natural in a national economy, and the South derived real benefits from its role in the form of increased job opportunities, payrolls, and taxable assets. On the other hand, this subordinate economic status imposed grave penalties on the South. As late as 1910 some 62 percent of its workers were engaged in the extractive industries—agriculture, forestry, animal husbandry, fishing, mining—as compared with 11 percent in New England and 14 percent in the Middle Atlantic states. Throughout the country, these industries paid the lowest wages of all, and the wages of Southern workers were even lower than the national average.

In wealth, living standards, and general welfare the Union was more a "house divided" now than when Lincoln first used the phrase. In 1880 the estimated per capita wealth in the South was $376 as compared with a national average of $870. No Southern state came within $300 of the national average nor within $550 of the average outside the South. In 1900 the national average in per capita wealth stood at $1,165, and in the South the average was $509. Per capita income of the same year in the South Atlantic and East South Central states was less than 50 percent of the national average. Little wonder that the region was noted for its "poor whites" and its "poor blacks" as well. Poverty was a characteristic of the regional economy. Closely related to that poverty was a lag in education, libraries, public health, and living standard.

The New South represented a striking shift in the geography of political power. In the seventy-two years between Washington and Lincoln, Southerners held the Presidency for fifty years and the title of Chief Justice of the Supreme Court for sixty years. They furnished more than half the Justices, nearly half the men of Cabinet rank, and more than half the Speakers of the House of Representatives. During the next half-century, by contrast, no Southerner save Andrew Johnson served as President or Vice President, and the South furnished only 14 of the 133 Cabinet members, 7 of the 31 Justices of the Supreme Court, and 2 of the 12 Speakers of the House. From the power and glory of the eighteenth and early nineteenth centuries the South had fallen to a lowly state. In the process of reunion it had become the frontier of a new order that was expanding southward as well as westward.

Suggestions for Reading

C. B. Dew has a "Critical Essay on Recent Works" in C. V. Woodward, *Origins of the New South, 1877–1913** (1971), a general study first published in 1951. P. M. Gaston, *The New South Creed: A Study in Southern Mythmaking** (1970), is well described by its title. On sectional reconciliation, P. H. Buck, *The Road to Reunion, 1865–1900** (1937), is still valuable. W. J. Cash, *The Mind of the South** (1941), contains provocative interpretations of the New South period, assessed in C. V. Woodward, *American Counterpoint: Slavery and Racism in the North-South Dialogue** (1971). By the latter author, see also *The Burden of Southern History** (1960).

On the sectional settlement of 1877 C. V. Woodward, *Reunion and Reaction: The Compromise of 1877 and the End of Reconstruction* (1951), is challenged in part by K. J. Polakoff, *The Politics of Inertia: The Election of 1876 and the End of Reconstruction* (1973). President Hayes' Southern policy is treated in K. E. Davison, *The Presidency of Rutherford B. Hayes** (1972). Republican efforts in the South are examined in V. P. DeSantis, *Republicans Face the Southern Question: The New Departure Years, 1877–1897* (1959), and S. P. Hirshon, *Farewell to the Bloody Shirt: Northern Republicans and the Southern Negro, 1877–1893* (1962).

The plight of Southern black people is freshly illuminated by R. L. Ransom and Richard Sutch, *One Kind of Freedom: The Economic Consequences of Emancipation** (1977), and from a different view by Robert Higgs, *Competition and Coercion: Blacks in the American Economy, 1865–1914** (1977). G. M. Fredrickson, *Black Image in the White Mind* (1971), has much to say on racism in this period. C. V. Woodward, *The Strange Career of Jim Crow** (3rd, rev. ed., 1974), emphasizes legal segregation, and H. N. Rabinowitz, *Race Relations in the Urban South, 1865–1890** (1978), shows how exclusion preceded segregation. The struggles of blacks and their friends are admirably treated by J. M. McPherson, *The Abolitionist Legacy: From Reconstruction to the NAACP** (1975), and with emphasis on the blacks' side by August Meier, *Negro Thought In America, 1880–1915: Racial Ideologies in the Age of Booker T. Washington** (1963). L. R. Harlan, *Booker T. Washington: The Making of a Negro Leader, 1856–1901** (1972), is first rate, as is his *Booker T. Washington: The Wizard of Tuskegee* (1983). An important interpretation of the whole subject is Joel Williamson, *The Crucible of Race: Black–White Relations in the American South since Emancipation* (1984).

Much is added to our understanding of politics in the New South by J. M. Kousser, *The Shaping of Southern Politics: Suffrage Restriction and the Establishment of the One-Party South, 1880–1910*** (1974). In some respects he revises V. O. Key, Jr., *Southern Politics in State and Nation* (1949), but the latter is still useful on the nineteenth as well as the twentieth century. Paul Lewinson, *Race, Class, and Party: A History of Negro Suffrage and White Politics in the South* (1932), shows how the race issue has been exploited. Among biographies the following are of interest: J. F. Wall, *Henry Watterson: Reconstructed Rebel* (1956); F. B. Simkins, *Pitchfork Ben Tillman: South Carolinian* (1944); and C. V. Woodward, *Tom Watson: Agrarian Rebel*** (1938). D. M. Potter, *The South and the Concurrent Majority* (1972), provides insight on the ruling group, and C. N. Degler, *The Other South: Southern Dissenters in the Nineteenth Century*** (1974), on the opposition.

Industrial and business history of the South has not been developed as much as other subjects. Some aspects are covered in M. L. Greenhut and W. T. Whitman, eds., *Essays in Southern Economic Development* (1964). H. L. Herring, *Southern Industry and Regional Development* (1941), views the Southern type of industrialization critically and analytically. James Blicksilver, *Cotton Manufacturing in the Southeast: An Historical Analysis* (1959), is a general account and David Carlton, *Mill and Town in South Carolina, 1880–1920*** (1982), revises old interpretations. N. M. Tilley, *The Bright Tobacco Industry, 1860–1929* (1948), treats the South's oldest industry in this period. J. F. Stover, *The Railroads of the South* (1955), is the best book on the subject, and W. H. Joubert, *Southern Freight Rates in Transition* (1949), is helpful. A biography of the Southern industrial propagandist is R. B. Nixon, *Henry W. Grady: Spokesman of the New South* (1943).

Southern men of letters have furnished some of the most profound insights into the life of the South. Of special relevance to this period are some of the works of William Faulkner, particularly *The Hamlet*** (1940) and *Go Down Moses*** (1942).

*Available in paperback edition.

17
THE NEW WEST: EMPIRE WITHIN A NATION

After the Civil War the American people embarked on the taming and exploiting of an area greater than all the territory that had been settled since the landing at Jamestown in 1607. Up to this time the settlers of the trans-Mississippi West had occupied only its eastern and western fringes, in one tier of states beyond the Mississippi and in another tier half a continent beyond along the Pacific coast. Between these two frontiers, separated by fifteen hundred miles, lay 1.2 billion acres inhabited by only 1.5 million souls. A vast and fabulous expanse of ocean-like plains, it was a scene broken by spired and towering mountain ranges, grassy plateaus, painted deserts, and breathtaking canyons. Of all the American wests, this was the one that most completely captured the imagination of the world.

Americans had conquered many frontiers in the past, but the New West was different from all the others. The experience of the pioneers there was less like that of their forebears in settling the forested "wests" of the East and more like the adventures of nineteenth-century Europeans in Africa and Asia. America was a nation with a built-in empire, an empire disguised as a nation. What the English and the western Europeans had to seek "somewhere east of Suez," their American contemporaries, until the region was tamed and settled, might find somewhere west of the wide Missouri. The impulse behind this late-nineteenth-century quest was more than a desire for private gain. It partook of the strange drive that

was sending Western men and women into all the remote corners of the world, to impose their will upon people of color and to master exotic environments. If in Rudyard Kipling's Mandalay there were no Ten Commandments and the best was like the worst, so it was too in Deadwood Gulch and in a hundred mining towns, cow towns, and trading posts of the Wild West.

Subordination of the Indians

The Great Plains environment. The steady westward advance of the American frontier ground to a halt in Texas and Kansas and then (except for Utah, p. 282) skipped all the way to the Pacific coast. What stopped the pioneer was the forbidding new environment of the Great Plains. Abnormally dry, almost treeless, and mostly level, the plains had their own particular soil, weather, plant life, animal life, and human life. Writing of the Texas plains, Colonel Richard J. Dodge warned: "Every bush had its thorns, every animal, reptile, or insect had its horn, tooth, or sting, every male human his revolver, and each was ready to use his weapon of defense on any unfortunate sojourner, on the smallest, or even without the smallest provocation."

So harsh and uninhabitable did the plains at first appear that the Easterner wrote them off as wasteland

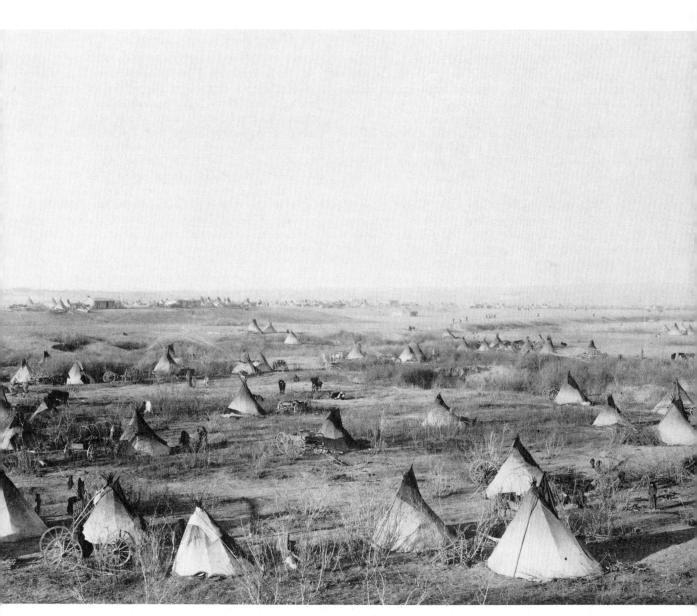

Sioux Indian camp, Deadwood, South Dakota

and until 1860 labeled the vast area on maps "The Great American Desert." Dry winds parched the throats of Easterners, cracked their lips, and made their eyes smart. Everything seemed different. There were chinooks, or warm mountain winds, northers, blizzards, and hailstorms, and all but the chinooks could bring distress or disaster. The rivers dried up unexpectedly, and when they flowed their waters were often unpalatable and sometimes treacherous. The slight rainfall, usually under fifteen inches a year, made traditional methods of farming impractical, and the new environment rendered useless many other traditions and familiar methods. The woodcraft and Indian craft that had enabled the frontiersman to master the humid, forested East were not adapted to the treeless, arid plains, and neither were his ax, his plow, his canoe, or his long rifle. And neither, for that matter, were some of his laws and institutions.

Once rebellion in the South had been put down, Americans turned anew to the taming of the Great Plains. Here they encountered rebels of a different and even more difficult breed.

The plains Indians. Of some three hundred thousand Indians left in the United States in 1865, more than two-thirds lived on the Great Plains. The frontiersman called them "wild Indians"—and so they were, in comparison with their sedentary cousins of the Eastern forests. The only mounted Indians the white man ever encountered, most of them were nomadic and nonagricultural. Above all, they were fierce, skillful, and implacable warriors—"the most effectual barrier," according to Walter P. Webb, "ever set up by a native American population against European invaders in a temperate zone." Against all comers—Spanish, French, English, and American— they had held their own as masters of the plains for two and a half centuries.

The Spanish had introduced horses into Mexico in the sixteenth century, and the animals had multiplied and spread northward over the plains in wild herds. Before then, the plains Indians had been miserable, earthbound creatures, hard pressed to earn a living and defend themselves. The horse revolutionized the life of the tribes and brought on the golden era of the plains Indians—an era that had about reached its peak when the Anglo-Americans first encountered them. The horse made the Indians more mobile and hence more nomadic than ever, less agricultural, more warlike, and, most important of all, far more effective buffalo-hunters. Estimates of the buffalo population of the Great Plains at the end of the Civil War range up to twelve million and more. The buffalo was even more indispensable to the plains Indians than the horse, for it provided them with food, clothing, shelter, and even fuel. Necessities, luxuries, ornaments, tools, bed-

ding, their very tepees—all were fashioned from the flesh, bone, and hide of the buffalo. The nomadic tribes moved back and forth across the plains with the great herds and organized their life and religion around the hunt. Whatever threatened the buffalo threatened their very existence.

Present knowledge about the great diversity of Indian cultures, languages, tribal alliances, and intertribal wars makes the old concept of a clear white-Indian conflict as outmoded as the old notion of civilization versus savagery. Each tribe had its own pattern of white-Indian relations, and tribes differed in the degree to which they adopted white ways, combined them with tribal ways, or sought to revive and maintain tribal traditions. They entered alliances with Anglos and Hispanics to fight enemy tribes. To picture them as entirely passive or the sole victims is false. And it does not increase understanding to foster white ancestral guilt and romanticize the red man.

Although their cultures varied from that of the peaceful tribes of the pueblos to that of fierce nomadic tribes, all the plains Indians shared the culture of neolithic man, using stone knives, stone scrapers, and bone awls as tools. The warriors carried bows and arrows and fourteen-foot, stone-tipped lances for hunting and warfare. Yet in combat the stone-age man asked no quarter of early industrial man. With his short three-foot bow and a quiver of two-score arrows or more, the Comanche would ride three hundred yards and get off twenty arrows with startling force and accuracy while the Texan was firing one shot and reloading his long and cumbersome rifle. Even the Colt six-shooter, with which the white man began arming himself in the 1840s, did not entirely overcome the Indian's advantage. As armor he carried a loosely slung shield made of buffalo hide so tough that it could deflect a bullet. The arrows he used against an enemy, unlike those he used in the hunt, were fitted with heads that came off in the wound when the shaft was withdrawn. The plains Indians lived on horseback, and in case of emergency even used their mounts as food. They could hang by a heel to one side of the horse and discharge arrows under its neck; they could execute intricate cavalry maneuvers controlled by a secret system of communications and signals that was the envy of white military experts.

Until the white man finally crushed the plains Indians, he was conscious of them mainly as warriors, as ruthless and dreaded enemies who sometimes held military supremacy in their own country. The Indian's conception of the conduct of war and the treatment of captives differed from that of the white man. His reputation for cruelty was probably as much deserved as his opponent's reputation for ruthlessness. The military struggle between the two races on the

Great Plains was marked on both sides by a peculiar ferocity and savagery.

White supremacy in the West. So long as Americans thought of the plains as the "Great American Desert" and as "one big reservation" for red people, conflict as well as contact between the races was rare. But in the 1850s the situation changed. Mass migrations got under way across the plains to Oregon; miners began to beg for protection; the Kansas and Nebraska territories were organized; and politicians demanded that the Indians be pushed aside to north and south to clear the way for transportation and settlement. In 1851 the federal government adopted a new Indian policy of "concentration," under which the chiefs of the plains tribes were persuaded to restrict their people to areas the white newcomers solemnly promised they would never violate. Caught between the mining frontier that, as we shall see, was closing in from the west, and an agricultural frontier advancing from the east, the plains Indian was soon to learn what the forest Indian had learned long before: trust none of the white man's promises, however solemn. The Indians were further embittered by the behavior of corrupt officials of the Indian Bureau of the Interior Department, who defrauded them of their land, and cheated them in trade, and by the treachery of a reckless breed of beaver-trappers, gold-prospectors, hunters, and outlaws. Then in 1858 and 1859 the Pike's Peak Gold Rush sent thousands hell-bent for Colorado and trouble, soon to be joined by deserters and draft-dodgers from the Union and Confederate armies.

Indian war broke out in Colorado about the time the Civil War was starting in the East. The immediate provocation was the effort of government officials to force the Arapaho and Cheyenne to abandon all claim to the area that had been granted them forever only ten years before. Many braves rejected the agreement made by their chiefs and took the warpath. After an intermittent warfare of pillaging, home-burning, and murdering that went on for more than three years, they sued for peace. Chief Black Kettle of the Cheyenne, after being assured of protection, was surprised and trapped by a force led by Colonel John M. Chivington on the night of November 28, 1864. Ignoring Black Kettle's attempts to surrender, the militia shot, knifed, scalped, clubbed, and mutilated men, women, and children indiscriminately. Chief Black Kettle and a few warriors escaped, but before a year had passed

Westering

Map labels: Blackfeet, Crow, Teton-Dakota, Chief Joseph's Rebellion 1877, Arapaho, Little Big Horn 1876, Nez Percé, Bannock, Fetterman Massacre 1866, Sioux, Snake, "Battle" of Wounded Knee 1890, Cheyenne, Crow, Chivington Massacre 1864, Navaho, Kiowa, Hopi, Zuñi, Red River War 1869-74, Apache, Comanche

Reservations in 1875
Reservations in 1900
--- Present state boundaries

the Cheyenne and Arapaho, as well as the Kiowa and Comanche, were compelled to surrender their claims and move on to more restricted areas assigned them.

Hardly had peace been restored to the Southwest in the fall of 1865 when war broke out in the Northwest. The bloody Sioux War of 1865–67 was brought on by many forces, but it was triggered by the demands of miners who had invaded the Sioux Country. In response to their request, the federal government announced its intention to build a road through the foothills of the Big Horn Mountains to connect the mining towns of Bozeman and Virginia City with the East. Such a road would spoil one of the Sioux' favorite hunting grounds, and Chief Red Cloud warned that it would be resisted. Sioux warriors ambushed a party of soldiers under Captain W. J. Fetterman near Fort Phil Kearny in December 1866 and slaughtered all eighty-two of its members.

The Chivington and Fetterman massacres, together with scores of minor battles and endless shooting scrapes, prompted the federal government to review its Indian policy in 1867. Easterners clashed with Westerners, humanitarian impulses with fire-and-sword military policies, and at last authority over the Indians was split between the Department of the Interior, which would placate them with gifts, annuities, and reservations, and the War Department, which was accustomed to punish with violence. The Westerner's disgust was reflected in a letter signed "Texas" in the Chicago Tribune: "Give us Phil Sheridan, and send Phil-anthropy to the devil." It is hard to say at times whether West or South was in fiercer revolt against the Eastern philanthropists. The East prevailed temporarily against the West as it had against the South, however, and sent out a Peace Commission of four civilians and three generals in the autumn of 1867 to end the Sioux War and to inaugurate a policy of "small reservations" to replace the old one of "concentration." The new policy meant that the Indians were to abandon their way of life, submit to segregation in small out-of-the-way reservations on land spurned by whites, and accept government tutelage in learning "to walk the white man's road." The Black Hills section of the Dakota Territory was to be set aside for the northern tribes. Poor lands in the western part of what is now Oklahoma, of which the five civilized tribes of the Southeast had just been defrauded on false charges of treason because of their

Confederate sympathies, were to be divided among the plains Indians of the Southwest.

The white man's policy toward the red man in these years contrasted strangely with his professed policy toward the black man, though both promised uplift by education. The same Congress that devised Reconstruction to bring equality and integration to the Negro of the South approved strict segregation and inequality for the Indian of the West. General William T. Sherman, the deliverer of the Southern slaves, was now in command in the West to enforce policy toward Indians.

But many Indians refused to renounce their way of life and enter meekly into the reservations. When they took the warpath in the summer of 1868, General Sherman unleashed his troopers and launched a decade of remorseless war against them. "I will urge General Sheridan to push his measures for the utter destruction and subjugation of all who are outside [the reservations] in a hostile attitude," Sherman wrote. "I propose that [he] shall prosecute the war with vindictive earnestness against all hostile Indians, till they are obliterated or beg for mercy." It took more than two hundred battles from 1869 through 1874 to restore peace. Sometimes called a war of "extermination," this, like other Indian conflicts, was not one-sided. A recent study finds that during the entire nineteenth century no more than five thousand Indians were killed, while the Indians killed some seven thousand soldiers and civilians in the same period. These figures, however, do not include indirect casualties caused by starvation and disease.

President Grant was persuaded early in his Administration to place under a dozen religious denominations the control of Indians living on reservations. Supported by government funds, agents chosen by religious bodies sought to educate, "civilize," and assimilate their charges. These actions became known unofficially as "Grant's Peace Policy." Indians refusing to settle on the reservations, however, were mercilessly subjected to the very unpeaceful policy of the United States Army. Coordination of the two policies

General Sherman: negotiating with the Sioux

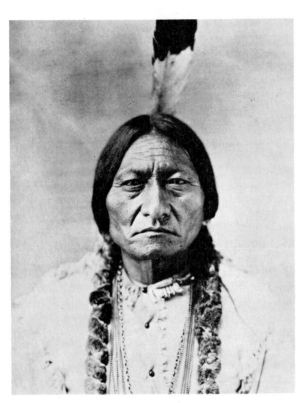

Chief Sitting Bull: compelled to surrender

served to remove most Indians from the path of white settlers and developers.

By the end of 1874 all seemed calm. Then in 1875, when government authorities permitted tens of thousands of gold-prospectors to crowd into the Black Hills, the Sioux and other northern Indians reacted violently. At the Battle of the Little Big Horn on June 25, 1876, the rash young General George A. Custer and 265 men were wiped out in the general's first, and last, stand in the new Sioux War. In spite of this victory, the Indians were compelled to surrender the following fall. Chief Sitting Bull and a few warriors fled to Canada, but, facing starvation, they were forced to sue for peace in 1881. The Nez Percé Indians of Oregon staged a rebellion that was repressed in 1877, and the survivors of this once-proud tribe were herded into a barren preserve in Indian Territory to be ravaged by disease and hunger. The last incident of the Indian wars was the sickening "Battle" of Wounded Knee in 1890, in which United States troops mowed down two hundred Dakota men, women, and children.

Long before the fighting ended, the near-extermination of the buffalo herds had hastened the collapse of Indian resistance. At first the indiscriminate shooting of buffalo was motivated by little more than the desire for "sport" or for the diversion of railroad hands and passengers, who might incidentally help to clear the tracks and curb a nuisance. But in 1871, when it was discovered that buffalo pelts and leather could be marketed at a profit, the slaughter was organized on a commercial basis. Now professional hunters and skinners working in teams stepped up the butchery. The advance of the railroads hastened the end of the herds as well as the subduing of the Indians. By 1878 the vast southern herd, the larger of the two main herds, had been wiped out. Five years later, when collectors tried to round up a few specimens of what had recently been the most numerous breed of large animals in the world, they found fewer than two hundred in all the West.

The slaughter of the buffalo, the expansion of railroads and settlers, and the pressure of the army did much to disintegrate the tribal culture of the Indians, but the humanitarian reformers waged a different kind of attack on that culture. They won their fight against physical extermination of the Indian only to substitute their own policy of relentless attack on Indian society, customs, and religion and on tribal unity and authority. This, they sincerely believed, was necessary to "civilize" the Indians and assimilate them into white civilization. As one of them put it, the object was "to get the Indian out of the blanket and into trousers . . . with a *pocket that aches to be filled with dollars.*" It was an article of faith among reformers that work, education, and the ownership of private property were the only way to salvation. They were especially opposed to tribal as against individual ownership of land.

Supported by humanitarian "friends of the Indian" and land-grabbers alike, the reform program was partly realized by the Dawes Act of 1887, which struck at tribal authority by authorizing the breakup of reservations and the "allotment in severalty" of small holdings to individuals. The land allotted was often unsuited to farming and the new owners unprepared to be farmers. Allotments were held in trust at first, but when final title was granted, four out of five of the holders were quickly fleeced of their property or lost it in other ways. The surplus of reservation tribal lands after allotments was put up for sale and much the greater part of it lost to the tribes. By the early years of the twentieth century the only considerable reservations remaining were those in the semiarid country of the Southwest.

Indians receiving allotments were to become citizens of the United States. Thus the oldest residents of the land became its newest citizens. But their government simultaneously deprived them of some of the basic rights of citizens. Those remaining on reservations were virtually imprisoned and pauperized. They were subject to the withholding of rations—those still entitled to them—in an effort to compel them to abandon tribal customs and loyalties. The government carried religious persecution to the point of espionage and force. The sacred Sun Dance, supreme expression of tribal unity, was outlawed as "pagan." The corruption of the Indian Bureau and its agents was checked by civil-service reform, but one meaning of this was that the misguided Indian policy was administered more effectively and destructively than before. The real trouble, according to John Collier, a reformer critic of a later generation, was not corrupt agents but "collective corruption, corruption which did not know it was corrupt, and which reached deep into the intelligence of a nation. It was such a collective corruption that dominated the plains-Indian record and nearly the whole Indian record of the United States."

The Era of the Bonanzas

Webb in *The Great Frontier* distinguishes between the "primary windfalls" and the "secondary windfalls" that are gleaned from any frontier. The primary windfalls are the first easy pickings—gold, silver,

furs—that are gained with little investment of energy or time. The secondary windfalls require more patience and expense. Usually the primary windfalls are grabbed up early in the game. The Spanish mined the precious metals in their quarter of the New World or seized them from the Indians in the sixteenth and seventeenth centuries, and the French gathered their bales of furs in Canada a little later. Entering the continent north of the gold and south of the furs, the Anglo-Americans were obliged to concentrate on secondary windfalls. Then late in the nineteenth century, after the frontier had become a prosaic matter of timber, corn, and cotton, they belatedly entered upon a fabulous phase of frontier history that for the rest of the world had faded into the mists of legend with the conquistadors and the Spanish treasure ships. The beaver pelts had been gathered, and we have seen what happened to the buffalo. But there remained the bonanzas of gold and silver and the lush grass left by the bison.

The miner's bonanza. There had been gold rushes from time to time in the East, but from 1804 to 1866 the five-state Appalachian gold field had yielded less

The Great Plains environment

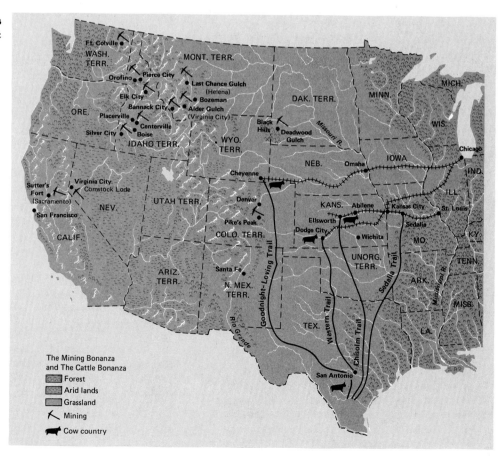

The Mining Bonanza
and The Cattle Bonanza
Forest
Arid lands
Grassland
Mining
Cow country

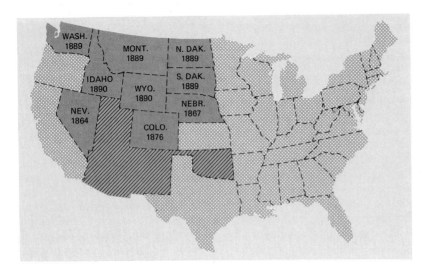

than $20 million. An entirely new scale was set by the California yield of $555 million in a single decade, 1848–58. In the 1860s and 1870s the turbulent gold rush of the forty-niners (see p. 292) was to be repeated with variations time and again in the mountain areas of Nevada, Colorado, Arizona, Idaho, Montana, and Wyoming. Since the Californians usually led the invasion of these areas, the mining frontier advanced eastward instead of westward. The Californians also developed the primitive technology of "placer" mining, by which "pay dirt" was washed in pans, "cradles," or sluice boxes. Armed with nothing more than a pick and shovel and a crude pan, the lucky prospector could gather up loose gold that had washed down through debris to bedrock. The richer deposits of gold, usually in deep-lying veins of quartz, could only be mined with machinery that was beyond the means of the prospector and had to await the corporation. During the sixties placer mining was more and more superseded by quartz mining.

The lure of the bonanza—even the hope of modest pay dirt—was enough to keep thousands of prospectors feverishly exploring gulches and canyons for three decades. Only the exceptional claim really paid off, but the promise of fabulous riches and the wild thrill of discovery seemed reward enough. After the discovery came the inevitable leak of the secret and the headlong scramble by other prospectors to stake a claim. One such rush in 1861 was described by a witness:

> As the news radiated—and it was not long in spreading—picks and shovels were thrown down, claims deserted and turn your eye where you would, you could see droves of people coming in "hot haste" to town, some packing one thing on their backs and some another, all intent on scaling the mountains through frost and snow, and taking up a claim in the new El Dorado. In town

there was a perfect jam—a mass of human infatuation, jostling, shoving and elbowing each other.

The prospectors' invasion of the interior was started by discoveries in Colorado and Nevada. During the summer of 1858 prospectors made a number of small strikes in the vicinity of what was later to become Denver. Rumors of these finds, wildly and perhaps deliberately exaggerated, spread rapidly through the frontier region and started a rush for the Pike's Peak country that fall. A new discovery in May 1859, followed by several smaller ones, had offered some justification for the excitement, but the great majority of fortune-hunters were doomed to disappointment.

In the meantime prospectors had struck it rich on the eastern slope of the Sierras in Nevada opposite the California fields on the western slope: the incredibly rich Comstock Lode, the biggest bonanza of them all! At the first rumor, a thundering stampede of fifteen thousand claim-stakers blanketed the Washoe district. But most of the gold and silver was locked in veins of quartz, and little mining could be done until quartz mills and mining machinery were brought in. Not until 1873, after heroic tunneling operations and giant engineering feats under the direction of John W. Mackay and his partners, was the greatest lode of silver and gold struck. From 1859 to 1879 the total output of the Comstock mines was $350 million, of which 45 percent was in gold and 55 percent in silver. No deposits of equal richness have ever been recorded in ancient or modern mining history.

Perched on the roof of this subterranean treasure house on the steep side of Mount Davidson, seventy-two hundred feet above sea level, was Virginia City, the most celebrated of the Western mining towns. Mark Twain, who arrived at the diggings in the early days, described the town in *Roughing It:*

> So great was the pack, that buggies frequently had to wait half an hour for an opportunity to cross

Last Chance Gulch, 1865

the principal street. Joy sat on every countenance, and there was a glad, almost fierce, intensity in every eye, that told of the money-getting schemes that were seething in every brain and the high hope that held sway in every heart . . . a dozen breweries and half a dozen jails and station-houses in full operation, and some talk of building a church. The "flush times" were in magnificent flower!

After Comstock one strike followed another in western Nevada. None was so rich as Comstock, but all served to attract an unstable population to the territory and to increase the demand for statehood. Eight days before the election of 1864 Nevada became a state and promptly furnished three electoral votes for Lincoln.

In the meantime the future states of Washington, Idaho, and Montana were the scene of gold rushes and flush times. During the years from Bull Run to Appomattox "yonder-siders" from California joined "pilgrims" from the East and seasoned prospectors from Nevada in stampedes to Orofino, Pierce City, Elk City, Boise, Placerville, Centerville, and Silver City. Some remained in Idaho as permanent settlers, but only fifteen thousand were living there in 1870. Many joined the great Montana gold rush around Bannack City, then jumped on to the spectacular diggings in Alder Gulch that produced $30 million of gold in three years, and ended up at Last Chance Gulch, where Helena was first laid out as a mining camp. A

few more strikes after the war turned up the last surface gold in Idaho and Montana; then the placer miners passed on, leaving ghost towns behind them. As in Nevada, the richest deposits lay in deep veins of quartz that could be reached only by expensive shafts

The lure of the bonanza: placer mining

and crushed only by heavy mills. Eastern capital moved in and opened up new mines in the seventies and eighties.

During the gold rushes a motley assortment of humanity accumulated on the mining frontier. The population of one camp was somewhat unscientifically classified as "Saxon, Celt, Teuton, Gaul, Greaser, Celestial, and Indian." The 206 souls of another camp were more carefully tabulated as 73 American white citizens, 37 Chinese, 35 British subjects, 29 Mexicans and Spaniards, 8 Negroes, and the rest assorted Europeans. Every camp of any size attracted its share of lawless outcasts—jailbirds, gamblers, prostitutes, deserters, desperadoes, stagecoach-robbers. And every town had to decide whether or not to let the outcasts take over. As one observer described life in Last Chance Gulch in 1864: "Not a day or night passed which did not yield its full fruition of fights, quarrels, wounds, or murders. The crack of the revolver was often heard above the merry notes of the violin. . . . Pistols flashed, bowie knives flourished, and braggart oaths filled the air." The United States government was far off and preoccupied with other matters, and its arm was not always long enough to reach into Nevada and Idaho. As a result the miners developed their own informal codes of law and their own informal means of enforcement. Throughout the region there was a loose resort to vigilantism, a more or less formalized lynch law intended to terrify the desperadoes. Though they were usually led by the elite with conservative purposes, vigilantes left a heritage of law defiance and mob rule.

In a grand finale at Deadwood Gulch in the Black Hills of what later became South Dakota the miners' frontier outdid itself in a lurid caricature of its reputation. The curtain was rung down in the 1870s on the rowdiest brawls, the wildest desperadoes, and the most vigilant vigilantes of them all. After the Black Hills rush the prospectors and their supporting casts trooped off the scene, leaving mining to heavy investors and engineers. The frontier's "primary windfall" of precious metals had been stripped off, though the serious business of mining had only begun.

The cattleman's bonanza. The windfall of the early cattlemen was almost as rich and free as that of the early miners. The cows harvested the free crop of grass, turned it into beef and hides, transported these commodities to market on the hoof, and obligingly dropped calves as replacements.

For a brief interlude between the passing of the Indian and the buffalo and the entry of the farmer and the barbed-wire fence, the Great Plains witnessed the most picturesque industrial drama ever staged—the drama of the open range and the cattle ranch. If the Southern planter could once claim that cotton was king, the Western cattleman could proclaim with equal fervor that grass was king. For the time being, at least, the plains were one limitless, fenceless, gateless pasture of rich, succulent, and ownerless grass that was there for the taking. Within an incredibly short period the herds of bison had been replaced and outnumbered by the herds of cattle.

The miner's invasion of the mountain and plains country came mainly from the Far West: the cattlemen, their animals, and their ranch culture invaded from the South. Herdsmen had acquired some of the cowboy's arts and lingo on their long trek across the Gulf states and the antebellum Southwest, but it was not until they had reached Texas and had begun to handle Spanish cattle from horseback that the craft took on its Mexican flavor and exotic style. A diamond-shaped area of the tip of Texas, with San Antonio at its apex, was the cradle of the future cowboy and his long-horned charges. The bulk of the cattle, a Spanish stock, grew up wild and were said to be "fifty times more dangerous to footmen than the fiercest buffalo." A tough, stringy, durable breed, wonderfully adapted to the plains, they multiplied so rapidly that they became a pest. Within just one decade the cattle population of Texas increased over 1,000 percent, and by 1860 cattle were estimated at nearly 5 million in that state alone.

Even before the Civil War Texas cattlemen had made a few inconsequential drives to Northern markets, and after the war inducements multiplied. During the 1860s the population of the United States increased 22 percent, while the number of cattle in the country decreased about 7 percent. But industrialization was piling up big meat markets in the cities and pushing the railroad out to the plains. At the end of the war cattle that brought $3 to $5 a head in Texas could be sold for $30 to $50 a head in Northern markets. Fantastic profits had recently induced speculators to bring Confederate cotton through armed ranks of blue and gray to Yankee mills, and Texans were not to be daunted by the mere twelve or fifteen hundred miles that separated them from the fabulous meat markets in the North. In 1866 they set forth on long drives north with more than a quarter of a million head during that year. Taking the most direct route to the nearest railhead, Sedalia, Missouri, the cattlemen fell into the hands of thieves along the wooded parts of their route. Thereafter they kept to the open plains. The first town founded for the specific purpose of receiving cows for shipment was Abilene, Kansas, established by J. G. McCoy (single-handedly, he implied) on the Hannibal and St. Joe Railroad in 1867.

Other cow towns followed—Wichita, Ellsworth, Dodge City—pushing farther and farther westward and southward with the railroad, an indispensable

Texas roundup

adjunct to the cattle kingdom. The Texas trails themselves pushed in the same direction toward the Texas Panhandle and eastern New Mexico and Colorado. The trails shifted during the years of the long drive, to take advantage of the best grazing and water supplies. Some of them—the Goodnight-Loving Trail, the Western Trail, and the Chisholm Trail—left broad, brown, beaten tracks across hundreds of miles of grasslands. Riders of the long drive, beset by heartbreaking misfortunes, watched helplessly as the weight of their droves dwindled on the way to market. Nevertheless, the cowboys drove more than 5 million head of cattle northward over these trails between 1866 and 1888, after which the trails faded out of the industry.

Not all the Texas cattle were sold directly for beef. Of the record drive of six hundred thousand in 1871 only half could find buyers and the rest spent the winter as "feeders" in the neighboring areas and corn states. It was mainly from this surplus of the Texas drives, many of them crossed with Hereford bulls to produce the white-faced hybrid, that the Great Plains area was stocked. Many herds were driven directly to the ranges of New Mexico, Arizona, Colorado, Wyoming, Montana, and the Dakotas to feed mining camps and railroad-builders and to supply the ranchers' demand for fresh stock. Some Eastern cattle, called "pilgrims" (as were the miners from the East), contributed slightly to the stocking of the plains. In the amazingly brief period of fifteen years, by 1880, the cattlemen and their ranches had spread over the whole vast grassland from the Rio Grande into Canada as well as up into the recesses of the Rockies. Between 1880 and 1890 cattle production on the plains increased from 10 percent to 21 percent of the total.

With the boom of the 1880s, the monarchs of the cattle kingdom became intoxicated with the magnificence of their domain and its immediate prospects. The depression of the seventies had been rolled aside, the Indians had been driven into reservations, the railroads were coming on, and neither the homesteader nor barbed wire had yet arrived in menacing quantity. Beef prices were soaring and the grass was growing higher by the hour. No wonder the cow king got a wonderful feeling that everything was going his way. His optimism spread abroad, and investors from the four corners of the earth rushed to the plains to seek their fortunes.

As a symbol of this spectacular adventure, the public took to its heart not the cow king but his hired hand, and there the cowboy has remained enshrined, his cult faithfully tended by votaries of screen and television. Known sometimes as "cowpoke" or "cowpuncher," names derived from an early method of prodding lagging critters with long poles, the cowboy is more popularly identified with the lariat and the branding iron. His picturesque accouterments—sombrero, spurs, long-heeled boots, chaps, gloves, and saddle, which he called his "workbench"—were strictly functional, not ornamental, and strictly adapted to life on horseback. There, indeed, much of his life was spent—eighteen hours or more a day during phases of the long drive. Each cowboy had a "mount" of from eight to fourteen horses, depending on the work he was doing and the class of horses. Normally a hardworking man of Spartan and sober habits, the cowboy has come to share with the sailor a public image derived from his rare escapades of frantic recreation after long ordeals. As for the cowboy's addiction to lethal six-guns, it was exaggerated.

Violence of the shooting-iron sort, however, was unavoidable in the open-range cattle kingdom. With millions of dollars' worth of property wandering at large on public lands, unfenced and poorly marked, rustlers found the temptation overwhelming. Since government was remote and undependable, cattlemen resorted to private associations for protection and self-government in matters of roundup, branding, and breeding. These associations sometimes furnished all the government there was. The sort of justice they dispensed and the methods they used were similar to the rough frontier government produced in the mining camps.

Even with free pasturage and virgin grassland, cattle-raising on the open range was extravagant and uneconomical. It exposed the herds to weather hazards, made adequate care of animals impossible and improvement of breeds difficult, encouraged rough and wasteful handling of cattle, and provoked costly and sometimes bloody range disputes. The approaching doom of the free range was further hastened by the expanding railroads and their loads of settlers, who staked claims and ran fences, and by the sheep-herders. But the cattlemen contributed to their own downfall. They resorted to land fraud, monopoly, and ruthless violence to protect their interests. They even adopted for their own use before homesteaders arrived that concrete denial of the open range, the barbed-wire fence: Charles Goodnight ran one all the way across the Texas Panhandle into New Mexico. Worse still, they overstocked and overgrazed the range.

The day of reckoning dawned in 1885, when beef prices started to tumble. On top of that, during the severe winter of 1885–86 up to 85 percent of the herds on the southern ranges either starved or froze to death. A bad drought the following summer scorched the grass and left the animals in poor condition. Then the legendary winter of 1886–87 fastened its cruel grip on the plains and brought panic to men as well as animals. When the thaw finally came, emaciated corpses of enormous herds were left stacked up against fences or piled deep in coulees. Loss of cattle in the northern plains was estimated to be 40 to 50 percent.

The disaster spelled the end of the great beef bonanza. It ruined large corporations and many individual ranchers and took the heart out of the open-range enterprise. There was little left of the reckless confidence with which cattlemen had greeted the great risks of the open range in its heyday. Open-range cattlemen were soon replaced by operators with the money to buy and fence in their own pasturage and monopolize water supplies. The steady retreat of investment to the security of privately owned land meant that the cattle industry was becoming a sober business instead of a high, wide, and dangerous adventure.

The Farmer Moves West

Ever since 1607 American farmers had been moving west to break new ground. But in the last three decades of the nineteenth century they occupied and brought under cultivation more land than in all the years before 1870. It might seem natural to attribute this rapid expansion to the free-homestead policy adopted in 1862 (see p. 403). Homesteading did work very well in the upper prairie frontier prior to 1880, but before we jump to the conclusion that free land explained the rapid multiplication of farms, however, it would be well to review that policy as a whole.

American land policy. The number of farms in the United States increased from some 2,000,000 in 1860 to 5,737,000 in 1900. And yet fewer than 600,000 homesteads were patented in those years, and they accounted for only 80,000,000 acres out of the more than 430,000,000 acres that were added to the total land in farms. Thus even if all the farmers who filed claims had been bona fide homesteaders, they would have accounted for fewer than one-sixth of the new farms and a little more than one-sixth of the added acreage. Actually, a great number of the so-called homesteads fell into the hands of large landholders and did not become farms until they were sold to settlers by speculators.

Nothing could have been further from the intention of the framers of the Homestead Act than the promotion of land monopoly. On the contrary, by distributing the bounty of free land among needy people they had hoped to defeat land monopoly. In practice, however, the great American promise of free land—a promise that was published around the world—turned out to be pretty much a delusion for the majority of new farmers. One trouble was that few prospective homesteaders could afford to take advantage of the opportunity, because they lacked the capital to transport their families and possessions to the public domain, stock up with expensive machinery, and stick it out for years until the farm became self-supporting. Fewer still understood the new type of agriculture required on the arid plains. Two-thirds of all homestead claimants before 1890 failed at the venture. Speculators hired people to stake out homesteads, falsely claim they had fulfilled the required conditions, and then turn over the land to their employer.

But the fundamental weakness of the Homestead Act was that it was not appropriate to much of the region where it applied. The law covered all public lands, of course, but not long after the act was passed the great bulk of public lands available for homesteading lay on the Great Plains and beyond. The Eastern congressmen who framed the law for the plains knew little about the needs of the people who were eventually going to live there. To the farmer back in the humid East a 160-acre tract seemed ideal for a family-sized farm—a good deal larger than the average, in fact. In the arid or semiarid West, however, a 160-acre tract was too small for grazing or dry farming and too large for irrigated farming. Of the last there was little anyway, so the great Western complaint was against the smallness of holdings. If the East persisted in writing laws for the West that did not work, said the Westerners, then the West was justified in ignoring or violating them.

In land policy, as in Indian policy, it proved difficult to reconcile the views of East and West—particularly since the Eastern outcry was against land monopoly and the Western demand was for larger and larger units of land. One attempt to adjust land policy to Western needs was the Timber Culture Act of 1873, which permitted homesteaders to add another 160 acres of relatively treeless land to their holdings provided they would plant trees on one-quarter of it within four years. The law failed to increase rainfall, however, and nine out of ten claimants are said to have made no serious effort to forest their holdings.

A more absurd law was the Desert Land Act of 1877, which offered 640 acres to anyone who would pay 25 cents an acre down and promise to irrigate the land within three years. Upon presenting proof of irrigation and paying an additional dollar per acre the claimant could close the deal. The trouble here was that the law required irrigation where no water was to be had. Cattlemen seized on the Desert Land Act to enlarge their holdings, but at least 95 percent of the "proofs" of irrigation were estimated to be fraudulent.

The Timber and Stone Act of 1878 permitted any citizen, or any alien with first papers, to buy at $2.50 an acre 160 acres of land "unfit for cultivation" and valuable chiefly for timber and stone. This act was as enticing an invitation to the timber barons as the Desert Land Act had been to the cattlemen. Using dummy entrymen to claim quarter-sections and deed them promptly to the corporation that paid them, lumber monopolists gobbled up vast empires of forest lands.

Taking advantage of cash sale and public auction of government lands, speculators moved in early and cornered the choice lands, the probable town sites, and lands along streams and roads to hold for high prices. When bona fide homesteaders finally arrived on the scene to stake out their claims, they usually had to choose from the less desirable and the poorly lo-

cated tracts or else pay the speculators' price. In addition to about 100 million acres bought from the federal land office, the entrepreneurs bought up another 100 million acres from shrinking Indian reservations that became available under the government's policy of concentration and 140 million acres from state land holdings. This accounted for some 340 million acres that were beyond the reach of homestead privileges.

Between 1850 and 1871 the federal government and the states had granted railroad corporations over 200 million acres of land to encourage construction (see p. 403), making the railroads the largest landjobbers of the West. Not all of this land was patented. But the form of the federal grants meant that many millions of acres in addition to the actual land granted were withheld from settlement. The railroad lands lay on both sides of the track, from twenty to forty square miles for every mile of track laid in the territories and up to twenty for every mile laid in the states. This land was not arranged in solid strips, however, but in alternate sections, checkerboard fashion. But the whole solid strip was commonly withheld from settlement until the railroad chose its right-of-way and decided which alternate sections to keep. Great belts of land on either side of the tracks were placed beyond the homesteader's reach. At one time or another some three-tenths of the area of the country, and a much greater proportion of the West, was forbidden to use.

Homesteaders were obliged either to accept areas remote from the rails or to pay the higher price the railroads asked. In 1887 this evil was alleviated by the Cleveland Administration (see p. 508), which threw open to settlement most of the land thus withheld.

The advance of settlement. The railroads became the principal colonizers as well as the biggest landowners of the New West. Rapid settlement along their lines meant larger revenues from passenger fares and freight charges and more land sales. Railroads and states sold settlers nearly six times as much land as the farmers were able to obtain by homesteading. Each Western road had its land department and its bureau of immigration, and each Western state its agency to advertise and exaggerate opportunities for settlers. Steamship companies with an eye to emigrant passengers joined in the campaign abroad; working with railroad agents, they plastered Europe with posters and literature in all important languages calculated to attract settlers to the "Garden of the West." The railroads provided what the Homestead Act had neglected: credit terms, special passenger rates, and agricultural guidance and assistance for prospective

purchasers and settlers. The success of the railroad colonizers was striking, and their campaigns in Europe infected whole countries with the "American fever." From Norway, Sweden, and Denmark, which were especially susceptible, peasants by the millions emigrated to the Northwest. By 1890 Minnesota had four hundred towns bearing Swedish names, and Irish and German colonies were sprinkled across Minnesota, Nebraska, and Dakota Territory. Whatever the shortcomings, frauds, and injustices of Western land policy, and whatever the delusions spread by promoters about a Land of Promise, all these evils should be viewed in comparison with realities in Europe. There productive land was almost totally unavailable save at prohibitive prices, and land ownership beyond the dreams of most rural people. Of some fourteen million Europeans who moved to America in the 1870s and 1880s many of them came with the hope of a farm of their own, most of them to stay in the belief that they had improved their lot.

As in the past, however, the states immediately to the east of the advancing frontier furnished a large proportion of the new settlers. In the 1870s some 190 million acres, an area equal to that of Great Britain

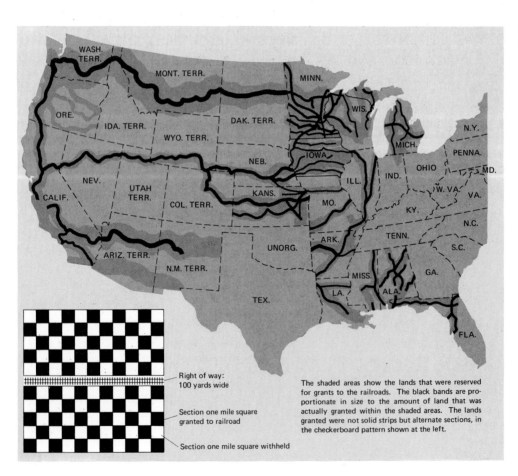

Federal grants to the railroads

The shaded areas show the lands that were reserved for grants to the railroads. The black bands are proportionate in size to the amount of land that was actually granted within the shaded areas. The lands granted were not solid strips but alternate sections, in the checkerboard pattern shown at the left.

Right of way: 100 yards wide

Section one mile square granted to railroad

Section one mile square withheld

Guthrie, Oklahoma, 1889: holding down a claim

and France combined, were added to the cultivated area of the country, mostly just to the west of the Minnesota-Louisiana tier of states. The line of settlement surged westward irregularly, first along the river valleys, rapidly along the growing railroad lines, and out over the rolling plains. A frontier in Kansas that had not budged perceptibly in two decades forged rapidly ahead in the seventies, and both Kansas and Nebraska had filled out to the edge of the semiarid plains by 1880. To the north the frontier advanced in a succession of three "Dakota Booms" roughly coinciding with three contemporaneous gold rushes. A demonstration of how to make a 100 percent profit in wheat-growing, put on by the Northern Pacific Railway after the Panic of 1873, started a rush that covered three hundred miles of the Red River Valley with "bonanza farms" ranging up to one hundred thousand acres in size. Farther north in Dakota Territory was the special province of James J. Hill, inspired colonizer of the Northwest and head of the Great Northern Railway. Hill planned and directed the settlement of thousands of pioneers along the tracks of his road to the Pacific. By 1885 all of Dakota east of the Missouri River was settled, and the population had increased 400 percent in five years. The mountainous territories to the west, except for the Mormon settlements of Utah, were slower in attracting settlers, but by the mid-eighties homesteaders in western Nebraska and Wyoming were challenging the cattlemen there.

Far to the south, in what was to become New Mexico and Arizona, a frontier of Mexican-American settlers moved north and west after the Civil War. Spreading out from their historic settlements along the upper Rio Grande that dated back to the sixteenth century, these Hispano sheepmen ran head on into expanding Anglo cattlemen. In violent clashes inspired by cultural and racial hostility, as well as economic conflict, the Hispano expansion came to a halt in the 1870s. Through the remaining years of the century, Mexican migrant laborers poured in from south of the border to work on railroads, mines, and cotton fields. Not until the twentieth century, however, did the wave of Mexican migration crest—a wave that was to make these people one of the largest minority groups in the country.

In the meantime farms in Texas more than doubled during the seventies. As both the Texas and the Kansas frontiers approached the semiarid country to the west, avid land-seekers began to eye the tempting lands of the Indian Territory between the two states. Egged on by railroad companies with actual or projected lines in the territory, agitators defied the troops guarding the boundaries, repeatedly invaded the territory, and besieged Congress with demands to throw the cowed and defeated Indian tribes out of their last refuge. Congress yielded to their demands and on April 22, 1889, threw open some 2 million acres of the Oklahoma District in the heart of the territory. At the signal, thousands of "Boomers" ("Sooners" had sneaked in earlier) riding on every conceivable vehicle, including fifteen trains with passengers jamming the roofs, swarmed into the district, staked it off in claims, and founded two cities—all within a few hours. Congress yielded to pressure again and created the Oklahoma Territory on May 2, 1890. In succeeding years one strip after another was opened—the largest, the 6 million acres of the Cherokee Outlet, in 1893—until the entire area of Oklahoma had been settled.

The superintendent of the census of 1890 discovered after the returns were in that something was missing: the long-familiar frontier. "Up to and including 1880," he reported, "the country had a frontier of settlement, but at present the unsettled area has been so broken into by isolated bodies of settlement that there can hardly be said to be a frontier line." In 1893 Frederick Jackson Turner, a young historian from Wisconsin, undertook to interpret the meaning of this development in a paper entitled "The Significance of the Frontier in American History." A devoted son of the West, Turner maintained that contact with the frontier fostered, among other things, a continuous rebirth and rejuvenation of democracy—a conclusion not always easy to reconcile with the way land was distributed and the frontier advanced.

New farms and new methods. The tribulations of the new pioneers of prairie and plain rivaled those of the Jamestown settlers in the early seventeenth century. Like the plagues that the God of Moses sent against the Egyptians, new calamities visited Western farmers with each season. Hardly had the winter blizzards ceased when melting snow brought flash floods to menace man and beast. Summer temperatures soared to 118°; drought and hot winds seared corn to crisp blades and whitened settlers' faces with the salt

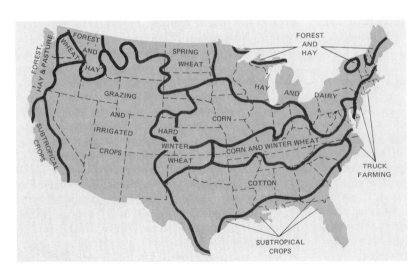

Agricultural regions of the United States

The frontier as innovator

of sweat. Worst of all were the grasshoppers, especially during the terrible plagues of the mid-seventies. The insects came in clouds that darkened the sun, cracked the limbs of trees with their weight, and covered the ground inches deep. Prairie fires, dust storms, marauding Indians, claim-jumpers, and rattlesnakes further chastened the spirit of the pioneers and discouraged all but the sturdiest.

Mrs. Abigail Scott Duniway, woman suffrage leader in the Northwest, described her own lot later in a pioneer community of Oregon: "To bear two children in two and a half years from my marriage . . . to sew and cook, and wash and iron; to bake and clean and stew and fry; to be, in short, a general pioneer drudge, with never a penny of my own, was not pleasant business for an erstwhile school teacher."

Gradually inventiveness and industry solved many of the problems of soil and climate and overcame the lack of wood and water. In their first few years the homesteaders lived in miserable sod houses, half buried in the prairie and roofed with slabs of cut turf. But later, when the railroad brought down the cost of lumber, they built frame houses. The problem of how to fence their land in a woodless, railless, stoneless region was solved by the invention of barbed wire. Of the several types devised, the most successful was patented by Joseph F. Glidden, an Illinois farmer, in November 1874. Joining forces with a wire-manufacturer, Glidden began mass production two years later, and by 1883 the Glidden factory was turning out six hundred miles of barbed wire every ten hours. Farmers and cattlemen strung it up as fast as it was produced.

The problem of water supply was harder to solve. The only reliable sources of supply lay far below the surface, too deep to reach by open, hand-dug wells. And even when a well was drilled, pumping the water up two hundred to eight hundred feet by hand was impractical. The obvious solution was to harness the free power of the winds and by 1880 scores of small firms were producing windmills adapted to this purpose.

To meet the problem of cultivating soil in semi-arid country without irrigation, Westerners developed the technique of "dry farming" where rainfall was at least ten inches per year. To break the tough soil of the plains and cultivate larger farms where labor was

Mechanized farming: Minnesota wheat

Plains farm: "harsh realities"

scarcer than ever, the farmer needed a new type of machinery. A revolution in farm machinery had started before 1860, and most of the basic patents had been granted by that year. But the mass production of machines came only after the Civil War.

The plow that most successfully broke the plains was devised by James Oliver of Indiana. After working on it for twenty-five years, by 1877 he had perfected the modern chilled-iron plow and smooth-surfaced moldboard. On bonanza farms in California before 1900 huge steam tractors were pulling sixteen plows, four harrows, and a seed drill, simultaneously breaking and planting as much as fifty acres a day.

Machine harvesting of wheat was improved in 1880 by a mechanical twine-binder that tied up the cut bundles. An even speedier device, used in drier parts of the West, was the header, which cut off the heads of the grain and left the stalk for pasturage or plowing under. The threshing machine was improved over the years by refinements that increased its capacity and efficiency, and in 1884 a blowing device was developed for stacking straw.

The soft winter wheat of the East could not withstand the rigors of the new climate and was replaced by a new variety imported from northern Europe and by Turkey Red from the Crimea. To mill the hard grain of the new varieties, the basic idea of the roller mill was borrowed from Hungary, and chilled-iron rollers were added by 1879. By the early seventies the storing, loading, handling, and transporting of wheat had all been reduced to mechanical processes.

The most striking results of mechanized farming were achieved in wheat production. An acre that had required 61 hours to farm by hand took only 3 hours to farm by machine, and where one man could farm only 7½ acres by old methods he could take on 135 acres in the nineties. Mechanization released men from drudgery and stupefying toil. On the other hand, in the very states where mechanization was most prevalent there was a remarkable growth of tenancy in the last two decades of the century and a corresponding decline in the percentage of farmers working their own farms. The farmers, like the placer miners and the range cattlemen, were destined in the late eighties for trouble and disenchantment with the Golden West. They fell victims to their own illusions.

The illusions of the farmer were part of a great national illusion dating from the early years of the republic. This was what Henry Nash Smith in *Virgin Land* has called "The Myth of the Garden"—the myth that the West was a realizable utopia, an agrarian Eden where free land and honest toil would produce a virtuous yeomanry and the good life. According to the myth, the West was the true source of national regeneration, the means of realizing the ideals of democracy and equality, and it was celebrated by poets, novelists, and historians alike. "All of the associations called up by the spoken word, the West," wrote the Western novelist Hamlin Garland in 1891, "were fabulous, mythic, hopeful." To the frontier West Frederick Jackson Turner attributed "that buoyancy and exuberance which comes with freedom." But the stark contrast between the hopes fostered by the myth and the harsh realities of experience could not escape even the dullest farmer. Far from utopian were the sod house, the dust storm, the grasshopper plague. "So this is the reality of the dream!" exclaims a character in a Garland novel. "A shanty on a barren plain, hot and lone as a desert. My God!"

To end on a note of defeat and disenchantment, however, would be to misrepresent the history of the last and most colorful of the nation's many wests. That adventure was too full of the "buoyancy and exuberance" that Turner celebrated to be fully characterized in terms of greed, oppression, and disappointment. The Western experience left a profound and lasting impact on the American mind and culture: in literature as reflected in Mark Twain, Bret Harte, or Willa Cather; in the arts as seen in painting, photography, and film; and in science as represented in the work of Clarence King and John Muir. In folklore, ballad, and story the legends of Billy the Kid, Wild Bill Hickok, Calamity Jane, and Buffalo Bill captured the popular imagination. They also captured the imagination of Europe. Buffalo Bill Cody landed his "Wild West Show" with hundreds of cowboys and Indians in England in 1887, opened with a command performance before Queen Victoria and Prime Minister Gladstone, and went on to tour Western Europe, a tour that was repeated annually into the following century. Cody himself was the hero of some 200 novels, and the "Original Buffalo Bill Library" contained more than 700 titles. Karl May, a German novelist who wrote 70 Westerns, was the favorite writer of both Albert Einstein and Adolf Hitler. Italian filmmakers alone released 130 western movies in 1964 and 1965. The West became and remained an international frontier of the popular imagination.

Suggestions for Reading

Frederick Merk, *History of the Westward Movement* (1978), is the fruit of a lifetime study. R. A. Billington, *Westward Expansion: A History of the American Frontier* (1967), stresses the Turner thesis, and T. D. Clark, *Frontier America: The Story of the Westward Movement* (2nd ed., 1969), disclaims the thesis. The thesis itself appears in an essay by F. J. Turner, "The Significance of the Frontier in American History," in his *The Frontier in American History** (1920). R. A. Billington, *America's Frontier Heritage** (1967), is a synthesis of recent thought on the subject. W. P. Webb, *The Great Plains** (1931), is a provocative study of regional culture and environmental influences, as is his *The Great Frontier** (1952, rev. ed., 1964). H. R. Lamar, *The Far Southwest, 1846–1912** (1966), is an excellent history of territories. J. C. Malin, *The Grassland of North America* (1947), brings agricultural and geographical science to the aid of historical understanding. Wayne Gard, *The Great Buffalo Hunt** (1959), is the best book on this dramatic subject, and R. G. Athearn, *Union Pacific Country** (1976), is best on another. The West as symbol and myth in American thought is brilliantly analyzed in H. N. Smith, *Virgin Land** (1950), and in European thought by R. A. Billington, *Land of Savagery, Land of Promise: The European Image of the American Frontier* (1981).

Three general histories of the Indians are recommended: W. E. Washburn, *The Indian in America** (1975); W. T. Hagan, *American Indians** (1961); and J. R. Swanton, *The Indian Tribes of North America* (1953). Two champions of the red man's rights have left moving accounts: H. H. Jackson, *A Century of Dishonor* (1881), and J. J. Collier, *The Indians of the Americas** (1947). On reform see F. P. Prucha, *American Indian Policy in Crisis: Christian Reformers and the Indians, 1865–1900* (1976), and R. W. Mardock, *Reformers and the American Indian* (1971). L. B. Priest, *Uncle Sam's Stepchildren: The Reformation of United States Indian Policy, 1865–1887** (1942), defends the reformers. H. L. Fritz, *The Movement for Indian Assimilation, 1860–1890* (1963), treats the philanthropists. Revealing books on military activities are R. G. Atherton, *William Tecumseh Sherman and the Settlement of the West* (1956); E. I. Stewart, *Custer's Luck** (1955); and C. C. Rister, *Border Command: General Phil Sheridan in the West* (1944). On white stereotypes, see R. F. Berkhofer, Jr., *The White Man's Indian: Images of the American Indian from Columbus to the Present** (1978).

On mining, the best reading on this period is R. W. Paul, *Mining Frontiers of the Far West, 1848–1880** (1963); D. A. Smith, *Rocky Mountain Mining Camps** (1967); and W. S. Greever, *The Bonanza West: The Story of the Western Mining Rushes, 1848–1900* (1963). C. H. Shinn, *The Story of the Mine* (1896) and *Mining Camps: A Study in American Frontier Government** (1885), are based on first-hand experience. For colorful reminiscences, see Mark Twain, *Roughing It** (1872), and Dan De Quille, *History of the Big Bonanza** (1876, reprinted 1947).

The cattleman's bonanza is briefly surveyed in E. S. Osgood, *The Day of the Cattleman** (1929). Maurice Frank, W. T. Jackson, and A. W. Spring, *When Grass Was King* (1957), is a roundup of scholarship. Lewis Atherton, *The Cattle Kings** (1961), is thoughtful and sympathetic. Also helpful are J. M. Skaggs, *The Cattle Trailing Industry: Between Supply and Demand, 1865–1890* (1973); G. M. Gressley, *Bankers and Cattlemen* (1966); E. C. Abbott and H. H. Smith, *We Pointed Them North** (1955); and R. R. Dykstra, *The Cattle Towns** (1968). Of the vast cowboy literature, Andy Adams, *The Log of a Cowboy** (1927), and J. F. Dobie, ed., *A Texas Cowboy* (1950), contain firsthand experiences; J. B. Frantz and J. E. Choate, *The American Cowboy: The Myth and the Reality* (1955), is a realistic analysis.

The plight of the farmers of the West appears grim in F. A. Shannon, *The Farmer's Last Frontier: Agriculture, 1860–1897** (1945), and more hopeful in G. C. Fite, *The Farmer's Frontier, 1865–1900** (1966). On the history of American land policy and its administration, two works of value are P. W. Gates, *History of Public Land Development* (1968), and R. M. Robbins, *Our Landed Heritage: The Public Domain, 1776–1936** (1942). The history of the new farm machinery is found in Waldemar Kaempffert, *A Popular History of American Invention* (1924), and R. M. Wik, *Steam Power on the American Farm* (1953). On a neglected minority see M. S. Meier and Feliciano Rivera, *The Chicanos: A History of Mexican Americans** (1972), and D. W. Meinig, *Southwest** (1971). The pioneer farm on the Western frontier is pictured in Everett Dick, *The Sod-House Frontier, 1854–1890* (1937). Vivid fictional accounts are Willa Cather, *O Pioneers!** (1913) and *My Antonia** (1918); O. E. Rølvaag, *Giants in the Earth** (1927); and Mari Sandoz, *Old Jules** (1935).

*Available in a paperback edition.

18
THE ORDEAL OF INDUSTRIALIZATION

The return of peace in 1865 had stimulated magnificent expectations among fortune-builders, profit-makers, and industrial entrepreneurs. "The truth is," Senator John Sherman wrote his brother General William T. Sherman, "the close of the war with our resources unimpaired gives an elevation, a scope to the ideas of leading capitalists, far higher than anything ever undertaken in this country before. They talk of millions as confidently as formerly of thousands." Their high hopes and expectations seemed justified by all they surveyed: half a continent to be developed; a built-in empire rich in coal, iron, oil, waterpower, lumber—most of the resources essential for great industrial power; a responsive federal government eager to further business interests; the greatest free-trade market in the world surrounded by a high protective-tariff barrier; and European immigrants swarming in to provide cheap labor. Surely the stage appeared to be set for the "heroic age" of industrial enterprise that has been glorified in legend.

Americans believed then and have continued to believe that their economy set the pace and outstripped all others in its rapid rate of industrial growth in the late nineteenth century and after. Furthermore, those on the victorious side of the Civil War chose to believe that it not only achieved moral aims but material wonders as well and played an important part in stimulating what they considered to be the unequaled speed and efficiency of American industrial progress.

In recent years, however, students of comparative growth have questioned the validity of that faith. They point out that because of rapid population growth in the United States its gross national product increased faster than in nations of Europe, but that in growth measured by product per capita the American economy did not take the lead. And production and distribution per capita are more closely related to individual welfare than is gross production. The legend of American economic superiority needs to be revised in some respects.

However unavoidable the Civil War may have been, it was more devastating and exhausting than any European war between 1815 and 1914. On balance it probably did more to retard than to stimulate growth in the national economy. The same may be said of some of the very natural endowments once thought to have been unique American advantages. The high rate of natural increase in population, for example, produced a larger percentage of nonworkers, higher investment in child-rearing and new households, as well as retarded savings and lower per capita income. The millions of immigrants provided cheap labor (and again, low per capita income), but not well-adjusted, educated, or geographically distributed labor—or labor highly endowed with "the Protestant work ethic." The very size of the country, whose vast expanse was the pride of patriots, contrasts unfavorably with the compact location of factories, resources,

Central Pacific rail-head

and markets in Europe and points up American disadvantages. Where a one-hundred-mile railroad was adequate there, it took one thousand miles of rails to do the job here. Far-flung raw materials and settlements deprived manufacturers of usable capital, slowed the movement of capital, created problems of management, curbed technological innovation, and produced conflict and frustration with local jurisdictions, jealousies, and corrupt governments.

Whether because of these or other deterrents and handicaps, American economic growth in product per capita during the famous age of enterprise lagged behind that of European leaders such as Germany, France, and Sweden, though it remained above that of Great Britain. It is the economic paradox of the period 1880–1914, when Americans were exploiting their fabulous natural resources and developing mass production and were assumed to be leading the world, that their country instead remained at about the average level of growth per capita maintained in northwestern European countries. Of course, it should be remembered that the leading countries had a very high rate and that Western Europe was increasing its industrial power enormously in those years. To have kept up with the average in such a race was a remarkable achievement.

Size and numbers and rate of population increase did count heavily in gross national product and sheer value of manufactured goods, and the United States looked better in comparative growth on those terms. In 1860 the United States was a second-rate industrial country, lagging behind the United Kingdom and perhaps France and Germany. But by 1890 the United States had stepped into first place, and the value of its manufactured goods almost equaled the combined production of all the three former leaders. Between the eve of the Civil War and First World War, American manufacturing production multiplied twelve times over. The growth rate of national product in those years was consistently higher than that of any other technologically advanced nation. In sheer size there was surely something "heroic" about the scale, if nothing else.

The Railroad Empire

"The generation between 1865 and 1895 was already mortgaged to the railways," reflected Henry Adams, "and no one knew it better than the generation itself." This was the generation that planned, built, financed, and made the first attempts to control the most extensive railroad network in the world. The headlong haste and heedless ethics of its experience

Railroad workers: spanning the continent

are caught in the national expression "railroaded through." No one, not even the enemies of the railroad, could be found in that age to deny its importance. Everyone believed it was the key to mass production and mass consumption, to the utilization of natural resources and the creation of a national market, and to the binding together and settlement of a two-ocean land mass. The railroad dominated the imagination, the politics, the economy, and the hopes of a generation, and the outsized cowcatcher and smokestack of the old-fashioned steam locomotive might well be taken as the symbol of the age. The poet William Ellery Leonard, who was born in 1876, entitled an autobiographical work *The Locomotive-God*, and the popular ballad-makers lavished a devotion on the iron horse they had formerly reserved for the flesh-and-blood steed and the sailing ship.

Building the network. The laying of rails went forward in fits and starts. Slowed by the Civil War, total mileage of rails increased from 31,000 to 53,000 in the 1860s. In spite of depression, the 1870s added 40,000 miles of new rails. The 1880s, the great decade of railway expansion, opened with some 93,000 miles and ended with 166,000, an increase of more than 73,000 miles in ten years. By the end of the century the United States had a total of nearly 200,000 miles, or

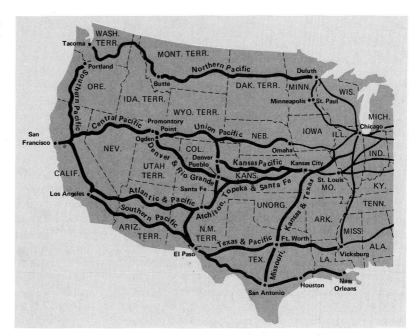

more than all Europe including Russia. In the meantime the ungainly little "bullgine" with the disproportionate funnel had evolved into a giant that could master mountain and plain, a giant that dwarfed any foreign make of locomotive. Greatly improved by the Westinghouse air brake and other inventions, the trains carried more passengers in 1900 than they did in any year of the decade beginning in 1932.

To build this vast railway network was an undertaking comparable in magnitude to the construction of a navy, and for the United States it was even more costly and was thought to be more essential to the national interest. European governments assumed a large part of the responsibility for building and running their railroad establishments as readily as for their military establishments. In America, apart from a few state-owned roads of antebellum origin, initiative and management were left primarily in the hands of private enterprise. Even by 1880, before half the network was completed, an investment of more than $4,600 million had gone into the nation's railroads. By 1897 their stocks and bonds totaled $10,635 million as compared with a total national debt of less than $1,227 million. Edward Kirkland, economic historian, concludes that the handling of railroad finances had "a greater effect upon the economy than the management of the national finances." Since such huge sums were far more than private American investors could supply, promoters turned to foreign investors and to local, state, and federal governments. Foreign investment reached its peak earlier, but in 1898 Europeans, mainly British, owned $3,100 million worth of American railroad securities, about one-third of the whole.

While public enthusiasm for railroad-building was at its height, government at all levels thrust credit and resources upon the railroad-promoters. Villages, towns, cities, and states came forward with extravagant support in the form of bonds and other commitments. The federal government lent approximately $65 million to six Western railroads and extended even more important aid through grants of public land. In all, Congress committed 175,000,000 acres of the public domain, of which the railroads actually received more than 131,000,000 acres. In addition they received 49,000,000 acres from the states. These grants made a substantial contribution toward paying for the railroad investment. Their main value to the railroads was not the cash they brought from sales but the credit and security they supplied for bond issues. Although government subsidies were often obtained through bribery and were responsible for much corruption, the policy of subsidizing the railroads with grants of public land was probably justified in the long run. By attaching conditions to the land grants that obliged the railroads to furnish cheap transportation for mail and military shipments, the government has enjoyed substantial savings over the years. Actually, less than 10 percent of the railroad mileage of the country was built with federal land grants. And most of that mileage was on the roads built across the Great Plains, where investment was slow in yielding returns and where some form of public credit was essential.

The transcontinental lines called for the most heroic efforts and attracted some of the ablest—and some of the most unscrupulous—enterprisers. The completion of the Union Pacific-Central Pacific in 1869 (see p. 403) realized the antebellum dream of spanning the continent with rails, and within the next quarter of a century four more lines flanked the original one, two on either side: the Southern Pacific and the Santa Fe to the south and the Northern Pacific and the Great Northern to the north. Each line excited intense rivalries and ambitions in the cities they connected and the sections they served, as well as among the railroad-builders and promoters.

Railroads east of the Mississippi, with exceptions such as the New York Central, were built mainly to serve local needs and to promote the interests of particular cities. Hundreds of small lines using a variety of gauges were built after the Civil War. The South alone had four hundred companies averaging not more than forty miles apiece. One task of the postwar generation was to fill in the gaps between lines and to weld them into an integrated national network. Through consolidation by lease, purchase, or merger, nearly two-thirds of the country's railroad companies were absorbed by the other third. In 1880 alone, 115 companies lost their identity, and between 1880 and 1888 some 425 companies were brought under control of other roads. The Pennsylvania Railroad by 1890 was an amalgamation of 73 smaller companies and some 5 thousand miles of rails. By 1906 two-thirds of the nation's mileage was operated under 7 groups.

In tandem and often in close alliance with the expanding railroads went the development of other communication and transportation services. Besides providing the means of a more modern postal system, the railroads were tied in with the development of the nation's telegraph network, dominated by the Western Union Company, and later with the growth of the telephone network. As a rule the railroads permitted the telegraph companies to use their right of way for poles and lines, and transported their equipment and personnel without charge in exchange for free telegraphic service in operating the roads. By the end of the century the railroads operated nearly all the country's domestic steamship lines, and typically the railroad stations were the central points of the new urban transportation systems.

The managerial revolution. The lives of the entrepreneurs and financiers who built the transcontinentals and welded together the great railroad systems—colorful figures like Collis P. Huntington, Thomas A. Scott, Jay Gould, and James J. Hill—make fascinating reading. Of more profound importance than these individuals, their manners and morals, however, was the revolution their operations brought about in the scale, management, and character of business enterprise. Up to their time the traditional business firm normally handled a single economic function in one geographic area and was managed by the owners or members of their families. By the 1890s, however, the great railroad systems were not only the largest business enterprises in America but the largest in the world. A single railroad system out of the thirty

largest in that decade managed more workers, handled more funds, and used more capital than the most complex government organizations, including the Postal Department or the combined national military establishments of that time.

Neither the owners and their families nor the investment bankers and financiers had enough qualified members to provide the great corps of managers required by operations of this complexity and scale. To fill this need railroads recruited salaried professional managers selected for skill and experience rather than family or money, and organized them in a hierarchical bureaucracy. Where in traditional firms owners managed and managers owned, in the new system management became separated from ownership. Where once the "invisible hand" of market and prices prevailed, now the "visible hand" of the specialized manager took charge. As pioneered by the railroads, this form of modern business enterprise became the most powerful institution in the American economy and its managers the most influential group of decision makers. It also became the model of modern business enterprise at home as well as in all developed countries. But unlike Europe, where government and public enterprise were main sources of administrative experience and training, in the United States private enterprise was the predominant source.

As the managerial revolution developed, the railroads modernized their technology and services. Steel rails replaced iron rails, and safety precautions such as double tracks, block signals, automatic couplers, and air brakes were standardized, as were time zones and track gauges. On November 18, 1883, the American Railway Association divided the continent into four time zones and millions of citizens set their watches accordingly—in spite of outraged advocates of "God's time." And on the last night in May 1886, the Southern roads moved one rail three inches nearer to the other to comply with the national standard gauge of 4 feet 8½ inches. Some results of these changes were tangible improvements, including more reliable, more punctual, and cheaper transportation. In the last half of the century, real passenger charges fell 50 percent and freight rates much more.

Competition and disorder. In spite of all these improvements, the American railroads were in serious difficulties. The construction boom of the eighties resulted in a network of railroads much greater than was needed at the time. Managers resorted to ruinous competitive wars, offering fantastic "rebates" and secret rates to secure the traffic of big shippers and overcharging outrageously where they had no competition. They employed all manner of rate jugglery and deception and trusted neither customer nor competitor. Under such conditions competition, instead of being "the life of trade" and a benefit to the enterprise as well as to the public, proved a curse to both. In their efforts to curb piratical rate-cutting and blackmail, competitors tried treaties, solemn agreements, and traffic "pools," but these proved difficult to enforce and were always breaking down. Demoralization of the industry was a serious threat.

If the railroad industry could not set its own house in order, then order would have to be imposed from outside. The state governments took the initiative and made the first experiments in regulation and control. Their laws and commissions are often attributed to the "Granger movement," the work of a farmers' organization (see pp. 512–13), and associated with the Middle West. But the movement to regulate railroads was limited to no one class or section. Merchants, wholesale dealers, and manufacturers were more prominent and effective than farmers in pressing for regulation in several areas. In particular they resented rate and service discrimination between persons and places. Small individuals resented bigness and the power it gave the railroads over legislatures, governors, and judges and correctly accused some roads of using bribes and free passes to corrupt or influence public officials.

Popular resentment of abuses found expression in numerous state laws. In 1869 Massachusetts established a commission to supervise railroad activities and investigate grievances. Within the next ten years a dozen more states established commissions modeled on that of Massachusetts. Several state legislatures in the Middle West adopted more thoroughgoing measures of regulation. The Supreme Court upheld the constitutionality of the legislation in the case of *Munn* v. *Illinois* (1877) and declared that when private property is "affected with a public interest" it "must submit to be controlled by the public for the common good" and that in the absence of federal policy states could lay down regulations. Railroads nevertheless waged relentless war against such legislation, which in some states was carelessly drawn and of limited effectiveness from the start. Then in the Wabash case of 1886 (*Wabash, St. Louis & Pacific Railway Co.* v. *Illinois*) the Supreme Court reversed earlier decisions and held an Illinois statute invalid on the ground that it was the exclusive power of Congress to regulate interstate commerce. With the states thus largely excluded, any effective regulatory action would have to be taken by the federal government.

A second spur to federal action in 1886 was the report of a Senate committee headed by Senator Shelby M. Cullom of Illinois, which denounced railroads sharply for the "reckless strife" of their competition and for "unjust discrimination between persons, places, commodities, or particular descriptions to traffic." Railroad-leaders themselves urged federal regulation, for they acknowledged the necessity for measures to end the anarchy in which they struggled. The Republican platform of 1884 had declared that "the principle of the public regulation of railroad corporations is a wise and salutory one." The Interstate Commerce Act, which eventually grew out of demands for regulation, was a milestone in American history, but it was not a triumph of radicals over conservatives or of the people over the corporation.

The Interstate Commerce Act, passed by large majorities in both houses of Congress and signed by President Grover Cleveland on February 4, 1887, forbade railroads to engage in discriminatory practices, required them to publish their rate schedules, prohibited them from entering pooling agreements for the purpose of maintaining high rates, and declared that rates should be "reasonable and just." The act placed enforcement in the hands of an Interstate Commerce Commission of five members, who were to hear complaints and issue orders to the railroads to "cease and desist." Vague and obscure in many sections, the act proved difficult to interpret, administer, and enforce. The commission found it virtually impossible to determine whether or not rates were "reasonable and just," proceeded cautiously, and leaned over backward to accommodate the complaints of the railroads. After a brief period in which some progress was made in reducing rate differentials and in stabilizing the industry, and in which railroad companies tried to obey the law, many of them began to evade the rules and return to their old practices. For enforcement of its orders, the commission had to appeal to the courts, and there the advantage was consistently with the railroads. As an assertion of the federal government's right to regulate private enterprise and as a precedent for more effective measures in the future, the Interstate Commerce Act was important. But it did not provide any immediate answer to the problem of cutthroat competition. It was a conservative measure, based on the belief that competition was beneficial rather than harmful and adopted mainly to alleviate the anxieties of the public.

Morgan and banker control. Within a year of the passage of the Interstate Commerce Act, the railroads began to return to the discriminatory practices that were now illegal. They were somewhat more secretive about rebates and blackmail competition, but it quickly became evident that the law had no teeth and that there was nothing to fear from the courts. With no effective government control, the industry appeared as anarchic as ever and management as quick to resort to speculative looting and stock-watering—issuing stock in excess of paid-in capital. After decades of waste, mismanagement, and folly, many railroads were in a shaky financial plight and in no condi-

J. Pierpont Morgan: a passion for order

Photo by Steichen, 1906
Collection, the Museum of Modern Art, Gift of A. Conger Good-
year. Reprinted with the permission of Joanna T. Steichen

tion to weather hard times. Railroad speculation and overexpansion had prepared the way for the panics of 1857 and 1873, and the first signal of the Panic of 1893 was the bankruptcy of the Philadelphia & Reading Railroad, on February 20. This panic was less closely connected with railroad overexpansion than the earlier panics. Railroad failures were not the only index of calamity, but by the middle of 1894 there were 192 railroads in the hands of the receivers. "Never in the history of transportation in the United States," reported the Interstate Commerce Commission at that time, "has such a large percentage of railway mileage been under the control of receiverships." About one-third of the total mileage of the country were foreclosed by the middle of 1898. To obtain the funds needed for reorganization, the distressed railroads turned to the bankers. The railroads received not only reorganization but a measure of control that neither they themselves nor the state and federal governments had so far been able to contrive.

Numerous bankers took part in the railway reorganizations of the nineties, but none took so prominent and conspicuous a part as J. Pierpont Morgan, the dominant investment banker of his time. For the quar-

ter of a century ending with his death in 1913, this tall, massive figure with piercing eyes and fiery nose was the very symbol of American financial power. Morgan began life near the top of the economic and social ladder, the son of a rich merchant from Hartford, Connecticut, who established a bank in London during the Civil War. He grew up with all the advantages of wealth, including a good education, travel and residence abroad, and study at the University of Göttingen in Germany. He established his firm and his family in New York during the seventies in princely fashion and began to collect treasures of art and rare books. Aboard his yacht or in the library of his home at 219 Madison Avenue the titans of industry and finance met at his call and submitted to agreements that made history in the world of business and sometimes in the world of politics as well. At such meetings he brought to bear his passion for order and his interest as a seller of securities. Morgan enhanced his reputation as a masterful peacemaker among railroads when in 1885 he intervened in a reckless war of blackmail competition between the New York Central and the Pennsylvania and persuaded them to abandon the destructive operation of parallel lines. It was natural that the managers of the sick railroads of the nineties should come to him, as to a famous surgeon, for the strong medicine and heroic surgery the bankrupt roads needed for recovery.

Other investment banking firms, such as Kuhn, Loeb & Company, employed the same methods as Morgan and charged huge fees for their services. First they ruthlessly pared down the fixed debt of the railroad, then assessed holders of the old stock for working funds, and next issued lavish amounts of new stock, heavily watered. To assure control along lines that suited them and to veto unwise expansion plans, the bankers usually installed a president of their own selection and placed members of their own firms on the boards of railroad directors. Between 1894 and 1898 the House of Morgan reorganized the lion's share of big railroads. Banker control was not the ideal solution or the final answer to the problems of competition and control, but it did curb prevailing anarchy and improved the management and efficiency of railroad service.

Industrial Empire

Carnegie and steel. The new industrial order of America was based on steel, and by 1870 the techniques of production, the supply of raw materials, and the home market were sufficiently developed to make the United States the world's greatest steel-producer. A cheap and practical process of making steel by forcing a blast of cold air through molten iron to clean it of impurities had been invented by Henry Bessemer, an Englishman, in 1857. A rival patent for the process was held by William Kelly, a Kentucky ironmaster who made the discovery before Bessemer, and a third patent on a vital process of refining steel belonged to Robert Mushet. The three patents were merged in 1866, and the following year the first steel rails in the country were rolled for commercial use. In 1867 the United States made 1,643 tons of steel ingots; in 1897 it made 7,156,957. In the meantime new discoveries of ore deposits in the fabulous Lake Superior district opened exciting prospects for the ironmasters. Government surveyors in 1844 had discovered the Marquette Range in Michigan, including "a mountain of solid iron ore, 150 feet high." In 1868 the rich Vermilion Range in Minnesota was discovered, and in 1875 it was tapped by a railroad. Within the next decade the Menominee, the Gogebic, and the Mesabi mines—all within close proximity to Lake Superior and cheap water transportation—were opened up. Together they constituted the greatest iron-ore district in the world.

These opportunities brought a multitude of entrepreneurs into the field of iron and steel in quest of profits. By 1880 there were 1,005 iron companies in the nation, all of them subject to the competitive struggle under which the railroads labored, with all its uncertainties, anxieties, and ruthlessness. Like railroad operators, the iron and steelmasters resorted to cutthroat tactics, price-slashing, and blackmail. Faced with large fixed costs, they sometimes ran their plants at a loss rather than let them remain idle. They sought rebates and unfair advantages and rushed into pools, combinations, and mergers to hedge against competition. Out of the melee emerged one dominant figure, Andrew Carnegie, the most articulate industrialist America ever had.

Quite untypical of industrial leaders of his day in several respects, Carnegie was of immigrant and working-class origin, a voluble speaker, a facile writer, and a religious skeptic. He came to the United States from Scotland with his family when he was thirteen years old and went to work immediately to earn a living. At seventeen he became a telegraph clerk in the office of Thomas A. Scott, then a rising official of the Pennsylvania Railroad, and won his employer's favor and confidence. His service with Scott, which lasted through the Civil War, not only brought valuable acquaintance with the foremost railroad and industrial leaders of the country but guided him in making shrewd and extremely profitable investments. With a salary of only $2,400 a year, he was receiving a millionaire's income from investments when he was twenty-eight years old. He was drawn into the iron business and then in 1872 into a venture for building a huge steel plant on the Monongahela River, twelve miles from Pittsburgh, a site with excellent river transportation and service from both the Pennsylvania and the B&O railroads. The new plant rolled its first rail in 1875.

Without pretense of engineering or technological skill, Carnegie was first of all a superb salesman with a genius for picking the right subordinates to supervise production. He was personally acquainted with all the railroad barons of the day and, as he said, simply "went out and persuaded them to give us orders." He did not have to remind them that steel rails lasted twenty times as long as iron. Drawing directly on his experience as an executive of one of the best managed railroads of the time, he put together the administrative structure for his steel works on that model. The supreme example of the industrial capitalist, Carnegie refused to permit his company to become a corporation, maintained it as a limited partnership, and retained a majority of the shares himself. Giving no hostages to the bankers, he used the firm's enormous profits to construct new plants, acquire raw materials, buy out competitors, and win fights with organized labor. His independent resources enabled him to go on building and spending, and lead the way in the development of integrated production. After hesitation about entering the ore business, he bought ore deposits in the Mesabi Range and ore ships on the Great Lakes, and he acquired docks, warehouses, and railroad lines to supply his great furnaces and mills with raw materials.

Carnegie had a remarkable gift for finding able lieutenants—men like Henry Clay Frick, Charles M. Schwab, and Alexander R. Peacock. He pitted these

Carnegie steel mill, Braddock, Pennsylvania

men against one another, rewarding the successful with shares and partnerships. Like other capitalists of his day, he benefited from pools, rebates, patents, and protective tariffs, but in time his power and resources became great enough to make him virtually independent of such devices. At the crest of his power he held the whole steel industry in his grasp except for steel finishing, which he had not entered. His trail to the top was strewn with ruined competitors, crushed partners, and broken labor movements including his bloody victory over labor at Homestead (see p. 470). Carnegie increased his annual production from 322,000 tons in 1890 to 3,000,000 tons in 1900. Over the same decade he and his lieutenants increased the annual profits of the Carnegie Steel Company from $5,400,000 in 1890 to $40,000,000 in 1900. Carnegie's own share of the 1900 profits was approximately $25,000,000.

In the meantime Pierpont Morgan turned his attention from railroads to steel, and the bankers challenged the industrialists for the control of heavy industry. The American Steel and Wire Company, the first big combination in steel, was constructed without his help. Then in the summer of 1898 Morgan swung his support to Judge Elbert H. Gary of Chicago and other Midwesterners who merged several big concerns to form the Federal Steel Company, second in size to Carnegie Steel. Quickly other mergers between hitherto competing steel firms sprang into being, "as if a giant magnet had moved over the surface of the industry," observed one historian. The next obvious move in the drive for mergers was to combine the combinations, that is, consolidate the whole industry into one vast supercorporation, the greatest in the world. Blocking that dream was the mighty Carnegie Steel Company and the known prejudice of its head against banker control. Even Morgan threw up his hands when it was proposed that he buy up Carnegie Steel outright; "I don't believe I could raise the money," he said. The new combinations for making finished steel products then decided in the summer of 1900 to produce their own raw steel, free themselves from dependence on Carnegie, and cancel their contracts with him. Carnegie's response was a cable from Skibo Castle, his summer home in Scotland, declaring open war: "Have no fear as to result. Victory certain." He proposed to go into the production of finished steel, which he had urged on his partners since 1898, and to drive all his competitors to the wall.

Alarmed at the prospect of a war that would place the new steel combinations in deadly peril and demoralize the whole industry, Morgan determined to buy out Carnegie and consolidate the supercorporation. After a night-long conference in the famous Morgan library, Charles M. Schwab agreed to take the matter up with Carnegie. The Scotsman scribbled a few figures on a scrap of paper, and Schwab took it to Morgan. The banker glanced at it and said, "I accept this price." There was no bargaining. The figure was nearly a half-billion dollars. In a few weeks Morgan pushed and pulled the big steel companies into combination and, on March 3, 1901, announced the organization of the United States Steel Corporation. The new concern brought under a single management three-fifths of the steel business of the country and was capitalized at nearly a billion and a half dollars.

Although U. S. Steel was never without competition within the industry, the uneasy popular sentiment about the gigantic deal was reflected in the words the humorist Finley Peter Dunne put in the mouth of his Irish saloonkeeper, "Mr. Dooley":

> Pierpont Morgan calls in wan iv his office boys, th' presidint iv a national bank, an' says he, "James," he says, "take some change out iv th' damper an' r-run out an' buy Europe f'r me," he says. "I intind to re-organize it an' put it on a paying basis," he says. "Call up the Czar an' th' Pope an' th' Sultan an' th' Impror Willum, an' tell thim we won't need their savices afther nex' week," he says. "Give thim a year's salary in advance."

Rockefeller and the trusts. An industrial giant of power and influence comparable to that wielded by Carnegie was John D. Rockefeller, who did for oil what the Scotsman did for steel. The two contemporaries were strikingly different in temperament and taste: Carnegie was exuberant and communicative, Rockefeller silent and taciturn; Carnegie was a skeptic and an agnostic, Rockefeller a Bible-class teacher and a devout Baptist. In their business methods and their achievements, however, there were many similarities. Both men showed the same astuteness in selecting lieutenants and putting them in the right jobs, the same abhorrence of waste and gambling, the same ability to transform depressions into opportunities for building, buying, and expanding. The Standard Oil Company, with Rockefeller its head, made ruthless use of railroad-rate discrimination, espionage, bogus companies, price-slashing, and other reprehensible practices. On the other hand, it had positive achievements to its credit, including improved and lower priced products, the elimination of waste, and efficiency in distribution.

Rockefeller was the outstanding American exponent of consolidation in industry. Of the trend toward consolidation he wrote:

> This movement was the origin of the whole system of modern economic administration. It has

revolutionized the way of doing business all over the world. The time was ripe for it. It had to come, though all we saw at the moment was the need to save ourselves from wasteful conditions. . . . The day of combination is here to stay. Individualism has gone, never to return.

By "wasteful conditions" he meant the glutted markets in crude and refined oil and the disorder, uncertainty, and wild fluctuation of prices and profits that attended free competition among thousands of small producers and hundreds of small refiners. Rockefeller hated free competition and believed that monopoly was the way of the future. His early method of dealing with competitors was to gain unfair advantage over them through special rates and rebates arranged with railroads. With the aid of these advantages Standard became the largest refiner of oil in the country. By the end of the 1870s the Standard Oil Company had created an "alliance," or cartel, of forty leading refiners of the country and held a majority of the securities of the members. In 1881 the alliance controlled nearly 90 percent of the country's oil refining capacity and could crush any remaining competitors at will.

A change in the technology of transportation—the completion of a long-distance pipeline for crude oil—triggered the decision of the Standard Oil alliance to solidify legal control and centralize management. Their railroad-rate advantages threatened by an independent pipeline that they were unable to stop, the alliance began construction of a huge interregional pipeline network of its own. The next problem was to establish a central authority with power to close down, modernize, or build refineries to take advantage of the new pipeline network. The solution was found in an old legal device put to new use—the trust. On January 2, 1882, the shareholders of the forty companies exchanged their stock for certificates of the new Standard Oil Trust. The board of nine trustees was given power to "exercise general supervision over the affairs of the several Standard Oil Companies." In three years the trustees consolidated refining capacity by reducing refineries it operated from fifty-three to twenty-two. They followed with the consolidation of crude oil buying and moved on to control of marketing at home and abroad. By the early 1890s Standard Oil completed the process of vertical integration through entering the production of crude oil as well.

The term "trust" was popularly and loosely applied to numerous industrial combinations that were formed after Standard Oil pointed the way, but it appears that in addition to petroleum, only seven were formed to operate in the national market, and two of those were short-lived. Of the successful trusts put together in the 1880s, all were in refining and distilling industries. The sugar and whiskey trusts did not move into national marketing, but cottonseed oil, linseed oil, and lead processing followed the Standard Oil example in this respect and others. In less than a decade after their formation they became fully integrated enterprises, organized according to the managerial revolution, and dominated their industries for decades.

The trust movement encountered popular suspicion and hostility from the start. The American creed, bred of an agrarian heritage, held that business should be organized in small units, that competition should be unfettered, and that opportunity should be open to all. The trusts were an affront to this traditional faith: they were gigantic, powerful, even awe-inspiring. To the public, the trusts were the product of an evil plot born of greed, and that was the way the cartoonists pictured them in the newspapers and journals and the way popular political leaders described them in their speeches in the eighties. The popular attitude was not without foundation, for the trusts often did use their enormous power to the detriment of both consumers and small businesspeople. Businesspeople adversely affected were among the most influential antitrust advocates. Even the big-business community, increasingly aware that mergers and trusts were not likely to stabilize and control industry, looked to the federal government for the answer.

As in railroad regulation, the state legislatures took the lead against the trusts. The laws they passed were never very effective, however, and the Wabash decision of 1886 limited the states here as it did in the regulation of railroads and left the problem up to the federal government. The growth of the trusts had stirred uneasiness in the East and the South as well as the West, and by the campaign of 1888 all political parties of significance had inserted antitrust planks into their platforms. In that year John Sherman of Ohio submitted an antitrust bill in the Senate, one of many similar bills introduced that year. Debate in Congress revealed concern for the interests of both the consumer and the small business-proprietor. It illustrated both the "folklore" of the old capitalism and apprehension about the new. The so-called Sherman Antitrust Act became law on July 2, 1890.

On the face of it the new act would seem to have spelled the end of every trust or trustlike combination. The opening sentence of the first section declares, "Every contract, combination in the form of trust or otherwise, or conspiracy, in restraint of trade or commerce among the several States, or with foreign nations, is hereby declared to be illegal." And the second section pronounces guilty of a misdemeanor "every person who shall monopolize, or attempt to monopolize, or combine or conspire with any other person or persons, to monopolize any part of the trade or commerce among the several States, or with foreign nations." The word "person" was specifically defined to include corporations, and the act fixed penalties, as the Interstate Commerce Act had not, for violations.

Efforts to enforce the act during the 1890s were not very vigorous, and clever lawyers found loopholes and various ways of evading its provisions. Some trusts merely reorganized as huge corporations, while others pointed the way to the future by finding refuge in holding companies—that is, giant financial structures that held enough stock in member companies to control their policies. In the first five years after the act was passed, twenty-five new combinations came into being. The fact is the public wanted the benefits of large-scale enterprise without the evils of big-business and monopoly—a dilemma never fully resolved.

The course of Standard Oil from trust to holding company illustrates the trend. The company formally abandoned the trust agreement of 1882 under an Ohio court order in 1892, but in practice the same nine men who had served as trustees continued to conduct the business of the member companies for five years after the trust was formally dissolved. Charged with evading the court order, the trust reorganized as a holding company under the laws of New Jersey, which permitted corporations of that state to own and control corporations of other states. The Standard Oil Company of New Jersey simply increased its stock some tenfold and exchanged it for stock of the member companies. These in turn elected directors of the New Jersey company, who carried on in the place of the old trustees. With concentration of control unimpaired and power enhanced instead of diminished, Standard made money as never before. In the eight years following its reorganization as a holding company, annual dividends on its stock varied between 30 and 48 percent.

The upward surge and eventually the downward turn of mergers throughout the economy reflected both the conditions of the nation's financial markets and the United States Supreme Court's interpretations of the Sherman Antitrust Act. In 1895 the court dealt a heavy blow to the law by its decision in the case of *United States* v. *E. C. Knight Company*, which was charged with furthering monopoly by selling out to the American Sugar Refining Company. Although the sale rounded out one of the most complete monopolies in the country, the court decided that it did not violate the antitrust act. It reasoned that manufacturing was not "commerce" within the meaning of the law, and that monopoly of manufacturing without "direct" effect on commerce was not subject to regulation by the federal government. With this encouragement and economic incentives, consolidation in the dominant industries went forward with a rush in the

next five years. The movement reached its peak in 1899, when 1,207 firms disappeared and merger capitalization rose to $2,263 million. Then in 1898 and 1899 the Supreme Court ruled clearly and precisely in two cases that any combination of business firms formed to fix prices or allocate markets violated the Sherman Antitrust Act. After that lawyers usually advised corporate clients to abandon such efforts. The merger movement declined temporarily after the formation of U. S. Steel in 1901.

The technology of centralization. The management of a vast railroad network, a continent-wide industry, or an international market required a new technology of control and communication. American inventors outdid themselves to meet these demands. The number of patents issued to inventors jumped from fewer than two thousand a year in the 1850s to more than thirteen thousand a year in the 1870s and better than twenty-one thousand a year in the 1880s and 1890s. In those days the typical inventor was not a trained engineer in an industrial or a university laboratory but an individual tinkerer who frequently operated on a shoestring.

Such a man was Christopher L. Sholes, printer and journalist from Pennsylvania and Wisconsin, who invented a typewriter in 1867. He sold his rights to the Remington Arms Company, which put the typewriter on the market in 1875. The year Sholes invented the typewriter, E. A. Callahan of Boston developed a superior stock ticker. In the summer of 1866 Cyrus W. Field employed new techniques to repair and improve his transatlantic cable, broken since 1858, and stock quotations crossed the ocean. Numerous other inventions, including the adding machine (1888), quickened the pace of business transactions.

None of these inventions, however, could rival the importance of the telephone. This was the work of Alexander Graham Bell, a Scotsman who was educated in Edinburgh and London, emigrated to Canada in 1870, when he was twenty-three, and then to Boston two years later. As a teacher of speech to the deaf, he formed the ambition to "make iron talk"—to transmit speech electrically. His experiments over three years resulted in the magnetoelectric telephone. He transmitted the first intelligible sentence on March 10, 1876, and a year later conducted a conversation between Boston and New York. The inventor and his supporters organized the Bell Telephone Company in 1877 and promptly plunged into law suits to defend their patent. The most formidable challenger was the Western Union Telegraph Company, which had originally spurned an opportunity to buy the patent for the "scientific toy" for a mere $100,000. Western Union settled out of court and left the field to Bell and his company, which continued to win hundreds of suits, improve the telephone, buy out competitors, and expand facilities. In 1885 the directors of Bell, led by Theodore N. Vail, organized the American Telephone and Telegraph Company. By 1900 it had become the holding company for the whole system, with some thirty-five subsidiaries and a capitalization of a quarter of a billion dollars.

Among the numerous social consequences of the new technology of communications—telegraph, cable, telephone, ticker-tape, typewriter—was the emergence of a new social class. This was the white-collar clerical worker, the fastest growing part of the urban labor force in the late nineteenth century. Although a majority of the new workers were male, the clerical services also opened up employment opportunities for female high-school graduates and added many women to the labor force.

The use of electricity for light is justly linked with the name of Thomas Alva Edison, who outdid his contemporary Bell as an inventor. The son of a Canadian who settled and prospered in Ohio, Edison grew up without formal schooling. He became a telegraph-operator and while still quite young made some very profitable inventions to improve transmission. He then established himself as a businessman-inventor and built his own "invention factory," forerunner of the modern industrial-research laboratory, at Menlo Park, New Jersey, in 1876. There in 1877 he invented the phonograph, and in later years his laboratories turned out hundreds of inventions or im-

Thomas Alva Edison: hundreds of inventions

provements, including the storage battery, the motion-picture projector, an electric dynamo, and an electric locomotive. The incandescent light required a vacuum bulb with a durable filament. Edison made one that burned for forty hours in 1879 and improved it until it was commercially practicable. With the backing of J. Pierpont Morgan he organized the Edison Illuminating Company and moved to New York City to install an electric-light plant. On September 4, 1882, in the presence of Morgan, Edison threw a switch and the House of Morgan, the New York Stock Exchange, the New York *Times*, the New York *Herald*, and smaller buildings in lower Manhattan began to glow with incandescent light.

Edison's plant used direct current, but in order to transmit electricity any distance its voltage had to be stepped up and then stepped down again. For this purpose alternating current and transformers were necessary. George Westinghouse of Pittsburgh, who had invented the railroad air brake in 1869, developed a power plant and a transformer in 1886 that could transmit high-voltage alternating current efficiently, safely, and cheaply over long distances.

For this type of current to be converted into mechanical power, an alternating-current motor had to be developed. In 1888 Nikola Tesla, a Hungarian engineer who immigrated to the United States in 1884, invented such a motor. Westinghouse and his associates bought the patent, improved it with the aid of Tesla, and dramatically demonstrated the practicability of alternating current by illuminating the Columbian Exposition at Chicago in 1893 and by harnessing the might of Niagara Falls and transmitting the power over the countryside. While American industry continued to depend mainly upon steam and water for power until the end of the century, the shift to electrical power had already begun, and factories no longer had to hover around waterfalls and coal supplies. They were now ready for the electrical revolution that came in the twentieth century.

Laissez-Faire Conservatism

The Gospel of Wealth. A survey of private fortunes conducted in 1892 revealed that there were 4,047 millionaires in the United States. These were largely new fortunes; very few of them dated from before the Civil War, when a millionaire was a rarity, though most of them came from well-to-do backgrounds. Only eighty-four of the millionaires of 1892 were in agriculture, and most of those were cattle barons. The fortunes of the new plutocracy were based on industry, trade, railroads. The new plutocrats were the

Andrew Carnegie: the duties of wealth

This, then, is held to be the duty of the man of wealth: To set an example of modest, unostentatious living, shunning display or extravagance; to provide moderately for the legitimate wants of those dependent upon him; and, after doing so, to consider all surplus revenues which come to him simply as trust funds, which he is called upon to administer, and strictly bound as a matter of duty to administer in the manner which, in his judgment, is best calculated to produce the most beneficial results for the community—the man of wealth thus becoming the mere trustee and agent for his poorer brethren, bringing to their service his superior wisdom, experience, and ability to administer, doing for them better than they would or could do for themselves.

From Andrew Carnegie, *The Gospel of Wealth and Other Essays*, 1901.

masters and directors of the economic revolution that was changing the face of American society.

To say that these men were conservative is to put a strain on customary usage of the word, for conservatives are usually opposed to change and devoted to tradition. Yet these men flouted tradition and preached progress. To confuse customary usage further, they adopted the slogan "laissez faire," which was traditionally the doctrine of Jeffersonian and Jacksonian liberals. In one of the strangest reversals in the history of political thought, the new conservatives of wealth took over virtually the whole liberal vocabulary of concepts and slogans, including "democracy," "liberty," "equality," "opportunity," and "individualism," and turned it against the liberals. In short, they gave an economic and material turn to ethical and idealistic concepts. Man became economic man, democracy was identified with capitalism, liberty with property and the use of it, equality with opportunity for gain, and progress with economic change and the accumulation of capital. God and nature were thus in league with the Gospel of Wealth.

The new doctrine was conservative, however, in the sense that it was bent on defending the status quo, conserving the privileges by which vast accumulations of wealth were gained, and preventing government interference with those privileges. The laissez-faire conservatives naturally found comfort in classical economics, and those who had heard of them found special fascination in the biological theories of Charles Darwin and the sociological theory of Herbert Spencer, an English philosopher. Spencer applied biological concepts, especially the concept of natural selection, to social principles and justified the unimpeded struggle for existence on the ground that "survival of the fittest" made for human progress. State interference in behalf of the weak would only impede progress. Spen-

cer was more readily acclaimed and more widely admired in America than in England. "The peculiar condition of American society," wrote the preacher Henry Ward Beecher to Spencer, "has made your writings far more fruitful and quickening here than in Europe." By 1903 more than 368,000 volumes of Spencer's works had been sold in the United States. Professors, clergymen, and intellectuals, as well as businessmen, were captivated by the new philosophy.

The most articulate and influential American exponent of Herbert Spencer's doctrines was Professor William Graham Sumner. The son of an immigrant artisan from England, he was educated for the ministry at Yale and later attended European universities. After a few years in the pulpit his interests shifted to the study of public affairs, and in 1872 he accepted a professorship in political and social science at Yale, where he spent the rest of his life. A prodigious scholar, he mastered all the social sciences of his time, several natural sciences, and a dozen or more languages. His numerous writings included not only learned contributions to the founding of the new field of sociology but essays that commanded nation-wide attention on virtually every public issue of his time. More consistent than most adherents of laissez-faire, Sumner vigorously opposed protectionism and imperialism. On essentials of the Gospel of Wealth, however, he wrote in an essay called "The Concentration of Wealth: Its Economic Justification":

> What matters it then that some millionaires are idle, or silly, or vulgar. . . . The millionaires are a product of natural selection, acting on the whole body of men to pick out those who can meet the requirement of certain work to be done. . . . They get high wages and live in luxury, but the bargain is a good one for society.

Henry George: the nature of property

What constitutes the rightful basis of property? What is it that enables a man justly to say of a thing, "It is mine"? From what springs the sentiment which acknowledges his exclusive right as against all the world? Is it not, primarily, the right of a man to himself, to the use of his own powers, to the enjoyment of the fruits of his own exertions? Is it not this individual right, which springs from and is testified to by the natural facts of individual organization—the fact that each particular pair of hands obey a particular brain and are related to a particular stomach; the fact that each man is a definite, coherent, independent whole—which alone justifies individual ownership? As a man belongs to himself, so his labor when put in concrete form belongs to him....

If production give to the producer the right to exclusive possession and enjoyment, there can rightfully be no exclusive possession and enjoyment of anything not the production of labor, and the recognition of private property in land is a wrong.

From Henry George, *Progress and Poverty*, 1879.

By the time it had become fully elaborated, the Gospel of Wealth and its corollaries of social Darwinism included many propositions widely accepted. Among them were the following: (1) that the American economy was controlled for the benefit of all by a natural aristocracy and that these leaders were brought to the top by a competitive struggle that weeded out the weak, the incompetent, and the unfit and selected the strong, the able, and the wise; (2) that politicians were not subject to rigorous natural selection and therefore could not be trusted to the same degree as businessmen; (3) that the state should confine itself to police activities of protecting property and maintaining order and that if it interfered with economic affairs it would upset the beneficent effect of natural selection; (4) that slums and poverty were the unfortunate but inevitable negative results of the competitive struggle and that state intervention to eliminate them was misguided; (5) that the stewardship of wealth obliged the rich to try to ameliorate social injustice.

In the Supreme Court the Gospel of Wealth found institutional support of great prestige and incomparable value. Under the persistent tutelage of Justice Stephen J. Field, the Court had been converted by the late eighties to the view that Herbert Spencer's *Social Statics* coincided remarkably well with the will of the Founding Fathers and the soundest moral precepts of the ages. Interpreting the "due process" clause of the Fourteenth Amendment as a protection of corporate interests, the Court proceeded to declare state regulatory measures unconstitutional on the ground that they deprived corporations of property without due process of law. By the end of the century, the Court's laissez-faire interpretation of the Constitution had gone far toward debarring the states from the exercise of ancient police powers for the protection of the public interest and the welfare of workers.

Social critics and dissenters. The Gospel of Wealth and the Darwinian apology for unrestrained capitalism did not meet with universal acceptance. The dissenters rejected the survival-of-the-fittest concept of social progress and found a place for ethical values in economic theory, as well as a need for governmental intervention to restrain the strong and protect the weak. A strong religious impulse often motivated the nonclerical as well as the clerical critics of social Darwinism.

Lester Frank Ward, one of the founders of sociology in America, was an outspoken critic of Spencer's theories. Ward took a job in a Washington bureau in 1865, after service in the Union army, and remained in government work for some forty years. Largely self-educated, he compensated for his impoverished background by astonishing feats of learning. He mastered ten languages and several fields of science in addition to sociology, and, when he finally found acceptance in academic life, he titled a course he gave at Brown University "A Survey of All Knowledge." His first book, *Dynamic Sociology* (1883), was a prodigious work of fourteen hundred pages that was not easily or widely read. He never achieved the acclaim or the influence his conservative rival, Professor Sumner, did. Ward pointed out that there was a difference between animal and human economics. Bears have claws, but humans have intelligence. Darwinian laws governed the former, but the human mind transformed the environment of human economics and substituted rational choice for natural selection. This was as it should be, for nature was terribly wasteful in its crude methods of evolution. For competition to survive, government regulation was necessary. Ward believed in social planning and had great faith in education. "Thus far," he wrote, "social progress has in a certain awkward manner taken care of itself, but in the near future it will have to be cared for." This, he said, should be done by social engineers, scientific planners, and managers of society.

A second self-taught social philosopher of the age, and one of the most original economists of the time, was Henry George, author of the famous book *Progress and Poverty* (1879). Born in Philadelphia, George traveled in the Orient and in 1868 settled in California, where he had ample opportunity to observe the land speculation, land monopoly, and social distress that played so important a part in his economics. Addressing himself to the problem of unequal distribution of wealth, he inveighed against the "shocking contrast between monstrous wealth and debasing want." Wealth is produced, he concluded, by applying labor to land, and capital is the surplus above the cost of labor. Labor therefore creates all capital. But capitalists, by withholding advantageous land sites until their value has been enhanced by labor, improvements in production, and speculation in adjacent areas, reap a profit out of all proportion to their contribution. This profit George called the "unearned increment." Since land should no more be monopolized than air and sunshine, George's solution was to tax land in such a fashion as to appropriate the unearned increment. This was to be done by a "single tax," which would make other taxes unnecessary. After 1885 he put aside the hope that this would result in common ownership of the land by the people. George's book and his lectures won him a political following at home and abroad and enabled him to make a strong showing as candidate for mayor of New York in 1886.

Another political aspiration born of a book was the Nationalist movement; this time the book was Edward Bellamy's *Looking Backward* (1888). The most successful of several utopian novels published during the eighties, Bellamy's book "looked backward" to the benighted 1880s from the collectivized society of the year 2000 A.D. By that time selfishness has been eliminated by the abolition of corporate property and the nationalization of industry. Competition is seen to have killed nineteenth-century society and its individualism. "Competition," says the protagonist, "which is the instinct of selfishness, is another word for dissipation of energy, while combination is the secret of efficient production." The utopian remedy was one big trust, bloodlessly achieved, and mandatory male service in an industrial army in place of wage competition. Women were promised a better place in this brave new world. Bellamy's attack on the ethic of "survival of the fittest" appealed to a wide variety of people. Nationalist clubs and periodicals advocated municipal ownership of utilities and public ownership of railroads. As agrarian reform mounted in the nineties, however, the Nationalists tended to join the farmers' parties and abandon their own organization.

From the viewpoint of a later day, the debate over laissez-faire doctrine and social Darwinism appears confused and paradoxical. If free competition was the goal of laissez faire, the industrialists who hated competition and sought to restrain it would seem to have embraced the wrong doctrine. If social Darwinism taught hands off by the government, those who sought subsidies, protection, and favors from the government again seemed inconsistent. But insofar as these doctrines were useful for the defense of the status quo and the discouragement of efforts to reform or change society by conscious purpose the conservatives were right in embracing them and the radicals in rejecting them.

The House of Labor

Man and the machine. In the long run industrialization raises the living standard and increases the opportunities of labor, but around the world labor has discovered that the revolution that establishes industrialization comes at heavy cost and that the worker's adjustment to the machine and the factory way of life is often painful and difficult. In America the labor shortage that had persisted since colonial times had kept the level of wages higher than the level that prevailed abroad; and yet American workers had their full share of troubles in the grim iron age of industry.

Many of the changes in his way of life the worker had to make were hard to understand and painful to accept, for they meant loss of status and surrender of independence. The skilled craftsman who owned the tools he used was likely to be an individualist who took pride in the quality of his product and enjoyed a strong bargaining position. The new factory discipline offered a humbler role and a lower status. In the factory the worker surrendered his tools, nearly all the creative pride he took in his product, most of his independence, and much of his bargaining power. He became the tender of a machine that set the work pace and the employee of owners whom he probably never met and never saw. The craftsmanship that had been the skilled worker's source of pride and security was no longer of any significance, for his place at the machine could be taken by an unskilled worker. The growing impersonality of his relations to his work and his employer and the ever increasing size of the industrial organization meant a sacrifice in security,

Women workers, National Cash Register Company

identity, and the satisfactions that bestow meaning and value on work.

Adjustment would have been easier had the change been less swift and the workers better prepared. But the mechanization and expansion of the factory system hit a breathtaking pace during the 1880s. Between 1880 and 1890 the total capital invested in the production of machinery increased two and a half times, and the average investment in machinery increased 200 percent for each establishment and 50 percent for each employee. Manufacturers, with their capital tied up in new machinery, were driven to seek a rapid return on their investment, generally at low prices in a highly competitive market. Real wages actually rose, but hard-pressed employers often made economies at the expense of the unskilled factory workers, who suffered from working conditions that impaired their safety, their comfort, and their health. While some states had enacted factory laws, the great body of legislation that now protects factory workers had not yet been written in the eighties and nineties. Employers thought nothing of using detectives and armed force to thwart the organization of labor unions. In "company towns," where all houses, stores, and services were company-owned,

employers subjected workers to endless harassments and petty tyranny. There was nothing but the urging of conscience and the weak protest of labor to keep employers from cutting costs at the expense of their workers.

After the 1880s occurred a large shift into the paid labor force among married women. In 1890 more than 90 percent of women over thirty-five were married, and up to that time the vast majority of them remained unemployed outside the home. Then rather suddenly they began to take jobs in large numbers and go "out to work." The change in employment followed a sharp decline in the birth rate. Between 1860 and 1890 the number of children under five per thousand women dropped nearly a third, while at the end of the century women were having half the number of children they were bearing at its start. The amount of home labor required of them decreased with the size of the family. In the workplace women accepted wages strikingly lower than those men were paid for comparable work and were often blamed by employers as well as by male employees for lowering the general wage level by taking jobs they did not "need." Organized labor made only weak gestures in behalf of women, often cutting them out of the kind of jobs held by unionized men. Without union help, women had few means of overcoming low pay, exploitation, and terrible work conditions—all of which resulted in a mortality rate more than double that of non-wage-earners.

The average weekly wages of common laborers remained less than $9 throughout the nineties, and farm laborers got less than half that amount. After the depression of the seventies, however, there was a fairly steady increase in real wages—for those who had jobs. The rise in real wages helps explain labor's relative indifference to socialism. Among other explanations that have been offered are mobility through the labor force and mobility through the ethnic ghettos, but more information is needed about the condition and mentality of labor. The millions who suffered unemployment during the depressions of the last three decades of the century were not even enumerated, much less assisted, by the government. The most insistent demand of organized labor was for the eight-hour day, but the main result was the adoption of a federal law passed in 1869, and amended in 1892, limiting the work day of federal employees to eight hours. In private industry, however, most workers continued to work a ten-hour day and a six-day week, and in steel and other industries they worked even longer. The accident toll taken by the rapid rate of change in unfamiliar machinery and by heedless negligence, and the damage done to workers' health by poor ventilation and lighting, dust and fumes—in so far as the facts were known at all—were charged off as the cost of progress.

A special handicap of American labor was its lack of homogeneity. The working class was fragmented by race and color, as well as by geography, philosophy, concepts of organization, style of protest, and national origin. Some formed exclusive groups to protect their own privilege and to keep underprivileged groups at bay. Between 1882 and 1900 there were fifty strikes waged against the employment of black labor. Blacks sometimes served as strikebreakers, thereby increasing the resentment of white workers.

Immigrants formed a large segment of the American labor force, except in the South, where few of them settled. There had been immigrant workers from the start in the United States, and while the percentage in the labor force remained about the same after the Civil War, immigrants were coming in greater numbers and from different parts of Europe, mainly the southern and eastern countries. Nineteenth-century immigration reached high tide in the 1880s, when nearly 5¼ million immigrants arrived, 2½ million more than had come in the seventies and 1½ million more than were to come in the nineties. Set apart by language and culture, accustomed to lower wages and living standards, the newcomers often concentrated as ethnic groups in certain industries—Irish in building construction, Germans in brewing and furniture, Italians in street and sewer work, Slavs in anthracite, Jews in the garment industry. Native workers often looked down on them with contempt and spoke of work for which they were suited as "foreign jobs." Both the Knights of Labor and the AFL called for immigrant restriction. The new immigrants crowded into the coal-mining and steel industries, with each wave pushing the earlier comers a step up the ladder. The bitterest and most implacable labor opposition to immigrants was directed at the Asiatics, particularly the Chinese of California. Supported by labor organizations in the East, the Californians persuaded Congress in 1882 to suspend admission of Chinese immigrants for ten years.

Unions and strikes. For a long time the attitude of American labor toward unions and collective bargaining was typically that of the skilled artisan or the small shopkeeper. Native workers, and many immigrants as well, were reluctant to abandon the American dream of rising higher and higher in the social scale. Instead of accepting the new industrial order and its conditions, they looked back nostalgically to the past and longed for the good old days. Longings of this sort found expression in such slogans as "every man his own master" or "every man his own employer." Labor unions remained very weak throughout the nineteenth century, embracing not more than 1 or 2 percent of the total labor force and less than 10 percent of the industrial workers.

During and after the Civil War the typical national trade union was designed primarily to protect the status of skilled workers. In 1866 William H. Sylvis, an iron-molder of Pennsylvania, attempted to unite the trade unions into a single organization called the National Labor Union. This organization, of which Sylvis became president in 1868, bore no resemblance to modern labor unions. It was led by visionaries and idealists who did not believe in strikes and who were unconcerned with the immediate needs of working people, apart from the eight-hour day. Sylvis stressed long-range reforms and humanitarian demands, and admitted farmers' societies and advocates of women's rights as members. The organization formed the National Labor Reform party in 1871, and after a feeble showing in the election of 1872 the new party went to pieces.

With many of the same generous impulses and naive assumptions, the Noble and Holy Order of the Knights of Labor was founded in 1869. A secret fraternal order with high-flown titles and elaborate rituals, the Knights sought to unite all labor and welcomed all "toilers" of whatever color, race, nationality, or craft, whether skilled or unskilled. They excluded only

Women delegates, Knights of Labor

gamblers, bankers, lawyers, doctors, liquor-dealers, and a few others—apparently on moralistic grounds. Utopian and nostalgic in many of their views, the Knights frowned on the use of the strike and promoted dreams of restoring the past. Their labor program, however, included demands for a federal bureau of statistics, equal pay for both sexes, the eight-hour day, and the abolition of child and prison labor. In practice they acted like a labor union. The two hundred or more consumer and producer cooperatives the Knights founded elicited great enthusiasm but little profit. Many of their political demands resembled those of contemporary farmers' organizations, for they included paper money, an income tax, abolition of the national banking system, and prohibition.

The Knights grasped one important fact of the new economy: that the consolidation of industry made necessary the consolidation of labor. They founded their General Assembly in 1878 with a view to centralizing control over labor in order to combat the monopolistic power of corporations. In 1879 they elected Terence V. Powderly as their Grand Master

Workman. The dominant figure in the Order during the years of its power and influence, Powderly was described at a labor convention in 1886 as elegantly dressed in "double-breasted, black, broadcloth coat, stand-up collar, plain tie, dark trousers and narrow small shoes," surrounded by "horny-fisted sons of toil" and acting "like Queen Victoria at a national Democratic convention." Powderly constantly preached against strikes, and yet it was as a result of strikes in 1885–86 that the Order made its most sensational gains. These were spontaneous revolts rather than organized strikes, but under their stimulus membership soared from about one hundred thousand to over seven hundred thousand. The strength of the Order quickly ebbed after the upheavals of 1886. It lingered through the 1890s but with declining membership and influence.

In the meantime the American Federation of Labor, founded in 1881, was hammering out a labor philosophy more closely related to the realities of the industrial economy and more in harmony with the future. Rejecting the utopian radicalism of the Knights of Labor, the AFL foreswore political goals for economic objectives. Instead of embracing the brotherhood of all workers, it devoted its attention to gaining concrete benefits for skilled workers organized along craft lines. It was a loose alliance of national trade unions, each of which retained a large amount of autonomy, with jurisdiction over its own affairs and with the power to call its own strikes. By 1900 the AFL did not hesitate to acknowledge the strike and the boycott as legitimate means of collective bargaining. These principles had been formulated by 1881 and reaffirmed when the AFL was reorganized in 1886.

As its first president the AFL elected Samuel Gompers, who retained the office for nearly forty years. An immigrant boy, born in London in 1850, Gompers grew up in the trade-union movement. Under the impact of his experience in America he gradually put aside his earlier leanings to socialism and slowly shaped a more conservative approach to the problems of labor. He felt that labor should accept the economic system and should try to win for itself a respectable place as a "legitimate" group within that system, as legitimate as business or the church. And to do so, he argued, labor would have to struggle day by day for higher wages and lower hours. Gompers strove to impose order by resolving jurisdictional disputes between unions and by consolidating local unions in state and national federations. The AFL grew as the Knights declined; by 1902 its membership topped the million mark.

Labor's struggle to win acceptance and to improve its lot was marked by an extraordinary number of strikes and lockouts, conflicts that sometimes flared into bloodshed, particularly in time of depression. In July 1877 a series of wage cuts and abortive strikes provoked an upheaval of insurrectionary violence along the trunk lines of three big railroads. In the first show of violence, along the B&O, federal troops were called in after a mob intimidated state militia. In Pittsburgh the community joined the strikers against the Pennsylvania Railroad and destroyed $5 million worth of property before being dispersed with heavy loss of life. Other disturbances broke out in Philadelphia, Harrisburg, Reading, Scranton, Buffalo, and Toledo, and farther west in St. Louis, Chicago, and San Francisco. Scores of people lost their lives, and property valued at millions of dollars went up in flames. The courts clamped down, the police became more ruthless, and the public began to withdraw its sympathy from the labor movement. Another upsurge of labor militancy occurred during the mid-eighties. With the Knights of Labor at the peak of their strength, labor solidarity materialized in general strikes, sympathetic work stoppage, and nationwide boycotts and political demonstrations. During 1886, a climactic year in labor history, 610,000 workers were unemployed because of strikes, lockouts, or shut-

Samuel Gompers: higher wages, lower hours

downs due to strikes, more than three times the average of the five preceding years. Then on May 4, during an anarchist demonstration against police brutalities at Haymarket Square in Chicago, a bomb was thrown that killed a policeman and fatally wounded six other persons. A jury found eight anarchists guilty, and four were hanged, though the identity of the bomb-thrower was never established. The incident smeared parts of the labor movement, especially the Knights, with the charge of anarchism and subjected labor to public suspicion and hostility.

Resort to violence was common in the turbulent nineties, but often labor was merely replying to force with force. In the remote Coeur d'Alene district of Idaho, company guards and miners fought it out in 1892 with rifles and dynamite until at last federal troops came in, crushed the strike, and turned the miners' jobs over to strikebreakers. At Carnegie's Homestead steel plant in Pennsylvania the same year, thirty-eight hundred members of the Amalgamated Association of Iron and Steel Workers struck over wage cuts and working conditions. As a preparation for breaking the strike, Henry C. Frick, the manager, imported three hundred Pinkerton detectives. When they arrived at the plant on barges, the strikers resisted and a gun fight ensued that resulted in the death of seven detectives and nine strikers, the wounding of a much larger number, and the surrender of the detectives. The sufferings of the workers stirred great public sympathy, a sympathy that was not entirely alienated by the attempt of an anarchist, who had no connection with the strike, to assassinate Frick. In the end, however, the strike failed miserably, and its failure heralded the end of unionism in the steel industry for many years to come.

The great depression that started in 1893 (see p. 516) brought on a new wave of wage cuts, layoffs, and strikes. More workers were thrown out of work by strikes in 1894, a year of exceptional unemployment and labor violence, than in any previous year. The most important strike of that year, and of many years to come, was the big railroad strike centering in Chicago. It originated not among railway workers but among factory workers in George M. Pullman's "model" company town just south of Chicago. The workers were driven to desperation by five wage cuts in one year and no reduction in the high rents charged for company houses. The Pullman workers had recently joined the new American Railway Union, headed by Eugene V. Debs and frowned on by the older Railway Brotherhoods of the AFL. Although Debs urged caution, his union voted to refuse to handle Pullman cars if the management would not accept arbitration of the strike. Pullman rejected all arbitration, and the General Managers Association came to his aid by dismissing switchmen who boycotted his cars. The union then struck against the railroads, and by the end of June 1894 nearly all railroad workers on roads west of Chicago were on strike.

Acting for the railroads, the General Managers Association then appealed directly to the federal government to intervene with armed force and end the strike. There had been no violence so far, and federal intervention with troops was a move that Governor John P. Altgeld strongly opposed. Railroad lawyers had no trouble persuading President Cleveland and Attorney General Richard Olney that intervention could nevertheless be justified on the ground that the strike had obstructed the delivery of United States mail. Actually, the railroads themselves refused, against the union's wishes, to attach mail cars to trains that did not include Pullman cars. Nevertheless, Olney secured an injunction against the union, and on July 4 Cleveland sent some two thousand troops to Chicago to enforce the injunction and protect the mails. After the troops arrived, the union completely lost control of the situation, and mobs of looters destroyed cars and burned and stole property. Twelve people were killed and many arrested at the scene, but none was a striker. The effect of the troop action was to break the strike, a result that Olney, by his own confession, intended to accomplish. The mood of labor at this time is suggested by the narrow defeat of a socialist demand for the collective ownership of the means of production in the AFL convention of 1894. The vote suggests that there were limits to labor's relative indifference toward collectivism (p. 468).

The failure of the Pullman strike had important consequences for the future of American labor. Debs and other union officials were tried and sentenced to jail for contempt of court in disobeying the injunction against the union. The Supreme Court in upholding the sentence gave the use of the injunction in labor disputes a prestige it had never before enjoyed. And the government in suggesting that a strike might be construed as a conspiracy in restraint of trade under the Sherman Antitrust Act placed a powerful weapon in the hands of management for use against unions. Another unforeseen consequence of the Pullman strike and the Court's decision was to bring into national prominence for the first time the name of Eugene V. Debs. Within a few years he became the foremost leader of the socialist movement in the country, a position he held during the years when that movement enjoyed its greatest strength.

Any realistic account of the ordeal of industrialization in America will tell of heedless waste and ruthless exploitation, of cutthroat competition and consolidation. Whatever economic progress came out of the grim struggle—and undoubtedly much was gained—was purchased at a high cost in brutalized labor, wasted resources, and deterioration in business and public ethics. Historians who emphasize the necessity for industrialization and the advantages ultimately derived from it remind us that the costs of industrialization have never been low and that when reckoned in human suffering and social turmoil the price has been even more appalling in other countries than in the United States. And in all fairness, the American ordeal should be judged in comparison with that of England, which preceded it, and that of Russia, which came after it. In neither case does the American record, as bad as it was, suffer by comparison.

Suggestions for Reading   New insights are provided by A. D. Chandler, Jr., *The Visible Hand: The Managerial Revolution in American Business* (1977), and Glenn Porter and H. C. Livesay, *Merchants and Manufacturers: Studies in the Changing Structure of Nineteenth Century Marketing* (1971). For comparative evaluation see T. C. Cochran, "The Paradox of American Economic Growth," *Journal of American History*, LXI (1975), 925–942. Glenn Porter, *The Rise of Big Business, 1860–1910** (1973), and E. C. Kirkland, *Industry Comes of Age: Business, Labor, and Public Policy, 1860–1897** (1961), are surveys of superior quality. A briefer sketch is S. P. Hays, *The Response to Industrialism: 1885–1914** (1957). J. A. Garraty, *The New Commonwealth, 1877–1890** (1968); R. H. Wiebe, *The Search for Order: 1877–1920** (1968); and T. C. Cochran and William Miller, *The Age of Enterprise** (1942), contain excellent chapters. William Miller, ed., *Men in Business** (1952), has illuminating essays. Louis Galambos, *The Public Image of Big Business in America, 1880–1940: A Quantitative Study of Social Change* (1975), assesses public opinion.

The railroad establishment of the period is described in G. R. Taylor and I. D. Neu, *The American Railroad Network, 1861–1890* (1956). The importance of railroads to the economy is questioned by R. W. Fogel, *Railroads and American Economic Growth: Essays in Econometric History** (1964). Railroading in the West is treated in R. E. Riegel, *The Story of the Western Railroads** (1926), and R. C. Overton, *Burlington West* (1941) and *Gulf to Rockies** (1953); in New England by E. C. Kirkland, *Men, Cities and Transportation*, 2 vols. (1948); and in the South by J. F. Stover, *The Railroads of the South, 1865–1900* (1955). On consolidation and management see E. G. Campbell, *The Reorganization of the American Railroad System, 1893–1900* (1938). T. C. Cochran, *Railroad Leaders, 1845–1890* (1953), emphasizes their attitudes and problems. Light on government regulation comes from Lee Benson, *Merchants, Farmers, and Railroads* (1955); Gabriel Kolko, *Railroads and Regulation, 1877–1916** (1965); and G. H. Miller, *Railroads and the Granger Laws* (1971).

On technological developments, Lewis Mumford, *Technics and Civilization** (1934), is suggestive. H. J. Habakkuk, *American and British Technology in the Nineteenth Century** (1962), is a comparative study. An authoritative work of reference is Charles Singer et al., eds., *A History of Technology*, Vol. V: *The Late Nineteenth Century, c. 1850 to c. 1900* (1958). Waldemar Kaempffert, *A Popular History of American Invention*, 2 vols. (1924), is full of interesting detail. Heavy industry and manufacturing generally are treated in V. S. Clark, *History of Manufactures in the United States from 1607–1928*, 3 vols., Vol. II (1929). H. C. Passer, *The Electrical Manufacturers, 1875–1900* (1953), reveals much about technical change and economic growth.

On the steel industry, Andrew Carnegie, *Autobiography* (1920), and J. F. Wall, *Andrew Carnegie* (1970), are highly informative. Oil and Rockefeller are the subject of exhaustive studies, including Allan Nevins, *John D. Rockefeller*, 2 vols. (1940); R. W. Hidy and M. E. Hidy, *Pioneering in Big Business, 1882–1911: History of the Standard Oil Company, New Jersey* (1955). For contrasting points of view on Rockefeller, see Earl Latham, *John D. Rockefeller: Robber Baron or Industrial Statesman?* (1949). See also H. F. Williamson and A. R. Daum, *The American Petroleum Industry, 1859–1959*, 2 vols. (1959–63). Jonathan Hughes, *The Vital Few** (1966), is another study of big-business leaders, as is Saul Englebourg, *Power and Morality: American Business Ethics* (1980). The trust and early regulatory legislation are most fully treated in H. B. Thorelli, *The Federal Antitrust Policy* (1955). See also Arnold Paul, *Conservative Crisis and the Rule of Law: Attitudes of Bar and Bench* (1969).

The business philosophy of laissez faire is perceptively treated in E. C. Kirkland, *Business in the Gilded Age* (1952) and *Dream and Thought in the Business Community, 1860–1900* (1956), and by R. G. McCloskey, *American Conservatism in the Age of Enterprise, 1865–1910* (1951). Richard Hofstadter, *Social Darwinism in American Thought** (1944, rev. ed., 1959), should be compared with Robert Bannister, *Social Darwinism* (1979); see also Sidney Fine, *Laissez Faire and the General Welfare State: A Study of Conflict in American Thought, 1865–1901** (1956). The authority on Henry George is C. A. Barker, *Henry George* (1955). See Samuel Chugerman, *Lester F. Ward: The American Aristotle* (1939), J. L. Thomas, *Alternative America: Henry George, Edward Bellamy, Henry Demarest Lloyd* (1983), and Arthur Lipow, *Authoritarian Socialism in America: Edward Bellamy and the Nationalist Movement* (1982), are recommended.

A useful brief survey is Henry Pelling, *American Labor** (1960). On social history see H. G. Gutman, *Work Culture & Society in Industrializing America** (1976), Melvyn Dubofsky, *Industrialism and the American Worker** (1975), and David Montgomery, *Workers Control in America* (1979). On the Knights of Labor, see N. J. Ware, *The Labor Movement in the United States, 1860–1895* (1929), and on its great rival see Harold Livesay, *Samuel Gompers and Organized Labor in America** (1978), and Philip Taft, *The A. F. of L. in the Time of Gompers* (1957). On trade unionism and reformers see G. N.

Grob, *Workers and Utopia* (1961). An important study is Lloyd Ulman, *The Rise of the National Trade Union* (1955). On women see Alice Kessler-Harris, *Out to Work** (1982). On the South see M. A. McLaurin, *Paternalism and Protest: Southern Cotton Mill Workers and Organized Labor, 1875–1905* (1971). Autobiographies of the two foremost leaders of labor are T. V. Powderly, *Thirty Years of Life and Labor, 1859–1889* (1890), and Samuel Gompers, *Seventy Years of Life and Labour*, 2 vols. (1925).

Industrial life and business struggles have been the subjects of such novels as Henry James, *The American** (1877); John Hay, *The Breadwinners** (1883), an antilabor work; W. D. Howells, *The Rise of Silas Lapham** (1885), the study of a businessman; and Theodore Dreiser, *The Financier** (1912) and *The Titan** (1914), portraits of industrial tycoons. Edward Bellamy, *Looking Backward, 2000–1887** (1888), is a utopian novel that started a reform movement.

*Available in a paperback edition.

19
THE URBAN SOCIETY

For a nation of cities to have been nourished on a long antiurban tradition is one of the paradoxes of America. Antiurbanism ranged from fear and revulsion to deep alienation and revolt from the cities. It was not a product of popular culture, which more often celebrated urban life, but of some of the most talented and influential intellectuals of the eighteenth and nineteenth centuries. Thomas Jefferson spoke of cities as "pestilential" and as "sores," and his friend the distinguished scientist Benjamin Rush compared them to "abscesses on the human body," and called them "reservoirs of all the impurities of a community." A favorite metaphor of the next generation was the city as "cancer." The antiurban outcry continued with Emerson, Thoreau, Hawthorne, Melville, and Poe—drowning out the few defenders such as Whitman—and was carried into the twentieth century by Henry Adams, Henry James, and William Dean Howells. Urban America enjoyed no mystique of attachment such as the Greeks professed for their city, the *polis*, or the affection French writers felt for Paris. No simple explanation is possible, but one reason was that the Founding Fathers, their children, and their grandchildren were almost completely rural by birth, by breeding, and in outlook. The grandchildren and great-grandchildren as well as later immigrants had only recently moved to town.

America Moves to Town

The pull of the city. In 1790, the year of the first census, only 3.35 percent of the population lived in towns of eight thousand or more. By the end of the nineteenth century ten times that percentage, a third of the population, was classified "urban" by this definition. The cities grew with the nation, of course, but after about 1820 they grew much faster than the nation. Between 1800 and 1890 the population of the entire country increased twelvefold, but over the same period the urban population multiplied eighty-seven fold. In 1800 there were only 6 cities with more than eight thousand people; by 1890 there were 448, and 26 of them had a population greater than one hundred thousand. More striking still was the rise of the American metropolis, the big city of more than half a million. The ancient world produced only two of that size, Rome and Alexandria, and western Europe had only two by the beginning of the eighteenth century, London and Paris. By 1900 there were six cities that large in the United States, and three of them had a population of over a million. Rapid urbanization was not limited to this country, but the pace was faster in the United States than in Europe. The New World metropolis grew at a pace unprecedented in history.

474

Urban transport, 1891

Chicago more than tripled its size between 1880 and 1900, when it had more than 1½ million, and New York grew from not quite 2 million to nearly 3½ million in those two decades. Buffalo, Detroit, and Milwaukee more than doubled, and St. Paul, Minneapolis, and Denver more than quadrupled their size. The surge of people from country to city spoke more eloquently of national preference than did the antiurban tradition of the intellectuals.

Urban growth was very unequally distributed, and some parts of the country did not really participate in the movement significantly until the twentieth century. In fact, half the entire urban population in 1890 was in the North Atlantic states and only 7.7 percent was in the South Atlantic states. More than half the nation's city-dwellers lived in the five states of New York, Pennsylvania, Massachusetts, Illinois, and Ohio. Four-fifths of them lived north of the Ohio and Missouri rivers. While by 1900 six out of ten people in the North Atlantic states and three out of ten in the Middle West lived in cities, scarcely one out of ten was an urbanite in the South. Urbanization affected all parts of the country, even the most remote, but in some parts toward the end of the century it was less an immediate experience than a distant and powerful lure.

The drain on the countryside was especially noticeable in the Middle West and the North Atlantic states. Some of it was due, as in the past, to the lure of the West. But the pull of the city was growing stronger and stronger. Between 1880 and 1890 more than half the townships of Iowa and Illinois declined in popula-

tion, and yet both states gained substantially in total number of inhabitants. Rural decline was even greater in the North Atlantic states, where the flight to the city had long been in progress. In New England 932 out of the total of 1,502 townships, including two-thirds of those in Maine and New Hampshire and three-fourths of those in Vermont, declined in population during the eighties. Thousands of farms were abandoned, houses were left to decay, and scores of villages were completely deserted. Yet in that decade New England, largely through the growth of its cities, actually gained 20 percent in total population. As early as 1890 the number of industrial wage-earners in the whole country almost equaled the number of farm-owners, tenants, and farm laborers combined.

Rural defenses against the lure of the city reached a new low in the eighties and nineties. The seventies and the nineties were the worst decades of agricultural depression (see Chapter 20), when everything seemed to go wrong with the farming economy. Crop prices were lower, debts greater, mortgages heavier, and more workers were displaced by machines than ever before. At the same time the glamour and attraction of the city were enhanced by the glitter of the new electric lights, as well as by the telephones, the trolley cars, and a thousand other wonders. The city was the only place one could enjoy such amenities, for they did not begin to penetrate the countryside and soften the contrast with urban comforts to any extent until well into the twentieth century. The contrast between rural ills and urban attractions made farmers regard their harsh lot and isolation as even

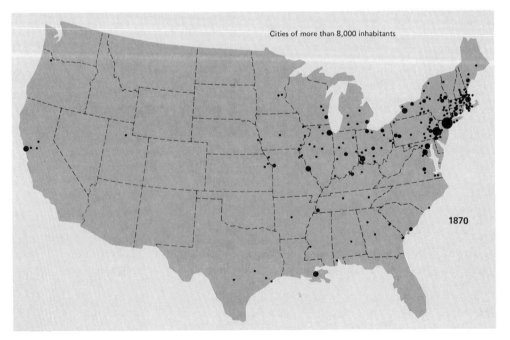

America moves to town, 1870

Cities of more than 8,000 inhabitants

1870

Telephone exchange: urban wonder

more intolerable than ever before, as indeed they were. Many farmers resorted to political rebellion for relief. A great many others simply moved to town.

Cities did not simply increase in number and expand in size; they changed in character, in pattern, and in structure, and all rather suddenly. Until about 1870 the downtown business section huddled around a harbor with factories, banks, slaughterhouses, and retail houses side by side. Surrounding them were both slum streets as well as streets of wealth and fashion. Beyond them stretched acres that mixed residential, industrial, and commercial neighborhoods indiscriminately, with boarding houses next to prosperous homes and a row of houses for downtown workers a block away. It was the era of "walking cities," when nearness to work was all important. There was no central city of poverty with an outer rim of affluence. Classes, races, and ethnic groups

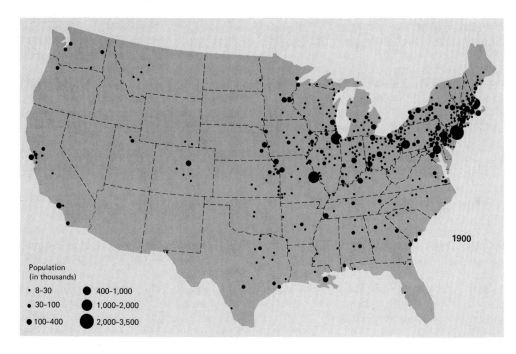

America moves to town, 1900

1900

Population
(in thousands)

- 8–30
- 30–100
- 100–400
- 400–1,000
- 1,000–2,000
- 2,000–3,500

were jumbled together to a degree unknown later, all in proximity to business and industry.

The segregated city of modern times, with a core of poverty and rings of rising affluence, developed swiftly after 1870. The changes were brought on by street railways, job locations, housing prices, racial prejudice, and class distinction. The result was a highly fragmented city tightly structured along economic lines. Smaller cities were identified by their economic specializations. There were beer cities, steel cities, textile towns, glass towns, even a candy town: Hershey, Pennsylvania. Albany concentrated on shirts, Troy on collars, Bridgeport on corsets and machine tools; Richmond and Durham made cigarettes, Tampa cigars, Tulsa petroleum, and Dayton was famous for producing cash registers—the very symbol of the urban culture. City people were tied together by the cash nexus, bound into an economic web, and lived under the absolute dictatorship of the clock.

Out west most of the mining towns—the gold, silver, copper, lead, coal, and oil towns—vanished with the depletion of their mineral resources. Hundreds of "paper" towns with thousands of lots laid out for sale by speculators and boomers died aborning without an inhabitant. At least sixty-two of more than a hundred such "cities" in Los Angeles County, one of which sold some 4,000 lots before it was discovered to be "most easily accessible by means of a balloon," vanished without a trace. Those that did flourish in the West, with few exceptions, were founded as commercial enterprises, mainly the work of railroad and real estate promoters.

City lights and cesspools. The new technology and the factories probably produced more discomforts and inconveniences than comforts and amenities for most of the city-dwellers of the late nineteenth century. But to the outsider the advantages and attractions were more readily apparent. First among these were the bright lights that were replacing the dim gas lamps in the streets and the kerosene lamps and gas jets indoors. Cleveland and San Francisco led the way in 1879 by installing brilliant electric arc lamps in their streets, and their example was quickly followed in cities across the country. The noisy, sputtering arc lamp was impractical for indoor use, but for that purpose the incandescent light bulb patented by Edison in 1880 (see p. 463) became available in a few years and spread as swiftly as the growth of power plants permitted. In 1882 there were only thirty-eight central power stations in the whole country, but before the end of the century there were three thousand. Improved lighting not only made cities safer at night but enabled factories to run night shifts, proved a boon to theaters and other amusement houses, and extended the hours of libraries, shops, and schools.

Cincinnati trolley, 1890

Electrical power provided the answer to a city problem that was even more pressing than that of lighting—the problem of moving vast numbers of people rapidly through the streets and the replacement of the walking city by the "streetcar suburbs." The expansion began in the seventies with streetcars pulled by horses. Streetcars broke down the self-contained economies of outlying towns and bound the suburbs to the cities. Construction of cheap housing, typically of the three-decker style, and expansion of public utilities and services extended the suburbs until they dwarfed the old central cities and transformed the character of both city and suburb. The transformation and the expansion were greatly increased when electric trolley cars began to replace horse cars in the late eighties. The first practical electric cars were developed in Richmond, Virginia, in 1887, and suburbs were extended everywhere the trolley car spread. What relief of congestion they provided came at the cost of increased segregation according to income and class in suburban residential patterns.

Technology and invention were slower to yield solutions to city problems that were traditionally assigned to the public domain, such as street-paving, water supply, and sewage disposal, and in these matters progress was halting. In the seventies the streets even of the larger cities were poorly paved—usually with cobblestones or granite blocks along the eastern seaboard, with wooden blocks in the Middle West, and with gravel or macadam in the South. Brick became popular as pavement in the mid-eighties, especially in cities where it was manufactured. The national capital in 1878 set the pace in adapting asphalt to street-paving, the method that eventually proved the favorite.

Water supply and sewage disposal lagged far behind the demands and needs of mushrooming city populations. The typical urbanite of the seventies relied on the rural solution of individual well and privy or cesspool: Washington had fifty-six thousand cesspools in the mid-seventies, and Philadelphia even more. Baltimore in the eighties smelled "like a billion polecats," according to H. L. Mencken, and a Chicagoan said in his city "the stink is enough to knock you down." Improvement was slow, and large cities of the East and South depended to the end of the century mainly on drainage through open gutters. Pollution of water supplies by sewage as well as by the dumping of industrial waste accounted in large measure for the wretched public-health records and staggering mortality rates of the period. The number of public waterworks multiplied more than fivefold in the eighties, but filtering and purification were slow to be adopted. Throughout the nineties the American city remained poorly prepared to accommodate the hordes that continued to pour in upon it.

The immigrant and the city. The cities grew at the expense of the European as well as the American countryside and village. For the pull of America was felt in Europe more powerfully than ever before, and the great majority of the immigrants crowded into the nation's cities. Like the new native city-dwellers, the immigrants were also country people. In spite of the distance they had come, they were usually no more familiar with city ways and city life than Americans fresh from the farm, and for the immigrants the uprooting was even more of a shock and a bewilderment.

The immigrants were often thought of as the primary cause of the urban crisis. Actually, the percentage of foreign born in the total population remained about the same; the immigrants came from much the same social classes as they always had; and they came for the same old reason—to better their lot. A much larger percentage of the new immigrants than previously returned to their native lands, and there were other significant changes. For one thing they began to come in far greater numbers than ever before. From 1850 to 1880 about 2½ million had arrived per decade, with the rate falling off a bit in the sixties but picking up again in the seventies. Big passenger ships, built for the purpose, altered immigration in many ways. In the eighties the number more than doubled, with nearly 5¼ million arriving during that decade, and with nearly 3¾ million more landing in the next. For another thing immigrants showed a

greater tendency than ever to congregate in the large Eastern cities and less disposition to disperse over the countryside. This concentration naturally made them more conspicuous. And finally there came a shift to what was called "new" immigration—from southern and eastern Europe—as contrasted with the "old" immigrants from northern and western Europe. The old immigrants had come typically from Britain, Ireland, Germany, or one of the Scandinavian countries, and they were usually Protestant. The new immigrants were Italians, Austrians, Hungarians, Poles, Serbs, and Russians; they were Catholic or Jewish in religion and had habits and ways that appeared outlandish to older Americans. Immigrants of the new type had made up only 1.4 percent of the total immigration of the sixties and less than 20 percent in the eighties; but in the nineties their proportion suddenly climbed to more than 50 percent and in the next decade to more than 70 percent. This increasing proportion of new immigrants coincided with, and provided stimulation for, two tendencies: (1) an increasing concern over the ills of urban life and (2) an increasing tendency to stress racial differences. Because of this coincidence, the new immigrants were blamed for many serious city problems that had little to do with racial or national origin.

There could be no doubt, however, that the foreigner and the immigrant had become conspicuous in American life. By 1890 one-fourth of the Philadelphi-

Immigrants: the pull of America

ans and one-third of the Bostonians and Chicagoans were of foreign birth, and in Greater New York four out of five residents were of foreign birth or foreign parentage. Of the male population of the eighteen largest cities in the country there were two and a half times as many of foreign birth or foreign parentage as there were of the older American stock. New York City had half as many Italians as Naples and two and a half times as many Irish as Dublin. The newcomers tended more than the "old" immigrants to huddle together clannishly by nationality. Jacob Riis, a New York journalist and reformer who had emigrated from Denmark in 1870, pictured a map of Manhattan in 1890 colored according to races and nationalities:

> Between the dull gray of the Jew, his favorite color, and the Italian red, would be squeezed in on the map a sharp streak of yellow, marking the narrow boundaries of Chinatown. Dovetailed in

Sources of immigration, 1871–1910

with the German population, the poor but thrifty Bohemian might be picked out by the sombre hue of his life. . . . Dots and dashes of color here and there would show where the Finnish sailors worship their *djumala* (God), the Greek pedlars the ancient name of their race, and the Swiss the goddess of thrift.

Less colorfully, Jane Addams described the map of Chicago:

> Between Halsted Street and the river live about ten thousand Italians—Neapolitans, Sicilians, and Calabrians, with an occasional Lombard or Venetian. To the south on Twelfth Street are many Germans, and side streets are given over almost entirely to Polish and Russian Jews. Still farther south, these Jewish colonies merge into a huge Bohemian colony, so vast that Chicago ranks as the third Bohemian city in the world.

Slums and palaces. The city of that period grew without plan, with a minimum of control, guided mainly by the dictates of industrial enterprise and private greed. Even with an alert and informed citizenry and an honest and efficient municipal government a city would have faced staggering difficulties, and few cities could boast either asset.

One product of the haphazard growth was the city slum, an old evil that took on new life in 1879 with the invention, in New York City, of the "dumbbell" tenement house, so named for the shape of its floor plan. Designed to get the maximum return for the landlord, the new tenement was no better than a barracks honeycombed with rooms, many of them with no direct access to light or air. Lacking sanitary facilities, privacy, or health precautions, these tenements rapidly degenerated into human pigsties, vile smelling and vermin infested. According to Jacob Riis, in 1890 half the city's population lived in them.

William Dean Howells, a realistic novelist, admitted in 1896 that from a distance the tenement might sometimes appear picturesque:

> But to be in it, and not have the distance, is to inhale the stenches of the neglected street, and to catch the yet fouler and dreadfuller poverty-smell which breathes from the open doorways. . . . It is to see the work-worn look of mothers, the squalor of the babes, the haggish ugliness of the old women, the slovenly frowziness of the young girls.

In the worst of the tenement slums crime and prostitution flourished, and organized gangs operated securely within their protection. In years when the homicide rate in England and Germany was less than half that in the United States and when the rate in

Europe was declining, the rate in the United States was increasing, and lawlessness was growing at an alarming pace. Extremes of human misery and degradation had become common sights.

In the eighties and nineties the gulfs between social classes were dramatically emphasized rather than concealed. The economist Thorstein Veblen, in his *Theory of the Leisure Class* (1899), hit on the expression "conspicuous consumption." Displaying habits of consumption that were competitive as well as conspicuous, Chicagoans sported liveried servants and dwelt in lavish palaces built in plain view. The contrast with conspicuous poverty was glaring and unconcealed; squalor and splendor paraded the same streets. The palaces of the wealthy that lined New York's Fifth Avenue were paralleled a few blocks away by the desolation of Shantytown, inhabited by Irish paupers and goats and stretching along the East Side for sixty blocks or more. In the same year in which Jacob Riis published his shocking study of the slums, *How the Other Half Lives* (1890), Ward McAllister published his *Society As I Have Found It* (1890), lovingly recounting the extravagances of New York's Four Hundred, the self-elected social élite. One exploit of this set was the Bradley Martin costume ball, staged in the Waldorf Hotel at a cost of $368,200. It took place on February 10, 1897, when thousands of unemployed roamed the street, and was attended by guests decked in costumes costing as much as $10,000. Scenes of this sort help to explain the violence in the rhetoric of Populism and other protest movements of the nineties.

Howells, in a poem called "Society" (1895), compared the violent social contrasts of his day with "a splendid pageantry of beautiful women and lordly men" playing and dancing upon a magnificent floor that barely covered the crushed and bleeding bodies of the oppressed:

> And now and then from out the dreadful floor
> An arm or brow was lifted from the rest,
> As if to strike in madness, or implore
> For mercy; and anon some suffering breast
> Heaved from the mass and sank; and as before
> The revellers above them thronged and prest.

The Awakening
of the Social Conscience

The city was a shock to the American conscience, not merely because of violent contrasts, abuses, and evils, but because the national conscience had taken shape in an agrarian culture and a rural past. So had national values, ideals, morals, folkways, and political institutions. American country folk or European peasants who emigrated were repelled as well as fascinated by the city; they accepted it and rejected it at the same time. Their feelings were torn and their consciences were bruised by the experience.

The challenge of the bosses. Probably the most flagrant offense against public morals in the last quarter of the nineteenth century was the corruption of

The immigrant and the boss

What tells in holdin' your grip on your district is to go right down among the poor families and help them in the different ways they need help. I've got a regular system for this. If there's a fire ... any hour of the day or night, I'm usually there with some of my election district captains as soon as the fire-engines. If a family is burned out I don't ask whether they are Republicans or Democrats, and I don't refer them to the Charity Organization Society, which would investigate their case in a month or two and decide they were worthy of help about the time they are dead from starvation. I just get quarters for them ... and fix them up till they get things runnin' again....

Another thing, I can always get a job for a deservin' man. I make it a point to keep on the track of jobs, and it seldom happens that I don't have a few up my sleeve ready for use...

And the children—the little roses of the district! Do I forget them? Oh, ·no! They know me, every one of them, and they know that a sight of Uncle George and candy means the same thing. Some of them are the best kind of vote-getters.

From William L. Riordon, *Plunkitt of Tammany Hall*, 1905.

---

city government. At least it got more attention than other offenses. Since the Federal Constitution is silent about cities, they had to derive their authority and frame of government from state charters. These charters were the work of legislatures generally composed of rural and small-town representatives who were fearful of the urban menace and sought to constrain it by denying city governments authority and saddling them with inappropriate legislative machinery and weak executives. The result was an urban power vacuum into which moved party machine organizations dominated by unelected political bosses. The bosses provided the necessary government by means that were often illegal and corrupt, if highly functional. A promising combination of circumstances provided an open invitation to corrupt government. The rapid growth of cities had made necessary the large-scale expansion of public utilities of all sorts—water, gas, transportation, electricity—as well as the construction of public buildings, sewage systems, docks, street and sidewalk pavement. For this work a multitude of valuable contracts, franchises, monopolies, subsidies, and privileges had to be granted. Such prizes were worth fortunes, and there were plenty of operators ready with the price.

Not surprisingly, the cities were excessively burdened with debt. Yet for all their heavy expenditures they often received wretched service from the utilities they subsidized and were cynically and repeatedly defrauded by the unelected public servants. "With very few exceptions," wrote Andrew D. White, president of Cornell, "the city governments of the United States are the worst in Christendom—the most expensive, the most inefficient, and the most corrupt." And

James Bryce, a generous but well-informed English critic, pronounced city government "the one conspicuous failure of the United States," far more serious, in his opinion, than the shortcomings of state and federal government.

Never in America had a more colorful set of politicians wielded such power as the great bosses of this period. With a disposition toward large girth, shiny hats, and heavy jewelry, the boss played the role of a freehanded spender, the Robin Hood of the masses. High in the annals of bossdom are the names of "Honest" John Kelley and Richard Croker of New York, Christopher L. Magee and William Finn of Pittsburgh, Ed Butler of St. Louis, "King" James McManes of Philadelphia, and "Czar" Martin Lomasney of Boston. Revenue flowed into their coffers from office-seekers, contractors, public utilities, railroads, prostitutes, gamblers—anybody who happened to need protection or favors. Even pushcart-peddlers and garbage-collectors paid tribute to New York's Tammany. Boss McManes, as head of Philadelphia's gas trust, had 5,630 public jobs at his disposal.

The city boss and his lieutenants in the wards and precincts found their most reliable supporters among the immigrants. These new voters certainly had no monopoly on ignorance and apathy, and many of them were intelligent and useful citizens. But they were usually unaccustomed to the ballot, unpracticed in the ways of democracy, and bewildered by city life in a strange land. Moreover, the great majority of them were unskilled laborers who lived close to the margin of existence and were often in need of a job and a friend. The boss dealt primarily in jobs and votes. He had sometimes sprung from the immigrant

**The immigrant
in the city**

community himself, shared its sense of solidarity, knew its leaders by name, and remained one of them. The immigrants responded to him with group loyalty and devotion. They knew him as a man who "got things done," a man to whom they could always take their troubles. The boss made it his business to know their needs and to give them tangible evidence of his interest in them. His favors took the form of getting them jobs, intervening with the law in their behalf, bailing them out of jail, paying burial money, distrib-uting free coal, and handing out Christmas baskets. In short, he performed services for which there was as yet no public agency and which no one else was ready to perform.

Irish politicians were especially adept at these arts, and it was a prevailing conviction that, as one writer put it, "The function of the Irishman is to ad-minister the affairs of the American city." A glance at the names heading the roster of bosses supports this conviction. One of them put his political theory in these words: "I think that there's got to be in every ward a guy that any bloke can go to when he's in trouble and get help—not justice and the law, but help, no matter what he's done." Theodore Roosevelt, who studied the matter, concluded that urban reform-ers would have to create social agencies to fulfill the role the boss played before they could replace him.

As the reformers found out for themselves, after a little experience, many "good" people supported the bosses and machines—educated, respectable, mid-dle-class people who had been natives for at least three generations. Some of these "good" people were busi-nessmen who were quite willing to cooperate with the machine to secure the favors, privileges, and exemp-

tions they desired. Other respectable citizens voted regularly, if regretfully, for the machine because of their sincere devotion to the national party with which the machine was identified and their desire for a party victory. In short, city machine and city boss were buttressed by some of the strongest as well as by some of the weakest elements of the population. Any-one who undertook to change the system would need to be very powerful indeed.

Humanitarians and reformers. The conscience of the middle class was eventually stirred to indigna-tion and action by the misery and degradation of the city. But first the middle class had to discover what poverty was. Early humanitarians and reformers did not understand the poor—the "depraved classes," as they called them. Attributing their plight to moral shortcomings, they sent agents of the Charity Organi-zations Society to discover which of the poor were "deserving." But it was the young social workers, nearly all of them women, patiently investigating and visiting the sweatshops and tenement firetraps, who began to establish contact between the middle class and the working class.

Inspired by English social-reform literature and a visit to Toynbee Hall in the slums of London, Jane Addams, the most famous American woman of her time, took up the settlement-house idea and estab-lished Hull House on Halsted Street in Chicago in 1889. She wished, she said, "to share the lives of the poor" and to make social service "express the spirit of Christ." One such house had already been established in New York in 1886, and in the next ten years some fifty or more were founded in Northern and Eastern cities. They offered a variety of services, maintained playgrounds, nurseries, club rooms, libraries, and kindergartens, and conducted classes in various subjects. But perhaps of more significance was the education they provided for the young middle-class social workers who came to live in the slums to gain firsthand knowledge of the workers' problems. By bringing them together with women of a very different class—poor, uneducated immigrants—the experience proved of importance to American women's history. Within a few years the settlement houses had become the spawning ground of women reformers. Among them were Lillian Wald, founder of the Henry Street Settlement in New York, Florence Kelley, leading spirit in the National Consumers League, and Frances Perkins, with a great future as a Progressive leader.

On the political front the battle for municipal reform began under leaders recruited from the solid and substantial middle class. These included Seth Low and George William Curtis in New York, Richard Henry Dana, Jr., and Nathan Matthews, Jr., in Boston, and Joseph W. Folk in St. Louis. Good-government clubs, committees, commissions, and reform organizations for municipal improvement proliferated rapidly in the eighties. Every city of any size had one such organization, and the larger cities had several. One of the most prominent was the National Civil Service Reform League, founded in 1881, which published the magazine *Good Government* to promote its prime object, the merit system for city employees. In the early stages these organizations wasted a good deal of time in mass meetings that drafted wordy resolutions and accomplished nothing except to make the reformers look ineffectual if not ridiculous. Cynics called the good-government people the "goo-goos," but they made their influence felt in practical reforms.

The National Municipal League was launched on a wave of public interest in 1894, and within two years more than two hundred branch leagues were founded. The League put forward as its program a model city charter that embodied such advanced reforms as the short ballot, greater freedom from state interference, limited franchise for utilities, separate city and state elections, the merit system, government by experts, and, above all, more authority for the mayor. Not a leader in municipal reform, the League merely reflected the results of reform movements that had been tried out in cities all over the country. It was slow to endorse two of the most important structural reforms, the commission and later the city manager plan. In 1880 only one of the nation's twenty-three principal cities was dominated by the mayor, but by 1900 there were twelve. In 1894 the embattled hosts of reform in New York overthrew Boss Richard Croker and elected William L. Strong mayor, though Tammany returned to power after a brief period. Reform-

ers in Chicago, Boston, and St. Louis also scored significant victories over their machines in the last years of the century.

All these were mere structural reforms inspired by the model of business efficiency, however, and their inadequacy was pointed up by the program of social reforms carried out by Mayor Hazen Pingree of Detroit, Mayor Samuel M. "Golden Rule" Jones of Toledo, Mayor Josiah Quincy of Boston, and Mayor Thomas L. Johnson of Cleveland. Their social reforms provided laws protecting working-class interests and included municipal ownership of utilities, unemployment relief, the eight-hour day, and a minimum wage. Reforms of this type, overlooked by the good-government reformers, attracted popular support that structural reforms often lacked. Their proponents were called "reform bosses" when they used machine methods and played politics with jobs and contracts.

The rights of women. Women reformers responded to the social problems of the city, as we have seen, but another of their preoccupations was the plight of their own sex in a male-dominated society. Their bill of grievances, well documented and long-standing, included political disfranchisement, legal discrimination, economic exploitation, cultural and educational deprivation, and domestic drudgery. If blacks had their "place," women had their "sphere," and to many women its limitations seemed increasingly oppressive. Woman's sphere was The Home, and beyond its walls she ventured, save on religious missions, only at the risk of breaching "the cult of true

New York City settlement house

womanhood"—piety, purity, submissiveness, and domesticity.

The Victorian family undoubtedly proved an important source of personal security against urban disorder for both the working class and those above them, but it came at a heavy cost to women. It was difficult if not impossible to reconcile women's right to equality with the demands made upon women by the institution of the family in nineteenth century America. The principle of equality denied a difference, while the practice of wifehood and motherhood demanded a difference in the roles of men and women. The demand was for the subordination of the wife. Personal achievement and self-fulfillment required attitudes of competitiveness and self-assertion and job opportunities usually denied her.

For a growing number of middle-class women technology—gas lighting, domestic plumbing, manufactured ice, and improved furnaces, stoves, washtubs, and sewing machines—provided some escape from the domestic treadmill. For others cheap domestic servants from the immigrant ships furnished release. New women's colleges and older men's colleges turned coeducational were graduating larger numbers of women—2,500 a year by 1890. But they were educated to fill places that, save for underpaid teaching, did not yet exist. Like their sisters who were venturing out of the "sphere," they found themselves in a society that had no use for them.

What organizations women then had were chiefly devoted to "self-culture." Founded in 1882, the Association of Collegial Alumnae remained small and exclusive for a long time, limited in 1889 to the graduates of the fourteen colleges that met their rigorous standards. At the opposite extreme of inclusiveness was the sprawling General Federation of Women's Clubs. Organized in 1890, it federated hundreds of clubs, had 150,000 members by 1900, and was soon to top a million. Mainly limited to "self-culture" and entertainment, most members were middle-aged, middle-class, conservative women. The General Federation took pains to avoid antagonizing the cautious rank and file, many of them antisuffragists, and did not endorse woman suffrage until the eve of victory. The leaders of the Federation were usually suffragists, however, and their movement furnished the hard core of feminism. Split into two organizations, the militant National and the conservative American associations, since the struggle over black suffrage in the 1860s, the rival groups resolved their differences and merged as the National American Woman Suffrage Association in 1890.

A new generation of women leaders had arrived by this time, though veterans like Susan B. Anthony, Elizabeth Cady Stanton, and Lucy Stone were still on the scene. Like them, Anna Howard Shaw met working women as equals, but she was an exception. "The younger women," as historian Eleanor Flexner writes, "were not, for the most part, distinguished by the breadth of their social views." This was true of Carrie Chapman Catt, May Wright Sewall, Rachel Foster Avery, and Harriet Taylor Upton. They reflected the drift of their times toward conservative views on labor and race relations and were more concerned with decorum in pressing their cause. Rejecting their radical origins, the new feminists also turned away from the disturbing and fundamental questions that their contemporary, Charlotte Perkins Gilman, asked in her book *Woman and Economics* (1898). Instead they narrowed their objectives to suffrage, submerged all women's rights in the political struggle, and as a consequence came to exaggerate the value of the ballot as the sovereign remedy for women's ills.

By 1890 seventeen states and territories had given women limited suffrage in school elections, but not until that year did Wyoming enter the Union as the first state with full suffrage for women. Three more underpopulated Western states followed suit, Colorado in 1893 and Utah and Idaho in 1896, but not for fourteen years did another state adopt woman suffrage. Congress gave formal hearings to pleas for a federal woman suffrage amendment, but neither house reported the bill favorably after 1893, and the question disappeared from Congress as an issue for twenty years. Women kept up their campaigns for state action, waging hundreds of them, many heroically under adverse conditions. Among their arguments were some that appealed to nativism and racism. The 1893 convention of the Woman Suffrage Association urged suffrage with literacy instead of sex qualifications, since there were "more white women who can read and write than all negro voters; more American women who can read and write than all foreign voters." For all that they continued to be rewarded with defeat after defeat until the First World War.

The conscience of the church. The church community was eventually to respond both in faith and in works to the human needs and social problems of city and industry. But in 1876, as Henry May has observed, "Protestantism presented a massive, almost unbroken front in its defense of the status quo." Slums, depressions, and unemployment were but necessary steps to progress, and suffering was the lot of humanity in good, orthodox theology. Religion was a spiritual and individual, not a social, concern, and salvation came through the striving of the individual with sin and conscience, not through social welfare and betterment. The churches, middle class in outlook, were dedicated to the early social creed of individualism and laissez faire, and the mightiest preachers of that era expressed these attitudes forcefully and repeatedly. There was no better exponent of laissez faire and social Darwinism than Henry Ward Beecher in his Brooklyn pulpit.

Revivalism and professional revivalists were usually powerful propagators of the old-time religion—orthodox fundamentalism—and had very little or no social awareness. Throughout the eighties and nineties the annual revival was a regular feature of the program of Methodist, Baptist, Presbyterian, Congregational, and smaller churches. The most famous of the professional revivalists was Dwight L. Moody, an impressive figure of two hundred eighty pounds who got his start with a successful campaign in Britain during the seventies. Returning to America in 1875, he set out with Ira D. Sankey, his equally weighty singer, to "evangelize the world in this generation." Moody brought into play all his great executive and publicity talents to attract huge crowds and with forceful and colloquial sermons converted sinners by the thousands in all parts of the United States. His popularity continued unflagging until his death in 1899. Moody and another famous revivalist, T. DeWitt Talmage, along with numerous imitators, set a record for professional revivalism in America. Whether as a result of their work or the growth of population, Protestant churches grew rapidly in the last two decades of the century, increasing their membership from somewhat over 10 million to almost 18 million.

In spite of this growth, clergymen complained constantly that the working people were drifting away from the church. Moved either by the pulpit's lack of sympathy for their plight or by the elegance of the clothing they saw in the pews, working people found the churches of the older Protestant denominations less suited to their tastes than they once had been. Large working-class districts in the cities were without church facilities of any kind. Some of the poor and the lowly, as they had in the past, sought solace in new sects founded to restore the lost purity or the original doctrine of the old sects. Many of these "holiness" people were recruited from the Methodist, Baptist, and other Protestant churches. Usually originating in the country and then moving to the city, a dozen or more pentecostal and millennial sects sprang up in the eighties and nineties.

A new sect of a different sort was the Church of Christ, Scientist, usually called Christian Scientist, which was chartered by a small group of the followers of Mary Baker Eddy in 1879. The prophet of the new faith was born in 1821 to a New England family of the pious, humble sort to which Joseph Smith, the Mormon prophet (see p. 255), had been born fifteen years earlier. Inspired by the help she received from a faith healer for her own rather complex health problems, she developed the belief that "disease is caused by

Mary Baker Eddy: prophet of a new faith

mind alone." At the end of Eddy's long life in 1910, adherents of her church numbered a hundred thousand, her book *Science and Health* (1875) had sold four hundred thousand copies, and her estate was appraised at more than $2½ million.

Addressing its appeal to the downtrodden, the Salvation Army invaded America in 1879 under the command of George Railton and seven women officers. Founded the year before in London by William Booth, it was born of his desire to reach the city poor. Using revivalist methods and brass bands to attract crowds, the uniformed army and its lassies preached repentance in the streets and sent "slum brigades" into the tenement districts to bring relief as well as the gospel to the poor. Also of English origins was the Young Mens Christian Association, first imported in the 1850s. After the Civil War the YMCA grew rapidly and built inexpensive residential hotels that were also religious, cultural, and recreational centers in the larger cities.

It would have been impossible for the Catholic Church to ignore the working class and the social problems of the city. Since the "new" immigration was overwhelmingly Catholic, working class, and urban, the American Catholic Church of the late nineteenth century became more than ever the church of the city, the worker, and the immigrant. The number of Catholics in the country increased from over 6 million to more than 10 million in the last two decades of the century. Responsibility for training and adjusting the new Americans to their country compelled the Church to adjust its social policy to urban needs and persuaded James Gibbons, then in Rome to be installed as cardinal, to defend the cause of American labor before the Holy See in 1887. American Catholics found some support for their social policy in the loyalty of their communicants, which contrasted with the defection and alienation of the masses of which European Catholics complained. The papal encyclical *Rerum Novarum*, of May 1891, enunciated social ideals and responsibilities for Catholics that gave additional sanction to the social views of the Americans.

In the meantime a small group of Protestant clergymen, at first responding as individuals to the social crises and labor struggles of the seventies, eighties, and nineties, had begun to shape a reinterpretation of their religion that in later years came to be known as the Social Gospel. Turning away from the traditional emphasis on spiritual and moral concerns, the new gospel stressed the social and pragmatic implications of Christian ethics and called for good works in social reform and betterment. The Reverend Josiah Strong's book *Our Country* (1885), which sold half a million copies in twenty years, has been called the *Uncle Tom's Cabin* of the movement. But Washington Gladden, a Congregational minister who wrote *Applied Christianity* (1886), was probably the most influential leader. Next in importance was R. Heber Newton, a liberal New York Episcopalian and an advocate of more sweeping reform. The Episcopal Church, the most aristocratic denomination and yet the one most influenced by the mildly socialistic doctrines then gaining attention in the parent Church of England, took most readily to the new gospel, while the Methodist Church, traditionally the church of the common people, tended to cling to rural individualism and resisted the Social Gospel at first. With a similar following and the additional restraint of such wealthy benefactors as John D. Rockefeller, the Baptists nevertheless moved earlier toward the Social Gospel under the inspiration of Walter Rauschenbusch. By 1895 the influence of the Social Gospel was being felt throughout American Protestantism and in secular thought as well. Its main impact, however, was not to come until the following century.

The Spread of Learning

Public schools and mass media. The national determination to educate everybody was best reflected in the growth of public schools, which increased at an unprecedented speed after 1870. Free education for all became a foremost article in the American faith, and the schools were unfairly expected to solve all of democracy's problems, from poorly cooked meals to poorly adjusted races. Growing cities expected the schools to take over many functions that parents, police, and priests had once performed and along the way to Americanize the children of the new immigrants. In 1870 only $69 million, or an average of about $15 per pupil, was spent on public education, while in the first school year of the new century $250 million, or nearly $23 per pupil, went into the school budget. By 1900 all but two of the states outside the South had compulsory school-attendance laws of some sort, and both the average school attendance and the length of the average school year had increased markedly. There were only one hundred sixty public high schools in the whole country in 1870, but by the end of the century there were more than six thousand. The cities, with a more concentrated school population and better transportation than rural communities, reaped the greatest benefits from the public-school expansion. More and more of them extended public schools to include kindergartens, normal schools, night classes, and adult and vocational education.

Under the sway of new theories of education the public schools gradually put aside the old authoritarian ways of the drillmaster and disciplinarian in the one-room country school. Just as the preceding generation imported the progressive doctrines of Pestalozzi, the new generation brought from Germany the theories of Johann Friedrich Herbart, who believed that education could be made into a science. The Herbartians encouraged the abandonment of corporal punishment and the teaching of "practical" subjects such as manual training.

Private schools still held on, particularly in the Eastern states, and certain ethnic and religious groups resisted being integrated into a uniform public-school system. Unable to win public support for their own educational efforts, the Catholics in 1884 determined upon an elaborate expansion of their parochial schools. The program was mainly designed to educate the immigrants of that faith in the cities, and most of the schools were located in New England and the Middle Atlantic states.

The federal government had made a gesture of assistance to public schools in 1867, when Congress laid the foundation of a bureau of education, but the Blair Bill for federal aid distributed according to the proportion of illiterates in a state was defeated in the 1880s. Since support of the schools was left to local communities, improvement and growth varied widely with the distribution of wealth. In general, the rural districts lagged behind the urban areas and the West and South behind the East. But the South had a staggering burden of special disadvantages. In the first place it had about twice as many children per adult as the North, and it had considerably less than half the per capita taxable wealth with which to educate them. At the century's end the schools of the South were still miserably supported, poorly taught, and wholly inadequate, and as poor as the average school was, the schools for blacks were far below that. Efforts to bring up the average in the next decade were largely confined to the white schools.

In spite of the physical growth of the educational plant and the millions of dollars poured into public education, the average American adult by the turn of the century had only about five years of schooling. Illiteracy had been reduced, however, from around 17 percent in 1880 to about 11 percent twenty years later. For all the faddism and quackery, in spite of the low-paid teachers and the attempt to saddle them with all the problems of democracy, the public schools continued to increase in number and grow in popular esteem.

The popular faith in education and the craving for its benefits were reflected in other ways as well. One of these was the highly popular Chautauqua movement, which was started in 1874 at Lake Chautauqua, New York, by Methodist laymen as a camp meeting for training Sunday-school teachers. The idea spread over the country as a sort of informal adult-education movement. It retained its pious, middle-class emphasis on temperance and morality and often made use of Methodist camp-meeting grounds. Small-town audiences sweated earnestly through long lectures on science and religion, thrilled to the illustrated travel lectures of John L. Stoddard, or relaxed with James Whitcomb Riley and Swiss bell-ringers. To supplement the summer meetings a home-study circle was formed in 1878, and ten years later a Chautauqua College began to offer correspondence courses and hand out degrees via the postman.

In the larger cities culture was displayed in magnificent palaces with neoclassical fronts and sweeping staircases that opened to the public in the 1870s: the Metropolitan Museum of Art in New York and the Boston Museum of Fine Arts in 1870, the Philadelphia Museum of Art in 1876, the Art Institute of Chicago in 1879. Conceived by their founders as democratic enterprises to diffuse refinement among the people, they also diffused an association of the idea of art and culture with the munificence of private wealth and power. As displayed in the luxurious museums, art and culture was seen as something that filtered downward from a distant past, from overseas, and from elite and wealthy custodians.

These years also brought a dramatic expansion of public libraries. Librarians laid claim to professional standing in 1876, when they organized the American Library Association. State and local tax money was tapped, and private donors began to put large amounts into library-building: Andrew Carnegie, the most munificent of them, launched his library benefactions at Pittsburgh in 1881. In the 1890s six library buildings costing more than a million dollars had been either started or completed. The most splendid were the Boston Public Library and the New York Public Library, both opened in 1895, and the Library of Congress, the largest and most costly in the world, opened in 1897. By 1900 there were more than nine thousand public libraries in the country, with a total of more than 45 million volumes.

The repetitive theme of "more and more and more" that drums through all phases of American life in the eighties and nineties was nowhere so striking as in journalism, especially in periodicals. In the last fifteen years of the century the number of periodicals published increased by twenty-two hundred, most of them devoted to trades and special interests. More striking was the increase in the number and circulation of periodicals for the general reader. There were only four such monthly magazines in the country in 1885 with circulations of a hundred thousand or more, and they were usually priced at 35 cents a copy. Twenty years later there were twenty such magazines with an aggregate circulation of more than 5½ million, and all but four of them sold at 10 to 15 cents a copy. The 10-cent monthlies created a vast new reading public. More than price was involved in the expansion, however. The older journals, such as the *Century*, the *Atlantic*, and the *North American Review*, were sedate, leisurely, rather aloof, and upper class in appeal and sympathy. The new 10-cent competitors, such as *Munsey's*, *McClure's*, and the *Cosmopolitan*, were lighter in tone, with shorter articles and many illustrations. News-mindedness was an innovation of *Public Opinion* (1886), *Current Literature* (1888), and the *Literary Digest* (1890), and reform-mindedness was the theme of the *Forum* (1886) and *Arena* (1889), as well as the older *Nation* (1865) and *Independent* (1848).

Growing cities, increasing literacy, and expanding population combined to create greater and greater markets for newspapers and to heighten the temptation to vulgarize the product in order to exploit the potential market. The number of daily papers, largely confined to the cities, more than doubled, and the number of weekly and semiweekly papers increased more than 50 percent between 1880 and 1900, while subscribers increased even more rapidly. The growth of daily newspapers came as follows:

Year	Number of Dailies	Total Daily Circulation
1860	387	1,478,000
1870	574	2,602,000
1880	971	3,566,000
1890	1,610	8,387,000
1900	2,226	15,102,000

By the end of the century the United States had more than half the newspapers in the world. Two technological innovations speeded up the expansion: the linotype machine and the half-tone photograph. Two other potent influences were at work to change the character of American newspapers: one was advertising, which surpassed sales as a source of revenue in the nineties, and the other was the mass audience. To reach the masses the news columns became more sensational and vulgar. The father of the new school of journalists was Joseph Pulitzer, who bought the New York *World* in 1883 and ran its circulation up from fifteen thousand in 1883 to over a million by 1898. The assault on privacy and taste was continued and intensified by his imitator, William Randolph Hearst of the New York *Journal*.

The higher learning. For all the crassness and materialism that earned for it the name of "Gilded Age," the period could boast of substantial advances in higher education and scholarship. There was obviously much room for improvement. American colleges of 1870, even the better ones, were likely to be strongly sectarian, provincial, and undistinguished. The typical college professor of that year was harshly, but not very unfairly, described as "a nondescript, a jack of all trades, equally ready to teach surveying and Latin eloquence." The traditional curriculum, designed for the training of ministers, did not permit specialization or allow time for research. Library and laboratory facilities were inadequate, and the natural sciences were neglected. There were no graduate schools and no professional schools beyond theological seminaries and the engineering and military academies. Collegiate pedagogy, like the Victorian family, was heavily authoritarian, with emphasis upon rules, discipline, rote learning, and recitations.

With Harvard in the vanguard and with Charles W. Eliot at its head, a small group of academicians undertook to reform the old collegiate order. The reforms they made were not universally acknowledged to be improvements in their day, nor are they yet, but they were widely if slowly imitated. One of them was the elective system, which resulted in a proliferation of

City Room, *New York World*

courses and subjects from which the student chose as fancy dictated. Additional reforms, such as an increase in the number of science courses and in the use of the laboratory method of instruction, were taken up rapidly, as were discussion periods as substitutes for rote recitation. Among other changes slowly adopted were the decline of authoritarian norms and traditional curricula and a decrease in the proportion of clergymen on boards of trustees and in presidents' offices.

Accompanying these changes and reflecting the shift to a secular and scientific emphasis was an increase in German influence in academic circles. During the nineteenth century more than nine thousand Americans studied at German universities, all but about two hundred of them after 1850. In the 1880s some two thousand Americans were studying in Germany. The Johns Hopkins University, opened in Baltimore in 1876 with an inaugural address by Thomas Huxley, the Darwinian, was an expression of both English and German influence. Nearly all the faculty of the new university had studied in Germany, and the policies pursued by President Daniel Coit Gilman expressed many of the academic ideals of that country's universities. Among these were a stress on research and graduate study and a shift from the attitude that professors and students were mere conservers of learning to the attitude that they were searchers and advancers of knowledge. The new emphasis implied an increase in the scholar's stature, freedom, and prestige. Inspired more or less by the example of Johns Hopkins, fifteen major graduate schools or departments had been established by the end of the century.

Nearly three thousand students registered in American graduate schools in 1890, as compared with a mere handful two decades before. The professional scholars founded scores of learned societies in the seventies and eighties: the Archaeological Institute of America (1879), the Modern Language Association (1883), and in the next ten years the historians, economists, mathematicians, physicists, and psychologists, to mention only a few, followed suit. Learned journals and books equal to Europe's best began to appear in America, and American-trained scholars began to acquire international reputations.

Medical and legal education was still primitive in the seventies and eighties. None of the schools of medicine or law required a college degree for admission, and the typical medical school turned its graduates loose on a helpless public after only a few months of haphazard lectures. Both medical and legal degrees could easily be bought. Between 1876 and 1900 eighty-six new medical schools were founded, but the Johns Hopkins Medical School, opened in 1894, was the first to require a college degree for admission and

the first to have a full-time teaching staff. By the end of the century many states had established boards of medical examiners that tightened license requirements, and the schools themselves began to raise their standards in response. Comparable improvement in law schools was to come only later.

This was an era prolific in the birth of new institutions of higher learning, both public and private. In the last two decades of the nineteenth century the total number of colleges and universities in the country increased by nearly one hundred fifty, though many of them had no valid claim to academic status and were often short lived. Ten new state universities, all of them coeducational from the start, were founded between 1882 and 1895. In the East, where coeducation was slower to win acceptance, several women's colleges were founded: Vassar in 1861, Smith in 1871, and Bryn Mawr in 1885, while several of the older men's colleges opened affiliated women's colleges nearby. Numerous land-grant colleges, taking advantage of the Morrill Act of 1862, sprang up to teach both agricultural and mechanical arts. A fraction of the new industrial and commercial fortunes of the age went into the founding of universities bearing the names of Cornell (1868), Vanderbilt (1873), Hopkins (1876), Tulane (1884), Stanford (1885), and Clark (1887). The University of Chicago (1891) was one of the few that did not take the name of its benefactor, in this case John D. Rockefeller.

The history of higher learning of this period was not, however, purely a story of expansion and improvement. A mistaken conception of democracy led to the assumption of equality among all academic pursuits and justified the teaching of courses in almost any subject, however trivial. Institutions became overexpanded, overcrowded, and absurdly bureaucratized. A misguided deference to the opinions of alumni, sports enthusiasts, and the unlettered public generally led to an anarchical confusion of values and distortions of academic purpose. For the first time in recorded history institutions of higher learning assumed the function of providing mass entertainment in spectator sports, particularly football, and the comparative distinction of a university came to depend on its success in pursuing these enterprises.

The business leaders who replaced the clergymen on the college boards of trustees were slow to acknowledge the status claimed by the new scholar and were sometimes quite unable to distinguish between their relation to faculty members and their relation to "other employees." The trustees of seven well-known universities approved a statement published in the Chicago *Tribune* in 1899 to the effect that college professors "should promptly and gracefully submit to the determination of the trustees" in deciding what should be taught, and that "if the trustees err it is for the patrons and proprietors, not for the employees, to change either the policy or the personnel of the board." During the 1890s nine prominent faculty members were dismissed for presuming to express their opinions on such subjects as labor, railroads, and currency. Though there was no legitimate excuse for these gaucheries, we must remember that America was trying to spread learning far more widely than had ever been attempted before.

Arts, Letters, and Critics

Artists and their work. In matters of taste the Gilded Age has acquired and in part deserved a deplorable reputation. Whether it was because the molders of fashion were insecure in their social position or new to their wealth or for some other reason, their taste ran to excesses in all things—in their clothing, their jewelry, and their houses, in interior décor and exterior ornament. They overloaded their rooms with bric-a-brac, their dresses with bustles, and their houses

The Brooklyn Bridge: daring and magnificent

with gingerbread. They had no trouble finding architects, painters, and sculptors of the sort who would cater to their preferences, but the work these people left behind need not detain us.

Beneath the crass surface and behind the clutter of imitative art, however, there were genuinely original and creative spirits at work in the land. Artists, engineers, architects, sculptors, and painters honestly faced the realities of the new urban, industrial society, contrived original and powerful answers to its problems, and contributed much to the urban vitality of the era. It was the new city that gave them both their challenge and their opportunity. The bold spirit with which they met the challenge and seized the opportunity is caught in a statement by a Georgia-bred architect, John Wellborn Root, who did his work in Chicago:

> In America we are free of artistic traditions. Our freedom begets license, it is true. We do shocking things; we produce works of architecture irremediably bad; we try crude experiments that result in disaster. Yet somewhere in this mass of ungoverned energies lies the principle of life. A new spirit of beauty is being developed and perfected, and even now its first achievements are beginning to delight us. This is not the old thing made over; it is new. It springs out of the past, but it is not tied to it; it studies the traditions, but is not enslaved by them.

One achievement of the age that was daring and magnificent enough to meet Root's description was the Brooklyn Bridge, a suspension such as had never before been built, with granite towers 276 feet high and with a central span of 1,600 feet. Sketched by John A. Roebling, who died before construction began, the great bridge was completed by his son Washington A. Roebling in 1883. A product of the new industrialism down to the last of the nineteen strands of steel cable and the last riveted girder, the bridge soared out of the soot and slums of Manhattan, monumental proof that the new society could produce a thing of beauty out of its materials. In the same city a landscape architect named Frederick L. Olmsted demonstrated that it was not necessary for a city to be the seat of an absolute monarch in order to create spacious, lovely, and exquisitely designed parks, such as Central Park, Olmsted's masterpiece. It was not his only great park, however, for he designed many more and left scarcely a major city in the country untouched by his influence.

The architect whom Root singled out to illustrate the new spirit in American art was Henry Hobson Richardson. Born in New Orleans, educated at Harvard and abroad, Richardson was a man of gargantuan ambitions and appetites, full of zest for any problem and equally ready to design churches, railroad stations, department stores, libraries, office buildings, anything. "The things I want most to design," he said, "are a grain elevator and the interior of a great river steamboat." His massive granite structures created a style and defined an architectural era. Although he died in 1886 at the age of forty-eight, he left his buildings scattered across the country from Trinity Church in Boston to a monument on the Wyoming plains.

The problem of the skyscraper, called into being by the fantastic extravagance of unplanned city growth and overcrowding, could not be solved by masonry. What was required was a steel skeleton for support and walls reduced to mere fireproof curtains instead of supporting buttresses. With contributions from engineers and steelmasters as well as architects, Chicagoans achieved a solution in the Tacoma Building in 1888. With the arrival of the electric elevator, the age of the skyscraper begins, and with that age the name of Louis Sullivan is intimately associated. Ranking with Richardson as one of the giants of the period, Sullivan was a capricious genius who commanded the respect of the ablest critics: Frank Lloyd Wright referred to him as *Der Meister*. Sullivan revealed the inner conflicts of his generation's adjustment to the city when he characterized the skyscraper as "profoundly antisocial."

It is curious that Chicago, which contributed so many new and original architectural techniques, should also have been the host and creator of the White City at the Columbian Exposition of 1893, which represented a return to Renaissance classicism and other traditional styles. Although Daniel H. Burnham of Chicago supervised the building, the White City was mainly the work of Easterners, particularly the firm of Charles F. McKim, William R. Mead, and Stanford White. The architects were assisted by the most famous American sculptor of the period, Augustus Saint-Gaudens, and by Olmsted, whose landscaping included the lovely lagoon surrounded by gleaming white-plaster buildings. The ephemeral dream city was undoubtedly an impressive spectacle, but Sullivan, who designed the only nonclassical structure in the Exposition, regarded it as "an appalling calamity" whose influence would "last for half a century." What he feared was a reversion to the academic, classical models of architecture; in the "Federal" style sponsored by McKim, Mead, and White in the national capital and elsewhere in the ensuing era, Sullivan's fears were justified. On the other hand the example of a city intelligently planned for comfort and beauty stimulated the "city beautiful" movement, and under Burnham's guidance Washington, Cleveland, San Francisco, and Manila made impressive achievements in the art of city-planning.

Some of the fine arts in what Lewis Mumford has called the "Brown Decades" were creditably served by American artists. John La Farge, a gifted interior-decorator and art critic, executed thousands of stained-

... one might enumerate the items of high civilization, as it exists in other countries, which are absent from the texture of American life, until it should become a wonder to know what was left. No State, in the European sense of the word, and indeed barely a significant national name. No sovereign, no court, no personal loyalty, no aristocracy, no church, no clergy, no army, no diplomatic service, no country gentlemen, no palaces, no castles ... nor ivied ruins; no cathedrals, nor abbeys, nor little Norman churches; no great Universities nor public schools—no Oxford, nor Eton, nor Harrow, no literature, no novels, no museums, no pictures, no political society, no sporting class—No Epsom nor Ascot!

From Henry James, *Hawthorne*, 1879.

glass windows and won the admiration of Richardson, for whom he did the windows of Trinity Church in Boston. Winslow Homer, a serious illustrator, occasionally struck the note of greatness in his paintings of the weather-beaten ruggedness of common life. But to find American painters who deserve to rank with their European contemporaries one must turn to Thomas Eakins and Albert Pinkham Ryder. Eakins worked in relative obscurity outside fashionable currents and left a house full of unsold paintings at his death. A friend of Walt Whitman, whose portrait he painted, he had a salty contempt for pretense and loved to paint boxers, oarsmen, and surgeons at their work. Ryder was a painter of the sea and the night and has been compared with Melville in the symbolic and lyrical qualities of his art. Among his great symbolic paintings are *Death on a Pale Horse*, *The Flying Dutchman*, *Jonah*, and *Macbeth and the Witches*—all eerie, mystic, and tragic.

Beginnings of realism. In letters as in arts the post-Civil War decades have had a poor reputation. Their writers have been tagged with the "genteel" label and condemned for complacency and blindness to the glaring faults of their society. Their reputation for shallowness, complacency, and prudery is not wholly unjustified, but the age was often as blind to its literary merits as to its social faults. It sometimes overlooked and sometimes misunderstood its best talent. Contemporaries of Emily Dickinson, the greatest American poet of the age, and one of the subtlest, never even heard of her, for she lived the life of a recluse and published very few poems before her death in 1886. They mistook Mark Twain, their greatest satirist, for a funny man and a writer for boys. They hardly had time to appreciate the pioneer naturalist Stephen Crane, who died in his twenties. They were misled by the surface mildness of William Dean

Howells, their major critic and leading realist, and they misunderstood (when they did not neglect) Henry James, their greatest artist. But any age that should produce Dickinson, Twain, Howells, and James should command respect and serious attention.

More completely and richly than any other writer, Mark Twain, who was christened Samuel Langhorne Clemens, embodied in his life and writings the sprawling diversity, the epic adventures, the inner tensions, and the cross-purposes of post-Civil War America. A Southerner by birth and heritage, he became a Westerner while the West was wildest and settled in New England to live out his life. He was a

Mark Twain: American satirist

child of the frontier and, like his America, a country man who moved to the city, a provincial who was thrust into a strange new world. His literary record of the experience documents a whole epoch. "I am persuaded," the playwright George Bernard Shaw wrote Mark Twain, "that the future historian of America will find your works as indispensable to him as a French historian finds the political tracts of Voltaire."

Mark Twain's American odyssey started in Missouri on the banks of the Mississippi, where the East bordered on the West and the South overlapped the North. He joined the Confederate army when the war broke out, but, after a trivial accident that involved no fighting, he gave up the war and joined his brother in the Far West. He recorded his adventures in the Nevada mining camps in *Roughing It* (1872) and gave the period a name that has stuck in *The Gilded Age* (1873), a broad political and social satire. His boyhood and his later experience as a pilot on the great river found expression in two of his works, *The Adventures of Tom Sawyer* (1876) and *Life on the Mississippi* (1883). But he surpassed all his other work in *The Adventures of Huckleberry Finn* (1884), a masterpiece of American literature. A composite of satire and nostalgia, it dips deeper into irony than was characteristic of the age, for it aligns the sympathies of every decent reader with Huck, the river rat, against civilization itself and fixes the primitive, superstitious Nigger Jim as one of the most memorable figures in American fiction. Mark Twain wrote a great deal more, but like the miners of his Nevada adventure and America itself, he was a spendthrift with his resources and could not always tell the stuff that glittered from real gold.

Howells, the friend of Twain and the generous friend of every creative spirit in letters of his time, was even more prolific. He wrote thirty full-length novels and five volumes of short stories, not to men-

tion an endless stream of literary criticism. In his time he was rightfully called the dean of American letters and the foremost exponent of American realism. Rejected by a later generation that unfairly associated him with complacency and materialism, Howells deserves better from the present perspective. In mid-life he reached a turning point marked by his reaction to the Haymarket executions in 1886, against which he conducted virtually a one-man protest among the intellectuals. The experience coincided with his reading of Tolstoy and Henry George, and he began calling himself a socialist and demanding a sterner realism that would confront the injustice and suffering of industrial society under plutocratic control. Though he was inclined to deal in abstractions, his fiction began at once to reflect his views. *Annie Kilburn* (1889) is an indictment of social injustice and the inadequacies of charity in a New England community, and *A Hazard of New Fortunes* (1890), the best expression of Howells' new phase and the climactic work of American realism, centers around a violent strike. *A Traveler from Altruria* (1894) is a utopian novel that exposes and attacks social injustice.

Henry James continued to develop as a writer after Howells and Twain began to decline. His wonderfully productive life carried over into the twentieth century, though the bulk of his work appeared before 1900. Unlike Howells and Twain, he was not interested in the common people. His typical subjects are Americans and Europeans of cultivated minds, usually in a cosmopolitan setting. *The American* (1877), *The Europeans* (1878), and *Daisy Miller* (1879) are treatments of national attitudes in transatlantic society. This was only the beginning of four decades of writing that included such masterpieces as *The Portrait of a Lady* (1881), *The Ambassadors* (1903), and *The Golden Bowl* (1904). Henry James was the most completely dedicated and probably the most wholly fulfilled American writer and artist of his time.

The age affords posterity one unflattering but fascinating portrait of itself drawn by a philosopher-historian who stands in a class by himself: Henry Adams, descendant of the two Presidents whose name he bore. All serious students of the period must make their own acquaintance and their own peace with this querulous and opinionated critic. His main writing dealt with the history of another period, that of Jefferson and Madison. But his novels *Democracy* (1880) and *Esther* (1883) and more particularly his autobiographical *Education of Henry Adams* (1918) and *The Degradation of the Democratic Dogma* (1919) are the keys to his incisive critique. It was characteristic of him that he had the first two books published anonymously and the last two posthumously. Having mastered those, one is then better prepared to find Adams, in *Mont-Saint-Michel and Chartres* (1913), searching the monuments of the Middle Ages for their meaning to modern America, and projecting lines of change from the year 1200 to the year 1900.

After the end of the century and near the end of his life, Henry Adams looked back philosophically over the American experience since the Civil War. He was astonished at how much history had been telescoped into that brief span of years and how frightfully the pace of change had accelerated. At the outset of the period, in his youth, his fellow citizens were still grappling with stone-age tribes on the Great Plains and debating the issue of African slavery in their midst. America had been a land of villages and farms, a provincial outpost of Western civilization. But now, as he steamed into New York Harbor in 1902, remembering his return from Europe in 1868, he searched in vain for landmarks of the earlier era. "The outline of the city became frantic in its effort to explain something that defied meaning," he observed. Titanic, uncontrollable forces "had exploded, and thrown great masses of stone and steam against the sky. . . . A Traveller in the highways of history looked out of the club window on the turmoil of Fifth Avenue, and felt himself in Rome, under Diocletian. . . . The two-thousand-years failure of Christianity roared upward from Broadway, and no Constantine the Great was in sight." Henry Adams' fellow Americans, less troubled by historical perspective and premonitions of things to come, called the spectacle "progress" and greeted the dawn of the twentieth century with a confidence that was apparently unbounded.

Suggestions for Reading General works of value include Daniel Boorstin, *The Americans: The Democratic Experience** (1973); Alan Tractenberg, *The Incorporation of America* (1982); D. W. Howe, ed., *Victorian America** (1976); and J. B. Jackson, *American Space: The Centennial Years, 1865–1876** (1972). Cities in this period are studied in Blake McKelvey, *The Urbanization of America, 1860–1915* (1963). Selected cities are subjects of F. C. Jaher, *The Urban Establishment: Upper Strata in Boston, New York, Charleston, Chicago, and Los Angeles** (1982); C. M. Green, *American Cities in the Building of the Nation* (1956); S. B. Warner, *Streetcar Suburbs** (1962) and *The Urban Wilderness: A History of the American City** (1972). Morton and Lucia White write engagingly of *The Intellectual Versus the City** (1962).

Contemporary sources on urban slums and poverty include Jacob Riis, *How the Other Half Lives** (1890), *The Children of the Poor* (1892), and *The Battle with the Slum** (1902); see also Josiah Strong, *The Twentieth Century City* (1898), as well as Jane Addams, *Twenty Years at Hull House** (1910). A good history of American attitudes toward poverty is R. H. Bremner, *From the Depths: The Discovery of Poverty in the United States** (1956). A sensitive analysis of immigration is Oscar Handlin, *The Uprooted** (1951). Another is Philip Taylor, *The Distant Magnet: European Emigration to the U.S.A.* (1971). On the new immigrants see particularly I. A. Hourwich, *Immigration and Labor* (1922); on their reception in the United States consult Barbara Solomon, *Ancestors and Immigrants** (1956), and John Higham, *Strangers in the Land** (1955) and *Send These to Me: Jews and Other Immigrants in Urban America** (1975). M. A. Jones, *American Immigration** (1960), is an expert synthesis. And Stephan Thernstrom, *The Other Bostonians** (1973) is important.

On the boss, the machine, and the reformer a contemporary account, James Bryce, *The American Commonwealth*, 2 vols. (1888), is a classic. For reformers of the period, see Gerald McFarland, *Mugwumps, Morals and Politics, 1894–1920* (1975). A muckraker who deals with this period informatively is Lincoln Steffens, *The Shame of the Cities** (1904). Later studies of value are F. J. Goodnow, *Municipal Problems* (1907); C. W. Patton, *The Battle for Municipal Reform: Mobilization and Attack, 1875–1900* (1940); A. B. Callow, Jr., *The Tweed Ring* (1966); and Seymour Mandelbaum, *Boss Tweed's New York* (1965). On these and other aspects of the period, J. A. Garraty, *The New Commonwealth, 1877–1890** (1968), is good reading.

On women's rights and the suffrage movement see W. L. O'Neill, *Everyone Was Brave: The Rise and Fall of Feminism in America** (1969); Eleanor Flexner, *Century of Struggle: The Woman's Rights Movement in the United States** (1959); A. S. Kraditor, *The Ideas of the Woman Suffrage Movement, 1890–1920**(1965); and C. N. Degler, *At Odds: Women and the Family in America from the Revolution to the Present* (1980).

A general history is Sidney Ahlstrom, *A Religious History of the American People** (1972). The reaction of the Protestant churches to social problems is discussed in several books, notably H. F. May, *Protestant Churches and Industrial America** (1949); A. I. Abell, *The Urban Impact on American Protestantism, 1865–1900* (1942); and C. H. Hopkins, *The Rise of the Social Gospel in American Protestantism, 1865–1915** (1940). On evangelists, see B. A. Weisberger, *They Gathered at the River: The Story of the Great Revivalists and Their Impact upon Religion in America** (1958), and J. F. Findlay, Jr., *Dwight L. Moody: American Evangelist, 1837–1899* (1969). On the Catholics there is a fine brief account in J. T. Ellis, *American Catholicism** (1956), and a longer study in Theodore Maynard, *The Story of American Catholicism** (1941). Allan Johnson's long sketch of Mary Baker Eddy in the *Dictionary of American Biography* is helpful on the origins of Christian Science. W. W. Sweet, *Revivalism in America: Its Origins, Growth and Decline** (1944), is a useful survey. Churchmen as social activists are portrayed in P. J. Frederick, *Knights of the Golden Rule: The Intellectual As Christian Social Reformer in the 1890s* (1976).

The history of public education receives vigorous reinterpretation in L. A. Cremin, *The Transformation of the School: Progressivism in American Education, 1876–1957** (1961). A. E. Meyer, *An Educational History of the American People* (1957), is a useful reference work. On the South see C. W. Dabney, *Universal Education in the South*, 2 vols. (1936). R. O. and Victoria Case, *We Called It Culture: The Story of Chautauqua* (1958), is the best account of that movement. F. L. Mott, *A History of American Magazines, 1885–1905* (1957), is an exhaustive and excellent history. The newspapers are treated in W. G. Bleyer, *Main Currents in the History of American Journalism* (1927), and B. A. Weisberger, *The American Newspaperman* (1961).

The history of higher learning has been surveyed by Frederick Rudolph, *The American College and University, A History** (1962), elaborated upon by L. R. Veysey, *The Emergence of the American University** (1965), and much illuminated by Richard Hofstadter and Walter Metzger, *The Development of Academic Freedom in the United States* (1955), and Hugh Hawkins, *Between Harvard and America: the Educational Leadership of Charles W. Eliot* (1972). For a stiff and amusing indictment see Thorstein Veblen, *Higher Learning in America* (1918). R. H. Shryock, "The Academic Profession in the United States," *Bulletin of the American Association of University Professors* (Spring 1952), is most important.

On the graphic arts there are several studies of value, notably Lewis Mumford, *The Brown Decades: A Study of the Arts in America, 1865–1895** (1931); John Kouwenhoven, *Made in America: The Arts in Modern Civilization** (1948); and O. W. Larkin, *Art and Life in America* (1949, rev. ed., 1960). On architecture, see Leland Roth, *A Concise History of American Architecture** (1979), and J. M. Fitch, *American Building: The Historical Forces that Shaped It** (1966), and on the growth of cities, Christopher Tunnard and H. H. Reed, *American Skyline* (1955).

Literary history in this era is treated by H. N. Smith, *Democracy and the Novel* (1978); Larzer Ziff, *The American 1890s: Life and Times of a Lost Generation** (1966); Jay Martin, *Harvests of Change:*

American Literature, 1865–1914 (1967); Everett Carter, *Howells and the Age of Realism* (1954), who discusses Howells' contemporaries as well; and Kermit Vanderbilt, *The Achievement of William Dean Howells: A Reinterpretation* (1968). E. H. Cady, *The Realist at War* (1958); K. S. Lynn, *William Dean Howells* (1971); and V. W. Brooks, *New England: Indian Summer, 1865–1915* (1940) and *The Confident Years, 1885–1915* (1952), are full of biographical incident. Alfred Kazin, *On Native Grounds** (1942), starts his account at 1890 but has two illuminating chapters on that decade. Some good biographies are Justin Kaplan, *Mr. Clemens and Mark Twain** (1966); Ernest Samuels, *Henry Adams: The Middle Years* (1958) and *Henry Adams: The Major Phase* (1964). H. M. Jones, *The Age of Energy: Varieties of American Experience, 1865–1915* (1971), contains essays on the cultural scene.

*Available in paperback edition.

20
STALEMATE, AGRARIAN REVOLT, AND REPUBLICAN TRIUMPH, 1877-1896

Like other aspects of American life between Reconstruction and the Progressive Movement, politics in the Gilded Age has suffered from harsh criticism. Compared with the Civil War and Reconstruction in their more heroic aspects, the politics of the postwar generation appears evasive, materialistic, tawdry, and cynical. And compared with the politics of the era after 1900—the progressivism with which many of the critics more-or-less identified—the Gilded Age is pictured as complacent, irresponsible, indifferent to social injustice, and unwilling to use the powers of government to redress grievances and control an unmanaged economy. Caught between the two comparative models, the interlude has been traditionally represented as a period of apostasy from the ideals of the past and failure to anticipate the goals of the future. And for good measure it is freely blamed for the social and economic evils to which the twentieth century is heir.

Granted its numerous shortcomings, the politics of the Gilded Age deserves to be considered in its own right rather than, in Howard Mumford Jones' words, "as an imperfect prophecy of twentieth century America." Or for that matter as the failed fulfillment of Civil War ideals. Emerging from the searing experience of the great war and plunging directly into massive industrialization, urbanization, and immigration, Americans of that confusing era sought stability and equilibrium ahead of social idealism. They had had their fill of headlong ideological crusades and the

politics of zealous causes under national leadership. They took refuge in community and organizational loyalties rather than ideological commitments. If the political leaders of the time shunned great issues of social injustice and inequality and avoided civic activism, they were restrained by more than wealthy patrons, for they had to deal with an electorate that, outside the South, was the most completely democratized in the western world. Moreover, it was an electorate that turned out and voted and participated to a greater extent than in any previous or subsequent period in American history. In view of the constraints and issues, it is not surprising that the political life under these rules attracted leaders of great skill, but none of true greatness.

The Business of Politics

The party equilibrium. Politics in the post-Reconstruction period was more a business than a game, a highly competitive business with the two major parties as the evenly matched competitors. The Democrats managed to elect only one of their candidates President (for two non-consecutive terms) in the fifty-two years between 1860 and 1912. And yet this gives a misleading impression of the relative strength of the Democratic and Republican parties. Actually, there was an extraordinarily narrow margin of differ-

498

Coxey's army

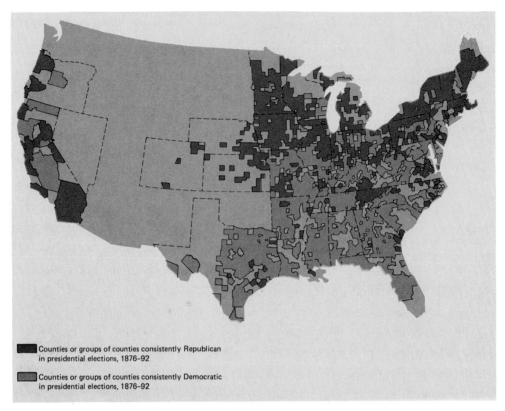

Counties or groups of counties consistently Republican
in presidential elections, 1876–92

Counties or groups of counties consistently Democratic
in presidential elections, 1876–92

The consistency of the vote, 1876–92

ence in the popular vote the two parties polled in the two decades following 1876. In none of the presidential elections from 1876 to 1892 did the Republicans carry a majority of the popular votes, and in only one, that of 1880, did they receive a plurality—but even that plurality was less than one-tenth of 1 percent. In three of the five elections, in fact, the difference between the popular votes for the two major-party candidates was less than 1 percent, and in 1876 and 1888, even though the Democrats received a popular majority, they lost the election. In the Electoral College votes, on the other hand, majorities ranged from 1 in 1876 to 132 in 1892. The narrow margin between victory and defeat encouraged the laissez-faire tendency of politicians, the tendency to avoid social issues and take few chances.

The Republican party was a loose alliance of regional and interest groups with different and sometimes conflicting interests. The basic regional alliance was between the Northeast and the Middle West—an alliance that had been consolidated in 1860 and had fought and won the Civil War. It hung together afterward partly because of wartime loyalties and memories of the heroic days of Lincoln, when the party had emancipated the slaves and saved the Union. Two other large groups traced their attachment to the party back to the Civil War: the freedmen and the Union army veterans. The blacks remained loyal to the party

of emancipation and continued to send one or two congressmen to Washington from the South, but after the Republicans abandoned them in 1877 the political power of the freedmen diminished rapidly. On the other hand the political significance of the war veterans increased as the Grand Army of the Republic grew as a pressure group and as Congress responded with larger and larger pensions for veterans. Economic conflict and political rivalry opened breaches in party unity. Republican policies such as high tariffs, sound money, and favors for railroads pleased some Eastern business interests, but Western grain-growers often resented those policies and threatened revolt. The noisiest quarrel within Republican ranks was the running war between the Half-Breeds, led by James G. Blaine of Maine, and the Stalwarts, led by Roscoe Conkling of New York. These factions reflected personal loyalties and alliances rather than significant differences of opinion or principle, though they differed somewhat in style. Stalwarts clung to old issues of the South, while Half-Breeds sought a new coalition reflecting changed conditions. Conkling's followers more openly pursued the spoils of office, but both factions wanted all the spoils. Empty as were their battles, however, they sometimes determined the choice of American Presidents.

The post-Reconstruction Democratic party was even more regional than the Republican. Its most reliable sources of support were the South and the machine-dominated cities of the Northeast. And the disparity of outlook and interest between the provincial, Protestant cotton-farmers of the South and the underprivileged, Catholic, immigrant, industrial workers of the big cities was almost as great as that between the impoverished blacks of the South and middle-class whites of the North who supported the Republican party. The Democrats also received support from Northeastern merchants and bankers who opposed the protective tariff and favored contraction of the currency—"sound-money" men, they called themselves. Other business interests favored inflation and tariff. The leaders of the party in the South, some of them of Whig background, preferred to be called Conservatives, and were often called Bourbons by their opponents. They had much in common with the dominant Democratic leaders in the Middle West, who were also business-minded conservatives and were also known as Bourbons. Rank-and-file Democrats, farmers, industrial workers, and small businessmen in the West, the South, and the East, were often restive and sometimes rebellious under such leaders.

The major economic issues over which the old parties divided, each under conservative leaders, were differences over tariff and monetary policies. Ethnic, religious, and cultural issues often took precedence over economic issues. Not that there was any lack of important economic and social issues. One has only to recall the recurrent industrial crises and depressions of the period and the desperate plight of the victims. But if they got a hearing in the political arena, it was through small third parties. The major parties preferred to avoid such issues (and so, apparently, did the majority of the electorate). In the North the Republicans "waved the bloody shirt," accusing the Democrats of rebellion and treason, and in the South the Democrats invoked the menace of "Negro rule" and called for white supremacy. Yet the rate of voter turnout was unusually high in these years.

"The American, like the Englishman," observed James Bryce in 1888, "usually votes with his party, right or wrong, and the fact that there is little distinction of view between the parties makes it easier to stick to your old friends." Party allegiance during these years was in fact remarkably rigid. In Indiana, for example, thirty-two counties remained unswervingly Republican from 1876 to 1892, and thirty-nine counties stuck as unswervingly with the Democrats, with neither group varying more than 3 percent. In spite of much population mobility, only twenty-one counties shifted parties at all, and with third parties in the picture neither of the major parties could muster a reliable majority in those counties until 1896. The same pattern had prevailed for years: two-thirds of the Democratic counties had been voting Demo-

cratic since 1844, and over four-fifths of the Republican counties had gone down the line for the old party since its founding in 1856. These rigid loyalties carried Hoosier voters right through war and peace, through a wide variety of candidates and policies, and through all the economic and social upheavals of the passing years.

Except in periods of hard times, party identifications seemed less determined by economic issues such as tariff and currency, which were handled in Washington, than by cultural, religious, and ethnic issues, which were resolved at the local or state level of politics. Struggles between prohibition and the "saloon power," between Sabbath observance and "desecration," or between public and parochial schools reflected religious and cultural values close to the grass roots. Democrats, calling for "laissez-faire" on cultural issues at the local level as well in economic issues at the national level, were described as the "Party of Personal Liberty." Their message was "leave us alone." Republicans of this period, on the other hand, being more inclined toward public intervention in private life as well as in the private sector of the economy, were sometimes called the "Party of Piety." Voters took their party identification seriously, because they did not take their religious and cultural values lightly.

Neither party was strong enough, however, to rely for victory on the allegiance of certain states or parts of states that could be counted "in the bag." There were always the "doubtful states"—that is, states with enough shifting voters to turn the tide either way. These states were thought to be Connecticut, New York, New Jersey, Ohio, Indiana, and Illinois, but the key states were New York and Indiana. In the 1880s the Republicans had to carry New York and all three of the doubtful Midwestern states to elect their candidate President. Since the whole contest hinged on a few states, it is no wonder that they commanded great bargaining power, absorbed most of the "slush funds" from the campaign treasuries, and gained desirable offices for their politicians. The strategic importance of the few doubtful Midwestern states also helps to explain why five of the six Republican candidates for President from Grant to McKinley came from those states, including four from Ohio and one from Indiana. And as a running mate for their Midwestern candidate, the Republicans almost invariably chose a man from New York. The Democrats, on the other hand, usually reversed the regional order, though they picked their nominees from the same doubtful states. Their presidential nominees usually came from New York—in four contests they nominated incumbent or former governors of that state—and their vice-presidential nominees from Ohio, Illinois, or Indiana. In 1876, 1880, and 1884 the second place on the Democratic ticket went to the "strategic" state of Indiana.

The spoilsmen and the reformers. From Grant to McKinley the power and influence of the presidential office remained at low ebb. No President between 1865 and 1897 enjoyed the advantage of having his own party in control of both houses of Congress throughout his tenure of office, so rapidly did control seesaw back and forth between the evenly matched parties. But more than that, the Presidency was slow in recovering from the blows struck by Congress in its bitter fight with President Johnson and from President Grant's continual acquiescence in the domination of Congress. For an entire generation, congressional supremacy and presidential subordination remained the rule. Senator John Sherman of Ohio, himself a perpetual aspirant to the office, wrote that the President "should be subordinate to the legislative department" and should merely "obey and enforce the laws." Ordinarily the President did not even have a voice in preparing the annual budget, and he was certainly not given the staff or the money to play the role of a real chief executive. To a large degree, Congress itself took care of administration. As Leonard D. White, a leading administrative historian, puts it, "The established course of the public business went on its appointed way, for the most part without requiring or inviting the collaboration of the man who sat in the White House."

Politics was really controlled by oligarchies of party bosses, many of them United States senators, who headed state machines and commanded armies of henchmen whom they paid off with public offices. In addition to Senators Blaine and Conkling, there were such potentates as Senator Zachariah Chandler,

Marcus Alonzo Hanna: industrialist turned politician

the boss of Michigan, and Senator John A. "Black Jack" Logan of Illinois, a power in the Grand Army of the Republic. The patronage system rested on three principles: appointment for political considerations, congressional control of appointments, and rotation of officeholders. The system stressed personal loyalty and the "spoils" of political victory. The spoilsmen sometimes sold offices to the highest bidder, but more regularly they distributed them among faithful workers for service rendered and systematically taxed the holders for "contributions." After the Civil Service Reform Act of 1883 (see p. 506) began to curb patronage as a source of revenue, a new type of boss then began to replace the old flamboyant "stump politician," a quieter, more efficient "desk politician," who worked hand in glove with the lobbyists of public utilities, railroads, industries, and manufacturers. Matthew Quay, who kept a card index of the foibles of Pennsylvania politicians; "Easy Boss" Tom Platt, who eventually succeeded Conkling in New York; Arthur P. Gorman, the friend of business in Maryland; Henry G. Davis and his son-in-law Stephen B. Elkins, who ran respectively the Democratic and Republican parties of West Virginia; and Marcus Alonzo Hanna, Ohio industrialist turned politician, were bosses of the new type.

A group of liberal reformers called Mugwumps by their deriders kept up a running crusade against patronage and corruption in office for two decades. Earnest and élitist, the Mugwumps held high social position and conservative economic views, usually Republican. Foremost among them was George William Curtis, scholarly editor of *Harper's Weekly*, whose cartoonist Thomas Nast made a career of ridiculing and caricaturing the corrupt. Carl Schurz, who called Curtis "the intellectual head, the guiding force" of the movement, was himself a hero of the Mugwumps. Another of the luminaries was E. L. Godkin, editor of the *Nation*. Devoted to laissez-faire principles and unconcerned over the deeper ills of the economy, the reformers of this school confined their economic program to tariff reform and sound money and fixed their hopes on achieving honest and efficient government through civil-service reform. Spoilsmen sneered at "snivel service," and Senator Conkling described the reformers as "the dilettanti and *carpet knights* of politics" and accused them of "canting self-righteousness." The influence of the Mugwumps was largely confined to the literate upper class, for they were isolated from the mass of voters by their attitudes and their social position.

The various reform movements of the period were not on speaking terms with one another, or they spoke different languages. Grangers, Greenbackers, and Alliancemen of the West and the South (see pp. 512–14) demanded reforms in the currency, banking, and credit systems that chilled the blood of Eastern reformers. Agrarian reformers were at the same time divided among themselves: Northerner against Southerner, Republican against Democrat. Both the urban Mugwumps and the rural agrarians had trouble understanding the impulses and strivings of labor reformers. The cause of reform, its forces divided and mutually suspicious, languished and faltered through the eighties.

The Conservative Ascendancy

Hayes in the White House. We have already seen how the means used to elect Rutherford B. Hayes cast widespread doubt on his title to the Presidency (pp. 414–16). He did not strengthen his position when he announced that he would not run for reelection. Hayes was never an astute politician, but he did not lack courage and determination. From the start of his Administration he set out resolutely to redress the balance between the executive and legislative branches and regain for the Presidency some of the powers that Congress had preempted, particularly the powers of appointment and removal of officeholders.

The nominations for the Cabinet that he sent to the Senate were his first challenge to congressional dominance, for they included names unwelcome to the bosses—notably the name of Carl Schurz for Secretary of the Interior. "Hayes has passed the Republican party to its worst enemies," said Senator Zach Chandler. The Senate balked and refused confirmation on the whole list at first but later yielded to the President. An old device that the House used to coerce the President was the "rider," a piece of legislation the President had to approve in order to secure the needed appropriation to which it was tied. The Democratic majority of the House used the rider repeatedly in an attempt to force Hayes to accept the repeal of Reconstruction laws providing federal protection of elections. Determined to resist the pressure and make the executive "an equal and independent branch of the Government," Hayes vetoed seven such bills, compelled acceptance of his independence, and gained a clear-cut victory over congressional encroachment.

Hayes struck at the spoils system in its most powerful entrenchment, the New York Custom House Ring, the center of Senator Conkling's machine. A commission appointed by the President in 1877 and headed by John Jay of New York investigated the Custom House patronage system and reported that it was "unsound in principle, dangerous in practice,

demoralizing in its influence on all connected with the customs service," and ridden with "ignorance, inefficiency, and corruption." Conkling's lieutenants, Collector of the Port Chester A. Arthur and naval officer Alonzo B. Cornell, refused to clean up the corruption and declined to resign. At Conkling's demand the Senate refused to confirm appointment of the successors whom Hayes nominated, but the President stubbornly persisted, dismissed Arthur and Cornell while the Senate was in recess, and eventually filled their places with men of his own choice. He was trying to build his own machine to overcome Conkling's. Hayes had won a battle, but not a war. His orders that officeholders not be assessed for political contributions or required to do political campaigning were ignored. His promise of "thorough, radical and complete" civil-service reform remained unfulfilled, but a reasonable start had been made.

Economic crises and social protest in the worst years of the depression caught the Hayes Administration without a policy and without real comprehension of what was happening. The first great industrial conflict in our history started with a strike on the B&O Railroad in July 1877 (see p. 470). The strike spread spontaneously and rapidly throughout all sections save New England and the South, affecting two-thirds of the railroad mileage in the country. At the request of four state governors, Hayes set the fateful precedent of using federal troops to intervene in a strike and restore order. The President incurred additional ill will from labor, especially on the West Coast, by vetoing a bill passed in 1879 to restrict Chinese "coolie" immigration. He vetoed the bill because it violated the Burlingame Treaty of 1868, but after the veto he began negotiations for a new treaty with China. The Treaty of 1880 acknowledged the right of restriction, and in 1882 Congress passed a bill putting an end to Chinese immigration for the following decade.

Monetary policy in politics. The President also took the unpopular side in a series of debates over national currency policies that divided both parties during his Administration. Hayes held that the duty of the government was to maintain the value of currency and that the only way to do this was by the demonstrated ability of the Treasury to redeem currency at face value in gold. While tight money appealed to industrial workers, whose real wages were thereby protected from inflation, agrarian spokesmen believed that it was the duty of the government to manage the currency so as to prevent or correct injustice and to relieve distress and suffering. While this was by no means the only explanation for the agricultural distress of the time, the farmer was right that crop prices were falling and that monetary policy was related to this decline.

The first clash between Hayes and the discontented occurred over a movement to repeal the Specie Resumption Act of 1875, which obliged the Treasury to resume the redemption of legal-tender notes in specie at full face value by January 1, 1879, and to reduce the number of greenbacks in circulation. Though offset by increased issuance of national bank notes, the measure contracted the currency and at the same time appreciated its value, the two things most complained of by farmers and debtors. Advocates of repeal, called Greenbackers, argued that fulfillment of the act would further depress prices and increase the burden of private and public debt. They denounced as outrageous the proposal to redeem war bonds that had been bought with greenbacks worth less than 40 cents to the dollar with currency worth 100 cents to the dollar. A National Greenback party had polled an insignificant vote in the election of 1876, but in the following year the movement gained recruits from labor and additional support from farmers and in February 1878 reorganized as the Greenback Labor party. In the fall elections the new party polled a remarkable total of 1,060,000 votes and elected fourteen representatives to Congress. Resisting all pressure, much of it from his own party, Hayes clung to the policy of resumption and supported Secretary of the Treasury John Sherman in building up a gold reserve to redeem the currency. Two weeks before the deadline of January 1, 1879, however, greenbacks became worth their face value in gold and no run on the gold reserve developed. Resumption was an accomplished fact. The Greenbackers nominated James B. Weaver of Iowa for President in 1880, but their issue was dead, and they attracted little attention.

Inflationist sentiment, by no means dead, found a new outlet in the movement for the free coinage of silver just as the greenback cause was becoming hopeless. Once again Hayes took the more unpopular side. The silver question was to become one of the most hotly debated issues in the history of American politics during the next two decades, but before 1875 it attracted no popular interest. The official government ratio of sixteen to one—sixteen times as much silver in a silver dollar as there was gold in a gold dollar—had undervalued silver ever since the gold rush of 1849 had lowered the price of gold. As a consequence, silver-miners sold their product commercially rather than offer it to the Treasury at a loss, and silver dollars virtually disappeared from circulation. Foreseeing a drop in silver prices, a few monetary experts persuaded an ill-informed Congress to abolish the coinage of silver dollars and put the country on the gold standard in 1873. New silver mines in Nevada, Arizona, and Colorado soon flooded the market, and the price of silver began to drop. Miners then discovered that the Treasury rejected their product and that their Eu-

ropean market had been reduced by widespread adoption of the gold standard abroad. Denouncing demonetization of silver as the "Crime of 1873," urban publishers in the Midwestern and Middle Atlantic states, not Western miners, started the demand that free coinage at the old ratio be restored. Inflationists eventually took up their cry because they saw in silver a means of halting currency contraction, getting cheaper money, raising crop prices, and securing debtor relief.

So rapidly did the silver movement spread that by the fall of 1877 an overwhelming majority of the lower house of Congress voted for a bill for the "free and unlimited coinage of silver" introduced by Representative Richard "Silver Dick" Bland of Missouri. The Bland bill would have stopped the sale of government bonds for gold and driven that metal out of circulation, since it would have produced silver dollars worth less than 90 cents (and still falling in value) and made them legal tender. Yet the bill commanded so much support in both houses that Hayes knew it would be passed over his veto. Before the Senate acted, however, Senator William B. Allison of Iowa amended and weakened the bill, and in that form it was passed over Hayes' veto in February 1878. The Bland-Allison Act deprived the inflationists of their objective of "unlimited coinage" and substituted the requirement that the Treasury buy not less than $2 million and not more than $4 million worth of silver per month and coin it into dollars. The act did not have the effects that the conservatives feared and the inflationists desired. For one thing the government consistently purchased the minimum amount of silver required by the act and stood ready to redeem the silver coin and notes in gold. And for another, the depression lifted in 1879, gold flowed in from abroad, and crop prices improved temporarily for reasons other than monetary policy. Silverites were to return to the battle in stronger force, but for more than a decade they made no change in the law.

In spite of the unpopularity of his stand on silver and his quarrels with Congress, Hayes ended his Administration on an upswing of confidence and respect. Ordinarily such an upturn would have overcome his announced intention to retire, but no such movement developed. His party virtually ignored him, and he became scarcely more than a spectator during the struggle to nominate his successor.

The Garfield tragedy. The Republicans brought their bitter feuds to the Chicago nominating convention under the banners of rival candidates. The Stalwarts were united under Conkling's leadership to name Grant for a third term. The Half-Breeds were determined to nominate Blaine; and Secretary of the Treasury John Sherman maneuvered to make himself

Republican National Convention, Chicago, 1880

available as a compromise candidate. When it became clear that none of the three could marshal a majority, the Blaine and Sherman forces joined on the thirty-sixth ballot and nominated Congressman James A. Garfield of Ohio. Garfield had managed Sherman's campaign and led the anti-Grant forces at the convention. To conciliate the defeated faction, the convention then nominated Conkling's lieutenant, Chester A. Arthur, the deposed spoilsman of the New York Custom House, for Vice President.

Prospects for revenging Governor Tilden by nominating him in 1880 looked promising to the Democrats, but at the last moment Tilden declined to run for the Presidency again. The party nominated instead General Winfield Scott Hancock, a Pennsylvanian and a Union hero in the Battle of Gettysburg. Hancock had no political experience, but his nomination was an effective answer to the charge of disloyalty that was so often thrown at his party. His running mate was William H. English, from the ''doubtful'' state of Indiana. Taking charge of his own campaign, Garfield stressed the tariff issue effectively and made protection the basis of a broadened party coalition. The Republican managers did the most decisive work of the campaign in the doubtful states of Ohio, New York, and Indiana, using large amounts of money to carry Indiana by a bare seven thousand votes and New York by twenty thousand. Garfield won by a plurality of less than forty thousand popular votes in the country at large, though his electoral vote was 214 to 155 for Hancock.

President Garfield's brief tenure in the White House began with embarrassments, continued with party feuds, and ended in tragedy. A handsome, massive figure of a man, with a reputation for courage under fire in the war and for resourcefulness as party-leader in the House, Garfield was not without integrity. Under the extraordinary pressures of his new office, he moved cautiously and skillfully in the construction of his Cabinet to consolidate his control. Acknowledging his obligations to Blaine for vital help in the presidential nomination, he made the senator from Maine Secretary of State. Then refusing to bow to the dictates of the Stalwart leader Conkling, Garfield moved to assert presidential authority by naming

James A. Garfield: reputation for courage

Chester A. Arthur: wealthy, easygoing, elegant

for Collector of the Port of New York the leading opponent of Conkling in that state. This precipitated a showdown in which Conkling and his friend the newly elected Senator Tom Platt were the losers.

At the very height of the furor over spoils and corruption, on July 2, 1881, Charles J. Guiteau, a crazed and disappointed office-seeker, shot the President in the back. With a bullet lodged in his spine, Garfield was incapacitated for eleven weeks before his death on September 19. Then Stalwart Vice President Chester A. Arthur was sworn in as President and assumed control.

The Arthur interlude. The new President was a wealthy, easygoing man with expensive tastes, elegant clothes and carriages, and twenty years of experience as a spoilsman in the Conkling camp of New York politics. His first year as President did little to dispel the fear that Garfield's martyrdom had been in vain and that the spoils system was there to stay. Arthur did not turn over patronage to his fellow Stalwart Conkling, as many expected, but after Blaine's resignation from the Cabinet the President did prosecute with vigor those charged with post-office frauds, one of whom claimed to have provided the money for carrying Indiana for Garfield and Arthur. The guilty men escaped punishment, and the President's efforts not only failed to win over the reformers but provoked party feuds and gave Democrats ammunition for the off-year campaign. The fall elections of 1882 drove his party from control of the House of Representatives and gave the Democrats a majority of nearly a hundred seats.

One cause of the Democratic landslide was the nation's shock over Garfield's assassination and revulsion against the system of patronage and spoils associ-

ated with the tragedy. Popular indignation put new power behind the demands of the small band of reformers who, having fought the spoilsmen since the 1860s, had in 1881 organized the National Civil Service Reform League, with George William Curtis as president. It was ironic that "Chet" Arthur, long the very symbol of spoils politics, should be cast in the role of civil-service reformer, but he firmly told Congress that "action should no longer be postponed" and promised his full cooperation. In January 1883 large bipartisan majorities in both houses of Congress passed a Democratic bill sponsored by Senator George H. Pendleton of Ohio. The Civil Service Act (often called the Pendleton Act) established a bipartisan Civil Service Commission of three members, appointed by the President with Senate confirmation, who were to administer competitive examinations and select appointees on the basis of merit and an apportionment among the states according to population. Arthur demonstrated his good faith by naming as head of the commission Dorman B. Eaton, an outstanding reformer who drafted the act, and appointing two prominent friends of reform as the other commissioners. Shrewdly designed to make it acceptable to spoilsmen in Congress, the Pendleton Act affected only about one-tenth of the federal employees at first. But it empowered the President to expand the proportion of jobs "classified" or subject to the merit system. By the end of the century 40 percent of the jobs were so classified, the civil service was securely established, and centralized presidential control was reversing the decentralizing pull of the spoils system and Congress.

While the Civil Service Commission was the most important achievement of the Arthur Administration, it was not the President's only assertion of independence and conscience, nor his only praiseworthy effort. Two such efforts, both of them futile as it turned out, were in response to the problem of a surplus accumulated in the United States Treasury by excessive tax revenues. The solution favored by Congress was to spend the surplus in lavish appropriations for river and harbor improvements and pork-barrel handouts. In order to win Half-Breed support, Arthur vetoed one such bill, only to have Congress pass it over his veto. His efforts in tariff reduction amounted to little. As an incidental means of reducing the Treasury surplus, Arthur's naval-construction program was more successful. The navy had deteriorated since the Civil War to a collection of wooden antiques with cast-iron guns and rotten hulls. It did not boast a steel vessel or a rifled gun afloat. The Arthur Administration awakened Congress out of its indifference and started the construction of new fighting ships. The three cruisers begun in his Administration had numerous defects, but he is properly credited with sweeping away barriers of ignorance and clearing the way for a modern navy. In this as in other ways Arthur proved worthier of the office he held than anyone had reason to believe when he took it.

Changing the conservative guard. The chances of Arthur's succeeding himself as President in 1884, never very strong in any case, were greatly weakened by the Democratic tidal wave of 1882, in which he lost control of his own state. Blaine remained the dominant figure in the Republican party, and his nomination seemed more and more likely as the convention approached. Ignoring the reformers and overriding the Arthur supporters, the Blaine men nominated their candidate without difficulty and named John A. Logan, favorite son of Illinois, for Vice President. The Yankee Mugwumps promptly decided to bolt the party provided the Democrats nominated the rising hope of the reformers, Grover Cleveland, governor of New York.

Cleveland's rise in New York politics had been recent and rapid. Elected mayor of Buffalo in 1881, he accepted the Democratic nomination for governor in 1882 and won an easy victory because of the split in the Republican party of the state. A burly figure of two hundred forty pounds, determined jaw, and hard eyes, he was known for his rugged honesty and his habits of hard work and thrift. As reformer Cleveland was a thoroughgoing conservative, a believer in sound money and a defender of the right of property. As governor he enhanced his reputation for scorn of popularity by vetoing a popular bill reducing the fare on Jay Gould's elevated railroads in New York City to 5 cents. Similarly, he risked the wrath of labor by vetoing a bill limiting the working day of New York streetcar-conductors to twelve hours, and with even greater recklessness he defied "Honest" John Kelley, boss of Tammany Hall. Businessmen, middle-class taxpayers, and reformers of the Mugwump school admired the independence and integrity of Cleveland. The nomination of Blaine and the promise of Mugwump support made Governor Cleveland the logical standard-bearer for the Democrats in 1884. He was nominated with the aid of state bosses and financed in his campaign by corporate wealth. His running mate was Thomas A. Hendricks, yet another available candidate from the shifting counties of Indiana.

The presidential campaign of 1884 was one of the most sensational and frenzied in our history. "The public is angry and abusive," wrote Henry Adams. "Every one takes part. We are all doing our best, and swearing like demons. But the amusing thing is that no one talks about real interests." Actually Blaine made some 400 speeches stressing protective tariff as support for high wages. Cleveland said little at all during the campaign. Popular attention and the press focused on the private life and personal morals of the candidates. Democrats and Mugwumps took the initiative by reviving charges (see p. 414) that had deprived Blaine of the nomination in 1876 and by publishing additional evidence that Blaine had been guilty of underhanded deals with railroad-promoters. George William Curtis declared that the issue was "moral rather than political." Thereupon the Republicans retaliated with evidence that Cleveland was the father of an illegitimate son. The campaign deteriorated into scandalmongering that became more and more irresponsible.

Cleveland had to carry New York to win the election, and the extreme closeness of the contest in that state concentrated attention on a number of intangible factors, particularly those affecting the Irish electorate, any one of which might conceivably have been decisive. Whatever the explanation, the tide turned narrowly in Cleveland's favor. In addition to all the Southern states, he carried the doubtful states of Indiana, New Jersey, Connecticut, and New York—the last by a plurality of a mere 1,149 votes. His share of the votes in the country as a whole was only slightly greater than Blaine's. Mugwumps and reformers rejoiced at the victory, but it is a mistake to conclude that a moral crusade had defeated Blaine, who came very near winning. Actually, he polled about the same percentage of the total vote as Garfield had in

Grover Cleveland: stubborn conservative

1880 and a larger percentage than the Republican candidates were to poll in 1888 and 1892. At any rate, the long Republican rule was at an end, and the Democrats were back in power for the first time in twenty-four years.

Cleveland in command.

No one could be sure of the new President's views on any of several leading issues, but everyone could be sure he was a conservative. His inaugural address promising adherence to "business principles" bore this out, and so did his Cabinet appointments, which included representatives of the most conservative and business-minded wing of the party in the East and South. The new Administration signified no break with the past on fundamental issues.

If there was any policy to which Cleveland had a clear commitment, it was civil-service reform, and it was over this issue that he came near to wrecking his administration. He came to office with two masters to please: the Mugwump reformer and the hungry spoilsman of his own party with an appetite for office whetted by twenty-four years of anticipation. The President's first moves delighted the reformers. Defying the Democratic bosses and spoilsmen, he retained in office some able Republicans and personally examined applications for office far into the night. Party-leaders besieged the President with patronage demands and insisted that he accept their definition of civil-service reform, which, according to one senator, "meant turning out of office of Republicans and putting honest Democrats in their places"—*all* their places. The party press thundered against his "ingratitude." Within a few months he yielded to pressure, and Republican heads began to roll. Carl Schurz wrote, "Your attempt to please both reformers and spoilsmen has failed," and Cleveland broke with the Mugwumps. By the end of four years he had removed about two-thirds of the 120,000 federal officers. He did increase the list of classified jobs to 27,380, nearly double the number when he took office, but he filled the Civil Service Commission with weak and incompetent men.

In the role of Treasury watchdog and thrifty steward of public funds, Cleveland showed more consistency than he did as civil-service reformer. For one thing, he rebuked a pensions racket run by a powerful lobby for Union veterans of the Civil War. Agents of this lobby used private bills to push through Congress thousands of dubious claims, hundreds of them obviously fraudulent. Previous Presidents, who feared the Grand Army of the Republic, had always signed these bills, but Cleveland called a halt and took to investigating individual claims himself, vetoing many of them, often with sarcastic comment. In January 1887, Congress passed a Dependent Pension Bill that provided a pension for all honorably discharged disabled veterans who had seen as much as ninety days of service if they were unable to work, regardless of the cause of their disability. The President defied the wrath of the GAR and its half-million members and vetoed the bill.

Cleveland believed that, except in rare circumstances, the President should confine himself to the execution of the laws. But by his pension vetoes and his stand against congressional patronage powers, and later on tariff reform, he strongly reasserted the integrity and independence of the executive branch and began to curb the long dominance of an imperial Congress. In spite of the storms of social protest in the mid-eighties, Congress enacted little legislation of lasting significance, and the President's influence upon that was largely negative. His Secretary of the Interior, L. Q. C. Lamar, showed initiative in compelling railroads and cattle barons of the West to give up 81 million acres of public lands that they illegally withheld from settlement. But Cleveland himself deserves no credit for what was probably the most important act passed during his Administration, the Interstate Commerce Act of 1887 (see p. 457). He regarded the whole idea with suspicion and signed the bill reluctantly and "with reservations."

The tariff in politics.

In his fight for tariff reform, however, Cleveland took a more forthright stand that may have contributed to his defeat for reelection. The issue was as old as the republic, but since the Civil War it had taken on a new importance and complexity and was treated with caution and evasiveness by politicians of both parties. The tariff acts of the Civil War had been justified on the grounds that high internal war taxes on American industries put them at a competitive disadvantage that had to be offset with protective tariff duties to enable Americans to compete with foreign manufacturers on equal terms. Beginning with modest rates of 18.8 percent on dutiable goods in 1861, a succession of acts raised the average to 40.3 percent in 1866. No politician at the end of the war would admit publicly that these rates were anything but a temporary expedient. But, while the American producers were soon relieved of the burden of internal war taxes, the protective tariff remained unrepealed. The protected industries quickly adjusted to the prices, dividends, and profits made possible by a measure of freedom from competition from abroad. Producers who enjoyed or desired these advantages organized to press their desires on Congress. Politicians learned the great power of the tariff lobbies, and both major parties, the Republicans explicitly and the Democrats for a time tacitly, accepted the principle of protection—though with dissent in each party, more among Democrats than among Republicans.

From time to time a President would make a gesture of reform, but Congress would regularly respond with jugglery that left the situation unchanged or made a mockery of reform. The Tariff Act of 1870 reduced the duties on coffee, tea, spices, and other articles not produced in this country but left the protective duties virtually unaltered. Regulars joined reformers in 1872 and actually effected a reduction of 10 percent in the protective duties, but the cut was quietly restored three years later on the ground that the Panic of 1873 had reduced federal revenues. Two Democratic bills for reform in 1876 and 1878 never got out of committee. President Arthur's efforts on tariff reform came to naught in 1883.

Cleveland hesitated for three years to take an aggressive stand. He knew that a minority of some forty Democratic congressmen had combined with Republicans to defeat tariff-reform bills in 1884 and 1886, and Democratic leaders assured him that an all-out fight on the issue would split the party and lose the next election. Finally deciding, however, the President devoted his entire annual message of December 1887 to the tariff question. He made a slashing attack on the injustice, inequity, and absurdity of existing rates, ridiculed the need to protect century-old "infant industries," and denounced high rates as "the vicious, inequitable and illogical source of unnecessary taxation." The House of Representatives, with a Democratic majority, responded by adopting a bill sponsored by Roger Q. Mills of Texas and favoring the South. Far from radical, it did place such raw materials as lumber, wool, and flax on the free list and made moderate reductions of about 7 percent in rates for finished goods. The House gave 240 hours to discussion of the bill, 51 working days, and public interest did not seem to lag. The Republican-controlled Senate then rejected the Mills bill, as expected, and adopted a highly protective substitute bill. The deadlock of tariff reform produced the first clear-cut economic issue between parties since Reconstruction and provided the leading issue of the 1888 election.

For their presidential candidate the Republicans chose Benjamin Harrison of Indiana, whose chief attractions were that he came from a doubtful state and that he was the grandson of former President William Henry Harrison, "Old Tippecanoe," of log-cabin and hard-cider fame. A senator of national reputation, Harrison proved to be an effective campaigner in spite of his chilly personality. His running mate was Levi P. Morton, a wealthy New York banker. The Democrats naturally renominated President Cleveland, and for their vice-presidential candidate they chose the elderly and ailing ex-senator Allen G. Thurman of Ohio.

The campaign for Cleveland's reelection was handicapped by halfhearted and ineffective leadership. By contrast, the Republican campaign had a vigorous leader in Senator Matt Quay, boss of a ruthless machine in Pennsylvania. Quay collected and spent a huge campaign fund. Republican strategists made telling use of this fund to purchase votes and rig elections in Indiana and New York. The winning party proved to have a more effective organization and staged a better campaign.

In spite of much talk about tariff reform, the election did not turn on that issue alone. Cleveland actually carried the manufacturing states of New Jersey and Connecticut, and the Democrats gained ground in Michigan, Ohio, and California, normally protariff states. Cleveland polled a plurality of almost one hundred thousand popular votes, but Harrison won the electoral vote 233 to 168. It was an extremely narrow victory for the Republicans. As usual, the outcome had hung on a few evenly divided states—Indiana, New York, Rhode Island, and Ohio—in all of which the tariff issue played a part, and Harrison had carried them all, each by a few thousand votes. Prominent factors in what was probably the most corrupt presidential election of national history up to that time appear to have been trickery in Indiana and New York and division within the Democratic party.

Harrison and the surplus. President Harrison's political obligations to Blaine dictated his appointment as Secretary of State, and other appointments paid off political debts. John Wanamaker, a wealthy Philadelphia merchant, became Postmaster General and turned over the Post Office patronage to spoilsmen. In spite of his commitment to civil-service reform, Harrison watched the process in silence.

For the first time since 1875 the Republicans in 1889–91 held the Presidency and a majority in both houses of Congress. Each majority was extremely slight, however, and under existing House rules the Democratic minority could frustrate the majority by simply not answering roll call, thereby depriving the House of a quorum. Speaker Thomas B. Reed of Maine earned the title of "Czar" by sweeping aside the rules over the indignant protest of the minority, strengthening party responsibility, and running House proceedings with an iron will. Under Reed in the House and the protectionist Senator Nelson W. Aldrich of Rhode Island in the Senate, the Republican majority won the name of the "Billion Dollar Congress" for its generosity in spending the Treasury surplus largely created by tariff revenues. The Republican legislative program included a new tariff bill, a federal election law, a silver purchase act, and an antitrust measure, all of which moved through Congress simultaneously, with supporters of one measure bargaining with or frustrating supporters of another.

Among those frustrated were advocates of an election law to protect voters' rights. Managed in the House by Henry Cabot Lodge of Massachusetts, the bill would enable a hundred voters in any city or district to petition for investigation of fraud or irregularities in an election and provide for ultimate federal enforcement of rights. It was aimed mainly at protecting black Republican voters, and Southern whites denounced it furiously as a "force bill" to restore "Negro rule." City bosses and some Westerners and business interests did not like the bill either. It passed the House but was blocked in the Senate by a filibuster. In order to get on with the stalled tariff bill, action on the election bill was postponed. When the Senate took up the bill later, Republican senators from the silver-mining states joined the Democrats in killing the election reform bill and displacing it with a bill for the free coinage of silver.

With the balance of power in their hands, silver champions stalled the tariff bill further. They had been promised that the Republican party would "do something for silver" in return for support of the tariff. The measure that was finally contrived to fulfill this commitment was the Sherman Silver Purchase Act, named for the senator from Ohio. It was designed to replace the Bland-Allison Act of 1878 (see p. 504), which had fixed in dollars a minimum amount of silver that the federal Treasury had to purchase each month. Under this law the Treasury had put about $378 million in silver into circulation without relieving the scarcity of currency. The Sherman Act fixed the amount of silver to be purchased in ounces rather than dollars: 4½ million ounces per month, approximately the amount of national production of the metal in 1890. The silver was to be paid for in Treasury notes of full legal-tender value, which could be redeemed in either gold or silver at the discretion of the government. As it turned out, the government chose to redeem the notes only in gold, and as the price of silver dropped the Treasury was required to spend fewer and fewer dollars to purchase the specified number of ounces. The act produced no more currency expansion than its predecessor had. The product of weak and shifty statesmanship, it pleased neither side and contributed nothing of importance toward solving the currency problems of the nation.

Another reform act passed about the same time, also bearing the name of the Ohio senator, was the Sherman Antitrust Act of June 1890 (see pp. 461–62). Although many congressmen were absent when the vote was taken, the act was adopted with only one vote against it in the Senate and none in the House. Although the law was no sham and had wide support, it had little effect during the following decade, for no administration during those years showed much interest in enforcing it.

The most controversial and, as it turned out, the most politically costly achievement of this productive Republican Congress was the tariff act that took the name of William McKinley of Ohio. Secretary of State

Blaine intervened to press his doctrine of reciprocity on a protectionist and suspicious congressional majority. Accepted in principle, the reciprocity clause only empowered the President to place tariff duties on certain goods from Latin America if those countries did not lower rates on American imports. The McKinley Act increased selectively an already high tariff scale. It placed raw sugar on the free list, but granted American sugar-growers a compensatory bounty of 2 cents a pound. As a gesture to farmers, duties were raised on agricultural products, though few of them needed protection. Explaining the bill's faults, McKinley freely admitted that they were necessitated by politics rather than economics.

In order to please Union veterans of the Civil War, Harrison appointed as commissioner of pensions James "Corporal" Tanner, a pensions lobbyist who indicated his purpose with the slogan, "God help the surplus!" He favored "an appropriation for every old comrade who needs it" and quickly added millions to the pension budget before the embarrassed President removed him. Congress assisted the veterans' cause, however, with the Dependent Pension Act of 1890, similar to the one Cleveland had vetoed in 1887, which recognized claims from virtually everyone connected with the Union war effort with a record of ninety days' service, a disability from any cause, and an honorable discharge. Their widows and children helped swell the pension rolls.

The Billion Dollar Congress did wonders in taking care of the Treasury surplus. The prohibitive tariff rates set by the McKinley Act reduced income, and the combination of excessive pensions and silver purchases increased expenditures. Still in a mood of generosity and still finding some of the surplus left, Congress hastily devised more handouts in the form of subsidies to steamship lines, lavish pork-barrel bills for river and harbor improvements, enormous premiums for government bondholders, and the return of federal taxes paid during the Civil War by Northern states. These handouts and the onset of depression wiped out the surplus in the Treasury by 1894, and the Treasury-surplus problem has never troubled the United States since.

The first Congress of the Harrison Administration promoted the interests of politicians and business leaders—that is, if they belonged to the right party or were engaged in the right business. To other interests, particularly farmers and small businesspeople (with the exception of Northern veterans), Congress appeared a wasteful dispenser of favors to the privileged. In the congressional elections of 1890 Republicans were overwhelmed by a revolt that penetrated traditional strongholds in Ohio, Michigan, Illinois, Wisconsin, and Kansas, even Massachusetts. Any attempt to attribute Republican losses of 1890 to reaction

against national policies of the party such as the McKinley Tariff is embarrassed by the fact that in some states the swing against the party *preceded* passage of the tariff act. In these and other states defection among religious and ethnic groups was tied to unpopular Republican positions on local cultural issues regarding prohibition, school regulations, and Sunday blue laws. Republicans were reduced to 88 seats in the House of Representatives, the smallest number in thirty years, while the Democrats took 235 seats. Republicans hung on to a small majority in the Senate. But the election of 1890 ran up danger signals for conservative leaders of both the old parties. A depression was on the way, and a third-party revolt was shaping up.

The Agrarian Revolt

The decline of agriculture. The spirit of revolt flamed up most fiercely in the agricultural sections of the South and the West, and it was fed by acute economic distress and a deep sense of grievance. American farmers reached a low point in their history in the 1890s. The past was not the golden age they sometimes dreamed of, but they had certainly been better off before and were to be better off in the future. But ever since the 1860s agriculture had been slipping backward, and they suspected the government of indifference, if not hostility, to their interests. They searched everywhere for the causes of their plight and the cure for their troubles. Some of their guesses were shrewd and accurate, but they overlooked some of the causes of their troubles.

They were caught up in an international crisis that afflicted agriculture in many parts of the world and provoked rebellion abroad as well as at home. The crisis for producers of export staple crops resulted from a revolution in communication and transportation that created a worldwide market for agricultural products. Ships first steamed through the Suez Canal in 1869, the year locomotives first steamed across the North American continent. The network of railroad and steamship lines was swiftly paralleled by a network of telegraph and telephone lines and transoceanic cables that linked continents and tied the world together.

Forced to compete in a world market without control over output, American farmers watched the prices of their product decline decade after decade. It did not seem fair: the more they grew, the less they earned. Prices of other goods declined too, but farmers said they had to buy expensive farm machinery in a protected market and sell their crops in an unprotected market. As the gap between income and expenses widened, farmers were increasingly forced to borrow money to cover the gap. They were therefore chronically in debt, and debtors always suffered most keenly from deflationary monetary policies, such as those the government had pursued ever since the Civil War. Contracting the amount of currency in circulation resulted in lowering the price that crops brought and increasing the difficulty of paying off debts. Farmers in debt had reason for opposing contraction and demanding expansion of currency.

It was no wonder that agrarian discontent was most bitter in the South and the West, for the growers of the staple crops of those sections were most vulnerable to the tight money market and the interest rates they had to pay for credit. The price of cotton and wheat had been falling steadily for two decades. From 1870 to 1873 cotton had averaged about 15.1 cents a pound; from 1894 to 1898 it dropped to an average of 5.8 cents. Over the same period wheat prices dropped from 106.7 to 63.3 cents a bushel, and corn from 43.0 to 29.7. These were market prices, after transportation and warehouse charges had been paid, not the lower prices the farmer received. In 1889 corn was actually selling for 10 cents in Kansas, and farmers were burning it for fuel. Georgia farmers were getting 5 cents a pound for their cotton at a time when economists were estimating that it cost about 7 cents a pound to produce. During several of these years the nation's farmers were running a losing business. Western farmers were kept going sometimes by the appreciation of land values and Southern farmers mainly by sheer habit and the momentum of generations, for in the South land values were declining as well as crop prices.

The ills of agriculture were reflected in the growing number of mortgages (not always an evil) and tenant farmers. Nearly a third of the country's farms were mortgaged by the end of the nineties. In Kansas, Nebraska, North Dakota, South Dakota, and Minnesota there were by 1890 more mortgages than families. In the Southern states mortgages were far fewer, but only because land was such a drug on the market that it could not be mortgaged. The South's substitute was the lien system, the worse credit system of all (see p. 425). Fewer and fewer farmers owned the land they worked, and more and more labored for a landlord, often an absentee landlord. The number of tenant farms increased from 25.8 percent of all the farms in 1880 to 35.3 percent at the end of the century, and were to rise even higher.

Understandably, the farmer blamed others for these woes. In the farmer's view the railroads were the archenemy, and the offenses attributed to them were by no means wholly imaginary, though sometimes exaggerated. The complaint that it took one bushel of wheat or corn to pay the freight on another bushel

was no exaggeration. The chief complaints of rate discrimination came from the South and the West, where rates were frequently two or three times what they were between Chicago and New York. Railroads favored large over small shippers and one locality over another, and flagrantly dominated politics and legislatures. The national banks were also a natural target for agrarian abuse, for they refused to lend money on real estate and farm property, manipulated banknote currency against agricultural interests, and were indifferent to seasonal needs for money for the movement of crops.

Few could deny the validity of the complaint that the farmer bore the brunt of the tax burden. Stocks and bonds could easily be concealed from the view of the tax-collector, but not livestock and land. Railroads and corporations could pass the taxes on to the consumer, but the farmer could not pass on taxes. There was no federal income tax at that time. The tax laws, like the bank laws, worked to the farmer's disadvantage. And so did the tariff. The injustice was all the harder to bear for those who believed that the tariff bred trusts and the trusts levied tribute on the consumers of all types of goods. Antitrust and antimonopoly feeling ran high in all farmer organizations. While those few who spoke of a "conspiracy" were on the wrong track, the many were right who contended that they had a number of legitimate grievances against a system that worked so consistently to their disadvantage.

In the late eighties and early nineties natural calamities came one on top of another with stunning impact. They are not to be confused with the deeper causes of the farmer's revolt, but they added to the feeling of despair—droughts on the plains that not merely damaged the crops but destroyed them; floods in the lower Mississippi Valley that not merely destroyed the crops but left the land unusable; grim, blizzard-bound winters on the high plains that destroyed not merely domestic animals but wild ones as well and threatened even the survival of the human inhabitants. Less spectacular, but contrasting sharply with the new urban way of life, was the loneliness, the drudgery, and the isolation of rural life in America in those years. This was the ancient lot of farmers, but the growing glitter of the city made it less tolerable than ever, especially when coupled with the grinding, ceaseless pressure of economic ills and grievances. To Thomas E. Watson of Georgia, who was to whip agrarian wrath into a frenzied crusade, the farmers of his region seemed to move about "like victims of some horrid nightmare . . . powerless—oppressed— shackled."

Agrarian protest. There was nothing irrational about the farmers' impulse to organize and protest against their lot. The Patrons of Husbandry, organized

Granger poster

in local "granges" and better known as the Grangers, served as a model for later and more powerful movements. Founded in 1867 by Oliver Hudson Kelley, a government employee in Washington who was moved by the plight of Southern farmers, the Grange grew slowly until the pinch of depression quickened interest in the early seventies. By 1874 the estimated membership was about 1½ million, and growth continued into the next year. In 1875 the Grange was strongest in the Middle West, the South, the Southwest, and the border states of Missouri and Kentucky.

Seeking to eliminate the profits of the middleman, Grangers founded cooperatives for buying and selling, for milling and storing grain, even for banking and manufacturing. These enterprises often suffered from inexperience and lack of capital, but some of them flourished and saved their members money. Membership fell off rapidly after 1875, but the Grangers left their imprint upon law and politics. They actually received more credit than they were due for the so-called Granger laws that were adopted in the early seventies by Midwestern states to regulate grain elevators and railroads. Eight "Granger cases" came before the Supreme Court in 1877, and in *Munn* v. *Illinois*, the most significant of them, the Court upheld the "police power" of state regulation (see p. 457). Curtailed and hampered by subsequent decisions, the

right of the public to control great corporations nevertheless held securely in the future.

Of the several farmers' organizations that succeeded the Grange after it subsided in political prominence, by far the most important and powerful was the National Farmers Alliance and Industrial Union, originally known as the Southern Alliance. Originating in 1877 in a frontier county of Texas, the Alliance grew slowly until it launched a crusade of rapid expansion in 1886 under the energetic leadership of Dr. Charles W. Macune. The culmination of the movement was Macune's subtreasury system, a plan for government warehouses where farmers could deposit nonperishable crops and receive greenbacks up to 80 percent of the market value of the crops deposited. The loan was to be secured by the crops and repaid when crops were sold, thus enabling the farmer to hold the produce for a favorable market. It was the most inspiring idea of the movement, but it was never realized.* Other demands of the Alliance's Ocala Platform of 1890 included the abolition of national banks, a substantial increase in the amount of currency in circulation, free coinage of silver, a federal income tax, reduction of tariff rates, the direct election of senators, "rigid" control of railroad and telegraph companies—and, if that did not work, government ownership of both.

The Farmers Alliance established its own extensive press supported by hundreds of local weekly papers and organized a lecture bureau that sent recruiters and cooperative founders all over the South and into the West. Farmers, tenants, and landowners joined up by the hundreds of thousands. At its peak in 1891 the Alliance probably had two million members. An affiliated but separate Colored Farmers' National Alliance and Cooperative Union probably had about a quarter million members. The expanding Farmers Alliance formed a coalition with the declining Knights of Labor and took firm hold in Kansas and the Dakotas, but it struck a snag in attempts to merge with the Northwestern Alliance with headquarters in Chicago. This was a small, largely paper organization with few members and weak leaders who had little sympathy with Southern radicalism. They had little claim to a place in the agrarian revolt and opposed the Populist party to the end. Yet they and their superficial silver crusade have been mistaken by some historians as the essence of Populism.

Though the Alliance, like the Grange, professed to be strictly "nonpolitical," it was clear that its demands could be realized only by political means.

---

*Some components of the subtreasury idea, though not the essential feature of popular control over the currency, were embodied in the New Deal measure of 1933 creating the Commodity Credit Corporation.

*Now the People's Party says to these two men, 'You are kept apart that you
may be separately fleeced of your earnings. You are made to hate each other
because upon that hatred is rested the keystone of the arch of financial despotism which enslaves you both. You are deceived and blinded that you may not
see how this race antagonism perpetuates a monetary system which beggars
both....'*

*The conclusion, then, seems to me to be this: the crushing burdens which
now oppress both races in the South will cause each to make an effort to cast
them off. They will see a similarity of cause and a similarity of remedy. They
will recognize that each should help the other in the work of repealing bad
laws and enacting good ones. They will become political allies, and neither
can injure the other without weakening both. It will be to the interest of both
that each should have justice. And on these broad lines of mutual interest,
mutual forbearance, and mutual support the present will be made the step-
ping-stone to future peace and prosperity.*

From Thomas E. Watson, *The Arena*, 1892.

Using their demands (similar to the ones adopted
later that year at Ocala) as a yardstick, Southern
Alliancemen required all Democratic candidates in
the 1890 elections to "stand up and be measured." As
a result, the Alliance seemed at the time to have come
near taking over the Democratic party in the South,
for it elected four governors, secured control of eight
legislatures, and elected forty-four congressmen and
three senators who were pledged to support Alliance
demands. Instead of working within one of the old
parties, Alliancemen in the West hastily set up independent third parties, the names of which differed
from state to state, and nominated their own candidates. Their most striking successes were in Kansas,
where they elected five congressmen and a senator; in
Nebraska, where they took control of both houses of
the legislature and elected two congressmen; and in
South Dakota, where they elected a senator. In other
Western states their vote came largely at the expense
of the Republicans and accounted in part for the large
number of Democratic congressmen elected in 1890.
The election served notice on both old parties that the
farmers were on the march.

The Populist crusade. Their successes in 1890
inspired Westerners with the ambition to form a national third party to promote Alliance ideas. Southerners hung back, however, in order to try out their
plan of working within the Democratic party. They
were quickly disillusioned, for all the Southern Democratic congressmen elected on an Alliance platform,
with the exception of Tom Watson, entered the Democratic caucus and voted for a conservative anti-Alli-
ance Georgian for Speaker. Thereupon Watson, red-
headed and a rebel by temperament, left his party and
became the "People's party" candidate for Speaker

with the support of eight congressmen from the West.
Thus the new party, often called the Populist party,
had a congressional delegation before it had a national
organization. The National Alliance, however, under
the leadership of President Leonidas L. Polk of North
Carolina, was moving rapidly in the Populist direction. On February 22, 1892, a huge Confederation of
Industrial Organizations met at St. Louis, attended by
delegates from the Knights of Labor, the Nationalists,
the Single-Taxers, Greenbackers, Prohibitionists, and
other reform groups, but dominated by delegates from
the National Alliance. The delegates officially
founded the People's party and called for a convention to nominate a ticket for the presidential election
of 1892.

Shortly before the convention met in Omaha on
July 4, the Populists were deprived of their strongest
candidate by the death of Polk. The party nominated
the old Greenback campaigner of 1880, General James
B. Weaver of Iowa, for President, and, to balance the
Union general with a Confederate one, chose General
James G. Field of Virginia as his running mate. The
platform emphatically reiterated Alliance principles
on money, credit, transportation, and land and
evoked the wildest enthusiasm for its planks on government ownership of railroads and monetary reform.
The fervor and violence of Populist rhetoric is illustrated by the following excerpt from the preamble to
the platform, written and delivered by Ignatius Donnelly of Minnesota, Populist writer and orator:

> . . . we meet in the midst of a nation brought to
> the verge of moral, political, and material ruin.
> Corruption dominates the ballot-box, the legisla-
> tures, the Congress, and touches even the ermine
> of the bench. The people are demoralized.

Kansas House of Representatives, 1893: a militant pose

Eastern conservatives were frightened by the Populist tone and built up a distorted image of the movement as an insurrection of hayseed anarchists or hick communists. The nicknames that the hostile metropolitan press bestowed on Populist leaders lent themselves to such propaganda—names such as Lemuel H. "Calamity" Weller of Iowa, Congressman "Sockless" Jerry Simpson of Kansas, Governor Davis H. "Bloody Bridles" Waite of Colorado, and orator James H. "Cyclone" Davis of Texas—not to mention the advice of Mary E. Lease of Kansas to "raise less corn and more hell." While it is true that some of the Populist leaders were provincial and ill-informed and tended to oversimplify issues, it is only fair to recall that the plight of the people for whom they spoke was desperate. We must recall also that their conservative opponents, better educated as a rule, entertained absurd monetary and economic theories of their own and talked wildly of conspiracies and subversives themselves. To their credit it should be remembered that the Populists were the first important movement in this country to insist that laissez-faire economics was not the final solution to industrial problems and that the federal government had some responsibility for social well-being.

The first task of the Populists was to bridge the cleavages between parties, sections, races, and classes that kept apart the forces of reform that they wished to unite. First they sought to revive the old agrarian alliance between South and West. Second, they felt that both the Republicans and the Democrats were bent on keeping natural allies divided and sought to replace the old parties with a third party. Third, they

Mary E. Lease: Populist firebrand

The Agrarian Revolt **515**

tried to unite farmers of the South who were divided by racial barriers, and some of the whites and blacks worked hard at the effort. Finally, the Populists sought to create an alliance between farmers and labor. The Populists enjoyed some success with all four of these alliances, but sectional animosities were kept alive by the bloody-shirt issue, old party loyalties were hard to break, racial antagonism was inflamed by white-supremacy propaganda, and farmers did not always see eye to eye with the laborers particularly on currency inflation. In view of all these handicaps the Populists made a surprisingly good showing in their first appearance at the polls. They cast a little more than a million votes for their presidential candidate and also elected ten representatives, five senators, three governors, and some fifteen hundred members of state legislatures. But it was obvious that they had a long way to go to establish a real national base for their movement.

The Depression and the Silver Issue

Cleveland and the silverites. The Democrats and the Republicans conducted their 1892 campaigns with more sobriety than usual. Cleveland, the choice of conservative Democrats, was nominated by the first ballot of his party's convention, and, in spite of efforts to draft an ailing Blaine, Harrison was the nominee of the Republicans. Adlai E. Stevenson* of Illinois became Cleveland's running mate, and Whitelaw Reid, editor of the New York *Tribune*, was the Republican nominee for Vice President. Cleveland improved his poll of 1888, and 1884 as well, winning 5,555,426 votes to 5,182,690 for Harrison, and 277 electoral votes to Harrison's 145. The Democrats carried not only the doubtful states of New York, New Jersey, Connecticut, and Indiana but the normally Republican states of Illinois, Wisconsin, and California. It was not quite a landslide, but it was the most decisive victory either party had won in twenty years.

President Cleveland moved back into the White House and surrounded himself with a thoroughly conservative Cabinet of Easterners and Southerners who were as completely out of touch with the radical discontent of the country as he himself. Almost immediately the financial panic of 1893 shattered his peace and ushered in the worst depression the nation had experienced up to that time. The panic had actually started ten days before Harrison left office, when

*Grandfather of the Democratic candidate for President in 1952 and 1956.

the Philadelphia & Reading Railroad went bankrupt and the New York Stock Exchange was shaken by the greatest selling spree in its history. Two months after Cleveland's inauguration the market collapsed. Banks called in their loans, and credit dried up. Unstable financial conditions abroad, especially the failure of Baring Brothers of London in 1890, had started a drain on the gold reserve that became increasingly severe after 1893. One great railroad after another—the Erie, the Northern Pacific, the Union Pacific, the Santa Fe—went down in failure. "Mills, factories, furnaces, mines nearly everywhere," reported the New York *Commercial and Financial Chronicle* in August, "shut down in large numbers, and commerce and enterprise were arrested in an extraordinary degree." By the end of the year five hundred banks and more than fifteen thousand business firms had fallen into bankruptcy. Populist Donnelly's apocalyptic picture in 1892 of "a nation brought to the verge of ruin" seemed about to be translated into reality.

Learned economists still argue about the causes and remedies of depressions, and there can be no doubt that the causes of the depression that settled over the country in 1893 were highly complex. But President Cleveland had a simple explanation and a remedy, and never did a dogmatist cling more tenaciously to his theory, or refuse more stubbornly to compromise with opponents in his own party. His explanation was that the Sherman Silver Purchase Act (see p. 510) had caused the depression, and his remedy was to repeal the act and maintain the gold standard at all costs—that is, continue to redeem all United States Treasury notes in gold. The economic consequences of Cleveland's remedy do not appear to have been decisive one way or the other, but the political consequences were disastrous. No issue since slavery had divided the people more deeply than silver. It disrupted Populism, and caused a revolution in the Democratic party that overthrew conservative control.

The trouble was that Cleveland's theory clashed head on with a theory held with equal dogmatism by the silverites. According to them, the cause of the economic disaster lay in the "Crime of '73" that demonetized silver, and the remedy lay in the free and unlimited coinage of silver at a ratio of sixteen to one of gold. The arguments and the sources of support for the silver movement acquired new strength and additional recruits. The admission of six new Western states—Montana, North Dakota, South Dakota, and Washington in 1889 and Idaho and Wyoming in 1890—brought reinforcements to the silverites in Congress, especially in the Senate. In the meantime American silver-producers suffered additional reductions in their market from the demonetization of silver in Europe and India and became more desperate for relief through free coinage in the United States. At the same time debtor agrarians saw free coinage of silver as one hope of relief from deflation and currency contraction and increased their cry for "free silver." In place of the inadequate relief provided by the Sherman Silver Purchase Act, they demanded unlimited and free coinage.

Cleveland stubbornly insisted, on the other hand, that the Sherman Act was the cause of the trouble and demanded its repeal. The only way to restore confidence and prosperity, he held, was to maintain the gold standard, and that required the maintenance of a gold reserve of $100 million in the Treasury. There was a case to be made in favor of the gold standard in the 1890s, but there were many causes for the drain on the gold reserve, and there were many causes of the depression other than the threat to the gold standard. But under relentless pressure by the President, Congress finally repealed the Sherman Act. Cleveland got his way by relying on Republican support and splitting his own party.

Repeal of the Sherman Act seemed to have no effect, for the drain on the gold reserve continued unabated, and so did the depression. Business confidence was not restored, and the hoarding of gold increased. The Treasury surplus that the Billion Dollar Congress had been so eager to spend was no more. Holders of gold and silver certificates, doubting the ability of the government to maintain the gold standard, started a run on the Treasury; and panic in Europe caused continual withdrawals. The President resorted to a series of highly unpopular bond sales to recoup the gold reserves. The third bond sale, in February 1895, caused the greatest indignation of all. This time the President yielded to the demand of J. Pierpont Morgan that the sale be kept private, and the syndicate of bankers that handled the loan drove a hard bargain for their services and were accused of making large profits, though Morgan refused to reveal how much. The bond issue yielded over $65 million to the government, half of it from Europe, and the bankers scotched some of the drain on the gold reserve. Nevertheless, another issue was necessary in January 1896. The four bond sales did save the gold standard, but they did not stop the decline of the gold reserve or restore prosperity. Each one further intensified the silverites' hatred of the President. These bond sales enhanced Cleveland's reputation for courage but not for wisdom: they failed to cure the depression, and they led to political disaster.

The politics of depression. The blight that had been familiar to farmers for years now began to fall on the factory and the city. Railroad construction fell off drastically, dividends halted, and investment in all business declined sharply. Bankers, businessmen, and employers seemed stricken with a failure of nerve.

They laid off workers, cut wages, closed factory doors, and swelled the army of the jobless. Visitors to the "dream city" at the Chicago Exposition in 1893 wondered at the miles of sleeping men who lined the tracks of the elevated railway. "What a spectacle!" exclaimed Ray Stannard Baker, a cub reporter, "What a human downfall after the magnificence and prodigality of the World's Fair."

The year 1894 was the most brutal of the depression. Between 2½ and 3 million, perhaps as many as one out of five workers, were thought to be unemployed, but no one really knew, and the unemployed felt that no one in the government really cared. Some cities provided a little work relief, but this was wholly inadequate, and when hungry men turned to the federal government they were met with cold indifference or angry rejection. Jacob S. Coxey of Massillon, Ohio, a well-to-do businessman who was a Populist and was quite untypical of his class in other ways, proposed a plan of federal work relief on public roads to be financed by an issue of $500 million in legal-tender Treasury notes. The "good roads" bill was designed to end the depression by providing monetary inflation and internal improvements as well as work relief for the unemployed. When Congress refused to pass it, Coxey declared, "We will send a petition to Washington with boots on." "Coxey's Army" marched peacefully from Massillon to the Capitol, picking up sympathizers on the way, including a few visionaries and eccentrics, and paraded into Washington on May Day, about five hundred strong. They were cheered by crowds, but Coxey and his lieutenants were arrested by the police, and some fifty people were beaten or trampled. No fewer than seventeen "industrial armies" started for Washington in 1894, and some twelve hundred men arrived. They were peaceful and sober as a rule, but it was the obvious sympathy they stirred over the country that frightened the government, even President Cleveland, into the mistaken idea that a spirit of rebellion threatened to bring on mob rule.

Not only the government but private employers resorted to violence in countering labor protest. An extraordinary number of strikes, some fourteen hundred in all, occurred during 1894, many of them provoked by wage cuts. More than 660,000 people were thrown out of work by strikes or lockouts. Management countered by using violence, employing secret police, or securing injunctions from friendly courts. In the Pullman strike of July, as we have seen (p. 471), the federal government used troops of the regular army to crush the workers. Cleveland earned as much hostility from labor by his use of troops as he had from agrarians by his sale of bonds.

In the meantime, the only serious piece of reform the second Cleveland Administration undertook was the reform of the tariff. To fulfill their campaign

The Supreme Court and the income tax: the government's argument

Richard Olney

Richard Olney:

The constitutional objection [is] nothing but a call upon the judicial department of the government to supplant the political in the exercise of the taxing power; to substitute its discretion for that of Congress.... It is inevitably predestined to failure unless this court shall, for the first time in its history, overlook and overstep the bounds which separate the judicial from the legislative power—bounds, the scrupulous observance of which it has so often declared to be absolutely essential to the integrity of our constitutional system of government.

James C. Carter:

Nothing could be more unwise and dangerous—nothing more foreign to the spirit of the Constitution—than an attempt to baffle and defeat a popular determination by a judgment in a lawsuit. When the opposing forces of sixty millions of people have become arrayed in hostile political ranks upon a question which all men feel is not a question of law, but of legislation, the only path of safety is to accept the voice of the majority as final.

From Pollock v. Farmers' Loan and Trust Co., 157 U.S. 429, 1895.

pledges, the Democrats did put through the House a bill, framed by William L. Wilson of West Virginia, containing modest reductions in the tariff. But in the Senate the protectionists of both parties fell upon it with six hundred amendments that restored many of the old rates. The Wilson-Gorman Act, which Cleveland allowed to become law without his signature, did not fulfill the Administration's promises of tariff reform. The only sop to reformers was an amendment, slipped in by the agrarians and deplored by the President, that provided for a small income tax of 2 percent on incomes over $4,000. The Supreme Court, which shared Cleveland's unpopularity as an agency of reaction, promptly declared the income tax unconstitutional by a vote of five to four. For relief of suffering among the unemployed, on the farms, and in the cities, for restoring credit, and for assisting industry afflicted by depression, Cleveland's Administration refused to take any responsibility beyond maintaining the gold standard.

In the fall campaigns of 1894, the Republicans capitalized on the spirit of despair over the depression. They identified their party with prosperity and recovery through the Republican program of tariff and sound currency. This time they avoided the cultural and religious issues that had hurt them in 1892 and appealed effectively to the industrialized Northeast and the developing Midwest. Governor William McKinley of Ohio proved the hero of the Republican campaign. The elections of 1894 were a triumph for Republicans, who recouped their losses of the previous election and took control of the House with a majority of 140 seats. Many prominent Democrats

went down to defeat. In twenty-four states no Democrat at all won national office and only one each in six others. New York, Illinois, and Wisconsin returned to the Republican fold and so did most of the Plains states where Populism had taken hold. Populists increased the vote they polled in 1892 by 42 percent but were disappointed in the results and suffered losses in offices held. In all, the elections of 1894 brought about the largest congressional gains and one of the most widespread political realignments in the nation's history. It was this election and not that of 1896 that marked the fall of the Democrats and the beginning of the long Republican ascendancy.

The Democratic party was, in fact, in the midst of a revolution almost as profound as that of 1860, when North and South wings split into two parties. Again it was a sectional split, but this time it was the Northeast Democrats who were isolated instead of the Southern. West and South joined hands in the name of the free coinage of silver, but silver merely served as a symbol for dozens of other sectional issues. And Grover Cleveland became the personification of the Northeastern conservatism against which the two agrarian regions were in revolt. Never since Andrew Johnson had a President been so detested and abused by members of his own party as was Cleveland.

Early in 1895 prominent Democrats in the South and West set to work systematically to use the silver issue as a means of taking over control of their party and unseating Cleveland and the conservatives. With financial support from the silver-miners, they held silver conventions all over the South and West to which they invited Populists and urged them to give

The Supreme Court and the income tax: the argument that prevailed

Joseph H. Choate

up their more radical demands and "come down to silver." They distributed great quantities of silver propaganda, such as Ignatius Donnelly's *The American People's Money* (1895) and the famous booklet by William H. "Coin" Harvey, *Coin's Financial School* (1894). In the latter, "Professor Coin" laid bare the "conspiracy of Goldbugs," proponents of the gold standard, and "proved" that the free and unlimited coinage of silver was the panacea for all economic ills. The work of the silver Democrats against Cleveland was so effective that after the state conventions in the summer of 1896 no state Democratic organization south of the Potomac and only three west of the Alleghenies remained in the hands of the President's friends. There was no longer any doubt that the silverites would be able to wrest control of the national Democratic convention from Cleveland.

McKinley and gold versus Bryan and silver.

Nor was there any doubt that the Republican convention would nominate William McKinley of Ohio when it met at St. Louis in June. McKinley's nomination had been assured not only by his popularity but by the systematic and patient work of his devoted friend Marcus Alonzo Hanna, who retired from business in 1895 to devote full time to fulfilling his ambition of putting McKinley in the White House. McKinley's nomination rolled forward as planned on the first ballot, and Garret A. Hobart, a relatively unknown corporation lawyer from New Jersey, balanced the ticket with an Easterner. A protectionist platform

was obviously called for, since McKinley's name had become synonymous with high tariff. McKinley was for the gold standard, but held open the possibility of an international bimetallic agreement. The only doubt was how explicit the plank on the gold standard should be. Hanna had already decided upon a forthright endorsement, but he cleverly hung back at the convention and permitted himself to be "persuaded" by Eastern delegates to accept the statement that "the existing gold standard should be preserved." Upon the adoption of the gold plank, Senator Henry M. Teller of Colorado led a small group of Western silver Republicans from the hall, and they withdrew from the party.

Eastern Republicans had reason to doubt McKinley's firmness on gold. In the political lingo of the battle of standards, politicians were classified as "Goldbugs," "Silverbugs," or "Straddlebugs," and the Ohioan was often classed with the third group. He had voted for both the Bland-Allison Act and the Sherman Silver Purchase Act, was a moderate on silver, and held out hopes for international bimetalism. In 1896, however, he accepted his party's decision for gold. He was an experienced and skillful politician who had served in Congress from 1876 to 1891, with the exception of one term, and had been governor of Ohio for two terms, completing the second in 1895. A kindly, impressive-looking man, McKinley had won his place of national political prominence on his own and acquired a mass following. The campaign caricature of McKinley as the spineless puppet of the millionaire boss had no foundation in fact, for the evidence is that Hanna constantly deferred to his friend and respected his wishes.

The Democratic convention at Chicago exhibited more disorder and spontaneity that the Republicans had endured at St. Louis. Cleveland-supporters, still full of fight, arrived from the East to clash with red-hot silver orators from the South and the West amid a din of hisses and catcalls and rebel yells in which only the leather-lunged could make themselves heard. But the Easterners had neither the strength to control the convention nor a suitable candidate to put before it, and the agrarian rebels rode over them roughshod. They adopted a platform strongly influenced by Governor John P. Altgeld of Illinois, the friend of the Pullman strikers and the pardoner of the Haymarket-riot anarchists. The platform, which denounced virtually everything Cleveland stood for, also struck out fiercely at the protective tariff, the national banks, trusts, and the Supreme Court; it demanded an income tax and, most important of all, free coinage of silver at the ratio of sixteen ounces of silver to one of gold.

Altgeld was disqualified as a candidate by foreign birth, and the convention had passed over Congressman Richard P. "Silver Dick" Bland, the most prominent contender. At a strategic moment of the platform debate a handsome young ex-congressman, William Jennings Bryan of Nebraska, captured the attention and the imagination of the silver forces with a speech that mounted to a thrilling peroration: "You shall not press down upon the brow of labor this crown of thorns, you shall not crucify mankind upon a cross of gold." Bryan was nominated on the fifth ballot, and, to balance the ticket, Arthur Sewall of Maine, a banker and businessman who opposed the gold standard, was nominated for Vice President.

While he was only thirty-six and little known in the East, Bryan was already widely known as a peerless orator in the West and the South, where he had been campaigning for three years to prepare the revolt of the silver forces. Bryan had some naive ideas about money and harbored suspicions of the East, "the enemy's country," as he once called it. He was no radical, and his ties were with the simple agrarian past rather than with the complex future. But conservatives were wrong to dismiss him as a one-idea fanatic. He had an intuitive grasp of the deep mood of protest that stirred the West and South, and he expressed that mood in a moral appeal to the conscience of the country. His real service was to awaken an old faith in social justice and to protest against a generation of plutocratic rule.

In their next maneuver, the silver-leaders of the "revolutionized" Democrats persuaded the Populist party, which held its convention in St. Louis after the Democratic convention had met, to make Bryan its candidate as well. The proposal deeply divided the Populists, who neither wanted to split the reform forces with a separate ticket nor give up their own party identity. Western Populists were eager to nominate Bryan, but Southern members, less devoted to

William Jennings Bryan: an old faith in social justice

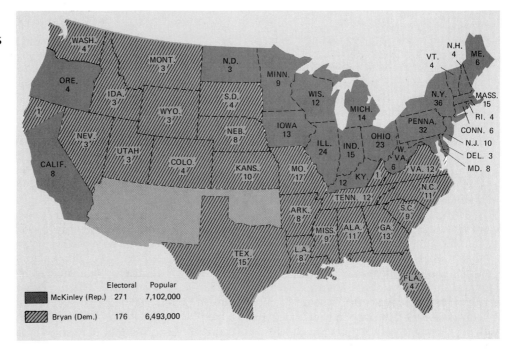

The election of 1896

	Electoral	Popular
McKinley (Rep.)	271	7,102,000
Bryan (Dem.)	176	6,493,000

silver, wanted a separate Populist ticket and no compromise. Bryan's nomination was at last secured when Senator William V. Allen of Nebraska, chairman of the convention, told the Southerners that the Democrats had agreed to withdraw Sewall and accept Thomas E. Watson as their vice-presidential nominee if the Populists would nominate Bryan. Southern radicals bitterly resisted fusion with the Democrats, whom they had been fighting for four years. But when their hero Watson agreed to compromise, they reluctantly consented and nominated Bryan and Watson. Only later did they learn that the Democrats refused to withdraw the banker Sewall.

Two more parties were created out of bolters from the old parties. The National Silver Republicans endorsed the Democratic candidates. Later on, the gold Democrats, with encouragement and financial support from Hanna, organized the National Democratic party and nominated a separate ticket that was intended to contribute to Bryan's defeat.

The contest between McKinley and Bryan in 1896 has taken on the legendary character of the combat between Goliath and David—except that it turned out quite differently. Bryan played the David role admirably—the lone youth armed with nothing but shafts of oratory pitted against the armored Gold Giant and all his hosts. Actually, reformers of many schools rallied to Bryan's cause, including Henry George of the Single-Taxers, Edward Bellamy of the Nationalists, W. D. P. Bliss of the Christian Socialists, and Eugene V. Debs of the Railway Union, all of whom campaigned for him. Samuel Gompers of the AFL endorsed silver but not Bryan. Bryan's chief

reliance, however, was upon his own voice. In a campaign without precedent at that time, he traveled eighteen thousand miles by train, made more than six hundred speeches, and talked to some 3 million people. He spoke not only of silver but of the price of crops, the cost of mortgages, the need for credit, and the regulation of railroads. The powerful popular

William McKinley, 1896: front porch in Canton

response to his campaign aroused great hopes for victory.

It also aroused a hysterical wave of fear among conservatives and facilitated Hanna's collection of campaign funds. He exacted tribute from every great trust, railroad, and bank with any stake in the outcome and built up a treasure chest of at least $3.5 million—as against a mere $300,000 at Bryan's disposal. Hanna spent the money lavishly but shrewdly, sending out propaganda by the ton and the carload and speakers by the battalion. He also transported trainloads of people, some 750,000 in all, from representative groups, all expenses paid, to hear McKinley read well-prepared speeches from his front porch in Canton, Ohio. From there McKinley set the tone and directed the strategy of his campaign. The press assisted Hanna with blasts of ridicule and charges of socialism and anarchism against Bryan. The Philadelphia *Press* described the "Jacobins" of the Chicago convention as "hideous and repulsive vipers." President Cleveland called them "madmen" and "criminals," and the New York *Tribune* referred to Bryan as a "wretched, rattle-pated boy."

The combination was too much for the resources of Bryan. He polled 6,492,559 votes, more votes than any victorious candidate had ever polled before, nearly a million more than Cleveland polled in 1892, but it was still not enough. McKinley won with 7,102,246 votes, a plurality of 609,687, and an electoral vote of 271 to 176. Bryan did not carry a single state north of the Potomac or east of the Mississippi above its juncture with the Ohio. He did not even carry the farming states of Iowa, Minnesota, and North Dakota. What is more significant, he carried no industrialized, no urbanized state. This may well be the main reason for Bryan's defeat. In spite of widespread unrest among labor, Bryan did not win labor's support, which might have given him victory. He really had little to offer either labor or the cities. He was the first Democratic candidate to lose New York City since 1848, and the largest city to give him a plurality was Troy, New York. Like many other American reformers of his day, he had something of significance for the present, but his true ties were the past. McKinley and Hanna may not have been looking very far into the future, but they clearly had a firmer grip on the present. They also had an appeal for labor, and they evidently won the confidence of the urban middle class. Their victory at the polls meant more conservatism and yet another businessman's regime.

The aftermath of '96. The election was followed by a brief revival of the economy and three years later by the end of the long depression. The upturn had little if anything to do with the saving of the gold standard or the victory of McKinley. The price of wheat had started to climb before the election, though hardly enough to have influenced the outcome. But in 1897 the European wheat crop fell off 30 percent, and American farmers doubled their exports of the previous year. Prices continued to rise, and the whole economy began to revive. Discoveries of gold in Australia and Alaska revived the flow of gold into the country, and gold production was further increased by discoveries of pay dirt in South Africa and the development of the cyanide process for extracting the metal from ore. The inflation that the agrarians and silverites had demanded came, ironically enough, not through silver but through gold. The influx of gold and capital stimulated industrial expansion, and that in turn touched off a boom in iron and steel.

With a Republican majority in both houses, McKinley called a special session of Congress in the spring of 1897. The Wilson-Gorman Tariff of 1894 was already high enough for most protectionists, but Congress passed a bill framed by Nelson Dingley of Maine, which raised duties to an average of 52 percent and included reciprocal trade provisions. Lacking a Senate majority for a gold standard until after the 1898 election, McKinley avoided action until gold was flowing in and silver sentiment was waning. But in his annual message of 1899 he called for legislation, and Congress adopted by a party vote the Gold Standard Act, which he signed on March 14, 1900. The act declared that the gold dollar was henceforth the sole standard of currency, thus writing an end to a generation of controversy, but without producing any significant economic effect, either good or bad.

One significant but often overlooked result of the election of 1896 and the return to prosperity was the demoralization of the Populist movement. Fusion with the enemy party and abandonment of principle for the sake of silver had demoralized the Populists and all but destroyed their party. "The sentiment is still there, the votes are still there, but confidence is gone," thought Tom Watson. The following decade was to see a new upsurge of reform, but it was achieved under urban, not rural, leadership. Nineteenth-century agrarian radicalism made its last significant bid for leadership of a national reform movement in 1896.

Suggestions for Reading   The political history of this period is treated by H. W. Morgan, *From Hayes to McKinley: National Party Politics, 1877–1896* (1969), Morton Keller, *Affairs of State: Public Life in Late Nineteenth Century America* (1977), and by R. O. Marcus, *Grand Old Party: Political Structure in the Gilded Age, 1880–1896* (1971). A revisionary estimate of politicians is D. J. Rothman, *Politics and Power: The United States Senate, 1869–1901* (1966). On the nineties, see H. U. Faulkner, *Politics, Reform and Expansion, 1890–1900* (1959), and L. P. Beth, *The Development of the American Constitution, 1877–*

1901 (1971). Richard Hofstadter, *The Age of Reform: From Bryan to F. D. R.* (1955), takes a dim view of Populism, and R. Hal Williams, *Years of Decision: American Politics in the 1890s** (1978), is generous to the Republican party. Paul Kleppner, *The Cross of Culture: A Social Analysis of Midwestern Politics, 1850–1900* (1970) and *The Third Electoral System, 1853–1892: Parties, Voters, and Political Cultures* (1979); R. J. Jensen, *The Winning of the Midwest: Social and Political Conflict, 1888–1896* (1971), emphasize cultural politics.

Key biographies are Harry Barnard, *Rutherford B. Hayes and His America* (1954); Allan Peskin, *Garfield, a Biography* (1978); T. C. Reeves, *Gentleman Boss: The Life of Chester Alan Arthur* (1975); D. S. Muzzey, *James G. Blaine: A Political Idol of Other Days* (1934); Allan Nevins, *Grover Cleveland: A Study in Courage* (1933); H. J. Sievers, *Benjamin Harrison: Hoosier Statesman* (1959); and R. E. Welch, Jr., *George Frisbie Hoar and the Half-Breed Republicans* (1971). (On Bryan and McKinley, see below.) See also J. G. Sproat, *The Best Men: Liberal Reformers in the Gilded Age** (1968).

On the politics and issues of reform see Gerald McFarland, *Mugwumps, Morals and Politics, 1884–1920* (1975), and Robert Kelley, *The Transatlantic Persuasion: The Liberal-Democratic Mind in the Age of Gladstone* (1969). Ray Ginger, *Age of Excess** (1965), is an interpretive study. Civil-service reform is the subject of three excellent works: L. D. White, *The Republican Era: 1896–1901* (1958); P. P. Van Riper, *History of the United States Civil Service* (1958); and Ari Hogenboom, *Outlawing the Spoils* (1961). Pensions for veterans are treated by M. R. Dearing, *Veterans in Politics: The Story of the G. A. R.* (1952). Monetary controversies of the period are examined in Milton Friedman and A. J. Schwartz, *A Monetary History of the United States, 1867–1960** (1963); Irwin Unger, *The Greenback Era: A Social and Political History of American Finance, 1865–1879* (1964); W. T. K. Nugent, *Money and American Society, 1865–1880* (1968); and Allen Weinstein, *Prelude to Populism: Origins of the Silver Issue, 1867–1878* (1970).

A challenging book on Populism is Lawrence Goodwyn, *Democratic Promise: The Populist Movement in America* (1976). Agricultural conditions and movements are authoritatively examined in F. A. Shannon, *The Farmer's Last Frontier: Agriculture, 1860–1897** (1945). For light on farmers' organizations, see J. D. Hicks, *The Populist Revolt** (1931); Norman Pollack, *The Populist Response to Industrial America** (1962); W. T. K. Nugent, *The Tolerant Populists: Kansas Populism and Nativism* (1963); and Theodore Saloutos, *Farmer Movements in the South, 1865–1933* (1960). A suggestive survey is C. C. Taylor, *The Farmers' Movement, 1620–1920* (1953).

The depression of the nineties and its political repercussions are intelligently discussed in S. T. McSeveney, *The Politics of Depression: Political Behavior in the Northeast, 1893–1896* (1972); J. E. Wright, *The Politics of Populism: Dissent in Colorado* (1974); and P. H. Argersinger, *Populism and Politics: William Alfred Peffer and the People's Party* (1974); and economic causes of the trouble in F. B. Webeg, *The Background of the Panic of 1893* (1929). The serious student will be fascinated by source materials in Hamlin Garland, *Main-travelled Roads** (1891), for agrarian ills; W. H. Harvey, *Coin's Financial School** (1894), and Ignatius Donnelly, *The American People's Money* (1895), for silver propaganda; and H. D. Lloyd, *Wealth Against Commonwealth** (1894), for an exposure of monopoly. Scholarly studies of labor protest are D. L. McMurry, *Coxey's Army** (1929), and Almont Lindsey, *The Pullman Strike** (1943). On the latter event, see also Harry Barnard, *"Eagle Forgotten": The Life of John Peter Altgeld** (1938), and Ray Ginger, *Altgeld's America—The Lincoln Ideal Versus Changing Realities** (1958).

On the crisis of 1896, many books already mentioned are relevant. In addition, see Stanley Jones, *The Presidential Election of 1896* (1964); J. R. Hollingsworth, *The Whirligig of Politics: The Democracy of Cleveland and Bryan* (1963); and P. W. Glad, *McKinley, Bryan, and the People* (1964). The best biographies are H. W. Morgan, *William McKinley and His America* (1963); Lewis Gould, *The Presidency of William McKinley* (1980); and P. E. Coletta, *William Jennings Bryan, Political Evangelist, 1860–1908* (1964) Vol. I of three. Bryan's own account, *The First Battle* (1897), is worth consulting. Still the best book on McKinley's great friend is Herbert Croly, *Marcus Alonzo Hanna* (1912). Agrarian leaders prominent in 1896 are pictured in C. V. Woodward, *Tom Watson: Agrarian Rebel** (1938), and F. B. Simkins, *Pitchfork Ben Tillman: South Carolinian** (1944).

*Available in a paperback edition.

21
EMPIRE BEYOND THE SEAS

The United States was not born in isolation, nor with any bias against expansionism. On the contrary, the long colonial experience was lived out in the midst of international rivalries. Independence itself was painfully won and precariously defended by taking shrewd advantage of those rivalries. Expansionism was a fundamental policy in the new nation's negotiations with foreign powers. Louisiana, Florida, Texas, New Mexico, California, Oregon, the Gadsden Purchase, and the Alaska Purchase—in fact the acquisition of all the continental area of the country beyond the original colonies—are dramatic evidence of expansionism, vigorously and steadily pursued.

After about a century, ending in 1867 with the purchase of Alaska, the nation lapsed into what might almost be called isolationism, though a better term would probably be withdrawal, or preoccupation. At any rate, the United States called a halt to territorial expansion for a quarter of a century or more. Then suddenly expansionism reawakened in a new form—overseas expansion—and concern over foreign affairs revived. A war with Spain, though not itself prompted by expansionism, actually brought overseas possessions, colonies, millions of colonial subjects, protectorates—a whole empire. A republic became an empire, a country long preoccupied with internal affairs turned its attention outward. One phase of isolationism ended, and with it one phase of American innocence.

Withdrawal and Return

The period of withdrawal. The United States' withdrawal from world affairs was not due to any lack of advocates of aggressiveness. William H. Seward, Secretary of State under Lincoln and Johnson, proposed, among other things, intervention in Korea, acquisition of the Hawaiian Islands, and adventures in the Caribbean. He could muster no support for these undertakings, however, and only with difficulty persuaded Congress to accept the Alaska bargain offered by Russia. Moved by scheming friends, President Grant devised a treaty for the annexation of Santo Domingo, though the Senate rejected it in 1870. Other expansionists agitated in vain for the annexation of Canada, for intervention in the Cuban rebellion in 1868–78, for securing a naval station in Samoa in the seventies, and for grabbing naval harbors in Haiti during the eighties. The standard arguments against such schemes were that it was against American principles to govern without the consent of the governed, that we should abstain from foreign entanglements, avoid large naval commitments and expenditures, and refrain from absorbing peoples of alien race and tradition. One name for this policy was "continentalism"—the idea that the nation should acquire no territory outside its continental limits.

Preoccupation with domestic concerns did not blind Americans entirely to opportunities and temp-

524

Americans in Peking

At last! *A determined effort to break England's hold on the commerce of the world, and give
America a chance*

tations abroad. The Administrations of Garfield and Arthur sought to advance limited and overlapping goals of prestige, markets, and security, especially in the Caribbean and Central America. Reciprocal trade agreements with countries of these areas were made with a view to exerting economic influence over approaches to the proposed isthmian canal region. Arthur's Secretary of State, Frederick T. Frelinghuysen, pointed out that this would confer "upon us and upon them [Puerto Rico and Cuba] all the benefits which would result from annexation were that possible." Less typical of that period, but suggesting expansionist impulses to come, were the negotiation of a treaty with Korea in 1882 opening up that country to the non-Asian world, and the United States participation in the Berlin Conference of European powers on trade rights in the Congo in 1884–85.

The fact remains, however, that Americans in the seventies and eighties were mainly preoccupied with their built-in empire of the West and their economic colonialism in the South, absorbed in political and economic problems of a domestic character, largely content to stay at home. When Cleveland became President in 1885 the State Department had only sixty employees, including clerks. Secretaries of State were usually political appointees with little knowledge of foreign affairs. Until the 1880s the United States navy was an obsolete and antiquated collection of wooden ships that provoked foreign ridicule. The American merchant marine had virtually disappeared from the seas, and the army was reduced to a handful of Indian-fighters. America still enjoyed—complacently took for granted—nature's marvelous boon of security, which was not only effective but relatively free. Wide oceans, weak neighbors, and rivalries that kept

its potential enemies divided accounted for this blessing of free security. No other great nation enjoyed it. When foreign policy disputes flared up in America during this period, the heat they generated was greatly intensified by the sudden expansion of the tiny circle normally involved to include an uninformed and excitable public in times of crisis. This plus the old habit of relying upon free security help explain the tendency of the United States to engage in heated disputes with foreign powers in which its threats and boasts were out of all proportion to its military strength.

Some of these disputes were with Great Britain, then the mightiest power in the world, and any such dispute was likely to become a game between the major political parties. The game was to see who could "twist the lion's tail" the harder and who could thereby curry the most favor with the Irish and other anti-British elements. One of the disputes during Cleveland's first Administration was merely a renewal of the perennial bickering over fishing rights along the coasts of British North America. Off the western shores of the continent the United States and Canada were simultaneously embroiled in another dispute— this one over the fur-seal industry in and out of the Bering Sea. The United States advanced an arrogant claim to exclusive jurisdiction over the Bering Sea with the contention that the seals were domestic animals that had wandered out of bounds. The American position was in obvious conflict with the traditional policy of "freedom of the seas." A court of arbitration rejected the American claims and prescribed regulations for the industry that were put into effect by both governments.

The only other embroilment to ruffle the relatively calm waters of foreign affairs during Cleveland's first Administration occurred in the Samoan Islands of the remote South Pacific. The splendid harbor of Pago Pago on Tutuila Island had stirred the interest of naval officers of the United States and other countries. In 1878, after rejecting the proposal of annexation or guardianship made by a Samoan chieftain, the Hayes Administration negotiated a treaty granting the United States the right to establish a naval station at Pago Pago. Germany and Great Britain secured similar treaties the following year, granting them naval-station rights in the same harbor and elsewhere. Competition among the traders of these three nations, and the intrigues of their consuls with rival native chieftains, precipitated a tropical squall of international temper in the mid-eighties. Alarmed by the threat of bloodshed, Cleveland called a conference among the three powers that met in Washington in the summer of 1887 but accomplished nothing. Conditions grew worse when Germany set up a new regime in the islands, and seven warships anchored at Samoa prepared for hostilities. A sudden storm of hurricane force in Apia Harbor brought peace unexpectedly by sinking all but one of the warships on March 15, 1889, less than two weeks after Cleveland's term ended. Harrison's Administration worked out a tripartite protectorate of the islands with Germany and Great Britain.

In spite of all these flurries and alarms, little had happened down to 1889 to divert Cleveland from his determination, announced in his first annual message to Congress in 1885, to adhere to "the tenets of a line of precedents from Washington's day, which proscribe entangling alliances," and to oppose "acquisition of new and distant territory or the incorporation of remote interests with our own." Yet the old tradition of isolation, abstention, and withdrawal was near its end, for America was now about to plunge into world affairs and abandon its tradition of "continentalism."

Manifest Destiny, new style. Historians have long had difficulties in agreeing over the nature and causes of this momentous change. Some have seen it as a more or less temporary "aberration" induced in large part by chance and coincidence and inspired by humanitarian impulse. Another historian contends that overseas expansion was simply an ongoing extension of continental imperialism. Still another has stressed popular psychological frustration brought on by social and economic crises of the nineties that found release in the aggressiveness of war and overseas adventures. Sensational journalism has been credited with stirring mass hysteria to an uncontrollable pitch. The discussion at times recalls the claim that the British Empire was founded in a fit of absent-mindedness. The fact remains that by the end of the century the United States found itself with colonial possessions on opposite sides of the globe and new military commitments in Asia. Something of importance had happened to American history that is linked to more than chance and passing moods.

It is best to avoid simplification, for numerous interests were involved and many causes were at work. To point out that some of these have been over-emphasized is not to deny that they were contributory. Among influences probably exaggerated was the idea of social Darwinism propagated by the English sociologist Herbert Spencer and spread by American disciples. Darwinism might best be thought of as a rationalization of the new style of Manifest Destiny rather than its inspiration. The same could be said of various theories of racial superiority and inferiority, some of which had been around a long time. Of growing popularity among the elite was a cult of Anglo-Saxon superiority with the concept of a breed endowed by nature to rule, an idea of obvious usefulness to white Americans who looked to England as a model. Religiously inclined exponents of racial superiority believed it had a divine sanction. One of these was Josiah Strong, who declared in his popular book *Our Country* (1885) that the Anglo-Saxon was "divinely commissioned to be, in a peculiar sense, his brother's keeper." Of more importance than this book in turning America toward expansionist sentiment were Protestant missions established abroad. These increased fivefold in the last thirty years of the century, and in the last decade the number of missionaries in China doubled to more than a thousand. The Protestant missionaries were the first converts to the new definition of the American mission, which was that the republic was destined not merely to serve passively as a model to less fortunate countries but to spread the national example abroad.

Such a mission could hardly be accomplished with an antiquated navy. Surely one explanation for the decision of Americans to plunge into overseas expansion is that they acquired the physical means to do so in the shape of a modern navy. In 1883 Congress authorized construction of three cruisers and in 1886 two battleships, the *Maine* and the *Texas*. This construction was still guided by the concept of the navy as a defensive force, but the Naval Act of 1890, which authorized the building of three more battleships, the *Indiana*, the *Massachusetts*, and the *Oregon*, all heavier and more powerful ships, announced the government's intention to have a navy that could meet a potential enemy anywhere on the high seas. Before the end of the century the United States had moved from twelfth to third place among naval powers. Thereafter the big-navy advocates began to reap the cumulative benefits of an expanding fleet: new bases and coaling stations, an even larger navy to protect the additional bases, and more bases to accommodate the larger navy.

The foremost exponent of navalism in his time was a historian, Captain Alfred T. Mahan, author of *The Influence of Sea Power upon History* (published in 1890 but delivered as lectures at the new Naval War College in 1886) and *The Interest of America in Sea Power* (1897). "Whether they will or no," wrote Mahan in 1890, "Americans must now begin to look outward." He advocated a program of mercantile imperialism that included building up foreign markets, expanding the merchant marine, constructing a navy to protect it, and acquiring overseas bases for the navy. His writings were rather more of a reflection than a cause of events, but his influence was felt in shaping naval policy in Washington and his ideas were seized upon by an elite group earnestly promoting what they called "the large policy" of expansionism. Including Theodore Roosevelt and Henry Cabot Lodge, as well as Captain Mahan, this group has been portrayed as a powerful, influential cabal.

The larger picture, however, would take into account the arrival of a new generation and a new world scene. The central experience of the previous generation had been the Civil War. They had had their fill of war and humanitarian crusades. They were not interested in Grant's efforts to take Santo Domingo, or in Spain's suppression of Cubans in the 1870s. The new men of the nineties, lacking such experience, looked out on a world teeming with imperialist adventures of other nations. European powers were carving up Africa and Asia, snatching island kingdoms in the Pacific, and looking for opportunities in the western hemisphere. The predatory powers moved in on the crumbling dynasty of China from bases already established in Asia: the French from Indochina, the British along the Yangtze Valley, and the Russians from Siberian possessions. Japan felt cheated when, after its victory over China in 1894–95, it received only Formosa (now called Taiwan) as booty. Americans began to wonder if they were not falling behind the times and whether they would ever be able to protect their interests and markets if they did not enter, even belatedly, into the imperialist adventure and "take up the white man's burden" along with the rewards and plunder that went with it. Some, including Theodore Roosevelt, believed that foreign adventures might divert angry farmers and workers as well as a distraught nation from preoccupation with economic ills.

Economic interpretations of American expansionism have provoked the most controversy, and emphasis on them has seesawed up and down. It has long been understood by historians that the depression of the nineties aroused concern over the need for foreign markets to absorb the surplus products of the American economy as well as the need for acquiring new markets to keep the wheels of industry turning or start them up again. Special interest in the China market had increased since 1895. For a generation or more historians gave economic motives primary emphasis. Then in the mid-1930s Professor Julius Pratt showed that most business leaders opposed intervention in Cuba and war with Spain for fear this would retard economic recovery that was under way in 1897. He did point out that once the war started business sentiment quickly and enthusiastically supported it. Further thoughts on this last point have led later historians to the reflection that the temporary timidity in the business community in 1897 and early 1898 have not eliminated economic motives from a satisfactory explanation of expansionism of the 1890s.

The New Diplomacy

American bellicosity. James G. Blaine, Secretary of State under Harrison, made the break with the old tradition. Blaine had served briefly in the same office eight years earlier under Garfield and revived the tradition of earlier Republican expansionism under Seward and Grant. Like them he also sought naval bases in Santo Domingo and Haiti, though with no more success. His followers expected him to pursue a "spirited policy" in keeping with his nickname of "Jingo* Jim." Actually Blaine exerted a moderating influence in several instances, including the settlement of the Samoan incident with Germany and Great Britain held over from the previous Administration. The three-power protectorate over the islands to which he agreed was, however, without precedent and constituted one of the first steps toward overseas expansion.

---

*The word was originated in England and popularized in America by a jingle printed in the Detroit *News* during the fisheries dispute with Great Britain and Canada:

> We do not want to fight
> But, by jingo, if we do
> We'll scoop in all the fishing grounds
> And the whole Dominion, too.

Closer to Blaine's interests was Latin America, especially the promotion of United States trade with sister republics, the obtaining of naval bases in the Caribbean, and the construction of an isthmian canal. Eight years earlier he had urged calling an international conference of the American republics, and the idea materialized when he became Secretary of State for the second time. Delegates arrived in the fall of 1889 and were treated to a six-thousand-mile barnstorming tour of the country, but when they settled down to consider Blaine's proposals on trade and arbitration treaties they could not agree. All they would accept was the setting up of an information center, which later became the Pan-American Union. More than a half-century was to pass before Pan-American conferences would finally accept the sort of agreements Blaine tried to effect in 1889.

In the early nineties a new martial spirit in America found expression in a succession of chauvinistic outbursts; "jingoism" it was called. Irresponsible talk of war with Italy occurred in American newspapers over the lynching of eleven prisoners of Italian origin, in March 1891, charged with murder in New Orleans. The dispute was settled by American payment of indemnity to the Italian government a year later. A much more serious outburst almost brought the United States to the point of war with Chile, a republic with not one-twentieth its population, but with a strong navy. In October 1891, when a party from the cruiser *Baltimore* went on shore leave in Valparaiso, a mob of Chileans killed two of the American sailors and injured seventeen others. President Harrison inserted a sword-rattling passage in his an-

"That's a live wire, gentlemen!"

nual message to Congress and followed this with another message to Congress virtually inviting it to declare war at a time when the apologies he had
demanded from Chile were hourly expected. Chile
fortunately capitulated with apologies and indemnities, and the war scare passed over.

The bellicose mood of the jingo editors and politicians did not pass over, however. Rather, it continued to mount during the nineties. "The number of
men and officials in this country who are now mad to
fight somebody is appalling," said the anti-imperialist
editor of the *Nation*, E. L. Godkin, in 1894. "Navy
officers dream of war and talk and lecture about it
incessantly. The Senate debates are filled with predictions of impending war and with talk of preparing for
it at once." The irresponsible warmongering of the
period was indeed appalling, though it should be remembered that nineteenth-century Americans knew
nothing of the total wars to come. They regarded the
Civil War as an exception and still thought of war as a
heroic affair filled with splendor and glory. It was an
illusion slow to die.

Even the antiexpansionist Cleveland was not
immune to the new spirit, as he showed in his handling of relations with Britain in the dispute over the
boundary between British Guiana and Venezuela. It
was an old dispute that went back into the colonial
history of Venezuela, but the discovery of gold in the
disputed territory, combined with a bit of Venezuelan
propaganda suggesting that British aggression was a
challenge to the Monroe Doctrine, stirred up the
Anglophobia and pugnacity of the jingo editors of the
United States. In 1895 Cleveland had his Secretary of
State, Richard Olney, demand that Great Britain conform to the Monroe Doctrine, as broadly interpreted,
by submitting the boundary dispute to arbitration.

Olney accompanied this demand with the truculent
assertion that the United States today "is practically
sovereign on this continent, and its fiat is law upon
the subjects to which it confines its interposition."
The tone of the note, coupled with his request for a
quick reply, gave it the flavor of an ultimatum.

The British foreign minister, Lord Salisbury, took
his time in replying, and when he did reply four
months later he repudiated Secretary Olney's interpretation of the Monroe Doctrine and flatly refused to
submit the dispute to arbitration. After receiving this
rebuff, Cleveland sent a special message to Congress
deploring "a supine submission to wrong and injustice
and the consequent loss of national self-respect."
Defusing the situation by delay, he asked that he be
authorized to appoint a commission to determine the
boundary and that the commission's decision be enforced at whatever cost. Privately he intended settlement by arbitration. Congress promptly complied, and
war sentiment mounted. "Let the fight come if it
must," wrote Theodore Roosevelt, who hoped to participate personally. "I rather hope that the fight will
come soon. The clamor of the peace faction has convinced me that this country needs a war." The risk
was altogether disproportionate to the American interest at stake, but it was not at all disproportionate to the
chauvinistic mood of the day. Fortunately Britain saw
fit to back down. Suddenly finding itself in trouble in
South Africa with no ally in Europe on which it could
count for support, Great Britain decided to court a
friend instead of making an enemy in the New World.
It switched to a conciliatory tone and signed a treaty
with Venezuela providing for arbitration, which
turned out to be mainly in its favor. The upshot of the
incident was to enhance American nationalist feeling,
but paradoxically it also ushered in an era of Anglo-
American understanding.

The Hawaiian question. When it came to expansion overseas, Cleveland clung consistently to traditional views and stood firm against the annexation of
Hawaii. American interest in these islands dated back
to the China trade in the late eighteenth century.
Traders were followed by American missionaries, who
converted the native Polynesians to Christianity in
the second quarter of the nineteenth century, and the
missionaries were followed by American sugar-growers. Efforts to annex the islands under President Pierce
and again under Secretary Seward failed, but in 1875 a
reciprocity treaty was signed opening a free market in
the United States to Hawaiian sugar-planters. Sugar
production in the islands multiplied tenfold in the
next twenty years in response to the free American
market. So dependent did the industry become on this
market, however, that when the McKinley Tariff of
1890 admitted other foreign sugar on the same terms

and subsidized domestic producers, the blow precipitated an economic crisis in the island kingdom and contributed to a political crisis.

King Kalakaua, the next to last of the reigning family, had been forced by the white business community in 1887 to accept a new constitution that curbed his power, made his ministers responsible to the legislature, and brought the legislature under control of the propertied classes. The dissolute old king was succeeded in 1891 by his sister Liliuokalani, who made it apparent that she was determined to overthrow the constitution her brother had accepted, shake off white control, and restore royal prerogatives. In January 1893 a committee of businessmen-revolutionaries demanded that she abdicate. Thereupon United States Minister John L. Stevens, an annexationist whom Blaine had picked for the office, requested that marines be sent ashore from the cruiser *Boston* and raise the American flag. The queen then capitulated, as she said, "to the superior force of the United States of America." A month later, on February 15, Harrison sent to the Senate a treaty annexing the islands. It might have gone through then and there had it not been for the declared preference of Cleveland, who was to begin his second Administration in a few days, that the matter be held over until his inauguration. As soon as he became President again he dispatched a special commissioner to investigate the situation in the islands. The commissioner's report convinced Cleveland that the great majority of the natives supported the queen. Cleveland therefore not only withheld the annexation treaty but insisted that it was his duty to restore "Queen Lil." The revolutionary provisional government refused to step down, however, and continued to rule, biding its time until a more imperialist-minded Administration came to power.

Cleveland's firm resistance to annexation, as compared with Harrison's receptive attitude, helped to make the question something of a party issue. The Republican platform of 1896 contained a plank favoring Hawaiian annexation, and though McKinley had previously shown no interest in the matter he was quickly won over after he became President in March 1897. Comparing him with Cleveland, commissioners from Hawaii reported that there was "the difference between daylight and darkness." On June 16, 1897, Secretary of State John Sherman signed a treaty of annexation and McKinley sent it to the Senate. Congress was strongly interested in Hawaii and alarmed by the interest Japan was manifesting in the islands, but the sentiment against overseas expansion was still too strong to be overcome, and the treaty languished for more than a year without action. Only in July 1898, after the war with Spain had opened the floodgates of expansionism, was Hawaii annexed.

War with Spain

The Cuban crisis. The expansionists and imperialists did not cause the war with Spain. They merely exploited it for their own purposes. The war itself grew out of deplorable conditions in Cuba that seemed intolerable to an aroused popular sentiment in the United States. Spanish misgovernment of the island had given rise to numerous revolts and a Ten Years' War, 1868–78, that brought little relief for Cuban ills. A new civil war broke out in February 1895. As in the case of the Hawaiian revolution, American tariff policy contributed to the uprising, for the tariff law of 1894, by imposing a duty on raw sugar, had added economic suffering to political discontent. Both the Cubans and the Spanish used savage methods. The Cubans systematically destroyed sugar mills, cane fields, and other property. Early in 1896 the Spanish commander, General Valeriano Weyler, resorted to the brutal policy of "reconcentration." This meant driving the entire population of large areas of Cuba—including women, children, and old people—into cities and towns fortified with barbed wire and under armed guard. Left without food or sanitation, the prisoners fell victim to famine and disease. Within two years more than two hundred thousand, or approximately one-eighth of the total population, were commonly believed to have been wiped out.

The American press exaggerated the Spanish atrocities, but the sufferings of the rebels were horrible enough in any case to arouse deep sympathies among Americans. The sufferings, moreover, were those of a neighbor, and they were incurred in a fight for independence from a manifestly unjust imperial ruler. Little more was required to whip up popular sympathy for the Cuban patriots and animus against Spain, especially in years when the public mind was as susceptible to jingoism as it had recently proved to be in far less serious disputes with Chile and Great Britain. Indications were abundant that influential Americans were "spoiling for a fight," and the Cuban junta that established itself in New York to dispense propaganda, solicit aid, and arouse sympathy was not without support. Those with long memories recalled that the United States had expressed great interest in Cuba since the early years of the century and since 1823 had implicitly regarded European control of the island as unnatural.

One strong ally of the interventionists was the "yellow press" of New York City. Led by William Randolph Hearst's New York *Journal* and Joseph Pulitzer's New York *World*, which were currently engaged in a war for circulation, the press sent a corps of reporters and artists to cover the Cuban conflict and supply the papers with vivid human-interest stories and pictures. The barbarities of the Spanish were played up and the atrocities of the Cubans glossed over, with the result that the newspaper coverage constituted powerful propaganda for the rebel cause. Waves of sympathy for the insurgents swept the country, but three years of sensationalism in the yellow press did not move the public to war with Spain.

American businessmen did not originally share the interventionist sentiment, though important segments of the business community became converts before the intervention. Protestant religious journals and both Republican and Democratic newspapers clamored loudly for intervention and war, though they insisted that they did so on purely humanitarian grounds and disclaimed any desire to annex Cuba or gain territory. Theirs was a moralistic aggression, with imperialism disavowed. Outright imperialists, including Roosevelt, Lodge, and Mahan, were also for war, but for the express purpose of conquest, expansion, and military glory. Two contrasting sets of aggressive impulses, both frustrated in the nineties, sought outlet in an idealistic crusade for Cuban freedom. One set embraced the impulses of protest and humanitarian reform; the other embraced the impulses of national self-expression, aggressiveness, and expansion. The convergence of these two groups in support of intervention in Cuba goes far toward explaining why Americans worked themselves up into a mood for war with Spain.

American intervention. When Grover Cleveland was President, he had opposed intervention in Cuba on every front. He had resisted pressure from Congress to accord the insurgents belligerent rights, had sought to suppress gun-running into Cuba from the States, and had tendered his good offices to Spain to settle the colonial war. In the summer of 1896, however, Cleveland underwent a change, and in his last annual message to Congress he came near to laying down a rationalization for America's intervention. McKinley tried to curb the jingoes and halt the drift to war, but a major concern of his was to maintain unity in a Republican party coalition divided over Cuban policy. Six months after he took office a satisfactory settlement seemed to be in the making. A change of government in Spain brought in a prime minister who recalled General Weyler and offered Cuba a considerable measure of self-government in local affairs. The offer proved unacceptable, however, since the Spanish in Cuba opposed rule by native Cubans and the insurgents refused to settle for anything short of complete independence. Further hopes for a peaceful solution were disrupted by a series of fateful incidents, or accidents, that brought relations between the United States and Spain to the breaking point.

The first incident was the publication on February 9, 1898, of a stolen private letter from the Spanish minister in Washington, Dupuy de Lôme, who indiscreetly described President McKinley as "weak and a bidder for the admiration of the crowd" and said that the Cuban rebels should be suppressed by force. The tone of the letter suggested that Spain was not negotiating seriously. Dupuy de Lôme resigned before his government had time to respond to Washington's inevitable request for his recall. Then, six days later, the battleship *Maine*, recently dispatched to protect American residents in Havana and appease jingoes at home, blew up in Havana harbor with a loss of two hundred sixty officers and enlisted men. The Spanish government hastened to offer condolence and propose a joint investigation. An investigation by American naval officers reported that the *Maine's* bottom plates had been thrust inward, indicating an external explosion, but the cause of the tragedy was never discovered. It is highly improbable that the Spanish government would have plotted such an act, but the jingo press held Spain guilty and raised the cry "Remember the Maine!" Before the report of the *Maine* explosion was completed, Congress unanimously voted a defense appropriation of $50 million, and on March 19 Senator Redfield Proctor of Vermont delivered a speech painting the shocking conditions he had found in Cuba during a recent unofficial visit. His calm tone, his reputation for moderation, and his matter-of-fact manner convinced many who had heretofore been skeptical of the lurid stories in the yellow press that action was indeed necessary.

On March 27 McKinley proposed to Spain a peaceful settlement in which it would abandon its reconcentration policy at once, grant an armistice until October 1, and enter into peace negotiations with the insurgents through his offices. He followed this proposal with a telegram apparently saying that independence would be the only satisfactory outcome of the peace negotiations. The American position was not stated with clarity. Spain was confronted with a cruel dilemma: if it rejected McKinley's demands it faced a disastrous war, and if it complied with them it faced a revolt that might overturn the government and possibly the throne. Spanish appeals for support from European powers won sympathy, but the only tangible response was a visit to President McKinley by the ambassadors of six powers who begged him not to intervene with armed force. Despairing of European aid, Spain replied on March 31 to McKinley's proposals by agreeing to abandon reconcentration and to grant an armistice upon the application of the insurgents. It did not promise Cuban independence but volunteered to submit to arbitration the question of who was responsible for sinking the *Maine*. Spain followed up on April 9 by declaring a suspension of hostilities on its own without waiting for the insurgents to take the initiative. The following day the American minister in Madrid cabled that he believed Cuban independence and a solution satisfactory to all could be worked out during the armistice.

Spain had gone far toward meeting the President's demands, but not so far as conceding independence. The President's insistence on this point made war inevitable. The day after receiving his minister's cable, April 11, McKinley sent a warlike message to Congress. He alluded in passing to Spain's concessions to American demands, but did not stress them. There was, it is true, ground for doubt that the Spanish government could make good its promises and evidence that it was stalling. Congress paused only to debate whether it should recognize the insurgent government as well as the independence of Cuba, decided on the latter only, and adopted the resolution on April 19 by a vote of 42 to 35 in the Senate and 311 to 6 in the House. An amendment to the resolution, which was prepared by Senator Henry M. Teller of Colorado and adopted at the same time without dissent, renounced any intention of annexing or governing Cuba and promised to "leave the government and control of the Island to its people." The Teller Amendment proclaimed American righteousness and abstention with respect to Cuba but, as the author of the resolution carefully pointed out, left the country a free hand "as to some other islands" that also belonged to Spain. Spain responded by declaring war on April 24, and Congress followed suit the next day. The American declaration of war was made retroactive to April 21, since the President had established a blockade of the Cuban coast on April 22.

The little war. Within ten weeks of the declaration of war the fighting was over and the victory assured. For the country at large—and the readers of headlines in particular—it could not have been a more "splendid little war," as John Hay described it, or one conforming more completely with the romantic imagination of the budding imperialists. The whole war seemed to have been fought to the stirring music of "The Stars and Stripes Forever," the battle song of the war, played by a marine band in dress uniform. Even

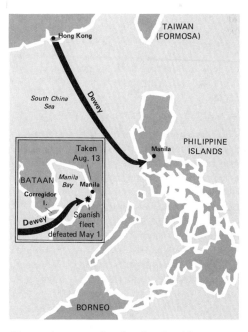

Dewey's campaign in the Pacific, 1898

the participants chose to remember it in the manly prose of Richard Harding Davis or in the heroic sketches of Frederic Remington, two of the numerous writers and artists who "covered" the story of one of the best-publicized wars in history. The Spanish-American War was, in short, the most popular of all American wars. Disillusionment takes a bit of time, especially among noncombatants, and this war was over even before weariness could set in—save among combat troops.

The most hardened skeptics were thrown off balance less than a week after the war started by Commodore George Dewey's dazzling naval victory in Manila Bay on the opposite side of the globe. In accordance with a navy war plan of 1896, Dewey had been ordered two months earlier to move his squadron to Hong Kong and be prepared for action. On receiving news of the war and his final instructions, Dewey had immediately steamed out of Hong Kong, slipped through the straits of Boca Grande during the night of April 30, and at dawn opened fire on the weak and inferior Spanish squadron at Manila. Before breakfast, and without losing a man, he had sunk the whole fleet to the last of its ten ships. Dewey had crushed Spanish power in the Pacific.

Unfortunately the army was not as well prepared as the navy, but the public did not learn about that until later. The account of the expeditionary force to Cuba that the public read and gloried in was the sort supplied by the debonair reporter Richard Harding Davis:

> It was a most happy-go-lucky expedition, run with real American optimism and readiness to take big chances, and with the spirit of a people who recklessly trust that it will come out all right in the end, and that the barely possible may not happen. . . . As one of the generals on board said, "This is God Almighty's war, and we are only His agents."

That was one way of putting it. At least Davis was accurate about the expedition's optimism and recklessness. The army, with only some twenty-six thousand men at the start of the war, had no adequate plans, equipment, or supplies. The War Department was crippled by antiquated methods, incompetent administration, and years of neglect. General William R. Shafter, a three-hundred-pound Civil War hero, presided over the chaos at Tampa preceding the embarkation of the expeditionary force. Transportation broke down and confusion reigned. Thousands of volunteers who rushed to the colors eager for glory could not be supplied with guns, tents, or blankets. With hopeless inefficiency they were clad in woolen uniforms for a summer campaign in the sweltering tropics. Food was inadequate, and sanitation was con-spicuously wanting. Over the expeditionary force there spread the stench of dysentery and illness and eventually the horror of plague, the yellow jack. Newspapers exaggerated all this sensationally, and the public found a scapegoat in Secretary of War Russell A. Alger. General Nelson A. Miles broadcast the myth of "embalmed beef" on which his troops were allegedly poisoned. The great losses came after the war from malaria, typhoid, and yellow fever.

Fortunately the Spanish blundered even more badly than the Americans. Among other things they obligingly immobilized their Cuban naval power, a small force of four cruisers and three destroyers under the command of Admiral Pascual Cervera, in Santiago Harbor, where it was immediately blockaded by a vastly superior fleet commanded by Admiral William T. Sampson. The blockade ended the threat to the landing of the expeditionary force, and after much backing and filling and countermanding of orders a force of some eighteen thousand regulars and volunteers got under way from Tampa, partly equipped and only partially trained. The most publicized unit of volunteers was the Rough Riders, commanded by Colonel Leonard Wood, who was loudly supported by Lieutenant Colonel Theodore Roosevelt, second in command. The landing force blundered slowly ashore on June 20 and established a beachhead at Daiquiri, a few miles east of Santiago.

Having some two hundred thousand troops in Cuba, the Spanish might have destroyed the Americans utterly. But they had only about thirteen thousand men at Santiago and were so handicapped in transportation that they could not bring their superior forces to bear and so unfortunate in military leadership that they could not employ what power they had at hand to their best advantage. Another handicap, of

The Cuban campaign, 1898

course, was a hostile population in rebellion. Even so they came near inflicting a disaster upon the invaders. The American objective was to capture the ridges, known as San Juan Hill, that dominated Santiago and then to take the town in whose harbor Admiral Cervera was blockaded. So poorly was the command organized, however, that the American units were largely without coordinated control in their attack. It was in the capture of Kettle Hill, a flanking outpost of San Juan Hill, that Theodore Roosevelt established his reputation for martial zeal and heroism. Later he was to describe the attack volubly and frequently as a "bully fight" that was "great fun," something of a rollicking skylark. Actually the fight, in which his was by no means the only part, was a pretty desperate and bloody affair marked by a reckless display of courage and a great many needless casualties. The capture of the heights proved decisive in the land fighting, for Santiago was now closely invested. But the American troops were believed to be in a dangerous plight. On July 3 Roosevelt wrote Lodge, "We are within measurable distance of a terrible military disaster," in desperate need of reinforcements, food, and ammunition.

On that very morning, however, Admiral Cervera hoisted anchor and steamed out of Santiago Harbor to face his doom for the honor of Castile. He knew perfectly well that he was far outclassed and outgunned by the four United States battleships awaiting him just outside the harbor, but he gave battle rather than surrender without a fight. The American battle line opened up with its thirteen-inch guns, and one after another the Spanish ships went down gallantly, guns ablaze. It was all over in a few hours, with four hundred enemy killed or wounded and with only one American killed. The next day was the Fourth of July, and orators had not had such an opportunity since the day after Gettysburg and Vicksburg.

Victory at sea left the Americans in command of Caribbean waters and rendered the besieged Spanish ashore in Santiago virtually powerless. General Shafter nevertheless decided to continue the siege rather than attempt assault. Meanwhile he quarreled with the naval command over aid from the sea, waited for General Miles to bring up army reinforcements, and watched his troops deteriorate from heat, fever, and want of supplies. One very minor and indecisive battle, the last of the campaign, occurred on July 10–11, just before Miles arrived with reinforcements. Faced with inevitable defeat, the Spanish command agreed on July 16 to the terms of surrender, which included turning over nearly 24,000 prisoners to be shipped back to Spain by the Americans. It remained, however, to carry out the planned occupation of Puerto Rico by General Miles, who embarked from Cuba on July 21 on that mission.

The Puerto Rico operation came off far more smoothly and bloodlessly than the Cuban campaign. The island had not suffered the devastation that Cuba had experienced. The inhabitants readily collaborated with the invading forces, and native volunteers, who made up about half the Spanish garrison, deserted en masse. Augmented by a stream of reinforcements from the United States, Miles' army of 17,000 met little opposition. His campaign was well planned and aggressively conducted. By August 12, when an armistice ended the fighting, he had, with the loss of only four dead and some forty wounded, overrun the island and isolated the only remaining armed resistance of consequence in the fort of San Juan.

While these operations were in progress in the Caribbean, American military forces were in action on the opposite side of the globe. Immediately after the news of Dewey's naval victory in Manila Bay, preparations were under way in Washington to dispatch army expeditionary forces for landing at Manila and reducing Spanish resistance ashore. There was never any question of ordering Dewey to withdraw without completing what he began. While he awaited arrival of the troops, warships of Germany, Britain, France, and Japan dropped anchor in Manila Bay to watch developments with interest. American troops first landed the last day of June and built up strength to take the fortified city. Their commanders avoided recognition of the insurgent Filipino forces under Emilio Aguinaldo, who rightly believed he was to be deprived of fruits of his previous victories over the Spanish. Out-gunned on sea and land, the Spanish put up largely token resistance and, after a battle costing Americans five dead and forty-five wounded, surrendered Manila and 13,000 troops on August 14.

Spain had sued for peace on July 18, but negotiations on the terms of an armistice were not concluded until August 12. The agreement finally dictated by President McKinley called for an immediate ceasefire, word of which did not reach Manila until after the battle. Spain gave up sovereignty over Cuba, leaving its fate to be settled by the Americans and the insurgents. The future of the Philippines was to be decided at a peace conference to meet in Paris on October 1, 1898.

The White Man's Burden

Mr. McKinley and his decision. The armistice deliberately left open the question of the disposition of the Philippine Islands. They had scarcely figured at all in the war motives of most Americans, who, in Reinhold Niebuhr's phrase, were bent on fighting a "pure-minded war." To seize those possessions and to rule them by force without consent of their inhabitants would be to violate both the humanitarian motives that prompted the war and the oldest and profoundest American political traditions. Knowing these things in their hearts, whether they admitted them or not, the imperialist-minded minority scarcely dared hope at the onset of the war that their dreams would materialize. As it turned out they were on the eve of sensational success.

Hawaii was the first sign. In the spring before the war a joint resolution for annexation gained strong support in Congress but was stalled in part by the crisis with Spain. But in the excitement of the Dewey and Sampson victories the traditional arguments were swept aside and the "large policy" of Hay, Lodge, Mahan, and Roosevelt prevailed. The New York *Tribune* maintained that Hawaii was "imperative" as a halfway station to the Philippines, and another expansionist argued later that the Philippines were imperative as an outpost for Hawaii. President McKinley gave strong support to annexation. On June 15 the House of Representatives, and on July 6 the Senate, adopted a joint resolution annexing Hawaii. The large policy was now on the way to further enlargement.

The enlargement was facilitated by the conscience of President McKinley. He advanced his insights in the form of such epigrams as, "Duty determines destiny," but he did not answer the New York *Evening Post's* query, "Who determines duty?" At any rate the destiny of the Philippines was becoming pretty manifest as McKinley's epigrams and actions multiplied. Even before Dewey's victory was confirmed he ordered a force to capture and hold Manila, and before the end of May Lodge was writing Roosevelt, "The Administration is now fully committed to the large policy that we both desire."

The commercial and industrial interests now helped swing the tide toward expansionism. Though they had opposed the war at first for fear of its effect on recovery and the gold standard, once the war started and news of the victories poured in and the potentialities of expansion for the advancement of trade became manifest, the business community swung about in support of the policies it had once opposed. Big business saw the Philippines as a key to the China trade and listened appreciatively to Senator Albert Beveridge's declaration that "the trade of the world must and shall be ours." Senator Marcus A. Hanna believed "we can and will take a large slice of the commerce of Asia. That is what we want."

At the same time the religious press, with the support of the missionary movement, stepped up support for the "imperialism of righteousness." Annexation would further the cause of world evangelization, extend the blessings of civilization and sanitation, and "civilize" more of the heathens. A more cynical approach to imperialism was that of editor Henry Watterson, who proposed to "escape the menace and peril of socialism and agrarianism" by means of "a policy of colonization and conquest." One popular way of thinking, however, was to attribute imperialism to a determinism of some sort: the hand of God, the instinct of race, the laws of Darwin, the forces of economics and trade—anything but responsible decision. Though many Americans seemed willing to surrender to imperialist policies, few would admit they did so because they wanted to.

McKinley revealed his intentions pretty clearly by the choice of commissioners he sent to negotiate with Spain at the peace conference held in Paris. Three of the five peace commissioners were open and avowed expansionists. Another indication was his seizure of Spain's island of Guam—whose inhabitants mistook the American bombardment for a salute and apologized for having no ammunition with which to return it. In his instructions to the peace commissioners the President took the moral position that "without any desire or design on our part" the United States had assumed duties and responsibilities that it must discharge as became a nation of noble destiny. He instructed the commissioners in October with regard to the Philippines that "duty requires we should take the archipelago."

John Hay, who had recently become Secretary of State, cabled the delegation in Paris to hold out for the whole of the Philippine Islands. The Spanish commissioners resisted the demand to the point of risking a renewal of hostilities. The talks continued for two months. McKinley stuck to his position that we should "not shirk the moral obligation of our victory" but made one concession, an offer to pay $20 million for the Philippines. The Spanish capitulated, and the treaty was signed December 10, 1898. By its terms Spain was to give up control over Cuba and surrender Guam, Puerto Rico, and the Philippine Islands to the United States.

There is little reason to doubt the sincerity of the reasons for his decision that the President offered a year later, though some critics have questioned his candor. The reasons he gave were that it would be cowardly and dishonorable to give the Philippines back to Spain, "bad business and discreditable" to let France or Germany seize them, impossible to leave them to their own devices since they were unfit for self-rule, and absolutely necessary to follow the humanitarian impulses to "civilize and Christianize" the Filipinos by taking possession of their land. What McKinley had in mind in his reference to the designs of European powers on the Philippines was that in November 1897, Germany landed troops at Kiaochow, and a Russian fleet anchored at Port Arthur. The following March the two European powers forced

Captured insurgents, Philippines

China to sign agreements giving Germany exclusive rights in Shantung province and Russia exclusive rights in Manchuria. Japan had occupied Korea, and France was established in Kwangchau Bay.

The debate on the Philippines. The treaty with Spain committed the United States to imperialism in the Far East and the Caribbean. But first the treaty had to be ratified by the Senate, and the question of ratification precipitated a debate that spread far beyond the Senate chamber and cast more light on the issues of annexation than had the President's speeches and the expansionists' slogans. After the drums of war were silenced and the people began to think more soberly, it became apparent that there was formidable opposition to the President's policy, perhaps enough to defeat it. Far more opposition came from Democrats than from Republicans, and the sentiment was strong enough to unite even such Democratic extremes as Bryan and Cleveland. But prominent members of McKinley's own party, including Speaker Reed of the House and Senator George F. Hoar of Massachusetts, broke with the Administration over the question, as did Senator Eugene Hale of Maine. To the very last it was doubtful whether the President could muster the two-thirds of the Senate required for consent to ratify his treaty.

Even before the treaty was signed an Anti-Imperialist League was organized that attracted the support of many distinguished men. As president, the league elected George S. Boutwell, formerly Grant's Secretary of the Treasury and later Republican senator from Massachusetts. Among the vice presidents were such contrasting figures as Grover Cleveland and Samuel Gompers, Andrew Carnegie and Carl Schurz, John Sherman and Charles Francis Adams. Intellectuals, novelists, and poets rallied to anti-imperialism in great numbers, among them President Eliot of Harvard and President David Starr Jordan of Stanford, along with William James, William Dean Howells, William Graham Sumner, Hamlin Garland, William Vaughn Moody, and Mark Twain. In a bitter satire Mark Twain assured his countrymen that the "Blessings-of-Civilization Trust" had the purest of motives. "This world-girdling accumulation of trained morals, high principles, and justice cannot do an unright thing, an unfair thing, an ungenerous thing, an unclean thing," he wrote. "It knows what it is about. Give yourself no uneasiness; it is all right."

Anti-imperialists tended to be elderly and have old-fashioned values and principles, but some of their arguments showed remarkable prescience. George Boutwell foresaw a war with Japan as a consequence of American expansion in the western Pacific, and following that the rise of a warlike China in potential alliance with Russia that would turn against American holdings. A favorite argument was based on the doctrine of the Declaration of Independence: no government without the consent of the governed. We had fought the Revolution for that principle and had intervened in Cuba on the same ground; how could we now shamelessly adopt the doctrines we fought to overthrow? Or, as Senator Hoar put it, how could we "strut about in the cast-off clothing of pinchbeck emperors and pewter kings?" Other objections were that the Asiatic people could not be assimilated into our tradition, that imperialism would lead to militarism and racist dogma at home, that overseas expansion was unconstitutional and inconsistent with the Monroe Doctrine. Opponents of empire in the South and West never fully understood those in the Northeast. Southerners viewed the new imperialism as a revival of carpetbaggery and warned of the difficulties of reconciling races of contrasting color and heritage. Racist arguments were used both for and against imperialism though mainly for it.

The imperialist-minded defenders of the treaty revived with new assurance their old arguments of naval strategy, world power, and commercial interests and incorporated the moralistic line of McKinley on duty, destiny, humanitarianism, and religious mission. In the latter vein Senator Beveridge declared, "It is God's great purpose made manifest in the instincts of our race, whose present phase is our personal profit, but whose far-off end is the redemption of the world and the Christianization of mankind." Senator Lodge dismissed the consent-of-the-governed argument as of no account because that principle had been ignored or violated before, notably in the Louisiana Purchase, in order to advance the national interest. He emphasized and exaggerated the supposed economic advantages of the Philippines: their resources, their trade, and their relationship to the international struggle for China and its trade. He stressed the political expediency of keeping the islands: they were not ready for self-government, would lapse into anarchy, or would be seized by more ruthless powers.

In the meantime the Senate continued its deliberations, the outcome still in doubt. Before the end of the debate the anti-imperialists were confused by a strange maneuver and strategic blunder of William Jennings Bryan. Although he was a strong opponent of the acquisition of the Philippines, he decided that the Senate should approve the treaty to assure peace and should leave the future disposition of the islands to be decided at the polls. He undoubtedly believed that this move would provide him with a winning issue in the presidential election of 1900, but he miscalculated. Approval of the treaty presented the voters with a *fait accompli*. Bryan's advice won some Senate votes over to the side of the Administration, though not enough to assure victory. On February 5, 1899, the very day before the final ballot was set, the drama of the decision was complicated and intensified by the arrival of news that the Filipinos had taken up arms in open revolt against the United States. There could be no more doubt of their desire for freedom or that the United States was now in the same position formerly occupied by discredited Spain. The effect of this news is impossible to estimate. The issue remained in doubt until the roll call the next day recorded fifty-seven in favor of the treaty and twenty-seven against—two more than the necessary two-thirds majority.

In the meantime the American army remained in control of Cuba, and the government refused to withdraw until the Cubans incorporated into their constitution a permanent treaty with the United States, the so-called Platt Amendment, proposed by the United

States Senate in 1901. This limited the power of Cuba to make treaties, borrow money, or change certain policies established by the occupation forces and required the sale or lease of lands for a naval base. More important, the United States was granted the right to intervene at will "for the preservation of Cuban independence" and "the protection of life, property, and individual liberty." Having no choice, Cuba submitted.

The motives that prompted America to "take up the white man's burden," as Rudyard Kipling urged it to do, were even more complex than the motives of the war that prepared the way for the decision. Part of the motivation was fear, the fear of appearing silly and playing the fool in the eyes of the world. Part of it was an uglier impulse of aggression. "The taste of empire is in the mouth of the people even as the taste of blood in the jungle," said the Washington *Post*.

Beyond the Philippines. What the other great imperial powers of the world were currently doing to China was a cause more of alarm than of emulation. Even before the Cuban war, John Hay had pressed upon President McKinley the common interest of the United States and Great Britain in forestalling exclusion from the China trade. Now the trade opportunities promised in the Far East by the acquisition of Hawaii and the Philippines were threatened by the impending dissolution of China and its partition among imperial powers. A small pressure group of American exporters interested in the China trade added their influence to that of Britain to move the State Department into action.

To meet the problem, Secretary Hay sent his "Open Door" notes to Great Britain, Germany, and Russia in September 1899 and later to Japan, Italy, and France, inviting them to agree to three principles: (1) that no power would interfere with the trading rights of other nations within its sphere of influence,

(2) that Chinese tariff duties (which gave America most-favored-nation rights) should be collected on all merchandise by Chinese officials, and (3) that no power should levy discriminatory harbor dues or railroad charges against other powers within its sphere. Great Britain agreed conditionally, Russia equivocated, and Germany, France, Italy, and Japan agreed on condition of full acceptance by the other powers. It was a chilling response, but Hay saved face by blandly announcing that since all powers agreed on the American proposals, their assent was considered "final and definitive." Since Russia had not agreed, and Britain only with conditions, and since the others made acceptance conditional on full acceptance by all powers, Hay's claims were not very impressive. His proposals at this point did not undertake to preserve the territorial integrity or independence of China.

In May 1900, two months after Hay announced his interpretation of the response to the Open Door notes, the Boxers, an organization of fanatical Chinese patriots, incited an uprising that took the lives of 231 foreigners and many Christian Chinese. In June the Boxers began the siege of the legations in Peking and cut the city off from the outside world for a month. The Western powers and Japan then sent in a military force, to which the United States contributed five thousand troops. This expeditionary force relieved the besieged legations on August 4.

During the Boxer Rebellion crisis, Secretary Hay labored successfully to prevent the spread of war, limit the extent of intervention, assure the rapid withdrawal of troops, head off the extension of foreign spheres of influence, and keep down punitive demands on China. On July 3, 1900, Hay issued a circular stating it to be the policy of the United States "to seek a solution which may bring about permanent safety and peace to China, preserve Chinese territorial and administrative entity," and protect all trade rights mentioned in the Open Door notes in all parts of the empire. This was an important extension of American policy in the Far East. Although only Great Britain, France, and Germany responded favorably to Hay's circular, its effect was to help soften the punitive terms imposed on China. Unwilling to risk the general war that might be precipitated by a struggle to divide China, the intervening powers were persuaded to accept indemnity in money rather than territory. The United States' share of the reparations was $25 million, more than enough to settle the claims of its nationals. In fact, the United States returned a balance of more than $10 million, and the Chinese government, as a gesture of gratitude, placed the money in trust for the education of Chinese youth in their own country and in the United States.

McKinley's vindication of 1900. It was Bryan's mistake, in planning to make the election of 1900 a popular referendum on imperialism, to believe that the anti-imperialist sentiment of the great debate of 1898–99 could be sustained or even revived, much less strengthened. Nearly two years were to pass between the ratification of the treaty and the presidential election, and by that time much water had passed under the bridge. Empire was no longer a dangerous menace to tradition and a decision that had to be worried out; it was an accomplished fact to which the people were growing accustomed. They did not like the war that was being waged to suppress Emilio Aguinaldo and his Filipino patriots, even though censorship kept some of its worst aspects from them. That war was to drag on for three years, during which the United States was to use more men to suppress freedom in the Philippines than it had used to bring freedom to Cuba. And the new American rulers were to repeat in grotesque imitation the tortures and brutalities of their Spanish predecessors. But all that was taking place on the other side of the widest of oceans. When pressed, people admitted, "Peace has to be restored."

At home there were plenty of distractions to divert a burdensome conscience. The most important one was the gradual return to prosperity. The war itself served as an additional stimulus. Business regained its nerve, trade quickened, and the economy bustled into activity.

As the farmers and laborers sloughed off the burden of depression, their radicalism declined. The new imperialism and patriotism also had a dampening effect on radicalism in labor and agrarian movements. "The Spanish War finished us," wrote Tom Watson of the Populist party. "The blare of the bugle drowned the voice of the reformer." The war, coupled with returning prosperity, mounting racism, and the legacy of the Populists' demoralizing fusion with Bryanism in 1896 (see pp. 520–22), did just about finish the party. In the 1900 campaign it split into two feuding factions, neither of which could make a substantial showing. Many of the Populists of the Southwest and Middle West were attracted to the new Social Democratic party, which was founded in 1900 and nominated Eugene V. Debs of Pullman-strike fame as its presidential candidate.

Although McKinley's policies had little to do with the revival of the economy, he was billed as "the advance agent of prosperity," and he prospered politically with the return of good times. With a Cabinet that was even more conservative than he was himself, McKinley's first administration had proved as willing and cooperative as the business community could have hoped. The Dingley Tariff of 1897 raised the rates to a new high, and the gold standard was now safe.

The presidential nominees of the two major parties in 1900 were pretty much a foregone conclusion. The Republicans had no hesitation about McKinley, but only with some difficulty did they settle upon the military hero and New York governor, Theodore Roosevelt for Vice President. The Democrats returned to Bryan and picked the Silverite Adlai E. Stevenson, who had been Vice President during Cleveland's second term, for second place. The Democratic platform stressed imperialism as the "paramount issue" and on Bryan's insistence revived the demand for free silver. His strategy of uniting silverites of West and South with gold men of the Northeast in a coalition against imperialism came to grief. Bryan soon discovered that he had two fairly moribund issues on his hands and therefore shifted his emphasis to monopoly and special privilege.

Bryan, in a poorer showing than he had made in 1896, lost his own state of Nebraska, as well as Kansas, South Dakota, Utah and Wyoming—all silver states he had carried before. The election neither revived the silver issue nor provided a mandate on imperialism. Even if the voters opposed imperialism, they could express their disapproval only by voting against prosperity. Republican leaders acknowledged that Americans had lost their appetite for further colonial expansion. To the majority of voters in 1900 McKinley meant prosperity rather than imperialism or gold, and with him conservatism was triumphant once more.

Suggestions for Reading

C. S. Campbell, *The Transformation of American Foreign Relations, 1865–1900** (1976), is a readable and reliable narrative. More briefly, R. L. Beisner, *From the Old Diplomacy to the New, 1865–1900** (1974), assesses conflicting interpretations, and M. B. Young, *American Expansionism: The Critical Issues* (1973), assembles and edits key interpretive essays. Scholarly controversy over expansionism has been shaped by A. K. Weinberg, *Manifest Destiny: A Study in Nationalist Expansionism in American History* (1935), and J. W. Pratt, *Expansionists of 1898: The Acquisition of Hawaii and the Spanish Islands* (1936). Economic influences are debated by Walter Le Feber, *The New Empire: An Interpretation of American Expansion, 1860–1898** (1963); W. A. Williams, *The Tragedy of American Diplomacy** (rev. ed., 1972); E. R. May, *American Imperialism: A Speculative Essay* (1968); and D. F. Healy, *U.S. Expansionism: Imperialist Urge in the 1890s** (1970).

More specific aspects of foreign affairs are treated by Harold and Margaret Sprout, *The Rise of American Naval Power, 1896–1918* (1939); D. M. Pletcher, *The Awkward Years: American Foreign Relations under Garfield and Arthur* (1962); J. A. S. Grenville and G. B. Young, *Politics, Strategy, and American Diplomacy: Studies in Foreign Policy, 1873–1917* (1966); C. S. Campbell, *Anglo-American Understanding, 1898–1903* (1957); W. A. Russ, Jr., *The Hawaiian Republic (1894–98) and the Struggle to Win Annexation* (1961), and T. J. Osborne, *Empire Can Wait: American Opposition to Hawaiian Annexation, 1893–1898* (1981).

On the Spanish-American War a short account is H. Wayne Morgan, *America's Road to Empire: The War with Spain and Overseas Expansion** (1965), and also Morgan, *William McKinley and His America* (1963). Contrasting treatments are found in E. R. May, *Imperial Democracy: The Emergence of America as a Great Power** (1961), and P. S. Foner, *The Spanish-Cuban-American War and the Birth of American Imperialism, 1895–1902*, 2 vols. (1972). Military history is enriched by G. A. Cosmas, *An Army for Empire: The United States Army in the Spanish-American War* (1971), and S. C. Miller, *Benevolent Assimilation: American Conquest of the Philippines* (1982). Naval aspects are treated in R. S. West, Jr., *Admirals of the American Empire* (1948). Margaret Leech, *In the Days of McKinley* (1959), throws light on the war as well as the election of 1900. On the influence of newspapers see C. H. Brown, *Correspondents' War: Journalists in the Spanish-American War* (1967), and J. E. Wisan, *The Cuban Crisis as Reflected in the New York Press, 1895–1898* (1934).

Far Eastern affairs are handled in M. B. Young, *Rhetoric of Empire: American China Policy, 1895–1901* (1968), and T. J. McCormick, *China Market: America's Quest for Informal Empire, 1893–1901** (1967). On the opposition to American imperialism see R. L. Beisner, *Twelve Against Empire: The Anti-Imperialists, 1898–1900* (1968); E. B. Tompkins, *Anti-Imperialism in the United States: The Great Debate, 1890–1920** (1970); and R. E. Welch, Jr., *Response to Imperialism: The United States and the Phillipine-American War, 1899–1902* (1979).

*Available in a paperback edition.

1901–1945

THE NATIONAL EXPERIENCE

In the celebrations that marked the turn of the twentieth century, Americans expressed pride in the extraordinary growth of the nation, in its wealth, and in its strength. They declared their confidence in an ever more glorious future marked by personal comforts, technological marvels, exemplary democratic institutions, and world renown. The progress they had made to date and the progress they believed lay ahead generated the ebullient spirit of the time.

Some men and women questioned that self-congratulatory mood. In 1899 the Chicago Conference on Trusts had heard spokesmen for labor, for agriculture, for small enterprise, and for the common people condemn the irresponsible wealth and power of the large corporations that dominated every basic industry. During the first decade of the new century, as in the last decade of the old, the blatant evidence of rural and urban poverty provoked persistent criticisms of American society. So too did the prevailing prejudice and discrimination against non-whites, non-Protestants, and women of whatever race or religion, who enjoyed no genuine equality of opportunity. Other critics lamented the continuing waste of the continent's land and minerals and water, and called for controls over further use of the national bounty of wealth and beauty. A few prescient men and women, alarmed by developing rivalries among the great powers of the world, the United States among them, sought means for settling international disputes peacefully.

Yet as the century turned, even the critics, with few exceptions, shared the confidence of the contented. They believed that intelligent men and women, animated by conscience, could and would enlist social energies, private and public alike, to remove the "excrescences of privilege" that were diminishing the country's potential. That was the objective of progressivism. Then the nation, already rich and powerful, would realize the best hopes of its founders. The progressives' moral fervor was not radical, for they themselves, again with few exceptions, did not much question the existing political and economic systems. They intended not to revolutionize but to improve society; they would reform in order to conserve.

Though the fervor of the reformers outstripped their achievements, during the first two decades of the century the cities and states and the

544

federal government took first steps toward taxing and regulating business, alleviating poverty, and protecting natural resources. At the same time the affairs of the world touched American interests more and more closely. By 1917 the war that began in Europe in 1914 had directly engaged the nation. That awful contest ended, like efforts for domestic reform, in at best a fractional victory. During the disenchanted years that followed, a mood of superficial contentment settled on most of the country. National confidence focused on material achievements, but those, too, had their critics, and below the surface of complacency the familiar problems, some of them undiagnosed, lay unresolved.

The crash of 1929 and the ensuing depression, the longest and most severe in American history, again exposed those problems and challenged the strength and resilience of the American people and their institutions. In the new pursuit of reform and the search for recovery, the moralism of the early century gave way to a tough, sometimes grim, often adventurous spirit of experimentation. The New Deal of the 1930s brought the agenda of reform closer to completion, though not to its conclusion. It also demonstrated the creative potentialities of an expanded federal government. Disinclined though Americans were to venture again into world affairs, the second great war of the century posed threats to national security that culminated in 1941 in the Japanese attack on Pearl Harbor. Over the next four years, the booming wartime economy, prompting a modest redistribution of income, fulfilled many of the materialistic expectations of most white Americans. Yet even while waging a war against racism, the United States had yet to resolve its own racial problems. And it had yet to assure to women the rights of men, or to erase the blight of poverty.

When the war ended the United States had become the strongest nation in the world, possessed of a technological marvel, a dreadful weapon, the atomic bomb. Yet the horror of that weapon seemed to exceed the nation's ability to bear responsibility for world peace and order. Victory had generated afresh the confidence of Americans in themselves and in their nation, their democratic institutions, and the appeal of those institutions to other peoples. The validity and the durability of that confidence would be tested soon again.

22
THE PROGRESSIVE MOVEMENT AND THE SQUARE DEAL

When the twentieth century began, the prodigious material developments of the preceding several decades (see Ch. 18) had transformed society. Yet almost all of those in positions of authority or influence in government, industry, the professions, even labor and farm organizations had been born during the years before the Civil War when the United States was still primarily a rural country. By 1901 the nation had changed profoundly, as had its problems, which were often perplexing to men and women who had grown up in an earlier age. Some Americans were nostalgic for that past as they remembered it. Others rejoiced in modernity but were eager to control its course and effects. Both of those attitudes pointed, though in different ways, to the desirability, even the exigency, of altering conditions as they had become.

As Americans were increasingly aware, they had yet to accommodate to the social and cultural changes stimulated by industrial and urban growth. They had yet to adjust their laws and their techniques of government to an age of large and complex private organizations. Americans had yet to recognize the international implications of their national wealth. They had yet to fulfill their national promise of individual liberty, opportunity, and dignity for all men and women.

The unprecedented productivity of the economy made comfort potentially available to all Americans. That possibility in turn highlighted the striking contrasts between the few and the many, the white-skinned and the dark, the urban and the rural—the striking contrast between national aspiration and national achievement. Out of an awareness of that contrast, out of the tensions of material development, out of a consciousness of national mission, there emerged the efforts at adjustment and reform that constituted the progressive movement, a striving by men and women of good will to understand, improve, and manage the society in which they lived.

National Wealth and the Business Élite

During the first two decades of the twentieth century the number of people in the United States, their average age, and their average per capita wealth all increased. In that period total national income almost doubled, and average per capita income rose from $450 to $567 a year. Though by the standards of the 1980s about 40 percent of Americans were then poor, growth in and of itself gave confidence to a generation who tended to measure progress in terms of plenty.

There were some 76 million Americans in 1900, some 106 million in 1920. Advances in medicine and public health, resulting in a declining death rate, accounted for most of the increase. It was accompanied

Population 1900

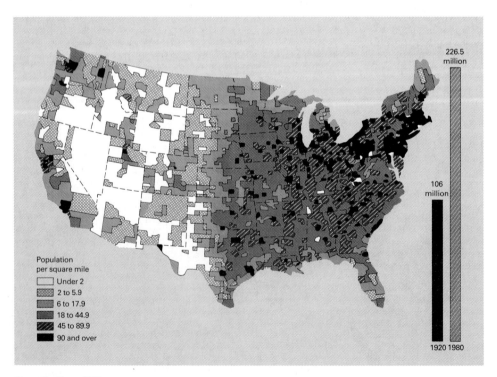

Population 1920

by a continuing movement of people within the United States. In the West the rate of growth was highest—along the Pacific slope, population more than doubled. But growth occurred everywhere, especially in the cities, where it proceeded six and a half times as fast as in rural areas. The cities, in the pattern of the past (see pp. 479–80), absorbed almost all of the 14.5 million immigrants who came largely from central and southern Europe in the years 1900–15. Usually swarthy and unlettered, ordinarily Catholics or Jews, these newcomers differentiated the cities further and further from the patterns of life that rural America remembered and revered. By 1920 more Americans lived in cities and towns of over 2,500 people than in the countryside.

Spurred by the pace of private investment, the nation recovered from the depression of the nineties. During the first two decades of the century, capital investment rose over 250 percent and the total value of the products of industry rose 222. But not all groups shared equally in national wealth. Though unemployment became negligible, the richest 2 percent of Americans in 1900 owned 60 percent of the nation's wealth, a condition that persisted with little change for two decades.

Those families were at once the agents and the beneficiaries of the process of industrial expansion and consolidation. Corporate mergers and reorganizations had given a dominant influence to a few huge combinations in each of many industries—among others, railroading, iron and steel and copper, meatpacking, milling, tobacco, electricals, petroleum, and, by 1920, automobiles. As early as 1909, 1 percent of all the business firms in the nation produced 44 percent of all its manufactured goods. The consolidators had become the richest and in some ways the most powerful men in the United States. They guided the process of investment. They controlled the boards of directors of the great American banks and industries. They interpreted the startling growth of industry as a demonstration of their own wisdom and their optimism about the economic future of the United States. Beyond all that, they were developing, as were the experts whom they hired and consulted, an identification with the entirety of the national economy—the enormous national market, the need for national corporate institutions to reach it, the consequent need for energetic, professional management on a vast scale. Those insights contrasted with the parochialism of smaller institutions and of rural America, and with the traditional (and rewarding) faith of the American folk in their own ability to run their affairs and in their own local institutions. The growth of the great corporations raised questions about scale and control as troublesome as were the questions raised by the related problems of poverty and wealth.

The "leaden-eyed." The magnificence of American wealth contrasted sharply with the sorry lot of the American poor, whom society, as the poet Vachel Lindsay put it, had made "oxlike, limp, and leaden-eyed." In 1910 the nonagricultural laboring force consisted of more than 30 million men and 8 million women, most of whom worked too long and earned too little. Between one-third and one-half of the industrial population lived in poverty. Their children ordinarily left school to find work—only one-third of the American children enrolled in primary schools completed their courses; less than one-tenth finished high school.

Work for men, women, and children was arduous. Those engaged in manufacturing were on the job between 44 and 55 hours a week—on the average over 52 hours. Industrial accidents were common and conditions of work unhealthy and sometimes despicable. Usually workers had to suffer their disasters alone. Employer-liability laws, where they existed, were inadequate; there was no social insurance against accident, illness, old age, or unemployment, nor were

Textile worker

"Sweating" in Tenements, 1905

The workers, poor, helpless, ignorant foreigners, work on ... in filth unspeakable, in the presence of all contagious and other diseases, and in apartments in which the sun enters only at noon or never at all. In such an apartment I attended a woman ill with tuberculosis, finishing trousers.... Three years of life in this apartment killed the woman.... As soon as a little child can be of the least possible help, it must add to the family income by taking on a share of the toil.

From Anne J. Daniel, "The Wreck of the Home," quoted in James T. Patterson,
America's Struggle against Poverty, 1901.

there child-care centers where women workers could safely leave their children. Indeed child labor remained common throughout the country. And the slums, where most workers lived, were as bad as they had been in the 1890s.

New kinds of mobile slums were developing, the slums of migratory workers—some immigrants, some native Americans, some blacks and Chicanos—who were leaving submarginal small farms to follow the wheat harvest north from Texas or to pick fruits and vegetables along the West Coast. So, too, the mining and lumbering camps of the South and West offered to workers only a life of drudgery, brutality, danger, and poverty.

Complacency and dissent. The inequities in American society evoked a variety of responses ranging from the complacent to the outraged. Most of the well-to-do—the business élite and the professional men who identified with them and served them—believed as they long had that success was a function of virtue and poverty evidence of sin. As the century turned, they were satisfied with existing conditions, and they remained fixed in their belief in minimal government. Other self-respecting men and women of the comfortable middle class harbored some anxieties about their own futures but few doubts about the merit of American institutions.

But there was a minority alike of the rich and of the comfortable who were receptive to the messages of protest and the efforts at particular social remedy that characterized the early years of the new century. That receptivity reflected in part a dread of drastic change and of the kind of radical agitation that had punctuated the 1890s. Still, apart from those fears, the center of American consciousness was slowly acquiring a new conscience. It produced a growing understanding of the efforts of some of the less-privileged to improve their lot, a sympathy for the protests of the best-informed against the inequities of American life, and, though rarely, a tolerance for the outrage of that small minority of Americans who were committed to rapid and radical social improvement.

Organized labor. The craft-union movement, well launched in the nineties, made significant gains during the early years of the twentieth century. Membership in the affiliates of the American Federation of Labor rose from 548,000 in 1900 to 1,676,000 in 1904 and, in the face of strong resistance from employers, to about 2,000,000 by 1914, though even then some 90 percent of industrial workers remained unorganized. The unions and the railroad brotherhoods continued to strive for the bread-and-butter objectives Samuel Gompers and their other leaders had defined earlier. Especially in the building and metals trades, they were able to win from management agreements providing for collective bargaining, higher wages, shorter hours, and safer conditions of work.

The craft unions were effective but in some respects selfish agencies of change. Though they excited opposition from business-managers not yet prepared to grant labor any voice in industrial decisions, they had little quarrel with the concentration of industrial power. The American Federation of Labor did demand the right to organize workers into national trade unions, consolidations that would parallel the consolidations of capital. In order to organize, labor needed to be unshackled from state and federal prohibitions on the strike and the boycott—and needed, too, state and federal protection from antiunion devices. The unions welcomed legislation setting standards of safety and employer liability, but otherwise they preferred to rely on their own power, rather than on the authority of the state, to reach their goals. They continued to distrust the federal government, for it had so often in the past assisted in breaking strikes, and they were eager to enlarge their own power even at the expense of those they had no intention of organizing. So it was that Gompers and his associates persisted in opposing legislation on wages and hours.

Collective bargaining, even when possible, assisted only union members, and the craft unions were generally unconcerned with the unskilled bulk of the labor force. Indeed Gompers, along with other labor-leaders, looked down on the unskilled, particularly on those who were women or immigrants. Craft-leaders feared that management would hire unskilled and unorganized immigrants and blacks to replace skilled workers (though in fact skilled workers were competing less with the unskilled than with an advancing technology and mechanization). This fear intensified prejudices against Asians, blacks, and southern and eastern Europeans—prejudices that fed growing sentiments for the restriction of immigration and for racial segregation. Organized labor condoned Jim Crow and sparked the agitation that led in 1902 to the renewed exclusion from the United States of Chinese immigrants and in 1907 to the effective exclusion of the Japanese.

Outsiders. Scorned alike by management and by the unions, the immigrants swelling the American labor force had to learn to help themselves. They continued, as in earlier decades, to receive unsystematic assistance in finding employment from urban political machines eager for their votes. Further, each new wave of immigration brought to the United States candidates for the meanest jobs. Their availability permitted their predecessors to climb a notch higher in the hierarchy of the work place. So it was during the first decade of the century in the needle trades in New York City where men and women from southern Italy took over some of the underpaid and arduous piece work that had fallen in the 1890s to eastern European Jews who moved up to become cutters or other skilled workers with accompanying increases in pay. The experience of those immigrant Jews revealed the need of every immigrant group to organize for its own self-protection and mutual benefit. The Jewish families in New York were able to survive financially only if wives and sometimes children added their earnings to those of husbands and

fathers, and to survive emotionally only because of the support they derived from their culture and their community. In the hostile new environment they entered, their language and religion set them apart, to be sure, but also provided them with a world of their own in which in time they could begin to prosper. Their own newspaper spoke to their hopes and their interests as no general metropolitan daily would or could. Their own unions, especially the International Ladies' Garment Workers Union, fought for their rights. Their own muscle combated the anti-Semitism of their neighbors, including the police. They provided their own theater, their own literature, and gradually their own bourgeoisie. Though they also learned older American ways, they were determined to sustain their culture as one part of a pluralistic society in which other cultures would also flourish.

In New York City, as elsewhere, that was the aspiration, too, of Italians and Poles, Greeks and Bohemians, Chinese and others, outsiders all, whose labor drove American shops and factories to ever higher levels of production and profit. The large majority of workers needed extraordinary courage and stamina to face the toil, the poverty, and the prejudice of a society eager to use but loath to include them.

American blacks. Within that majority were numbered the 10 million American blacks, of whom almost 90 percent still lived in the South. In 1910 almost a third of all blacks were still illiterate; all were victimized by the inferior facilities for schooling, housing, traveling, and working that segregation had imposed upon them. Worse still, the incidence of lynchings (over 1,100 between 1900 and 1914) and race riots remained high, dramatized by mass killings in Atlanta in 1906 and by riots in Abraham Lincoln's own Spring-

For the rights of working women

field, Illinois, in 1908. As racist concepts spread in the North as well as the South, American blacks experienced their worst season since the Civil War. A few black intellectuals, led by W. E. B. DuBois, a Harvard Ph.D., in 1905 organized the Niagara movement. Abandoning the program of Booker T. Washington, DuBois and his associates demanded immediate action to achieve political and economic equality for blacks. With some support from informed whites, the Niagara movement was transformed in 1909 into the National Association for the Advancement of Colored People. But the NAACP, though a hopeful portent for legal redress of black grievances, was some years from becoming an influential instrument of reform.

American women. With varying success women, too, intensified their struggle for political, economic, and social status equal to that of men. Sarah Platt Decker, president of the General Federation of Women's Clubs, converted the energies of that middle-class organization to agitation for improving the conditions of industrial work for women and children (see p. 485). That was also the objective of the Women's Trade Union League and Florence Kelley's National Consumers' League, which sponsored state legislation for minimum wages and maximum hours. In New York City, the International Ladies' Garment Workers Union, financed in part by wealthy matrons, conducted a prolonged strike in 1909 that won limited gains in spite of opposition from employers and police. The Triangle Shirtwaist Company in New York City did not agree to the union's demand for better wages or for safer conditions of work. The company's stubborn parsimony accounted for the tragedy that

occurred in 1911 when fire broke out on its premises and resulted in the death of 146 employees, mostly young women, who could not escape from the building. Official investigations following the episode led ultimately to new factory laws and immediately to broader support for the ILGWU, which by 1914 had become the third-largest union in the AFL.

The contributions of women to various movements for social justice demonstrated their creative and organizational abilities, abilities that most Americans—men and women alike—still viewed as inferior to those of men. But women, though exploited by industry, were by no means inferior. To put a stop to the exploitation, social feminists sponsored special factory laws to protect women from hazardous conditions and overlong hours of work. In so doing, they often contended that women needed special care because they were physically frailer than men. But no man worked as hard or accomplished as much for the settlement-house movement in the United States as did Jane Addams at Hull House in Chicago or Lillian Wald at Henry Street in New York. Indeed, those extraordinary women trained a younger generation, both men and women, to understand the problems of poverty and to combat the circumstances that caused them.

Women also served among the officers and troops in the war against whiskey. The Women's Christian Temperance Union, strongest in rural America, was an unequaled force in the growing demand for the prohibition of the manufacture and sale of alcoholic beverages. Prohibition, an issue of continuing political importance during the first three decades of the twentieth century, aligned (with exceptions of course) rural, native-born, fundamentalist Americans against

The new demand of women for political enfranchisement comes at a time when unsatisfactory and degraded social conditions are held responsible for so much wretchedness and when the fate of all the unfortunate, the suffering, and the criminal, is daily forced upon woman's attention in painful and intimate ways. At the same moment, governments all over the world are insisting that it is their function, and theirs alone, so to regulate social and industrial conditions that a desirable citizenship may be secured....

Governmental commissions everywhere take woman's testimony as to legislation for better housing, for public health and education, for the care of dependents, and many other remedial measures, because it is obviously a perilous business to turn over delicate social experiments to men who have remained quite untouched by social compunctions and who have been elected to their legislative position solely upon the old political issues. Certainly under this new conception of politics it is much easier to legislate for those human beings of whose condition the electorate are "vividly aware."

From Jane Addams, "The Larger Aspects of the Woman's Movement," 1914.

The woman's movement rests not alone on her larger personality, with its tingling sense of revolt against injustice, but on the wide, deep sympathy of women for one another. It is a concerted movement, based on the recognition of a common evil and seeking a common good....

In our present stage of social evolution it is increasingly difficult and painful for women to endure their condition of economic dependence, and therefore they are leaving it. This does not mean that at a given day all women will stand forth free together, but that in slowly gathering numbers, now so great that all the world can see, women in the most advanced races are so standing free....

The banner advanced proclaims "equality before the law," woman's share in political freedom; but the main line of progress is and has been toward economic equality and freedom.

From Charlotte Perkins Gilman, *Women and Economics*, 1898.

---

their urban, immigrant, Catholic countrymen. Yet in cities as well as small towns, women expressed a special interest in protecting families against the profligacy of alcoholic breadwinners, and most urban prohibitionists came to view their objective as a scientifically valid effort to improve human life by controlling part of it. If they were naive about the ability of the state to govern private behavior, they were more sophisticated than their critics realized in their recognition of the dangers of addiction to any drug, alcohol included.

It was primarily urban women who absorbed the more unconventional messages of Charlotte Perkins Gilman, Emma Goldman, and Margaret Sanger. Gilman, eager to free women from the burdens and constraints of rearing a family and caring for a house, proposed communal arrangements for child care and domestic chores. She influenced fewer women than did Goldman and Sanger, who had begun to advocate free and open instruction in birth control. Birth control, they argued, by gradually reducing the size of the working force, would soon enhance the ability of laborers to bargain with capitalists. Interest in birth control, however, spread largely among women who recognized the physical, social, and psychological advantages of family planning and who were eager to be freed from the demands of the ordinary American home. Under their auspices, the National Birth Control League in 1915 began its attempt through education and lobbying to effect the repeal of state and federal laws that forbade as obscene the dissemination of information about birth control. But like the NAACP, the NBCL was still many years from becoming an effective political force.

The effectiveness of women as individuals—more and more, for example, were attending college and entering the professions of law and medicine—was matched by the effectiveness of the collective demand for women's suffrage. In the second decade of the new century the suffrage movement gained strength under the quiet leadership of Carrie Chapman Catt, president of the American Women's Suffrage Association, and Alice Paul, the more militant head of the new Congressional Union. In 1914 the General Federation of Women's Clubs at last enlisted its significant support for the cause, which was also attracting more and more of those many men who, eager to democratize voting, saw women's suffrage as one part of their program. Indeed, suffrage as an issue came to absorb much of the energy of feminism, to stand out as the central goal of American women. Between 1910 and 1914 they won the ballot in six states and were moving close to the national victory they sought.

Protest and Reform

Prosperous farmers.   The new century brought unparalleled prosperity to American farmers. As domestic and world markets revived, the prices of farm products and the value of farm land just about doubled within a decade. The farmer was still suspicious of bankers, of industry and middlemen, of cities and foreigners. But prosperity tempered farmers' hostilities, softened their rhetoric, turned them from outright attack to flanking maneuvers by which they sought to procure for themselves a larger share both of

urban culture and comforts and of the business profits of agriculture.

Farm organizations continued to press for political reforms designed to give voters a stronger and more direct voice in government. The reforms, they hoped, would help them obtain public policies that would aid agriculture—better roads and marketing facilities, cheaper credit, technical advice on planting and cultivation, more and cheaper electric power, assistance to cooperatives, lower taxes on land, and tariff adjustments that would facilitate sales abroad. Those practical goals, some of which entailed special privileges for farmers, challenged the special privileges and the superior power big business had long enjoyed.

In Washington farm spokesmen continued to urge the creation of agencies to monitor the growth and the practices of the great consolidations. Reflecting the agrarian bias against monopoly, they also urged the enforcement of the languishing antitrust laws. Some farm leaders believed that federal programs of assistance should extend to labor. Thus the objectives of farm politics sometimes merged with the objectives of urban reformers.

Radical critics.   But there remained little of the agrarian radicalism of the 1890s and less of anarchism, which had begun to decline as a cult before the assassination of McKinley revived old, middle-class fears for the safety of the Republic. The radicalism of the early century took other forms.

Socialism consistently gained adherents, especially in the cities, though one strong group flourished for a time in Oklahoma. Most socialists were not proletarians but middle-class, sometimes even quite comfortable, native Americans, though another influential group consisted of New York Jewish immigrants. Intellectuals like Max Eastman and John Reed gave to the Socialist party a brilliant style but recruited few followers. Moderate party leaders like Morris Hillquit in New York and Victor Berger in Milwaukee stood for peaceful, democratic means to effect reform and gradually acquire for the state private means of production, beginning with natural monopolies in such industries as transportation, communications, and utilities. Their program had only a limited appeal to American workers. Most of them still harbored some faith in the American dream of success, at least for their children, and skilled workers identified their interests not with socialist doctrines but with the strategy of trade unionism.

Eugene V. Debs, the engaging head of the Socialist party and its continual candidate for President, employed a stirring rhetoric that mixed Jeffersonian and Marxist principles. But even he was no revolutionary. Nor were the almost one million Americans who supported him in 1912, the year of the party's largest vote.

Suffrage: central goal of American women

Eugene V. Debs: a stirring rhetoric

Further, Debs stood with the moderates in 1913 in expelling from the party's national executive committee "Big Bill" Haywood, who at times advocated industrial sabotage and revolution.

In 1905 Haywood and others had founded the Industrial Workers of the World, the "Wobblies." Determined to organize the most destitute Americans—itinerant farm workers, Western miners (many of whom were immigrants), the primarily immigrant textile workers of the Northeast, and others whom the AFL ignored—the IWW unhesitatingly employed the strike to obtain recognition of industrial unions (unions of all employees in a plant or mine regardless of skills). The industrial union had earlier support from the Knights of Labor and the American Railway Union, and later was advanced by the Congress of Industrial Workers (CIO) of the 1930s. But the AFL preferred trade unions, objected to any dual unionism—that is, to competition between unions for membership—and feared the IWW would give all labor a bad name. IWW rhetoric suggested sympathy for recourse to violence, though the violence of IWW strikes arose largely because of the force with which management resisted. The very appearance of violence disturbed the middle class. Native Americans, moreover, interpreted the combination of the radicalism of the IWW and the union's large immigrant membership as proof of the old stereotype of the immigrant radical. Accordingly, from the time of its founding the IWW knew continued repression from government as well as management. Even occasional victories, as in the Lawrence textile strike of 1912, provided only temporary hopes for the movement's survival.

The growing repression of the Wobblies and the socialists revealed the essential conservatism and ethnocentrism of American culture. The champions of meliorative reform shared those biases with those who opposed any change. But the meliorists, the progressives, in contrast to the stand-patters, advocated reform precisely because they believed that the preservation of American institutions depended on altering them sufficiently to remove the most disturbing injustices in American life.

Politics had not created those injustices, but politics did reflect and sustain them, so politics might also help gradually to erase them. The early twentieth century witnessed a flowering of ideas that politics might implement, ideas that in one way or another struck against the thoughtless behavior and special privileges of the wealthy and their allies, against the selfishness that was generating the corrosive discontent of moderate and radical dissenters alike.

Art and literature of protest. Those ideas took shape as artists, journalists, and social workers exposed the conditions of filth and misery that violated the ideals of middle-class Americans. Realistic literature and art, candid and conscientious journalism, reached the hearts of ladies and gentlemen of good will and helped enlist them in the causes of reform.

Theodore Dreiser, an immigrant's son schooled in poverty, used his powerful novels to describe the barren life of the poor "as simply and effectively as the English language will permit." His *Sister Carrie* (1901), *Jennie Gerhardt* (1911), *The Financier* (1912), and *The Titan* (1914) revealed the human tragedy of inadequate wages, of insecure, hopeless, mechanical existence. Most of Dreiser's characters, driven by greed or

IWW and militia, Lawrence, Massachusetts, 1912

Dangers in The Jungle

Let a man so much as scrape his finger ... in the pickle-rooms, and ... he would have a sore that would put him out of the world; all the joints in his fingers might be eaten by acid.... Of ... all those who used knives you would scarcely find a person who had the use of his thumb.... They would have no nails— they had worn them off pulling hides.... There were men who worked in the cooking-rooms, in the midst of steam and sickening odors ...; in these rooms the germs of tuberculosis might live for two years.... Other men ... worked in tank-rooms full of steam, ... in which there were open vats upon the level of the floor, their peculiar trouble was that they fell into the vats.... Sometimes they would be overlooked for days, till all but the bones of them had gone out to the world as Anderson's Pure Leaf Lard!

From Upton Sinclair, *The Jungle*, 1906.

sex to bestial violence, tried to fight their way into more splendid circumstances, but Dreiser made it poignantly clear how great were the odds against them, how cruel the cost of success, how sorry the lot of those success left behind. Frank Norris, a lesser talent than Dreiser, made his novel *The Octopus* (1901) a vehicle for condemning the inhumane policies of the Southern Pacific Railroad. In spite of the evils he recounted, he professed a faith that "all things . . . work together for good," but he continued his indictment of wealth in *The Pit* (1903). Jack London, a socialist, was optimistic only about the ultimate triumph of those who had lived, as he had, in "the unending limbo of toil." His fellow socialist and novelist Upton Sinclair, writing *The Jungle* (1906) in a similar vein, showed how those who labored in the poisonous world of the Chicago packinghouses "hated their work . . . the bosses . . . the owners . . . the whole place, the whole neighborhood." The poet Carl Sandburg railed at the stockyards and at "Pittsburgh, Youngstown, Gary—they made their steel with men."

Realistic painters, representatives of the "ash-can school," produced canvases that one of their number, John Sloan, called "unconsciously social conscious." Sloan, Robert Henri, William Glackens, George Luks, and others, experimenting with new brush techniques and new relationships of form, found compelling subject matter in dirty alleys, dank saloons, and squalid tenements—"chapters out of life," which they interpreted with beauty that expressed the sorrow and injustice of an experience previously unrecorded in fashionable galleries.

The art of men like Sloan, Sandburg, and Dreiser, for whom social criticism was often a secondary purpose, supplemented and sharpened the message of outraged authors of a deliberate literature of exposure. Social workers, sociologists, and economists recited the facts of poverty in the magazine *Charities and the Commons*; in reports like *The Tenement House Problem* (1903); in books like Robert Hunter's *Poverty* (1904), Father John A. Ryan's *A Living Wage* (1906), John Spargo's *The Bitter Cry of the Children* (1906), Walter Rauschenbusch's *Christianity and the Social Crisis* (1907), and Frances Kellor's *Out of Work* (1915). Those documents demonstrated that between half and two-thirds of all working-class families had incomes too small to buy food, shelter, and clothing—incomes that left nothing for recreation or education, little even for union dues or church contributions. No thoughtful reader of those works could any longer believe that poverty was a function of sloth or moral turpitude; clearly there was something wrong with a society that permitted so much misery while it pretended to a Christian ethic and a generous standard of living.

But humanitarian striving, effective though it was, influenced fewer Americans than did the hortatory, often sensational, journalism of exposure. *McClure's* set the pace for inexpensive, middle-class magazines. It published Ida M. Tarbell's devastating account of the business methods of the Standard Oil Company, Lincoln Steffens' exposés of the role of respectable citizens as well as ward politicians in the corrupt government of a dozen cities and states, Burton J. Hendrick's disclosures of the fraudulent practices of various insurance companies, and Ray Stannard Baker's indictments of railroad mismanagement, labor-baiting in Colorado, and race discrimination in the South. Though other "muckrakers" (the phrase was Theodore Roosevelt's) sometimes enlivened their work with willful exaggerations, they had no need to distort. The bare facts stirred the awakening conscience of middle-class Americans.

Experts and intellectuals. Meanwhile, American intellectuals were formulating the attitudes and techniques on which reform was to rely. These new attitudes, taken together, suggested the need for skepticism about rigid, formal systems of thought. They suggested also the importance of rigorous, dispassionate inquiry as a foundation for knowledge and of constant testing of hypotheses and modification of them on the basis of experience. These principles, derived from the methods of science, were expected to yield ideas for social action. Indeed for the innovative proponents of the developing philosophy of pragmatism, the value of any idea depended on its utility for the thinker and society.

Among the influential intellectuals of the early century, none better stated the case for enlightened skepticism than did Justice Oliver Wendell Holmes, Jr., who recognized that the prejudices of judges often determined their interpretations of the law. Explaining the divergences between law and ethics, Holmes questioned the propensity of courts to upset the decisions of popularly elected legislatures. Though he understood the fallibility of the majority, he preached judicial restraint, for he understood also the judiciary's fallibility and its tendency to traditionalism and arrogance.

The artificiality and formalism of prevalent theories of social Darwinism invited the attack of William James and John Dewey, the fathers of American pragmatism. A psychologist as well as a philosopher, James emphasized the vagaries and the resilience of the mind, and warned against imprisoning intellectual creativity within arbitrary or mechanistic systems. For him the truth of an idea depended on its consequences. Dewey conceived of philosophy as an instrument for guiding action, an instrument he himself used in advocating experimentation in education and government. Tolerance and freedom of belief and of expression, Dewey noted, were essential if ideas were to enjoy a competitive chance to prove their merit.

Thorstein Veblen continued to strip away the façade of contemporary institutions as he had in the nineties. His *The Theory of Business Enterprise* (1904) explained the cultural and economic importance of the machine process, and his *The Instinct of Workmanship* (1914) showed that wasteful and destructive monopolistic practices frustrated man's basic drive to create. Veblen's uncompromising analyses contained insights from which reformers, economists, and sociologists—"social engineers"—were then and later to borrow freely and with reward.

Other less angry and less probing students of contemporary economic institutions directed attention to reform. The writings of John R. Commons on labor, Jeremiah W. Jenks on industry, and William Z. Ripley on railroads were characteristic of moderate, but perceptively critical, scholarship. These experts, often counselors to state and federal regulatory or investigatory commissions, understood that business-managers were not ordinarily bad but that they were too often timid or unimaginative. With Ripley, the economists Henry C. Adams, Richard T. Ely, and Simon Patten viewed human beings not as the creatures of deterministic forces but as the makers of beneficent change. They urged that the principles of management be applied to government and that the state be empowered to solve the public problems business could not.

Reform in the cities and the states. Democratic government had failed most blatantly in American cities. Now municipal-reform organizations, many of them founded in the nineties, succeeded gradually in winning home-rule charters and permission to regulate franchises or to provide for public ownership of vital services. The experiments of Galveston, Texas, with a commission form of government, and of Staunton, Virginia, with a city-manager, demonstrated how efficient these substitutes for an aldermanic system could be. Over a hundred cities had copied them by 1910. Their concern for efficient government took into account the usefulness for public institutions of the methods of professional private management. It also reflected the desire of the urban middle class to reduce their tax burden by cutting city budgets and to decrease the influence of immigrants by abolishing the election of aldermen from wards that contained large foreign-born constituencies. Those concerns complemented the purpose of reformers animated primarily by a desire to root out corruption and to assist the poor. Such men and women drew inspiration from the examples set by mayors like Hazen Pingree of Detroit and Samuel "Golden Rule" Jones of Toledo.

Those developments impinged continually on state government, partly because urban reform could not proceed without improvements in state laws. A wave of reform in the Middle West began in Wisconsin with the election of Robert M. La Follette as governor in 1900. "Battle Bob," who set precedents for the entire region, had tried for years to overcome the regular Republican machine. A loyal party man, he built his own faction of those who shared his worries about the special advantages the state had given many corporations, about high property taxes, and about rising prices. He attracted both a rural and an urban following that was essentially middle class in its background and aspiration. Before he became United States senator in 1906, La Follette made his administration a model of honesty and efficiency, established a fruitful liaison between the government and the state university, whose distinguished faculty included many valuable advisers on public policy, and overcame the opposition of the Old Guard in the legislature. At the governor's urging, Wisconsin passed laws providing for a direct primary, civil service, restrictions on lobbying, conservation, state control of railroads and banks, higher taxes on all corporations

(previously undertaxed), and the first state income tax. Wisconsin had become, as Theodore Roosevelt later said, "the laboratory of democracy."

Progressive government came also to states as diverse, for some examples, as Iowa, Minnesota, the Dakotas, Oregon, Arkansas, Mississippi, Georgia, and South Carolina. Progressive administrations in those states moved, with variations in each case, to institute programs like La Follette's, though in the South the democratization of politics followed the disfranchisement of blacks and many poor whites.

Progressivism won similar victories in Northern industrial states, where much of the impetus for reform came from the middle class of the suburbs as well as the cities. In New Jersey the "New Idea," a local version of progressivism, arose among prosperous suburbanites who were fighting to prevent valuable rapid-transit and other franchises from falling into exploitative hands, to empower a state commission to regulate commutation fares, to extract taxes from corporations (instead of from real estate alone) to defray the costs of public schooling. Objectives like those, along with the characteristic middle-class hostility toward machine politics, brought the New Idea into alliance with the reform mayor of Jersey City, who had built his strength among the workers he befriended. In 1904 the resulting coalition of independent Republicans began to convert New Jersey into a progressive community. In 1910 the state elected a Democratic governor, Woodrow Wilson, and during his administration a bipartisan coalition of progressives completed the program of the New Idea.

New York, Michigan, California, and Ohio, all states with important industrial centers, had political experiences not unlike New Jersey's, though none elected a governor who was so quickly and dramatically successful as Wilson. In the states, as in the nation, progressives looked to a strengthened executive to provide equitable and intelligent solutions for the social and governmental problems of the time. The reformers distrusted legislatures and the interest groups that influenced them; they also distrusted the traditionally conservative courts; but they trusted the people to elect able governors. However transient and frail that faith, reform in the industrial states led to a salubrious restructuring of government and to major improvements for the working force, which cast some of the crucial votes for progress. Before 1915, twenty-five states passed employer-liability laws; five limited the use of injunctions preventing strikes or boycotts; nine passed minimum-wage laws for women; twenty granted pensions to indigent widows with children; others restricted hours and conditions of work.

Progressive attitudes and motives. The strivings of the progressives revealed a great deal about the progressives themselves—their faith in democratic processes, their hostility to large aggregations of private power, their confidence in public regulatory agencies, their belief in efficiency, their humanitarian and moralistic temper. Yet they were a diverse group, and their movement was a concatenation of similar but independent movements. In rural areas, it borrowed much from Populism, and it retained an agrarian flavor modified by time, experience, and prosperity. The traditional middle class of small towns and villages remained skeptical about science, big business, and strong government but often confident about the beneficent possibilities of Prohibition and devices of direct democracy. In the cities, the poor were increasingly conscious of the need to remedy their lot by political action. Still progressivism was more visible as a political expression of the attitudes of liberal intellectuals and lawyers, journalists, and business executives who believed in professionalism in public as well as private life. They often distrusted the masses but counted on an elite to govern in behalf of all people. Such middle-class men and women were both good-hearted and worried. They mobilized partly because they had gained a better understanding of the urgency of social reform, partly because they saw that change was needed if they were to preserve the things they valued. Violence, trembling below the surface of society, threatened the comfortable middle-class world. But the middle class had a chance to remove the inequities that bred disquiet. Further, the state (as those middle-class Americans viewed it) and especially expert agencies created by the state would mediate the tensions between rich and poor, the powerful and the weak.

Rural or urban, many professional and white-collar men and women, many proprietors of small businesses, felt their status and their well-being threatened by the advancing power of big business, big city machines, and—more rarely—big labor. They had to organize to protect themselves and their standing. Mostly native Americans, they resented the immigrant or second-generation political boss. Mostly gentlefolk of modest means and often of old family, they resented the purchased prestige and paraded vulgarity of the newly rich. Though some of them were bureaucrats, successful servants of big business and finance, more of them were the victims of bigness. Where labor unions were strong, as in California, they became targets for the attack on power. More often the attack was pointed toward corporations that dealt directly with many customers—monopolies or near-monopolies selling transportation, utilities, and food—or that were saddled (sometimes unjustly) with especially bad reputations.

Some managers of large corporations realized that reform sentiment might work to their own advantage. Such men, eager to protect the industrial stability they had achieved, worried about the possibility of renewed competition. They recognized that limited and benign federal regulation—for example, of railroading, lumbering, banking, or the manufacture of pharmaceuticals—could restrict the sharp practices of their smaller but aggressive business rivals. Public policy, in that view, instead of being permissive or anti-monopoly, had the potentiality of providing positive guidance for industrial behavior, guidance compatible with the interests of big business. Spokesmen of big business who were also reformers—distinctly a minority of their kind—acted either in pursuit of selfish advantage, or out of a sense of social obligation, or in some cases out of both motives.

Whatever their motives, many Americans who considered themselves progressive reasoned from the unstated, paradoxical premises that were characteristic of their thought. They had a sense of their own special status—whether of wealth or social standing or talent—which they felt they deserved. They also believed in representative government and in the agencies it created. They reconciled those beliefs with the comforting assumption that candidates sympathetic to them would win the confidence of the people. In that assumption, honest businessmen had little to fear from federal regulation of industry, for the regulators would appreciate the problems of those they regulated. Indeed, urban progressives believed that the growth and prosperity of industry, properly disciplined, was essential to the national interest.

The progressives, men and women of many stripes, included many middle-class people, but not all—or even most—middle-class people were progressives. Those who were, were the most socially conscious, perhaps the most anxious, but also, by and large, the younger, the better educated, and the more adventurous. They drew much of their inspiration from the most dynamic national exponent of their spirit and purpose, President Theodore Roosevelt. Without Roosevelt, progressivism would doubtless have happened, but it would not have been nearly so exciting.

The Republican Roosevelt

In September 1901 McKinley died, the third President to be assassinated in less than forty years. His successor, Theodore Roosevelt, whom Mark Hanna had called "that damned cowboy," had set his political course for the White House long before McKinley's death. "It is," wrote Roosevelt, "a dreadful thing to come into the Presidency this way; but it would be a far worse thing to be morbid about it." The gift of the gods to Roosevelt—at forty-two the youngest chief executive in American history—was joy in life, and for seven years he brought that joy to his office.

The son of patrician parents, a graduate of Harvard, an accomplished ornithologist and an enthusiastic historian, Roosevelt chose early in life to make

Theodore Roosevelt: joy in life

politics his career, for he wanted to rule—and he chose to work not as an independent but as a loyal Republican, for he wanted to win. He served successfully, with occasional time out as a rancher in the Dakotas, as an assemblyman in New York, a United States Civil Service commissioner, a New York City police commissioner, Assistant Secretary of the Navy, colonel of the celebrated Rough Riders, and governor of New York. Senator Thomas C. Platt, the long-time boss of the state Republicans, developed serious apprehensions about Roosevelt's successful ventures in reform and managed in 1900 to get him out of New York by arranging his nomination for Vice President, a position Roosevelt accepted with somewhat resigned grace but with characteristic vigor.

Roosevelt and his office. As a campaigner Roosevelt displayed the qualities that were to give him during his Presidency an enormous influence with the people. To the Americans who acclaimed him he was many wonderful things—policeman, cowboy, hero in arms, battler for the everlasting right. He was that toothy grin, that animal energy, that high-pitched voice exhorting the worthy to reform. Roosevelt was also a learned man, receptive to the advice of the men of ideas whom he brought to Washington.

A skilled politician, Roosevelt made the Presidency a great office and used it boldly. He conceived of the President as "a steward of the people bound actively and affirmatively to do all he could for the people." He set out therefore as President to define the great national problems of his time, to propose for each a practicable solution, to win people and Congress to his proposals, and to infuse the executive department with his own dedication to efficient administration and enforcement of the laws.

Roosevelt summoned to federal service a remarkable group of advisers and subordinates. The President's example and support inspired them; his reorganizations of federal agencies gave scope to their talents. They included, among others, Elihu Root, McKinley's Secretary of War whom Roosevelt continued in that office and later made Secretary of State; William Howard Taft, Root's successor in the War Department; Chief Forester Gifford Pinchot and Secretary of the Interior James R. Garfield, both eminent conservationists.

In filling dozens of lesser federal offices, Roosevelt assured his own control of his party. He manipulated patronage so deftly that Mark Hanna had lost control of Republican affairs months before he died in February 1904. By that time Roosevelt, profiting also because he was the incumbent, could count on the support of every important state delegation to the forthcoming national convention. He could rely, too, on the influential party-leaders, for he had satisfied the most urgent demands of the liberal wing without offending or frightening the stand-patters.

Attack on the trusts. Roosevelt, always a gradualist, fashioned a circumspect domestic program, which he dressed in a pungent rhetoric. At the outset of his Administration he indicated that he would accept the advice of the Old Guard in the Senate on tariff and monetary policies, matters about which they were most sensitive. He was himself much more worried about the problems of industrial consolidation. The "absolutely vital question," Roosevelt believed, "was whether the government had power to control" the trusts. The Supreme Court's decision in the E. C. Knight case (1895) suggested that it did not (see p. 462). Seeking a modification of that interpretation, Roosevelt in 1902 ordered his Attorney General, Philander C. Knox, to bring suit for violation of the Sherman Act against the Northern Securities Company.

The President had chosen his target carefully. The Northern Securities Company was a mammoth holding company for the Northern Pacific, the Great Northern, and the Chicago, Burlington, & Quincy railroads. A battle for the stock of the Northern Pacific, key to control of transportation in the Northwest, had led in 1901 to panic on Wall Street. The antagonists made peace by creating the Northern Securities Company for the immediate purpose of quieting the market and for the ultimate purpose of monopolizing the railroads of a rapidly growing region. The contestants had been the titans of finance: J. P. Morgan and Company, the Rockefeller interests, James J. Hill, and E. H. Harriman. The panic they had brought on, a calamity for many brokers, drew attention to their ruthless speculation. The holding company they formed, in which 30 percent of the stock represented only intangible assets, worried the farmers of the Northwest, who, suspicious as ever of monopolies, expected freight rates to soar.

While several states initiated legal action against the holding company, Roosevelt began his preparations in secret. Announcement of the federal government's suit stunned Wall Street. Morgan, with the arrogance of an independent sovereign, tried in vain to have his lawyer settle things with the Attorney General. His failure, like Roosevelt's attack, symbolized a transfer of power from lower New York to Washington. In 1903 a federal court ordered the dissolution of the Northern Securities Company, a decision the Supreme Court sustained the next year. Roosevelt wrote that it was "impossible to overestimate the importance" of the case.

The government proceeded against forty-four more corporations during Roosevelt's term in office. In 1902 action began against the "beef trust," so unpopular with sellers of livestock and buyers of meat.

Equally unpopular were four defendants in cases started in 1906 and 1907, the American Tobacco Company, the Du Pont Corporation, the New Haven Railroad, and the Standard Oil Company.

Roosevelt's revival of the Sherman Act won him a reputation as a "trust-buster," but he never believed that the fragmentation of industry could solve the nation's problems. He had, he felt, to establish the authority of the federal executive to use the antitrust law in cases of monopoly or flagrant misbehavior. Trust-busting, however, was in his view inappropriate in the case of most enterprises that had reduced the cost of production and had won for the nation the industrial leadership of the world. The growth of industry was, he argued, natural, unavoidable, and beneficial. Breaking up corporations whose only offense was size would be impossible unless the government also abolished steam, electricity, large cities, indeed all modern conditions. The need was for continuous, informed, and expert regulation, which only the federal government could properly undertake.

The Square Deal. In December 1901 Roosevelt made his first modest recommendations to Congress for creating the efficient system of control on which, he believed, the orderly development of industrial life depended. The President, like many of the consolidators, had an organizational and a national rather than a local view of economic problems, and a confidence in expert management rather than in popular sentiment. Where some consolidators of that mind looked to the federal government to enhance its authority in order to further their needs, Roosevelt favored that enhancement in order to advance what he considered the public interest. Yet his was not primarily an adversary stance. The public interest, as he saw it, did not call for federal punishment of business but for federal regulation to prevent the abuses of predatory business, and thereby to encourage the productive energies of responsible business.

Roosevelt asked first for an act to expedite antitrust prosecutions, which Congress passed in 1903. Without opposition it then also enacted his proposal for forbidding the granting or receiving of rebates, a practice that powerful shippers had forced upon unwilling railroads. The railroads had wanted the protection they received, as did most shippers. More serious opposition developed to Roosevelt's major objective, the creation of a new Department of Commerce and Labor with a Bureau of Corporations empowered to gather and release information about industry. Such a bureau was essential if the government was to learn what businesses to regulate and how. On that account, conservative Republican senators blocked Roosevelt's bill, though many congressmen preferred it to more stringent measures then under consideration. The President saved his bill by announcing that John D. Rockefeller was secretly organizing the opposition to it. The culprit was actually one of Rockefeller's subordinates, but the purport of Roosevelt's charge was accurate, and the consequent public clamor accelerated the passage of the controversial law.

The new act gave to the Bureau of Corporations authority to investigate significant public issues, as that bureau did, for example, in finding the facts on which Roosevelt later based his hydroelectric policy. For its part, the Bureau of Labor, also primarily a fact-finding agency, demonstrated its usefulness to Roosevelt and to workers by its fair reporting during the strike of anthracite-coal miners that began in May 1902 and lasted until October. The managers of the Eastern coal-carrying railroads that owned most of the mines would not negotiate with the union, the United Mine Workers, which was demanding recognition, an eight-hour day, and a 10 to 20 percent increase in pay. Labor's orderly conduct and willingness to arbitrate won growing public approval, particularly after the intransigent owners, speaking through George F. Baer, the president of the Reading Railroad, insisted that "God in his Infinite Wisdom has given control of the property interests" to the directors of large corporations. This attitude invited public antagonism at a time when fuel was short and the days were growing chilly.

Roosevelt, sympathetic to the workers and worried about the coal shortage, had hesitated to enter the dispute only because his advisers felt that he lacked the legal authority. Early in October he summoned the mine-operators and John Mitchell, the union chief, to the White House. Mitchell again offered to submit to arbitration, but the owners remained obdurate. Indeed, they demanded that the President issue an injunction and, if necessary, use the army to end the strike. Their "arrogant stupidity" provoked Roosevelt instead to let them know indirectly that he was prepared to use troops to dispossess them and produce coal. With this kind of intervention in the offing, Mark Hanna, Elihu Root, and other conservative men quickened their efforts for peace, enlisted the help of J. P. Morgan himself, and persuaded the mine-owners to accept a compromise settlement. By its terms the miners resumed work, and a commission appointed by the President arbitrated the questions at issue. In March the commission awarded labor a 10 percent raise, a reduction in working hours to nine and in some cases eight per day, but not recognition of the union. The owners in return received a welcome invitation to raise coal prices 10 percent. Roosevelt was the first President to bring both labor and capital to the White House to settle a dispute, the first to get them both to accept the judgment of a commission appointed by the executive, the first to coerce the owners of a crucial industry by threatening to take it over. All this contrasted vividly with the course of the federal government during the Pullman strike (see p. 471).

In other labor episodes, Roosevelt insisted on the open shop for government-workers and resisted not only radical unionism but even the principle of the union shop in industry. He believed, as he put it, in "the right of laboring men to join a union . . . without illegal interference." This was less than Gompers advocated, but it was more than most businessmen or conservative politicians were yet willing to concede. It was a position characteristic of Roosevelt—advanced but not radical, cautious but not timorous.

His purpose during the coal strike, Roosevelt explained during the campaign of 1904, had been to give both sides a "square deal." The phrase became a familiar label for his Administration, and for his intention to abolish privilege and enlarge individual opportunity. His "natural allies," he said, were "the farmers, small businessmen and upper-class mechanics," middle-class Americans "fundamentally sound, morally, mentally and physically." Like him, they abhorred extremes; like him, they judged in moral terms. They warmed to Roosevelt's fusillades against those he later called the "malefactors of great wealth." They accepted and cheered his image of himself as a champion of fairness.

The election of 1904. That was the basis of his campaign. It was the basis, too, for his appointment to office of qualified men from minority groups—blacks, Catholics, Jews, Americans of Hungarian and German and Irish extraction. His appreciation of the inherent dignity in every human being encouraged him to invite to the White House Booker T. Washington, the Negro educator who doubled as an adviser on patronage. Yet like almost all Americans of his generation, Roosevelt believed that black men and women were lesser people than whites. Washington did not again receive an invitation to the White House. Much worse, in 1906 the President revealed a cruel prejudice by discharging without honor black troops who refused to reveal the names of a few of their fellows who had allegedly shot up the antiblack town of Brownsville, Texas. That hasty and unjust decision reflected the racism of the army, which Roosevelt shared. American blacks properly resented the ruling, but it was not reversed until 1972.

In 1904, an election year, there was a convenient compatibility between Roosevelt's conscience and the needs of politics. That did not detract from his conscience, though it manifestly strengthened his campaign. He took no chances. A new pension order, making age alone a sufficient qualification for eligibility, held the GAR to the GOP. The official platform contained standard Republican platitudes about the tariff and prosperity, sops to the Old Guard, as was the lackluster nominee for Vice President, Senator Charles W. Fairbanks of Indiana. Taken together, the platform and the ticket strengthened the basis of the successful Republican coalition of the late 1890s. But the real platform was Roosevelt's record, and the real issue was the man.

That made things difficult for the Democrats. As Bryan complained, Roosevelt had captured his banner. The Republicans now marched as the party of reform. Conservative Democrats returned to the formulas of Grover Cleveland's days, to a platform emphasizing strict construction of the Constitution and a candidate—Judge Alton B. Parker—chosen for his safe views and close ties to New York wealth.

Parker conducted a dull campaign until the vision of impending defeat persuaded him to charge that Roosevelt's campaign-manager, George B. Cortelyou, was blackmailing corporations for contributions. Cortelyou, who had been Secretary of Commerce, had indeed had access to the findings of the Bureau of Corporations, but he neither resorted to blackmail nor needed to. Wealthy Republicans, loyal party men in spite of their reservations about Roosevelt, had responded without stint to the usual appeals for funds. Parker's charges reminded the electorate that Roosevelt's campaign was well endowed but served otherwise only to provoke from the President an indignant denial. Indeed, Roosevelt directed his party treasurer to return any contributions that had come from predatory wealth. The treasurer ignored the order, just as the voters by and large ignored Parker's accusations. Roosevelt could have won without much financial support. In a landslide victory, he received 57.4 percent of the popular votes (7,628,461) to Parker's 37.6 percent (5,084,223), and 336 electoral votes to the Democrat's 140.

Roosevelt and Reform

Government and business. When Congress convened in December 1904, the progress of reform in Washington and in the states was gathering momentum. President now in his own right, Roosevelt took advantage of the mandate he had helped to create. His prime objective was railroad regulation. Decisions of the Supreme Court had stripped the Interstate Commerce Commission of authority over railway rates or rebates, which the roads continued to grant in spite of the government's efforts to enforce the antirebate act of 1903. The only feasible remedy was to give the com-

mission power to set reasonable and nondiscriminatory rates and to prevent inequitable practices. Farmers and small businessmen and their representatives were demanding that remedy. Some railroad managers saw advantages in dealing with a single federal authority rather than with many state commissions, but even they preferred final decisions to rest with the conservative judiciary rather than with the ICC. Further, most railroads, their privileged customers, and the devotees of conservative economic theory opposed federal rate-making, which would for the first time in American history give the national government authority to determine prices, the sacrosanct prerogative of private enterprise.

For Roosevelt, laissez-faire theory was not sacred, but moral corporate behavior was. In 1904 and 1905 he urged Congress to endow the ICC with the power to adjust rates against which shippers had complained. During the long debate that ensued, Roosevelt advanced his purpose skillfully. Concentrating on the railroad issue, he gave up a tentative plan for a downward revision of the tariff, which agrarian Republicans as well as Democrats favored. The President had never considered the tariff a vital matter, for in his opinion it was not a moral question. It was, however, an issue that divided his party. So, rather than risk division, he conceded to the Old Guard on tariff reform. At least partly on that account, the House of Representatives passed the President's railroad bill by an overwhelming margin.

Handling the Senate was more difficult, for the Old Guard delayed a vote while the railroads underwrote a national publicity campaign, which Roosevelt answered in a series of vigorous speeches. In 1906 he outmaneuvered his opponents and, after few modifications, the Hepburn Act carried. It gave the ICC the authority upon complaint from a shipper to set aside existing rates and to prescribe substitutes, subject to court review. As it worked out during the next several years, the courts did not overrule the commission. The act was less than the most vocal critics of the roads had wanted, for they advocated the physical valuation of railway properties as the proper basis for rate-making. But the act was just what Roosevelt was after. It was a keystone in his intended system of continuous, expert federal regulation of American industry.

Congress in 1906 passed several notable laws. One was an employer-liability act for the District of Columbia and all common carriers. Another was a pure-food-and-drug bill, whose chief exponent was Dr. Harvey W. Wiley of the Department of Agriculture. For several years this measure, twice approved by the House, had faltered. Now a series of articles by Samuel Hopkins Adams exposed the dangers of patent medicine, aroused public opinion, and speeded the enactment of the legislation, though appropriations for its enforcement remained inadequate for two decades.

In a similar way, the publication of Upton Sinclair's *The Jungle*, with its description of the scandalous conditions in meatpacking houses, led Roosevelt to order a special investigation. This confirmed Sinclair's findings and precipitated the passage of a federal meat-inspection law. The act revealed the crosscurrents of purpose that characterized the cautious reform of the Roosevelt era. Sinclair had hoped to obtain remedy for the exploited workers, but the statute ignored them. Progressive senators like Beveridge of Indiana had wanted the packers to pay for federal inspection, but the legislation left the cost with the government, and Congress in later years appropriated stingy sums for enforcement. The large packers, in some cases before the act was passed, in all cases thereafter, preferred unitary federal inspection to irregular and uneven inspections by the many states in which they had plants. The packers also expected that federal inspection would discipline small establishments that could not afford sanitary methods. But those small concerns continued to function in intrastate commerce. Further, though the large packers were eager to retain and enlarge their European markets, Roosevelt threatened that goal by publishing reports about conditions in the meat industry. For his part, the President, who turned to the whole issue rather late, used his influence to keep the House of Representatives, where the packers had interested friends, from subjecting meat inspection to broad judicial review. All in all, then, the legislation, like the Hepburn Act and the Pure Food and Drug Act, constituted at best a partial victory for each of the various principals involved. The laws improved the structure of federal relationships in the industries affected, but they were at best, as Roosevelt said, not an ultimate reform but a first step toward a purpose that might require many more. A first step, he believed, was far better than none at all.

In 1906 Roosevelt also sent Congress a series of recommendations, addressed in large part to social reform, on which it did not act. Labor problems were much on his mind. He proposed the abolition of child labor and an effective workmen's-compensation law. The National Association of Manufacturers had won a number of victories in its drive to cripple unions by obtaining injunctions against strikes and boycotts, the unions' most effective weapons. The NAM was also exhorting legislators to oppose all labor legislation. Fighting back, Gompers and his associates submitted to Roosevelt and the Congress a Bill of Grievances voicing their traditional demands, especially for relief from injunctions granted under the Sherman Act. The American Federation of Labor struck politically

as well, campaigning in 1906 against congressmen unfriendly to labor, most of whom were Republicans. Caught between his growing sympathy for labor's goals and his partisan loyalties, Roosevelt endorsed all Republican candidates but exhorted them to mend their ways.

New programs and the Old Guard. The gulf between the President and the Old Guard widened in 1907 and 1908. They especially differed over conservation. In 1902 Roosevelt, an ardent conservationist, had spurred the passage of the Newlands Act, which set aside a portion of receipts from the sale of public lands for expenditures on dams and reclamation. Pushing on, largely on the advice of Gifford Pinchot, he had withdrawn from private entry valuable coal and mineral lands, oil reserves, and waterpower sites. He had proceeded vigorously against cattlemen and lumbermen who were poaching on public preserves. These policies offended the Western barons who had become rich by exploiting the nation's natural resources (see pp. 444–45). In 1907 their representatives attached a rider to an appropriation bill for the Department of Agriculture that prevented the creation of new forest reserves in six Western states without the consent of Congress. Roosevelt had to sign the bill, for the department had to have funds, but before signing he added 17 million acres to the national reserves. He later vetoed bills that granted waterpower sites to private interests but that did not provide for federal supervision of waterpower development.

In 1908 Roosevelt called a National Conservation Congress, which forty-four governors and hundreds of experts attended. It led to annual meetings of governors and to the creation of state conservation commissions. Congress, more and more hostile, ignored recommendations for river and flood control made by the Inland Waterways Commission, which Roosevelt appointed, and refused to provide funds to publish the report of another of his boards, the Country Life Commission, which advocated federal assistance for rural schools, roads, rural electrification, and farmers' cooperatives. Yet Roosevelt had succeeded in making the conservation of human and natural resources an issue of the first importance to thousands of Americans. He believed in the preservation of threatened species and of areas of great natural beauty. He believed just as strongly in conservation for use. In protecting natural resources from ruthless private exploitation, he intended to assure their use to meet the needs of both his own and later generations. Further, he shared the spirit of progressive reform that stressed the ability of the human mind and will to alter and improve the environment. Conservation provided an obvious laboratory for testing that belief.

Roosevelt's general policies jarred many businessmen who blamed him for the financial panic that occurred in the autumn of 1907 and for the brief depression that preceded and followed it. The basic causes of the slump were beyond his control. Productive facilities had expanded beyond the country's immediate capacity to consume, but the differential would probably have led to no serious trouble if the nation's banking and monetary systems had been stronger and if financiers had not been guilty of speculative excesses. Panic began only after depositors learned that several New York trust companies had failed in an expensive attempt to corner the copper market. As runs began on these and other (sound) banks, some had to close and all had to call in loans from creditors in New York and throughout the country. J. P. Morgan, at his most magnificent in this crisis, supervised a pooling of the funds of the leading Manhattan banks to support the threatened institutions. Undoubtedly this action prevented general disaster.

Morgan and his fellows could not have succeeded without assistance from the Treasury Department, which moved government deposits into threatened New York banks. The complex maneuvers depended in part on the purchase by the United States Steel Corporation of controlling shares of stock in the Tennessee Coal and Iron Company. That transaction, however, was unthinkable if there was any danger that it might lead immediately to an antitrust suit. So informed, Roosevelt, without making "any binding promise," urged Morgan's associates to proceed.

Though the panic quickly subsided, it had demonstrated the urgency of financial reform. It was ridiculous for a great nation in a time of crisis to have to fall back on Morgan or any other private banker.

And it was vital to relax the general monetary stringency that intensified the crisis. Both the President and his detractors endorsed the action of Congress authorizing a commission, with Senator Nelson Aldrich as chairman, to study and report on monetary and banking policy.

Roosevelt meanwhile had condemned the "speculation, corruption and fraud" that contributed to the panic. His messages to Congress of December 1907 and January 1908 disclosed his zeal for further reform. Indeed, he now favored measures that he would have considered radical a few years earlier—measures that seemed far too sweeping to the conservatives who dominated Congress. After repeating many of his earlier recommendations, the President called for federal incorporation and regulation of all interstate business, federal regulation of the stock market, limitation of injunctions against labor, compulsory investigation of labor disputes, extension of the eight-hour law for federal employees, and imposition of personal income and inheritance taxes. He went on to castigate the courts for declaring unconstitutional a workmen's-compensation law and to condemn "predatory wealth" for its follies and its unscrupulous opposition to "every measure for honesty in business." Roosevelt in private warned that a revolution would break out if rich men and blind judges made the lot of the worker intolerable. Without reform, capitalism could not survive.

The social reforms to which Roosevelt gave increasing emphasis in his last years in office depended for success on the political reforms he had been pursuing. Power, he knew, was the essence of politics. For him, political reform meant the shift of power from private hands, not accountable to the public, toward government; from states and localities, lacking broad jurisdictions, toward Washington; from the unrepresentative Supreme Court and from an inexpert and inefficient Congress toward the President—who was representative of all the people and positioned to command expert counsel. Those changes, Roosevelt believed, necessary in themselves, would also enhance prospects for progressive social goals.

He did not invent those goals, but he gave them effective expression, put the dignity of his high office at their service, and converted to them the thousands who felt the vitality of his person. All this he did with a faith in the progress that conserves, a conviction that the holder of power has an obligation to promote justice and enforce orderly and moral behavior, and a confidence in his own ability to handle power to those ends. Those beliefs and that confidence also guided his foreign policy.

Roosevelt and World Power

Power, empire, and responsibility During the first decade of the twentieth century, more and more Americans, including those who considered themselves progressives, subscribed to a new doctrine of manifest destiny (see p. 527). Along with that concept there grew up other ideas about the international role of the United States. The writings of Alfred T. Mahan, the experience of the Spanish War, and awareness of the swelling ambitions and power of Germany and Japan persuaded an influential minority of Americans of the importance of naval preparedness and national defense. Some, like Roosevelt, Root, and Senator Henry Cabot Lodge, also believed that every powerful nation had a stake in world order and an obligation to preserve it, that a great country like the United States could not escape involvement in international affairs.

Roosevelt as President continually reminded Americans of the oneness of the world. Nineteenth-century progress in transportation, communication, and production, he warned, had created situations of potential chaos in which only the availability of power and, when necessary, the application of force could establish a tolerable equilibrium.

He therefore preached preparedness to the frequently reluctant public. For Roosevelt, preparedness was not simply militarism. It entailed, too, the preservation and development of natural and human resources. Sharing the Anglo-Saxon bias of his time, Roosevelt urged Americans of old stock to increase their birth rate. But all Americans, regardless of national origin, could contribute, he maintained, to national well-being if they saw to their physical fitness and cultivated clear minds, clean souls, and brave hearts.

High character and the strenuous life were not in themselves enough, for preparedness ultimately involved the size, equipment, and leadership of the military services. The President heartily supported the reform of the outmoded army organization that Secretary of War Root had begun to plan under McKinley. Root set up an Army War College, demanded rigorous tests for the promotion of officers, and in 1902 asked Congress to authorize the creation of a general staff and the incorporation of the state militia into the regular army. Congress rejected the plan for the militia, but approved a general staff that began to direct the modernization of the army.

Roosevelt also demanded the construction of a modern navy strong enough to protect American interests and to further his "large view" of national obligations. The United States, he realized, could no longer depend on the British fleet for protection. It had to keep pace with the building programs of Japan and Germany and with rapid changes in naval technology. Before Roosevelt left office, Congress acceded to his constant prodding. The navy and army profited, too, from the enthusiastic recognition the President gave to military service and to dedicated and imaginative commanders like General Leonard Wood and Commander William S. Sims.

A strong nation, in Roosevelt's view, had the duty of imposing civilization and justice in the backward territories it ruled. In the Insular cases of 1900 and 1901, the Supreme Court held that inhabitants of the recently acquired American empire were not American citizens and did not have a right to the liberties guaranteed by the Constitution unless Congress expressly conferred them. Except for Hawaii and Alaska, which were destined for statehood, the Court's rulings left the determination of colonial policy to the Roosevelt Administration. It adopted a variety of expedients. The navy administered Guam and Tutuila, where it had coaling stations. Puerto Rico elected its own house of delegates, though its decisions had to be confirmed by a council and executed by a governor appointed in Washington. The American protectorate in Cuba ended in May 1902 with the inauguration of the first government under Cuba's new constitution. The next year, however, a formal treaty between Cuba and the United States provided for American intervention in the event of a foreign threat or domestic disturbance. Insurrection in Cuba in 1906 persuaded Roosevelt to exercise the right of intervention. After three years the Americans withdrew their troops but retained a major naval base at Guantanamo and continued to exercise a monitory influence over Cuban policy. Earlier, the President had insisted that in return for the rights accorded by the Cuban treaty, the United States had a moral duty to aid the Cuban economy by granting special tariff rates to Cuban sugar, a concession he wrung from protectionist congressmen after a stiff legislative struggle in 1903.

He was unable, in spite of repeated attempts, to obtain tariff concessions for the Philippines. Those islands presented a number of difficult problems. Occasional episodes of cruelty by the American army during the suppression of the independence movement (see p. 538) had whetted native resentment. That resentment began to abate (though for a brief time the revolt continued) when Congress in 1902 passed an organic act for the Philippines, when Roosevelt abolished the office of military governor, and when William Howard Taft, the first civilian governor, proclaimed a general amnesty. A patient proconsul, Taft got along well with the elected assembly and furthered municipal home rule, improvements in public health, civil affairs, education, and transportation. He was successful, too, in delicate negotiations with the Vatican and with Catholic friars in the islands for the purchase of lands that the Church claimed but the Filipinos held and deserved to keep. Like Roosevelt and Root, Taft believed the Philippines would not be ready for independence for many years. Though native patriots and American anti-imperialists remained impatiently committed to that goal, Taft's benign administration gradually won the confidence of the islanders, assisted the development of their economy, and helped them prepare for ultimate self-government. Still, the inability of Roosevelt and his associates to understand the urgency of sentiment for self-government among subject peoples made American policy,

as it developed, indistinguishable from the imperialism of European powers.

Policing the Caribbean. Roosevelt's foreign policies, like his colonial policies, were derived from his assumption that it was "incumbent on all civilized and orderly powers to insist on the proper policing of the world." This was, of course, a highhanded assumption, which Roosevelt defended when he had to by arguing that only with stability could there be justice. An imperious manner characterized his methods as well as his objectives. As President, he believed, he had to conduct foreign policy himself, for in that field the Congress and "the average American" did not "take the trouble to think carefully or deeply."

Stretching his constitutional authority to its limits, Roosevelt intervened to preserve stability and American hegemony in the Caribbean, where, with Mahan, he felt the United States could not afford a rival. Like other small states in that area, Venezuela had borrowed money in Europe, which Cipriano Castro, its prodigal dictator—Roosevelt considered him a "villainous little monkey"—lacked either the means or the will to repay. In December 1902 England, Germany, and Italy, demanding payment for their citizens, blockaded Venezuela and fired on one of its ports. Venezuela asked the United States to arrange arbitration, to which England and Germany agreed. But a German ship again bombarded a port, and later Germany briefly opposed referring the dispute to arbi-

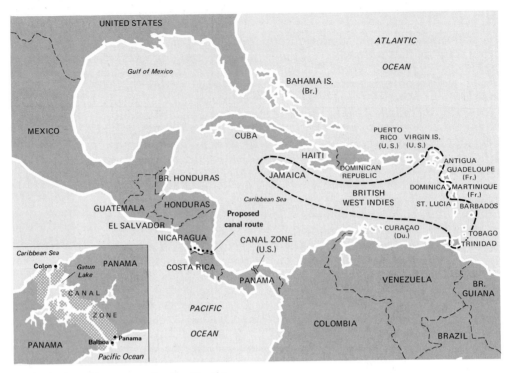

UNITED STATES

ATLANTIC

OCEAN

Gulf of Mexico

BAHAMA IS.
(Br.)

MEXICO

CUBA

PUERTO
RICO VIRGIN IS.
(U.S.) (U.S.)

HAITI

ANTIGUA
GUADELOUPE
(Fr.)

DOMINICAN
REPUBLIC

JAMAICA

DOMINICA MARTINIQUE
(Fr.)

BR. HONDURAS

BRITISH
WEST INDIES

ST. LUCIA BARBADOS

Caribbean Sea

GUATEMALA HONDURAS

**Proposed
canal route**

EL SALVADOR

CURAÇAO
(Du.)

NICARAGUA

CANAL ZONE
(U.S.)

TOBAGO
TRINIDAD

Caribbean Sea

Colon

PANAMA

COSTA RICA

*Gatun
Lake*

VENEZUELA

BR.
GUIANA

CANAL

PANAMA

ZONE

PACIFIC

OCEAN

COLOMBIA

BRAZIL

PANAMA

Balboa Panama

Pacific Ocean

International interests in the Caribbean

tration. Roosevelt implied to the German ambassador that the United States would insist on that solution. The President did not intend to permit Germany or any other European power to use the excuse of debt collection for establishing a foothold in the Caribbean. He was determined to make that region an American area of influence.

The best way to keep Europe at home, the President believed, was to keep order in the Caribbean. That purpose gave Roosevelt a flimsy pretext for incontinent behavior in Panama. In December 1901 the Senate approved the second Hay-Pauncefote Treaty by which England acknowledged the right of the United States alone to build and fortify an isthmian canal, so long an American dream. Such a canal would facilitate intercoastal shipping and would make it easier for the navy to move from ocean to ocean. The preferred route had at one time been through Nicaragua, where a sea-level canal could be built, but the commission of experts that Congress had authorized had come to prefer a lock canal through Panama, which would provide the cheapest and shortest route between the coasts of the United States. Accordingly, in June 1902 Congress directed the President to negotiate with Colombia for the acquisition of a strip of land in Panama, provided that the old French canal company, which had begun work decades earlier, agreed to sell the United States its titles and equities in the area on reasonable terms. Members of the American commission had valued the French holdings at not more than $40

million, only half of the company's own official estimate, but the company gratefully accepted the revised figure.

With that matter settled, Roosevelt pressed Colombia to surrender control of the land in return for $10 million and an annual rental of $250,000. A treaty to that effect was rejected by the Colombian government, which wanted more money and greater rights of sovereignty in the zone. Roosevelt, outraged at what he considered "blackmail," though the Colombian request was scarcely that, let it be known privately that he would smile upon insurrection in Panama. Predictably, in November 1903 insurrection occurred (if it had not, the President was prepared to ask Congress for authority to take the zone from Colombia). The United States aided the revolutionists and immediately recognized the new, independent Republic of Panama, which promptly accepted Roosevelt's terms for a canal zone.

Roosevelt later boasted that he "took Panama," and most Americans at the time condoned his behavior. But the episode was a national disgrace. There was even suspicion of scandal. Agents of the French company, eager to unload their otherwise worthless assets, had influenced the State Department and members of Congress to favor the Panama route and had helped to foment the insurrection. Roosevelt's ruthless pursuit of his own interpretation of national advantage was no more ethical than was their pursuit of profit. Yet he argued that he had stamped out lawlessness in Colombia and disorder in Panama. Thus he used his insistence on stability in the Caribbean as a rationalization for imperialism.

He did have a clear strategic purpose—the control of the Caribbean as one essential part of national defense. That purpose imbued his message to Congress of December 1904, in which he announced that the United States would not interfere with Latin American nations that conducted their affairs with decency, but that "brutal wrongdoing" might require intervention by some civilized power, and that the United States could not "ignore this duty." The Monroe Doctrine told Europe to stay out of the Americas; the Roosevelt Corollary asserted that the United States had a right to move in. In 1905 Roosevelt interceded in Santo Domingo to end the cycle there of debt, revolu-

tion, and default. He imposed American supervision of customs collections and finance and established a trust fund to repay the European-held debt. The convention containing those terms was blocked in the United States Senate, which was growing restive under the President's single-handed conduct of foreign affairs, but Roosevelt substituted an executive agreement and protected his policy until the Senate accepted a modified treaty in 1907.

The balance of power. The international police power that Roosevelt arrogated to the United States he expected other civilized nations to exercise elsewhere—Japan in Korea, England in Egypt and India. Stable and prosperous nations, however, had in his view no right to proceed against one another. World order depended on their restraint and on the shifting balances of their power. British restraint preserved the growing Anglo-American entente during a dispute about the Alaskan boundary. Canada in 1902 claimed Alaskan lands that cut off newly discovered Canadian gold fields from the sea. Roosevelt rightly judged the claim weak, but he wounded Canadian sensibilities by his blustering refusal to arbitrate (for, he said, arbitration usually resulted "in splitting the difference"). To help Canadian officials save face, in 1903 he submitted the issue to negotiation but instructed the commissioners he appointed to concede nothing. He also took pains to inform London of his order. The single English commissioner voted with the three Americans against the two Canadians, thereby straining temporarily the bonds of empire but serving both the merits of the issue and the cause of transatlantic friendship.

As he contemplated the balance of power in Europe, Roosevelt was grateful for England's friendship, dubious about Russia's immediate strength (though he recognized its great potential), and more and more anxious about Germany. Had the Kaiser had the "instinct for the jugular," Roosevelt thought, he would have kept a sharp eye on Russia. As it was, Germany was more jealous of France and England, and the Kaiser entertained "red dreams of glory" that might disrupt Europe and thus the whole world.

Aware of the network of European alliances that would engage every major continental power in a contest between any two, the President worried about the tensions that flared in 1905 over French and German rivalry in Morocco. The Kaiser secretly asked Roosevelt to persuade England not to support France. The President at first hesitated, for, as he said, the United States had "no real interest in Morocco." It did have a major stake in preserving peace, however, and Roosevelt carried on the difficult negotiations that brought all parties, including the United States, to a conference at Algeciras, Spain, in January 1906.

Roosevelt's instructions to the American delegates revealed his concern about German ambitions and his conviction that the entente cordiale between France and England preserved the essential balance of power in Europe. Though American participation had little effect on the outcome of the conference, at which France won a diplomatic victory, Roosevelt's role was nevertheless significant. He had served peace. Furthermore, he had demonstrated to Europe and to the American people, many of whom criticized his departure from the course of isolation, that the President of the United States recognized the nation's legitimate interest in any European crisis.

In Asia, Roosevelt judged, slumbering China was of no account, but to prevent dislocations of power he accepted the prevailing fiction of its territorial integrity, and he gave lip service to the principle of the Open Door. He was little interested in Chinese markets, but to stabilize the Orient politically he counted on a balance between Russia and Japan. He welcomed an Anglo-Japanese defensive alliance of 1902, which committed both signatories to preserve the status quo in Asia. In 1904, when the Russo-Japanese War began, he feared that a Russian triumph would be "a blow to civilization," but the elimination of Russia's "moderative influence" on Japan would be equally unfortunate. That possibility seemed imminent after Japan's initial naval and land victories and the outbreak of revolution in Russia. Though Roosevelt was partial to the Japanese, he intensified his effort through mediation to arrange a peace that would preserve an equilibrium. Proceeding without the knowledge of Congress, he worked secretly and deftly through personal friends in the diplomatic corps of Japan, Germany, and Great Britain. By the summer of 1905 Russian distress and Japanese financial infirmity brought both belligerents to accept a peace conference at Portsmouth, New Hampshire.

The President's brilliant diplomacy continued at the conference, which produced a settlement that suited his purpose and earned him a Nobel Prize for Peace. Japan took over the southern half of the island of Sakhalin, Port Arthur, and the South Manchuria Railroad, but Manchuria remained legally a part of China, where the Open Door in theory still permitted all nations to trade and invest. Russia retained effective control over northern Manchuria and all of Siberia, the source of its basic weight in Asian politics. The Japanese failed to get the huge indemnity they had wanted, which made the treaty and Roosevelt the object of considerable public criticism in Japan. But the Japanese government was satisfied, particularly because the United States, like Russia, had recognized Japan's primacy in Korea.

Also in 1905 Taft and Japanese Foreign Minister Taro Katsura reached an agreement by which the United States acknowledged Japan's occupation of Korea and Japan disavowed any ambitions in the Philippines. This, too, was a victory for the President's realistic and essentially cautious diplomacy. Though he sometimes sounded fierce, he never undertook ventures beyond his means to execute them. The United States, he knew, lacked the means to interfere in Korea, and Japan had to be kept friendly or it could easily conquer the Philippines, which Congress would not arm.

Japanese-American relations might have remained excellent had it not been for the problem of immigration. In 1900 Tokyo agreed to deny passports to emigrant laborers bound for the United States. But Japanese workers continued to make their way to the

West Coast through Hawaii, Mexico, and Canada. In California anti-Japanese feeling rose. In 1906 San Francisco segregated Asian school children. The proud Japanese protested officially to Washington. Roosevelt assured them that he had no sympathy with the "outrageous agitation" of the Californians. He could not, however, silence the yellow press or the "idiots" in the California legislature. Yet he was unwilling to ask the Japanese to concede any racial inferiority. The State Department resolved the crisis by negotiating the "Gentlemen's Agreement" of 1907, an official but informal understanding that bound both countries to stop direct immigration between them.

This crisis focused attention on the whole immigration question. In large degree Roosevelt shared the common prejudice against the unrestricted entry of southern and eastern Europeans and Asians. Still, he feared that a general debate about immigration in 1906 would complicate relations with Japan and possibly divide the Republicans, some of whom were urging enactment of a literacy test for immigrants. He recommended the appointment of a fact-finding commission, a solution that would delay debate, appease the restrictionists, and, he believed, throw light on a complex subject. In 1907 Congress authorized such a commission. Its members, under the chairmanship of Senator Dillingham, approached their task with a formidable bias for the restriction of immigration.

Besides provoking a debate on immigration policy, the Japanese-American crisis stirred up loose talk of war. The President was apparently worried in 1907 about Japan's intentions. His anxiety may have been contrived to stir Congress into pushing ahead with the naval building program. There was no genuine need for alarm, although years later Roosevelt said that he had detected "a very, very slight undertone of veiled truculence" in Japan's communications. "It was essential," he then decided, "that we should have it clearly understood by our own people especially, but also by other peoples, that the Pacific was as much our home waters as the Atlantic." He sent the battle fleet around the world to make his point clear.

Had Japan been belligerent, it could have demolished the American ships that entered Tokyo Bay. Instead it welcomed them heartily. Yet Roosevelt believed their presence curbed any Japanese urge toward aggression and was therefore "the most important service" he ever rendered to peace. It certainly exemplified one of his favorite adages: "Speak softly but carry a big stick." Good will rather than fear led the Japanese ambassador to propose a declaration of friendship. In the Root-Takahira Agreement of 1908, the United States acknowledged Japan's special interest in Manchuria, and both nations promised to uphold the status quo in the Pacific and to respect the Open Door and China's territorial integrity.

Prospects for American commerce and investment in China, the objectives of the Open Door, remained important to the Department of State, but the President, according to his own account, was concerned primarily with the balance of power in the Pacific. "A council of war never fights," Roosevelt wrote in his *Autobiography*, "and in a crisis the duty of a leader is to lead." As President he personally conducted the nation's foreign policies, acting sometimes with skill, sometimes with daring, sometimes with scant regard for the opinion of public or Congress or for the rights or sensitivities of other nations. His magisterial manner and imperialistic ventures set potentially dangerous precedents that his critics deplored. Still, as he asserted, the United States had become part of an interdependent world; the use of force could keep isolated trouble spots from erupting into general war; power was a pervasive element in world affairs and the United States had a vital interest in preserving the balance of power in Europe as well as in Asia. As Roosevelt saw it, the United States, a powerful nation, had also an obligation to keep its power in a state of readiness and, when necessary, to use it intelligently but with restraint.

The election of 1908. No harm came from the concentration of power in one man's hands, Roosevelt observed, "provided the holder does not keep it for more than a certain, definite time, and then returns it to the people from whom he sprang." An American President, he believed, should serve only two terms. So he had announced in 1904 that he would not run again, and, though he gloried in his office, he resisted the strong sentiment for his renomination in 1908 and used his power in the party to ensure the nomination of William Howard Taft, whom he had selected as the man most able to continue his policies.

The President's endorsement and Taft's own excellent reputation kept the party united. With the tide of progressivism rising, the Democrats turned again to Bryan, who ran with more prudence but less vigor than before. He had the support of the leaders of organized labor, who applauded the Democratic plank urging the restriction of injunctions, and he made what he could of an attack on the Republican tariff. But Taft polled 52.0 percent of the popular vote and carried the Electoral College 321 to 162.

Taft's identification with Roosevelt accounted for his nomination and assisted his election. In 1901 Roosevelt had inherited a conservative administration. Increasingly he had enlisted with reform. When he bowed out in 1909, off to hunt in the African jungles, a majority of Americans had come to adulate him and to approve, or at least to accept, his policies. It remained to be seen what Taft would do with his inheritance.

Suggestions for Reading

GENERAL

G. E. Mowry, *The Era of Theodore Roosevelt** (1958), provides a comprehensive account of the developments during the first twelve years of this century. A more recent synthesis informs O. L. Graham, Jr., *The Great Campaigns** (1971). There is a stimulating interpretation of progressivism in R. Hofstadter, *The Age of Reform* (1955), and another in E. Goldman, *Rendezvous with Destiny** (1952), which should be compared with C. Lasch, *New Radicalism in America, 1889–1963* (1965); A. Ekrich, *Progressivism in Practice* (1974), J. W. Chambers, *The Tyranny of Change** (1980); and J. D. Buenker, *Urban Liberalism and Progressive Reform* (1973). S. P. Hays, *The Response to Industrialism** (1957), and R. H. Wiebe, *The Search for Order: 1877–1920** (1966), offer interpretations suggested by their titles. Others of interest are in W. L. O'Neill, *The Progressive Years: America Comes of Age** (1975); L. L. Gould, ed., *The Progressive Era** (1973); and D. M. Kennedy, ed., *Progressivism: The Critical Issues* (1971).

PROGRESSIVISM

Among the best places to begin reading about progressivism are the lucid studies of the underprivileged and their champions in R. H. Bremner, *From the Depths** (1956), J. T. Patterson, *America's Struggle Against Poverty* (1981), and R. Lubove's *The Progressives and the Slums* (1962) and *The Professional Altruist: The Emergence of Social Work as a Career, 1880–1930** (1965). See, too, A. Davis, *Spearheads for Reform: The Social Settlements and the Progressive Movement, 1890–1919** (1967). Two of the champions revealed their concerns in J. A. Riis, *How the Other Half Lives** (1890), and Jane Addams, *Forty Years at Hull House** (1935). The contributions of the churches receive analysis in H. F. May, *Protestant Churches and Industrial America* (1949). P. Taft, *The A. F. of L. in the Time of Gompers* (1957), provides an account of the trade unions as does B. Mandel, *Samuel Gompers, A Biography* (1963). On Jewish immigrants in New York the best treatment is in I. Howe, *World of Our Fathers** (1976), while the classic general interpretation of the immigrants' experience is in O. Handlin, *The Uprooted** (3rd ed., 1973). Contrasting accounts of the struggle for women's rights are in W. L. O'Neill, *Everyone Was Brave: The Rise and Fall of Feminism in America* (1969), and D. M. Kennedy, *Birth Control in America: The Career of Margaret Sanger** (1970). Also important on the subject of women are A. Kraditor, *The Ideas of the Women's Suffrage Movement, 1890–1920* (1965), and L. Banner, *Women in America** (1974). On American blacks, see L. Harlan, *Booker T. Washington* (1972); C. F. Kellogg, *NAACP** (1970); E. Rudwick, *W. E. B. DuBois** (1969); B. J. Ross, *J. E. Spingarn and the Rise of the NAACP** (1972); and N. Weiss, *The National Urban League, 1910–1940* (1974). There are good accounts of dissident radicals in P. Renshaw, *The Wobblies* (1967); M. Dubofsky, *We Shall Be All: A History of the Industrial Workers of the World* (1969); D. Shannon, *Socialist Party in America* (1967 ed.); and J. P. Diggins, *The American Left in the Twentieth Century* (1973). Among the important interpretations of progressive intellectuals, besides the volumes listed in the preceding paragraph, are D. Aaron, *Men of Good Hope* (1951); M. White, *Social Thought in America: The Revolt Against Formalism** (1949); D. W. Noble, *The Paradox of Progressive Thought* (1958); S. Fine, *Laissez Faire and the General-Welfare State** (1956); J. Weinstein, *The Corporate Ideal in the Liberal State, 1900–1918** (1969); S. Haber, *Efficiency and Uplift: Scientific Management in the Progressive Era, 1890–1920* (1964); and H. F. May, *The End of American Innocence** (1959). These should be read in conjunction with the contemporary works mentioned in the text and with such revealing autobiographies as those of Lincoln Steffens and William Allen White. Progressive ferment and achievement in various regions, states, and cities have had excellent treatment in C. V. Woodward, *Origins of the New South, 1877–1913** (1951); D. Thelen, *The New Citizenship, 1885–1900* (1972), on the rise of La Follette; G. E. Mowry, *The California Progressives* (1951); R. E. Noble, *New Jersey Progressivism Before Wilson* (1947); R. M. Abrams, *Conservatism in a Progressive Era: Massachusetts Politics, 1900–1912* (1964); H. L. Warner, *Progressivism in Ohio, 1897–1917* (1964); S. Hackney, *Populism to Progressivism in Alabama* (1969); and R. F. Wesser, *Charles Evans Hughes: Politics and Reform in New York, 1905–10* (1967).

ROOSEVELT AND HIS ADMINISTRATION

The best introduction to Theodore Roosevelt remains his autobiography, which can be profitably supplemented by reading in his voluminous collected works and his published letters, E. E. Morison, ed., *Letters of Theodore Roosevelt*, 8 vols. (1951–54). E. Morris provides a glowing account in *The Rise of Theodore Roosevelt** (1979), as does D. McCullough in *Mornings on Horseback** (1981). Two good

---

572 *The Progressive Movement and the Square Deal*

biographies are G. W. Chessman, *Theodore Roosevelt and the Politics of Power* (1968), and W. H. Harbaugh, *Power and Responsibility** (1961). J. M. Blum, *The Republican Roosevelt** (1954), focuses on Roosevelt as politician and President; L. L. Gould, *Reform and Regulation: American Politics, 1900–1916** (1978), contains a contrasting interpretation; and H. K. Beale, *Theodore Roosevelt and the Rise of America to World Power** (1956), offers an analysis of Roosevelt's foreign policy, as does F. W. Mark, *Velvet on Iron* (1982). G. Kolko, *The Triumph of Conservatism** (1963) and *Railroads and Regulation, 1877–1916** (1965), attributes the reforms of the progressive era largely to conspiratorial big-business leaders; R. H. Weibe, *Businessmen and Reform* (1962), emphasizes division of opinion about reform issues within the business community, and A. Martin, *Enterprise Denied: Origins of the Decline of American Railroads, 1897–1917** (1971), reveals business resistance to reform. On the ambiguities of progressive politics, see J. M. Blum, *The Progressive Presidents** (1980), which also deals with Woodrow Wilson. Among other special studies of important public policies, some of the most rewarding are E. L. Peffer, *The Closing of the Public Domain* (1951), which should be supplemented by Gifford Pinchot's autobiography, and S. P. Hays, *Conservation and the Gospel of Efficiency** (1959); O. E. Anderson, Jr., *The Health of a Nation* (1958); R. Esthus, *Theodore Roosevelt and the International Rivalries* (1970); and W. La Feber, *The Panama Canal** (1978). There is a wealth of good autobiography by and biography of the men around Roosevelt. Besides those autobiographies noted earlier, Robert La Follette's is important, and among the most instructive biographies are J. Braeman, *Albert J. Beveridge* (1971); N. W. Stephenson, *Nelson W. Aldrich* (1920); P. C. Jessup, *Elihu Root*, 2 vols. (1938); D. E. Anderson, *William Howard Taft* (1973); R. Lowett, *George W. Norris: The Making of a Progressive* (1963); and D. P. Thelen, *Robert M. La Follette and the Insurgent Spirit** (1976).

*Available in a paperback edition.

23

PROGRESSIVISM: RETREAT AND RESURGENCE

Republicans celebrating the inauguration of William Howard Taft in March 1909 had no cause for complacency. Their party had won four successive presidential elections, and its national leaders had preserved the alliances on which its majority rested. But the partners in those alliances—the Old Guard, Midwestern townspeople, urban progressives, and Western agrarians—were growing uneasy with one another. The Democrats, secure in the South and in many Northern cities, were gaining strength among labor unions and farmers. In 1906 and 1908 the Republicans had lost seats in the House of Representatives, and in 1908 they had also lost several governorships. If they hoped to remain in power, they would have to satisfy their restive factions and close ranks against their opposition.

Insurgency

A cautious President. Taft, the new President and head of the party, had excellent intentions. A kindly, learned man, he saw the need for social-welfare legislation, understood the purposes of the Roosevelt reforms, for which he had worked with skill, and meant to keep his promise to preserve and further his predecessor's program. He was also a loyal Republican who hoped to strengthen his party, which in his opinion

was the only fit instrument of government. In a placid time he might have done well.

He was, however, seriously handicapped for the job he had to do. Taft was almost a caricature of the fat man—genial, usually easygoing. He was also both indecisive and untrained in politics. His career had been on the bench and in appointive administrative offices. He had no instinct for manipulation, no nerve for controversy. His reluctance to use the full powers of the Presidency grew out of his interpretation of the Constitution, which led him to believe that he should not interfere in the course of legislation. He was uncomfortable in the company of those who did not share his background of old family, personal means, and Eastern education. He preferred talking with Nelson Aldrich to conversing with La Follette, whom he considered one of the party's troublemakers.

The President was by nature and conviction a conservative whose highest confidence was in the law as he and other judges had shaped it. The bench, he believed, was the appropriate arbiter of social issues. He was antagonistic toward labor unions and suspicious of direct democracy, because he did not trust the majority to make laws. He was also cautious about enlarging the power of the executive for fear that it might encroach upon the traditional authorities of the other branches of government.

Taft was not unresilient. He accepted the need for change. But he did not particularly like it, and he

Preparedness parade

did not at all like to be rushed. Yet he came to his office when the progressives were in a hurry. And they expected him, on the basis of his commitment to Roosevelt's programs, to keep pace with them. He preferred an easier pace, an advance in which each forward step was measured carefully against the footprints trailing through the past.

An Old-Guard tariff. Taft began boldly by calling a special session of Congress to revise the tariff. His campaign speeches had suggested that he preferred a moderate downward revision. Republican representatives of manufacturing interests were still wedded to high protectionism, but Midwestern farmers and their party spokesmen were convinced that the Dingley duties (see p. 522), by protecting the trusts from foreign competition, were sustaining artificial prices for manufactured goods. Furthermore, as proponents of the "Iowa Idea" argued, Europeans had to sell in the American market in order to earn dollars to buy American agricultural surpluses.

The Western progressives counted on the President's support in getting the tariff lowered, but even before the special session got under way they experienced their first disappointment. Taft appointed a Cabinet of conservatives, five of them corporation lawyers. He also turned down young George Norris of Nebraska and other insurgents in the House of Representatives who appealed for his support in their effort to restrict the power of the Speaker, "Uncle Joe" Cannon of Illinois, an arch-Tory and protectionist. And when debate on the tariff began, Taft made no gesture in behalf of the revision he had advocated.

The House of Representatives passed a tariff bill that made modest concessions to reform. It reduced some duties and imposed an inheritance tax graduated from 1 to 5 percent.

In the Senate, however, the Old Guard carried the day. The Finance Committee struck out the in- heritance tax, made over eight hundred amendments to the House bill, and even slightly increased the average rates of the Dingley Tariff. On the floor of the Senate, progressives attacked the swollen tariff schedules one by one and joined the Democrats in urging an income tax. Taft's intercession fostered a compromise that set a 2 percent tax on corporate income and assured passage of a constitutional amendment authorizing a personal income tax. But the compromise little affected the tariff itself. A conference committee of the two houses made modest changes in a number of schedules, but most of those revisions benefited manufacturers rather than farmers or consumers.

The Payne-Aldrich Act as it finally passed was a triumph for the protectionists. During the struggle Taft had alienated the insurgent Midwesterners and their constituents. In September, in a series of implausible speeches he scolded the progressives who had voted against the tariff, which he declared the best the party had ever enacted.

A divided party. When Congress met again in 1910, the insurgents made common cause with the Democrats and passed a resolution transferring much of Speaker Cannon's authority to the House Rules Committee. The insurgents then joined the Democrats to amend Taft's railway bill, though the President made support of that bill a test of party loyalty. Taft's measure empowered the Interstate Commerce Commission to fix rates on its own initiative. But it established a Court of Commerce with broad powers of review over the commission's decisions, thereby giving the traditionally conservative judiciary a determining veto. The bill also permitted railroads to acquire competing lines. The Democratic-progressive coalition supported the first of those three provisions, attacked the others, and succeeded in eliminating the third. It further amended the bill to bring telephone and telegraph companies under the commission's jurisdiction and to provide for the physical valuation of railway properties as a basis for determining fair rates.

In the Senate Aldrich eliminated the provision calling for physical valuation and preserved the Commerce Court by making a trade with the Democrats. In return for their help on the railway bill, he agreed to the admission of Arizona and New Mexico, which were sure to elect four Democratic senators in 1912. This was a Pyrrhic victory: it saved the Administration's face, but it did not long prevent a physical-valuation law (which Congress passed early in 1913), and it precipitated open warfare within the Republican party. The insurgents had defied the President, who had unwisely raised the question of party regularity. Now he retaliated by denying them patronage and starting a campaign to defeat them in the fall elections of 1910.

Meanwhile Taft had got caught up in a damaging controversy. With his approval, his Secretary of the Interior, Richard A. Ballinger, had reopened to private sale millions of acres of public land and many valuable waterpower sites that Gifford Pinchot, Roosevelt's trusted friend, had previously arranged to have closed. Pinchot, still chief forester of the United States, learned that Ballinger had been instrumental in selling certain government coal lands in Alaska to a wealthy syndicate controlled by J. P. Morgan and David Guggenheim. Pinchot took the case to Taft, who ruled for Ballinger on every count and urged Pinchot to drop the issue.

The indignant Pinchot supplied material for two magazine articles attacking Ballinger. He also made his case in a letter that was read to the Senate. Taft had no choice but to dismiss him, though he knew that in so doing he would seem to oppose Roosevelt's conservation policies and possibly antagonize the Colonel. His worst fears materialized. A joint congressional committee in 1910 exonerated Ballinger, but Louis D. Brandeis, counsel for the opposition, revealed that Taft and his Attorney General had tampered with evidence they sent to Congress. Though Taft was an effective conservationist, Brandeis' argument hurt his reputation. The political damage was compounded when Pinchot greeted Roosevelt after the Colonel emerged from the African jungles. In the future Roosevelt always saw the matter Pinchot's way.

The election of 1910. Taft felt that Roosevelt's friends had plotted to cause a rupture between him and their hero. After Roosevelt's triumphant return to New York, the insurgents set out to enlist his help. Roosevelt, who was temperamentally incapable of remaining out of politics and who was sensitive to a coolness on Taft's part, now decided that his principles needed defending. He embarked on a speaking tour during which he endorsed the Administration but gave stronger praise to the insurgents. At Osawatomie, Kansas, invoking the spirit of John Brown, Roosevelt announced his New Nationalism, a program of social welfare, federal regulation of business and industry, and direct democracy. In that address he frightened conservatives by attacking the courts for having invalidated progressive labor legislation.

The friction within the Republican party contributed to its losses in the elections of 1910. The Democrats in many states managed to identify themselves with progressivism and to identify the Republican tariff with the rising cost of living, a particularly sensitive issue among city-dwellers. The Democrats won several governorships, including those of New York and New Jersey, which had been safely Republican for many years. For the first time since 1892, the

New states, 1896–1912

A case for bigness

If the anti-trust people really grasped the full meaning of what they said, and if they really had the power or the courage to do what they propose, they would be engaged in one of the most destructive agitations that America has known. They would be breaking up the beginning of a collective organization, thwarting the possibility of cooperation, and insisting upon submitting industry to the wasteful, the planless scramble of little profiteers. They would make impossible any deliberate and constructive use of our natural resources, they would thwart any effort to form the great industries into coordinated services, they would preserve commercialism as the undisputed master of our lives....

It is said that the economy of trusts is unreal. Yet no one has ever tried the economies of the trust in any open, deliberate fashion. The amount of energy that has had to go into repelling stupid attack, the adjustments that had to be made underground—it is a wonder the trusts achieved what they did to bring order out of chaos, and forge an instrument for a nation's business.

From Walter Lippmann, *Drift and Mastery,* **1914.**

Democrats elected a majority to the House of Representatives. The Republicans' loss of New York and the defeat of Senator Beveridge in Indiana saddened Roosevelt. The Democratic victories over Old Guard candidates in the East and the victories of progressive Republicans in the West repudiated Taft. Overall, the returns suggested that only an insurgent could save the Republicans in the presidential election of 1912, but the Old Guard, tense and defensive, prepared to resist the temper of the time.

Taft's political operatives began in 1911 to strengthen their factions in the North and to wrap up the Republican organizations in the South. At the same time, La Follette set out to recruit support for his own candidacy, which many progressives endorsed. Some of them, however, privately hoped to draft Roosevelt, whose personal appeal remained strong even after his announcement that he had retired from politics.

A divisive foreign policy. During the year Taft succeeded in intensifying party discord and stirring the Colonel to action. In January 1911 the President submitted to Congress a reciprocity agreement with Canada. It put on the free list many agricultural products, including important raw materials for industrial use, and some manufactured goods. Western progressives, fearing the competition of Canadian farmers, opposed the measure. So did most high-tariff advocates, who objected to any breach in the wall of protection. Together they rejected the agreement. But Taft called a special session in April during which the Democrats, delighting in the discomfort of the Republicans, helped Administration forces to put the

measure through. The Canadians, however, disturbed by the prospect of economic competition and Americanization, in September repudiated the agreement. Another tariff debate had produced only more wounds. The Democrats kept them open, with help from Republican insurgents, by passing a series of bills reducing specific schedules—"pop-gun" tariffs that the President systematically vetoed.

Taft's foreign policy also aroused opposition. His Secretary of State, Philander C. Knox, intended to use American economic power to promote American influence, a strategy that departed from Roosevelt's balance of power approach. Knox negotiated treaties with Nicaragua and Honduras providing for the assumption of their European-held debt by American investors and for the appointment of Americans to direct their finances and thus assure the collection of those debts. Though the Senate rejected the treaties, Knox pursued his policy throughout the Caribbean with considerable success. He and Taft also emphasized the possibilities for American investments in China. At the instigation of the State Department, American bankers agreed to join in various commercial projects there, including an international railway consortium.

Roosevelt disapproved of that "dollar diplomacy." He had urged Taft to abandon commercial competition with the Japanese in China. It was more important, the Colonel argued, to cultivate Japanese friendship and to arrange a clearer understanding about Japanese immigration.

Roosevelt also opposed arbitration treaties that Taft negotiated with France and England. Taft was confident that international problems could be solved by courts of law. In the summer of 1911 he submitted to the Senate treaties with France and Great Britain that bound the signatories to arbitrate all differences "susceptible of decision by the application of the principles of law or equity." Those treaties excited the hopes of the thousands of Americans who considered them an important step toward avoiding wars. But Roosevelt denounced the arbitration of questions involving "territory" or "national honor," and he cooperated with like-minded senators who succeeded in amending the treaties so drastically that the President scrapped them. Taft was dismayed by the outcome and offended by Roosevelt's scathing language.

The road to revolt. Roosevelt in turn was offended by Taft's antitrust policies. The Supreme Court in 1911 in the Standard Oil and American Tobacco cases found that the corporations were monopolies guilty of violating the Sherman Act. Yet the decisions also pronounced the "rule of reason," which held that only unreasonable restraints of trade were unlawful. That was a necessary corollary to antitrust law, for an undiscriminating application of the Sherman Act would weaken the structure and impede the functioning of American business. But whereas Taft was content to have the Court define reasonableness, Roosevelt believed that an administrative agency should make that judgment and should base it on considerations of economic efficiency and business behavior.

This difference of opinion was exemplified in the case of the United States Steel Corporation, then the largest of all holding companies, which Taft chose to prosecute. Roosevelt, who considered the company guiltless, concluded that Taft had acted largely to embarrass him, for the prosecution, which resulted ultimately in an acquittal, and the congressional hearings that it provoked, publicized Roosevelt's negotiations of 1907 with J. P. Morgan (see p. 565).

Taft's antitrust and foreign policies gave Roosevelt a chance to rationalize what he would undoubtedly have done anyway. In February 1912 he announced that his hat was in the ring. A furious battle for the Republican presidential nomination was under way.

The struggle was really between Roosevelt and Taft, who denounced each other with unrestrained vehemence. Though La Follette remained in the race, most of his supporters of 1911 deserted him for Roosevelt. Now just as progressive and vastly more sophisticated and popular than La Follette, Roosevelt had in his New Nationalism formulated a program that promised to distribute the abundance of industrialism, while both promoting and controlling the institutions that had made that abundance possible. Roosevelt stood an excellent chance of winning the election. Taft had no such chance, but his dander was up, and the Old Guard cared more about nominating him, defeating Roosevelt, and dominating the party than about beating the Democrats.

The Taft forces, moreover, had in their hands the party apparatus through which they could control the convention. In some states Roosevelt's supporters managed to pass legislation establishing preferential primaries for the nomination, but in the end only thirteen states held such elections. They gave 36 delegates to La Follette, 48 to Taft, and 278 to Roosevelt—an overwhelming mandate for the Colonel. Taft, however, controlled the South, New York, and the crucial national committee, which with its affiliates disposed of 254 contested seats at the convention. With a cynical disregard for the merits of the contestants, it allotted 235 of the contested seats to Taft delegates. The rigged convention then renominated the President on the first ballot.

The Bull Moose. Before the balloting took place, most of the Roosevelt men bolted, crying fraud. In August they reconvened as delegates of the new Progressive party. To that convention there came social workers, feminists, intellectuals, and industrialists attracted by Roosevelt's personality and program, and Republican politicians disenchanted with their factional rivals—all imbued with a revivalist spirit. Roosevelt, "strong as a Bull Moose," told them they were standing at Armageddon battling for the Lord and accepted the nomination they tendered with thundering unanimity.

The Progressive party was hastily and inadequately organized. Roosevelt probably knew in his heart that by splitting the Republican party he was assuring the election of a Democrat. He and Taft, however, had gone too far to turn back toward compromise. The split was much more than just a personal falling out. Taft's adherents by and large stood for the status quo. Some, to be sure, were of a progressive mind but were unwilling to break with their party. Many were genuinely frightened by Roosevelt's advocacy of the recall of state judicial decisions by referendum, a proposal that in their view would substitute the fickle and untutored will of the majority for the presumed majesty of the courts. For the most part they

Spring, 1912

stayed with Taft because they considered him and his sponsors safe, whereas they considered Roosevelt, along with his friends and his platform, downright alarming.

The Bull Moose platform was incontestably adventurous, a charter of progressive reform for its own time and for years to come. It advocated the familiar devices of popular democracy—presidential primaries, women's suffrage, the initiative and referendum, and popular election of United States senators. It advocated, too, a comprehensive social-welfare program—conservation of natural and human resources, minimum wages for women, the restriction of child labor, workmen's compensation, social insurance, a federal income tax,* and the limitation of injunctions in labor disputes. Finally, in keeping with Roosevelt's ideas about the restructuring of government, it called for expert federal commissions to adjust the tariff and to regulate interstate business and industry. Party and candidate alike stood for social justice and popular rule, and stood, too, for the application of efficiency to the management of public problems, an objective attractive at once to many progressives and to many men of affairs. As it developed, however, they faced formidable competition as champions of reform from a united and inspired Democratic party.

*The Sixteenth Amendment, which provided for an income tax, was already before the states, as was the Seventeenth, providing for popular election of senators. Both were ratified in 1913.

"Strong as a Bull Moose"

Progressivism at Zenith

Woodrow Wilson. The Democratic candidate in 1912 had found his way into politics by an unusual route. Woodrow Wilson, the son of a Southern Presbyterian minister, had abandoned a brief and unrewarding career in law for one in education. After earning his doctorate at The Johns Hopkins University, Wilson taught history and political science at Bryn Mawr, Wesleyan of Connecticut, and Princeton, his own alma mater, of which he became president in 1902. He first won national attention for his writings, especially his earliest book, *Congressional Government* (1885), which criticized the weakness of the executive and the inefficiencies of Congress and praised the British parliamentary system. As president of Princeton Wilson initiated a number of celebrated educational reforms, but he lost his battle with faculty members and wealthy alumni over plans for a graduate school. That struggle brought on his resignation but also gave him a reputation as a champion of democracy in education.

Wilson resigned in 1910 to accept the Democratic nomination for governor of New Jersey. He had always had political ambitions; now he owed his nomination to Democratic machine leaders who were impressed, as were his wealthy New York friends, by his stature and his presumably conservative economic views. But during the campaign Wilson adopted the program of New Jersey progressives: As governor he made a brilliant record that put New Jersey in the van of progressive states (see p. 558) and put Wilson in the lead for the Democratic presidential nomination.

In 1912 the Democrats, like the Republicans, were caught in a momentous struggle over selecting a candidate. Wilson had offended his conservative sponsors, who now helped organize a movement to defeat him. His opponents were particularly successful in the South, where they captured most of the state delegations. In the East, the city machines, alarmed by Wilson's treatment of their counterparts in New Jersey, embarrassed him by publicizing sections of his *History of the American People* (1902), which disparaged the new immigrants. In the farming West, moreover, the favorite candidate was Champ Clark, the folksy "Ol' Hound Dawg" of Missouri. Bryan Democrats there rightly judged that Wilson was not one of them.

During the national convention at Baltimore Bryan, probably more to further his own ambitions than Wilson's, took the floor to castigate any candidate supported by Tammany. Tammany had just moved New York into the Clark column, thus contributing to his majority. But it took a two-thirds vote to nominate, and Wilson's floor-leaders gradually

made the deals that turned the convention their way. One of those deals assured the vice-presidential nomination to Thomas R. Marshall of Indiana, a politician best remembered for his fetching assertion that what the country needed was "a good five-cent cigar." On the forty-third ballot Wilson won a majority of the votes; on the forty-sixth, the nomination.

The election of 1912. The basic contest in 1912 was between the Democrats and the Progressives. Certain of the South, assisted elsewhere by the Republican schism, the Democratic leadership took pains to preserve party unity by placating the factions that had opposed Wilson and by appealing to the urban ethnic groups that had long sustained the party's political machines. But Wilson, though the odds were with him, could not take Roosevelt for granted. He had to meet the challenge for progressive votes.

In many respects the Bull Moose and Democratic platforms were similar, but there were several significant differences between them. Where the Progressives endorsed a protective tariff, the Democrats called for sharp downward revision. Where the Progressives demanded powerful federal regulatory agencies, the Democrats emphasized state rights.. The Democrats did not spell out a broad social-welfare program, but they did advocate limiting the use of injunctions against labor unions. The party's continuing insistence on that issue held the allegiance of Gompers and most of his associates in the American Federation of Labor. Moreover, farmers responded enthusiastically to Democratic promises to make loans for agriculture cheaper and more readily available.

More than the platforms, the attitudes of the candidates marked the differences between the parties. Roosevelt's New Nationalism assumed that the consolidation of the economy was inevitable and healthful. He welcomed big business but demanded big government to supervise it and to promote the welfare of nonbusiness groups. The political theorist Herbert Croly expressed these ideas forcefully in *The Promise of American Life* (1909), an influential book that helped Roosevelt and like-minded people articulate their principles. It demanded positive, comprehensive federal planning for the national interest and for social reform.

Wilson had reached dissimilar conclusions. There lingered in his mind a complex of ideas he had cherished since youth. He was a devout Presbyterian who held human beings individually responsible to God for their actions. Guilt in business affairs, he believed, was also personal guilt. Where a corporation misbehaved, his instinct was to punish its officers as the Lord punished sinners. He was more the stern prophet than the vigorous promoter. He was also convinced that laissez-faire principles of economics would work if only the state would protect and encourage competition. It should, he felt, act as a handicapper resolved to make the race equitable at the start and as a policeman determined to keep the runners in their lanes. An enemy of political and business corruption, a believer in popular democracy, a proponent of regulation to prevent industrial abuses, Wilson, a progressive in the tradition of rural America, was uncomfortable with Croly's formulations.

Another able intellectual, Louis D. Brandeis of Massachusetts, helped Wilson organize his developing ideas. The great corporations, Brandeis argued, controlled credit, raw materials, and markets. They prevented competition and guarded their own inefficient methods, excessive profits, and overcapitalized values.

The election of 1912

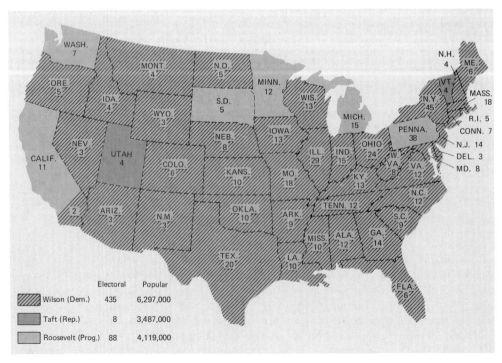

		Electoral	Popular
	Wilson (Dem.)	435	6,297,000
	Taft (Rep.)	8	3,487,000
	Roosevelt (Prog.)	88	4,119,000

They had corrupted government, Brandeis went on, and had to be prosecuted and broken up. He also urged that the rules of competition be defined by law and that federal programs be launched to provide credit for small and new businesses. His ideas and the data with which he supported them confirmed Wilson's own theories, which the candidate set forth in the program he called the New Freedom.

Roosevelt's plans, so Wilson said, would result in "partnership between the government and the trusts." The Democratic alternative would ensure a free economy and preserve free government. "Free men," he asserted, "need no guardians." Indeed, they could not submit to guardians and remain free, for submission would produce "a corruption of the will."

Wilson called for "regulated competition" in preference to "regulated monopoly." He feared that individuals were being "swallowed up" by great organizations, and he condemned what he considered "an extraordinary and very sinister concentration in . . . business." He demanded "a body of laws which will look after the men . . . who are sweating blood to get their foothold in the world of endeavor." Roosevelt called Wilson's program "rural Toryism." In a sense it was. But Wilson affirmed the hopes of the farm, of the small town, of middle-class America. His party, furthermore, retained the allegiance of the South and of urban ethnic groups that had long voted Democratic.

Wilson won a telling victory, though he polled only 41.9 percent of the popular vote. Roosevelt received only 27.4 percent and Taft only 23.2. In the electoral count Wilson led his rivals 435 to 88 and 8, and the Democrats carried both houses of Congress. The Democrats, who ran best in the areas of their traditional strength, had needed the Republican division to win. The returns were just as clearly a triumph for reform. Taft's miserable showing revealed the voters' disdain for standpat government, while the dissatisfaction with existing conditions was evidenced by the nearly one million votes for Socialist candidate Eugene V. Debs and by the remarkable support won by the Bull Moose party in its initial test.

It was also remarkable that so lively a contest produced a turnout of voters that, as in other presidential elections of the first decades of the century, fell short of the percentage of eligibles who had voted in the 1880s and 1890s. Apart from those voters who had been disfranchised in the South, many other Americans were obviously either preoccupied with questions that politics did not address or persuaded that the choices politics offered made little difference. Yet the degree of voter participation never alone measured the significance of elections, for politics had never been wholly rational. In 1912 there was a choice. At the least, the election signaled the resurgence of reform that marked Wilson's first term in office.

A Democratic tariff. Wilson realized that he could work most efficiently through his own party. Though he had come to recognize the power inherent in the Presidency, he also considered himself a party-leader in the English style, with the right to hold party members in Congress to his programs and, if necessary, to appeal over their heads to the electorate. From the first he set out to unite the Democratic factions, to use his united party to legislate, and to endow it with a record and reputation that would make a majority of Americans prefer it to any rival.

Wilson, however, had neither the temperament nor the experience to get along with professional politicians. A tense and angular man, he was incapable of displaying good fellowship he did not feel. But he knew his limitations and compensated for them by selecting a group of skilled advisers. Among others they included Bryan, the new Secretary of State, influential as always with the agrarian liberals; Albert S. Burleson, Postmaster General, a veteran Southern congressman popular among the party regulars on the Hill; Secretary of the Treasury William G. McAdoo, a progressive businessman who had the confidence of those who had made Wilson's nomination possible; Joseph P. Tumulty, the President's private secretary, a young Irishman wise in the ways of machine politicians and professional journalists; and Colonel Edward M. House, an urbane Texan who attached himself to Wilson and became his "second personality." Though House had neither title nor office, he quickly acquired important responsibilities as a liaison man between the President and leaders of the party, of American finance, and of the Congress, as well as between the President and foreign heads of state.

Informed and assisted by his subordinates, Wilson made his own major decisions and gave a personal stamp to his executive leadership. Right after his inauguration he called a special session of Congress to fulfill the Democratic pledge of tariff revision. He dramatized the session and his intended role by appearing personally, as had no President since Jefferson's time, to address the Congress. He had already begun a fruitful cooperation with the committees responsible for tariff recommendations. In May 1913, only a month after the President's address, the House passed a bill reducing average *ad valorem* rates about 11 percent; adding a number of consumer goods to the free list; and eliminating the protection of iron, steel, and various other products of the trusts. To make up for the attending loss in revenue, the bill levied a modest graduated income tax, which ratification of the Sixteenth Amendment had legalized two months earlier.

The test of Wilson's leadership came in the Senate, where the Democrats had a majority of only three votes. Democratic senators from sugar- and wool-pro-

Edward M. House: urbane Texan

duducing states were reluctant to leave those products on the free list where the House had placed them. Wilson urged them to vote with their party, but they wavered, and lobbyists for protection tried to exploit the chance for logrolling. The President then called on public opinion to "check and destroy" the "intolerable burden" of "insidious" lobbyists. His statement helped to initiate an investigation of the private interests of all senators, some of whom, it developed, stood to profit personally from the protection of wool and sugar. With a refreshed sensitivity to public opinion, all but two Democrats voted for the party's bill. It kept sugar and wool on the free list and reduced the general level of rates another 4 percent. It also, thanks to the efforts of progressives in all the parties, doubled the maximum surtax on personal incomes.

The tariff of 1913, the Underwood-Simmons Act, removed an accumulation of privileges and, without abandoning protection, reduced previously swollen schedules. It modified the federal tax structure by shifting some of the burden to those best able to bear it, a significant precedent for the future. It was a convincing demonstration that the Democrats could achieve the goals of the New Freedom, and it was an acknowledged triumph for Wilson's leadership.

Banking reform. Pressing his gains, the President had urged the special session of Congress to correct the nation's anachronistic money and banking system. The Panic of 1907 (see p. 565) had underscored the inflexibility of currency and the inelasticity of credit. The events of the panic also suggested that financial power was concentrated in the hands of a small group of Eastern private bankers. That situation had been the subject of investigation by a House committee chaired by Congressman Arsène P. Pujo. Its findings, later popularized in Louis Brandeis' *Other People's Money* (1914), persuaded many progressives that there existed a "money trust."

Southern and Western farmers had long assumed that there was a bankers' conspiracy against their interests and had long agitated for monetary reform. By 1913 the bankers themselves were in favor of reform, but of their own kind. The experience of the panic and the report of Aldrich's Monetary Commission (see p. 565) led most of them to advocate central control of the banking system and the creation of a currency responsive to, and partly based on, the expansion and contraction of commercial paper—that is, loans that banks made to business.

The bankers, taking as their models the Bank of England and the controversial Second United States Bank, wanted a central bank to be authorized by the government but privately controlled. They also wanted it to issue currency on its own liability. The conservative Democrats modified those proposals by replacing a single central bank with a number of regional banks supervised by a federal board that bankers would control. This modification, the plan Wilson at first favored, failed to satisfy the party's progressive and agrarian factions. To meet their minimum demands, the President agreed that the government should appoint the supervising board and that the bank notes issued by the new system should be obligations of the United States.

Those concessions fell short of the program advanced by Southern farmers. They called for a prohibition of interlocking directorates, for public control of the regional banks, for permitting reserve banks to discount agricultural paper, and for preventing the use of commercial paper as a basis for currency. Bryan mediated their differences with Wilson, who met them part way. The President conceded the discounting of agricultural notes and promised later to take care of interlocking directorates. In return, the militants supported the rest of the bill, which the House passed in September 1913.

There was resistance again from conservatives in the Senate. Wilson overcame some of it by another appeal for party responsibility and by a timely use of patronage. Again taking his case to the people, he asserted that bankers were trying to defeat the measure by creating artificial fears of impending panic. Although Senate conservatives managed to increase the percentage of gold reserves required for the issue of bank notes and to reduce the authority of the Federal Reserve Board, the Democrats were sufficiently united to pass the bill without further changes in December 1913.

The Federal Reserve Act was the most important statute of Wilson's Administration. The Federal Reserve Board and the regional Reserve Banks gave the United States its first efficient banking system since the time of Andrew Jackson. Their power over currency and credit put into responsible hands the means to provide the flexibility of short-term credit that was so badly needed. Though private banking interests dominated the regional banks with their large powers, the regulatory authority of the board assured a greater degree of public control over banking than ever before. Indeed, the act remedied almost all the deficiencies in American banking and currency that informed observers then recognized. Without the new system the country could not have adjusted to the financial strains of the First World War. There was still need to ease long-term agricultural credit and (though it was not yet understood) to endow public authorities with effective instruments to modulate the business cycle. But the new law was an impressive structural reform. Americans of all points of view and parties applauded it and the President's "great exhibition of leadership" in guiding it through Congress.

The New Freedom and the trusts. When Congress met in regular session in 1914, Wilson presented his program for regulating industry. He asked Congress for legislation to make it impossible for interrelated groups to control holding companies, to create a commission to help dissolve corporations found in restraint of trade, and to define unfair business practices.

Those recommendations, too strong for conservatives, did not satisfy either labor-leaders, who urged the exemption of unions from the Sherman Antitrust Act, or Bull Moosers, who advocated a strong regulatory agency. Louis Brandeis had moved closer to the Bull Moose point of view, and he now drafted a bill that Wilson supported. It created a Federal Trade Commission to prevent the unlawful suppression of competition. The measure passed, but only after Southern conservatives had helped the Republicans amend it to provide for broad court review of the commission's order, a review that soon proved to be debilitating.

A companion measure, the Clayton Bill, was also amended before enactment. As the House passed it, it followed the prescriptions of Wilson's message, defined unfair practices, and forbade interlocking directorates. Senate conservatives modified that prohibition by exempting instances that did not tend to decrease competition. That standard failed to assure prosecution of the largest holding companies. It was also in the Senate that friends of labor added to the bill a statement declaring that labor was not to be considered a commodity, a mere article of commerce. The House had earlier included a clause exempting labor unions and farm organizations from antitrust prosecutions, but only when those groups were lawfully pursuing legitimate aims. As the courts were to interpret the Clayton Act, the reservation about legitimate aims canceled the exemption.

The antitrust laws of 1914 failed to prescribe business conduct to the extent Wilson had sought, and they failed to give unions the freedom of activity Gompers had urged. The Federal Trade Commission, moreover, had less power than many progressives had recommended. But the weaknesses of the legislation were not immediately apparent, and the laws seemed to constitute another, though limited, victory for the Administration. In less than two years Wilson had reached the major statutory goals of his New Freedom.

The voters responded favorably in the elections of 1914. Superficially the Democrats suffered that year, for the Republicans made sizable gains. But the Democrats retained control of both houses of Congress. The collapse of the Progressive party helped the Republicans in the Northeast, where they made their best showing. Elsewhere the Democrats picked up progressive support, and in the new Congress that sat in 1915 and 1916 Southern and Western farmers had a larger voice than they had had before. The returns convinced perceptive Democratic strategists that they could carry the nation in 1916 only by winning the progressives of the West. Once more, reform had won a mandate.

In behalf of progress. As Wilson saw it, the interests of legitimate business did not conflict with the need for social reform. His appointments to the Supreme Court, the Federal Reserve Board, and the Federal Trade Commission had on the whole been conservative. After the election he adjusted to the demands of congressional and national politics. He encouraged reform Democrats, who in 1916 succeeded in passing the Federal Farm Loan Act and the Child Labor Act. On matters of international trade the President came to respect the program of the Progressive party for the promotion of American business. He endorsed legislation permitting firms engaged in export trade to combine to meet foreign competition, and he supported an act in 1916 creating a nonpartisan, expert tariff commission designed to prevent the dumping of unprotected goods on the American market.

In 1916 Wilson also practically ordered Congress to establish the eight-hour day at ten-hour pay for railway labor. Congress responded with the Adamson Act. In this case the President acted largely to prevent a threatening strike that would have tied up shipping of war materials for France and England, but his intercession won plaudits from organized labor. Labor leaders and reformers had earlier found convincing evidence of Wilson's progressive intentions in his nomination of Louis D. Brandeis, the first Jew to gain the office, as Associate Justice of the Supreme Court.

The Wilson of 1916 had moved a long way from his position of 1912 toward that of Roosevelt and the Bull Moose. In endeavoring to promote both business and social welfare, the President revealed his faith, a characteristically progressive faith, in a dynamic but humane capitalism, and in the role of government in fostering those concerns. He had a right to boast that the Democrats had opened their hearts to "the demands of social justice" and had "come very near to carrying out the platform of the Progressive Party" as well as their own.

Wilson and Moral Diplomacy

The force of moral principle. The conditions of world affairs had changed only superficially between 1901, when Theodore Roosevelt took office as President, and 1913, when Wilson and Secretary of State Bryan brought a different perspective to American foreign policy. Wilson and Bryan were guided by attitudes they shared with many progressive Americans, particularly rural reformers, social workers, and Protestant Social Gospelers. "The force of America," the President said during one crisis, "is the force of

moral principle." Moral principle, as he interpreted it, involved a duty to work for peace both by example and through diplomacy. It also involved obedience to the law. Wilson and Bryan felt that they had a mission to teach semideveloped countries to live according to the kind of legal and constitutional system that existed in the United States. They believed that that system was not only especially efficient but especially ethical. They believed, too, that there was a definable body of international law that moral nations should obey in their relations with one another. And they placed their hope for peace, as well as for American commercial interests, in that law rather than in systems of alliances or in defensive or deterrent military buildups.

Those attitudes led Wilson and Bryan to distrust the career men in the navy, the army, and the State Department, whom they considered conventional and even cynical. The President and the Secretary of State were willing to risk offending the experts in order to strike out along new diplomatic paths. Bryan launched his program in 1913 and 1914 by negotiating treaties with Great Britain, France, Italy, and twenty-seven lesser powers. Those treaties provided for submitting all disputes among the signatories to permanent commissions of investigation. For one year, while investigation proceeded, the parties to the treaties promised that they would neither go to war nor increase their armaments. At the end of that year they could either accept or reject the findings of the investigation, but Bryan expected the "cooling-off" period to remove the chance of war.

In a similarly benign spirit Wilson in 1913 withdrew American support from the Chinese railway consortium that Taft had helped to arrange (see p. 578). The United States, Wilson said, could not be a partner to foreign interference in Chinese affairs. He also recognized the new Republic of China, the first major recognition that government received.

The most imminent threat to China's national integrity was Japan, whose relations with the United States had deteriorated because of the troublesome race issue. Wilson had characteristic Southern prejudices about race. During his Administration there was increasing segregation of blacks within the federal service. Never an enemy of Jim Crow, Wilson made no effort to dissuade California politicians who were determined in 1913 to prohibit Japanese from owning land in their state. On the President's advice, they passed a statute that achieved that end indirectly, and without violating American treaty obligations. But the Japanese were nonetheless humiliated. Their ambassador protested to the State Department; there were anti-American disturbances in Japan; and the Joint Board of the Army and Navy, deeming war probable, advised Wilson to move warships into Chinese and

Philippine waters. The President resorted instead to conciliatory diplomacy. The ensuing exchange of notes eased the crisis and ended talk of war, but the issue remained unresolved, and the Japanese remained understandably resentful.

That resentment contributed to a new controversy in 1915. The preoccupation of European powers with the war then raging on their own continent gave Japan a chance to make twenty-one extraordinary demands of China. Had China agreed to the treaty containing the demands, it would have become a political and economic dependency. American protests, supplemented by pressure from England, persuaded the Japanese temporarily to moderate their terms. The episode revealed how tenuous the balance of power in Asia had become. It also disclosed Bryan's commitment to conventional national policies and to American commercial interests. The United States, Bryan warned Japan in a portentous note, could not recognize any agreement impairing the Open Door policy, the treaty rights of Americans, or the political or territorial integrity of China.

Confusion in Latin America. As in Asia, so in Latin America, Wilson intended to abandon "dollar diplomacy" with its attendant intrusions on the sovereignty of weak nations. He also hoped to cultivate the friendship of Latin American peoples and to help them achieve a higher standard of living and a more democratic government. He began convincingly by negotiating a treaty with Colombia providing both apology and indemnity for Roosevelt's Panamanian adventure. But Roosevelt's friends in the Senate prevented approval of that treaty, and the Administration's benign purposes soon produced policies that seemed imperialistic to those countries they were designed to assist.

A combination of circumstances made moral diplomacy difficult. The small nations in and around the Caribbean were, as they had long been, impoverished and turbulent. Unwilling to have the United States government assume and service their debts, Wilson relied on private bankers, whose motives he suspected. Like Roosevelt, he would not permit turmoil in the area to breed revolutions or European intercessions that might endanger the approaches to the isthmus. Consequently he turned to American troops and, like Taft, to American dollars to keep order. Since the local forces of order were often also the forces of reaction, Wilson at times resisted reform. Further, he let Bryan send to the Caribbean area "deserving Democrats" lacking any qualifications for diplomacy except faithful party service.

Yet the President tended to attribute qualities of justice and legality to the reactionary government Bryan supported in Nicaragua and to the protectorates the Administration established in Santo Domingo and Haiti. Wilson never fully appreciated how closely his policies resembled "dollar diplomacy" or the intensity of the anti-American feeling those policies provoked.

The President also plunged into Mexican affairs. During the late nineteenth century, large landholders, the army, the hierarchy of the Church, and foreign investors had sustained a dictatorial government in Mexico that had suppressed the landless, uneducated, impoverished peasants and workers. In 1911 a revolution, in this phase instigated by a middle class seeking greater opportunity, overthrew the government, but in 1913 General Victoriano Huerta engineered a *coup d'état* that restored a reactionary regime under his domination. The revolutionists, who called themselves Constitutionalists, continued to resist under Venustiano Carranza, their able and implacable leader. Though his forces controlled much of the country, the major European powers recognized the Huerta government.

Americans with financial interests in Mexico urged Wilson also to do so, but the President would have no formal dealings with a government of assassins. He therefore refused to appoint an ambassador to Mexico. He did, however, send a series of special agents, whose reports intensified his dislike for the

Wilson: "I am going to teach the South American republics to elect a good man!"

regime but also led him erroneously to believe that the United States could decree a solution to its neighbor's problems.

Wilson followed a policy of "watchful waiting" until October 1913, when Huerta, supported by British oil interests, proclaimed himself military dictator. The President then demanded that Huerta retire. The United States, he assured the Mexicans, sought no territory but only the advancement of "constitutional liberty."

To cut off the dictator's support, Wilson promised to protect British property if a Constitutionalist victory endangered it. He also, in 1914, drove through Congress a law repealing the exemption from tolls for American coastal shipping using the Panama Canal. That exemption, as the British had argued, violated an Anglo-American treaty that pledged the United States not to discriminate against British shipping using the canal. In full agreement, Wilson timed his action also to serve his Mexican policy. The danger of war in Europe made the British particularly solicitous of American friendship, and in March 1914 they withdrew their recognition of Huerta.

Meanwhile Wilson had told Carranza that the United States would join him in war against Huerta if he would keep the revolution orderly. Opposed to any American interference, Carranza rejected the indiscreet offer. But, since he needed the arms that an American embargo denied all Mexicans, his representatives assured Wilson that he would respect property rights. Somewhat skeptically, the President lifted the embargo in February 1914.

Intervention in Mexico. Soon thereafter Wilson seized an excuse for intervention. On April 10, 1914, an Huertista colonel arrested some American sailors who had gone ashore at Tampico. Though the Mexicans immediately apologized, they refused to make a formal salute to the American flag. On that pretext Wilson prepared to occupy Vera Cruz, Mexico's most important port. On April 20 he asked Congress for authority to use military force "to obtain from General Huerta . . . the fullest recognition of the rights and dignity of the United States."

The next day, before Congress could act, Wilson ordered the navy to seize Vera Cruz in order to prevent a German merchant ship from landing arms for Huerta. Both Americans and Mexicans were killed in the action that followed. While American newspapers predicted war and Wilson ordered war plans drawn up, the Constitutionalists as well as the Huertistas denounced the violation of their national sovereignty.

Fortunately both countries accepted an offer of mediation from Argentina, Brazil, and Chile. The resulting proposals were never signed by the Constitutionalists, who had become the dominant faction in

Mexico. Huerta abdicated in July, and Carranza marched into Mexico City in August 1914, angry with the United States and disdainful of Wilson.

During 1915 the revolution in Mexico reached high pitch. Violence sometimes accompanied reform. The destruction of private property and attacks on priests and nuns excited American demands for intervention, especially among Catholics, Republicans eager to embarrass Wilson, and jingoes spoiling for a war. The President resisted that pressure, partly because he respected Carranza's objectives, partly because he dared not let embroilments in Mexico tie his hands in the crisis then developing with Germany. In October 1915 he recognized the Constitutionalists as the *de facto* government.

Within a few months Pancho Villa, a champion of the peasants, created a new crisis. An opponent of Carranza, Villa had earlier won some support from Wilson. In January 1916, however, Villa murdered a group of Americans whom he had removed from a train in Mexico. In March he killed nineteen more during a raid on Columbus, New Mexico. Again there were demands in the United States for war, but Wilson tried to contain the situation. He ordered an expe-

Pancho Villa

dition to cross the border and punish Villa but to avoid engaging the Constitutionalists.

The futile pursuit of Villa aroused Mexican tempers. In April Carranza insisted the Americans leave his country. Wilson refused. When Villa brazenly raided Texas, the President called up the national guard for service on the border and commissioned plans for a full-scale invasion. Twice there were serious skirmishes between American and Constitutionalist soldiers. Carranza, however, needed to devote his full energies to his domestic affairs, and Wilson had growing problems in Europe. Both men, moreover, genuinely desired peace. In July 1916 they agreed to appoint a joint commission to resolve their differences. Although Carranza later rejected its decision, the danger of war had passed. In January 1917 Wilson called the troops home, and two months later he granted the Constitutionalists *de jure* recognition.

In the balance Wilson's restraint outweighed his moralism. In attempting to impose American standards upon the Mexicans, the President offended those he wanted to help. But he also succeeded in withstanding the demands for war that he had inadvertently fanned. He succeeded most of all in grasping the need for reform in Mexico. The American people in varying degree shared his confusions and his distaste for the excesses of revolution. Most of them, however, also shared his reluctance to permit disagreement and discord to grow into war.

Problems of Neutrality

War in Europe. In August 1914 a crisis within the empire of Austria-Hungary provided the match to light the fire of war in Europe that had been brewing for more than a decade. Ambitious Germany dominated the alliance of the Central Powers, including Austria-Hungary and Turkey. On the other side were the western powers, France and England, their ally, Russia, and soon also Italy, a partner bought by promises of more lands.

Though most Americans had known that war was threatening, they were shocked by the outbreak of hostilities and unprepared to face the problems war imposed on them. Relieved that war seemed so far away, they had yet to learn that distance alone could not insulate the United States. Most progressives tended to believe that selfish commercial rivalries had moved the European nations toward disaster. They believed, too, that the United States could serve the world best by concentrating on further reform at home, by setting a noble example of peace and democracy. Even those who were not progressives were slow

to recognize the intensity of nationalistic emotions that war bred, slower still in seeing how those emotions blocked a return to peace. Americans, like other peoples, had no experience with the shocks of total war, calculated brutality, and mass hatred.

The Administration's initial statements of policy gave official sanction to attitudes that prevailed throughout the nation. Wilson expressed his faith that the United States could play "a part of impartial mediation," and he urged Americans to be "neutral in fact as well as in name." But impartiality of sentiment was impossible. Many Americans of various national origins identified themselves with the loyalties of their forebears. The German- and Irish-Americans particularly supported the Central Powers, as did Czechs, Slovaks, Serbians, and others from Austria-Hungary. British-Americans favored the western Allies. The similarities between British and American speech and institutions, furthermore, fostered widespread sympathy for England. Wilson himself had long been an admirer of England's culture.

Belligerents in both camps tried to enlist American emotions. The Germans circulated stories alleging that the British blockade was causing mass starvation; the British published accounts of atrocities allegedly committed by German soldiers. Both sides exaggerated, but propaganda won few converts. The course of the war itself, however, made a deeper impression. Germany's invasion of Belgium in August 1914, which violated a treaty pledging Germany to respect Belgian neutrality, offended many Americans. Propaganda could not erase that evidence of German ruthlessness, and evidence was to come of German intrigue against the United States. The Allied cause gradually gained adherents, though very few even among them favored American participation in a war across the Atlantic.

Neutral rights. While Wilson remained firm in his purpose to be neutral in fact, he upheld neutral rights to trade and to the use of the ocean. Those traditional objectives of American diplomacy had, the President believed, a clear basis in law and morality. His standards for defining neutral rights were "the existing rules of international law and the treaties of the United States." But those rules were uncertain, especially under the unprecedented conditions created by the tactics of the submarine, the novel weapon on which Germany counted heavily. Particularly with Germany, but also with England, troubles arose over Wilson's interpretations of American neutral rights.

The British, who controlled the seas, were determined that the Allies alone should receive munitions and other essential war materials from the United States. They therefore established a tight blockade of Germany and narrowly limited the kinds of goods that American ships could carry to neutral ports from

Central Powers
Allied Powers
Neutral nations

which they could be sent on to Germany. The British also diverted suspect shipping to their own ports, confiscated many cargoes, interfered with American mail in order to intercept military and economic information, and ultimately forbade British subjects to do any business with American firms "blacklisted" for violating British rules.

Wilson protested often and vigorously against these and other British practices that infringed upon traditional neutral rights. The British, engaged in total war, considered him peevishly legalistic. But, since they had to have American supplies, they made the basic objective of their diplomacy "the maximum blockade that could be enforced without a rupture with the United States."

The success of that policy owed much to the increasing good will Americans felt for England. It owed something, too, to the growing importance of war production for the American economy. Allied demands for war materials stimulated American heavy industry and provided a market for American agriculture. Indeed, with a wise solicitude the British even provided funds to help stabilize the price of cotton at a level satisfactory to the Democratic South.

There were no international rules against selling war materials to the Allies. And if Wilson had refused to permit such sales, he would have indirectly aided the Central Powers. Nor were there any rules to prevent American bankers from making loans to finance Allied purchases. Bryan at first maintained that such loans violated "the true spirit of neutrality," but early in 1915, when the Allies were desperate for funds, he partially reversed himself. Before the end of that year the State Department had approved enormous loans, arranged by American financiers, without which England and France could not have continued to buy the materials they had to have. Thereafter the United States had something of a stake in preventing a German triumph.

The Germans, who were unable to transport supplies through the British blockade, protested against American sales of war materials to the Allies and against British interpretations of maritime law. They also sent out submarines to destroy Allied shipping. These U-boats created the issue on which German-American relations ultimately foundered.

The submarine issue. Submarines could not operate according to the traditional rules governing the conduct of ships bent on destroying commerce. Their effectiveness depended upon surprise. They could not warn their prospective targets before attacking them or remove crews or passengers from stricken ships. Yet Wilson insisted that the Germans observe traditional international law.

The submarine issue arose in February 1915, when Germany proclaimed a war zone around the British Isles. Enemy ships, Germany warned, would be sunk on sight, and neutral ships would be in danger of misidentification. In a sharp reply Wilson called the sinking of merchant ships without visit and search "a wanton act." The destruction of an American ship, he declared, or the loss of American lives on belligerent ships, would be regarded as "a flagrant violation of neutral rights." It would be an offensive act for which he would hold Germany to "strict accountability." His note expressed the horror most Americans felt toward the barbarity of modern weapons. It left the Germans with a choice between abandoning their strategic plan or risking American antagonism.

They chose to take the risk. In April 1915 an American went down aboard a British ship. On May 1 an American ship was torpedoed. Six days later the Germans sank the British passenger liner *Lusitania*, and with it died more than 1,200 men, women, and children, 128 of them Americans whom the Germans had warned not to embark. That sinking shocked the nation. A minority wanted to break off relations with Germany, which in their view was guilty of "murder," as Theodore Roosevelt put it. Most Americans of that mind hoped soon to see the United States at war. At the other extreme, those who sympathized

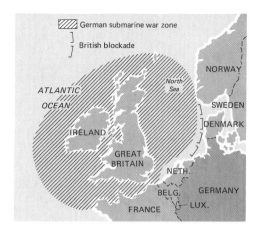

The war at sea

with Germany and those who considered war the worst possible calamity were eager to arbitrate the issue, if necessary to prohibit travel on the ships of belligerents. The majority of Americans were angry but anxious to avoid hostility. Like Wilson, they hoped the problem could be negotiated away.

"There is such a thing," the President told one audience, "as a man being too proud to fight. There is such a thing as a nation being so right that it does not

Neutral in fact

The New York Times.

EXTRA
5:30 A.M.

VOL. LXIV...NO. 20,923. ••••• NEW YORK, SATURDAY, MAY 8, 1915.—TWENTY-FOUR PAGES. ONE CENT In Greater New York, Elsewhere Jersey City and Newark. | THREE CENTS.

LUSITANIA SUNK BY A SUBMARINE, PROBABLY 1,260 DEAD; TWICE TORPEDOED OFF IRISH COAST; SINKS IN 15 MINUTES; CAPT. TURNER SAVED, FROHMAN AND VANDERBILT MISSING; WASHINGTON BELIEVES THAT A GRAVE CRISIS IS AT HAND

SHOCKS THE PRESIDENT

Washington Deeply Stirred by the Loss of American Lives.

BULLETINS AT WHITE HOUSE

Wilson Reads Them Closely, but Is Silent on the Nation's Course.

HINTS OF CONGRESS CALL

Loss of Lusitania Recalls Firm Tone of Our First Warning to Germany.

CAPITAL FULL OF RUMORS

Reports That Liner Was to be Sunk Were Heard Before Actual News Came.

Special to The New York Times.
WASHINGTON, May 7.— Never since that April day, three years ago, when word came that the Titanic had gone down, has Washington been so stirred as it is tonight over the sinking of the Lusitania. The early reports told that there had been no loss of life, but the relief that these advices caused gave way to the keenest concern late this evening when it became known that there had been many deaths. Although they are profoundly reticent, officials realize that this tragedy, involving the loss of American citizens, is likely to bring about a crisis in the international relations of the United States.

It is pointed out that the sinking of the Lusitania is the outcome of a series of incidents that have been the

The Lost Cunard Steamship Lusitania
X Where the First Torpedo Struck.   XX Where the Second Torpedo Struck.

Cunard Office Here Besieged for News; Fate of 1,918 on Lusitania Long in Doubt

Nothing Heard from the Well-Known Passengers on Board—Story of Disaster Long Unconfirmed While Anxious Crowds Seek Details.

List of Saved Includes Capt. Turner; Vanderbilt and Frohman Reported Lost

LONDON, Saturday, May 8.—5:30 A.M.—The Times Bureau has received from the British Admiralty at Queenstown a report that all the torpedo boats and tugs and armed trawlers, except the Heron, which went out from Queenstown to the relief of the Lusitania have returned.

Saw the Submarine 100 Yards Off and Watched Torpedo as It Struck Ship

Ernest Cowper, a Toronto Newspaper Man, Describes Attack, Seen from Ship's Rail—Poison Gas Used in Torpedoes, Say Other Passengers.

SOME DEAD TAKEN ASHORE

Several Hundred Survivors at Queenstown and Kinsale.

STEWARD TELLS OF DISASTER

One Torpedo Crashes Into the Doomed Liner's Bow, Another Into the Engine Room.

SHIP LISTS OVER TO PORT

Makes It Impossible to Lower Many Boats, So Hundreds Must Have Gone Down.

ATTACKED IN BROAD DAY

Passengers at Luncheon—Warning Had Been Given by Germans Before the Ship Left New York.

Only 650 Were Saved, Few Cabin Passengers

QUEENSTOWN, Saturday, May 8, 4:28 A.M.—Survivors of the Lusitania who have arrived here estimate that only about 650 of those aboard the steamer were saved, and say only a small proportion of those rescued were saloon passengers.

Official Confirmation
WASHINGTON, May 8.—A dispatch to the State

---

need to convince others by force." In that spirit he began his negotiations. It did not matter, he told Berlin, that the *Lusitania* carried munitions as well as passengers. That was a secondary consideration. The United States was concerned with the "sacred . . . rights of humanity," particularly "the right to life itself." The sinking was an "illegal and inhuman" act, and Wilson demanded an apology and reparations. Since submarines could not be used without violating "principles of justice and humanity," he also by implication demanded that they should not be used at all. And by identifying neutral rights with "sacred" human rights, he charged a difficult issue with needless emotional electricity.

The extremists were dissatisfied. Roosevelt called the President "yellow." Bryan, who had urged Wilson to adopt the principles of the "cooling-off" treaties, considered the notes to Germany too harsh. Sadly he resigned from the Cabinet, to be replaced by Robert Lansing, a New York lawyer with a talent for diplomatic phraseology. As he and the President continued to negotiate, the Germans met them part way. They

would not admit the illegality of the sinking, but in February 1916 Germany offered an apology and an indemnity. By and large the American people were relieved. As Lansing put it, they desired only honorable friendship.

Peace with honor. As long as the war continued, however, the submarine issue might involve the United States. The national interest as well as the interests of the besieged people of Europe impelled Wilson to attempt to arrange a peace. He had sent Colonel House to Europe in January 1915 to investigate the possibility of mediation, but House had found the Germans adamant in their decision to hold Belgium and to destroy England's naval power. In October, however, House concocted a plan for peace, which Wilson approved. They intended to force Germany to negotiate by warning that otherwise the United States might enter the war on the Allied side. If the Germans were agreeable to negotiations, House hoped to bring them to reasonable terms at the conference table. Again, failure, according to the plan, would invite American participation in the war. In London in January and February 1916 House made progress toward his goal. But the enterprise collapsed when Lansing tried to revise American policy toward the submarines.

Wilson and Lansing had decided to ease the submarine issue by attempting to persuade the Allies not to arm their merchantmen. In that event the U-boats could issue warnings before attacking. The Germans welcomed the idea, for their purpose was not to kill sailors but to destroy cargoes and bottoms. To their advantage, just as House was completing his negotiations in England, Lansing suggested that Allied merchantmen be disarmed. The British of course refused. Lansing had earlier suggested to the Germans that if the Allies declined, Germany might declare unrestricted submarine warfare against all armed ships. In February 1916 the Germans made precisely that declaration. But Lansing then reasserted Wilson's original submarine policy and announced that the United States would not warn Americans against travel on armed ships. "Strict accountability" still applied.

The Roosevelt Republicans prepared to make a major campaign issue during 1916 of the embarrassment the President had caused the Allies. At the opposite pole of opinion, Bryan, La Follette, and other agrarian progressives saw a "sort of moral treason" in letting American citizens create crises by sailing on endangered ships. Resolutions forbidding such travel failed in Congress only because Wilson exerted all his influence to defeat them.

One month later, in March 1916, a German submarine without warning torpedoed an unarmed French steamer, the *Sussex*, which was carrying some American passengers. The President's policy seemed to have failed. But he did not retreat from his principles. After much reflection, in April he sent Germany an ultimatum. Unless it immediately abandoned "its present method of submarine warfare," the United States would "sever diplomatic relations." The Kaiser's advisers decided that since they lacked the submarines to conduct a useful blockade of England, it was more important to keep the United States neutral. In May Germany acceded to Wilson's demand. Submarines would observe the rules of visit and search, the Germans said, but they might remove that limitation unless the United States compelled England to obey international law.

In spite of the threat that Germany might revert to its earlier tactics, most Americans were again relieved. Unaware of the reasons for the German decision, they felt that the President had avoided war, maintained justice, and conquered the submarines with his pen. They did not realize that Wilson's ultimatum and the German response left an American decision about going to war up to Germany. For if that

nation resumed unrestricted submarine warfare, Wilson had committed himself to belligerence. Nevertheless, in 1916 the *Sussex* pledge seemed to promise peace with honor—a happy formula for a campaign year.

Americanism and preparedness. As the war went on, it revealed to Americans as well as to Europeans the terrors of organized brutality and the dangers of organized passions. Intelligence and decency and orderliness gave way before the strains of continual fear. Though the United States was far from the fields of battle, even here the timid sought some symbol that would protect them from the disturbances around them. Others seized the chance to create nationalistic symbols they could use for their own selfish ends. The most avid foes of labor unions underwrote a campaign to equate the open shop with "Americanism." Those who distrusted blacks or Catholics or Jews now did so in the name of Americanism. It was a word that the opponents of women's suffrage used, a word used also by the advocates of a literacy test for immigrants. The Senate blocked an amendment to enfranchise women, and Congress in 1915 passed a bill establishing a literacy test. Wilson vetoed it, pointing out that it abridged the traditional right of asylum and tested education rather than talent.

The President resisted the spirit of frightened conformity that Roosevelt exalted in the name of Americanism. The name, however, had a political magic no politician could safely ignore, and Wilson himself used it to describe his foreign policy. In 1915, condemning the sabotage of munitions production for the Allies, he attributed it to extremists among the German- and Irish-Americans. Calling on all others to dedicate themselves to the national honor, the President planned to make his version of Americanism the keynote of his campaign for reelection.

The position Wilson and his party took on preparedness also accorded with the middle-of-the-road attitudes of most Americans. Even after the war began, they tended, like the President, to consider arms and munitions the unnecessary tools of evil men. Again like the President, they had an instinctive dislike for widespread military training and a large standing army, neither of which had any place in the American tradition. That tradition persisted, in spite of the nature of modern war, in defining the militia and a citizen-soldiery as proper safeguards for national security. Four months after the sinking of the *Lusitania*, Wilson expressed a popular sentiment when he said he saw no need "to stir the nation up in favor of national defense."

Moved by the possibility of war in Europe and Mexico, a vocal minority began to preach the need to prepare, pointing out that it took time to produce weapons and to train armies and navies for twentieth-century warfare. Theodore Roosevelt led these advocates of preparedness. He was sometimes too strident to be convincing, but more moderate men gradually put their ideas across. Preparedness became a political issue, and Wilson's advisers warned him that he had better do something about it.

In July 1915 the President instructed the armed services to make plans for expansion. In November, asking for much less than they had recommended, he proposed a volunteer army of four hundred thousand men who were to serve only a few months in each of several successive years. Even this modest proposal met opposition from rural liberals in Congress, most of them Democrats, some of them with great influence. Preparedness also incurred the hostility of a passionate peace party, its membership recruited not least from among women who saw all war as a needless exercise of raw masculinity. To win support for his program, Wilson went on a speaking trip that took him halfway across the continent. During that tour he came out for a "navy second to none."

Yet in 1916 the President had to make concessions to his opponents. Still close to the middle of the road, he first rejected the War Department's plan for creating a large reserve force under the regular army, and he appointed a new Secretary of War, Newton D. Baker, a progressive with a reputation for antimilitarism. Wilson and Baker then worked out a compromise that satisfied the Congress. The resulting statute of May 1916 doubled the regular army but left the national guard still largely independent of the authority of the War Department. The President's influence helped, too, to carry a measure accelerating the building of a strong navy.

The agrarians scored one success: in the face of Administration opposition, they fashioned the revenue legislation to pay for the defense program. It increased surtaxes on personal income and put new taxes on inheritances. Those best able to pay would have to foot the bill for preparedness.

The Democrats had given the preparedness issue a progressive stamp and had identified their party with national defense. The measures fell short of the demands of the armed services, but they met the most urgent requirements of a nation that still hoped and expected to remain at peace.

The election of 1916. For the Republicans one major problem in 1916 was how to reassimilate the Progressive party. Roosevelt had kept it alive largely to further his own ambitions, but the Old Guard would not countenance his nomination on the Republican ticket, and the Colonel cared more about defeating Wilson than about nursing old grudges. In order to regain Bull Moose votes, the Republicans selected a candidate with a progressive record, Charles Evans Hughes. He had been a successful reform governor of New York and in 1912, as an Associate Justice of the Supreme Court, had stayed neutral in the party split. He was an able man and a strong candidate whose cause may have been hurt rather than helped by Roosevelt's obsessive attacks on Democratic foreign policy.

Election of 1916

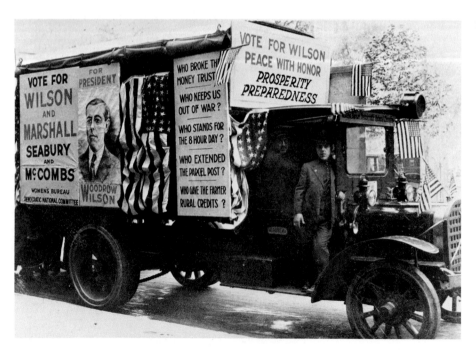

Although Wilson had planned to run on the issues of Americanism and progressivism, foreign policy became a central factor in the campaign. The party-managers realized that their most effective slogan would be: "He kept us out of war." Its effectiveness grew as Hughes explained that he would have been tougher on Mexico and Germany than Wilson had been. The President himself told the voters that he was "not expecting this country to get into war," and Democratic propagandists advertised: "Wilson and Peace with Honor? or Hughes with Roosevelt and War?"

There were, of course, other issues. The Irish-American and German-American extremists embarrassed Hughes by supporting him openly; but he failed to repudiate them publicly, while Wilson deliberately attacked them. The Democrats had made a progressive record that was persuasive with those from the defunct Bull Moose who could not yet tolerate the idea of voting Republican again.

By and large, rural America voted for Wilson, as did labor, the liberals, and most intellectuals. That coalition was still tenuous, but it foreshadowed the profile of Democratic hegemony years later. In 1916 the contest was so close that it hinged on the ballots in California and Minnesota, which were counted only after early Eastern returns had put Hughes ahead. Hughes went to bed election night thinking that he had won. But the South and the West reversed the verdict. Wilson received 49.4 percent of the popular vote to Hughes' 46.2 percent and carried the Electoral College 277 to 254. Peace and progressivism had helped to put Wilson across again, but his victory had also depended upon traditional Democratic loyalties and the continuing Republican division.

The Road to War

Wilson knew how uncertain was the nation's hold on peace. Before election day the British had tightened their regulations on neutral trade, and the Germans had intensified their submarine campaign against the Allies. Either Wilson had to find ways to end the war or else he would have to sacrifice peace or honor—or both.

The President planned to send a dramatic note to the belligerents. He was ready, his draft said, to pledge the "whole force" of the United States to end the "war of exhaustion and attrition" and to keep the future peace. The draft asked each side for "a concrete definition" of its war objectives. It also demanded an immediate peace conference. Wilson intended to employ every pressure short of war to assist

the more reasonable side. While he was still reworking his draft, in December 1916, the German chancellor announced his government's readiness to negotiate.

The offer hid a calculating spirit. The Germans made the gesture out of confidence of impending victory. Masters of the eastern front, where the Russians were collapsing, the Germans expected to smash France and England if their terms were rejected. They had also secretly decided that, if negotiations failed, they would resume unrestricted submarine warfare. And their secret terms were harsh—they would insist on territory along the Baltic, in the Congo, and in Belgium, France, and Luxembourg.

Slowly Wilson discovered the truth. He dispatched the note he had been drafting, but the Germans replied that they wanted no neutral at the peace table. The Allies publicly rejected the President's proposal but privately let him know they would negotiate if the German conditions were reasonable. Then in January 1917 the Germans revealed their greedy terms and announced that their submarines would sink at sight all ships, belligerent or neutral.

For several weeks Wilson would not admit that he had either to surrender his principles or go to war. He broke off relations with Germany, but he told Congress he wanted no conflict. He remained outwardly temperate even after learning on February 25 that Germany was plotting against the United States. That day the British communicated to Washington secret orders of the German foreign minister, Arthur Zimmermann, which they had intercepted. Those orders told the German minister to Mexico that, in the event of war with the United States, he should invite Mexico and Japan to join the Central Powers and promise Mexico its lost lands in the Southwest as war booty—a shocking prospect to Americans.

Wilson had meanwhile pressed his interpretation of neutral rights. He had asked Congress for authority to arm American merchant vessels and to employ any other means that might be necessary to protect American ships and citizens at sea. To win votes for his proposal, he made the Zimmermann note public on March 1, 1917. A wave of anti-German sentiment swept the country, but the Democratic House of Representatives withheld the broad authority the President wanted, and in the Senate a dozen antiwar progressives talked a stronger bill to death.

That "little group of willful men," as Wilson called them, struggled in vain. The Zimmermann note had dissolved the myth that the war was strictly European. The President on his own ordered the merchantmen armed, and on March 18, two weeks after his second inauguration, U-boats sank three American ships. Moreover, the first Russian revolution established a limited monarchy and a responsible parliament, temporarily destroying the despotism that had made Americans reluctant to associate with the Allied cause. And the Allies could no longer fight without American men, money, and material. The combination of events convinced even the most ardent peace advocates in the Cabinet of the necessity for war.

Wilson was agonized by a conclusion he could not escape. War, he allegedly told one confidant, "would overturn the world we had known," lead to "a dictated peace," require "illiberalism at home." Sadly he predicted that "the spirit of ruthless brutality" would enter the very "fibre of our national life." His pain was shared by most progressives, for progressivism had based its faith on the peaceful, reasonable improvement of the lot of humanity in a world of quiet and intelligence. It was also, however, a moral faith, and in the view of Wilson and other progressive intellectuals, Germany had violated moral principles. It had forced war on France and Belgium. It was bent on conquest. Whatever the definitions of neutral rights, so Wilson had concluded, no one was immune from German aggression, and there could be no real peace while it went unpunished.

With those thoughts in mind, Wilson on April 2 addressed the special session of Congress he had summoned. On April 4 the Senate by a vote of 82 to 6, and on April 6 the House of Representatives by a vote of 373 to 50, passed a resolution recognizing the existence of a state of war with Germany.

The decision of the German General Staff to resume unrestricted submarine warfare had rested on the calculation that American belligerency would cost Germany less than continuing shipments of American supplies to the Allies. That decision, as the Germans expected it would, led to the American declaration of war, for Wilson and his supporters had staked the grandeur of the nation and supposedly the rights of humanity on his policies. If Americans had not been allowed to travel upon the ships of belligerents, if American bankers had been forbidden to make loans to England and France, if the United States had surrendered its historic commitment to neutral rights, if Wilson's rhetoric had been more disciplined, the crisis of war would not have developed as it did. But American business interests would not have abandoned their markets without protest. Indeed Wilson sought a settlement that would serve American interests. With the failure of his efforts at mediation, war provided another path to that goal. As important, the sense of national greatness that had been growing since the 1880s precluded an easy acceptance of limitations on the country imposed by any foreign power. Wilson gave a special cast to American pride and sensitivity, but those sentiments were not his alone. Most important, though no one of the great powers of Europe was uninvolved in the contest for supremacy that brought on the war, the Germans did precipitate the war and pursue it without the delicate and deliberate care for American sensibilities that the British cultivated. Further, had the Germans prevailed, they intended to impose upon Europe and much of the rest of the world a Carthaginian settlement. German intentions, as well as the special conditions of war-making that guided German maritime strategy, created the problems that American policy-makers found no way to resolve, in the end, short of war itself.

New York American

WAR WITH GERMANY

BAKER | Gibbons Prays God May Guide | Austria and Turkey Hope to | HOUSE

Suggestions for Reading

GENERAL

The best general account of the Taft years and of the breakup of the Republican party is in G. E. Mowry, *The Era of Theodore Roosevelt** (1958). A. S. Link, *Woodrow Wilson and the Progressive Era** (1954), covers the succeeding years to the American entry into the war. Both books are challenged by Gabriel Kolko, *The Triumph of Conservatism** (1963). Also useful are relevant parts of Eric Goldman, *Rendezvous with Destiny** (1952), and Richard Hofstadter, *The Age of Reform: From Bryan to F. D. R.** (1955). An older book of G. E. Mowry, *Theodore Roosevelt and the Progressive Movement** (1946), contains a more detailed account—and less friendly to T. R.—than that in the same author's later work.

PROGRESSIVES AND REGULARS

A case for Taft is set forth in P. O. Coletta, *The Presidency of William Howard Taft* (1973), and D. E. Anderson, *William Howard Taft* (1973), which should be compared with the Roosevelt biographies listed in connection with the preceding chapter and with A. T. Mason, *Bureaucracy Convicts Itself* (1941); J. L. Holt, *Congressional Insurgents and the Party System, 1909–1916* (1967); and L. L. Gould, *Reform and Regulation: American Politics, 1900–1916** (1978). For an understanding of progressive social ideas, see the books suggested in the previous chapter. It is also essential to read Herbert Croly, *The Promise of American Life* (1909); Walter Weyl, *The New Democracy* (1912); and Walter Lippmann, *Drift and Mastery* (1914). See also Otis Graham, Jr., *Encore for Reform: The Old Progressives and the New Deal* (1967). Two significant studies of progressive thought, besides those referred to in the previous chapter, are Walter Johnson, *William Allen White's America* (1947), and C. B. Forcey, *The Crossroads of Liberalism* (1961). There are no comparable studies of conservative thought, but that subject gets useful treatment in Richard Leopold, *Elihu Root and the Conservative Tradition** (1954). Useful in the context of its title is Walter and Marie Scholes, *The Foreign Policies of the Taft Administration* (1970).

WILSON

The outstanding work on Wilson is A. S. Link's multivolume biography. Two brief studies of Wilson are J. M. Blum, *Woodrow Wilson and the Politics of Morality** (1956), and J. A. Garraty, *Woodrow Wilson* (1956). See, too, the comparison of Roosevelt and Wilson in J. M. Cooper, Jr., *The Warrior and the Priest* (1983). Of the special studies of Wilson's diplomacy, the best are A. S. Link, *Wilson the Diplomatist* (1957); N. G. Levin, Jr., *Woodrow Wilson and World Politics** (1968); and P. Devlin, *Too Proud to Fight: Woodrow Wilson's Neutrality* (1974). There are keen analyses of the issues of American foreign policy in R. E. Osgood, *Ideals and Self-Interest in America's Foreign Relations** (1953), and E. R. May, *The World War and American Isolation 1914–1917* (1959). W. A. Williams, *The Tragedy of American Foreign Policy* (1962), presents the most influential interpretation of the dominance of economic considerations. Other important monographs include D. G. Munro, *Intervention and Dollar Diplomacy in the Caribbean, 1900–1921* (1964); R. E. Quirk, *An Affair of Honor: Woodrow Wilson and the Occupation of Vera Cruz** (1962); P. E. Haley, *Revolution and Intervention: The Diplomacy of Taft and Wilson with Mexico, 1910–1917* (1970); R. W. Curry, *Woodrow Wilson and Far Eastern Policy, 1913–1921* (1968); Ross Gregory, *The Origins of American Intervention in the First World War** (1971); D. M. Smith, *The Great Departure: The United States in World War I, 1914–1920** (1965); and J. M. Cooper, Jr., *The Vanity of Power: American Isolationism and the First World War, 1914–1917* (1969). Of the various studies of the Wilsonians, one is indispensable: C. Seymour, ed., *The Intimate Papers of Colonel House*, 4 vols. (1921–28), for which an important corrective will be a new edition of the House Papers by Wilton Fowler. Also useful, particularly on domestic issues, is A. T. Mason, *Brandeis: A Free Man's Life* (1946). J. A. Garraty, *Henry Cabot Lodge* (1953), presents an understanding account of one of Wilson's foremost antagonists. The literature on Wilson and his time has been richly expanded with the continuing publication of his letters and papers under the editorship of A. S. Link.

*Available in a paperback edition.

24
WAR AND
ITS SEQUEL

The American nation was unprepared for the First World War. To begin with, the country had no clear sense of purpose. Many German- and Irish-Americans were unreconciled to fighting on the side of the Allies. Smaller groups of pacifists saw no excuse for any fighting, and some progressives believed that the United States had no business involving itself in what they considered to be a struggle between European imperialists. The majority of Americans were in full accord with the decision to go to war, but they were confused about its origins and objectives. Like the President, they had hoped to remain neutral. Like the President, they regarded the submarine issue as a matter of morality. They had little, if any, understanding of world politics.

Indeed, the moral temper of the times led Americans to seek utopian rather than realistic reasons for the actions to which they were committed. To accommodate that temper, and to convert the dissenters, Wilson defined American war aims in idealistic terms. The spirit of his war message and later addresses was noble as well as persuasive. It helped transmute the fervor of progressivism into the selfless bravery of the "great crusade." But it also turned some fervor into frenzy, and it led Americans to expect a paradise that no war could give them. The failure to achieve that expectation tinged the persisting frenzy of the immediate postwar years with bitterness and vindictiveness.

The United States was also unprepared for the total mobilization demanded by modern war and for the special strengths required to fight a war overseas. The nation lacked the necessary army, the plans and facilities to raise it, the guns and tanks and airplanes to equip it, and the ships to transport it. Even the tools and the organization to produce the materials of war were wanting. In every respect—emotional, economic, military—mobilization was urgent but erratic.

The Armed Forces
on Land and Sea

Selective service. The President and his military advisers agreed that conscription was the only efficient and democratic way to recruit a large army. Yet the Speaker of the House and the Chairman of the Military Affairs Committee, both Democrats, led the opposition to the Administration's selective-service bill. Many of the bill's opponents considered conscription a threat to democracy. Others had a romantic attachment to the tradition of voluntary military service. But if war had ever been romantic it was no longer so, and selective service, as Wilson argued, spread the obligation to serve among all qualified men without regard to their social position, a desirable

598

At the front

Attention!

ALL MALES between the ages of 21 and 30 years, both inclusive, must personally appear at the polling place in the Election District in which they reside, on

TUESDAY, JUNE 5th, 1917

between the hours of 7 A.M. and 9 P. M. and

Register

in accordance with the President's Proclamation.

Any male person, between these ages, who fails to register on June 5th, 1917, will be subject to imprisonment in jail or other penal institution for a term of one year.

NO EXCUSE FOR FAILURE TO REGISTER WILL BE ACCEPTED

NON-RESIDENTS must apply personally for registration, at the office of the County Clerk, at Kingston, N. Y., AT ONCE, in order that their registration cards may be in the hands of the Registration Board of their home district before June 5, 1917

Employers of males between these ages are earnestly requested to assits in the enforcement of the President's Proclamation.

Signed,

BOARD OF REGISTRATION
of Ulster County
E. T. SHULTIS, Sheriff
C. K. LOUGHRAN, County Clerk
Dr. FRANK JOHNSTON, Medical Officer

The army's top command was strictly professional. Bypassing General Leonard Wood, an intimate of Roosevelt, Wilson made General John J. Pershing head of the American Expeditionary Force and gave his decisions consistent support. "Black Jack" Pershing, a laconic, stern West Pointer, pursued two controversial policies. He refused to send troops into battle until they had completed their training, and he insisted on preserving a separate identity for the American Expeditionary Force, though the French and British were impatient for reinforcements and eager to merge American units with their own.

The war in the west. In the fall of 1917 German offensives routed the Italians and destroyed the Russian army. The Bolshevik Revolution of November removed Russia from the war and left the western front, manned by war-weary French and British troops, exposed to the full attack Germany was certain to mount the following spring. The alarmed Allies created the Supreme War Council to direct their resistance and urged Pershing to supply men, trained or untrained. But Pershing still declined. In the spring, however, as the Allied lines crumbled before a furious German offensive, Wilson agreed to the appointment of French Marshal Ferdinand Foch as supreme commander, and Pershing put his four available divisions at Foch's disposal.

Foch and Pershing

---

contrast to the Union draft during the Civil War. The House passed the bill in May, but only after mollifying American mothers by raising the minimum draft age from nineteen, which the army recommended, to twenty-one.*

In the Senate the Republicans wasted three weeks in a futile effort to force the Administration to accept the volunteer division Theodore Roosevelt was organizing. Roosevelt and his admirers believed that even though his troops were half-trained they would make up the deficiency in dash. Wilson prudently preferred professional to political generals. The Selective Service Act finally passed by the Senate left Wilson free to dispose of volunteer units as he saw fit, and he saw fit to reject Roosevelt's.

Early in June 1917 over 9 million men registered quietly with the local officials whom the War Department authorized to supervise the draft. Before the war ended, over 24 million had registered and almost 3 million had been inducted into the army. There was little significant opposition to conscription, and the drafted troops fought as heroically as the 2 million volunteers who enlisted in the various armed services.

*It was necessary in 1918 to lower the minimum age to eighteen.

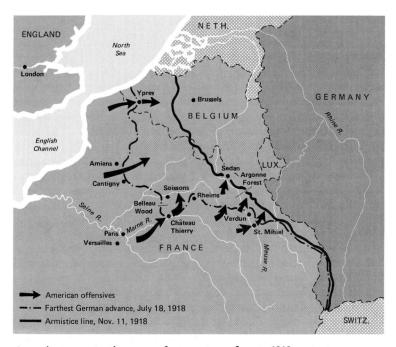

American operations on the western front, 1918

During May 1918 the Germans pushed the French back to the Marne River, only fifty miles from Paris. Foch then called up one American division and a few regiments of marines who met the Germans at Chateau Thierry, carried the intensive battle there, and in June drove the enemy out of Belleau Wood.

Gambling for a quick victory before more American forces could reach France, the Germans in July struck at the sector of the Marne between Rheims and Soissons. Here some eighty-five thousand Americans helped to turn the attack, and eight divisions of Yanks participated in the French counteroffensive that cleared out the sector early in August. The American First Army under Pershing then took over the southern front near St. Mihiel and routed the Germans there in an independent offensive in September. Late that month Pershing attacked the German lines between Verdun and Sedan. This Meuse-Argonne engagement produced a costly but crucial American victory. Along with the success of French and British forces on the northern and central fronts, it defeated the German army and set the stage for an armistice (see p. 608).

The triumph exacted extraordinary expenditures of nerve and flesh, for in some respects the First World War was the most ghastly in history. Casualties ran high, particularly during offensives, and American troops, along with their allies and foes, suffered a heavy incidence of shell shock, a form of battle fatigue, and of tuberculosis, a companion of the poison gas and the mud, cold, wet, and filth of the trenches. For most soldiers the war was an awful combination of fear, drudgery, and exhaustion.

The signal exceptions were the aviators. Their craft were simple and slow, their tactics rudimentary. Yet the new knights of the air wrote a chapter of military history in their man-to-man combat in the skies, and American aces dramatized for their countrymen the potentialities of aerial warfare.

In the trenches: American reinforcements

"I got within fifty feet of the German machine-gun nests when a bullet plowed through the top of my skull.... As I lay there I could plainly see the German gunners and hear them talking.... They reloaded their gun and turned it on me. The first three bullets went through my legs and hip and the rest splashed up dust and dirt.... That night ... one of my comrades ... who later in the battle was himself killed, crawled out and started to carry me back to the lines.... The Germans ... turned their guns our way.... Thinking it impossible for him to get me to the lines alone, he piled up a half-dozen bodies of my poor dead 'buddies' and barricaded my position. There I remained for several hours longer.... The boys piled up around me were my own camp-mates whom I knew.... Back of the lines the surgeons came out ... and ... exclaimed, 'What, ain't you dead yet?'" (Joyce Lewis)

"I dove down beside that road ... and recognized those Boche helmets! In a twinkling I was passed them ... and came diving down upon them from the rear. I just held both triggers down hard while the fiery bullets flew streaming out of the two guns.... I had a vague confused picture of ... rearing horses, falling men, running men, general mess.... I found myself trembling with excitement and overawed at being a cold-blooded murderer, but a sense of keen satisfaction came too. It was only the sort of thing our own poor doughboys have suffered so often." (Hamilton Coolidge)

"Side by side I have Americans, English, Scotch, Irish, and French, and a part in the corners are Boche. They have to watch each other die side by side. I am sent for everywhere—in the ... operating-room, the dressing room, and back again to the rows of men.... Of course, some only stay twenty-four hours, because they send them away just as fast as it is possible, for even this cellar is too dangerous a place to be in. The cannon goes day and night and the shells are breaking over and around us.... I have had to write many sad letters to American mothers. I wonder if it will ever end." (Florence Bullard)

From Frank Freidel, *Over There*, 1964.

The Yanks had reached France just in time. The Allies needed the new manpower to stop the Germans' gamble for victory—a gamble that would probably have succeeded had reinforcements failed to appear. Yet the Americans, indispensable during the last months of war, and gallant and effective then, arrived only after the Allies had held the Germans for almost four terrible years. Over 50,000 Americans died in France, but the war took the lives of 3 million English, French, and Russian soldiers. The role of the American army was both relatively small and absolutely vital.

The war at sea. So too was the role of the American navy. In all but one respect the war at sea had been won by the success of the British navy in bottling up the German fleet. As the British Admiralty admitted, however, the German submarines also had to be brought under control. During 1917 U-boats

sank more than twice the tonnage of shipping that the Allies and Americans built that year. Hard pressed to supply themselves, the British could not guard the American lines of supply to Europe, and the Americans could not afford to risk transporting an army aboard ships unprotected from enemy submarines.

The United States navy had the ships and the men to take over the patrol of the Western Hemisphere and to assist the English in patrolling the waters around the British Isles. But the Allies lacked the antisubmarine vessels to root the U-boats out of the ocean. An American plan proved to be at least as important as the ships themselves. Admiral William S. Sims, the ranking American naval officer in Europe, was the primary exponent of the idea of using destroyers and other men-of-war to escort convoys of merchantmen across the Atlantic. Though British skippers preferred to sail alone rather than to proceed in formation under naval command, Sims in the summer of 1917 overcame their objections and the resistance of the British Admiralty. By the end of 1917 the use of convoys had cut shipping losses in half.

The escorted convoys and the patrolling American destroyers were so effective that not one American soldier was lost in transit to Europe. The bridge of ships to France carried the troops and supplies that the Germans had expected to destroy, and the miracle of transportation turned the tide of war. That great American achievement was possible only because the British also provided bottoms for men and equipment, and only because the Yanks at the front could use Allied cannon, tanks, and airplanes.

The Home Front

Problems of production. By themselves the eventual prodigies of American war production would have been too little and too late for victory. Since there were no precedents for economic mobilization, the Administration had to feel its way along in creating agencies to supervise production and distribution and to allocate vital goods and services. When war came, the army did not even have information about the uniforms and shoes it would need. There was no inventory of national resources, no adequate plan for priorities or for stockpiling critical materials. Most of the first nine months of the war were spent in learning about mobilization, and in tooling up for production.

The lost time was especially serious for the aviation program. American planners were so slow in designing and manufacturing aircraft that American aviators had to fly in British and French machines all through the war. The situation was almost as desperate in the production of artillery and tanks. The building program for transports and cargo vessels collapsed completely, and the government had to rely on ships seized from neutrals or purchased from private industry.

These and other difficulties spurred the Senate Military Affairs Committee to investigate the conduct of the war. As 1918 began, the Democratic chairman of that committee asserted publicly that the military effort had been impeded by waste and inefficiency. Republican senators, joined by several Democrats, urged that a war cabinet of three distinguished citizens be set up to exercise the powers the Congress had conferred upon the President. If that measure had passed, Wilson would have become a figurehead. Even as it was, the Senate committee was close to assuming the role of its predecessor that had harassed Lincoln during the Civil War.

The President, however, had begun to address the problems of mobilization. Neither during 1917 nor later, moreover, did any scandal taint the administration of the war. Aware of the threat from the Senate, Wilson prepared a bill giving him sweeping authority to reorganize and manage all executive agencies. This measure, which Senator Lee S. Overman sponsored, passed Congress in April 1918 and enabled the President to complete his own plans.

Economic mobilization. Those plans were imbued with characteristically progressive hopes that the war would hasten the emergence of a cooperative commonwealth in which industry would substitute productive efficiency for the mere pursuit of profits, and government and business would work together in the public interest. In fact, business groups dominated public policy. Eager for efficient management of the economy, Wilson turned to the efficient managers of industry and finance. They had the experience and talents he needed. Able and patriotic men, they nevertheless remained alert to the interests of the firms they had left, which they naturally identified with the public good. Consequently, wartime economic management resulted in continuing boons to business rather than in federal monitoring of private enterprise in the manner that earlier regulatory efforts had contemplated. During the war, in spite of new taxes, corporate profits rose to three times their prewar level.

Agriculture also profited. In the spring of 1917 England, France, and Italy urgently needed food. Stretching the mandate of the Council of National Defense, which Congress had authorized the year before, the President established a food-control program in May under Herbert C. Hoover, who had acquired an international reputation as director of the Belgian Relief Commission. Wilson also asked Congress for emergency authority over agricultural production and distribution. The Lever Act of August 1917 granted him that authority, together with limited power to control the prices of certain scarce commodities. Wilson at once created the Food Administration. With Hoover at its head, that agency controlled prices to stimulate the production of wheat and pork, managed the distribution of those and other foodstuffs, and persuaded the public to observe meatless and breadless days. To that last objective, as to the selling of war bonds, American women contributed impressive energy. The success of Hoover's policies made possible the feeding of the nations fighting Germany and a 25 percent increase in the real income of American farmers.

The mobilization of industry proved less successful. The General Munitions Board, another offshoot of the Council of National Defense, showed itself incapable of coordinating the conflicting demands of the American armed services and the Allied purchasing commissions. Consequently, in July 1917 Wilson appointed a War Industries Board with authority to pass on all American and Allied purchasing, to allocate raw materials, to control production, and to supervise labor relations. The WIB, however, failed to elicit the full cooperation either of industry or of the armed services. In March 1918 the President rewrote its charter and named a new chairman, the wealthy and influential Democrat Bernard M. Baruch, who utilized the organizational structure of the nation's trade associations, common to many industries by that time. Through that arrangement businessmen thereafter dominated WIB policy, including arrangements for price-fixing. As one result big business gained economic power, but the WIB was also able to speed conversion to war production. The agency was helped in its task by a reorganization of the general staff of the army into functional divisions, each under an experienced officer selected without regard to seniority. Nevertheless, both government and business remained hesitant and ambiguous about the proper role of the modern state in wartime.

As in agriculture and industry, so in fuel, transportation, and labor, peacetime practices faltered under the stress of war. To relieve the critical coal shortage, the Lever Act empowered the President to fix the price of coal high enough to encourage operators to work marginal mines. In August 1917 he established the Fuel Administration under Harry A. Garfield, president of Williams College. Though the agency was unpopular with producers, enough coal was mined to meet the nation's needs. Snarls in railway transportation, however, impeded coal deliveries, and for four days in January 1918 Garfield closed all East Coast plants that used coal for any but vital purposes.

That emergency order underlined the crisis in railroading. The roads had tried to handle the extraordinary wartime traffic on the basis of voluntary cooperation, but in the absence of unified authority delays became worse and worse, and the snow and freezing weather of December 1917 precipitated a collapse of internal transportation. With congressional approval, Wilson therefore established the United States Railway Administration under William G. McAdoo. Exercising an even greater authority than Baruch had over industry, McAdoo and his associates, mostly railroad men, improved the railways' equipment, strengthened their finances, and adjusted their operations to the demands of war.

Labor and inflation. In April 1918 the President created the National War Labor Board to help resolve labor disputes and prevent attendant losses in production. Under the joint chairmanship of former President Taft and Frank P. Walsh, a labor lawyer, the WLB heard more than twelve hundred cases and forestalled many strikes, but it lacked the jurisdiction and the information it needed to set labor policies for the entire country. To remedy that deficiency, Wilson in May 1918 appointed the War Labor Policies Board under Felix Frankfurter, a young law professor who had been the War Department's labor adviser. The WLPB surveyed national labor needs and practices and standardized wages and hours. At its recommendation, the President created the United States Employment Service, an agency that placed almost 4 million workers in essential war jobs.

While keeping the country free from serious strikes during the last months of the war, the government's manpower agencies and policies also advanced some peacetime objectives of social reformers and union-leaders. Industry hired 40,000 more women. Membership in the American Federation of Labor grew more than 50 percent, reaching over 3,200,000 by 1920. The government demanded an eight-hour day for war industry wherever it could and insisted on decent working conditions and living wages. Even though the cost of living rose, booming wages and full employment permitted an increase of 20 percent in the average *real* income of blue-collar labor, considerably less than the increase in corporate and agricultural profits.

War worker

The federal agencies that exercised the mediating authority in the wartime economy served the interests primarily of industry but also of agriculture and labor. The agencies did not, however, lessen the conflicts among those major interest groups, nor did they operate according to peculiarly scientific principles. Rather, the various wartime agencies represented their own constituencies whose interests continued to conflict. The superficial reconciliation of those conflicts through administrative rulings bought cooperation at the price of favor, kept the machinery of war going, but charged the costs in the form of accelerating inflation to unrepresented individuals. Between 1916 and 1919 salaried workers suffered a 22 percent loss of purchasing power. Prices rose during 1917 to 31 percent above the level of 1913 and during 1918 to 59 percent above that base.

Propaganda, public opinion, and civil liberties. The growth of federal power gave some of the wartime agencies a dangerous authority over the minds of citizens. A week after war was declared, Wilson created the Committee on Public Information to mobilize public opinion. George Creel, chairman of the CPI, worked out with newspapermen a voluntary censorship that kept the public reasonably well informed while safeguarding sensitive information. He also hired hundreds of artists and writers to mount a propaganda campaign without precedent in American history.

The CPI stressed two major points. One argued, as Wilson did, that the United States was fighting only for freedom and democracy. The other maintained that the Germans were all Huns, diabolic creatures perpetrating atrocities in an effort to conquer the world for their lust and greed. The releases of the Creel committee intensified the unreasoning attitudes of a nation at war. They hinted that German spies had an ear to every wall. Often they carried antiunion overtones, labeling as treason all work stoppages, whatever their real cause. More often they implied that all dissent was unpatriotic and that pacifists and socialists had hidden sympathies for the enemy.

This propaganda helped to sell war bonds, combat absenteeism in the factories, and reconcile some doubters to the war. But the price was high. The attitudes the CPI encouraged were the same as those fostered by private vigilante groups like the National Protective Association, which cultivated a kind of war-madness. All dissent became suspect. There were continual spy scares, witch hunts, even kangaroo courts that imposed harsh sentences of tar and feathers. The innocent victims were usually German-Americans or antiwar radicals. The orgy of hatred had its ridiculous as well as its outrageous side. Americans stopped playing German music and stopped teaching

or speaking the German language; they called sauerkraut "liberty cabbage"; and in Cincinnati they even removed pretzels from the free-lunch counters of saloons.

It was essential, of course, to protect the country from espionage and sabotage, but wartime legislation and its administration exceeded reasonable bounds. The Espionage Act of 1917, which Wilson requested, provided penalties of up to twenty years in prison and a $10,000 fine for those who helped the enemy, obstructed recruiting, or incited rebellion within the armed services. One section gave the Postmaster General authority to deny the use of the mails to any publication that in his opinion advocated treason or forcible resistance to the laws. The Trading-with-the-Enemy Act, which Congress passed in October 1917, added sweeping authority to censor the foreign-language press.

In 1918 Congress went still further. The rising hysteria was stimulated by the demands of the Attorney General and by the antipathy toward the Industrial Workers of the World. Copying state statutes, Congress passed the Sabotage Act and the Sedition Act, which empowered the federal government to punish any expression of opinion that, regardless of whether or not it led to action, was "disloyal, profane, scurrilous or abusive" of the American form of government, flag, or uniform. Subsequent systematic persecution effectively destroyed the Wobblies, and in one characteristic case, Eugene V. Debs was sentenced to prison for expressing his revulsion against the war.

The recklessness of Congress in stocking such an arsenal had its source in the frenzy of the people. Timid in the face of public opinion, state and federal officials and judges made a mockery of the right of freedom of speech and belief. Just as those administering the draft subjected conscientious objectors to needless humiliations, often imprisonment, so those administering the espionage, sedition, and other wartime laws made conformity a measure of loyalty. The mails were closed to publications whose only offense was a statement of socialism, a plea for feminism, or anti-British bias. People were haled into court who had done no more than criticize the Red Cross or the financing of the war or who had merely declared that war was contrary to the teachings of Jesus Christ. Of over fifteen hundred arrests for sedition, only ten were alleged to be for actual sabotage. The government's own immoderation and its failure to control private vigilantes shocked men and women of good will and good sense, blemished the Administration's war record, and exaggerated passions that long outlived the crisis itself.

Politics in wartime. Those exaggerated passions sometimes found expression in partisan, sectional, and factional politics. Though Wilson expressed the wish that politics might be adjourned for the duration, wartime problems raised conflicts of interest and irresistible opportunities to pursue partisan advantages. The Republicans, determined to prevent the Democrats from getting all the credit for American successes, criticized the conduct of the war. But that criticism, much of it valid, hurt the Democrats less than did the behavior of a few Southerners in key congressional posts who consistently voted against war legislation.

Southern agrarians and Western progressives demanded heavy income, inheritance, and excess-profits taxes to prevent war profiteering. Conservatives, in contrast, preferred federal borrowing and excise or sales taxes of various kinds. They argued that future generations should share the cost of a war fought in the national interest and that taxes on consumption would help check wartime inflation. The Administration took a middle position. In all, the war cost about $33.5 billion, of which $10.5 billion was raised by taxes, the balance by Treasury borrowing. Secretary of the Treasury McAdoo had intended taxes to carry a larger share, but the soaring cost of the war upset his calculations. As it was, wartime taxes were heavier than they had ever been in the United States. The Revenue Act of October 1917 imposed new and larger excise and luxury taxes, a graduated excess-profits tax on business, and increased estate and personal income taxes. It raised the maximum surtax on income to 63 percent, and the Revenue Act of 1918 lifted it and the excess-profits tax still higher.

The revenue measures passed during the war attempted to place a heavy but equitable burden on those best able to carry it. Nevertheless they prospered. During the war years some 42,000 new millionaires emerged, and the number of taxpayers in the $30,000–$40,000 bracket tripled. The newly rich and the middle class also complained. Especially in the Northeast, Republican politicians won middle-class support by contending that the agrarian Democrats were deliberately punishing the nation's industrial regions. By 1918 the tax issue was being hotly debated by the affluent who had once supported less expensive progressive policies.

The Republicans also made gains among Midwestern farmers who had defected to the Democrats in 1916. The Lever Act empowered the Administration to control the price of wheat but not the price of cotton, and the Western farmers resented the larger profits of their Southern brethren and blamed the Democratic policies that had created the inequity.

The Democratic coalition of 1916 was hurt by other issues as well. Southern votes were crucial in overriding Wilson's veto of an act of 1917 establishing a literacy test for immigrants. The urban laboring force found the Southerners' support of prohibition even more exasperating. Advocates of the prohibition of the manufacture and consumption of alcoholic beverages achieved their goal during the war. First, a section of the Lever Act limited the production of whiskey, and a section of the Selective Service Act limited its sale near army camps. Later, in December 1917, Congress adopted the Eighteenth Amendment—the Prohibition Amendment—and submitted it to the states for ratification (completed in January 1919).

Prohibition offended many Irish-, German-, and Scandinavian-Americans who were also dubious about Wilson's foreign policies. While most of them did not openly oppose the war, they questioned the virtue of the Allied nations and they resented the domestic pressures for conformity that sometimes seemed to denigrate their native lands.

For their part, Northern liberals, disturbed by the Administration's threats to civil liberties, were also irritated by Southern resistance to the woman-suffrage amendment, which senators from Dixie blocked to Wilson's disappointment. As he had learned from the suffragists, democratic principles included the right of women to vote. But only in January 1919 did Congress remove the injustice of limiting suffrage on the basis of sex. (Ratification followed in August 1920.)

As the coalition of interests that had elected Wilson in 1916 fell apart, the Republicans effected a powerful reorganization of their party. They approached the elections of 1918 (see p. 608) with more confidence than they had had in a decade, and their campaign threatened not only Democratic control of Congress but the program for a liberal peace on which Wilson pinned his most fervent hopes.

Constructing the Peace

Wilson's program. During the war, sentiment for a liberal peace developed on both sides of the Atlantic, especially in England and the United States. The plans of various humanitarian groups differed in detail, but they usually advocated four common principles: the substitution of an international organization for the alliance system, the substitution of arbitration for armaments, the institution of self-government among all peoples, and the avoidance of seizures of territories and of demands for reparations.

Wilson embraced these objectives. In 1916 he publicly advocated the idea of a league of nations. In 1917 he began to meditate seriously on the components of a generous peace—a peace without victory. Soon after the United States declared war, he assigned the task of preparing detailed peace plans to Colonel House and a staff of experts. While they were at work, the President in a series of addresses spelled out his own goals, which reflected the principles that had previously characterized his New Freedom and his neutrality policies.

It was necessary, Wilson believed, to remove the military party, including the Kaiser, from authority in Germany, to divest Germany of power over other peoples, to establish democratic self-government in Germany and among each of the national groups rescued from its domination or the domination of its allies. It was necessary then to bring all nations into a world parliament whose collective democratic judgment would guard the peace. "Peace," he said, "should rest upon the rights of peoples, not the rights of governments—the rights of peoples great or small . . . to freedom and security and self-government and to . . . economic opportunities."

This grand vision underestimated the role of power in world affairs and the selfishness of nations torn by war. Indeed, Wilson exacted from the Allies no commitment to a liberal peace. By his own choice the United States had fought not as one of the Allies but as an "associated" belligerent, with the others but not of them. This was the Administration's way of paying tribute to the questionable tradition of avoiding "entangling alliances." Wilson chose, too, to avoid facing squarely the punitive intentions of the Allies, intentions that they had recorded in secret treaties. He simply ignored the existence of those treaties, with their clauses providing for the division of German, Austrian, and Turkish territories and for the exaction of huge indemnities. In so doing he surrendered the opportunity to insist that America would help the Allies only if they agreed to give up those plans.

The course of revolution in Russia focused the attention of the world on the problems of peace. After taking over the government in November 1917, the Bolsheviks moved to capitulate to Germany in a separate peace. They also set out, in the midst of ruthless civil war, to solidify their hold at home and to advance the communist revolution elsewhere. In order to embarrass the Allies, they disclosed the terms of the secret treaties they found in the czar's archives. Both David Lloyd George, the British prime minister, and Wilson countered by reasserting their dedication to a just peace.

In January 1918, while the war was still raging, Wilson announced his celebrated Fourteen Points. They expressed his belief in the inextricable interconnections among free trade, democratic institutions, and human liberty. Five were broad: open diplomacy, by which he meant an end to secret agreements; free use of the seas in peace and war; the reduction of armaments; the removal of barriers to free trade; and an impartial adjustment of colonial claims. Eight points pertained to the principle of national self-determination: German evacuation of Russian territory; the restoration of Belgian independence; the return to France of Alsace-Lorraine (which Germany had conquered in 1870); the establishment of an independent Poland; and the autonomous development of each of the peoples of Austria-Hungary and European Turkey. The fourteenth and crowning point called for forming "a general assembly of nations" to afford "mutual guarantees of political independence and territorial integrity."

Those objectives conflicted not only with the ambitions of the Allies but with the attitudes of many Americans. Though there was much enthusiasm for the President's ideals, there was also opposition from those who wanted protective tariffs, from those who resisted internationalism of any kind, and particularly from those whose war-born hatreds demanded revenge, a march on Berlin, and gallows for the Kaiser.

The armistice and the election of 1918. The President was by no means soft. In October 1918, as the Allies drove through the German lines, the German high command urged the chancellor to propose an armistice to Wilson on the basis of the Fourteen Points. During the ensuing exchange of notes, Wilson took a position charitable enough to lead the Germans on, but firm enough to make them admit defeat. This satisfied all the Allied chiefs of state and military commanders except Pershing, who urged unconditional surrender. The British and French, exhausted by four years of war and frightened by the westward surge of Bolshevism, were eager for an armistice so long as it gave them security.

Aware of those views, Wilson demanded withdrawal of German forces from all invaded territory and immediate cessation of aerial and submarine warfare. When the Germans acceded to those conditions, which were designed to make renewed hostilities impossible, Wilson on October 23 opened negotiations with the Allies and suggested to the Germans that reasonable terms would depend on their establishing a democratic government. This suggestion precipitated the overthrow of the Kaiser, who abdicated on November 9.

The Allied leaders chafed at the Fourteen Points; the British explicitly rejected the point on the freedom of the seas, and the French demanded reparations for civilian damages. They would have insisted on further changes had Colonel House not threatened to make a separate peace if they did not assent to the rest of the Fourteen Points, which were to be the basis for an armistice. The Americans for their part ultimately agreed to add terms forcing the Germans to withdraw well beyond the east bank of the Rhine and to surrender vast quantities of war materials, including their submarines.

Those were tough conditions. But even so the Republicans attacked the President's foreign policy, insisting, as Roosevelt put it, on dictating peace to the hammer of guns instead of to the clicking of typewriters. This demagoguery frightened many Democratic leaders who, with a congressional election coming on, were tempted to seek votes by flag-waving. But Wilson refused to let politics interfere with his carefully devised program. He yielded, however, to his advisers' demand for a blanket endorsement of all Democratic candidates. Angry himself at the onslaughts of men like Roosevelt, Wilson on October 25 urged the people to vote Democratic if they approved of his policies at home and abroad. The return of a Republican majority, he said, would be a repudiation of his leadership.

This appeal made Wilson's foreign policy more than ever a partisan issue. It infuriated the Republicans, and though it helped some Democratic candidates it did not prevent the Republicans from gaining control of both houses of Congress. Republican leaders later claimed that it was foreign policy that had determined the outcome. On November 11, 1918, only a few days after the election, men of all parties rejoiced at the news that an armistice had been arranged. Now, as Wilson turned to negotiating the terms for peace, he had to reckon with a Republican majority in the Senate, where partisanship could delay or even prevent approval of any treaty he submitted.

Negotiating Peace

The background of the Paris conference. Wilson failed to appoint any influential Republican to the American delegation preparing to leave for the peace conference at Paris. To advance his liberal program he chose to head the delegation himself, thus becoming the first President to go overseas on a diplomatic mission. Though his critics complained that he would slight his duties at home, his able performance at Paris justified his decision. Wilson named to the delegation Secretary of State Lansing and Colonel House, in his view obvious choices, and two others: General Tasker H. Bliss, a military expert, and Henry White, a career diplomat, ostensibly a Republican but in no sense a politician or a representative of the Senate. The delegation was to be Wilson's instrument, under his domination, but any advantage this control gave him during negotiations was overshadowed by the disadvantages inherent in slighting the Republicans.

Wilson also slighted public opinion. He had little talent for dealing with journalists, many of whom distrusted his official press representative, George Creel. Moreover, at the peace conference he had to yield to the other negotiators' insistence on secret sessions. The American press interpreted this decision as a violation of the principle of open diplomacy, even though there was no secret about the decisions reached at the conference. If Wilson's press relations had been better, American newspapers could have helped explain the President's difficulties to a public that did not fully understand the necessity for give-and-take.

Wilson had to bargain endlessly with the Allies, for their objectives often conflicted with his. He be-

Wilson in Paris

lieved that the Fourteen Points should guide the peace settlement. He did not expect a perfect peace, but he thought that a league of nations could continually improve the terms of a peace treaty, and he counted on enlisting the moral force of the world behind the league. His optimism grew during his tour of Europe before the conference opened. Crowds greeted him as a savior, and he mistook their gratitude for victory as an endorsement of his goals.

Actually, the peoples of Europe and Asia, with unimportant exceptions, supported the demands of their own spokesmen. Four of those men were, with Wilson, the major architects of the peace. There was the self-controlled and resourceful Count Nobuaki Makino of Japan, ambitious for territory that Britain had promised his country in return for Japan's joining the Allies; equally land-hungry was the cultured and adroit Vittorio Orlando of Italy; there was the perspicacious but shifty British prime minister, David Lloyd George, who had promised his electorate vast reparations; there was the French premier, Georges Clemenceau, cynical, tenacious, weary, aloof, determined to crush Germany forever. These men were bound by treaties to support one another's claims. Their armies, moreover, actually held most of the lands they planned to annex or assign.

Over large parts of the world neither they nor Wilson could exercise much influence. The Bolshevik Revolution had made Russia unwelcome at the conference, and it stood apart brooding, dissatisfied, potentially a mighty and ominous force. There was, furthermore, continuing war within its borders while the peace conference sat. British troops in the northern part of European Russia were trying to assist anti-Bolsheviks there, and in Siberia a Japanese army was pushing west with an eye to conquest. The United States also dispatched forces to both areas. The Bolsheviks, resenting the presence of foreigners, believed the British, Japanese and Americans were agents of counterrevolution, as some authorities in Washington, London, and Tokyo intended them to be.

Revolution and counterrevolution infected all of Russia's European neighbors. The empire of Austria-Hungary had simply ceased to exist in part because Wilson's demand for self-determination had stirred the nationalistic hopes of the various peoples of the area. In the territories it once had ruled, the quarrels of self-conscious ethnic groups, complicated by the conniving of communists, were forging the new states that were to mark the map of central and eastern Europe whether the men at Paris willed it or not. Within Germany the new republican government faced revolution at the borders, Red plots within, and a populace exasperated by a food shortage imposed by the continuing Allied blockade. In distributing American food supplies, inadequate at best, Herbert Hoover attempted to cut off the Left, particularly in eastern Europe. With the world in turmoil and Europe exhausted by war, the Paris conference had an unpropitious setting. With the Allies opposed to a liberal peace, moreover, the odds against Wilson's program were enormous.

The League of Nations. Wilson's plans for a charter for a league of nations included the disposition of former German colonies. In order to bring about an impartial and equitable settlement of colonial claims, as the Fourteen Points promised, Wilson hoped to put the German colonies under the guardianship of small neutrals like Switzerland and Sweden. Those neutrals were to be trustees for the league and were to help the backward colonial peoples to move toward independence.

The British and Japanese, however, would not surrender the territory in Africa and the Pacific that they had seized during hostilities. According to a secret treaty between them, German islands in the Pacific north of the equator were to go to Japan and islands south of the equator were to go to Australia and New Zealand. Wilson prevented the outright transfer of colonies by persuading the Allies to accept instead a system of "mandates," which obliged their holders to render annual accountings and theoretically to help subject peoples to stand alone. The compromise subjected the Allies to some surveillance in their administration of the territory they received. The mandate system was disingenuous, but Wilson felt that the league would gradually better it (though the League never did).

The concept of a league met opposition from the French, who wanted a military alliance of the victors against Germany. Japan further complicated Wilson's negotiations by demanding a statement of racial equality pledging member nations of a league not to discriminate against the nationals of other members. But the President had help from the Italians, who were pleased by his endorsement of the northern boundary they wanted, and from the British, who shared his hopes for the league. The racial pride of the Japanese was assuaged by their new mandates, and the French accepted the idea of a league after they realized that they could obtain their objectives elsewhere in the treaty. Wilson's draft served as the basis for the Covenant of the League of Nations, which the responsible committee approved and reported to the peace conference in February 1919.

It was a simple document. Each signer of the treaty was to have one vote in a Body of Delegates of the League. Larger authority rested with the Executive Council, which was to consist of representatives from the United States, the British Empire, France, Italy, Japan, and four states selected by the Body of Delegates. Decisions of the council required a unanimous vote except when a council member was itself a party to a dispute. The covenant also established a permanent secretariat, an international Bureau of Labor, and the mandate system. It provided for the admission of new members by a two-thirds vote of the delegates and for amendment by a three-fourths vote.

The main purpose of the League was to keep the peace. To that end the covenant obliged signatories, before they resorted to war, to submit disputes either to inquiry by the council or to arbitration by the Permanent Court of International Justice, which the council was to create. Member nations were to punish any breach of this article by severing economic relations with the offending state. The council, moreover, might recommend that members of the League contribute military and naval units to protect its principles. And the council was to advise on means of

America is going to grow more and more powerful; and the more powerful she is the more inevitable it is that she should be trustee for the peace of the world.... All Europe knew that we were doing an American thing when we put the Covenant of the League of Nations at the beginning of the treaty.... The most cynical men I had to deal with ... before our conferences were over ... all admitted that the League of Nations, which they had deemed an ideal dream, was a demonstrable, practical necessity. This treaty cannot be carried out without the League of Nations....

The rest of the world is necessary to us, if you want to put it on that basis. I do not like to put it on that basis. That is not the American basis. America does not want to feed upon the rest of the world. She wants to feed it and serve it. America ... is the only national idealistic force in the world, and idealism is going to save the world.... That is the program of civilization.

Need for the League

From Woodrow Wilson, Speech at Helena, Montana, September 1919.

---

ensuring that member nations lived up to Article 10, which Wilson considered the heart of the covenant. This article bound signatories "to respect and preserve against external aggression the territorial integrity and . . . political independence of all members of the League."

The League was not a superstate. It could only recommend, but not compel, the recruitment and use of military force. Its deliberations would not bind Germany or Russia until the victorious powers invited them to join. Those powers had sufficient authority, moreover, to use the League to try to perpetuate the status quo. But the covenant did create the first promising international organization in modern history. It also fulfilled Wilson's purpose of recognizing war and the threat of war as everybody's business and of providing a forum for the nations of the world to discuss problems that might lead to conflict. In his view, the covenant organized the moral force of the world.

Consequently the President was distressed by the opposition to the League that he confronted during a brief trip home. The essence of that opposition was Republican partisanship, but it fed on other attitudes as well. Many German-Americans still resented the war and its outcome. Many Irish-Americans believed Wilson should have insisted on Irish independence. The President pointed out that that was a question for England to resolve, but he was pointedly cool toward his Irish critics. He was even less patient with those Americans who viewed the covenant as an "entangling alliance," and hesitated to depart from what to them was a national tradition of isolation from Europe. Those and other sentiments bred susceptibility to the propaganda of Wilson's opponents.

On March 4, 1919, the day before the President returned to Paris, Senator Henry Cabot Lodge pro-

duced a round robin signed by thirty-seven Republican senators and senators elect, four more than were needed to defeat the treaty. It stated that the covenant was unacceptable and insisted that consideration of the League be deferred until after a treaty had been completed. In a speech that night, Wilson condemned the "careful selfishness" of his critics and their "ignorance of the state of the world." The covenant would be intimately tied to the treaty itself, he said. That interrelationship was essential for working out the problems of the conference, and the President was understandably annoyed. But his strong language intensified the partisanship that provoked it.

The Treaty of Versailles. Though Wilson would not separate the League from the treaty, he realized that the covenant would have to be modified to meet the suggestions of American moderates. The revisions the President sponsored on his return to Paris would certainly have been demanded by the Senate in any event. They defined procedures for withdrawal from the League, stated that the acceptance of mandates was optional, and excluded from the purview of the League domestic issues such as immigration and regional agreements such as the Monroe Doctrine. By reopening the question of the covenant, however, Wilson exposed himself to the bargaining of his associates, who once more pressed their demands for Europe and Asia. The President secured his revisions, but only at an inflated price.

Clemenceau, still determined to assure French security, insisted that Germany be dismembered. He urged that two states, a revivified Poland and a new Czechoslovakia, be set up on Germany's eastern border. He also asked for the creation of a Rhenish buffer state, to be splintered off from Germany's west, and for the cession to France of the Saar Basin, a bountiful source of coal and iron, as well as of Alsace-Lorraine. Wilson balked at those extreme demands. For ten days the conference stalled, but when Wilson threatened to leave, Clemenceau bowed to the proponents of compromise.

The treaty drew generous boundaries for Poland and Czechoslovakia, but it also arranged for the League to conduct a plebiscite to determine the disposition of a part of Silesia coveted by both Germans and Poles. The treaty gave Poland access to the sea through a narrow corridor that put some Germans under Polish rule, just as other German-speaking people became subject to Czechoslovakia. France received Alsace-Lorraine and temporary economic concessions in the Saar, but the League was to administer the Saar and after fifteen years was to conduct a plebiscite there. France could also occupy the Rhineland for fifteen years; after that time the area was to be demilitarized but left a part of Germany. The German army was limited to a token force.

Furthermore, Wilson and Lloyd George agreed to a special security treaty pledging their nations to assist France if it were attacked. Clemenceau realized that the United States Senate would probably reject the special treaty, but in that case the Rhineland could be occupied indefinitely. All in all, Clemenceau obtained as much safety for France as any treaty could reasonably provide.

The French and the English also pushed Wilson into accepting their demands for reparations in excess of what Germany could pay and in violation of the prearmistice agreement to limit payments to the cost of civilian damages. The President let the Allies include the cost of pensions, which later permitted the reparations commission to calculate that the Germans owed some $120 billion, the fantastic figure that had been the British objective. The reparations clause of the treaty, moreover, specifically attributed the cause of war to "the aggression of Germany," a phrase that rankled in German minds for years to come, however accurate it may have been. Along with the economic dislocations that grew out of the exorbitant reparations imposed on Germany, the war-guilt clause proved to be an emotional threat to future peace.

At the time, however, the President's troubles with Italy seemed more ominous. Before the conference Wilson had agreed to a northern frontier for Italy at the line of the Brenner Pass, which put two hundred thousand Austrians under Italian rule. This left him with nothing else to trade when the Italians also insisted on taking Fiume, an Adriatic port surrounded by Yugoslav land. When the Italians discov-

Europe in 1920

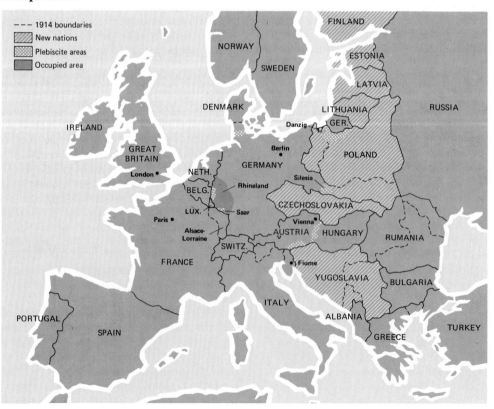

- – – 1914 boundaries
- New nations
- Plebiscite areas
- Occupied area

ered that all the powers were antagonistic to their claim to Fiume, they boldly marched into the city. Wilson appealed to the Italian people in the name of justice, but they, with their leaders, resented the President's miscalculated intrusion. The Italians left Paris in a rage, and, though they returned to sign a treaty that did not give them Fiume, the incident alienated Italian-Americans from Wilson's treaty and almost disrupted the conference.

The Japanese seized on the confusion to advance their own claims. They were seeking endorsement for their economic ambitions in China and for their assumption of the German leasehold at Kiaochow (Jiaozchou*) and of German privileges in the Shantung (Shandong) Peninsula. After the whole conference seemed about to disintegrate, Wilson accepted most of those claims though the Chinese opposed them. Many Americans, including two of the delegates, thought the President conceded too much, but he felt he had obtained a solution "as satisfactory as could be got out of the tangle."

The same could be said of the whole treaty that the victors and the vanquished signed at Versailles in 1919. It was punitive, but Germany had lost the war it

*The spelling in parentheses indicates the Pinyin Romanization of Chinese proper names.

had expected to win, and the Allies were less severe than the Germans would have been. The treaty followed the Fourteen Points as closely as world conditions permitted. Europe had a new map that approximated ethnic groupings. Negotiations had involved some compromises of the principle of self-determination and created some boundaries that conflicted with the military defense and the economic needs of the new states. But those difficulties and others could be negotiated later in the forum of the League. As Wilson had predicted, the League was inextricably part of the treaty, a "convenient, indeed indispensable" instrument. He had yet, however, to convert two-thirds of the Senate to his way of thinking.

The Struggle Over Ratification

The Senate and the treaty. Wilson brought the treaty home to a people initially predisposed in its favor. Though few Americans were familiar with the whole long document, most had learned something about the League, and millions were enthusiastic about it. But the people could not vote on the treaty. The question of its approval, and therefore the portentous question of what direction American foreign policy would take, were for the Senate to decide.

Of the ninety-six senators forty-nine were Republican, but only fourteen—as well as several Democrats—were irreconcilably against the League and the treaty. Those irreconcilables, many of them progressives, believed that the mission of the United States was to create a model society for other nations to emulate, not to get involved in international affairs. Indeed, they shared the distrust of foreigners so common among the American people. The other thirty-five Republicans intended not to reject the treaty but to make its adoption contingent on a number of reservations, of which the most significant had to do with Wilson's League of Nations. Twenty-three Republicans favored a list of strong reservations drafted and sponsored by Senator Lodge; twelve were willing to settle for milder reservations. Since only four of the forty-seven Democrats opposed the treaty, a coalition of Democrats and moderate Republicans would have commanded a majority vote. And a majority was all that was needed to settle the kind of reservations that would be demanded. Such a coalition, moreover, could probably have attracted the necessary two-thirds vote for approval. But the crucial coalition was never formed.

The Democratic leaders knew they had to make concessions to their opponents, but they felt that they also had to wait for instructions from the President. They never received those instructions, for Wilson refused to compromise an issue he considered both personal and moral.

It was Lodge who had made the issue personal. Lodge had endorsed the strategy of insisting on reservations; Lodge had packed the important Foreign Relations Committee with irreconcilables and strong reservationists. Lodge, the majority leader of the Senate, was determined to hold his party together and to win in 1920. Further, he honestly believed that the League as Wilson had planned it was a threat to national sovereignty. Lodge was not an isolationist, but he put his faith in armies and navies and the balance of power, the "large view" of his old friend Theodore Roosevelt, who had just died. A ruthless, often exasperating man, Lodge was also moved by mean considerations, including the prejudices of his many Italian- and Irish-American constituents. He was a formidable antagonist who hated Wilson as Wilson hated him.

Lodge's reservations struck the President as unnecessary and immoral. Wilson objected to the very idea of making the approval of the treaty subject to reservations. He also held that reservations would mean that the treaty would have to be renegotiated, though the British, the French, and the State Department did not think so. Two of the reservations would have made Congress the sole judge of whether the United States should accept a mandate and whether it should withdraw from the League. Two others reserved to the United States exclusive authority over tariff policy, immigration, and the Monroe Doctrine. As Wilson argued, the revised covenant already covered those issues. Another reservation exempted the United States from any decision of the League on which any member and its self-governing dominions had cast in the aggregate more than one vote. The American veto in the council, Wilson noted, made superfluous such an ungracious protest against the seats of the British dominions in the Body of Delegates. The President especially opposed the reservation on Article 10, which stated that the United States would assume no obligation to preserve the territorial integrity or political independence of any other country without the approval of Congress. To Wilson this would be a violation of the essential spirit of the League—the moral obligation to protect the peace of the world.

In the abstract Wilson may have been right, but the politics of the Senate made compromise necessary. Even if Lodge's reservations did make the United States seem timid and selfish, they would have damaged the League far less than would outright rejection of treaty and League alike. Senator Gilbert Hitchcock, the Democratic minority leader, advised Wilson to work out some sort of compromise with Lodge, as did Colonel House, Robert Lansing, Bernard Baruch, and many other friends of the President.

But Wilson would not listen, and as the days passed, the public tended to become bored with the whole question about which most voters were ill-informed. Wilson had advocated a degree of national involvement in foreign affairs greater, in all probability, than most Americans, after reflection, were willing to accept. The idealism of wartime was fading into the problems of the postwar period. Inflation, unemployment, and fears of Bolshevism reduced public enthusiasm for a generous peace and for a genuine internationalism.

The President's collapse. In order to arouse new enthusiasm for the League, Wilson set out in September 1919 on a speaking tour across the country. His train moved through the strongholds of isolationism, over eight thousand miles, stopping thirty-seven times for him to address the voters. As he proceeded through the Middle West to the Pacific Coast, then south, and then east, he was greeted by larger and larger crowds. But their applause did not change one vote in the Senate. Indeed, Wilson's attacks on his opponents stiffened their resolution to resist, and his absence from Washington impeded Democratic efforts to find a basis for compromise. The President's strenuous efforts taxed his limited strength without achieving his political purpose.

On September 25 Wilson spoke at Pueblo, Colorado. That night his head hurt mercilessly. Frightened by the President's exhaustion, his physician canceled the remainder of the trip. Back in Washington Wilson was too tired to work, too tense to rest. On October 2 he fell to the floor unconscious, the victim of a cerebral thrombosis, a blood clot in his brain.

The stroke did not kill the President, but it paralyzed his left side, thickened his speech, totally disabled him for almost two months, and prevented him thereafter from working more than an hour or two at a time. For six months he did not meet with the Cabinet. For six weeks he could not execute the minimum duties of his office. Though his mind was not injured he became petulant, suspicious, and easily moved to tears. He was unable to assess situations with accuracy. His collapse was a tragedy not only for himself but for a nation facing a momentous crisis in foreign policy.

On November 6, while Wilson was still bedridden, Lodge presented his reservations to the Senate. It was obvious that the Republicans had the votes to adopt them but not the two-thirds needed to approve the treaty after the reservations had been attached. The Democratic leaders hesitated to move without the President's consent, and he gave stringent orders on November 18 that they were to reject the treaty so long as it was subject to the Lodge reservations. They were then to move that the treaty be accepted either as it stood or with mild interpretive reservations of which Wilson approved. This order conceded nothing to the Republican moderates, who stood behind Lodge. Though nonpartisan friends of the League preferred accepting Lodge's reservations to rejecting the whole treaty, the Democrats on November 19 voted to reject the treaty with those reservations. Consequently the resolution to adopt the treaty as Lodge had modified it failed by thirty-nine to fifty-five. Lodge blocked debate of the interpretive reservations that the Democrats then proposed, and minutes later a resolution to approve the unamended treaty also failed, thirty-eight to fifty-three.

The final rejection. The moderate Republicans and the Democrats were stunned by what they had done and felt they had to try again. Furthermore, organizations representing some 20 million Americans petitioned for compromise and ratification. The same hope was voiced by the British and French press and by the British government. Influential Democrats without exception tried to persuade the President to relieve his party of the hopeless battle to defeat the Lodge reservations.

But Wilson would still not hear of concessions. Instead, on January 8, 1920, he wrote a blistering letter to his fellow Democrats. The majority of the people wanted ratification, he said. Let the Senate accept the treaty without tampering with it or else reject it. If there was any doubt about public opinion, Wilson warned, the issue could be resolved at the next election, which would be "a great and solemn referendum."

This was the counsel of a deluded man, for presidential elections turn on many issues, not just one. The Democratic party had been losing strength for three years, and the treaty, if the Senate rejected it again, would be impossible to resuscitate. Recognizing the folly of Wilson's position, Senator Hitchcock and other Democrats tried to work out a satisfactory compromise on the reservations. They failed, partly because the Republican irreconcilables warned Lodge against compromise, partly because Lodge himself probably did not want to rescue the treaty. The President, increasingly peevish, on March 8 again instructed the Democrats to hold the line.

His adherents prevailed. The Lodge reservations, only slightly modified, were adopted, this time with some Democratic help. On March 19, the day of the final test, half the Democrats voted to approve the treaty with the reservations. But twenty-three Democrats, twenty of them Southerners, did the President's bidding. Together with twelve irreconcilables, they voted against approval and thus prevented by a margin of seven the two-thirds majority needed for adoption.

There was to be no "solemn referendum." The Democratic presidential nominee in 1920, James M. Cox, supported the League, but sometimes with hesitation. The Republican plank on the treaty was deliberately vague, as was the Republican candidate, Warren G. Harding. Though Harding enjoyed the full support of both Republican isolationists and Republican internationalists, he chose to consider his smashing victory a repudiation of the treaty.

The Senate had made the telling decision. In rejecting both treaty and League, the Senate had for the while turned America's back to Europe. The rejection destroyed the best available chance for developing world peace. Perhaps the irreconcilables, the forceful spokesmen of isolation, could have defeated the treaty in any event, but it was not they who did so, though they helped. Wilson's stubbornness and Lodge's partisanship helped even more. Indeed, partisanship was the real culprit, and the outcome of the fight revealed how severely domestic politics could damage foreign policy.

The damage, in the end, affected the whole world, for without the United States the League became an instrument for preserving the status quo. Even if the United States had been a member, the League would probably have acted just about the way it did. But as it was, the League never had a chance to fulfill Wilson's vision. That vision, which rested on the moral intent of the President's peace program, was the most compelling image democracy then offered to the world. With the defeat of the treaty, the United States seemed to have renounced its claims to the imagination of people everywhere. The renunciation came just at the time when Bolshevism was advancing its revolutionary claims more effectively than ever before. The American retreat eased the way for both the advocates of reaction and the advocates of communism. It cost the United States the only available fruits of a gallant victory. It made a travesty of the noble effort to create a world safe for the ideals Wilson cherished.

Transition from War

Demobilization. When the war ended, the government had no plans for demobilization. It simply lifted the controls it had imposed on the economy during the war. In accord with public sentiment, it hastened the discharge of the soldiers, many of whom were unable to find jobs when they returned to civilian life. Though unemployment declined after February 1919, it persisted in troubled areas for another half-year, and it soured thousands of veterans who had expected a hero's welcome to include a job.

Immediately after the armistice the War Industries Board began to close up shop, confident that private industry would be able to switch back to a peacetime economy with no help or direction from the federal government. That was a miscalculation. While industry bid for new plants and machinery, consumers dug out their wartime savings to make the purchases they had long postponed. Inflation struck the country. During 1919 the cost of living climbed to 77 percent above prewar levels; during 1920, another 28 percent.

The government developed only piecemeal and inadequate remedies for unemployment and inflation. There was as yet no body of economic ideas to explain the need for overall federal policies that would ease the process of reconversion. Wilson, moreover, was preoccupied with peacemaking and hampered by an opposition Congress. Yet the Revenue Act of 1919 carried on the policy of progressive taxation, ensured the government the income it needed, and helped check inflation.

Both Congress and the public were anxious to settle the question of what should be done with the railroads, which the government was still running. Private management wanted them back, but labor had found that public administration was more generous and more efficient. An attorney for the railway broth-

erhoods, Glenn E. Plumb, proposed a plan for nationalizing the roads. The AFL supported the Plumb plan, but elsewhere it evoked little enthusiasm. Congress, in the Transportation Act of 1920, extended the tradition of mixed capitalism by turning the railroads back to their private owners while subjecting them to increased but deliberately benign supervision. In a similar spirit, the Water Power Act of 1920 set up a Federal Power Commission, consisting of the Secretaries of War, Agriculture, and the Interior, to license the building and operation of dams and hydroelectric plants. This clumsy arrangement by its very failure drew attention to the need for genuine public control of waterways.

Labor strife. In the years right after the war, the once-progressive fervor of Americans seemed to have spent itself. The nation's policy-makers, like the American people, turned more and more to the past. The Administration, which had sympathized with organized labor, now began to favor management. That reversal was prompted by several forces: Wilson's advisers were growing impatient with the strikes that continued to cripple the nation's industries, and management had launched a successful campaign to associate all unions with radicalism, about which the country at large was harboring hysterical fears.

The enforced wartime truce between labor and management ended in 1919. The unions then set out to consolidate their gains and to bring wages into line with the rising cost of living. And the National Association of Manufacturers and other management groups set out to reestablish the open shop, which they liked to call "the American way." Management propaganda extolled the beneficence of business and warned that unions and union demands were inspired by foreign and radical influences. Nevertheless, many of the first strikes after the war were successful, notably those of clothing, textile, telegraph, and telephone workers.

The most celebrated postwar strikes occurred in Seattle and Boston. In February 1919 the Seattle Central Labor Council called a general strike to support shipyard workers who had walked out in quest of higher pay and shorter hours. Those workers and others in Seattle, something of a wartime boom town, were also worried about postwar unemployment. Some of the local labor leaders were unquestionably radical, and a general strike was itself a radical technique, perhaps especially in the view of the residents of a city where the IWW had been active. But Mayor Ole Hanson grossly exaggerated the Red menace and used troops to stamp out the strike.

In Boston the police found that they could not stretch their prewar wages to cover postwar living costs. Denied a raise and restive because of other

Boston, 1919: Coolidge called out the guard

grievances, they secured a charter from the AFL and threatened a strike in August 1919. The mayor appointed a citizens' committee, which suggested that most of the policemen's demands, except recognition of their union, be granted. The police commissioner, however, a declared enemy of organized labor, rejected the suggestion and fired nineteen of the union's leaders. On September 9 the policemen went out on strike. Volunteer vigilantes were unable to control the gangs of looters who brought Boston to the point of anarchy. The American middle class was shocked and scared. But just then the governor of Massachusetts, Calvin Coolidge, called out the national guard to restore order. The strike failed, and many of the police were dismissed.

The whole episode was as unnecessary as it was lamentable. Coolidge could have supported the mayor and overruled the police commissioner before the strike began. Instead, he won a national reputation by putting down the strike. The American people knew little about the facts of the case, but they long remembered the governor's characteristic response to Gompers' request that the policemen be reinstated: "There is no right to strike against the public safety by anybody, anywhere, any time."

The AFL faced its crucial test in the steel industry. The secretary of its organizing committee, William Z. Foster, had been radical enough in his beliefs

for management to persuade the public that he was a Red. He was also a less than effective organizer. Still, the steelworkers had grave grievances. Most of them put in a twelve-hour workday in return for subsistence wages. After recruiting a substantial minority of workers, the union called a strike in September 1919, after management had rejected its demands for recognition, an eight-hour day, and decent pay. Episodes of violence punctuated the strike. Public opinion, misled by the steel companies' propaganda, condoned the widespread use of state and federal troops to prevent picketing. United States Steel alone used thousands of strikebreakers. In January 1920 the union gave up, thoroughly beaten.

Meanwhile, in November 1919, the bituminous-coal miners had walked out under the leadership of their new and colorful president, John L. Lewis, who was radical only in his pugnacious manner. A wartime agreement had governed wages in the mines, but the union claimed that the armistice had made that agreement inapplicable. As Lewis observed, there was no ceiling on the rising price of coal. The miners demanded a 60 percent wage increase, a six-hour day, and a five-day week. When the operators refused to negotiate, the miners prepared to strike. With Wilson's approval, Attorney General A. Mitchell Palmer ruled that the wage agreement was still in effect and obtained an injunction against the union. Lewis then called off the strike because, as he put it, "we cannot fight the government." Still the miners refused to go back to work until the government ordered an immediate 14 percent increase in pay and set up an arbitral commission, which ultimately awarded another 27 percent. The miners' other demands were denied.

Race hatred. Old prejudices, whetted by new fears, had also provoked a wave of persecution and violence that engulfed American blacks. In response to wartime labor shortages, several hundred thousand blacks had moved from the South to Northern industrial centers. Segregated there in urban slums, they were the continuing objects of the race hatred of their white neighbors, especially of unskilled workers who viewed blacks as competitors for their jobs. More and more blacks, for their part, educated by the experience of military service, by the war's avowedly democratic aims, and by the inequities they met in the North, began to demand rights long denied them, particularly higher wages, equal protection under the law, and the chance to vote and hold political office. Those were key goals of the increasingly militant National Association for the Advancement of Colored People and of its foremost leader, W. E. B. DuBois. Yet white supremacists were determined "to keep the Negro in his place," by force if necessary, and many of them applauded irresponsible statements of men like Congressman James F. Byrnes of South Carolina, who warned that the Reds were inciting a black uprising in the South.

Turning to terrorism, lynch mobs in the South made victims of more than seventy blacks in 1919, ten of them veterans in uniform. The new Ku Klux Klan (see p. 638), committed to the intimidation of blacks, gained some one hundred thousand members. In 1919 South and North alike saw the worst spate of race riots in American history to that time. Two of the most tragic occurred in Washington, D.C., where a majority of the offenders were white veterans, and in Chicago, where for thirteen days a mob of whites fought blacks in the black slums. Before the year ended, twenty-five race riots had resulted in hundreds of deaths and injuries and millions of dollars of property damage.

Most blacks resisted their attackers, as the NAACP advised them to, and liberal whites organized to fight intolerance and to lobby for antilynching laws, but by and large blacks were neither hopeful of remedy nor yet ready to campaign in their own behalf. Instead, by 1923 about half a million blacks had joined the Universal Negro Improvement Association of Marcus Garvey, a Jamaican black nationalist who proposed to create a new empire in Africa with himself on the throne. Garvey had a fundamental appeal to American blacks. Touching their traditional sensibilities, he used religious symbols and rituals in his

Race riot, Chicago, 1919

Marcus Garvey

organizational meetings. His attacks on the oppression of blacks were based upon Christian ethical standards. Though Garvey's scheme for empire collapsed, his movement met the powerful need of blacks for self-identity, racial pride, and an escape from a society that denied them dignity, opportunity, and even personal safety.

The Red scare. American radicals also felt the sting of old prejudices and new fears. There was, to be sure, genuine cause for concern over the spread of Bolshevism in Europe. In March 1919 Soviet leaders organized the Third International as an agency for world revolution, and during the rest of that year the communists made striking gains in Germany, Hungary, and along Russia's frontiers. The International fed on the postwar disintegration of eastern Europe—a disintegration the United States did little to check.

Within the United States, however, communism was feeble. In 1919 the Socialist party, its ranks depleted and its morale low, broke into three factions. Some forty thousand moderates retained the old name. One left-wing faction of about twenty thousand, almost all of them immigrants, formed the Communist Labor party. Another militant group of between thirty thousand and sixty thousand, also largely immigrant, joined the Communist party of America under native-born leaders. But the three groups together constituted less than half of 1 percent of the population.

During the war, public and private propaganda had generated hatred and fear of the Germans, and Americans had already begun to fight the shadows of their anxieties. In the postwar months they transferred much of this hate to the nation's immigrants, whom the suspicious middle class had long stereotyped as radical. Hysteria reached pathological proportions under the influence of business propaganda that branded all labor as radical, under the spur of politicians who exploited the mood of the nation for their own advantage, and under the stimulus of sporadic episodes of violence.

Scare headlines and legislative investigations of alleged Red activity kept the public edgy. In April the handiwork of a few lunatic radicals created near-panic when bombs were mailed to thirty-eight eminent citizens, including John D. Rockefeller, Justice Holmes, the Postmaster General, and the Attorney General. The Post Office intercepted all the bombs but one. In June there were several direct bombings. One weapon exploded in front of the Washington home of Attorney General A. Mitchell Palmer, damaging the building and dismembering his would-be assassin, an Italian anarchist.

The bombings of April and June had been plotted by dangerous criminals. They were not, however a part of communist strategy, for the leaders of international communism recognized that simple terror would be an ineffective weapon for overturning a strong capitalist state. But most Americans did not differentiate among radicalisms. They grew more frightened every day, and they saw Red in everything they feared or disliked.

The mood of the nation endorsed the witch hunts conducted by Attorney General Palmer. A Quaker, a progressive Democrat who had worked effectively for women's suffrage and labor reforms, an enthusiast for the League of Nations, Palmer had enjoyed a deserved reputation as a liberal until he took office in March 1919. Then he threw his department, especially the newly created Federal Bureau of Investigation, into a strenuous campaign against aliens and radicals. He may have been hoping to advance his candidacy for the Democratic presidential nomination in 1920. If so, he overreached himself. But he did succeed in violating the Anglo-American heritage of civil liberties.

Congress refused to pass a sedition bill that Palmer had drafted, but the Attorney General on his own authority ordered a series of raids, many against the remnants of the IWW, beginning in November 1919. During the first raid his agents arrested 250 members of the Union of Russian Workers and beat many of them up, but the Justice Department could find cause to recommend that only 39 of them be deported. In December Palmer cooperated with the

Labor Department in deporting 249 aliens to Russia,
most of whom had committed no offense and were
not communists. A nationwide raid on January 1,
1920, led to the arrest of some 6,000 people, many of
whom were American citizens and noncommunists.
They were herded into prisons and bull pens; some
were seized on suspicion only, taken without warrants from their homes, and held incommunicado.
The raids revealed no evidence of a grand plot. Nevertheless, outside of the small membership of the
incipient Civil Liberties Union, few Americans spoke
out against the highhanded tactics of the Attorney
General, the chief legal officer of the United States.

Still worried about preventing a revolution that
was not brewing, Palmer continued to warn the nation about Red plots. But the outbreak he predicted
for May 1, 1920, failed to materialize, and gradually
the public began to tire of his unfounded alarms. The
tide of Bolshevism had started to recede in Europe,
and Palmer and his imitators had made themselves
ridiculous. They could, of course, also be ruthless, as
was the New York legislature, which expelled five
innocuous Socialists, all properly elected members of
the Assembly. This travesty on the American elective
system evoked sharp denunciations, the most influential from Charles Evans Hughes. By the summer of
1920 the Red scare was largely over, the hysteria spent.
In September Americans were horrified by a bomb
explosion at the corner of Broad and Wall streets in
New York; but they accepted the episode for what it
was, the work of a crazed individual, not the product
of a Bolshevik conspiracy as Palmer maintained.

The Red scare left ugly scars. The constitutional
rights of thousands of Americans had been violated.
Hundreds of innocent people had been deported.
Many states had enacted sedition laws even more extreme than those passed during the war. And there
lingered a less strident but still pervasive nativism that
in the years ahead was to condone the new Ku Klux
Klan, an organization dedicated to the hatred of
blacks, Catholics, Jews, and foreigners. Nativism set
the stage for a major reversal of immigration policy,
which had for so many decades kept the gates of
America open to newcomers. In February 1921, over
Wilson's veto, Congress passed a law limiting the
number of immigrants in any year to 3 percent of the
foreign-born of each national group who had been living in the United States in 1910. Even this restrictive
quota, which just about choked off immigration from
Asia and central and southern Europe, was later to be
reduced (see p. 637).

Hatred of aliens and radicals made a mockery of
justice in the celebrated case of two Italians, confessed
anarchists, Nicola Sacco and Bartolomeo Vanzetti.
They were arrested, tried, and convicted for murdering two employees of a shoe company in South Brain-
tree, Massachusetts, during a payroll robbery in 1920.
Yet there was little conclusive evidence against them,
but after a trial that made a mockery of justice, they
were condemned essentially for their language and
their beliefs. The judge who conducted the trial referred to them privately as "those anarchist bastards."
Many Boston patricians felt the same way, and most
of them, including the presidents of Harvard and
M.I.T., approved the decision to deny a retrial. Felix
Frankfurter, the novelist John Dos Passos, the poet
Edna St. Vincent Millay, and other defenders of justice tried for six years to save Sacco and Vanzetti, but
they failed. The cause attracted attention throughout
the world and engaged the hearts of men and women
who were to provide liberal leadership in the years to
come. But in 1927, when Sacco and Vanzetti were
electrocuted, the wounds of the Red scare festered
again. The forces of respectability and conformity and
repression seemed to be united against justice and
decency and democracy.

The election of 1920. The Red scare drained away the vestiges of progressive zeal. Americans, weary of public matters great and small, withdrew to a private world of pleasure, entertainment, and sensationalism. The political parties reflected the nation's fatigue and selfishness. The confident Republicans met in Chicago, where the professionals who controlled the party intended to name a candidate they could manage. After six ballots, the bosses arranged for the nomination to go to Senator Warren G. Harding of Ohio. The convention selected Harding on the tenth ballot, and then the delegates, ignoring their orders, named Calvin Coolidge for Vice President.

Harding was a handsome, semieducated political hack with a modest talent for golf; a larger taste for liquor and poker; a complaisant disposition; an utterly empty mind; and an enduring loyalty to the Republican creed of 1890. He was one of the least-qualified candidates ever nominated by a major party. His platform fitted his creed. It promised lower taxes, a higher tariff, restriction of immigration, and—with opportunistic generosity—aid to farmers. It damned the League of Nations but called vaguely for an "agreement among nations to preserve the peace"—a phrase that made the isolationists happy and that Harding's wordy speeches did nothing to clarify.

The Democrats were at odds with themselves. The failure of President Wilson, in spite of his illness, to disclaim ambition for the nomination impeded the candidacy of his son-in-law, William G. McAdoo, probably the ablest of the hopefuls. Attorney General Palmer had begun to lose support before the convention met. And in any event the Democratic bosses, almost as powerful as their Republican counterparts, wanted no candidate who was identified with the Wilson Administration. They preferred Governor James M. Cox of Ohio, a good vote-getter and an opponent of Prohibition. The convention selected as his running mate Assistant Secretary of the Navy Franklin D. Roosevelt. The platform was pro-League (though it allowed for amendments to the covenant), and otherwise undistinguished. So, except in contrast to Harding, was the Democratic candidate.

The movement toward the Republicans, still the normal majority party, had begun in 1918 (see p. 606), and it quickened in 1920. Midwestern farmers, alienated by wartime controls, were now troubled by falling prices. Much of the once-progressive middle class had come to resent high taxes, inflation, and labor strife. Urban Democrats of the North were suspicious of Southern "drys," and Irish-Americans were hostile toward Wilson's foreign policy. Many independents could not forgive Palmer his behavior or Wilson his sometimes open endorsement of it.

All these factors combined to produce a Republican "earthquake." Harding received 61 percent of the

New voters, 1920

popular vote, which now included women, carried every state outside the South and also Tennessee, and led Cox by 404 to 127 in the Electoral College. The Republicans also swept the congressional elections, obtaining a majority of 22 in the Senate and 167 in the House of Representatives. Not only had the voters repudiated Wilson and internationalism, they had repudiated progressivism. They restored to power the Republicans who had stuck with the party when Roosevelt bolted in 1912. The party balance of 1896 prevailed again. Harding, for all his limitations, had caught the purpose of his constituency when he called for a return to "not nostrums, but normalcy."

Normalcy

All the advantages. Harding, his Secretary of State, Charles Evans Hughes, and the Republican majority in the Senate quickly buried the issue of the Treaty of Versailles. In his first message to Congress the President stated that the United States would have nothing to do with the League of Nations. Since the rejection of the treaty left the United States still technically at war with the Central Powers, the Senate passed again a resolution establishing a separate peace with Germany—a resolution that Wilson had vetoed. Harding signed it in July 1921, and Hughes then negotiated peace treaties with Germany, Austria, and Hungary. Like the resolution, these treaties claimed for the United States all the rights and advantages, but none of the responsibilities, of the Paris settlement.

The pursuit of advantages without responsibility—in Wilson's words "an ineffaceable stain upon . . . the honor of the United States"—also engaged the Harding Administration as a diplomatic partner to American oil companies. Harding's advisers, equating national interests with corporate interests, sought to fulfill corporate wishes. Pressure from oil companies persuaded the President to champion a treaty with Colombia, ostensibly designed only to indemnify that republic with $25 million for its loss of land and honor when Roosevelt assisted the Panamanian revolt. The treaty had been under consideration for several years, but Roosevelt's friends had blocked it while he still lived. In 1921, two years after his death, Colombia was preparing to withdraw all private rights to subsurface oil deposits. That possibility helped to move even Lodge to seek the good will that would permit Standard Oil to obtain concessions from the Colombian government. In April 1921 the Senate approved the treaty; Colombia ratified it in 1922; and American investments there, largely in oil, grew from about $2 million to $124 million by 1929. The State Department opened even richer prospects for profit by persuading the British to share with American companies the enormous oil fields of the Middle East.

The outstanding diplomatic venture of Harding's term was a 1921 conference on naval disarmament. At the time of Harding's inauguration, the Navy Department was urging the completion of the vast building program that had been launched five years earlier (see p. 594). But businessmen were impatient to cut federal expenses so that taxes could be reduced, and they grumbled about the cost of the program. Continued naval expansion, moreover, was provoking an armament race with two recent associates, Great Britain and Japan. Senator William E. Borah of Idaho suggested a three-power meeting on naval limitation, and large majorities in both houses of Congress endorsed that scheme in a resolution attached to the naval-appropriations bill of 1921.

This move was welcomed by the British, who were eager to terminate the defensive alliance made with Japan in 1902, an alliance that the dominions, especially Canada, disliked. The British also felt that the arms race was intimately associated with stability in the Far East. Harding proposed a conference on naval limitations on the same day the British called for a conference on East Asia. They agreed to discuss both matters at a single meeting in Washington.

The double agenda made it necessary to invite all the major naval powers—the United States, Great Britain, Japan, France, and Italy—as well as smaller powers with interests in the Far East—China, Portugal, Belgium, and the Netherlands. Everyone agreed that Bolshevik Russia, though a Pacific power, should be excluded, and its protests were ignored.

The delegates assembled on November 11, 1921, to commemorate the third anniversary of the armistice. The next day they heard an address by Secretary of State Charles Evans Hughes, who had been named presiding officer. He presented the conference with a detailed plan for naval disarmament. The United States was to scrap thirty capital ships—that is, battleships, battle cruisers, and aircraft carriers; the British were to give up twenty-three; Japan, seventeen. This destruction of more than 1,878,000 aggregate tons afloat, on the ways, or planned, would establish a capital-ship tonnage ratio among the three nations of 5:5:3. The ratio was to persist for ten years, during which the powers would observe a moratorium on the construction of capital ships. France and Italy were each to have one-third the tonnage allotted the United States and Great Britain.

Hughes' speech stirred the amazed delegates to cheers. The Japanese, however, disliked being on the short end of the ratio. They bargained successfully to keep their newest battleship, and they accepted the Five Power Naval Treaty only after the United States

On the Limitation of Armaments

and England had agreed not to fortify their possessions in the western Pacific. Another agreement, the Four Power Treaty, bound the United States, Great Britain, Japan, and France to respect each other's rights affecting insular possessions in the Pacific. It also specifically supplanted the Anglo-Japanese alliance.

Now Hughes pressed on to conclude a Nine Power Treaty that committed all the nations at the conference to observe traditional American policies in the Far East. They agreed to respect the territorial and administrative integrity and the independence of China and to uphold the Open Door.

The Washington treaties, as the British had intended, and as the United States later maintained, were integrally related to each other, and together they reduced tension in the Far East. Japan restored Shantung (Shandong) to China's sovereignty, withdrew from Siberia, and granted the United States cable rights on the former German island of Yap. The naval treaty, moreover, marked the first time in history that major powers had consented to disarm. Hughes had made a virtue of necessity, for he had really given up nothing he had any reasonable chance of getting from the parsimonious Congress.

Yet the Washington settlement also had shortcomings. It left the powers free to construct auxiliary naval vessels, such as destroyers, cruisers, and submarines, which were to prove vital weapons in the future. It provided no mechanism for consultations among the four major powers. All in all, it left the western Pacific a Japanese lake. Japan could build up its fleet, fortify its mandate islands, and encroach upon China, unless the United States and the other powers were prepared to defend their stated policies. The test of the settlement lay not in its terms but in whether or not the powers chose to honor them. As Wilson had asserted, peace was a matter of continual

negotiation and accommodation. And, as Roosevelt had preached, power was ever a factor in the affairs of nations.

Hughes had done remarkably well, but the spirit with which Americans greeted his accomplishment was ominous. In ratifying the Four Power Treaty, the Senate added a reservation asserting that the United States recognized "no commitment to armed force, no alliance, no obligation to join in any defense." Congress in 1922 and for years thereafter was unwilling to maintain the navy even at treaty strength. In short, the American people accepted words as realities, and the Washington settlement proved to be another case of seeking all the advantages and none of the responsibilities.

The best minds. Advantages rather than responsibilities were also the goal of the representatives of business and finance who shaped the domestic policies of the Harding Administration. The President had promised to recruit for government the "best minds" of the country. Hughes met that standard, as did Secretary of Commerce Herbert C. Hoover and Secretary of Agriculture Henry C. Wallace, who had long devoted himself to the cause of agricultural prosperity. But Wallace's influence was outweighed by that of Hoover, who used his department to promote the interests and enlarge the markets of American business. Hoover, in Harding's view, had proved his worth by acquiring a magnificent fortune. That was the President's surest criterion for finding the "best minds."

Foremost among Harding's advisers was Secretary of the Treasury Andrew Mellon, a reticent multimillionaire from Pittsburgh whose intricate banking and investment holdings gave him, his family, and his associates control, among many other things, of the aluminum monopoly. A man of slight build, with a cold and weary face, Mellon exuded sober luxury and contemptuous worldliness. "The Government is just a business," he believed, "and can and should be run on business principles."

Great businesses, as Mellon knew, thrive on innovation and expansion. Yet the only business principle he considered relevant to government was economy. With small regard for the services that only government could furnish the nation, Mellon worked unceasingly to reduce federal expenditures. Expenses had to be cut if he was to achieve his corollary purpose: the reduction of taxes, especially taxes on the wealthy. It was better, he argued, to place the burden of taxes on lower-income groups, for taxing the rich inhibited their investments and thus retarded economic growth. A share of the tax-free profits of the rich, Mellon reassured the country, would ultimately trickle down to the middle- and lower-income groups in the form of salaries and wages. Robert La Follette paraphrased that theory succinctly: "Wealth will not and cannot be made to bear its full share of taxation."

The quest for economy in government had some beneficial results. In 1921 Harding signed the Budget and Accounting Act, which improved the budgeting procedures of the federal government. It also served Mellon's purpose, for Harding's first Director of the Budget, Charles G. Dawes, a Chicago banker, made economy the touchstone of the budget that was presented to Congress in 1922.

Primarily to hold expenditures down, Harding opposed a veterans'-bonus bill that Congress debated in 1921, and he vetoed it when it passed the next year. Perhaps veterans did indeed deserve something more than gratitude from their country, but this bonus was little more than a raid on public funds supported by the American Legion, an energetic and increasingly influential veterans' pressure group. The newly created Veterans Administration was already taking care of the disabled. Veterans were not necessarily the neediest candidates for public assistance. Yet the veterans were simply acting in the spirit of the time when they continued to seek special advantages. Congress overrode a second veto in 1924 and granted a bonus in the form of paid-up twenty-year insurance policies, against which the veterans could immediately borrow limited funds.

Meanwhile, Mellon had advanced the tax program of the business community. In 1921 he urged Congress to repeal the excess-profits tax and to reduce the surtax on personal income from a maximum of 65 percent to 32 percent for 1921 and 25 percent thereafter. These proposals would have prevailed had it not been for the opposition of a group of Western Republican senators who joined with the Democrats to preserve the progressive principles of wartime revenue legislation. The Revenue Act of 1921 fell short of Mellon's goals. It held the maximum surtax on personal income at 50 percent, and it granted some tax relief to lower- and middle-income groups.

The Administration had better luck with its tariff policy. Following the tradition of their party, Republican leaders set out to restore the protective rates that had prevailed before 1913. Two developments eased their way. The spread of industry in the South had dispelled much of the traditional Democratic resistance to tariff protection. More important, farm representatives had concluded that they would profit from protective rates on farm products. This was a delusion, for the farmer really needed larger markets abroad, but there was no spirited debate on the tariff, as there had been in 1909.

Without significant dissent, Congress in 1922 passed the Fordney-McCumber Act, which reestablished prohibitive tariff rates. The act did instruct the Tariff Commission to help the President determine differences in production costs between the United States and other nations. And it did empower the President to raise or lower any rate by 50 percent, on the commission's recommendation. In practice, however, the commission was strongly protectionist, and of the thirty-seven rates that were altered during the life of the act, thirty-two were actually increased.

The Tariff of 1922 and its administration damaged foreign trade. By preventing Europeans from selling their goods in the United States, it made it impossible for them to buy American products, including agricultural surpluses, except by borrowing dollars and thus increasing the large debts they had incurred during the war. This was an unhealthy situation both for the United States and for Europe.

Nullification by administration. The restoration of tariff protection was only one part of a concerted effort by the Administration to restore the conditions of the nineteenth century. Wherever they could, Harding and his associates rolled back the accomplishments of the progressive movement.

The President could not tear down the apparatus that had been constructed for regulating business and industry, but he succeeded in rendering that apparatus useless by turning it over to the very interests it had been designed to regulate. His appointments to federal commissions, as Senator Norris said, "set the country back more than twenty-five years." They achieved "the nullification of federal law by a process of boring from within."

The Administration also stood aside while management continued its attack on labor unions and labor legislation. In 1922 Harding interceded to stop the violence that attended a nationwide coal strike. The report of the commission of inquiry he appointed revealed the pitiful, even desperate, state of life in the coal towns. The commission recommended various federal controls over the mining industry, but Congress and the Administration ignored the report. In the same year, the national Railway Labor Board approved a 12 percent reduction in the wages of railway shopmen, a decision that precipitated a strike that lasted two months. It ended only when the Attorney General got an injunction that forbade the union to picket or in any way to encourage workers to leave their jobs.

In this and other rulings the federal courts, acting in the spirit of the executive establishment, took ad-

vantage of the permissiveness of the Clayton Act (see p. 585). Contrary to Gompers' hopes, the injunction was still a handy instrument for breaking strikes. In the same spirit, the courts sustained "yellow-dog" contracts that bound employees not to join unions. The courts' hostility toward labor not only helped management's campaign for the open shop but destroyed social legislation designed to protect the poorest and weakest workers. The Supreme Court in 1922, in the case of *Bailey* v. *Drexel Furniture Company*, declared unconstitutional a federal statute levying a prohibitive tax on products manufactured by children. The Court had ruled earlier, in *Hammer* v. *Dagenhart* (1918), that federal laws to control child labor were an unconstitutional invasion of the police powers of the states. In the Bailey case, it said that Congress could not use its tax power to accomplish this unconstitutional purpose. The decision protected child labor, a common practice especially in Southern textile mills.

The Supreme Court was just as opposed to regulation of wages, hours, and working conditions. In 1923, in *Adkins* v. *Children's Hospital*, it held unconstitutional a District of Columbia statute establishing minimum wages for women. Ignoring the social and economic arguments for the act, the majority of the Court found it a violation of the freedom of women to contract to sell their labor as they pleased. The Adkins decision contravened the spirit of the Clayton Act, which asserted that labor was not a mere commodity. The decision also left labor defenseless, for neither federal nor state governments could insist on minimum standards of health and decency, and the attitudes of the courts denied the unions much of their opportunity to recruit membership or to strike for fair treatment.

The farmers fared better politically, but not economically, under the Harding Administration. In 1922 agricultural prices began to recover from their postwar slump, but the farmers were harassed by high interest charges on mortgages and by heavy taxes on land. Agricultural technology raised production and expanded surpluses even though the number of farms and of agricultural workers was steadily declining. And advancing industrialism continually reduced the farmers' share of the national income. Agriculture during the early 1920s was not generally impoverished, though segments of it were. But even the more privileged farmers were anxious about their future and resentful of their diminishing influence on American life. They were jealous, too, of the conveniences, especially electricity, automobiles, and entertainment, that were becoming more and more common in the cities.

In 1921 and 1922 the discontent of farmers generated considerable political force in the South and the Middle West, and the farm bloc in Congress won a series of victories. With few exceptions, however, the leaders of the farm bloc failed to understand the basic difficulties. They made their mark instead where the objectives of the fading progressive movement helped them to define their goals. Legislation in 1921 authorized the Secretary of Agriculture to compel commission merchants, grain merchants, and stockyard owners to charge reasonable rates. An act of 1922 exempted farm cooperatives from the antitrust laws, and Congress added a representative of agriculture to the Federal Reserve Board. In 1923 the Agricultural Credits Act established twelve Intermediate Credit Banks to make loans to cooperatives and other farm groups for six months to three years. The loans were to help cooperatives to withhold crops from the market when prices were temporarily low. These statutes strengthened the farmer's ability to conduct business, and they created instruments for controlling the middlemen who bought agricultural produce. But they did not ease the farmer's mortgage burden, and they helped the small farmer, sharecropper, and farm laborer not at all.

In the off-year elections of 1922, agrarian dissent carried anti-Administration candidates to victory in Republican primaries in most of the West. In November the resurgent Democrats reduced Republican majorities to eight in the Senate and eighteen in the House. And, of the Republicans who were elected, so many were disenchanted that the Administration no longer controlled Congress. The elections assured key committee assignments to strong men in both parties who were dubious about the Administration's program and methods. Those men, using Congress' power of investigation, soon exposed the Harding regime to publicity it could not afford.

The Harding scandals. The President of the United States sets the tone of his Administration. The first two decades of the twentieth century had been marked by McKinley's kindness, Theodore Roosevelt's strenuosity, Taft's decent ineffectuality, and Wilson's soaring idealism. Warren Harding brought to government the qualities of his own weak person. To his credit, he stopped the repression of dissent that marked the late Wilson years, and he pardoned Debs. But he was an ignorant, naive, confused man whose loose standards made him particularly vulnerable to his intellectual deficiencies and to the corrupt character of the hail-fellows with whom he instinctively surrounded himself.

Ruefully aware of some of his limitations, Harding once admitted he did not know whom to trust. Uncomfortable with the "best minds," he preferred the kind of tawdry companionship he had known in his native Marion, Ohio. The "Ohio gang" and their friends met continually with Harding at a house on K Street. There councils of state had an incidental but insinuating part in the rounds of poker and whiskey that made the President feel at home.

For two years the Ohio gang flourished. Early in 1923, however, Harding learned that the head of the Veterans Bureau had pocketed an impressive fraction of the $250 million his agency spent lavishly for hospitals and hospital supplies. Though Harding permitted the culprit to go abroad and resign, he was later exposed, tried, convicted, and sentenced to prison.

It also developed that Harding's Attorney General, Harry M. Daugherty of Ohio, had peddled his power for cash, but two divided juries in 1926 saved Daugherty from prison.

Secretary of the Interior Albert Fall was less fortunate. In 1921 he persuaded Harding to transfer to the Interior Department control over naval oil reserves at Elk Hill, California, and Teapot Dome, Wyoming. The next year Fall secretly leased Elk Hill to the oil company of Edward L. Doheny and Teapot Dome to the company of Harry F. Sinclair. But the leases could not be kept secret very long. In October 1923 a Senate committee under the chairmanship of Thomas J. Walsh, a Montana Democrat, began an investigation, which a special commission completed in 1924. The inquiries disclosed that Doheny had "lent" Fall $100,000 and that Sinclair had given the Secretary of the Interior a herd of cattle for his ranch, $85,000 in

Warren G. Harding: "This is a hell of a job."

cash, and $223,000 in bonds. In 1927 the government won a suit for cancellation of the leases. Though another remarkable verdict acquitted Doheny, Sinclair, and Fall of conspiracy to defraud the government, Sinclair was convicted of tampering with a jury, and in 1929 Fall was convicted of bribery, fined $100,000, and sentenced to a year in jail. He was the first Cabinet officer ever to go to prison.

Harding knew of only the earliest scandals. In June 1923, before setting out on a speaking tour through the West, the President unburdened himself to William Allen White: "My God, this is a hell of a job. I have no trouble with my enemies. . . . But my damned friends, my God-damned friends . . . they're the ones that keep me walking the floor nights!" Depressed and tired, Harding grew "nervous and distraught" as he traveled. Late in July, while in Seattle on the way home from Alaska, the President suffered acute pain. His doctor diagnosed it as indigestion, but other physicians in the party believed that Harding had had a heart attack, a diagnosis that was confirmed by a San Francisco specialist. On August 2, in a room at the Palace Hotel, Harding died, the victim of a coronary or cerebral thrombosis.

Vulgarity and scandal were the sordid fruits of normalcy, of a government that sought all the advantages of power but none of the responsibilities, of organized self-interest that sought special favors in bonuses, bounties, lower taxes, and higher tariffs. Pressure groups had gained advantages for big business even during the progressive years. After the war those interests dominated the federal government as they had not since the 1890s. The scandals passed, but the equation of national interests with privileged interests did not. That equation satisfied the "best minds" during the decade that followed the great war. It contradicted the best hopes cultivated before that war had begun.

Suggestions for Reading

THE WAR

The best study of the United States during the war is D. M. Kennedy, *Over Here: The First World War and American Society** (1980). There are adequate discussions of economic mobilization in B. M. Baruch, *American Industry in War* (1941) and *The Public Years* (1960), but more important are R. D. Cuff, *The War Industries Board* (1973), and the pertinent parts of O. L. Graham, Jr., *The Great Campaign* (1971). The relevant chapter of S. Ratner, *American Taxation* (1942), is useful on its subject. On congressional developments, see S. W. Livermore, *Politics Is Adjourned** (1966). On the administration of the War Department, D. R. Braver, *Newton D. Baker and the American War Effort, 1917–1919* (1966), offers considerable information; the Navy Department receives perceptive treatment in F. Freidel, *Franklin D. Roosevelt: The Apprenticeship* (1952). The most rewarding of the war memoirs is J. J. Pershing, *My Experiences in the World War*, 2 vols. (1931), but there are more useful accounts of military developments in E. E. Morison, *Admiral Sims and the Modern American Navy* (1942), and R. Weigley, *The American Way of War** (1973). There are a number of admirable studies of propaganda, censorship, and civil liberties in wartime, including, J. R. Mock and C. Larson, *Words That Won the War: The Story of the Committee on Public Information, 1917–1919* (1939); H. C. Peterson, *Propaganda for War* (1939); H. C. Peterson and G. C. Fite, *Opponents of War, 1917–1918* (1957); J. M. Jensen, *The Price of Vigilance* (1968); W. Preston, *Aliens and Dissenters: Federal Suppression of Radicals, 1903–1933* (1963); H. N. Scheiber, *The Wilson Administration and Civil Liberties, 1917–1921* (1960); and the classic Z. Chaffee, *Free Speech in the United States* (rev. ed., 1941).

THE PEACE

Students of peacemaking and of the American rejection of the peace treaty have at their disposal a voluminous literature that is continually growing. One excellent place to begin reading is in the penetrating analysis of H. R. Rudin, *Armistice, 1918* (1944). On the significance of the Bolsheviks in the fashioning of peace terms, see J. M. Thompson, *Russia, Bolshevism, and the Versailles Peace* (1966), and A. J. Mayer, *Political Origins of the New Diplomacy, 1917–1918* (1959) and *Politics and Diplomacy of Peacemaking* (1968). Two detailed accounts of the negotiations at Paris, which applaud Wilson's efforts, are D. F. Fleming, *The United States and the League of Nations, 1918–1920* (1932), and P. Birdsall, *Versailles Twenty Years After* (1941). On the United States and the Soviet Union, there are two superb volumes by G. F. Kennan, *Russia Leaves the War: The Americans in Petrograd and the Bolshevik Revolution* (1956) and *The Decision to Intervene: The Prelude to Allied Intervention in the Bolshevik Revolution* (1958). Also scholarly, and essential on its topic, is R. J. Bartlett, *League to Enforce Peace* (1944). There is a critical but persuasive analysis in T. A. Bailey, *Woodrow Wilson and the Lost Peace* (1944). The same author, in *Woodrow Wilson and the Great Betrayal* (1945), provides a trenchant study of the rejection of the treaty. Also significant on that subject are: R. A. Stone, *The Irreconcilables: The Fight Against the League of Nations** (1970); N. G. Levin, Jr., *Woodrow Wilson and World Politics** (1968); J. A. Garraty, *Henry Cabot Lodge* (1953); W. C. Widenor, *Henry Cabot Lodge** (1980); R. W. Leopold, *Elihu Root and the Conservative Tradition** (1954); and M. C. McKenna, *Borah* (1961). There are conflicting views about the conduct of government during Wilson's illness in E. B. Wilson, *My Memoirs* (1938), and J. M. Blum, *Joe Tumulty and the Wilson Era* (1951). Among the accounts of contemporaries friendly to Wilson, two of the most valuable are D. F. Houston, *Eight Years with Wilson's Cabinet, 1913–1920*, 2 vols. (1926), and Herbert Hoover, *The Ordeal of Woodrow Wilson* (1958). Two important unfriendly statements appear in H. C. Lodge, *The Senate and the League of Nations* (1928), and J. M. Keynes, *Economic Consequences of the Peace* (1919). Several of the books here listed cover the question of the League in the election of 1920, a subject further explored in J. M. Cox, *Journey Through My Years* (1946), and F. Freidel, *Franklin D. Roosevelt: The Ordeal* (1954).

THE RED SCARE

R. K. Murray, *The Red Scare** (1955), contains the most comprehensive narrative about the subject. It has to be supplemented, however, by the studies of civil liberties listed above and the perceptive biography by S. Coben, *A. Mitchell Palmer: Politician* (1963); the masterful analysis of G. L. Joughin and E. M. Morgan, *The Legacy of Sacco and Vanzetti** (1948); K. Jackson, *The Ku Klux Klan in the City, 1915–1930** (1967); the excellent studies of labor in I. Bernstein, *The Lean Years** (1960), and D. Brody, *Labor in Crisis: The Steel Strike of 1919* (1965); the analysis of blacks in A. I. Waskow, *From Race to Riot to Sit-In, 1919 and the 1960s* (1966), E. D. Cronon, *Black Moses** (1955), T. Vincent, *Black Power and the Garvey Movement* (1972), R. Burkett, *Garveyism as a Religious Movement* (1978), A. H. Spear, *Black Chicago** (1967), and N. I. Huggins et al., *Key Issues in Afro-American Experience*, 2 vols. (1971); and the penetrating treatments of nativism in J. Higham, *Strangers in the Land** (1955), and O. Handlin, *Race and Nationality in American Life* (1957) and *The American People in the Twentieth Century* (1954, 2nd rev. ed., 1966).

HARDING AND NORMALCY

W. E. Leuchtenburg, *The Perils of Prosperity, 1914–32** (1958), provides a crisp and thoughtful account of the Harding period. Also lively, but less judicious, is F. L. Allen, *Only Yesterday** (1931). There is a short but incisive evaluation of the Harding years in A. M. Schlesinger, Jr., *The Crisis of the Old Order** (1957), and a fuller narrative in J. D. Hicks, *Republican Ascendancy, 1921–1933* (1960). The economy and its problems receive able handling in G. Soule, *Prosperity Decade: From War to Depression, 1917–1929** (1947); but for a richer discussion of taxation and agriculture, respectively, the relevant chapters of R. E. Paul, *Taxation in the United States* (1954), and T. Saloutos and J. D. Hicks, *Twentieth Century Populism: Agricultural Discontent in the Middle West, 1900–1939* (1951), are particularly valuable. The Harding scandals get the treatment they merit in S. H. Adams, *Incredible Era* (1939); K. Schriftgiesser, *This Was Normalcy* (1948); and B. L. Noggle, *Teapot Dome** (1962). A. Sinclair, *The Available Man* (1965), tries to redeem Harding's reputation, as does R. K. Murray, *The Harding Era* (1969). Stimulating accounts of the Washington Conference are H. H. and M. T. Sprout, *Toward a New Order of Sea Power* (1946); J. C. Vinson, *The Parchment Peace: The United States Senate and the Washington Conference, 1921–1922* (1950); and T. H. Buckley, ed., *United States and the Washington Conference* (1970). Two biographies have given first-rate attention to the diplomacy of Harding's Secretary of State: M. J. Pusey, *Charles Evans Hughes*, 2 vols. (1951), and Dexter Perkins, *Charles Evans Hughes and American Democratic Statesmanship* (1953).

*Available in a paperback edition.

25
A NEW AGE OF BUSINESS

Calvin Coolidge believed in the kind of luck that Horatio Alger had immortalized. If a man worked hard, saved his pennies, respected the authorities, and kept his mouth shut, an invisible hand would contrive an occasion to make his reputation. Coolidge took no chances while he waited for his breaks. The son of a Vermont storekeeper, he worked his way through Amherst College, studied law in Northampton, Massachusetts, and entered politics there, winning successively those minor state offices on which undistinguished politicians build their careers. His patient course endeared him to the Massachusetts Republicans, who valued his unquestioning acceptance of things as they were, his unwavering preference for inaction, and his obvious personal honesty.

In 1919, twenty years after he first won public office, Coolidge achieved national prominence for his role in stopping the Boston police strike. His delay in dealing with that episode invited anarchy, but his friends used his new reputation to generate the boom that made him the Republican choice for Vice President. In that post Coolidge dispatched his ceremonial duties with quiet pleasure, warned Americans against the "Reds in Our Women's Colleges," and awaited his next break. When Harding died, Coolidge's luck had him at home, where his father, a notary public, administered the oath of office. The event was a blessing for the most privileged Republicans, for the accession of Calvin Coolidge gave them a new President who cloaked normalcy with respectability.

A New Cult of Enterprise

Coolidge and the business creed. Personally neat, even prim, deliberately laconic and undemonstrative in public (though given in private to temper and garrulity), Coolidge scrubbed the White House clean of the filth that Harding had left. Grace Coolidge, the new first lady, erased scandal with her natural dignity, charm, and warmth. The President chose two lawyers of impeccable integrity to prosecute the rascals in government. When the mounting evidence against the Attorney General forced his retirement in March 1924, Coolidge named to his place an eminent former dean of the Columbia Law School, Harlan Fiske Stone, whose appointment completed the shift from rascality to virtue.

In other respects Coolidge left the national government unaltered. As much as Harding, Coolidge subscribed to the creed of American business. "The business of America is business," Coolidge believed. "The man who builds a factory," he once said, "builds a temple. . . . The man who works there worships there." The President himself worshiped wealth and those who had it. Worldly possessions were for him evidence of divine election. He stood in awe of Andrew Mellon. He took a smug delight in his own eminence, but he was absolutely euphoric when his office commanded for him the deference of the rich. Coolidge, as William Allen White put it, was "sincerely, genuinely, terribly crazy" about wealth.

This passion coincided exactly with the theories of business spokesmen. There were, they preached, a superior few and an inferior many. And they were easy to distinguish, for "a man is worth the wages he can earn." Material success marked the élite, and to them the others should leave the important decisions about society. The 1920s witnessed a renaissance of the conservative dogmas of the 1880s, now clothed in new metaphors. Bruce Barton, a magnificently successful advertising man, gave the gospel its most popular phrasing in his best-seller of 1925, *The Man Nobody Knows*. To his infinite satisfaction, Barton, the son of a minister, discovered that Christ was a businessman. "Jesus," he wrote, ". . . picked up twelve men from the bottom ranks of business and forged them into an organization that conquered the world." The parables made incomparable advertisements; the gospel, an incomparable business school.

Coolidge was devoted to the dominant values of his time, to business, materialism, élitism, and their corollaries. If only the rich were worthy, it followed that government should beware the counsels of the majority. Since poverty was the wage of sin, government should not tax the virtuous rich in order to assist the unworthy poor. And since the rich best understood their own interests, government should not interfere with the businesses they ran, though it should help promote them both at home and abroad.

No devotee of laissez faire ever abhorred government more than Coolidge did. "If the Federal Government should go out of existence," he said, "the common run of people would not detect the difference . . . for a considerable length of time." Government's grandest service was to minimize itself, its activities, and its expenditures. So persuaded, Coolidge slept more than any other President in this century. He also said and did less when he was awake. "Four-fifths of all our troubles in this life," he told one agitated senator, "would disappear if we would only sit down and keep still." Silence, inactivity, gentility, complacency, and a shrewd political sense—those were the sum and the substance of the Coolidge calculus.

Productivity and plenty. The extraordinary prosperity of the 1920s cast a mantle of credibility over the doctrines of business and its representative President. It was easy for him and others of like mind to interpret prosperity as majestic proof of their beliefs. As the country came out of the short slump of 1921, unemployment became negligible except in sick industries like textiles and coal. By 1923 the average money wages of industrial workers were twice what they had been in 1914, and they continued to advance through 1928. Real wages rose, too, steadily though less dramatically. By 1928 they were about one-third

Calvin Coolidge: a smug delight

higher than they had been fourteen years earlier. Several factors accounted for those increases. Abundant, cheap energy in coal, oil, and waterpower kept down the costs of manufacturing and the goods it supplied. Many employers had begun to realize that higher wages removed one of the incentives that prompted workers to join unions and also provided purchasing power that swelled the market for industrial products. Wages stretched further as prices fell, especially the prices of food and of goods manufactured in industries where mechanization pushed productivity to new peaks.

The profits that came with mechanization invited investment in new plants and new tools. Investment was encouraged also by the growing national market, by the permissive climate of inactive government, and by Mellon's gradual success in persuading Congress to reduce taxes on large incomes. While investment provided the means for building more and more productivity into American industry, management was mastering new ways to use machinery and to organize production more effectively.

The American system of manufacturing that flowered during the 1920s had deep roots. It depended on the concept of continuous fabrication, by which raw materials entered a plant to emerge after multiple operations as finished products. That concept was at least as old as the first Lowell textile mills. It depended also on machine tools capable of producing standard, complex artifacts with interchangeable parts—the

Let us begin by asking why he was so successful in mastering public attention and why, in contrast, his churches are less so?... In the first place he recognized the basic principle that all good advertising is news. He was never trite or commonplace; he had no routine. If there had been newspapers in those days, no city editor could have said, "No need to visit him to-day; he will be doing just what he did last Sunday." Reporters would have followed him every single hour, for it was impossible to predict what he would say or do; every action and word were news....

Can you imagine the next day's issue of the Capernaum News, *if there had been one?...*

PROMINENT TAX COLLECTOR JOINS NAZARETH FORCES

MATTHEW ABANDONS BUSINESS TO PROMOTE NEW CULT
GIVES LARGE LUNCHEON

Every advertising man ought to study the parables of Jesus ... schooling himself in their language.... They are marvelously condensed, as all good advertising should be.... Jesus had no introductions. A single sentence grips your attention; three or four more tell the story; one or two more and the application is driven home.

From Bruce Barton, *The Man Nobody Knows*, 1925.

---

kind of tool and the kind of standardization that Eli Whitney had developed for guns a century before Coolidge's inauguration. More immediately, the American system of manufacturing depended on two recent and interrelated developments. One was the emerging profession of industrial engineering, with its concern for continuous process, improved machinery, specialization of jobs, and time-motion studies of performance. The other was an emerging cult of productivity, a rationalization of the glories of making and distributing and consuming ever more bountifully. Americans had long honored that objective, but never more avidly than in the 1920s.

The founding father of "scientific management" was Frederick W. Taylor. Born into a comfortable family in Germantown, Pennsylvania, in 1856, Taylor had to interrupt his gentleman's education at Harvard because of poor eyesight. Moving into an entirely different environment, he learned the trades of patternmaker and machinist and in 1878 went as a common laborer to the Midvale Steel Company. By 1885 he had earned his Master of Engineering degree at Stevens Institute; a year later he became chief engineer at Midvale. His driving concern was with making machines and their operatives produce more and faster. Those interests led him to establish his own consulting practice on production, on "systematizing shop management."

Taylor's system started with a close study of every step in manufacturing. By applying the resulting data,

by breaking the process of manufacturing into separate parts, and by specializing the function of the worker and machine involved in each part, he could substantially increase the rate of production. His classifications of jobs and of capacity, he believed, would lead also to higher wages as workers first met and then exceeded their calculated goals. The aim of every establishment, Taylor wrote in *Shop Management* (1911), should be to give each workman the highest grade of work of which he was capable, to call on each to turn out his maximum, and to pay each in accordance with his product. "This means," he argued, "*high wages* and *low labor cost.*" It also meant time-motion studies, discipline, pressure, and incentives for speedup. For Taylor efficiency was a fetish, but he got results. Before he died in 1915 (with a watch in his hand, John Dos Passos surmised), he had caught the attention of management and had aroused the fears of labor-leaders, who were learning that piecework and the speedup would grind profits out of workers' fatigue. In spite of those fears, Taylorism spread. It was praised by Louis Brandeis and other progressives—so often devotees of efficiency—and institutionalized by a Taylor Society.

Taylor was the philosopher of the machine process; Henry Ford was its commanding general. In 1911 Ford opened his plant at Highland Park, Michigan. There he and his fellow executives arrived at Taylor's principles along their own routes and began to turn out automobiles at prodigious rates. The Ford Motor

St. Louis: the fruits of industry

Company outsped all industry in specializing the tasks of men and machines. After 1913 it also applied the idea of continuous motion, using conveyor belts, gravity slides, and overhead monorails to feed the machinery by which workers stood. The modern assembly line turned out the Model T's that put America on wheels. As his production and market grew, Ford cut prices and increased wages. To be sure, the wages he claimed to pay did not reach all his workers, the speedup at the Ford company was notorious, and the company tolerated no unions. But the $5 day that Ford announced in 1914 seemed to mark the dawn of a new era, and so did Ford's staggering profits. In the mid-1920s Ford had become, in the phrase of Upton Sinclair, the Flivver King.

By that time Ford's production techniques had become standard in the automobile and other industries. The Model T was a very stark car, but America's machines were also producing more comfortable, more sumptuous, and more complex mechanisms. During Coolidge's tenure in office, for the first time in the history of any nation, a mass market developed for cars, for radios, for refrigerators and vacuum cleaners. There was, in a sense, no longer any problem of production. The available stocks of American raw materials, workers, machines, and techniques could saturate the nation, and much of the world, with the necessities and conveniences of modern civilization.

Businessmen, however, were interested in more than just the science of production. Their restrictive

Modern business enterprise

labor policies during the 1920s kept the rise in real wages well below the rise in profits. And they guarded their market jealously, trying to produce only as much as the market could absorb without a break in prices. Large firms in heavy industries had long since learned the importance of administered, noncompetitive pricing and had long since contrived the consolidations that made for industrial stability. During the 1920s the tendency toward consolidation proceeded at an accelerating tempo, in old industries as well as new. And, as consolidation advanced, managers became more and more skillful in governing costs, price, and output.

Indeed, professional business management came into its maturity in the 1920s. Before the war, business had integrated vertically, incorporating the stages of industrial activity from extraction through manufacturing, transportation, and marketing under unitary management, as in the steel and food industries. The combination of mass production with mass distribution accounted for the size and much of the efficiency of big business. After the war the growing professionalization of management increased that efficiency. At both senior- and middle-level positions, managers brought a new sophistication to their responsibilities. With increasing diversification of ownership, moreover, no stockholder or group of stockholders could any longer control the policy of most great corporations (the Ford Motor Company, still family-owned, was an exception and began to lose its share of market largely because of the superior management of its major competitors). Consequently, control of policy passed to management, and managers for their part refined corporate strategies. Large corporations moved to diversify their line of products and to enter international markets. Perhaps more important, managers of major enterprises achieved a new independence in planning expansion, diversification, and moderniza-tion by reserving portions of current profits for their own future investment, not the least in research and development. That strategy freed those planning it, among others General Motors and Standard Oil of New Jersey, from dependence for new investment on banks or capital markets in Wall Street or elsewhere.

Those developments disturbed Americans for whom the production of wealth for universal use was a more precious objective than the amassing of profits. The Nobel Prize-winning novelist Sinclair Lewis, in *Dodsworth* (1929), told of an automobile-manufacturer who was forced to sell out to a giant holding company, a fictional General Motors. Dodsworth, deprived of the satisfaction of producing cars himself, and unwilling to serve as a subordinate in a great corporation, sought vainly to find new satisfactions in the culture of Europe. But in the end he came back to the United States to embark on the manufacture of

Marketing home appliances

Thorstein Veblen: perceptive critic

mobile homes. He was the kind of business engineer who adhered to a commitment to production that Lewis felt ordinary business-managers were destroying.

Thorstein Veblen made the most devastating comparisons between those who made goods and those who made money. In *The Engineers and the Price System* (1921) and *Business Enterprise* (1923) he condemned businessmen for artificially curtailing output for the sake of profit—a practice he labeled "sabotage." He called for a revolution of technicians, of men committed to production, who would free industry of pecuniary restraints and use the machine process to provide plenty for humanity. There was a naiveté in Veblen's attitude toward competition, and a strong dose of Marxism. But his simplifications and nostalgia had both merit and influence. Whereas business-managers often planned only for profit, Veblen urged public planning for the general welfare. His message helped to bridge the space between the progressive era and the next era of reform.

Republican symbols: 1924. In the Coolidge era, however, the impulse for reform flagged. The spirit of that time saw no conflict between profits and productivity. It found a symbol in the person of Herbert Hoover, who seemed to have walked right out of American mythology. Son of an Iowa farmer, descended of pioneer stock, orphaned at ten, Hoover went west, worked his way through Stanford University, married a banker's daughter, and as an engineer in Asia earned his first million before he was forty. He was the hero of Belgian relief, the successful Food Administrator of Wilson's war Cabinet, and, in the opinion of one London newspaper, "the biggest man . . . on the Allied side" at Paris. By 1920 Hoover's name stood for personal success, for food for the hungry, and for rigor in administration. His reputation reached its height while he was serving under Harding and Coolidge as Secretary of Commerce.

To that office Hoover applied, as it were, the principles of scientific shop management. His department studied business trends, fought economic waste through its Office of Simplified Practice, and promoted American commerce and investment abroad. Concurrently it encouraged trade associations to sustain prices and profits by adjusting production to demand. Hoover personally organized the relief of victims of the Mississippi flood of 1927, exercised control over radio and the air waves, avoided associating with politicians, and harbored an ambition as broad and inconspicuous as his conservative blue suits. He stood at once for laissez-faire doctrines, "cooperative individualism," humanitarian endeavor, and quiet and humorless efficiency. Coolidge, increasingly jealous of Hoover's reputation, could barely tolerate "the wonder boy."

The President did not suffer any rival kindly. A shrewd political manipulator, he rapidly brought the machinery of the Republican party under his control. As the nominating convention of 1924 approached, he had only one possible opponent—not Hoover, who was biding his time, but Henry Ford. The Flivver King had run as a Democrat, and lost, in the race for senator from Michigan in 1918. His publicity men, who wrote much of what he signed, had begun in 1922 to suggest that he might be available as a Republican candidate for the White House. The prospect was both preposterous and alarming. Away from his machines, Ford was a ludicrous, semiliterate figure, the captive of folk prejudices. He was opposed to tobacco, liquor, and ballroom dancing. He had published and circulated anti-Semitic propaganda. He detested labor unions and Wall Street, both of which he felt were the tools of an international Jewish conspiracy. But this nonsense had an unfortunate appeal to the uneducated, and a third of those who were polled by *Collier's* in a straw ballot of 1923 named Ford as their first choice for President.

Ford's candidacy may not have been serious, though many people thought it was. He was, however, deadly serious in his proposal to take over the government dam, nitrate plant, and other facilities constructed during the war at Muscle Shoals on the Tennessee River. He proposed to purchase the nitrate works for less than 5 percent of what they had cost

*No doubt, individualism run riot, with no tempering principle, would pro-
vide a long category of inequalities, of tyrannies ... and injustices. America,
however, has tempered the whole conception of individualism by the injection
of a definite principle, and from this principle it follows that attempts at domination, whether in government or in the processes of industry and commerce,
are under an insistent curb. If we would have the values of individualism,
their stimulation to initiative, to the development of hand and intellect, to
the high development of thought and spirituality, they must be tempered with
that firm and fixed ideal of American individualism—an equality of opportunity. If we would have these values we must suffer its hardness and stimulate
progress through that sense of service that lies in our people.*

From Herbert C. Hoover, American Individualism, 1922.

the government, to lease the waterpower facilities for a hundred years for less than 10 percent of what it would cost the government to complete them, and to have the government pay him simply by issuing new paper money. In return, he hinted that he would be able to produce fertilizer for American farms at half its current price. As Senator Norris said, this was the "most wonderful real estate speculation since Adam and Eve lost title to the Garden of Eden."

Norris exposed and defeated the scheme, which would have destroyed his cherished plans for the public development of the Tennessee. Yet before the chimera vanished, Coolidge, after talking with Ford, recommended that Congress sell Muscle Shoals to private interests. Ford himself soon put an end to his presidential boomlet by announcing that the nation was "perfectly safe with Coolidge." There may have been no bargain, but the coincidence of events suggested that both men were trading in character.

It was a striking commentary on the times that Ford's nitrate project was even proposed. It was no less striking that Ford's candidacy seemed to be the only barrier to Coolidge's renomination. Robert La Follette and Hiram Johnson, dedicated, doughty old progressives, could muster between them only forty-four votes at the Republican convention that gave Coolidge over a thousand votes on its first and decisive ballot. Only a dozen years earlier almost half the Republicans had cast their lot with Theodore Roosevelt.

One Nation Divisible

For white Protestants only. The temper of the twenties was marked by narrowness and provincialism as well as by prosperity and complacency. The attitudes on which the Red scare had fed survived the passing of the scare itself. Among many Americans there lingered an intolerance of all "isms," a distrust of foreign nations, and a dislike, often bordering on

hatred, of people of foreign origin. Much of the farm community had long been susceptible to those feelings, and organized labor had endorsed the racial as well as the economic arguments of those who advocated that immigration be restricted.

In 1924 Congress adopted the recommendations of the Dillingham commission (p. 571) and passed the National Origins Act. This based annual immigration quotas temporarily on the proportion of descendants of each nationality resident in the United States in 1890 and limited immigration from outside of the Western Hemisphere after 1927 to 150,000 a year, selected on the proportion established by the census of 1920. Those quotas ended all but a trickle of immigration from southern and eastern Europe. The act, furthermore, included a provision that West Coast racists had been urging for years. It forbade the immigration of Asians, thus terminating the Gentlemen's Agreement (see p. 571) and insulting the race-sensitive Japanese. "It has undone the work of the Washington Conference," Charles Evans Hughes wrote, "and implanted seeds of . . . antagonism."

Asians, blacks, Catholics, and Jews were all victims of the prejudice based on the ethnic self-consciousness of white, Protestant Americans of older stock. Even many educated and comfortable people, who should have known better, attributed to race, religion, or national origin varying qualities of character and intelligence, always with the assumption that Americans of old stock were a superior breed. That kind of bigotry thrived even among college professors and more virulently among Southern whites, and it also appealed to the poorer and semieducated who lived or had grown up in rural or small-town America. That America, as the census of 1920 indicated, now contained a minority of the American people. Rural folk felt threatened. More and more they tended, as they had for at least half a century, to blame their personal disappointments on the growth of cities and industry and to express their anxieties in hostility toward those who peopled the cities.

The new Klan: politics of prejudice

Those prejudices were the stock in trade of the Ku Klux Klan, an organization founded in Georgia in 1915 on the model of its Reconstruction predecessor. It recruited only "native born, white, gentile Americans," and it gave them a sense of importance by admitting them to membership in a group dedicated to persecuting an alleged enemy within the country. It also gave them a uniform, a hierarchy, and a ritual.

In 1920 two professional fund-raisers organized a membership drive and arranged to share with local officers the profits from increased initiation fees and from the sale of uniforms and insignia. By 1925 membership approached 5 million. The Klan grew rapidly in cities like Portland, Oregon, Indianapolis and Denver where much of the inflowing population consisted of displaced rural folk who were still suspicious of urban ways of life. They were attracted not the least by the Klan's attacks on wickedness, on saloons and pimps and "deviants" of all kinds.

The Klan used floggings, kidnapings, cross-burnings, arson, even murder to terrorize whole communities. It was especially vicious in its treatment of Catholics. An Alabama jury acquitted a Klansman who had murdered a priest; a Klan mob burned a Roman Catholic church in Illinois; the Klan and its sympathizers attempted to crush parochial schools in Oregon; and in Oklahoma they inspired the impeachment of a governor who had declared martial law in a brave effort to rout the organization. Increasingly powerful in politics, the Klan held the balance of power in several states.

At its zenith in 1923 and 1924, the Klan by its very excesses attracted increasing opposition. In 1924 William Allen White, its implacable enemy, lost the Kansas governorship to one of the Klan's friends, but White's campaign set a sensible example. In some states the Klan began to fade, especially after "Dragon" David Stephenson of Indiana kidnaped and assaulted his secretary and connived to keep her from medical attention after she took poison. Convicted in 1925 of second-degree murder and sentenced to life imprisonment, Stephenson demanded a pardon from his fellow Klansman, Governor Ed Jackson. When Jackson refused, the vindictive "Dragon" opened a "little black box" whose contents provided evidence that sent one congressman, the mayor of Indianapolis, and various lesser officers to jail. Most important, the Klan, which had pretended to guard civic purity and feminine virtue, now stood exposed for what it was—corrupt, sordid, and licentious.

Prohibition. The Prohibitionists, who were always strongest in rural areas and particularly among fundamentalist sects, considered liquor an instrument of the devil. Unaware of the complex personal and social problems that provoke excessive drinking, they insisted that alcoholism was created by alcohol itself and by the saloon keepers who sold it. Whiskey and beer seemed to them, moreover, the potions of immigrants and political bosses, the poison of the corrupt city.

Ben Shahn, gouache mural for the Public Works Administration: New York speakeasy

The Prohibition Amendment of 1919 also drew strength from the belief of many Americans that legislation could somehow control personal behavior of all kinds. They were understandably eager to reduce drunkeness and the diseases and poverty it spawned. But before long only the most rabid or stubborn "drys" failed to recognize the difficulties of enforcement. The Prohibition commissioner, in his quest to prevent the manufacture, transportation, and sale of alcoholic beverges (defined by the Volstead Act of 1919 as one-half of 1 percent by volume), had to depend on a small force of agents who were often third-rate political appointees with neither the background nor the intelligence to resist bribes or needless violence. They simply could not police the millions of Americans who wanted to drink and who either made their brews at home or, more often, bought their beer or whiskey from the hundreds of "bootleggers" who earned an illegal, sometimes dangerous, but remunerative living supplying it.

Smugglers brought whiskey in across the Canadian border, or on fast boats from the Caribbean. To supplement the supplies of these "rum-runners," there were countless domestic distillers of illicit whiskey, much of it bad and some of it poisonous. It was easy to buy whiskey by the case, the bottle, or the drink. Indeed, "speakeasies," illegal saloons, did business in every major city, and obliging policemen and cab-drivers were glad to tell strangers where they were.

The traffic in bootlegging provided a new and rich source of income and influence for organized crime. In 1920 the most notorious gangland chief, "Scarface" Al Capone, moved to Chicago, where within seven years he had established a $60-million enterprise in whiskey, drugs, gambling, and prostitution. Capone applied the techniques of business management to crime, but with a difference. His private army of about a thousand gangsters, who were charged with protecting his domain, accounted for most of the one hundred and thirty murders in the Chicago area in 1926–27. Such was Capone's influence that not a single murderer was convicted. In New York, Philadelphia, Kansas City, and elsewhere, gangsters put high public officers on their payroll and transformed machine politics into agencies for crime.

Prohibition, manifestly unenforceable, had not created organized crime, but it had given gangland a vast privilege to exploit—a privilege that repeal of Prohibition would at least remove. Urban "wets," who had opposed Prohibition from the first, led the movement for repeal, supported by more and more former "drys." The most adamant foes of repeal were the moralists of the countryside who had failed to distinguish between liquor and crime and who identified both with immigration and the city.

Last-ditch fundamentalism. Rural hostility to urban culture also showed itself in matters of the mind. The unsophisticated have always fallen prey to antiscientism, partly because they do not understand the methods of science, partly because they resent many of the changes that science and technology bring about. Though most Americans admired the technological advances of the 1920s and recognized them as the products of earlier scientific strivings, some were distressed by the complexities and uncertainties of a machine civilization, by its speed, its capacity for destructive as well as constructive power, its overwhelming challenge to the ways of the "good old days." To those Americans science seemed threatening and mysterious. In the rural areas that modern culture had just begun to reach, Protestant fundamentalism seized on science as an archenemy.

The fundamentalists insisted that the Bible must be accepted as literal truth. More than sixty years after the publication of Darwin's *Origin of Species*, they still rejected the concept of biological evolution and attacked those who taught it. In the postwar years William Jennings Bryan a "dry," a fundamentalist, a folk hero of a kind, and now an old and frustrated man, enlisted in the antievolutionist crusade. Strengthened by his leadership, the antievolutionists scored partial victories in several Southern states. Bryan himself in 1925 assisted the lobby that pressured the Tennessee legislature into passing a statute making it illegal to teach in public schools any theory that denied the account of creation recorded in Genesis.

The American Civil Liberties Union, responding to this challenge to the freedom of inquiry, offered counsel to any Tennessee teacher who would test the law. More in amusement than in anger, John T. Scopes of the mountain town of Dayton lectured from a Darwinian text and was arrested. Among the lawyers who defended him were Clarence Darrow, the most famous pleader of the time, and Arthur Garfield Hays, a celebrated advocate of civil liberties. Assisting the prosecution was Bryan, who had been retained by the World's Christian Fundamental Association. The all-star cast in the Dayton "monkey trial" engaged the interest of the entire nation.

The prosecution contended that the only issue was Scopes' violation of the law, but the defense raised the question of the validity of the law itself. The case reached its climax when Bryan took the stand as an expert on the Bible. Joshua had made the sun stand still, the Commoner said; the whale had swallowed Jonah; if it was in the Bible, it was so. As Darrow pressed the cross-examination, Bryan revealed an invincible ignorance of modern learning.

Scopes was convicted for violating the law, but the state supreme court reversed the decision on a technicality, and the constitutionality of the statute could not be tested. (It was not repealed until the 1970s.) There was no longer any reason to test it. Bryan had admitted in his testimony that creation took centuries; a "day" in Genesis might be an eon. That admission cost the fundamentalists their argument, and the ridicule of Bryan's performance had lost them their cause.

But by 1925 the blind innocence of fundamentalism, together with the pernicious zeal of the Klan, had

Darrow and Bryan at Dayton: creation took centuries

estranged the ordinary citizen from the intellectual and had divided the underprivileged of the farms from the underprivileged of the cities. Protestant laborers had been set against Jewish and Catholic laborers, whites against blacks. Americans whom prosperity either did not reach or did not beguile had been sealed off into separate and often hostile groups.

The election of 1924. This estrangement made it difficult for the Democratic party to select a national candidate to oppose Coolidge in 1924. One of the two leading contenders was William G. McAdoo, who had won the acclaim of liberals for his administration of the railroads during the war (p. 604), but who had lost their favor by taking a job as counsel to Edward L. Doheny, one of the scoundrels of Teapot Dome. Yet McAdoo, ardently "dry" and equivocal about the Klan, held the support of the South and the West. His major rival, Alfred E. Smith, the governor of New York, was a "wet," a Catholic, and a Tammany man. The darling of the Eastern cities, Smith was anathema to the rural delegates in spite of his progressive record.

The convention met in New York's Madison Square Garden during an early summer heat wave. To the party's shame, a motion not to include a plank in the platform condemning the Klan by name passed by a margin of one vote. There followed a nine-day deadlock over the nomination. Through ninety-five ballots the hoarse voice of the aged Bryan vied with the raucous noise of the Tammany gallery, and the contest was relayed by radio to millions of American homes. The split in the party had become irremediable; the sweltering delegates had become exhausted. At last Smith and McAdoo withdrew by mutual agreement. On the 103rd ballot the convention nominated John W. Davis for President and Charles Bryan as his running mate. They were an unlikely brace. Davis, who had served as Solicitor General and briefly as ambassador to Great Britain during the Wilson Administration, was a cultivated gentleman and an eminent corporation lawyer identified with the House of Morgan. The liberals who disdained him could find small solace in Bryan's younger brother Charley. Wall Street and Nebraska could not be squeezed onto a single ticket, but the prolonged bitterness of the convention had made a saner choice impossible.

A third nomination stirred wider interest. The resurgence of reform candidates in the congressional election of 1922 had owed much to the Conference for Progressive Political Action, an organization of farm leaders, social workers, former Bull Moosers, and Socialists. Now the leaders of the Conference began to talk about running a separate ticket in 1924. The communists forced their hand by taking over the Farmer-Labor party and offering its nomination to "Battle Bob" La Follette. Then almost seventy, iron-

Robert La Follette, 1924: "Wisconsin Bolshevism"

gray, still the indomitable Daniel in the lion's den of "the interests," La Follette scorned the offer. That response prompted his supporters to form a new Progressive party, which named La Follette and the liberal Montana Democrat Burton K. Wheeler as its national candidates.

La Follette's candidacy attracted a host of tireless battlers for reform, among them Felix Frankfurter, John R. Commons, and Jane Addams. It was endorsed by the American Federation of Labor and, curiously, by the Socialists. La Follette stood for conservation, public ownership of waterpower, increased taxes on wealth, curbing the authority of the Supreme Court, limiting the use of injunctions in labor disputes, the popular election of judges, the direct election of Presidents, the end of child labor, and a national referendum on declarations of war. But he emphasized the evil of monopoly, ringing again the changes of his early campaigns in Wisconsin. The *Wall Street Journal* called his platform "Wisconsin Bolshevism"; the head of the Communist party in the United States called it "the most reactionary document of the year." Both statements were nonsense. The platform and the campaign were simply refurbished Grangerism, still appealing to many farmers, and the only haven for those who could stomach neither Coolidge nor Davis.

The Republicans ignored Davis and harped on La Follette's radicalism. They need not have worked so hard as they did nor have spent the millions they poured into the campaign, for the nation voted overwhelmingly to "keep cool with Coolidge." The President carried thirty-five states to Davis' twelve and La Follette's one, Wisconsin. Coolidge won 382 electoral votes to his opponents' 149. And his popular vote, over 15,000,000, exceeded the combined total of Davis, who polled fewer than 8,500,000, and La Follette, who had slightly more than 4,800,000. Prosperity and "Silent Cal" had enjoyed a major triumph.

Yet the new Progressive party had made a point, though it died in 1925 with La Follette. The point was simply that there was room in politics for dissent from the business creed. The lesson was not lost on the Democrats, who realized that they had to close ranks and reconstruct a coalition that welcomed men and women of all colors, all parentages, all sections. If the Democrats were to win in the future they would have to be "unequivocally the party of progress and liberal thought." That phrase was Franklin Roosevelt's, who saw small chance for a victory before 1932. When it came, at its core would be the combination of Davis and LaFollette voters.

Grandiose Illusions

The good life. Americans were optimistic during Coolidge's second term. The middle class in particular, more comfortable than ever before, experienced a sense of well-being. They admitted no limit to a personal success symbolized by material possessions. They neither liked nor trusted the "knockers," but preferred the "boosters," those with their eyes and hearts set on the rosy future.

Some of the boosters channeled their optimism into the expanding advertising profession. National advertising flourished in the twenties. It offered an attractive substitute for more painful forms of competition, like price-cutting, which, in any event, were being curtailed by trade agreements and informal arrangements among manufacturers. Advertising also helped identify brands for consumers, who were buying more and more of their goods in stores and producing fewer and fewer at home. Advertising men believed they were "inspiring citizens to live a more abundant life." They were creating new wants and encouraging discontent with possessions outmoded but not necessarily outworn. Advertisers sold the ingredients of the good life—health in orange juice, cleanliness in soap, popularity in deodorants, romantic love in voguish clothes.

As one General Motors executive put it, advertising had to make people "healthily dissatisfied with what they have. . . . The old factors of wear and tear . . . are too slow." Built-in obsolescence paved the road to business success. Manufacturing prettier, more comfortable cars than Ford did, changing models annually (while also meeting competitive standards in engineering), General Motors won primacy in the automobile industry largely by catering to luxury and fashion.

Advertising also created and sold reputations, both corporate and personal. Public-relations experts,

taking over the new game of ballyhoo as their own, fabricated heroes on demand. Some of the celebrated athletes of the 1920s, for example, owed part of their fame to sheer ballyhoo. To be sure, Bobby Jones in golf, Bill Tilden in tennis, Jack Dempsey in boxing, and Babe Ruth in baseball were athletes of genuinely heroic proportions. But their proportions were overdrawn, and cynical public-relations men learned to conceal the boorish behavior of Ruth, among others, by planting stories of fictitious noble deeds.

The prospering tabloid newspapers catered to a mass audience that delighted in sensationalism and hero worship. The art of sham was especially effective when it could concentrate on sex. It publicized the new heroes and heroines of the booming motion-picture industry—Rudolph Valentino, the Casanova of the silent films, whose untimely death broke thousands of adolescent hearts; Clara Bow, the "It" girl, whose curves and curls entranced a male multitude; Mary Pickford, the sweet charmer whom a plucky lad could more properly admire; and Charlie Chaplin, the incomparable clown.

In Hollywood's films and in magazines and popular fiction standard success stories followed classic forms—farm boys conquered the city while remaining pure, poor boys struggled and saved their way to wealth, nice boys met and married beautiful rich girls.

Bill Tilden: tennis hero

Valentino: Casanova of the silent film

The modern woman

The protagonist's gleaming teeth, curly hair, lithe muscles, humility, and hard work assured a happy ending. And ordinary Americans could do just as well through diligent use of the right toothpaste, hair lotion, and correspondence course. But the plot was used too often to boost sales and circulation, and it was beginning to wear thin. Just then a real hero revived the faith.

In the spring of 1927 there was startling news of a young man flying solo, eastward across the Atlantic, in a small monoplane. No one before had made that flight alone. The prayers of the nation followed Charles A. Lindbergh, Jr., to France. His safe landing set off a jubilee; Coolidge sent a cruiser to bring him home; New York extended ecstatic greetings. Briefly, sham and commercialism hid from authentic daring and clean-cut youth. Lindbergh took it calmly. After writing another stanza to his saga by marrying Anne Morrow, the daughter of a Morgan partner, he tried to escape the tabloids and the confetti. Myths need a foundation in truth, and the Lindbergh story had been as genuine as it was refreshing. When it faded from the headlines, myth fed once again on the exploits of hired muscle men who drew crowds to mammoth stadiums.

Advertising and public relations and ballyhoo, like the newspapers and magazines and radio that

carried them, exported urban ways to rural people. They disseminated a common set of symbols to diverse groups. They told farmers and laborers and suburbanites to admire the same success stories and buy the same cars and cosmetics. They told them all to spend their money to increase their comfort, to prove their mettle, to live "the good life." They en-

Lindbergh: eastward across the Atlantic

couraged installment buying to ensure the sale of an expanding national product. They helped Americans with rising wages to forget about the frustrations of their dull and routine jobs. The spurious self-esteem that sprang from possession and fashion would endure only so long as Americans could count on steady income and easy credit; but so long as prosperity lasted, advertisers gilded the promises of a commercial culture, the only brand of Americanism they really understood. This crass and transient boom was rooted in illusion, in calling things by the wrong names and then accepting the names as true. The illusions of public life were similarly deceiving.

The image of America abroad. The Coolidge Administration became involved in Latin-American affairs even though the President, like Harding before him, meant to avoid intervention and allow private interests to carry the burden of policy. Nevertheless, the Administration often succeeded only in obscuring national purpose and generating ill will among Latin Americans. Secretary of State Hughes, moved by a concern for peace and order, had helped bring about the peaceful settlement of several Latin American boundary disputes. During Hughes' tenure, the United States also sponsored a conference of Central American powers, which agreed to withhold recognition from any government established by a *coup d'état*. But this genuflection to stability ignored the realities of Central American politics, for where the government in power had complete control over elections, a *coup d'état* or revolution was the only means of ousting it.

In Nicaragua Coolidge acted unilaterally. First, in 1925, he withdrew a token force of marines from that nation, which then seemed capable of servicing its foreign debt and preserving its internal stability. But the appearance was deceptive. Almost at once revolution broke out, and Coolidge again landed the marines, in time some five thousand. Regrettably, in its quest for order and for commercial opportunity the United States chose to support the reactionary faction, whose identification with large landowners and American investors had helped provoke the revolution in the first place.

The marines contained the fighting, but they could not bring it to an end. American bankers were lending money to the conservative faction for the purchase of munitions in the United States, and the rebels were receiving some arms from sympathetic Mexico. Increasingly uncomfortable, Coolidge in 1927 named Henry L. Stimson as his personal emissary to negotiate a peace. Stimson succeeded in arranging an effective truce and an honest election, in which the rebel general triumphed. The marines, however, remained until 1933. They also remained in Haiti but in

1924 left the Dominican Republic, where President Wilson had sent them.

Though the United States had no territorial ambitions, Yankee investors were seeking bonanzas in Latin America, and Latin Americans resented the Yankee habit of intervening in their local affairs. At the Pan-American Conference of 1928 the Argentine delegation sponsored a proposal that "no American country have the right to intervene in any other American country." The United States succeeded in defeating the proposal but in doing so heightened the resentment. Late in 1928 the State Department concluded that intervention was not justified by the Monroe Doctrine or by the interests of American investors. But it was still not ready to announce that conclusion.

Latin American liberals continued to identify the United States with the forces of reaction. Even more than the Nicaraguan episode, developments in Mexico contributed to that view. In 1925 Plutarco Elias Calles, the new president of Mexico, revived the spirit of the revolution of 1910, which had for several years been in eclipse. He sponsored laws that permitted foreigners to acquire land only if they renounced the protection of their own government, and laws that defined all subsoil deposits as the inalienable property of the Mexican nation. Oil companies, American and other, were required to apply for a renewal of their concessions before 1927. Four large American companies refused. Their spokesmen in the United States, asserting that Mexico was on the road to Bolshevism, called for military intervention, but in January 1927 the United States Senate by unanimous vote passed a resolution demanding the peaceful settlement of all contested issues—by arbitration, if necessary.

Several months later Coolidge appointed a new ambassador, Dwight W. Morrow, with the overriding commission "to keep us out of war with Mexico." Morrow's patient negotiations led to a temporary relaxation of the Mexican land laws and restored friendly relations. Yet Morrow's admirable performance could not erase the hostility created by earlier American diplomacy. To reformers south of the border American amity was colored by oil.

Europeans resented a different kind of diplomacy of the dollar. During the First World War the United States had lent the Allies $7 billion and after the war another $3.3 billion. The recipients had spent their loans almost entirely on American military products and relief supplies. With the return of peace, they regarded the loans merely as one part of the total Allied resistance to Germany, an American contribution toward a victory to which Europeans had given a larger share of flesh and blood. So they were reluctant to repay either the loans or the interest on them. And even those who wanted to square accounts found it difficult to pay. The European nations had depleted their own reserves before borrowing from the United States, and now they found it impossible to replenish those reserves in an American market sealed off by the tariff.

The only way they could meet their obligations to the United States was to draw on the huge reparations that had been imposed on Germany at Versailles. But Germany lacked both the means to pay and the will to scrimp in order to exonerate a war guilt it did not really accept. In 1923 it defaulted, and French and Belgian troops occupied the Ruhr Valley. The Germans there cut down coal production, while the German government inflated its currency recklessly, and the resulting economic distress in both France and Germany seemed to forebode economic collapse and possibly even armed conflict.

The crisis commanded American as well as European attention. Earlier, Charles Evans Hughes had suggested that an international commission of experts, including Americans, be appointed to examine the whole reparations problem. The deadlock in the Ruhr now persuaded the French to agree. The committees that then met recommended what was called the Dawes Plan, in recognition of the participation of Charles Gates Dawes, who was soon to become Coolidge's running mate. That plan, which went into effect in 1924, arranged for an international loan to stabilize German currency and for a flexible, graduated scale of reparations payments. Five years later another American, Owen D. Young, headed a second committee, which substantially reduced the payments. The Allies, satisfied by these terms and concurrent European political agreements, withdrew their forces from the Ruhr and the Rhineland.

American money, however, played a more significant role in the European crisis than did either Dawes or Young. Between 1924 and 1931 Germany managed to meet its payments only because its government, its municipalities, and its banks and businessmen were able to borrow $2.6 billion in the United States. Those funds, loaned by private American bankers, were indispensable for the postwar reconstruction of the European economy, especially in Germany. The American investors who lent the money were performing a function, with expectations of profits of course, that was indispensable for the postwar social and political stabilization of Europe. But the network of private debt among the western nations that the loans constructed depended for its stability on the American prosperity that made possible the availability of money for investment overseas, in Latin America as well as in Europe. Indeed, in the course of the decade there grew up a complex of private international debt, potentially unstable, that paralleled the structure of intergovernmental debts spawned by the Great War.

Only the reparations collected from Germany by the Allies enabled them to keep up their payments on their war debts to the United States government. The interdependence of debts and reparations payments was obvious, but the United States refused to acknowledge it. Most Americans, moreover, most of their congressmen, and certainly their President rejected the notion that the debts had in any sense been offset by the Allied losses in battle. For Coolidge, as for most of his constituents, the debts were business obligations pure and simple. When the French proposed that the burden of governmental debt be eased, the President unhesitatingly turned them down. "They hired the money," he said. The spirit behind that phrase overshadowed all the efforts of Dawes and Young.

Deluded diplomacy. The Administration resisted the facts of international politics as strongly as it resisted the facts of international economics. Like most Americans, Coolidge believed in disarmament, not only because he knew that it would reduce federal expense, but because he presumed that it would assure peace. But he did not understand, or at least would not admit, the continuing importance of power in international affairs.

Further, the conventional men in control of the army and the navy husbanded their meager appropriations and resisted spending anything on airplanes and submarines, even though those weapons had clearly made traditional military tactics and strategy obsolete. The failure to develop aircraft infuriated General William ("Billy") Mitchell of the Army Air Service, whose bombers had sunk a battleship in 1921. In an oracular report two years later, he warned the authorities of the vulnerability of battleships. In 1925, after the navy's sheer incompetence had resulted in the destruction of a dirigible, Mitchell attacked his superiors in public and urged the creation of a separate air command. A court-martial suspended him from duty for five years. The flurry over the episode persuaded Coolidge to appoint a civilian board of inquiry under Dwight Morrow, but it shrugged off Mitchell's arguments. The Administration denied public funds to promote commercial aviation as well. By 1929 the productive capacity of the American aircraft industry had fallen to seventy-five hundred planes a year, little more than a third of the capacity available at the war's end. In the absence of responsible public policy, the United States alone of the major powers slept smugly through the morning of the air age.

Coolidge was less complacent about international naval competition. The Five Power Treaty had applied only to capital ships, and the signatories had continued to build auxiliaries. Late in 1924 Congress authorized the construction of eight cruisers. Hoping to avoid the expense of further construction and to end the naval rivalry, the President invited the powers to a conference in 1927. Italy, already infected by Mussolini's fantasies of military glory, refused to attend. So did France, unhappy with the small ratio it had already received at Washington and reluctant, in the face of Italian resurgence, to commit itself to further self-restraint. Coolidge, dedicated to a policy of isolation from European affairs, had failed to assess these obstacles to disarmament, always a difficult international objective. He failed also to negotiate a preliminary understanding with the British. As a consequence, the English-speaking delegates at the 1927 conference wrangled to no purpose, while the Japanese stood contentedly aside.

Coolidge had already retreated from an earlier, cautious gesture toward internationalism. The Permanent Court of International Justice called for by the League of Nations Covenant had been established in 1921. The purpose of this World Court was to adjudicate certain types of case, to render advice whenever the League requested it, and to arbitrate cases brought before it. Americans had long hoped for the development of a body of law that could be applied to international affairs, and in 1923 Harding, influenced by Hughes, recommended conditional American adherence to the court. Coolidge made the same recommendation in his first annual message. But, even though Hughes had drafted four reservations to the court's protocol to protect the United States from contact with the League itself, the isolationists in the Senate balked. After a long delay the Senate adopted a fifth reservation that would limit the court's right even to render advisory opinions to the League. Further, the court could give no opinion, without American consent, on any question in which the United States claimed an interest. In 1926 the Senate finally voted adherence to the court on those conditions. When the members of the court then tried to clarify the meaning of the reservations, Coolidge declared that clarification constituted rejection and that there was no prospect of American adherence to the court.* That denouement, followed by the failure of the naval-armaments conference, left the Administration's diplomatic record singularly barren.

During his last months in office, however, Coolidge's diplomacy won wide acclaim. Salmon O. Levinson, a Chicago lawyer, had been recommending that the great powers sign an agreement condemning war. Professor James T. Shotwell, who had been advancing the same suggestion independently, also proposed sanctions to enforce such an agreement. The idea of outlawing war caught the attention of many Americans, including William E. Borah, chairman of the Senate Committee on Foreign Relations. Shotwell urged it upon Aristide Briand, the French foreign minister, who promptly used it for his own purposes. In April 1927, in a gesture of good will to compensate for Franco-American friction over disarmament and war debts, Briand wrote an address to the American people in which he proposed a pact outlawing war. Coolidge was irritated by Briand's resorting to irregular channels to announce his scheme, but the popular enthusiasm for the proposal forced the President's hand. The State Department asked Briand to submit his plan formally.

Secretary of State Frank B. Kellogg now outflanked Briand. Intent on avoiding a bilateral agreement that would imply some sort of alliance between the United States and France, Kellogg recommended instead "an effort to obtain the adherence of all the principal powers of the world to a declaration renouncing war as an instrument of national policy." While Briand stalled, the Secretary of State circulated the draft of a declaration he had drawn up on his own. He also let it be known that the United States would consent to sign the pact in Paris. Briand then accepted the American scheme, and in August 1928 fifteen nations meeting in Paris endorsed a treaty by which they renounced war and promised to settle all disputes, whatever their nature, by "pacific means."

Americans were jubilant over the banishment of war—so jubilant that they tended to ignore qualifications made in diplomatic notes exchanged by the signatories. These set down reservations safeguarding France's interpretations of its own self-defense and Great Britain's obligations to its empire. In recommending ratification of the pact, the Senate Foreign Relations Committee reported that ratification would not, in its view, curtail the right of the United States to self-defense and to its own interpretations of the Monroe Doctrine, nor would ratification oblige the United States to take any action against a violator of the Kellogg-Briand pact. So interpreted, the pact won approval by a vote of eighty-five to one. But so interpreted, it was, in the words of Senator Carter Glass of Virginia, "worthless, but perfectly harmless."

For most Americans the Paris pact constituted a triumph. To declare perpetual peace without assuming the responsibility for preserving it suited the nation's mood. Now the nation could cut its expenditures, disarm, collect its debts, and trust to reassuring words for sunny safety. Yet the hocus-pocus that sold peace in multilingual print was not unlike the hocus-pocus that sold beauty in a bottle.

Get rich quick. Of all the grandiose illusions of the 1920s none was more beguiling than the prospect of easy riches. It rested on the simple faith that the value

---

*Both Hoover and Franklin Roosevelt later recommended adherence to the court on terms like those contemplated by Hughes. But the Senate declined.

of property would constantly increase, and that the investor who bought today could sell tomorrow at a handsome profit. Those who had property to sell nourished this faith, and they were helped by the ready credit that enabled speculators to borrow what they needed. The hucksters and the boomers, moreover, made the allure of speculation a favorite fantasy of the time.

For a while in the mid-twenties the quest for a bonanza drew thousands of Americans to ventures in Florida real estate. The population of Miami more than doubled between 1920 and 1925, and other Florida cities and resorts along the Atlantic and Gulf coasts also mushroomed. Florida's boomers pointed to the warm winter climate, the ready accessibility of their region to vacationers from the North, the prospect of an American Riviera. Imagination covered swamps and barren sands with towns and building lots. As the greedy rushed to buy the dream, a few who invested early and sold at the peak of the boom made fortunes. Their success lured others. Most of the transactions took the form of binders—agreements to buy property, which could be had for a fraction of the value of the property itself. The binders could be sold and sold again, each time for more money.

For every sale, of course, there had to be a buyer. The trade in binders was profitable only so long as someone came along to bid them up, and once people began to compare the dream with the reality the buyers were bound to disappear. The balloon began to deflate in the spring and summer of 1926. That fall it burst when a hurricane swept through the Miami area, destroying developments that had emerged from the dream stage, and wrecking the railroad to Key West. The grand plans of the boomers were laid away; the millions of dollars in speculative profits were wiped out; and the Florida craze was over.

But a much larger boom was already under way. During the prosperous twenties most of the gains from increased productivity and from the growing market for manufactured goods were funneled into corporate profits. And as profits rose, enhanced by Mellon's tax favors to business, so did the value of corporate shares. Initially that rise reflected a genuine increase in the worth of corporate properties and in the earning potential of the corporations themselves. In the mid-twenties, however, the price of stocks began to soar at a dizzying pace. Investors who were looking for securities that would give them a reasonably safe return now had to compete with speculators who were after overnight fortunes. To meet the demand for stocks, promoters organized investment trusts and multitiered holding companies whose only assets were hope and good will. They offered their new issues to eager buyers deluded by greed and by a naive confidence in the surging market. In 1923 new

capital issues totaled $3.2 billion; in 1927, $10 billion, much of it purely speculative. The volume of sales on the New York Stock Exchange leaped from 236 million shares in 1923 to 577 million in 1927 and to 1,125 million a year later.

Corporations themselves speculated. As the market rose, corporations found that they earned less by investing their reserves in new facilities than by putting them into brokers' loans—that is, loans that brokers made to their customers to enable them to gamble far beyond their cash resources. In "buying on margin," as this practice was called, customers relied on brokers' loans to cover most of the cost of their stock purchases. Brokers and customers alike expected that the growing value of the stocks would make it easy enough to repay the loans. Meeting the pressing demand for brokers' loans, or "call money," corporations emptied their surpluses into the money market, where they received staggering returns.

Instead of tempering the boom, public officials encouraged it. The Federal Reserve System had means to tighten credit—that is, to make loans more expensive. But it chose to use its power to keep interest rates low. It did so in order to discourage the import of gold from Europe, and thus to protect the value of European currency and also to facilitate American loans to Europe, then still in need of investment funds for economic rehabilitation and development. (If interest rates had gone way up, Europeans and Americans would both have tended to invest more of their money within the United States.) Even if the Federal Reserve had tightened credit, however, it could not have controlled the call-money market that the corporations were feeding, for speculators were willing to borrow at usurious rates to finance their march to riches.

In the absence of federal authority over either credit or the chicanery of promoters, the best weapon available to the government was simple candor. There was, however, none of that. Secretary of the Treasury Mellon knew exactly what was going on; indeed, he was himself deep in speculation. Yet whenever sober businessmen questioned the state of the market, he or his colleagues in the Administration invariably responded with soothing reassurances. And Coolidge went along. Early in 1927 William Z. Ripley, a Harvard economist, lectured the President on the prevalent "double-shuffling, honey-fuggling, hornswoggling and skulduggery." Coolidge, feet on desk and cigar in teeth, asked gloomily: "Is there anything we can do down here?" Ripley answered that the regulation of securities was the responsibility of the states, not of the federal government. Relieved, the President relaxed and put the incident out of his mind.

By the end of the year brokers' loans had reached nearly $4 billion. In January 1928 Coolidge reassured the dubious few by announcing that this volume of

It was lost ... because it was uprooted, schooled away and almost wrenched away from its attachment to any region or tradition. It was lost because its training had prepared it for another world than existed after the war (and because the war prepared it only for travel and excitement). It was lost because it tried to live in exile. It was lost because it accepted no older guides to conduct and because it had formed a false picture of society and the writer's place in it. The generation belonged to a period of transition from values already fixed to values that had to be created. Its members ... were seceding from the old and yet could adhere to nothing new; they groped their way toward another scheme of life, as yet undefined; in the midst of their doubts and uneasy gestures of defiance they felt homesick for the certainties of childhood.

From Malcolm Cowley, *Exile's Return*, 1951 ed.

loans was perfectly natural. Shortly thereafter Roy Young of the Federal Reserve Board, a close friend of Herbert Hoover, told a congressional committee that the loans were "safely and conservatively made." Those sanctions hastened the tempo of the boom and gave a Midas touch to 1928, an election year.

To Coolidge the ascending figures on the ticker tape were evidence of the nation's prosperity and of his own sagacity. He was as much honey-fuggled as hornswoggling. Like the brokers and speculators, he was at once the prisoner and the propagator of the grandiose myths that bemused the nation.

Nonconformity and Dissent

The Jazz Age. Some Americans, however, were repelled by materialism and its delusions. Disappointed by a progressive faith that seemed to have failed, they were alienated by the emptiness of business civilization. Some few thousands sought a solution in communism, but all kinds of radicalism recovered only slowly from the postwar repression, and the American communists during the 1920s spent their zeal in factionalism and debate. Most of the disenchanted were equally cynical about serving society and about striving for worldly success. Finding only futility in the past and the future, they chose to seek out the pleasures of the present, to live for their private selves and for immediate self-expression.

Those men and women, many of them young, were no more immoral or promiscuous than men and women had been before. But they dropped pretense. They revealed their impatience with traditional standards of conduct openly and often. One symbol of their protest was jazz, a serious idiom that owed its development to American musicians—particularly black

musicians. Other American artists, notably Martha Graham, contributed to the formative period of modern dance.

Jazz had other connotations, too—with its sensuality, its spontaneity, its atavistic rhythms, and with

Martha Graham

the sinuous and intimate dancing it inspired. Jazz was ungenteel, even un-Caucasian, above all uninhibited. It expressed not only protest and art of a kind but a controversial change in sexual mores.

That change sprang largely from the ways in which city living altered family life. The nuclear family of the city and suburb (man, wife, children) existed in a private world quite different from that of the kinship family of the country or of the immigrant community, where grandparents, aunts, uncles, and cousins provided support and where community was more common than aloneness. The very impersonality of middle-class life in the city obliged its inhabitants to meet and resolve the problems of their lives with neither help nor impediment. Not every marriage was equal to the challenge.

Increasingly, women demanded easier and more equitable divorces, and they struggled for equal rights to jobs, to income, to their own apartments, to cigarettes, to whiskey, and to sexual satisfaction in matrimony or sometimes outside it. Much of the energy of feminism concentrated on the birth control movement. That movement, so Margaret Sanger claimed, freed the mind from "sexual prejudice and taboo." Not the least of its functions was to increase the quantity and quality of sexual relationships. The incidence of premarital and extramarital sexual experience also rose, as it had been rising for two decades. To some extent, especially for young people, adventures in sex released part of a rebellion against the reigning culture and its neopuritanical code.

During the twenties, moreover, even the unrebellious were learning to understand the significance of sex in human nature. The most important contributions to that understanding were made by Sigmund Freud, whose doctrines had first reached America in the years before the war. After the war Freudian psychology rapidly became a national fad, ordinarily in vastly simplified and distorted forms. Freud himself,

while demonstrating that neurotic symptoms and behavior could usually be attributed to sexual origins, did not advocate promiscuity. His first concern was with creating a system of analysis that would enable doctors to help patients find the emotional sources of their disorders, behavioral or somatic. On the basis of that discovery sick people could then reconstruct their lives. His popularizers, however, often interpreted his works as a rationale for sexual freedom. The average American met Freudian ideas only in that sense.

A literature of alienation. "Society was something alien," Malcolm Cowley wrote about himself and his literary contemporaries of the 1920s. "It was a sort of parlor car in which we rode, over smooth tracks, toward a destination we should never have chosen for ourselves." Gertrude Stein called the young writers of the time "a lost generation." Those she referred to turned their backs on progress, on economics, on Main Street, and on Wall Street. "It was characteristic of the Jazz Age," said novelist F. Scott Fitzgerald, one of its high priests, "that it had no interest in politics at all." And the editor of *The Smart Set*, H. L. Mencken, wrote: "If I am convinced of anything, it is that Doing Good is in bad taste."

These men and their fellows detested the business culture. Many of them fled, some to Paris, others to Greenwich Village, still others to an impenetrable privacy of creativity. And they attacked the civilization they had left. Sinclair Lewis peopled the Middle West with confused men and women, trapped by their own futile materialism and unthinking gentility, narrow, unhappy, stifled. Lewis' *Main Street* (1920) and *Babbit* (1922) created satirical symbols of American life that persisted for a quarter of a century, not in the United States alone, but in Europe as well.

Sherwood Anderson exercised a large influence

Fitzgerald: novelist of the Jazz Age

tween self and society and the exacerbation of those tensions in the culture of the Deep South. Eliot's "The Love Song of J. Alfred Prufrock" (written in 1911, published six years later) made impotence the weary symbol of modern man. His *The Waste Land* (1922), probably the most emulated poem of the decade, provided a text in fragmentation and despair.

All these works revealed alienation and spoke of protest, but their authors were first, and most self-consciously, artists. So, too, were the other Americans who shared in the extraordinary literary renaissance of the period. They included an impressive number of talented black artists and authors, among them James Weldon Johnson, Countee Cullen, and Langston Hughes. Though some of the prose and poetry of the "Harlem Renaissance" repudiated black themes, much of it borrowed self-consciously from black culture, and the best of it, like the poetry of Hughes, ranked with the best work of white Americans.

The great outburst of artistic creativity had begun before 1920; it continued beyond 1929; but it came to a crescendo during the Coolidge era. In that time, the arts made a far more enduring mark on the nation than did politics. But the religion of art, then so prevalent, could be as futile as materialism itself. Alienation ordinarily denied social responsibility. The artists who rejected their national culture also accepted most of its claims. They turned away from the Coolidge era not because of its inequities but because of its superficial accomplishments. In contrast to the progressive intellectuals who had preceded them, they sought private escapes and private satisfactions, and they surrendered society to its shortsighted masters. This escapism deprived the nation of the assistance of many of its most imaginative minds.

Worse still, some Americans cast off democracy along with materialism. They agreed with the Mellons and the Fords and the Coolidges who believed that the business cult was the democratic ideal. They concluded that democracy necessarily generated a vulgar, selfish, pecuniary civilization. The critic Van Wyck Brooks, in his *The Ordeal of Mark Twain* (1920), wrote about the Gilded Age, with the twenties much in mind, as "a horde-life, a herd-life, an epoch without sun and stars," which condemned the artist, and the soul, to frustration. Eliot also scorned democracy and remained rootless until he found salvation in the church, as Brooks did in sentimentality. H. L. Mencken was more acid. He ridiculed not only Prohibition, the Ku Klux Klan, and censorship, but the whole American people, whom he considered a sodden, brutish, ignorant mob. Democracy, for him, was government by orgy. As for democracy as a theory, "all the known facts lie flatly against it." Irving Bab-

on his literary compatriots. A compassionate critic of small-town America, Anderson abandoned a business career, after a nervous breakdown in 1912 to devote himself to writing. His *Winesburg, Ohio* (1919) was a moving, autobiographical novel of alienation. Perhaps more important, he exemplified the religion of art, for he had escaped Babylon and had succeeded in his career of the spirit.

Seeking in art a distillation of experience, the young masters experimenting with literary form gave a new beauty and vitality to American letters. Encouraged particularly by Ezra Pound and Gertrude Stein and inspired by their prewar poetry, the novelists Ernest Hemingway and William Faulkner and the poet T. S. Eliot raised the national literary reputation to its all-time zenith. Hemingway's *The Sun Also Rises* (1926) and *A Farewell to Arms* (1929) expressed a deep revulsion against nineteenth-century standards of conduct and idealizations of war. In *The Sound and the Fury* (1929) Faulkner used Freudian insights and adventurous prose to expose the awful tensions bebitt, who formulated an aristocratic doctrine of the "inner check," had no patience with the "sickly sentimentalizing of the lot of the underdog," no confidence in social reform, no hope except in pseudo-Platonic comforts, and thus no real hope. The price of complacent materialism was alienation; and the bill of despair that went with alienation was ominously high.

Progressive hopes and failures. Yet disenchantment did not lead all critics to alienation. Some drew on the legacy of progressivism and on their own undaunted spirit to point out anew the paths toward a good society. John Dewey (see p. 557) continued to examine the practical consequences of social policies in *Human Nature and Conduct* (1922) and *Individualism Old and New* (1929). These books urged experimentation in education for selfless citizenship, and public rather than private planning for social rather than pecuniary goals. Charles Beard in his *The Rise of American Civilization* (1927) stressed optimistically the historical significance of economic change. A year later he called for social engineering, national planning, to organize advancing science and technology for the general good. John R. Commons (see p. 557) worked out theories and techniques for social insurance, and among his fellow economists Irving Fisher showed that the government had to manage the nation's money supply if it was to achieve desirable social and economic ends. William T. Foster and Waddill Catchings advanced even more novel ideas. They attacked the beliefs that savings flowed automatically into investment and that business cycles righted themselves. If the nation was to avoid depressions,

they insisted, government would have to resort to public spending when private investment faltered.

In public life, too, the progressive faith persevered, though it suffered major setbacks. Militant feminists, by no means satisfied with suffrage, now worked through the Women's party for the goal of total equality with men, a goal to be achieved through the proposed equal rights amendment to which Congress had yet to give serious consideration. Indeed, the militants lost influence during the decade after 1919. The League of Women Voters, however, a growing organization almost wholly of middle-class membership, reached a broader constituency in its efforts to educate the electorate about reform issues familiar to prewar progressives, including the protection of working women. But the League won no important legislative victories, partly because women, who did not vote in a bloc, shared the indifference to politics or the conservative bias of most men of the time.

So it was that in 1926, when Mellon again advocated tax relief for the rich, his dwindling opponents could find no telling argument against cutting taxes. Federal revenues were then more than ample for the costs of government, and no one had yet developed a cogent program for spending to improve the nation's housing, roads, and natural resources. Without difficulty, the Administration put through Congress a revenue act that cut in half the estate tax and the maximum surtax on individual incomes. Two years later Congress eased the tax on corporations. Mellon had carried the field.

Private utility companies were almost as successful. Sales of electric power doubled during the twenties, and ingenious promoters with very little cash managed to monopolize the industry by setting up complex holding companies. By the end of the decade ten utility systems controlled approximately three-fourths of the nation's light and power business. The promoters kept the cost of electricity unreasonably high and through financial sleight of hand manipulated securities at the expense of bewildered stockholders. They also carried on a massive propaganda campaign and financed a powerful lobby to beat back demands for public supervision and for public distribution of electrical power.

The reformers, led by George Norris, included Governor Smith of New York and his successor, Franklin Roosevelt, who advocated state ownership and operation of public power. Gifford Pinchot, governor of Pennsylvania, organized a survey in 1923 that paved the way to public rural electrification. Many municipalities built or acquired their own power plants, and Nebraska, Norris' home state, established a public power system.

Farm politics particularly exercised Washington during Coolidge's second term, when farmers stepped up their demands for a government marketing plan. Such a plan had first been suggested in the lean years right after the war. Now it became the basis for legislation sponsored by Senator Charles L. McNary of Oregon and Representative Gilbert N. Haugen of Iowa. At the heart of the proposal was a two-price scheme—a high domestic price and a low foreign price for staple crops. By purchasing farm surpluses, the government was to sustain a balance of supply and demand that would keep commodity prices at "parity" (see p. 678). In that manner the government would be underwriting the prosperity of the American farmers. The government would sell farm surpluses abroad for whatever price it could get, and any loss would be offset by an equalization tax levied on farmers or on those who processed and transported farm products.

Congress rejected the McNary-Haugen bill in 1924. But it passed a revised measure in 1927 and another one in 1928. Coolidge vetoed both versions. The bill, he said, would create a vast and clumsy bureaucracy, would improperly delegate taxing power from Congress to the administrators of the program, and would involve the government in trying to fix prices. Such prices, he argued, would be artificial and would encourage farmers to overproduce. Moreover, if the American government began to dump farm surpluses abroad, foreign governments would be bound to retaliate. The last two objections were undoubtedly sound, but Coolidge's concern for minimized government and a laissez-faire economy was unconvincing. After all, the government used the tariff, which was simply one kind of taxation, to aid industry. And the tariff, combined with the market-

ing practices of big business, led to artificial prices for manufactured goods. Those very prices kept farmers' costs high while their incomes lagged. Coolidge's vetoes, as the economist Rexford G. Tugwell put it, revealed "a stubborn determination to do nothing."

The debate over farm policy, like the debate over public power and taxation, highlighted the policy issue that dominated the late twenties: Was the federal government to be the handmaiden of business, the servant of the wealthy? Or was the government to build an equitable society in which all could obtain a fair share of the nation's wealth? Intellectuals like Dewey and Commons and politicians like Norris and Smith insisted on the second alternative. They were insisting that Americans, both in their private lives and in their conduct of public affairs, accept a responsibility that the spirit of the times rejected.

The election of 1928. Calvin Coolidge announced that he "did not choose to run" in 1928. He might have been persuaded to accept a draft, but the Republican convention nominated Herbert Hoover on its first ballot. Professional politicians had little liking for Hoover, who was never one of them, and Midwestern farmers had little enthusiasm for a man who had opposed the McNary-Haugen bill precisely as Coolidge had. But businessmen trusted Hoover; his reputation for efficiency and humaneness was at its peak; and his personal success more than compensated for his lack of public glamour.

Hoover stood stolidly on a platform that attributed good times to Republican rule, praised the protective tariff, endorsed Prohibition, offered only platitudes to labor, and warned farmers of the evil of "putting the government into business." In his campaign speeches Hoover emphasized the virtues of individualism and "the American system" of free enterprise. There lay the source of prosperity. "We in America," Hoover said, "are nearer to the final triumph over poverty than ever before in the history of any land. . . . Given a chance to go forward with the policies of the last eight years, we shall soon with the help of God be in the sight of the day when poverty will be banished from this nation."

The Democrats nominated Al Smith. Those who had kept the nomination from him in 1924 could no longer deny his claims. As governor of New York he had made a record for efficiency as compelling as Hoover's. He had reordered the state's finances and reorganized its administration. He had promoted public health and public recreation, workmen's compensation, and civil liberties. As a national candidate, Smith stood for public ownership of the principal power sites and generating plants, and he endorsed the McNary-Haugen Plan.

"Socialism," Hoover retorted. But Smith was no radical. Indeed, he, too, deferred to the temper of the time. He accepted the need for protective tariffs. He chose as his campaign-manager John J. Raskob, a Republican industrialist, identified with Du Pont and General Motors. The Democratic campaign may have reassured the conservatives, but it converted almost none of them, and it disappointed the liberals.

Raskob's appointment, furthermore, reopened the party wounds of 1924, for, like Smith, Raskob was a Catholic and a "wet." Rural America dug out its old suspicions of the city, booze, Tammany, and the pope. Particularly in the South, fundamentalist preachers associated Smith with all the old fears and hates. Smith explained that his religion had not and would not affect his policies, and his record confirmed his words. But the suspicious took their cue instead from his East Side accent, his brown derby, his open advocacy of repeal, his unabashed cityness. Hoover, for his part, made no convincing effort to dispel the religious issue.

As much as bigotry, prosperity defeated Smith, who could not counter Republican claims to credit for "the new era." He received only 87 electoral votes to Hoover's 444; some 41 percent of the popular vote to Hoover's 58. Five Southern states and all the border states went Republican. The Grand Old Party had won another landslide.

The returns, however, were not that unambiguous. Smith carried the dozen largest cities, which the Republicans had won handily four years before. The Democrats also cut into the traditionally Republican agricultural vote in the West. The farmers had doubts about prosperity, and in the cities the ethnic issue cut both ways, helping the Democrats in the urban North as much as it hurt them in the rural South. In 1928, as in 1924, the vote suggested the emergence of a new party balance and dramatized the need for Democratic unity and for a positive commitment to social reconstruction. But the prospects seemed poor, for the Coolidge era ended much as it had begun. Prejudice had divided the underprivileged, and prosperity had obscured public irresponsibility. Most Americans, as they had shown at the polls, were remarkably content. And confident, too. The stock market boomed as it awaited Hoover's inauguration and the nation's final triumph over poverty.

Suggestions for Reading

GENERAL

The outstanding general accounts of the Coolidge years and their implications are in A. M. Schlesinger, Jr., *The Crisis of the Old Order** (1957); W. E. Leuchtenburg, *The Perils of Prosperity, 1914–32** (1958); and John Braeman, ed., *Change and Continuity in 20th Century America: The 1920's* (1968). F. L. Allen, *Only Yesterday** (1931), has charm and flair; and J. D. Hicks, *Republican Ascendancy: 1921–1933* (1960), is sober. See, too, E. Hawley, *The Great War and the Search for a Modern Order** (1979). The most entertaining biography of Coolidge is W. A. White, *A Puritan in Babylon* (1938); but see also Donald McCoy, *Calvin Coolidge* (1967). Coolidge speaks often but rarely well in H. H. Quint and R. H. Ferrell, eds., *The Talkative President: The Off-the-Record Press Conferences of Calvin Coolidge* (1964). Still important is R. and H. L. Lynd, *Middletown** (1929).

BUSINESS ENTERPRISE

The economics of prosperity are described in George Soule, *Prosperity Decade: From War to Depression, 1917–1929** (1947); the institutions of business, in A. D. Chandler, Jr., *Strategy and Structure** (1962) and *The Visible Hand** (1977), and T. C. Cochran, *The American Business System: A Historical Perspective, 1900–1955* (2nd ed., 1957); the business creed, in J. W. Prothro, *The Dollar Decade: Business Ideas in the 1920's* (1954); and the techniques of advertising, in Otis Pease, *The Responsibilities of American Advertising* (1958). On the Ford Motor Company, its master, and the automobile industry in general, the preeminent works are Allan Nevins and F. E. Hill, *Ford: The Times, the Man and the Company* (1954) and *Ford: Expansion and Challenge* (1957). There is also an acid analysis in Keith Sward, *The Legend of Henry Ford** (1948). See, too, John Rae, *The Road and Car in American Life* (1971). The best introduction to F. W. Taylor is his own *The Principles of Scientific Management** (1907). Siegfried Giedion, *Mechanization Takes Command: A Contribution to Anonymous History** (1948), offers brilliant observations about technology, which is handled on a more elementary level in Stuart Chase, *Men and Machines* (1929). By far the fullest and best account of labor during the 1920s is in Irving Bernstein, *The Lean Years** (1960). See also Robert Zieger, *Republicans and Labor, 1915–1929* (1969). Two studies of the first rank on corporate concentration and on the business cycle, respectively, are A. A. Berle, Jr., and G. F. Means, *The Modern Corporation and Private Property* (1932, rev. ed., 1969), and Thomas Wilson, *Fluctuations in Income and Employment* (1948). E. A. Goldenweiser, *American Monetary Policy* (1951), deals expertly with its subject, as does J. Potter, *The American Economy Between the Wars* (1974).

IDEALS AND IDEOLOGIES

The works mentioned in the text, and other works of the authors noted there, provide a good point of departure for studying the artists and intellectuals of the 1920s. For that purpose, Malcolm Cowley, *Exile's Return** (1934), is rewarding; and so are Alfred Kazin, *On Native Grounds** (1942), and Edmund Wilson, *The Shores of Light** (1952) and *The American Earthquake** (1958). The outstanding anthology of the social and cultural expressions of the time is L. Baritz, *The Culture of the Twenties** (1969). There are useful interpretations in R. Nash, *The Nervous Generation* (1969), and R. Crunden, *From Self to Society* (1972). On black artists, see N. Huggins, *Harlem Renaissance** (1971), and E. Levy, *James Weldon Johnson** (1973). Among the helpful literary studies are Mark Schorer, *Sinclair Lewis** (1961); Grover Smith, Jr., *T. S. Eliot's Poetry and Plays: A Study in Sources and Meaning** (1956); Cleanth Brooks, *William Faulkner: The Yoknapatawpha Country** (1963); and H. D. Piper, *F. Scott Fitzgerald: A Critical Portrait* (1965). See also C. A. Fenton, *The Apprenticeship of Ernest Hemingway* (1954), and C. H. Baker, *Hemingway: The Writer As Artist** (1956). American anti-intellectuals and bigots receive their just rewards in N. F. Furniss, *The Fundamentalist Controversy 1918–1931* (1954); Don Kirschner, *City and Country: Rural Responses to Urbanization in the 1920's* (1970); Ray Ginger, *Six Days or Forever?** (1958), on the Scopes trial; J. M. Mecklin, *The Ku Klux Klan* (1924); and D. M. Chalmers, *Hooded Americanism** (1965). More sympathetic is W. B. Gatewood, Jr., ed., *Controversy in the Twenties* (1969). Among the engaging works on the ideology and politics of Prohibition, and on the crime it helped to spawn, are Andrew Sinclair, *Prohibition: The Era of Excess* (1962) and Herbert Asbury, *The Great Illusion* (1950). The case for Prohibition emerges in N. H. Clark, *Deliver Me From Evil** (1976). On women during the 1920s, see William Chafe, *The American Woman: Her Changing Social, Economic, and Political Roles, 1920–1960** (1972); J. S. Lemons, *The Woman Citizen: Social Feminism in the 1920's** (1973); and Lois Banner, *Women in Modern America** (1974).

PUBLIC ISSUES AND PUBLIC MEN

Two important accounts of major federal public policies in the period 1923–29 are in the pertinent parts of R. E. Paul, *Taxation in the United States* (1954), and Theodore Saloutos and J. D. Hicks, *Twentieth Century Populism: Agricultural Discontent in the Middle West, 1900–1939* (1951). Agricultural matters also receive useful treatment in J. D. Black, *Agricultural Reform in the United States* (1930), and M. R. Benedict, *Farm Policies of the United States, 1790–1950* (1953). On the campaign of 1924, there are telling studies in K. C. MacKay, *The Progressive Movement of 1924* (1947); E. A. Moore, *A Catholic Runs for President* (1956); and A. J. Lichtman, *Prejudice and the Old Politics* (1979). O. Handlin, *Al Smith and His America** (1958), is short and thoughtful, while M. and H. Josephson, *Al Smith: Hero of the Cities* (1969), is laudatory. For electoral trends, see D. Burner, *The*

Politics of Provincialism (1968). Among the autobiographies and biographies of other public men of the time, some of the more rewarding are B. C. and F. La Follette, *Robert M. La Follette*, 2 vols. (1953); F. Freidel, *Franklin D. Roosevelt: The Ordeal* (1954); A. Mann, *La Guardia: A Fighter Against His Times, 1882–1933** (1959); L. Levine's sympathetic study of Bryan, *Defender of the Faith* (1968); R. Lowitt, *George W. Norris: The Persistence of a Progressive* (1971); W. Harbaugh, *Lawyer's Lawyer: The Life of John W. Davis** (1973); Herbert Hoover, *Memoirs*, 3 vols. (1951–52); D. Burner, *Herbert Hoover** (1978); E. E. Morison, *Turmoil and Tradition: A Study of the Life and Times of Henry L. Stimson* (1960); and H. L. Stimson and M. Bundy, *On Active Service in Peace and War* (1948). The last two shed significant light on the foreign policy of the Coolidge years, on which R. H. Ferrell, *Peace in Their Time** (1952), J. H. Wilson, *American Business and Foreign Policy, 1920–1933** (1971); M. P. Jeffler, *The Elusive Quest: The U.S. and French Security* (1979); and C. S. Maier, *Recasting Bourgeoise Europe** (1975) are also useful.

*Available in a paperback edition.

26
THE END OF AN ERA

The United States met the new year of 1929 with a smile and a swagger. The national habit of confidence had grown during three decades in which both the reformers of the early century and the managers of the new age of business believed they were fashioning a national Eden. A college graduate of the class of 1901, fifty years old in 1929, could believe with them that they had succeeded. As evidence of success, he might point to the statutes left over from progressivism, the great war won, the apparent unlikelihood of future war, the excitement of new inventions, and the largess of good times. Not since the mid-nineties, not for a generation, had the nation suffered a serious depression.

President Hoover

Business plans. "I have no fears for the future of our country," the new President announced at his inauguration. "It is bright with hope." There was no nonsense about Hoover, none of T. R.'s boyishness or Wilson's dreaminess, none of Harding's incontinence or Coolidge's folksiness. The President was a serious man who kept in shape by playing medicine ball in the early morning. He would, most people thought, keep the nation in shape and lead it to ever higher plateaus of prosperity.

Hoover approached his office like a businessman with a business plan. He reorganized the inefficient presidential staff by creating a secretariat in which each member was assigned a specific place and duty. Government was to be neat. It was also to be respectable. Hoover appointed a Cabinet of men who stood for what the business community admired. Mellon continued as Secretary of the Treasury. The others, with one exception, were undistinguished. The exception was Secretary of State Henry L. Stimson, a conservative whose superior perceptions soon made him as uncomfortable as he was valuable.

Always active in pursuit of his own beliefs, Hoover, according to the solicitor of the Federal Power Commission, interceded to prevent private companies from being regulated rigorously. The President also proposed that the federal government withdraw its control from all public lands and from all new reclamation and irrigation projects. The states, he said, were "more competent to manage . . . these affairs." That was a debatable assertion, but it suited Hoover's purpose. In conservation, as in most other matters, he was determined to keep federal government small in both size and power.

Hoover's farm program reflected that determination. Still, he recognized the need for some aid to agriculture, and he summoned a special session of Congress to provide it. The President suggested that the best way to help American farmers would be to raise the tariff and to give them federal assistance in

Bread line, Christmas, 1931

marketing their produce—policies that would not, he said, undermine the farmers' initiative. In the Agricultural Marketing Act of 1929, Congress acted on Hoover's suggestions. It created a Federal Farm Board that was to be advised by committees representing the cooperative associations that marketed each of the major commodities. It also provided a revolving fund of $500 million from which the board could make loans to cooperatives to help them market their crops more effectively. Another provision, inserted by the farm bloc, permitted loans to be made to stabilization corporations "for the purpose of controlling any surplus." In other words, these corporations could influence prices so long as the Farm Board lent them enough money. But the Farm Board had no control over production. Consequently, not even generous loans for stabilization could long sustain prices if they should begin a major decline in the face either of gross overproduction or of adverse general economic circumstances. From the first, farmers were dissatisfied with the legislation of 1929.

They gained nothing at all from Hoover's proposal to give them more tariff protection. The President lacked the political skill to guide a tariff bill through Congress. In 1929 Congress put the matter aside. In 1930 industrial lobbyists and their friends in the Republican majority carried protection to its all-time high. The Hawley-Smoot Tariff of that year raised average *ad valorem* rates from about 32 percent to about 40 percent. It increased rates on some seventy farm products and over nine hundred manufactured goods. More than a thousand economists urged Hoover to veto the bill. It would, they pointed out, raise the cost of living, encourage inefficient production, hamper American export trade, including trade in agricultural surpluses, and provoke foreign bitterness and retaliation. Though those arguments were entirely correct, Hoover signed the measure. It reflected the continuing influence of business interests in Washington and their continuing shortsightedness.

The crash. Dramatic evidence of that shortsightedness had already appeared in the stock market, the barometer of prosperity. It soared during the early months of 1929, but unbridled speculation began to worry conservative financiers and the President too. He privately urged the New York Stock Exchange to curb the manipulation of securities, but with no success. Hoover would not ask Congress to interfere, for he "had no desire to stretch the powers of the Federal Government" that far. Instead he supported the Federal Reserve Board when it warned banks against making loans for speculative purposes, and he approved the board's 1 percent increase in the interest rate first in June and again in August 1929. But the

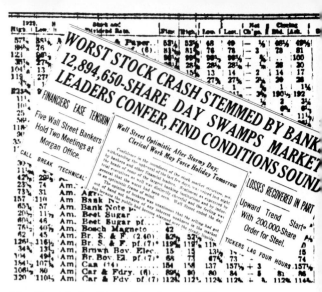

The *New York Times*: October 25, 1929

higher cost of funds for speculation did not check the speculative fever.

Gamblers in stocks paid no heed to other warnings. The first signs of danger began to appear during the summer of 1929. Residential construction, important for the many industries that supplied its needs throughout the nation, fell off more than a billion dollars; business inventories trebled; the rate of advance in consumer spending dropped some 400 percent. From June onward, industrial production, employment, and commodity prices declined steadily. Indeed, the August increase in the interest rate came at a time when legitimate enterprise could ill afford it.

Yet the stock market boomed on. Ignoring the evidence of industrial decline, undeterred by the advancing costs of brokers' loans, speculators bid shares to new peaks. The morning after Labor Day the New York *Times* average of selected industrial stocks stood at 452, up more than 200 points since early 1928. The market seemed strong, but it was sustained only by deluded confidence. In one week brokers' loans had risen $137 million, and New York banks had borrowed $64 million to carry the weight of speculation.

During September and most of October the market wavered, moving gently downward. Some days were worrisome, but none of the captains of finance in New York or their lieutenants in Washington voiced alarm. Then on October 24 security prices crumbled in a wave of frenzied selling. Panic was temporarily averted when a group of New York bankers met next morning at J. P. Morgan and Company and agreed to pool their resources to hold the market up. The senior Morgan partner assured reporters that the heavy selling had been "due to a technical condition," not to any basic cause. The following day President Hoover announced that "the fundamental business of the country . . . is on a sound and prosperous basis."

They were wrong. During the next fortnight the market shuddered to collapse. As values fell, all the bets made on a rising market paid off in panic. An uncontrollable decline swept past the support the bankers had organized. By mid-November the New York *Times* average had fallen to a shattering 224. In less than a month the securities listed on the New York Stock Exchange lost $26 billion—more than 40 percent—of their face value. Nor was the descent over. In July 1932 the *Times* average hit bottom at a mere 58.

Contrary to Hoover's assertion, the fundamental business of the country was unsound. Excessive industrial profits, along with skimpy industrial wages, were distributing one-third of all personal income to 5 percent of the population. Some two years before the crash, the annual rate of increase of national investment (as contrasted to speculation) had started downward, not the least because corporations and their executives had diminished expectations for profits from an economy in which purchasing power could no longer keep pace with productivity. That rate of increase of investment, as economists came to understand a decade later, had to continue to rise if economic growth was to be sustained. Since 1927 the shortage of purchasing power among consumers had had a particularly bad effect on the important automobile and construction industries. The falling market for homes and cars, expensive items, reflected the uneven distribution of American income and wealth that left even the middle class without sufficient cash or credit to continue the buying splurge of the earlier years of the decade. But in the 1920s the level of economic intelligence, like the level of both private

and public economic policy, was still relatively low. The surfeit of disposable income among the rich, together with the swollen profits of corporations, had encouraged speculation. When trouble came, the jerry-built corporate structures of many businesses, especially the utilities, toppled. Nor could the American banking system meet the strain, for bankers, though they had been aware of the loose practices of their profession, had long refused to discipline themselves.

Business had failed to keep its house in order. Even worse, it had persuaded the government to follow the unwise economic policies of the decade preceding the crash. The crash itself brought the sagging economy down. It wiped out savings and confidence alike. Money lost in the market could not be spent for new consumer goods nor invested in new enterprise. The mood of despair that settled over the nation also stifled renewal of private investment that might have encouraged recovery. It dispelled the confidence of Americans in the business élite. The dominance of businessmen and industrialists, in government and out, had brought, not a new Eden, but a panic that marked the onset of the most baleful depression in all history.

The Onset of Depression

The Hoover policies: first phase. Few of the leaders of American business and politics, either Republican or Democrat, had expected the crash. And when it came, very few of them understood what had caused it or foresaw the severity of the depression it was to bring. Most of them agreed with the head of Bethlehem Steel, who announced in December 1929 that "never before has American business been as firmly entrenched for prosperity as it is today." Most of them agreed also with Andrew Mellon, who recommended letting the economy run down to the depths, from which it would presumably recover automatically, as it had in the 1870s and 1890s. That policy would entail great suffering, but those who believed that the economy operated according to mechanical laws believed too in the inexorability of business cycles and in the wisdom of leaving them alone, suffering or no. "Liquidate labor," Mellon advised, "liquidate stock, liquidate the farmers."

Hoover knew better. Though he remained convinced that the economy was basically sound and that government should not interfere with business, he took steps to prevent the spread of depression. In a series of conferences he tried to persuade business-leaders to keep wages and prices up voluntarily. He called on the Federal Reserve to make it easy for business to borrow. He encouraged the Farm Board to provide funds to help the stabilization corporations in their efforts to sustain commodity prices. Above all, he hoped, by offering private advice and by making public pronouncements, to restore the nation's confidence in business.

Hoover welcomed the Tariff Act of 1930 (see p. 658), for he was convinced that business would be encouraged by a continuation of protection. To hearten businessmen further, he recommended, and Congress in 1930 provided, cuts in personal and corporate income taxes. The reductions gave the wealthy more disposable income to use for investment, but they gave lower-income groups, who paid little taxes anyway, no additional money to spend on consumption. In the absence of confidence in business, the investments were not forthcoming. Following Hoover's advice, Congress did make modest appropriations for public works. These gave some boost to the sick construction industry and to the heavy industries that supplied it, and indirectly to the workers who were employed in those industries.

But those efforts were too meager to check the contraction in private spending, investment, and employment that followed the crash. Both Hoover and the Federal Reserve Board opposed a rapid, deliberately inflationary expansion of currency and bank deposits, which the board might have attempted with some possible healthy effect. The President would not countenance any more spending, because he was determined to keep the federal budget balanced, or as close to balanced as possible. This, he believed, as did most Americans, was sound finance, and it was also an unshakable article of business faith. Large federal

deficits, like inflation, would have frightened the business community, which the President wanted to soothe. To that purpose, during 1930 the President continually applied the balm of official optimism. True, official gloom would have caused further alarm; but Hoover, while privately dubious, acted as if his conferences with business-leaders had succeeded, whereas wages and prices actually continued to decline.

The blight of depression. "We have now passed the worst," Hoover announced wishfully in May 1930, "and . . . shall rapidly recover." The statistics told a different story. In 1929 new capital issues in the United States, a rough yardstick of investment, had totaled $10 billion; in 1930 they dropped to $7 billion. As the depression deepened, the figure reached $3 billion in 1931 and $1 billion in 1932. Investment was discouraged by the decline in corporate profits, which fell off steadily from $8.4 billion in 1929 to $3.4 billion in 1932. At the same time, the rate of business failures rose—over 100,000 businesses went under in the period 1929–32. And banks were failing too. In 1929, 659 banks with total deposits of about $200 million closed their doors; in 1930, 1,352 banks with deposits of $853 million; in 1931, 2,294 banks with deposits of almost $1,700 million, at the rate of almost 200 a month. Each collapse erased the cash and savings of depositors, most of whom had no other resources.

By the last quarter of 1930, industrial production had fallen 26 percent below the 1929 level. By mid-1932 it was off 51 percent from that level. Unemployment mounted: 4 million in October 1930; nearly 7 million a year later; almost 11 million by the fall of 1932. Even those who kept their jobs were earning less and less. Between 1929 and 1933 the total annual income of labor dropped from $53 to $31.5 billion. Average manufacturing wages came down 60 percent, average salaries 40 percent. Farmers fared even worse:

Reginald Marsh, *Bread Line—No One Has Starved*, 1932

their income declined from $11.9 to $5.3 billion. In 1929 national income touched $81 billion; by 1932 it had shrunk to $49 billion.

Liquidation carried a frightful burden of human suffering. Thousands of middle-class families, their incomes dwindling, sometimes entirely gone, lost next their savings, then their insurance, then, unable to pay their mortgages, their very homes. The optimism of the twenties gave way to gloom and fear. The times were even harder on laboring men and their families. The lost job, the fruitless search for work, the shoes worn through and the clothes worn thin, the furniture and trinkets pawned, the menu stripped of meat and then of adequate nutrition, no rent, no joy, no hope; and finally the despair of bread lines— these visited every city, leaving in their path sullen men, weeping women, and hungry children. So, too, on the farm—vanished incomes, foreclosures, tenancy, migrancy, and with them, as in the cities, the death of self-respect.

Hoover had predicted the abolition of poverty in America. Instead, within two years there mushroomed around America's cities settlements of shacks built of empty packing boxes, where homeless men squatted, reduced to desultory begging. A new Eden? "Brother, can you spare a dime?"

The Hoover policies: second phase. In the congressional elections of 1930 the Democrats conducted a rousing campaign against Hoover, though they offered no clear alternatives to his policies. The intensification of depression hurt the Republicans, as depression had always hurt the party in power. Though Hoover had been by no means unenlightened, he was, by virtue of his office, the most exposed target for abuse. The Democrats made his name a synonym for hardship. A "Hoover blanket" was yesterday's newspaper; a "Hoover flag" was an empty pocket turned inside out. Rough tactics and national discontent produced a slim Democratic victory, the first since 1916. The Republican majority in the Senate was reduced to a single vote, leaving that body dominated by a coalition of Democrats and Western agrarians. The Democrats held a bare majority in the House when the new Congress met.

Hungry, sullen men

In December 1930 the Democratic minority of the old Congress used the rump session to develop a program for unemployment relief. Hoover, irritated by the Democratic campaign and appalled by its success, reasserted his own policies.

The President felt that relief was strictly a local problem. The cities, he insisted, with help from private charity, should and could take care of the needy. That was a fallacious assumption, for nowhere in the nation was there an adequate system of relief. Local

"Brother, can you spare a dime?"

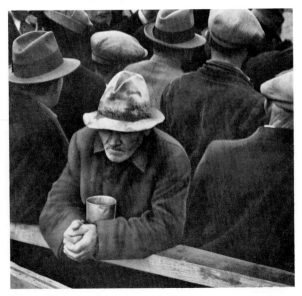

public funds in 1929 paid three-fourths of the cost of relief (by 1932, four-fifths), but the localities had neither the means to raise revenue nor the capacity to borrow to defray their mounting obligations. Their relief agencies and programs, moreover, had concentrated on helping unemployables, people unable to work. Local administrators had neither the experience nor the facilities to cope with mass unemployment, and private charity was incapable of meeting the nation's massive need for immediate relief.

As the winter of 1930–31 came on, cold and hunger moved into the homes of the unemployed. Relief payments were only $2.39 a week for a family in New York and even less in most other cities. Two Texas cities barred relief for blacks. Detroit, unable to tax or borrow, dropped a third of the needy families from its relief rolls; St. Louis cut off half, and children there combed the dumps for rotting food.

In October 1930 the President appointed an Emergency Committee for Employment under Colonel Arthur Woods. Though Hoover told the committee that relief was a local responsibility, Woods recommended a federal public-works program. The President rejected it, and in April 1931 Woods resigned.

Meanwhile Senator Robert Wagner, a New York Democrat, had introduced bills providing for federal public works and a federal employment service. Along with Wagner, Senator Robert M. La Follette, Jr., "Battle Bob's" son and successor, and Republican Senator Bronson Cutting of New Mexico urged federal spending for public works and relief. All this Hoover opposed on the ground that federal action was unnecessary.

Instead, in February 1931 Hoover expressed his continuing dedication to individualism, local responsibility, and mutual self-help. But in the face of depression, the virtues of economic individualism and private charity were outweighed by the needs of the helpless. The sheer shock of the depression and the pervasive ignorance about the causes of the business cycle impeded the search for remedies. Like others in government, the President was a captive of those circumstances as well as an honest man whose convictions had glued him to inaction.

Hoover's interpretation of the economic ups and downs of 1931 strengthened his convictions. Between February and June of that year the economic indexes rallied slightly, partly because of a normal seasonal upturn. The gains, though tiny, persuaded the President, and others bent on optimism, that recovery was under way. Then in the spring and summer of 1931 financial panic swept over Europe. The American crash had precipitated the collapse abroad by drying up the loan funds on which the European economy and the interrelated reparations and war-debt payments had come to depend. And the European collapse in turn drove foreigners to dump American securities in their scramble for dollars, thereby driving American stock prices down even further. Moreover, shortages in exchange forced one European nation after another to devalue its currency. This action disrupted international trade, and the prices of American agricultural commodities plummeted. Before the end of the summer, the indexes had resumed their decline. Again the depression deepened.

The depression, worldwide in scope, was provoking individual nations to pursue their separate advantages. The resulting scramble hurt them all, but none of the great powers, either in 1931 or for another decade, assumed and sustained the leadership that was required to bring about needed measures of cooperation. The United States was no exception.

The fault, Hoover concluded, lay in Europe. All the calamities since 1929, he came to believe, had originated in the Old World. The war had taxed the world economy beyond repair; the United States had regrettably become involved not only in war but in a morass of bad loans as well. European bankers had collaborated with their New York associates to create the easy-money conditions on which speculation had fed (see p. 647), and from that collusion was born the Panic of 1929. Then, just as recovery beckoned, European disaster in 1931 had reversed the gains so arduously won. This view of the causes of the depression reasserted the persistent myth of American innocence—even wounded innocence—for as Hoover saw the situation American business shared little of the blame; he himself shared none. Hoover's theory, moreover, excused him from embracing the domestic policies he had rejected, for if the basic cause of depression lay outside the United States the most appropriate action would be to ease the strains abroad and to protect the American economy from them.

Diplomacy in Depression

A set of good intentions. The foreign policies on which the Hoover Administration embarked in 1929 were marked by good will and peaceful purpose. The President and his able Secretary of State, Stimson, believed, as had their immediate predecessors, that the world had fought its last major war a decade earlier. Europe, they expected, could take care of itself, as could Asia and Latin America, with occasional advice from the United States. The aroused morality embodied in the Kellogg-Briand pact would prevent aggression and discourage militarism. Indeed Hoover expected the powers to put an end to their arms race in the very near future.

Initially Hoover and Stimson made some progress toward their benign goals. While still President-elect, Hoover had carried friendship to Latin America during a ten-week tour that publicized the "good neighbor" policy.* In Argentina he promised to abstain from intervention in the internal affairs of the nations south of the border. He kept his word. In 1930 Stimson announced that the United States henceforth would grant diplomatic recognition to *de facto* governments. Moreover, Hoover set about withdrawing the marines from Nicaragua, a task that was completed in 1933, and he arranged to remove them from Haiti.

In 1930 the President formally repudiated the Roosevelt Corollary to the Monroe Doctrine (see p. 569). A memorandum written by former Assistant Secretary of State J. Reuben Clark, which Hoover ordered published, denied that the doctrine justified American intervention in Latin America. Nor did Hoover regard the doctrine as a mandate for collecting the private debts of Americans. Some fifty revolutions or attempts at revolution shook the "good neighbors" of the hemisphere during his Administration. But he kept hands off, even though those disturbances often resulted in the repudiation of debts owed to American citizens and in the nationalization of their properties. Although the State Department fell into argumentative negotiations that ran on for many years, the

---

* A phrase later used by and ordinarily associated with Franklin Roosevelt.

United States did not resort to force. By abandoning protective imperialism, Hoover created an improved atmosphere in hemispheric relations.

This success contrasted with the Administration's diplomatic disappointments in Europe and its agonies in Asia. Intent on naval disarmament, Hoover welcomed the cooperation of Ramsay MacDonald, the head of the new Labor Cabinet in England. Their preliminary negotiations prepared the way for the multipower conference that met in London in 1930. There the Americans, the British, and the Japanese extended the "holiday" on the construction of capital ships, and American and British representatives evolved a formula for limiting the construction of cruisers, destroyers, and submarines. Naval experts of the English-speaking nations, however, deplored a compromise that increased Japan's ratio for cruisers and destroyers and gave it equality in submarines. In effect, this arrangement recognized Japan's primacy in the western Pacific. Japan would have accepted nothing less, and neither the Hoover nor the MacDonald government wanted to engage in an expensive naval race. Neither, moreover, considered Japan unfriendly. They confirmed, therefore, only what they had already conceded.

Even so, they failed to close the door on a naval race. The French, frightened by the militarism of fascist Italy, refused to limit their naval program unless the United States promised to help France in the event of aggression. Such a pledge was unthinkable to Hoover, the Senate, or the American people. When France and Italy would not subscribe to significant parts of the London treaty, the British insisted on adding a clause permitting England, the United States, or Japan to expand their fleets if their national security was threatened by the building program of some other power. This "escalator" clause made naval limitation conditional upon the self-restraint of a resurgent Italy and an alarmed France. Yet the Hoover Administration and the American people accepted disarmament as a fact.

Monetary diplomacy. When the panic struck European banks and security markets in 1931 (see p. 663), the focus of Hoover's diplomacy shifted to money. American investors, hard hit by the depression, cut off the loans to Germany that had so far enabled it to pay reparations for its part in the First World War. Without this source of income, the former Allies were unable to keep up payments on their debts to the United States. Even before the distressed German president appealed for help in the spring of 1930, Hoover had begun to think about a one-year moratorium on all intergovernmental debts and reparations payments. The idea was admirable, but Hoover said nothing about it until he had made

sure of congressional support, and he failed to consult the French. When he announced his proposal late in June, England and Germany endorsed it, but France held back, still hopeful of collecting reparations. The French also suspected that the American proposal was partly designed to enable Germany to pay back private debts it owed in the United States. During the two weeks before France endorsed the moratorium, the accelerated flight of funds from Germany forced widespread bank failures.

To his shock, the President discovered that Europe's distress directly embarrassed American banks. They had lent some $1.7 billion, on a short-term basis, without collateral, to central European banks, especially in Germany. Bank runs in Europe made those loans impossible to collect, and the solvency of the American banks that had made them was threatened. The loans were part of a complex network of obligations among banks in many countries. In order to stop demands for payments back and forth among them, Secretary Stimson and other American representatives in July 1930 negotiated an emergency "standstill" agreement. It was later extended to September 1931, and again to March 1933. The standstill agreements froze private debts just as the moratorium had frozen public debts. This gave financiers time to try to protect the banks of the Western world from bankruptcy, and time to delay putting pressure on borrowers for loans due.

But the freezing came too late to stop panic. Depositors, their confidence in banks shaken, demanded their money, which they intended to hoard. A run on the Bank of England, for decades the world's foremost symbol of financial stability, drained its gold and forced Great Britain off the gold standard in September 1931. That nation devalued the pound— that is, increased the cost of gold in terms of British currency—and established a special government fund to manage the value of the pound in terms of other currencies. By the end of 1931 every major power except Italy, France, and the United States was also forced off the gold standard, and each depreciated its currency and attempted to control its value in international exchange. These efforts at control were often designed to produce selfish advantages in trade, as were the prohibitive tariffs that invariably accompanied devaluation. Exchange controls and high tariffs actually impeded world trade and, worse still, gave rise to international suspicion and distrust.

Hoover had shown commendable initiative in arranging the moratorium and the standstills, but he never saw to the bottom of the problem. He failed to recognize that America's high protective tariffs impeded international commerce and invited foreign retaliation. And he would not support the cancellation of war debts. At the Lausanne Conference of

**On the Hoover
moratorium**

From Felix Frankfurter to Walter Lippmann, April 12, 1932.

1932, England and France finally admitted Germany's
bankruptcy and agreed to scale reparations down to
an insignificant sum provided that the United States
would scale war debts down equivalently. Most
American bankers favored that plan, as did Stimson,
who urged cancellation of "these damn debts." But
Congress, reflecting public opinion, would not even
consider a new debt commission, and Hoover, equivocal himself, demanded that the European nations
resume payments on their debts after the moratorium
expired. The debtor nations—except for Finland,
whose obligation was tiny—had no choice but to
default.

The defaults, like the demand that forced them
and the long stalemate over debts and reparations that
preceded them, engendered ill feeling on both sides of
the Atlantic. The resulting distrust weakened the will
of the democracies to cooperate in order to resist the
black forces gathering around them.

Fire bells in the Orient. Japan broke the peace of
the world. Since its victory over Russia in 1905, it had
dominated the economy of southern Manchuria, the
northeastern section of China. Tokyo was willing to
acknowledge China's political claim to the area so
long as that claim did not collide with Japanese military interests and economic privileges. During the late
twenties such a collision grew increasingly likely. In
China, Chiang Kai-shek (Jiang Jieshi) took over the
central government and broke with the communists
who had been his allies. Chinese nationalists hoped
soon to have the whole country under their control.
But the Russians still managed the Chinese Eastern
Railway and were developing its Pacific terminus, the
Siberian city of Vladivostok. Alarmed by the construction there, Japan resolved to reinforce southern
Manchuria. Here it confronted Chiang Kai-shek
(Jiang Jieshi), who was determined to yield nothing
further to any foreign power.

In the fall of 1931 the Japanese army in effect
took over the Tokyo government. In September Japanese troops occupied Mukden (Shenyang) and other
Manchurian cities and moved rapidly to establish
political control over the province. This violation of
the Nine Power Treaty and the Kellogg-Briand pact
was perfectly timed. China turned to the League of

The West was paralyzed

Nations for help, but the West was paralyzed by depression.

Even in good times Japan would probably have had little to fear. The British were opposed to any strong action in Manchuria. American public opinion, though it condemned Japan's behavior, was vehemently against any measures that might precipitate war. Hoover, anxious to avoid war at any cost, rejected Stimson's suggestion that the United States might have to cooperate with the League in imposing economic sanctions on Japan.

At Hoover's insistence, Stimson proceeded cautiously. He hoped at first to strengthen the civilian moderates in the Japanese cabinet and to persuade them to end the occupation of Manchuria. But in January 1932 the Japanese army drove on. Now Stimson resorted to moral condemnation, the only weapon Hoover would countenance. In identical warnings to China and Japan, he revived the doctrine Bryan had enunciated in 1915. The United States, Stimson warned, would not recognize any change brought about by force that impaired American treaty rights or Chinese territorial integrity. Japan scoffed politely.

Before the end of January the Japanese invaded Shanghai, bombarded the city, and killed thousands of civilians—all on the pretext that they were retaliating against a Chinese boycott. America's warning had proved no deterrent. Yet once again Hoover refused to consider economic sanctions. Stimson could turn only to sterner words.

In February he published a long letter to Senator Borah, in which he reiterated his nonrecognition doctrine and lamented the failure of other nations to endorse it. He also recalled the interdependence of the various Washington treaties of 1922. "The willingness of the American government to surrender its commanding lead in battleship construction and to leave its positions at Guam and in the Philippines without further fortification," Stimson wrote, "was predicated upon, among other things, the self-denying covenants contained in the Nine Power Treaty."

He hoped that his letter would encourage China, inform the American public, exhort the League and Great Britain, and warn Japan. But sentiment did China no good. Americans, like the League and its members, shared Hoover's determination to confine deterrence to words, and Japan was confident that neither the President nor his constituents were prepared to heed Stimson's counsel.

The Assembly of the League, with Japan abstaining, unanimously adopted a resolution incorporating the nonrecognition doctrine. A year later a League commission of inquiry named Japan the aggressor in Manchuria and called on the Japanese to return the province to China. They simply withdrew from the League, though they left Shanghai temporarily.

Stimson, a disciple of Theodore Roosevelt, believed that power and the will to use it were essential to world peace. The vast majority of Americans, including Congress, disagreed. Indeed, as Hoover understood, there neither would nor should have been any support for a war against Japan, or a policy that invited war. For its part, Congress early in 1933 passed a bill granting independence to the Philippine Islands, largely in response to pressure from American interests eager to raise the tariff barrier between themselves and their Filipino competitors. The measure, enacted over Hoover's veto, demonstrated that Congress was willing to throw the islands to the mercy of Japan, and it canceled the veiled warning in Stimson's letter to Borah.

The story was much the same in Europe, where the German Nazis were marching to power. At a World Disarmament Conference in Geneva in 1932, the French proposed that an international army be established and that all powers submit to the compulsory arbitration of disputes. Hoover countered with a plan for the immediate abolition of all offensive weapons and the reduction by one-third of existing armies and navies. But with the United States still unwilling to guarantee their security, the French were unimpressed by the arithmetic of arms reduction, and the conference adjourned in July with nothing accomplished. In 1933 Germany was Hitler's.

Good will and high moral purpose had no meaning in the Germany of the Nazis or the Japan of the Imperial Army. For those who hoped for disarmament and peace and the rule of law, the hour of peril was close. Neither the American people nor their leaders had brought the world to the edge of disaster, nor could they alone have prevented the collapse of order. But the foreign policies of the United States lacked the force to check depression or aggression.

The Depths of Depression

The Hoover policies: third phase. Hoover, William Allen White once said, was "constitutionally gloomy, a congenital pessimist who always saw the doleful side of any situation." The President took no joy in his office or in its potentialities for leadership. As he put it himself, "I can't be a Theodore Roosevelt." Grim and aloof, Hoover was nonetheless resolute. Just as he tried to halt the panic in Europe in 1931, so did he try to buttress the United States against the effects of that panic. By the fall of that year he had reached certain conclusions that were to shape his policies during the coming months. He intended to do everything he could to keep the nation on the gold standard, in his view an indispensable condition of economic health. The business and financial community shared that belief passionately, as it had for almost a century. The President also intended, again with ardor and with the blessing of men of means, to strive for economy and a balanced budget. He was prepared, however, to use federal funds and federal authority on an unprecedented scale to rescue the banks and industry from their troubles. The effects of their recovery, he thought, would reach down to the farmers and laborers, who were to receive little direct aid from the federal government.

The new Congress convened in December 1931. At Hoover's suggestion it appropriated $125 million to expand the lending powers of the Federal Land Banks. Also at his urging, but not until July 1932, it established a system of home-loan banks with a capital of $125 million for discounting home mortgages. The purpose of this scheme was to enable savings banks, insurance companies, and building-and-loan associations to obtain cash for the mortgages they held instead of having to foreclose them. The act not only helped to keep the assets of the lending institutions liquid but also, as Hoover said, spared hundreds of Americans the "heartbreaking . . . loss of their homes." And it set a significant precedent for more extensive legislation later on.

In February 1932 Congress passed the Glass-Steagall Act, as requested by the President. It freed about a billion dollars' worth of gold to meet the demands of Europeans who were converting their dollars to gold. This enabled the United States for the time being to retain enough gold to remain on the gold standard without putting controls on gold movements or on transactions in foreign exchange. Yet the continuing outflow of gold even further reduced bank reserves and thus the availability of bank loans to business. That situation further depressed prices and added to the burden of debts contracted when prices were high. To hold to the gold standard was in keeping with the theories of classical economics, with their emphasis on the automatic workings of domestic and international trade and of the business cycle. Yet now that mechanism spun the business cycle downward and helped depression feed upon itself.

In spite of the Glass-Steagall Act, moreover, many banks remained weak. To supplement their resources, Hoover in the fall of 1931 persuaded New York bankers to create a National Credit Association with a $500-million pool. But the halfhearted use of this fund doomed the effort to failure. The President then gave in to the urgings of Eugene Meyer, governor of the Federal Reserve Board and formerly head of the War Finance Corporation established in 1918. Meyer proposed reviving that agency in order to rescue Ameri-

can finance. Hoover, hoping that the psychological lift provided by this scheme would justify the cost of financing it, made it the keystone of his recovery policy in 1932.

In January Congress created the Reconstruction Finance Corporation with a capital stock of $500 million and the power to borrow three times that sum in guaranteed, tax-free bonds. It was authorized, as Meyer and Hoover had recommended, to lend money to banks and insurance companies and, with the approval of the Interstate Commerce Commission, to railroads. Most of the $1.5 billion the RFC disbursed before March 1933 went to banks and trust companies. The RFC, however, could lend funds only against adequate collateral, and it could not buy bank stock. Its loans increased bank indebtedness, but it could not satisfy the banks' basic need for new capital.

The RFC kept its transactions secret for five months, largely because Hoover feared that publicity would incite runs on the weak banks that were receiving the loans. More than half of the $126 million that the RFC disbursed during those months went to three large banks. One of them was the bank of Charles G. Dawes, who resigned as president of the RFC only a month before the loan went through. In July 1932 the Democrats in Congress, to Hoover's dismay, put through an amendment compelling the RFC to report its transactions. Thereafter the number of loans made to large institutions fell off.

The muddle of relief. Late in 1931 Hoover appointed a new committee on unemployment with Walter S. Gifford as its head. Gifford, the president of the American Telephone and Telegraph Company, agreed with Hoover that relief was the responsibility of local government and private charity. Yet Gifford could not convincingly defend this view. In January 1932 he confessed to a Senate committee that he did not know how many people were out of work; he did not know how many needed help, how much help they needed, or how much money localities were raising or could raise. But of one thing he seemed certain: the "grave danger" of taking "the determination of these things into the Federal Government."

The gravest danger, in the view of the President and most congressmen of both parties, was that the budget might be thrown further out of balance. Yet throughout 1932 the need for federal spending increased. In the words of Senator Edward P. Costigan, Colorado's progressive Democrat, "nothing short of federal assistance . . . can possibly satisfy the conscience and heart and safeguard the good name of America." With La Follette, Costigan introduced a bill granting a modest $375 million for relief, but the

Administration blocked it. Sensing the political importance of the issue, the Democratic leadership now began to press for direct federal aid to the unemployed and for deficit spending for public works.

Hoover insisted on limiting any relief program to RFC loans to localities and on limiting public works to self-liquidating projects, like bridges and housing, which could return enough income from tolls or rentals to pay back the initial cost of construction. But many states had nearly exhausted their legal authority to borrow from any source, and few projects had emerged from the drawing board. Consequently the President's restrictions put a low ceiling on spending.

Even so, Hoover endorsed a federal program without precedent in American history. After a partisan wrangle, on July 21, 1932, he signed a bill that authorized the RFC to lend $1.5 billion for local self-liquidating public works and $300 million at 3 percent interest to supplement local relief funds.

The relief loans, the President said, were to be based on "absolute need and evidence of financial exhaustion." That limitation kept them small. The governor of Pennsylvania asked for a loan of $45 million (three-fourths of the sum, he noted, that would allow the jobless in the state a mere 13 cents apiece a day for food for a year). The RFC let him have only $11 million (enough for little more than 3 cents a person a day). By the end of 1932 the RFC had allotted only $30 million for relief loans and even less for public works.

The outlook of the nation's farmers seemed as hopeless as that of the unemployed workers in the cities. Even before the depression destroyed the European market for farm commodities, the Federal Farm Board had recognized that it could never stabilize farm prices without some control over farm production. When in 1932 American prices followed world prices down to bewildering lows, the stabilization corporations made a brief but futile effort to brake the decline. They lost $354 million in market operations, accumulated huge stocks of unsalable commodities, and finally in the summer simply gave up. Wheat, which had brought $2.16 a bushel in 1919 and $1.03 in 1929, sank to 38 cents. Cotton, corn, and other prices suffered comparably. Farmers found themselves without enough income to meet their mortgage payments or even to buy food for their families. And certainly they lacked the money to buy manufactured goods, which still sold at prices sustained by industry.

The members of the Federal Farm Board urged Congress to do something about regulating acreage and production as a first step in setting up some sort of program for boosting farm prices. The only alternative was agricultural bankruptcy. Yet Hoover and Secretary of Agriculture Hyde rejected the idea of imposing federal controls on agriculture. Before the year ended, farmers were burning corn in Nebraska to keep warm, forming angry posses in Minnesota to prevent foreclosures, and joining Milo Reno's militant Farmers' Holiday Association in Iowa to block the shipment of produce until prices rose.

Moods of despair. Father John Ryan, the Catholic social reformer, despaired for the state of the nation. "I wish," he said, "we might double the number of Communists in this country, to put the fear, if not of God, then . . . of something else, into the hearts of our leaders." Communism had a particular appeal for the intellectuals who had been alienated by the culture of the Coolidge era, men like Malcolm Cowley and Sherwood Anderson. But the theories of Karl Marx had little appeal for the general public. The communists organized "hunger marches" in Washington and Detroit and preached revolution elsewhere, but Communist party membership was little more than one hundred thousand.

Though desperate Americans spurned communism, they gave way to hatred and violence. Farmers, brandishing shotguns to prevent foreclosures, defied the law to defend their homes. The president of the Farmers' Union damned the rich as "cannibals . . . who live on the labor of the workers." Some of the prosperous took out "riot and civil commotion insur-

I want to tell you about an experience we had in Philadelphia when our private funds were exhausted and before public funds became available....

One woman said she borrowed 50 cents from a friend and bought stale bread for 3½ cents per loaf, and that is all they had for eleven days except for one or two meals.

With the last food order another woman received she bought dried vegetables and canned goods. With this she made a soup and whenever the members of the family felt hungry they just ate some of the soup....

One woman went along the docks and picked up vegetables that fell from the wagons. Sometimes the fish vendors gave her fish at the end of the day. On two different occasions this family was without food for a day and a half....

Another family did not have food for two days. Then the husband went out and gathered dandelions and the family lived on them.

From Hearings Before a Subcommittee of the Senate Committee on Manufactures, 1932.

ance'' and began to suggest that the United States needed a fascist dictator like Mussolini.

In the spring of 1932 some fifteen thousand unemployed veterans converged on Washington from every region of the country. They announced that they planned to stay in the capital until Congress voted full and immediate payment of the bonus. The year before, over Hoover's veto, Congress had authorized loans up to 50 percent of the value of each adjusted service certificate (see p. 624). But those funds had been spent, and the unemployed veterans, like all other unemployed Americans, were in dire need of help. When the Senate voted down the bonus bill, half the veterans went home. But the rest had no place to

Anacostia flats, 1932

Unemployment has steadily increased in the U.S. since the beginning of the depression.... The number of persons totally unemployed is now at least 10,000,000.... The number ... next winter will ... be 11,000,000 ... one man of every four employable workers....

This percentage is higher than the percentage of unemployed British workers ... and higher than the French, the Italians, and the Canadian percentages, but lower than the German....

Eleven million unemployed means 27,500,000 whose regular source of livelihood has been cut off.... Taking account of the number of workers on part time, the total of those without adequate income becomes 34,000,000 or better than a quarter of the entire population.... It is conservative to estimate that the problem of next winter's relief is a problem of caring for approximately 25,000,000 souls....

And it is not necessary to appeal ... to class fear in order to point out that there is a limit beyond which hunger and misery become violent.

From *Fortune*, September 1932.

go and no way of getting there, so they camped in a muddy shantytown on Anacostia Flats and in vacant government buildings.

Their plight evoked the sympathy of the chief of the District of Columbia police, who treated them generously and intelligently. But their presence worried the Administration. Hoover, anxious to get rid of them, had Congress pass a bill that permitted them to borrow against their bonus certificates in order to get funds for transportation home. Still most veterans waited around after Congress adjourned. They hoped at least for a conference with the President.

Late in July the Administration ordered the eviction of all squatters from government buildings. In the ensuing melee, brought about largely by the small corps of communists among the veterans, two men were killed and several policemen wounded. Secretary of War Patrick Hurley had been looking for just such an incident. At his request, the White House now called in the army—four troops of cavalry and four infantry companies, with six tanks, tear gas, and machine guns. Under the personal command of General Douglas MacArthur (whose junior officers included Dwight D. Eisenhower and George Patton), the troops rode into Anacostia Flats, drove out the veterans and their families, and burned their shacks. Crowing over his triumph, MacArthur called the veterans "a mob . . . animated by the essence of revolution." The Administration published reports claiming that most of them had been communists and criminals.

Neither a grand jury nor the Veterans Administration could find evidence to support those charges. The bonus marchers were destitute men. Whether or not they merited special treatment, they deserved, as did unemployed Americans everywhere, compassion and assistance. They received first indifference and

veiled hostility, then vicious armed attack. That treatment appalled the nation.

With government callous and blundering, with the business élite defensive about the disrepute it had brought on itself, with depression still spreading, Americans began to fear that the whole political and economic system might collapse. Yet they waited patiently, as they had so often before in times of trouble, to see whether the presidential campaign would give them a vote for a brighter future.

The changing of the guard. In the summer of 1932 the Republicans renominated Hoover and his Vice President, Charles Curtis. A minority of the delegates to the convention were dissatisfied with the Administration's policies but were unwilling to repudiate the President. The convention was listless, for the delegates realized that the electorate, rightly or wrongly, blamed the party for the depression and regarded Hoover as the symbol of the party.

The Democrats, in contrast, sensed victory ahead. A majority of the delegates came to Chicago pledged to Franklin D. Roosevelt, who had been the front runner for the nomination since his easy reelection as governor of New York in 1930. He had the nerve for politics, the sense of fun, and the zest with people that had once made his distant cousin, Theodore Roosevelt, the most popular man in America. Franklin Roosevelt, moreover, had worked effectively with Tammany Hall, had made friends with the masters of other Northern machines, and yet had always preserved close relations with the Southern wing of the party. He closed the gap that had divided the party in 1924. Further, though conservative in his economic thinking, Roosevelt believed in positive, active, humane government.

Roosevelt stood to the left of his serious opponents. Their one hope was to organize a coalition to keep him from getting the two-thirds vote necessary for nomination. Al Smith, still a favorite of the machines, hoped to be nominated once again. Ambition had soured Smith's best instincts. When Roosevelt before the convention called for help for "the forgotten man at the bottom of the economic pyramid," Smith remarked testily, "This is no time for demagogues." But Smith lacked allies. The McAdoo faction still opposed him and now backed Speaker of the House John N. Garner. After Roosevelt had failed to win the necessary vote in three ballots, McAdoo, evening up the old scores of 1924 (see p. 641), switched California's delegation to the New York governor. This put Roosevelt across, and in return his lieutenants arranged second place on the ticket for Garner.

In a characteristically dramatic gesture, Roosevelt broke precedent by flying to Chicago to accept the nomination before the convention adjourned. "Let it . . . be symbolic that . . . I broke traditions," he told the cheering delegates. "Republican leaders not only have failed in material things, they have failed in national vision, because in disaster they have held out no hope. . . . I pledge you, I pledge myself to a new deal for the American people."

Roosevelt began to define that New Deal during his campaign. He was often deliberately vague and took pains to avoid offending any large bloc of voters. He hedged on the tariff. He made much of his party's demand for the repeal of the Eighteenth Amendment: Prohibition was still an important political issue in 1932, but it had no immediate bearing on the depression, which was the overriding concern of Americans. But he also set forth strong lines of attack on the nation's economic ills. At the Commonwealth Club in San Francisco, Roosevelt said that "government . . . owes to everyone an avenue to possess himself of a portion of that plenty sufficient for his needs, through his own work." In its dealings with business, government was to "assist the development of . . . an economic constitutional order." And such an order, he pointed out, demanded national planning.

Roosevelt's plans drew on the ideas reformers had nurtured throughout the twenties and promised assistance to the victims of depression. He called for strict public regulation of the utilities and federal development of public power. He advocated federal controls on agricultural production as a part of a program to support commodity prices and federal loans to refinance farm mortgages. He expressed interest in the schemes for currency inflation that agriculture-leaders were urging as a means to raise prices and reduce the weight of debt. He appealed to the business community by demanding cuts in government spending in order to balance the budget, but in the same speech he also promised to incur a deficit whenever human suffering made it necessary.

Roosevelt's oratorical flair and personal ebullience contrasted with Hoover's heavy speech and grim manner. The President emphasized his dedication to budget-balancing and the gold standard, defended his record, and charged his opponent with recklessness. The policies Roosevelt advocated, Hoover said, "would destroy the very foundations of our American system." If they were adopted, "grass will grow in the streets of a hundred cities, a thousand towns."

That rhetoric reflected Hoover's gloom. It obscured his own expansion of federal control, and it

Roosevelt in 1932: a real choice

exaggerated Roosevelt's intentions. Actually the Democrat's campaign disappointed many intellectuals who felt, as Walter Lippmann earlier had, that Franklin Roosevelt was "a highly impressionable person . . . without strong convictions. . . . a pleasant man, who, without any important qualifications for the office, would very much like to be President."

But there were significant differences between the two candidates and their ideas, between Hoover's pessimism and Roosevelt's effervescence, between Hoover's belief that the origins of the depression lay outside the United States and Roosevelt's belief that they were internal, between Hoover's impulse toward caution and Roosevelt's impulse toward experiment, between Hoover's identification with industry and finance and Roosevelt's identification with the forgotten and with the intellectuals and social workers who championed them. Hoover in his last campaign speech was right in associating Roosevelt with Norris and La Follette, right in asserting that the contest was between two philosophies of government. Both philosophies were fundamentally American, but Hoover's looked backward, while Roosevelt's looked cautiously ahead.

The people had a real choice when they went to the polls in November. Dismissing radicalism (the Socialists—rent by factionalism—polled 881,951 votes, the Communists, only 102,785), they swept the Democrats into office. Roosevelt won over 57 percent of the popular vote and carried the Electoral College 472 to 59. The Democrats also gained a large majority in both houses of Congress. The vote, a protest against the Administration, gave Roosevelt a clear mandate for change, though the nature of that change was clear neither to the voters nor the victor. Roosevelt lost only six states—Maine, New Hampshire, Vermont, Connecticut, Delaware, and Pennsylvania. He carried the agricultural West as well as the South; he carried the great cities by majorities larger than Smith's in 1928.

Depression had driven a majority of Americans of all backgrounds into the Roosevelt column. Among them, farmers and workers after twelve lean years could again expect to have some voice in Washington. The total vote repudiated business, its policies and its servants; threw out the Old Guard; and placed the direction of government in a new President who saw himself as a tribune of the people.

Suggestions for Reading

HOOVER AND HIS POLICIES

A. M. Schlesinger, Jr., *The Crisis of the Old Order** (1957), provides a critical and detailed analysis of the Hoover Administration and its problems as does the more generous account in D. Burner, *Herbert Hoover** (1978). Also critical, though the authors intend to be sympathetic, are H. G. Warren, *Herbert Hoover and the Great Depression* (1956), and J. A. Schwarz, *The Interregnum of Despair* (1970). The relevant chapters in J. D. Hicks, *Republican Ascendancy: 1921–1933* (1960), and J. H. Wilson, *Herbert Hoover** (1975), are unsympathetic and those in W. E. Leuchtenburg, *The Perils of Prosperity: 1914–32** (1958), lucid but brief. Two incisive works are A. Romesco, *The Poverty of Abundance: Hoover, the Nation, the Depression* (1965), and E. Rosen, *Hoover, Roosevelt and the Brain Trust* (1977). The most ardent defense of the Administration appears in Herbert Hoover, *Memoirs: The Great Depression, 1929–1941* (1952). On Hoover's foreign policies, there is significant material in the biographies of Stimson mentioned in connection with the preceding chapter, and in R. H. Ferrell, *American Diplomacy in the Great Depression: Hoover-Stimson Foreign Policy, 1929–1933* (1957).

DEPRESSION

All the volumes noted above of course deal with the depression. Its impact is also poignantly revealed in the pertinent parts of I. Bernstein, *The Lean Years** (1960); C. Bird, *The Invisible Scar* (1965); B. Sternsher, ed., *Hitting Home* (1970); and D. A. Shannon, ed., *The Great Depression* (1960). There are excellent descriptions of the stock-market crash in F. L. Allen, *Only Yesterday** (1931), and J. K. Galbraith, *The Great Crash, 1929** (1955). The skillful analysis of the latter should be compared with the also able view in T. Wilson, *Fluctuations in Income and Employment* (1948), with the important chapters on Hoover in H. Stein, *The Fiscal Revolution in America** (1969), and in C. P. Kindleberger, *The World in Depression, 1929–1939** (1973); and with the special view of central banking policy in M. Friedman and A. J. Schwartz, *The Great Contraction, 1929–1933** (1965). Within his excellent general study of American radical intellectuals, *Writers on the Left** (1961), D. Aaron discusses the influence of the depression on the spread of radicalism.

F.D.R. AND 1932

Franklin D. Roosevelt's governorship and first presidential campaign receive important treatment in A. M. Schlesinger's work, mentioned above, which is brilliant and panoramic on those subjects, and in F. Freidel, *Franklin D. Roosevelt: The Triumph* (1956), a work of outstanding scholarship. Less comprehensive but still useful are parts of J. M. Burns, *Roosevelt: The Lion and the Fox** (1956), and R. G. Tugwell, *The Democratic Roosevelt** (1957).

*Available in paperback edition.

27
THE NEW DEAL

During the winter of 1932–33, the despair born of depression gripped the United States ever more tightly. The four-month interval between the November election and the inauguration of March 1933 found Hoover without influence and Roosevelt without power. Hoover impeded any chance of collaboration with his successor by insisting on policies Roosevelt had condemned. In February, when the President called on Roosevelt to make a series of conservative declarations, he privately wrote a Republican senator, "I realize that if these declarations be made by the President-Elect, he will have ratified the whole major program of the Republican Administration." The incoming President, interpreting Hoover's invitation as a request for capitulation rather than cooperation, naturally rejected it, as he was, in any event, inclined to.

Without making public commitments to any program, Roosevelt awaited his day to take charge. Americans, worried and gloomy, also awaited the change of command, their anxieties deepened by an attempt upon Roosevelt's life by a madman in Miami, Florida, in February. The electorate had no sure sense of what a new deal might bring them, but they had clinching evidence that the old deal was ending in disaster.

The spreading panic was beginning to concentrate on one of the weakest links in the economy—the banking system. As the economy continued downward, more and more people played it safe by converting their savings to cash. The mounting pressure on financial institutions, the lines of depositors waiting to draw out their savings, the threat of further runs on the banks, led the governor of Michigan in mid-February to proclaim a bank holiday—that is, to order the temporary closing of the banks in his state. That act set off a chain reaction in other states. On the last day of Hoover's Administration, with banks shutting their doors across the land, the retiring President said, "We are at the end of our rope. There is nothing more we can do."

Franklin D. Roosevelt

His background. The new President was fifty-one years old. Like his distant cousin Theodore, he had come from a patrician background that gave him both a high sense of civic responsibility and a certain disdain for those whose chief achievement was making money. Like Theodore, Franklin Roosevelt was a man of charm, vivacity, and energy. He had been much influenced by Theodore, and their careers offered curious parallels. Both had made their political debuts in the New York legislature; both had served as Assistant Secretary of the Navy in Washington; both had

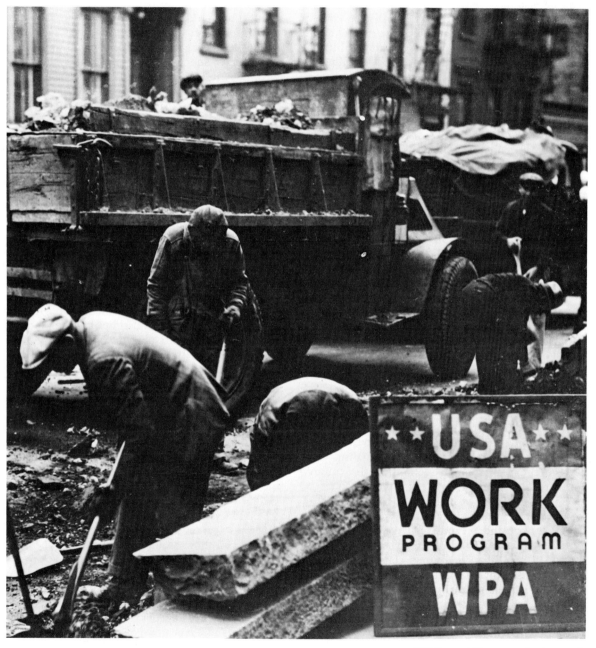

WPA: putting people to work

been governor of New York; both had been candidates for the Vice Presidency.

Unlike Theodore, Franklin was a member of the Democratic branch of the Roosevelt family. He was less of an intellectual than Theodore, but he was also less moralistic and evangelical. His urbane and conciliatory manner, indeed, led some observers to suppose him too compliant for hard responsibilities and decisions. But as second in command in the Navy Department during the First World War, he had been a resourceful executive. As candidate for Vice President in 1920, he had been a vigorous campaigner. In 1921 he had been stricken by poliomyelitis. That illness deprived him of the use of his legs; many thought it would end his public career. The determination of his comeback revealed an inner spirit that was not only gallant but tough. He had been an imaginative governor of New York; no state had taken so many positive measures to meliorate the effects of depression. His capture of the Democratic nomination in 1932 was the work of a seasoned politician.

The superficial affability of Roosevelt's manner concealed a complex personality—at once light-hearted and somber, candid and disingenuous, open and impenetrable, bold and cautious, decisive and evasive. Throughout his life he pursued certain public ends—especially the improvement of welfare and opportunity for the great masses of people—with steadiness of purpose; but the means he employed to achieve those ends were often inconsistent and occasionally unworthy. Yet his capacity to project the grand moral issues of his day—and his readiness to use the resources of presidential leadership to prepare the country for necessary action—enabled him to command the confidence of a great majority of Americans during his terms in office, despite the persistent opposition of a powerful minority.

His ideas. Roosevelt was a child of the progressive era. Theodore Roosevelt and Woodrow Wilson had been his early inspirations. Government seemed to him a necessary instrument of the general welfare, and he had no inhibitions about calling on the state to redress matters when "rugged individualism" left parts of the population or sections of the country without adequate protection. But the problems of 1933 were novel. Progressivism had been a gospel of social improvement rather than a program for economic growth, and progressives were no less baffled than conservatives by economic collapse. But, where faith in laissez faire constrained conservatives from taking positive government action, progressives like Roosevelt, with activist temperaments and an adventurous attitude toward social policy, were ready to invoke affirmative government to bring about economic recovery.

In economics, Roosevelt had leanings rather than theories. In his campaign for the Presidency, he had identified himself with two main ideas—action and planning. As to what should be tried, his views were sometimes incompatible.

Certain of his advisers had more clear-cut ideas. A group of college professors, mostly recruited from Columbia University, had served as his campaign brain trust. A book of 1932, *The Modern Corporation and Private Property*, by Adolf A. Berle, Jr., and Gardiner C. Means, provided one foundation for their analysis. The trend toward economic concentration, they contended, was irreversible. Already it had transformed great parts of the old free market of classical economics into "administered" markets, in which basic economic decisions were made, not by equations of supply and demand, but by the policies of those who ran the great corporations. In Berle and Means' opinion this change in the structure of the market rendered classical laissez-faire theory obsolete.

So persuaded, another Columbia economist, Rexford G. Tugwell, urged the President-elect to bold conclusions. If concentration was inevitable, Tugwell argued, then control over the nation's economic life could not be safely left in private hands. Such private control had brought about the depression. In the twenties the gains of economic productivity had gone into profits, savings, and speculation when they should have gone into a buildup of purchasing power through the payment of higher wages to workers and higher prices to farmers. The only way to operate the modern integrated economy at capacity, in Tugwell's view, was organized public planning.

Men like Berle, Tugwell, Means, and Raymond Moley, who acted as nominal head of the brain trust, were in a sense heirs of Theodore Roosevelt's New Nationalism. Their predisposition toward new institutions for central planning was reinforced by the views of those who, recalling America's last national emergency, the First World War, reverted to wartime economic agencies in the battle against depression. The Reconstruction Finance Corporation of the Hoover Administration was itself a revival of Wilson's War Finance Corporation (see p. 667). Now men who had once been associated with the War Industries Board, men like Bernard Baruch, Hugh S. Johnson, and George N. Peek, began to sponsor schemes of industrial and agricultural planning, though with little of Tugwell's zeal for accompanying social reform.

Not all those around Roosevelt accepted the virtues of national planning. Others close to him—especially Associate Justice Louis D. Brandeis of the Supreme Court and Professor Felix Frankfurter of Harvard—rejected the thesis of inevitable economic concentration. They distrusted the idea of central planning and advocated policies designed to encourage more competition. Still others, though these were more powerful in the Democratic party in Congress than in the President's immediate circle, were inflationists in the tradition of William Jennings Bryan. And others, like Lewis W. Douglas, whom Roosevelt was about to appoint Director of the Budget, were sound-money, laissez-faire Democrats deeply committed, like the Republicans, to the gold standard and the annually balanced budget. As now one, now another, of these groups exerted a telling influence, the resulting policies on occasion clashed.

Roosevelt, concerned more with action than consistency, presided benignly over the clash of debate and policy alike. Disagreement stimulated him, enabled him to compare the merits of competing arguments and personalities, and reassured him that crucial questions would come to him for decision. His choice of Cabinet members reflected his desire for a variety of views and his confidence that he could control advisers of divergent opinion. To the State Department he named Cordell Hull, a Tennessee Democrat who had sponsored the income tax amendment during the Wilson Administration but who was now cautious in his views except as a passionate foe of international trade barriers. Two vigorous progressive Republicans—Henry A. Wallace of Iowa and Harold L. Ickes of Illinois—were appointed to Agriculture and Interior; the first woman in history to go into the Cabinet, Frances Perkins of New York, a veteran social worker, became Secretary of Labor; and the other posts were filled largely by Democratic politicians.

The Hundred Days

The inauguration. On March 4, 1933, millions of Americans clustered around their radios to hear the new President deliver his inaugural address. "Let me assert my firm belief," Roosevelt began, "that the only thing we have to fear is fear itself." Then he assailed the business-leaders whose incompetence and misconduct, he said, had been largely responsible for the economic disaster. "This Nation asks for action, and action now," he concluded, adding that he would seek from Congress "broad Executive powers to wage a war against the emergency, as great as the power that would be given to me if we were in fact invaded by a foreign foe."

Action itself was quick to follow. Immediately after the inauguration, Roosevelt declared a national bank holiday and called Congress into special session. When Congress convened on March 8, it received at once a special message on the banking crisis and a draft of emergency banking legislation, on which Roo-

Lines of depression, 1933: "The end of our rope."

sevelt's advisers had collaborated with some of Hoover's outgoing Treasury staff. In less than eight hours the House and Senate shouted through the bill and returned it to the President for signature. The new legislation made it possible for banks to convert assets into cash. That liquidity permitted almost all banks to reopen, reassuring depositors who no longer withdrew their money in panic. The few insolvent banks were put under control of federal "conservators" who reorganized their affairs. The unprecedented combination of decision and speed in the passage of the act electrified the country.

Quick to seize advantage of the national mood, the President put forward a bill calling for the reduction of government expenses, including veterans' pensions. He followed his economy message with a call for the amendment of the Volstead Act to legalize light wines and beers. The prompt enactment of both the economy and the beer bills involved the defeat of the two most powerful lobbies in the nation's capital—the veterans and the prohibitionists. All this activity increased the national sense of exhilaration. "In one week," wrote Walter Lippmann, "the nation, which had lost confidence in everything and everybody, has regained confidence in the government and in itself."

Planning for agriculture. So far the Roosevelt program had been dashing in style but orthodox in content. Now, focusing on the problem of recovery, the President followed the path of the planners who

Plowing up the cotton

advocated using the power of the federal government to "rationalize" and to help to manage agriculture and industry. On March 16, Roosevelt sent to Capitol Hill a message calling for a bold national policy in agriculture. "I tell you frankly that it's a new and untrod path," he said, "but I tell you with equal frankness that an unprecedented condition calls for the trial of new means."

The condition was indeed unprecedented. The per capita cash net income of the American farmer had declined from $162 to $48 between 1929 and 1932. Because farm prices had fallen faster than industrial prices, the farmer's purchasing power was only about 60 percent of what it had been in 1929. The farmer's fixed charges—especially the burden of mortgage debt assumed at higher price levels—weighed more heavily than ever. Since the individual farmer saw no way to fight falling prices except to increase production, more produce was sent to market and prices were driven down faster and further. Some farmers, instead, burned their crops or threw them away.

The central idea in the Administration proposal was "agricultural adjustment." This plan aimed to increase farm income by controlling production; and it aimed to control production by offering benefit payments to farmers who agreed to regulate their plantings according to a national plan. The adjustment programs were to be financed by processing taxes collected at the flour mill or textile mill or packinghouse. No program would go into effect until a majority of farmers indicated they wanted it by voting in a referendum. The local administration of the plan was to be as much as possible in the hands of the farmers themselves. The ultimate object was to restore to farmers substantially the purchasing power they had had in 1909–14. That concept was known as "parity."

The agricultural-adjustment bill that emerged from conferences between the Department of Agriculture and leading farm organizations incorporated, in addition to benefit payments, a number of other approaches to the farm problem. It gave the government authority, for example, to maintain prices through loans on or purchase of nonperishable crops, which would then go into government storage; it also conferred authority to withdraw land from cultivation through leasing and to regulate the release of commodities for sale through marketing agreements and quotas. Through the use of those powers the government could not only prevent gluts on the market but could build up reserves against lean years, and, in the phrase of Henry Wallace, maintain an "ever normal granary." The inflationists in Congress added an important amendment giving the President power to issue greenbacks, to remonetize silver, and to alter the gold content of the dollar. In the meantime, the newly created Farm Credit Administration provided quick and effective mortgage relief.

While Washington laid its plans, trouble was mounting in the countryside. In late April a mob marched on a judge in Le Mars, Iowa, who had refused to suspend foreclosure proceedings, and nearly lynched him. The Farmer's Holiday Association, the most radical of the farmers' groups, renewed its threat of a farm strike. Alarmed by the rising agrarian wrath, the governor of Iowa called out the national guard and placed half a dozen counties under martial law.

Those developments speeded passage of the Agricultural Adjustment Act on May 12. It established the Agricultural Adjustment Administration and opened the New Deal's campaign to raise farm income. The first task was to cut down production in areas already overwhelmed by surpluses. Thus a carry-over from previous years of 8 million bales of cotton had driven cotton prices down to 5 cents a pound. Yet, by the time the act had passed, some 40 million acres had already been planted in new cotton. The only way to save the cotton-growers was to persuade them to plow under the planted crop in return for benefit payments. This the AAA proceeded to do in a whirlwind plow-up campaign of some 10 million acres in the spring and summer. Acting on the recommendation of the Farm Bureau and the Grange, the AAA dealt with the market glut in corn and hogs by buying and slaughtering some 5 million little pigs.

No one perceived more sharply the irony of destroying plenty in the midst of want than the men who ordered the job to be done. "To destroy a standing crop goes against the soundest instincts of human nature," said Henry Wallace. Yet industry, the Secretary of Agriculture pointed out, had in effect plowed under much of its potential output after 1929 by cutting down on production; how, in all logic, could agriculture be denied the same right of self-protection?

The terrible logic of scarcity worked. As production declined—aided, in the cases of wheat and corn, by the searing droughts of 1933–34—prices rose. Between 1932 and 1936 gross farm income increased by 50 percent, and cash receipts from marketing (including government benefit payments) nearly doubled. The parity ratio rose from 55 in 1932 to 90 in 1936. The chief beneficiaries were commercial farmers, owners of large holdings and recipients of a disproportionate share of benefit payments. Many owners of family-sized farms also benefited, though tenant farmers and share-croppers suffered (see p. 688). Their champions were forced out of the AAA which in other respects conducted its complex administrative operations effectively.

Planning for industry. Agricultural planning covered only the lesser part of the American economy. By 1933 American industry was employing some 5 million fewer workers than in 1929 and producing less than half the value of goods. Businessmen, striving to maintain a margin of profits, saw no choice but to cut

costs—that is, to lower wages and lay off employees. But the more wages and employment were reduced, the more mass purchasing power declined.

There was increasing agreement that the only way to stop the industrial decline was through joint planning by government and business. This view was backed not just by Tugwell, with his belief in public management of the economy, and by Johnson, with his memory of the War Industries Board. Powerful voices in business, especially the United States Chamber of Commerce, now urged that private trade associations be given authority to fix prices, divide markets, and "stabilize" industrial production. Recovery, they argued, depended on limiting the play of what Johnson called "the murderous doctrine of savage and wolfish individualism."

In the spring the Administration worked out its national-industrial-recovery bill, divided into two parts. The first part was designed "to promote the organization of industry for the purpose of cooperative action among trade groups" through codes of fair competition that granted exemption from the antitrust laws. An important provision—the celebrated Section 7a—sought to win labor support by offering federal guarantees of the right of trade unions to organize and bargain collectively. The second part of the bill provided for the establishment of a Public Works Administration with an appropriation of $3.3 billion. Roosevelt signed the bill on June 16, calling it "a challenge to industry, which has long insisted that, given the right to act in unison, it could do much for the general good which has hitherto been unlawful. From today it has that right."

Two agencies were set up under the National Industrial Recovery Act—the National Recovery Administration, with General Johnson as head, and the Public Works Administration under Harold L. Ickes. Johnson saw the NRA as a national crusade designed to restore employment and regenerate industry in an excitement of torchlight processions and giant rallies. Finding the negotiation of codes with specific industries disappointingly slow, Johnson came up in July with the idea of a "blanket code" in which cooperating employers would pledge themselves to observe NRA standards on minimum wages and maximum hours. The Blue Eagle, modeled on the Indian thunderbird, became the symbol of compliance. Briefly, in the revivalist atmosphere conjured up by Johnson, the Blue Eagle soared. Two million employers accepted the blanket code, and the great industries of the country began to accept special codes.

Protected from competition by those codes, managers were able to stop cutting prices and with them wages. But the codes also protected marginal firms that might best have been allowed to fail, as well as strong firms that could have produced at a profit at

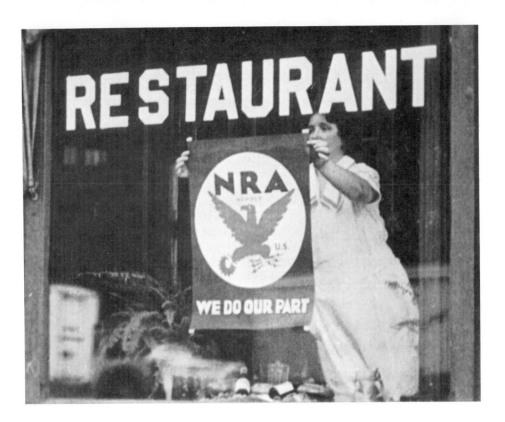

prices lower than those that tended to obtain. Further the codes decreased the probability of investment in new, improved facilities. Yet new capital investment would have helped to stimulate the overall economy.

Those liabilities were balanced in part by the attempts of the NRA to pursue some of the long-term objectives of American reformers. In the economic field, it hoped to bring about permanent reemployment by raising wages and shortening working hours. In the social field, it sought the abolition of child labor, an improvement of working conditions, an encouragement of labor organization, an extension of fair-trade practices.

Soon the NRA began to overextend its efforts. Instead of concentrating on codification in the major industries, it allowed itself to be tempted into setting up codes for local and service trades. There was good humanitarian reason for this effort, for these were the trades where the sweatshop was most deeply entrenched. But it involved the NRA in a host of petty enforcement problems, which at once distracted its energies and dissipated its credit. Johnson was reluctant to use the NRA's coercive powers, since he wanted to avoid a court test of the NRA's constitutionality. Consequently his chief reliance against those whom he denounced as "chiselers" was the compulsion of public opinion. So long as the nation felt itself in acute crisis, this compulsion worked. But as soon as economic conditions began to grow better, more and more employers tried to beat the codes.

Within the NRA, moreover, there was constant pressure from trade associations to use the code mechanism as a means of raising prices. Many businessmen felt that price-fixing would be an appropriate *quid pro quo* for their concessions on wages, hours, and collective bargaining. On the other hand, many inside the NRA and out argued that excessive price increases would defeat the whole policy of expanding purchasing power. They feared that price-fixing would turn the codes into a vehicle for the sort of monopoly Congress had tried to outlaw in the Sherman Act. An investigation by a special committee in 1934 under the chairmanship of Clarence Darrow, the criminal lawyer, seemed to substantiate the charge that the NRA had become the instrument of monopoly.

In the meantime the labor provisions in Section 7a had given a great stimulus to trade-union organization, and this embittered many employers. Hugh Johnson's unstable personality and his increasingly erratic course further complicated the NRA's existence. Roosevelt forced him out in the fall of 1934 and replaced him by a five-man board. By now the NRA had lost its allure. In 1933 nearly everyone had been for giving it a chance. By 1935 most people—except for the trade associations and the trade unions—were against it. When the Supreme Court finally declared the National Industrial Recovery Act unconstitutional in 1935, the Administration accepted the verdict with relief. From the outset it had been seeking other roads to recovery and reform.

If we could have perfect balance among all producing segments—agriculture, capital, industry, workers in industry ... there would be almost no limit to our consuming capacity.... All law, all administration ... should be directed toward that goal.... The essence of the New Deal is to point toward that balance....

That is the reason for NRA, AAA, PWA and all the loan and fiscal acts.... The most obvious, immediate way to erase the effect of the depression on wages and hours was the NRA project to decrease hours ... and to increase wages to maintain purchasing power....

We relied ... on PWA to activate the heavy industries ... and thus increase the total number of available purchasers. We relied on AAA to increase farm purchasing power ... and thus still further add to the number of purchasers. These added to NRA additions would so far increase volume that we thought ... the increased labor cost could be absorbed without much increase in price.... We also relied on the principle ... that many men with a little each is a far better market than one man with much, and all the rest with nothing.

National Planning and the NRA

From Hugh Johnson, *The Blue Eagle from Egg to Earth*, 1935.

The end of the Hundred Days. The AAA and the NRA set the pattern of national planning and were, in this sense, crucial measures of the early New Deal. But they by no means exhausted the achievement of the special session of 1933. During the Hundred Days after March 4, 1933, Roosevelt sent fifteen messages to Congress and saw fifteen major bills through to enactment.

Advocates of inflation, strongest in Congress but vocal also within the executive branch, were eager to relieve the burden of debt contracted when the price level was much higher. Since the closing of the banks and the Economy Act had a deflationary impact, the Administration looked, too, for means to induce a general price increase. Conservative officials, especially Budget Director Douglas, opposed anything that savored of inflation. In contrast, many Southern and Western congressmen demanded either a massive printing of greenbacks or an extensive monetization of silver. Those prospects had broad support among farmers and even some members of the business community. Roosevelt himself had no desire for currency inflation, but he was determined to bring about a rise of prices—not so fast as to absorb the increases in wages and farm income but fast enough to reduce the drag of debt on the economy. It seemed increasingly evident to him that the United States had to choose between the old gold standard and the price-raising policy, and he had no hesitation about the choice. On April 18, 1933, the President determined to abandon the gold standard officially by executive orders authorizing the control of the flow of gold from the United States. In a few weeks Congress confirmed the departure from gold by passing a resolution providing for the abrogation of the gold clause in public and private contracts.

In the meantime, the inflationist amendment to the Agricultural Adjustment Act (see p. 678) had bestowed a variety of monetary powers on the President. He protected the independence of American monetary policy by refusing at the London Economic Conference in July to peg the dollar at a fixed value in international exchange, and, when farm prices sagged in November, Roosevelt, always eager for action, embarked on a program designed to raise the level of prices, especially commodity prices, by Treasury purchases of gold. The program was of doubtful economic validity. But the exercise permitted Roosevelt to retain control of monetary policy at a time when both inflationists and bankers were demanding that he take action that he deemed positively harmful. By January 1934 the experiment had obviously failed to raise prices, but the pressure for inflation had abated. The Administration then stabilized the dollar at $35 for an ounce of gold, 59.06 percent of the pre-1933 gold value. Roosevelt also guided through Congress the Gold Act of 1934, which gave the Treasury large new authority in managing the value of the dollar abroad and the conditions of credit at home.

The gold policy, along with the banking and securities legislation of 1933–34, shifted the financial capital of the nation from Wall Street to Washington. The adventure in inflation and the Treasury's use of its new powers established a continuing policy of "cheap money"—that is, low interest rates. Those low rates made private borrowing more attractive and the financing of government borrowing less expensive. But the inducement to private or public investment proved inadequate, for the private sector still envisaged small opportunities for profit and the Administration still hesitated deliberately to incur heavy deficits. Like planning for industry, inflation and cheap money did not produce recovery. They did establish public authority over an area of economic activity that private power had previously dominated. That authority was expanded by a landmark act of 1935 that amended the Federal Reserve Act of 1913. The earlier statute had left most of the authority over the banking system with the regional Federal Reserve Banks, which were dominated by private bankers. The new law concentrated authority in the Board of Governors of the Federal Reserve System, the public agency in Washington, which now had direct control over the significant instruments affecting the volume of money and credit.

The Securities Act of 1933, a first step toward disciplining the practices of Wall Street, required full disclosure of relevant information in the issuance of new securities, and the Glass-Steagall Act, also of 1933, provided for the separation of commercial and investment banking in order to limit speculation by banks. Legislation in 1934 strengthened the Securities Act, and a further measure of 1935 established the Securities and Exchange Commission to prevent and punish misrepresentation and fraud in the securities business.

Other actions of the Hundred Days were designed at once to help the banks and to reduce the human cost of depression. The House Owners' Loan Act saved countless homes by providing means for the refinancing of mortgages. That refinancing, along with the similar operations of the Farm Credit Administration for agricultural mortgages, protected homes and farms from foreclosure and assisted banks and insurance companies as well. In return for mortgages that were not being paid, those lending institutions received government bonds that they could always convert to cash and on which regular interest payments were assured. Still another New Deal measure, the Federal Deposit Insurance Corporation, set up a system for the insurance of savings and demand deposits and thereby helped restore confidence in the banks. That restoration revealed the New Deal's commitment to saving capitalism while reforming it.

More precedent-breaking was the Federal Emergency Relief Act, which established for the first time a system of federal relief. Under the resourceful direction of Harry L. Hopkins, a New York social worker, the new relief agency rapidly supplied the states with cash for immediate assistance to the indigent unemployed. Hopkins the next winter began to experiment with "work relief"—jobs rather than handouts—a program that pointed toward the policies Congress endorsed in 1935.

Another measure of the Hundred Days linked work relief to the conservation of natural resources. This was the Civilian Conservation Corps, an organization that recruited young men between the ages of eighteen and twenty-five to work in the countryside. CCC camps were set up in all parts of the country, and CCC boys played a useful role in protecting and developing reservoirs, watersheds, forests, and parks. The dust storms of the early thirties, whirling up from the parched and eroded land of the Great Plains, emphasized the need for a revitalized national conservation policy. A "shelterbelt" of trees was planted along the one-hundredth meridian from Canada to Texas; other measures were undertaken to promote

Civilian Conservation Corps at work

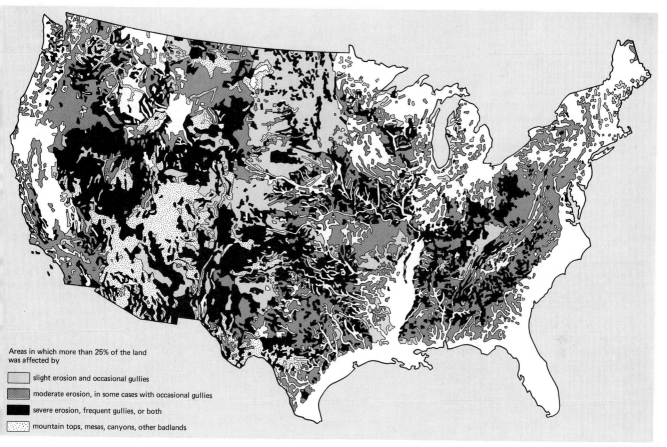

Areas in which more than 25% of the land
was affected by

slight erosion and occasional gullies

moderate erosion, in some cases with occasional gullies

severe erosion, frequent gullies, or both

mountain tops, mesas, canyons, other badlands

The extent of erosion, 1935

reforestation, to control overgrazing, and to encourage farmers to plant soil-improving crops and adopt other soil-conservation practices.

In some respects the most striking innovation of the Hundred Days was an effort to rescue an entire region. The Tennessee Valley was a conspicuous example of what later generations would know as an "underdeveloped" territory. Recurrent floods washed away the topsoil; the forests were thin and overcut; income was less than half the national average; and in the highland counties, over half the families were on relief. Only two out of every hundred farms had electricity. Yet the Valley also contained one of the most valuable power sites in the country, at Muscle Shoals, Alabama; and some people, especially Senator George W. Norris of Nebraska, saw in cheap electric power the means of transforming life in the Valley. But Norris' bills providing for government operation of hydroelectric plants had fallen under the vetoes of Republican Presidents.

Many factors—some opportunities, some problems—converged in the Valley: not only electric power and conservation but fertilizer production, flood control, inland waterways, and, above all, the hopeless cycle of human poverty. In a bold change of

perspective, Roosevelt now saw all these elements as parts of a single problem. The answer, he believed, was not a collection of separate and unrelated reforms but multipurpose development under the direction of a single authority. In April 1933 he called on Congress to establish "a corporation clothed with the power of Government but possessed of the flexibility and initiative of a private enterprise" charged with "national planning for a complete river watershed."

Despite the opposition of the power companies of the area, whose executives claimed that the Valley already had all the power capacity it could absorb for years to come, Congress passed the bill establishing the Tennessee Valley Authority in May 1933. The TVA proved to be one of the most dramatically successful of all New Deal undertakings. Seeking at every opportunity to win local collaboration under TVA director David E. Lilienthal's slogan of "grassroots democracy," the TVA built dams and powerhouses, cleared the rivers, replenished the soil, rebuilt the forests, and brought the magic of electricity into the farthest corners of the Valley. Grassroots democracy in the Valley proved to be for whites only. Without protest from Washington, local agencies working with TVA systematically excluded blacks from participation and benefits. Yet for whites at least the region vibrated with a new life. Soon visitors came from all over the world to inspect the result. No other New Deal agency had such an international impact.

The Struggle for Recovery

The conquest of fear. The Hundred Days induced a tremendous revival of confidence. In this revival the personality of the President himself played a basic role. As late as the 1932 campaign, Franklin Roosevelt had still been a hazy figure. Now his speeches, his radio "fireside chats," his twice-a-week press conferences made him seem almost a constant presence in the homes of Americans. He radiated energy, decision, and good cheer. His superb personal faith, along with the explosion of administrative inventiveness and political audacity in Washington, convinced the people that they had a chance to recover control of their economic destiny.

During 1933 Roosevelt enjoyed almost universal support. As the crisis receded, however, opposition began to emerge—first from the business community on Roosevelt's right, then in a clamor of discordant voices on his left. At the start his critics made little

dent in his popularity. The congressional election of 1934 provided an almost unprecedented national endorsement of the President's program. The Administration actually increased its strength in both the House and the Senate, and the Republicans were left with the governorship of only seven states. Many of the new Democrats came to Congress from urban districts and were especially responsive to labor and welfare concerns.

Critics, right and left. Roosevelt confronted the congressional session of 1935 with top-heavy majorities in both houses, but the policy momentum of 1933 had begun to slacken. Full economic recovery still seemed distant, and the voices of criticism were now speaking out with new confidence. The American Liberty League, an organization formed in 1934 by a group of conservative businessmen and politicians, offered the most active opposition on the right. On the left the most powerful of the new leaders was Huey Long of Louisiana.

As governor of Louisiana, Long had brought new roads and schools and textbooks to the state; but the price of his impressive program of social improvement was spreading corruption and repression. By 1935 he ruled his native state almost as a dictator. In national politics, Long's role was more that of a demagogue. His "Share Our Wealth" movement, which stressed heavy

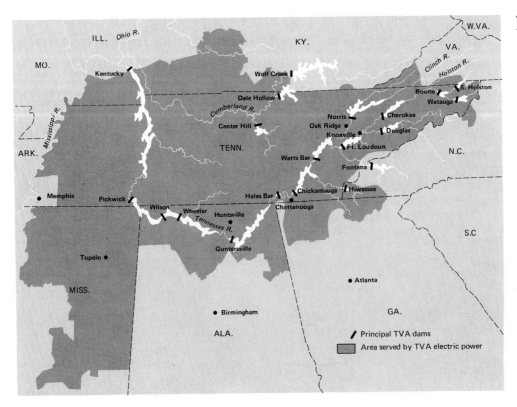

The Tennessee Valley Authority

Principal TVA dams

Area served by TVA electric power

The Liberty League and the New Deal

taxation of the rich and large handouts to the poor, reminded Americans of the need for social justice. But Long used his program primarily as a means of stirring existing resentments in the hope that the Kingfish, as Long fondly called himself, could be propelled into the Presidency.

Another rising leader was a California physician, Dr. Francis E. Townsend, who proposed a two-hundred-dollar monthly pension for all those over sixty who were to spend the money in the month they received it in order, so the theory went, to boost the economy. The aged had suffered deeply from the depression, and the Townsend Plan seemed for a while in 1935 to be developing genuine mass support. Both Long and Townsend were openly hostile to the New Deal. A third leader, Father Charles E. Coughlin, the famous "radio priest" of Royal Oak, Michigan, had originally endorsed Roosevelt but by 1935 was drifting into opposition. He established in that year the National Union for Social Justice, an organization that appealed especially to the nativist and inflationist traditions of the Middle West and to Irish-Catholics of the great cities. Coughlin's particular nostrum was the nationalization of the banks.

Long, Townsend, and Coughlin were hawking competing patent medicines for the nation's economic ills. But they drew their following from much the same audience—baffled and disoriented members of the lower-middle class who were seeking attention and protection. They drew, too, from rural Americans, many of them now removed to the cities, who resented the impersonality and unfamiliarity of industrialism and urbanism, and who neither understood nor accepted the nature of the modern industrial state. The emergence of the new movements signified a discontent that the President could not ignore.

Stalemate in 1935. Though the policies of the Hundred Days had ended despair, they had not produced recovery. The gross national product, though nearly $20 billion larger than in 1933, was still $30 billion less than in 1929. Four million more workers were employed in 1935 than in 1933, but 9 million were still unemployed. Roosevelt was still in economic trouble

Huey Long: "share our wealth"

In determining how far the federal government may go in controlling intrastate transactions upon the ground that they "affect" interstate commerce, there is a necessary and well-established distinction between direct and indirect effects. The precise line can be drawn only as individual cases arise, but the distinction is clear in principle....

If the commerce clause were construed to reach all enterprises and transactions which could be said to have an indirect effect upon interstate commerce, the federal authority would embrace practically all the activities of the people and the authority of the state over its domestic concerns would exist only by suffrance of the federal government....

There would be virtually no limit to the federal power, and for all practical purposes we should have a completely centralized government. We must consider the provisions here in question in the light of this distinction.

The question of chief importance relates to the provisions of the code as to the hours and wages of those employed.... It is plain that these requirements are imposed in order to govern the details of defendants' management of their local business. The persons employed ... are not employed in interstate commerce. Their wages have no direct relation to interstate commerce....

The authority of the federal government may not be pushed to such an extreme.

From the Majority Opinion of the United States Supreme Court by Chief Justice Charles E. Hughes, Schechter v. United States, 295 U.S. 495, 1935.

and, as the clamor of the demagogues and the fractiousness of the new Congress made clear, might well be in increasing political trouble. He needed a new forward thrust of policy if he was to maintain his control.

The Supreme Court further increased the pressure against the policies of 1933. For two years the Administration had delayed tests of the constitutionality of New Deal legislation, but now the dam was breaking. Early in 1935 the Court invalidated a provision of the National Industrial Recovery Act prohibiting interstate shipment of "hot" oil—that is, oil produced in violation of production quotas fixed by state laws. A few weeks later, the gold resolution of 1933, one of the foundations of the nation's monetary policy, barely escaped judicial veto in a bitter and somewhat ambiguous five to four decision. Then the Court, in another five to four decision, declared against the whole idea of a federal pension act for railroad employees. And on May 27, 1935, the celebrated "Black Monday" of New Deal annals, the Court in three sweeping decisions killed a farm-mortgage-relief act, rebuked the President for what it declared to be an illegal exercise of his removal power, and condemned the entire National Industrial Recovery Act as unconstitutional.

The NRA case, irreverently known as the "sick chicken" case, involved some Brooklyn poultry-dealers, the Schechter brothers, who had been charged with violations of the Live Poultry Code. The Court pronounced unanimously against the Recovery Act on two grounds: that it delegated excessive powers to the executive and that it ascribed to Congress powers of economic regulation that could not be justified under the commerce clause. This second objection was particularly devastating. The language used in the decision seemed to say that the Court regarded mining, manufacturing, agriculture, and construction as "essentially local" activities. In a press conference a few days later Roosevelt concluded, "We have been relegated to the horse-and-buggy definition of interstate commerce."

New directions in policy. In invalidating the NRA, the Supreme Court knocked out the keystone of the early New Deal experiment in national planning. The Court's action came at a time when Roosevelt himself was perhaps losing faith in the efficacy of national planning and when the New Dealers most identified with the planning idea were beginning to lose their political usefulness. Roosevelt, always the activist, turned to those best prepared to offer him a convinc-

The scope of congressional power: a broader view

From the Majority Opinion of the United States Supreme Court by Chief Justice Charles E. Hughes, National Labor Relations Board v. Jones and Laughlin Steel Corporation, 301 U.S. 1, 1937.

ing program of action. He found this program in the Brandeis-Frankfurter group (see p. 676).

During the Hundred Days, that group had played a subordinate role except in their influence on bank-ing and securities legislation. They disapproved of the NRA, both of the philosophy on which it was based and the program of national planning to which it led. In 1935 the group moved to the forefront. It influ-enced both the President and his program for that year. In a message to Congress on June 19, 1935, the President committed himself to the view that "with-out . . . small enterprises our competitive economic society would cease. Size begets monopoly." Roosevelt moved equivocally along the new lines, but the mounting hostility of business and the Court's con-demnation of the NRA pushed him on.

With the revival of Roosevelt's leadership, the 1935 session broke the log jam that had blocked action for months. The result was a stunning program of legislative achievement. A $4.8 billion relief bill had already passed in April. It gave Harry Hopkins the authority and some of the appropriations he had been seeking to establish the Works Progress Administra-tion and thus to pursue his belief that the solution for aid to the unemployed lay in work relief. Though his new program led to a small amount of made work,

known invidiously as "boondoggling," it also built roads, airports, and schools, improved parks and wa-terways, produced plays and concerts, maps and guidebooks, and sustained the morale and preserved the skills of millions of Americans unable through no fault of their own to find private employment. Where Hopkins' WPA specialized in light public works, Ickes' Public Works Administration, which shared the $4.8 billion, concentrated on heavy and durable proj-ects, ranging from dams and bridges to irrigation proj-ects and aircraft-carriers. The activities of the PWA not only gave some stimulation, albeit inadequate, to the national economy but permanently improved the national estate in many ways.

Meanwhile the elimination of the NRA had cre-ated an urgent need for new laws continuing elements of the NRA program. Thus the Wagner Labor Rela-tions Act, to which the President now gave his sup-port, replaced Section 7a of the National Industrial Recovery Act. The act outlawed unfair labor prac-tices, including the firing or blacklisting of employees for union activities. It also established the National Labor Relations Board to enforce its provisions, which provided more reliable guarantees for collective bar-gaining. The Public Contracts Act applied NRA wage and hour standards to firms doing business with the

Displaced agricultural workers

federal government. The Guffey Coal Act tried to put the NRA Coal Code into constitutional form. No one could be sure whether these laws would survive the Supreme Court, though they had been drawn up to avoid the more obvious defects of the National Industrial Recovery Act.

The defects of the Agricultural Adjustment Act also needed remedy. The crop limitation and support programs of the AAA operated to the disadvantage of tenant farmers and sharecroppers, especially in the South. Owners of the land they tilled took much of

that land out of cultivation in order to qualify for federal subsidies. The displaced tenants and croppers either drifted to the cities, where they had difficulty finding employment, or became migrant agricultural workers who followed the harvest from place to place. The dust storms of the Great Plains were forcing small farmers there to join the migration, primarily toward California. The poverty both of the migrants and of the croppers, who remained near starvation on the land where they had grown up, contrasted with the growing prosperity of the large landowners, the chief beneficiaries of the AAA. In 1935 Roosevelt first addressed the problem by establishing the Resettlement Administration, financed by part of the $4.8 billion relief appropriation. The RA was to rehabilitate tenants and small farmers, establish cooperative farm communities, and resettle farm families existing on submarginal land. The program never received adequate funds from Congress, as the President's Committee on Farm Tenancy reported in 1937. That report, an encyclopedia of agricultural distress, provoked Congress to reorganize the RA as the Farm Security Administration to provide financial help for tenants hoping to become landowners, to refinance small farmers, and to assist migratory workers. The new program assured many of the neediest farmers of federal aid, though never on the scale that the largest landowners enjoyed.

Works Progress Administration: light public works

Most important for the future, the Congress passed in August 1935 the Social Security Act, setting up the Social Security Board to operate both a national plan of contributory old-age and survivors insurance and a federal-state plan of unemployment compensation. Both programs, though at first limited in their coverage, provided the men and women they affected with a measure of protection against hazards and vicissitudes beyond their control. They started the government toward a permanent and inclusive system of social welfare. In addition, the Social Security Act, along with other measures of the session, helped further to consolidate a political alliance between the New Deal and organized labor.

Other acts of the 1935 session were designed to restore competition to the economy. The Public Utilities Holding Company Act limited each holding company after 1938 to a single integrated public-utility system unless it could make a convincing economic case for holding more than one system. The tax law of 1935, with its increased surtaxes and estate taxes and its substitution of a graduated for a uniform corporation income tax, sought to discriminate in favor of small business and the small taxpayer. The tax act of 1936, deeply resented by business, made an attempt to force management to distribute most corporate profits to shareholders. Once distributed, those profits would be subject to the high personal surtax rates. Most important, the forced distribution of profits would reduce the power of management and enhance the options of shareholders who might spend their larger incomes or seek alternative investments. Still another tax act in 1937 aimed to close the loopholes through which Andrew Mellon, Alfred Sloan, the du Ponts, and other rich Americans had been escaping taxes.

The New Deal's revenue acts fell short of their purpose. With the economy still lagging, the increased tax rates did not yield their potential revenue, nor did they effect their social objectives. Further, the states continued to rely upon sales taxes and other inequitable devices. Yet with the return of full employment after 1940, the revenue measures at last had their intended, progressive impact.

The philosophy of the New Deal.   Alike in its earlier and later emphases, the New Deal strove continuously for both economic recovery and social reform. The focus of policy shifted partly as a consequence of the change in national mood between 1933 and 1935. The desperation of 1933 seemed to demand sweeping economic measures; at the same time, it produced a large measure of political unity. The partial recovery of 1935 increased political disunity and decreased the desire for centralized economic control. By 1935 the New Deal had abandoned its early adventures in inflation. More important, while the New Deal had at first

Dust storm

Organized enterprise is obtaining an increasingly large proportion not only of national income, but of all savings and of all wealth.... Within the corporate structure itself the concentration is progressing....

This amazing concentration of the corporate ownership of wealth has been accompanied by a similar concentration of dividend distribution. The great and powerful business organizations which dominate the economic scene are owned by a numerically insignificant proportion of the total population.... Less than 1% of all American corporate stockholders are the beneficiaries of one-half of all the dividends paid in this country....

As the concentration proceeds, the flow turns away from organized business to government.... The inevitable and inescapable result of continued concentration in big business is the final triumph of big government....

If we are agreed ... that we want to preserve free enterprise ... it must be perfectly clear that any remedy that does not stop the steady progress of concentration will be utterly futile and will end only in an all-powerful government....

The only remedy to save a democratic economy is to be found in making the economy democratic.

From Senator Joseph C. O'Mahoney in *Final Report ... of the Temporary National Economic Committee*, 1941.

accepted the logic of the administered market and tried to devise new institutions to do what competition had once done to keep the economy in balance, the New Deal by 1935 was stressing a more competitive market and a more egalitarian distribution of income, wealth, and private power. It was politically more radical. Earlier the New Deal had sought government-business cooperation to achieve national objectives. Now the New Deal, persuaded that equitable competition could be restored only through rigorous government enforcement of the rules of the competitive game, was zestfully antibusiness in rhetoric. If "a concentration of private power without equal in history" was the great menace to the American economy, as Roosevelt told Congress in 1938, then the way out was a program "to stop the progress of collectivism in business and turn business back to the democratic competitive order." His basic thesis, Roosevelt said, was "not that the system of free enterprise for profit has failed in this generation, but that it has not yet been tried." In 1938 the antimonopoly drive picked up new speed with the appointment of Thurman Arnold as head of the Antitrust Division of the Department of Justice and with the establishment of the Temporary National Economic Committee, headed by Senator Joseph O'Mahoney of Wyoming, to survey the concentration of economic power.

The fight against economic concentration, however, constituted only part of the second phase of the New Deal. A new theory of recovery through the use of the federal budget was beginning to emerge within the Administration. The chief spokesman for this new view was Marriner Eccles of the Federal Reserve Board, who contended that, when the decline of private spending brought about a depression, it was the obligation of government to offset the decline by increasing public spending. Eccles felt that the deliberate creation of compensatory government deficits would stimulate capital formation and purchasing power until the consequent rise in national income produced enough revenue to bring the budget once again into balance. In 1935 these ideas were still tentative and unorthodox, even among New Dealers. The New Deal was spending large sums and was running budgetary deficits (the largest in the prewar years was $4.5 billion, in 1936); but it was doing these things in response to conditions, not to theories. Further, the deficits were too small to spur recovery effectively. In 1936 the English economist John Maynard (later Lord) Keynes gave Eccles' approach its first extended theoretical justification in his influential book *The General Theory of Employment, Interest, and Money*. Many of the younger New Dealers found Keynesian ideas increasingly congenial, and their alliance with the compensatory spenders was decisive in the final evolution of New Deal policies.

The 1936 Election

The estrangement of business. The emergence of big government and big labor in the early thirties meant that the business community no longer enjoyed unchallenged primacy in American society. Resentment over loss of status, resentment over government regulation and taxation, resentment over uncertainty and strain—all these emotions, joined in many cases to a sincere conviction that the New Deal was a first step toward a totalitarian state, gradually produced among many businessmen a state of bitter opposition to Roosevelt's Administration. In alienating those businessmen, the New Deal also discouraged them from new investment, but they had not invested while Hoover cultivated their interests and solicited their confidence. Further, had the New Deal ignored social problems, and had it used taxation not to redistribute income and reform business but instead to provide favors for business, the Administration would have surrendered the social interests of the whole people to the possibility, by no means certain, of a recovery beneficial primarily to the wealthy. Even if recovery had occurred under those conditions, it would have left unaltered the many injustices of American society in the twenties. New Deal social reforms may have involved some short-run economic and political liabilities, but, for the long run, Roosevelt's emphasis was indispensable for preserving democratic possibilities in the United States.

Still the attitude of the Supreme Court seemed to validate the notion of businessmen that the New Deal was using unconstitutional means to achieve unconstitutional objectives. When the Court returned in 1936 to its assault on the New Deal—vetoing the Agricultural Adjustment Act in January, the Guffey Coal Act and the Municipal Bankruptcy Act in May, and a New York minimum-wage law in June—its actions deepened convictions on both sides that an impassable gulf existed between the America of individualism and the America of reform. Hoover denounced the New Deal as an attack on "the whole philosophy of individual liberty." Some conservatives began to trace the New Deal to subversive foreign ideas—to fascism or, more generally and fashionably, to communism. At the height of the holding-company fight, and on occasion thereafter, rumors were even put into circulation that Roosevelt was a madman given to wild bursts of maniacal laughter.

The 1936 campaign. The "hate-Roosevelt" feeling, the conviction that the New Deal represented the end of the American way of life, permeated the conservative wing of the Republican party. Other Republicans, recognizing Roosevelt's popularity and, in many cases, agreeing with his policies, opposed Hoover's notion of making the 1936 campaign an all-out fight against the New Deal. This view prevailed in the Republican convention of 1936. The Republicans nominated Governor Alfred M. Landon of Kansas, a former Bull Moose Progressive, who, while conservative on matters of public finance, had shown himself tolerant of many aspects of the New Deal. Frank Knox, a newspaper-publisher from Chicago, was chosen as Landon's running mate. The Democrats meanwhile renominated Roosevelt and Garner. The forces of Coughlin, Townsend, and Long (Long himself had been assassinated in September 1935) coalesced in the Union party and nominated Congressman William Lemke of North Dakota for the Presidency.

At the start Landon took a moderate line, accepting New Deal objectives but arguing that only the Republican party could achieve them thriftily and constitutionally. In the later stages of the campaign, however, his line became almost indistinguishable from Hoover's. In a moment of last-minute desperation the Republican high command even decided to make an issue of the social-security program, which was due to go into effect on January 1, 1937. The Social Security Act, declared Frank Knox, "puts half the working people of America under federal control." The Republican national chairman said that every worker would have to wear metal dog-tags carrying his social-security number.

Such efforts were unavailing. Roosevelt conducted his campaign in a mood of buoyant confidence. He was aware, however, of the bitterness of feeling against him; and, in indignation over the social-security panic, he gave vent to bitterness of his own. "Never before in all our history have these forces [of selfishness and greed] been so united against one candidate as they stand today," he said. "They are unanimous in their hate for me—and I welcome their hatred." The election revealed that the attacks on Roosevelt had made little impression on the voters. In a victory without previous precedent in American politics, Roosevelt carried every state except Maine and Vermont. The Republicans were routed, and the Union party sank without a trace. In 1936, the celebrated Roosevelt coalition had emerged in its full strength. The coalition of 1936 included the farmers, West and South, who had supported the party in 1916. It included also the city machines and workers of all ethnic origins, most of whom had rallied to Al Smith in 1928. In 1936 increasing numbers of blacks in Northern cities were also voting Democratic, as they had never before. So were reform-minded intellectuals, as they had not consistently since 1916, and so was much of the middle class, its confidence revived since 1932, its debt to the New Deal considerable, and its previous Republicanism in eclipse. Though with continuing shifts of influence and support within it, that coalition was to dominate national elections, especially presidential elections, for a generation.

The Supreme Court Fight

The Court versus the New Deal. Roosevelt opened his second Administration by issuing a vigorous call for an extension of the New Deal. "I see one-third of a nation ill-housed, ill-clad, ill-nourished," he said in his inaugural address. But he faced a formidable roadblock in his determination to push ahead his reform program. That roadblock was the Supreme Court. By the end of its 1936 term the Court had heard nine cases involving New Deal legislation. In seven of those cases a majority of the Court had found the legislation unconstitutional, though three verdicts of unconstitutionality were by the narrow margin of five to four and two more by six to three. In addition, the Court, having in 1923 (*Adkins* v. *Children's Hospital*) denied the federal government power to set minimum wages, had now denied that power to the state of New York, thereby apparently saying that no power existed in the United States to outlaw the sweatshop.

So sustained and devastating a use of the judicial veto to kill social and economic legislation had never before occurred. Moreover, the minority, which in several cases had affirmed its belief in the constitutionality of the disputed laws, comprised by far the more distinguished members of the Court—Louis D. Brandeis, Benjamin N. Cardozo, Harlan F. Stone, and, on occasion, Chief Justice Charles Evans Hughes. "Courts are not the only agency of government that must be assumed to have a capacity to govern," Stone had warned his conservative brethren.

The whole future of the New Deal appeared uncertain. Such laws as the Social Security Act, the Wagner Act, and the Holding Company Act seemed the next candidates for execution by the Court. And, so long as the majority's narrow reading of the Constitution prevailed, there was little chance that the New Deal could take further steps to meet the problems of the forgotten third of a nation. During 1936 Roosevelt and his Attorney General, Homer Cummings of Connecticut, came to feel that, before anything else could be done, something had to be done about the Court. They considered and then dismissed the idea of a constitutional amendment, partly because of the difficulties of the ratification process, partly because the amendment itself would be at the mercy of judicial interpretation. In any case, the trouble seemed to lie, not with the Constitution, which they regarded as a spacious charter of government, but with the Court majority. They concluded that the best solution would be to do something directly about the personnel of the Court.

"Packing" the Supreme Court. In February 1937 Roosevelt sent a message to Congress calling for the reorganization of the federal judiciary. He contended that the Supreme Court could not keep up with its work burden, and that the interests of efficient administration required the appointment of an additional justice for each justice aged seventy or over. The argument about overcrowded dockets was disingenuous and gave the Court plan an air of overslickness from which it never recovered. Chief Justice Hughes was soon able to demonstrate that the Court had, in fact, been keeping abreast of its responsibilities. In two speeches in March, Roosevelt tried to wrench the debate back to the real issue. The Court, he said, had "cast doubts on the ability of the elected Congress to protect us against catastrophe by meeting squarely our modern social and economic conditions." His object was "to save the Constitution from the Court and the Court from itself." But protest against the measure was now too great to be diverted.

Those who had disliked the New Deal from the start found in the Court plan verification of their claim that Roosevelt was trying to destroy the American system. And many who had supported the New Deal were genuinely shocked both by the idea of "packing" the Court and by Roosevelt's circuitous approach to his objective. The proposal set in motion a bitter national debate. In Congress the Republicans held back and allowed dissident Democrats to lead the fight against the President. The measure might have carried with some modifications had not the Court itself suddenly changed its attitude toward New Deal legislation. On March 29, 1937, the Court in effect reversed its decision of 1936 and affirmed the constitutionality of a Washington minimum-wage law. Two weeks later it sustained the Wagner Act. Plainly the Court majority had abandoned the narrow ground of 1935–36; in Robert H. Jackson's phrase, it had retreated to the Constitution. The way had apparently been cleared for the New Deal without the appointment of a single new justice. And the resignation of one of the conservative justices in June, giving the President his first Supreme Court appointment, made his plan of enlarging the Court seem less necessary than ever. The bill was defeated, though Roosevelt could later claim with some justice that if he had lost the battle he had won the war. But the New Deal had lost momentum in Congress, where the Court fight both revealed and widened the rift between reform Democrats and the conservatives in the party.

Social and Economic Crises

The rise of the CIO. The Court battle had struck a blow at Roosevelt's prestige as well as at the unity of the Democratic party. And the surging militance of organized labor was creating new problems. The NRA had given the trade-union movement its first impetus to mass organization since the First World War. Under the leadership of John L. Lewis and the United Mine Workers, a great campaign had begun in 1933 to organize the unorganized in the mass-production industries. This campaign soon led to a major conflict within the labor movement itself. The American Federation of Labor was dominated by craft unions; under the craft theory, the automobile industry, for example, was to be organized, not by a single union, but by as many different unions as there were different crafts involved in making a car. But Lewis, as head of one of the few industrial unions in the AFL, thought instinctively in terms of organization, not by craft, but by industry. Moreover, craft unionism had failed to organize the basic industries, to which industrial unionism seemed peculiarly adapted. The consequence was a fight within the AFL between craft unionism and industrial unionism, culminating in the expulsion of Lewis and his associates in 1936 and their formation of a rival labor federation, the Congress of Industrial Organizations.

The CIO came into existence at a time when workers throughout the country, especially in the mass-production industries, were hungering for organization in unions of their own choosing. The spontaneous character of the labor uprising was shown in 1936 and 1937 by the development of a new strike technique, frowned upon by national labor leadership—the "sit-down strike," in which workers sat down by their machines in factories and refused to work until employers would concede them the right of collective bargaining. To many employers, the sit-down strike threatened property rights and smacked of revolution; its vogue led them to fight all the more savagely against any recognition of industrial unions as bargaining agents.

But the CIO pushed its organizing campaigns ahead vigorously, especially in automobiles and steel. There were shocking moments of violence. In May 1937 police shot and killed ten pickets outside the Republic Steel plant in Chicago. In Detroit, leaders of the United Automobile Workers were brutally beaten by company guards at Henry Ford's River Rouge plant. But the decision of General Motors to negotiate with the UAW in February 1937 and of United States Steel to negotiate with the Steel Workers Organizing Committee in March marked the start of a new era. The battle for collective bargaining was not yet wholly won. But the courage and spirit of working men and women in their determination to gain their rights gave a romance to the labor movement of the time that appealed to many Americans who were not themselves directly involved. Union membership, which had been less than 3 million in 1933 and barely over 4 million at the start of 1937, grew to 7.2 million by the end of the year and to 9 million by 1939.

The recession of 1937–38. The years 1935 and 1936 had been years of slow but steady economic improvement. So marked was the trend that leading bankers began to worry about inflation, though resources and labor were still widely underemployed. Under pressure from the bankers, the Federal Reserve Board tried to put on the brakes by raising interest rates in 1936 and 1937. This action had some effect. But it was less significant in arresting the upward swing than the decline between 1936 and 1937 in the federal government's net contribution to the economy. In 1936 the payment of the veterans' bonus of $1.7 billion on top of relief and public-works expenditures and the normal costs of government resulted in a net federal government contribution of $4.1 billion. In 1937 several factors—the collection of taxes under the Social Security Act as well as the attempt to reduce public spending and to move toward a balanced budget—resulted in a decrease of the net government contribution to $800 million, a drop of $3.3 billion in a single year. Private business spending, contained by the apprehensions of investors, did not fill the gap created by the contraction of public spending.

The collapse in the months after September 1937 was actually more severe than it had been in the first nine months after the crash. National income fell 13 percent, payrolls 35 percent, durable-goods production 50 percent, profits 78 percent. The increase in unemployment reproduced scenes of the early depression and imposed new burdens on the relief agencies.

The recession brought to a head a policy debate within the Administration. One group, led by Henry Morgenthau, Jr., the Secretary of the Treasury, had supported the policy of government retrenchment and favored balancing the budget as soon as practicable. Those steps, they believed, though historical evidence contradicted them, would restore business confidence and lift private investment. Another group, led by Hopkins of the WPA and Eccles of the Federal Reserve Board, urged the immediate resumption of public spending. Economists advising them and like-minded New Dealers could now buttress their case by reference to the theories of J. M. Keynes, which were gradually winning converts in Washington (see p. 690). Roosevelt himself favored for a while the first group; but, as the downward slide speeded up, he reluctantly accepted the necessity for spending. In March 1938 he announced a new spending program. Again too small to achieve its intended results, this program, which included as much as Congress would tolerate, did begin to reverse the decline. It sopped up some unemployment and by 1939 effected a gross national product larger than in 1937. The recession, however, killed Roosevelt's hope of attaining full economic recovery before the end of his second term.

1938 and the purge. The Court fight, the new aggressiveness of organized labor, and the resumption of the spending policy all tended to widen the gap between the liberal and the conservative wings of the Democratic party. The liberals were mostly Northerners, the conservatives mostly Southerners, and other events of 1938 hastened the alienation of the Bourbon Democrats from the New Deal. Southern employers were bitterly opposed to the Administration's Fair Labor Standards (or Wages and Hours) Act, which was passed in June 1938. They objected that its policy of setting minimum wages and maximum hours and outlawing child labor would increase labor costs. Southern planters were equally bitter against the Farm Security Administration and its activities on behalf of tenant farmers and sharecroppers. The release in August 1938 of a government report on economic conditions in the South and Roosevelt's description of the South as "the nation's No. 1 economic problem" seemed to express a determination to extend the New Deal into the South. Conservative Democrats in Congress prepared to resist; and the alliance between Southern Democrats and Northern Republicans, tentatively initiated in 1937 during the Supreme Court fight, began to harden in 1938 into a major obstacle to further New Deal legislation. The House Committee on Un-American Activities, dedicated under the chairmanship of Martin Dies of Texas to the harrying of radicals in and out of government, became an instrument of conservative retaliation against the New Deal.

The defection of the Southern conservatives raised difficult problems for the Administration. Roosevelt felt that many conservative Democrats had taken a free ride on the popularity of the New Deal; their refusal to support liberal policies, in his judgment, served to blur essential distinctions in American politics. "An election cannot give a country a firm sense of direction," he said in June 1938, "if it has two or more national parties which merely have different names but are as alike in their principles and aims as peas in the same pod." Accordingly he decided to make the New Deal itself an issue in the Democratic primary elections. In August he began to intervene personally in state primaries in the hope of replacing anti-New Deal Democratic senators and representatives with liberals. Such intervention was a striking departure from precedent, and his opponents were quick to denounce it as a "purge." The largely unsuccessful result of Roosevelt's efforts was a prelude to Administration setbacks in the general election: the Republicans gained seven seats in the Senate and eighty in the House.

The year 1938 marked the end of the forward thrust of the New Deal. The public demand for reform seemed to be slackening. Congress, now controlled by a conservative coalition, rejected the Administration's Lending Bill of 1939, a measure based on Keynesian principles. By that time the drift toward war in Europe was leading both the President and the people to shift their attention to foreign policy. In his state-of-the-union message in January 1939 Roosevelt had spoken significantly of the need "to invigorate the processes of recovery in order to *preserve* our reforms."

The American People in the Depression

The trauma of depression. The depression had been a severe shock to the American people—to their expectations, their values, and their confidence in themselves and their future. Mute evidence of a declining faith in their prospects was the sudden slowdown of the marriage and birth rates. Population grew at a rate of less than a million a year; the total population increase (to 131.7 million in 1940) was hardly more than half that of the preceding decade. In 1938 there were 1.6 million fewer children under ten than there had been five years before. With the increase in life expectancy (from fifty-six in 1920 to sixty-four in 1940), the proportion of people over sixty-five increased from 5.4 percent in 1930 to 6.9 percent in 1940. In the perspective of depression America began

The South: "the nation's No. 1 economic problem"

1938: the New Deal
was the issue

to look like an aging country, its future limited. The demographic trend led economic theorists to argue that the nation had reached "economic maturity" and could not hope to resume growth without aggressive government intervention.

Americans brought up in the tradition of the bright future and the happy ending found it hard to adjust to bread lines, government relief, and mass unemployment. Some fell into listlessness and apathy. Others, unwilling to concede that the old story had come to an end, flocked behind one or another of the social demagogues with their promises of miraculous deliverance. A few believed that depression was an inherent and ineradicable evil of the capitalist system and concluded that the only way out was to abolish capitalism.

Some of these, excited by the success of fascism in Italy and Germany, formed fascist groups, bearing such names as the Silver Shirts. In a vivid novel, *It Can't Happen Here* (1935), Sinclair Lewis showed how a 100 percent American fascist movement might take over the United States. But, though the American fascists diligently imitated many of the Nazi techniques and appeals (including anti-Semitism), they had little impact on American life.

More of those who despaired of capitalism turned toward Marxism. In 1932 just under a million Americans voted against the capitalist system. Most of the votes went to the Socialist party, a reformist group under the appealing leadership of Norman Thomas; but over one hundred thousand voted for the Communist party ticket. The communist movement, the more serious of the two, was controlled by a hard core of disciplined devotees, faithfully conforming to the turns and twists of the party line laid down in Moscow. Not all those who joined the party, however, were aware of its whole nature. At one time or another during the decade, a large number of people passed rather quickly through the movement, attracted primarily by the apparent idealism of communist promises but soon bored by the sectarian inflexibility of communist analysis or repelled by the ruthless dishonesty of communist performance, especially in Europe. Secret communists had some success in penetrating certain labor unions and even a few government offices, though without significantly influencing American policy.

The shake-up of the people. If depression induced despair, it also compelled change. In particular, it discredited and disrupted the structure of status and prestige that had ruled the United States in the twenties. The businessman had been the culture hero of the prosperity decade. In 1929 his New Era had exploded in his face. In the thirties his pretensions to wisdom were derided, his leadership rejected, and he himself often dismissed as a fool if not a crook. A midget perched impudently on the knee of the mighty J. P. Morgan at a congressional investigation became the symbol of the new skepticism about the wealthy.

People from outside the business community—especially politicians and intellectuals—were now in power. Still smarting from their own sense of inferior status in the twenties, they often took undue pleasure in rubbing the nose of the once-arrogant businessman in the mess he had helped create. And in their wake came a rush for status of the "forgotten men" of America—men who had been denied opportunities in the past because of their class or ethnic origin. The New Deal, by revising the structure of status, brought about profound social changes, including visible gains for previously disadvantaged ethnic groups, that diminished the attractiveness to Americans of radical ideologies.

The social revolution. Organized labor's rise to respectability typified the tendencies of the decade. In 1933 the presidents of the six great steel companies blanched and fled when Secretary of Labor Frances Perkins proposed to introduce them to William Green of the American Federation of Labor for a discussion of the NRA steel code. Four years later, when United States Steel signed up with the CIO, labor had achieved substantial recognition. The business community had reluctantly accepted the right of other groups to participate in national economic decisions. Even though the depression continued to restrict economic opportunity, members of once-marginal groups—not only wage-earners but tenant farmers, sharecroppers, old folks, and even intellectuals and women—now had larger chances for fulfilled lives.

The social revolution also enhanced the quality of life, particularly in the countryside. Though the Supreme Court knocked out the original AAA in 1936, the principle of national responsibility for the agricultural economy was established and reaffirmed in legislation of 1938. No other federal agency had such an impact on the quality of country life as did the Rural Electrification Administration. When it was founded in 1935, only about one farm in ten had power-line electric service, and these were mostly in the neighborhood of towns or cities. Through low-interest loans to cooperatives, the REA enabled farmers to build their own power lines and generate their own electricity. The spread of electricity transformed the countryside. Had distribution been kept in the hands of privately owned utilities, this expansion would not have taken place so quickly.

The ethnic revolution. Immigration substantially stopped in the thirties (except for refugees from fascism toward the end of the decade). The last wave of immigrants, mostly from southern and eastern Europe, in the earlier part of the century had not yet achieved full acceptance in American society; the upheaval of depression gave many Italians, Poles, South Slavs, and Jews their first opportunities. Where craft unions, for example, had often discriminated against the "wops" and the "hunkies," as against the blacks, the industrial unions of the CIO opened their doors to them. Similarly the New Deal gave them their first chance in politics and public service, as did many of the states, especially those that followed the example of the federal government with their own "little new deals."

Roosevelt himself had no patience with the old American attitude of superiority toward more recent immigrants. "Remember, remember always," he once told the Daughters of the American Revolution, "that all of us, and you and I especially, are descended from immigrants and revolutionists." Of the 214 federal judges appointed by Harding, Coolidge, and Hoover, only 8 were Catholics; of the 196 appointed by Roosevelt, 51 were Catholics. Political figures in the great cities, like Mayor Fiorello La Guardia of New York, acted as brokers in gaining recognition for ethnic minorities previously shut out from political preferment. Concurrently there was a notable decline in the foreign-language press and a more effective acculturation of ethnic minorities into American life.

Most striking of all, perhaps, was the rise in expectations of American blacks, for many years the victims of economic and political neglect. During the depression, the Negro was, in the phrase of the day, "the first man fired and the last man hired." And, though blacks had voted Republican since the Civil War, the Republican administrations had shown little concern for their welfare; black leaders had denounced Hoover as "the man in the lily-White House." Roosevelt brought to Washington an unprecedented sympathy for black problems. New Deal agencies generally conformed to local folkways that perpetuated segregation and discrimination within the CCC and in the distribution of work relief in the South, for two of many examples. But the New Dealers appointed many able blacks to senior administrative positions from which they were able not only to symbolize new opportunities for their race but to mount programs to assist their fellows. Roosevelt himself repeatedly denounced lynching, though he would not provide direct support to the Northern Democrats in the Senate who took the initiative in sponsoring bills to make lynching a federal crime. The New Deal did far less for American blacks than their circumstances warranted, but it did far more than had any administration since Reconstruction. By 1936 black voters had begun to shift to the Democratic party.

The American Indians also had a new champion in Washington, John Collier, the Administration's Commissioner of Indian Affairs. Collier, an experienced social worker, had long believed in the importance of preserving the cultural heritage of immigrant groups and of solving the social problems of poverty by community cooperation. Those concepts underlay his work as founder and guiding spirit of the American Indian Defense Association. In 1933, with the support of Secretary of the Interior Ickes, Collier began directly to influence federal policy. During his years in office, he forbade discrimination against Indian religious ceremonies, introduced instruction in Indian languages and culture in schools on reservations, doubled the proportion of Native Americans employed by his agency, and moved millions of dollars of New Deal funds into improving the Indian landed estate. The Indian Reorganization Act of 1934 explicitly recognized the right of Indians to organize "for the purpose of local self-government and economic enterprise," committed the federal government to promoting "the study of Indian civilization," created a special Court of Indian Affairs to remove Indians from the jurisdiction of the states, and perhaps most important, abandoned the division of Indian lands into individual parcels—the discredited policy of the Dawes Severalty Act of 1887 (see p. 438)—and pledged the government to a constructive program of Indian land use. Collier's sympathetic and creative management of Indian affairs did not outlast the New Deal, but he started the

John Collier: new champion of the American Indians

Eleanor Roosevelt and WPA workers

nation toward a belated rectification of centuries of injustice.

New Deal policies also mitigated, though they did not eliminate, discrimination against women. As they had during the 1920s, so during the 1930s educated women confronted formidable obstacles to entering the professions. A much larger number of women than ever before needed industrial or clerical employment in order to support themselves or to help support their families. Yet with the onset of depression, employers tended to discharge women before they discharged men, and during the 1930s women found it harder than did men to secure new jobs. Consequently many women dropped out of the working force. Those who remained ordinarily earned less than did men in similar positions and normally received no consideration for promotion to supervisory posts. New Deal policies provided partial remedies for those conditions. First the NRA codes and later the Fair Labor Standards Act at least set minimum wages for women as well as men. The WPA created some jobs for women clerical workers, teachers, and lawyers. And the CIO, flourishing under the New Deal, set out, as the AFL had not, vigorously to recruit women into industrial unions and thus to assure them of the gains obtained through collective bargaining.

The New Deal did succeed in recruiting women voters. The President and particularly his wife encouraged women to work for the Democratic party, as did their friend Molly Dewson, a leader of the National Consumers League. Dewson enlisted thousands of women in the precincts and helped to persuade the Democratic national committee to appoint eight women as vice-chairmen. In 1936 the Democratic convention required each delegate to the platform committee to have an alternate of the opposite sex, a reversal of earlier policy. Dewson also solicited federal patronage for women, who received more postmasterships than ever before and more recognition in major offices—in the Cabinet, where Frances Perkins was Secretary of Labor, on the bench, in executive positions with the WPA. Eleanor Roosevelt, the most visible and influential woman New Dealer, became a national symbol for advocates of social justice. Though feminism as a social movement remained subdued, her spirit heartened all women, workers and intellectuals alike.

The release of energy brought about by the New Deal, the invigorating sense that the "forgotten" man and woman could still make a place for themselves in American life—all this gradually began to heal the trauma of depression. The sense of America as an exhausted nation gave way to the image of a purposeful society capable of meeting its problems with energy and conviction.

In the twenties, the intellectuals who scorned the American present had turned to "debunking" the American past. In the thirties, when the American present was acquiring purpose and dignity, they began to read this purpose and dignity back into American history. The title of John Dos Passos' book *The Ground We Stand On* (1941) summed up the new attitude. "In times of change and danger," Dos Passos wrote, "when there is a quicksand of fear under men's reasoning, a sense of continuity with generations gone before can stretch like a lifeline across the scary present." Other skeptics of the twenties joined Dos Passos in taking a more affirmative view of American traditions. Van Wyck Brooks, who had once seen American culture as pinched and sterile, now portrayed it, in *The Flowering of New England* (1936) and succeeding volumes, as rich and abundant. Even H. L. Mencken, though he took small comfort in the America of the thirties, dedicated his main energies to bringing up to date his loving study of *The American Language* and to writing his own nostalgic recollections of an earlier America. The publication of a number of important biographies helped meet the new national desire to repossess the past in all its solidity. This impulse came into happy conjunction with the New Deal in the valuable series of state guidebooks produced by the WPA.

As never before in American history, the federal government, through the WPA especially, sponsored the arts—not literature only but architecture, the fine arts, music, dance and drama. Hallie Flanagan of Vassar presided over the strikingly successful Federal Theater Project. The plays she and her associates produced—some classics, some powerfully timely—reached thousands of Americans who had never before attended theater. Sponsored or not, much of the art of the time included a strong and self-conscious strain of social criticism. With a critical but constructive urgency artists rejected the mood of inwardness of the 1920s, attacked those like Thornton Wilder and T. S. Eliot who still worked in creative privacy, and often devoted themselves to political causes. Among others, the novelist Mike Gold and the playwright Clifford Odets wrote from the perspective of the far left; Edmund Wilson and James Agee, both less doctrinaire, moved a larger audience toward their causes; Ernest Hemingway moved still more readers with his socially conscious fiction.

The new pattern of American society. The recovery of American faith in the thirties both derived from and contributed to the capacity of the American people to reassert a measure of control over their social and economic destiny. In so doing, American society was countering the prevailing ideologies of the day. Both laissez faire and Marxism were philosophies of economic determinism with narrow views of social possibility. The New Deal, with all its improvisations, contradictions, sentimentalisms, and errors, did have the signal advantage of rejecting economic fatalism and of affirming a faith in intelligent experiment.

By Roosevelt's second term the essential pattern of the new society was complete for his generation. The American nation had renounced laissez faire without embracing socialism. Government had acquired the obligation to underwrite the economic and social health of the nation. The budget provided the means by which the government through the use of fiscal policy could compensate for a decline in private economic activity. The state had abandoned efforts aimed at the direct control of industrial production, but industry had to accept ground rules covering minimum standards of life and labor; and the state continued to intervene to maintain, in modified form, the free play of competition. Special areas of economic activity required more comprehensive government control—banking, transportation, public utilities, agriculture, oil. Human welfare was to be protected through various forms of public insurance. A collection of "built-in stabilizers"—minimum wages, unemployment compensation, farm-price supports, social-security payments—were to help secure the economy against future crashes like that of 1929.

Was the Roosevelt way possible? These measures involved more government intervention in the economy than some had thought the economy could stand and still remain free. This was the critical question raised by the New Deal—whether a policy of limited and piecemeal government intervention in economic life was feasible; whether a mixed system was possible that gave the state power enough to assure economic and social security but still not so much as to create an all-powerful dictatorship or so little independence as to remain uncorrupted by the large influence of powerful industrial, labor, and agricultural groups.

The New Deal especially assisted the American middle class. It protected their savings, homes, and farms. It opened the way to middle-class comforts and status for previously stigmatized ethnic groups and many clerical and blue-collar workers. But the New Deal also knew many failures. It did not achieve recovery. It did not sufficiently redistribute income and wealth, though it proposed more effectual policies than Congress would accept. It did not bring American blacks or women an equitable share in the country's social and economic life. It could not overcome the conservative social and regressive economic policies of most American states. It could not perma-

nently insulate its new regulatory agencies from the tendency of regulators to develop excessive sympathy for those they were supposed to control.

Those failures, clearer in retrospect than at the time, suggested that the particular middle way of the Roosevelt years would later need modifications. But to the question of the viability of any middle way, doctrinaires returned a categorical *no* through the decade. Ogden Mills stated the issue with precision for the conservatives: "We can have a free country or a socialistic one. We cannot have both. Our economic system cannot be half free and half socialistic. . . . There is no middle ground . . . between tyranny and freedom."

Golden Gate Bridge, product of the New Deal: rekindling confidence in America

In such sentiments, at least, the critics of capitalism agreed enthusiastically with the conservatives. "Either the nation must put up with the confusions and miseries of an essentially unregulated capitalism," said a radical weekly in 1935, "or it must prepare to supersede capitalism with socialism. There is no longer a feasible middle course." The proponents of individualism and the proponents of collectivism agreed on this if on nothing else: no regulated capitalism was possible, no mixed economy, no middle way between laissez faire and socialism.

But the New Dealers cheerfully rejected the conclusion. They believed that there was more on heaven and earth than could be found in any ideology. Roosevelt himself was blithe and humane in his undeviating rejection of any all-encompassing doctrine. He might have undertaken social experiments either more or less bold than those he chose. But his aim was consistent—to steer "slightly to the left of center," avoiding alike "the revolution of radicalism and the revolution of conservatism." The New Deal faith in intelligence, compassion, and experiment postulated that a managed capitalist order could combine personal freedom and economic growth. For the generation that lived through it, the decade of the New Deal, with all its confusion and recrimination, rekindled confidence in free society, not in America alone, but throughout the Western world.

Suggestions for Reading

GENERAL

The most comprehensive account of domestic developments, 1933–36, is in A. M. Schlesinger, Jr., *The Coming of the New Deal* (1959) and *The Politics of Upheaval** (1960). W. E. Leuchtenburg, *Franklin D. Roosevelt and the New Deal 1932–40* (1963), provides the best short account. There are valuable insights in J. M. Burns, *Roosevelt: The Lion and the Fox** (1956) and E. W. Hawley, *The New Deal and the Problem of Monopoly** (1966). P. Conkin, *The New Deal** (1967), criticizes Roosevelt and his policies from the point of view of the disenchanted revisionists of the 1960s and 1970s. Compare with J. M. Blum, *The Progressive Presidents** (1980), which is sympathetic. Caroline Bird, *The Invisible Scar* (1965), provides a lively account of the social impact of continuing depression.

MEMOIRS AND BIOGRAPHIES

Memoirs of the New Dealers and biographies based on their papers throw important light on Roosevelt and his problems. R. E. Sherwood, *Roosevelt and Hopkins: An Intimate History* (1948, rev. ed., 1950), provides a view of an important friendship and a favorable account of relief policies. Frances Perkins, *The Roosevelt I Knew* (1946), is significant for its compassion but must be compared with George Martin, *Madam Secretary: Frances Perkins* (1976); see R. G. Tugwell, *The Democratic Roosevelt* (1957) and *The Brain Trust* (1968), for retrospective reflections; *The Secret Diary of Harold L. Ickes*, 3 vols. (1953–54), for its gossip and atmosphere. On politics, two illuminating memoirs are J. A. Farley, *Behind the Ballots* (1938), and Edward Flynn, *You're the Boss* (1947). J. M. Blum, *Roosevelt and Morgenthau* (1970), recounts in detail the activities of the Secretary of the Treasury, one of the President's influential advisers. H. S. Johnson, *The Blue Eagle* (1935), presents a contemporary view of the National Recovery Administration. There is a valuable contemporary critique of the early New Deal in Raymond Moley, *After Seven Years* (1939); this may be supplemented by his retrospective *The First New Deal* (1966). In *Beckoning Frontiers* (1935), M. S. Eccles provides an important account of the evolution of economic policy. Samuel Rosenman writes as a close counselor to the President in his *Working with Roosevelt* (1952). J. J. Hutchmacher, *Senator Robert Wagner and the Rise of American Liberalism* (1968), is a telling study of a leading liberal senator. There is indispensable personal material in Eleanor Roosevelt, *This I Remember* (1949), and in J. P. Lash, *Eleanor and Franklin** (1971). F. Freidel has completed four volumes of his long biography of Roosevelt. Though there is no useful edition of Roosevelt's private papers, one source for study of the man and his times is Samuel Rosenman, ed., *The Public Papers and Addresses of Franklin D. Roosevelt*, 13 vols. (1930–50). Also important is M. Dubofsky and W. Van Tine, *John L. Lewis* (1977).

NEW DEAL POLITICAL THOUGHT

Students wishing to study New Deal political thought in the important works of the time should consult, as the text suggests, at least the following influential sources: A. A. Berle, Jr. and G. C. Means, *The Modern Corporation and Private Property* (1932, rev. ed., 1969), significant on economic concentration as is J. Burnham, *Managerial Revolution** (1941); M. S. Eccles, *Economic Balance and a Balanced Budget* (1940), significant on countercyclical spending; R. G. Tugwell, *The Battle for Democracy* (1935), and H. L. Ickes, *The New Democracy* (1934), both important on social goals and public planning, as is H. A. Wallace, *New Frontiers* (1934); and D. E. Lilienthal, *TVA* (rev. ed., 1953), on regional development. Two incisive books by Thurman Arnold—*The Symbols of Government* (1935) and *The Folklore of Capitalism* (1937)—well express the iconoclastic and deflationary side of the New Deal. For a revisionistic view, see Howard Zinn, ed., *New Deal Thought** (1966).

SPECIAL STUDIES

Outstanding studies of economic problems in the 1930s include the analytical T. Wilson, *Fluctuations in Income and Employment* (1948); K. D. Roose, *Economics of Recession and Revival: An Interpretation of 1937–38* (1954); and R. E. Paul, *Taxation in the United States* (1954). Some of the most useful of more recent works are Irving Bernstein, *Turbulent Years* (1970), which describes the labor movement as in one major case does S. Fine, *Sit-Down: The General Motors Strike of 1936–37* (1969). R. Lekachman, *The Age of Keynes** (1966) discusses the rate and range of acceptance of the ideas of the new economics, as does H. Stein, *The Fiscal Revolution in America** (1969). Significant, too, are R. Kirkendall, *Social Scientists and Farm Politics in the Age of Roosevelt** (1966); J. T. Patterson, *The New Deal and the States: Federalism in Transition* (1969); R. Lubove, *The Struggle for Social Security, 1900–1935* (1968); T. McCraw, *TVA and the Power Fight, 1933–1939* (1970); and M. Parrish, *Securities Regulation and the New Deal* (1970).

Among the stimulating works about social and intellectual currents are R. A. Lawson, *The Failure of Independent Liberalism, 1930–1941* (1971); R. Pells, *Radical Visions and American Dreams: Culture and Social Thought in the Depression Years* (1973); C. Alexander, *Nationalism in American Thought, 1930–1945* (1969); E. Purcell, Jr., *The Crisis of Democratic Theory** (1972); D. Meyer, *The Protestant Search for Social Realism, 1919–1941* (1960); and D. O'Brien, *American Catholics and Social Reform* (1965). For a thoughtful account of the appeal of communism and other radical ideas, see D. Aaron, *Writers on the Left** (1961); R. Crossman, ed., *The God That Failed* (1949); F. A. Warren, *Liberals and Communism: the "Red" Decade Revisited* (1966); I. Howe and L. Coser, *The American Communist Party* (1957); and B. Johnpoll, *Pacifist's Progress* (1970), on Norman Thomas. R. G. Swing, *Forerunners of American Fascism* (1935), offers a contemporary account of the lunatic right, which is modified in A. P. Sindler, *Huey Long's Louisiana* (1956), and D. H. Bennett, *Demagogues in the Depression* (1969), and challenged by T. H. Williams, *Huey Long** (1969) and A. Brinkley, *Voices of Protest** (1982). On the problems of blacks during the 1930s, see B. Sternsher, ed., *The Negro in Depression and War: Prelude to Revolution* (1969); R. Wolters, *Negroes and the Great Depression* (1970); H. Sittloff, *A New Deal for Blacks* (1978); D. T. Carter, *Scottsboro: A Tragedy of the American South** (1969); and J. M. Jones, *Bad Blood* (1981). On women, see William Chafe, cited after Chapter 26.

Samuel Lubell, *The Future of American Politics* (1952), identifies important political changes in the period; also revealing about politics are T. Lowi, *The End of Liberalism** (1969); G. McConnell, *Private Power and American Democracy** (1969); and B. Stave, *The New Deal and the Last Hurrah* (1970). G. Wolfskill, *The Revolt of the Conservatives* (1962), displays the reaction on the right, as does his volume with J. Hudson, *All But the People* (1969). The career of the ablest Republican senator of the era receives admirable treatment in J. T. Patterson, *Mr. Republican, A Biography of Robert A. Taft* (1972). On the Supreme Court fight, especially rewarding studies are R. H. Jackson, *The Struggle for Judiciary Supremacy* (1941); A. T. Mason, *Harlan Fiske Stone* (1956); and M. J. Pusey, *Charles Evans Hughes*, 2 vols. (1951). The same subject is treated by one of the masters of constitutional history, E. S. Corwin, in his *Twilight of the Supreme Court* (1934), *Court over Constitution* (1938), and *Constitutional Revolution, Ltd.* (rev. ed., 1946).

*Available in a paperback edition.

28
THE DECAY OF
THE PEACE

When Franklin D. Roosevelt became President, the American people were absorbed in gloomy domestic problems. The crusading internationalism of 1917 was a distant, and for most a distasteful, memory. The rejection of the League of Nations had been followed by growing disenchantment about the motives and results of the First World War; and the renewed American determination to go it alone in world affairs was only slightly tempered during the twenties by such symbolic gestures as the Kellogg-Briand pact and the Stimson Doctrine. Though the Republican Administrations sought to enlarge world markets for American products, they simultaneously undercut the policy of commercial expansion by raising tariffs and thereby denying foreign nations the opportunity to earn dollars for the purchase of American goods. After 1929 depression intensified tariff warfare and economic nationalism in both the United States and Europe. By 1933 isolationism, both political and economic, was the dominant American mood.

There were more and more signs, however, that the uneasy peace established after the First World War was in jeopardy. Japanese expansionism in East Asia was accompanied by German militancy in Europe. On January 30, 1933, Adolf Hitler became the new chancellor of Germany. In March, nineteen days after Roosevelt's inauguration, the Reichstag gave the Nazi leader dictatorial powers to carry forward his program of rearmament, anti-Semitism, and messianic nation-

alism. The German *Führer*'s fanatical resolve to overthrow the system established at Versailles in 1919 offered an ominous challenge to international order.

Roosevelt and World Affairs

Preparation for statesmanship. Few American politicians could rival Roosevelt in the breadth of his world experience. Between 1885 and 1931 he had made thirteen trips to Europe, and, though he had never visited the Far East, family tradition—his maternal grandfather had been active in the China trade—gave him a lively interest in Asia and especially in China. He had come of age when the United States, under Theodore Roosevelt, was first beginning to exercise the responsibilities of world power. As a young man, he was also greatly influenced by the strategic ideas of Admiral Alfred T. Mahan.

His service under Woodrow Wilson as Assistant Secretary of the Navy provided him varied experience in international affairs. He quickly perceived the catastrophic implications of the events of the summer of 1914. The young Roosevelt then made no secret of his desire to build up American naval power or of his passionate belief in the Allied cause. The war also placed his principles of strategy in a new setting. To Mahan's realism, Roosevelt now added Wilson's ide-

Hitler addressing the Reichstag

alism: the combination defined his own future approach to foreign affairs. He retained his sharp concern with the actualities of national power but now saw power in the context of international order.

During the twenties Roosevelt opposed the drift toward isolationism, condemned the Republican tariff policy, derided the pretensions of the Kellogg pact, and pleaded the case for international collaboration. But, as depression accentuated the isolationist mood, he announced in 1932 that in existing circumstances he no longer favored American participation in the League.

The Roosevelt style in foreign policy. Nevertheless Roosevelt named as Secretary of State Cordell Hull, an unregenerate Wilsonian and low-tariff man. "In pure theory," he once wrote Hull, "you and I think alike but every once in a while we have to modify principle to meet a hard and disagreeable fact!"

Roosevelt was far more ready than Hull to modify principle. Toward the State Department itself, the President's attitude was one of disdain. He instinctively understood the problems of military as of political leaders, but he was often impatient with the professional diplomat. Foreign-service officers, he tended to believe, represented a narrow social group and knew little of American life.

This attitude molded his own style in foreign affairs. His conduct of foreign policy was marked by imagination and also a certain dilettantism. He remained the brilliant amateur, better in the main than the professionals, bolder, more creative, more compelling, but often deficient in steadiness and follow-through. He tended toward personal diplomacy and used his own agents and emissaries to bypass the professionals. His basic preference, not always realizable in practice in these early years, was for direct negotiation among heads of state.

Uniting the Western Hemisphere

The good neighbor. "In the field of world policy," Roosevelt said in one of the scant references to foreign affairs in his inaugural address, "I would dedicate this Nation to the policy of the good neighbor—the neighbor who resolutely respects himself and, because he does so, respects the rights of others—the neighbor who respects his obligations and respects the sanctity of his agreements in and with a world of neighbors." Though this thought was evidently intended to be general in its import, its immediate sphere of application was Latin America. Soon the Good Neighbor

policy came to refer specifically to United States policy in the Western Hemisphere.

During the twenties Roosevelt and others of his generation, among them his old friend Sumner Welles, a former diplomat, had become critical of the policy of intervention. Yet, Roosevelt's Latin American policy got off to an ambiguous start. Welles went to Cuba as ambassador to get rid of the brutal Machado dictatorship. The dislodgment of Machado, however, eventually brought into power a revolutionary government that the United States declined to recognize. In response to the American attitude, a conservative regime received recognition. Though Roosevelt at the same time speeded up plans for withdrawing the marines from Haiti, Latin Americans in the fall of 1933 were suspicious of Washington.

From Montevideo to Buenos Aires. In that atmosphere the Seventh International Conference of American States met at Montevideo in December 1933. The United States, reversing its policy of five years before in Havana, now accepted (with minor qualifications) a proposal declaring that "no state has the right to intervene in the internal or external affairs of another." The Montevideo Conference, by establishing inter-American relations on the principle of nonintervention, much improved hemispheric relations.

The United States proceeded to show that it meant to live up to its Montevideo pledge. In May 1934 it abrogated the unpopular Platt Amendment, thereby abandoning its treaty right to intervene in the affairs of Cuba, but retaining the naval base at Guantanamo Bay. In 1934 in El Salvador, it abandoned the policy of nonrecognition of revolutionary governments in Central America. The establishment of the Export-Import Bank the same year provided a means of extending credit to Latin American states. The Panama Treaties of 1936 renounced the right to intervene in Panama and recognized Panama's joint responsibility in the operation and protection of the canal. A treaty of 1940 terminated United States financial controls in the Dominican Republic.

Relations with Mexico provided a test of the new policy. The hostility of the radical Mexican government toward the Roman Catholic Church in the early thirties had produced demands in the United States that Washington intervene in Mexico. The expropriation of foreign-owned petroleum companies renewed this pressure in 1938. Washington declined to intervene, however, confining its activities to urging the Mexican government to provide American owners their due compensation. A State Department memorandum of 1939 summed up the new attitude: "Our national interests as a whole far outweigh those of the petroleum companies."

Those national interests, in the State Department's interpretation, included increased trade with and investment in Latin America. Both the reciprocal trade treaties with Latin American states and the activities of the Export-Import Bank furthered those objectives. For Roosevelt, however, political considerations outweighed economic. As he understood, the friendship and cooperation of the Latin American states had strategic significance for the defense of the western hemisphere.

His policies by 1940 had inspired confidence throughout the hemisphere in the reality of the Good Neighbor policy. By December 1936, when Roosevelt himself attended the Inter-American Conference at Buenos Aires, the warmth of his reception attested 'to growing Latin American confidence in the colossus of the north.

Early Relations with Europe

The London Economic Conference. American relations with European nations had been bedeviled since 1919 by the question of war debts. Beset by depression, most European nations, except for Finland, began to suspend payment in 1933. War debts thereafter became a dead issue—except to the United States Congress, which retaliated in 1934 by passing the Johnson Act prohibiting loans to defaulting governments.

From the European viewpoint, war debts were only a part of the larger problem of world economic relations. Governments everywhere were building walls of protection in the hope of defending their national economies against the worldwide decline. Economic nationalism took more than one form. The Hoover version was nationalist in trade, internationalist in finance: Hoover thus advocated raising the protective tariff to new levels and at the same time argued that recovery depended on the restoration of a world gold standard. In this belief, he agreed to United States participation in an international economic conference favored by the gold-bloc nations and scheduled for London in the spring of 1933.

Roosevelt and the early New Dealers, on the other hand, though they recognized that the depression was worldwide, believed that recovery was to be achieved primarily through domestic planning. "I shall spare no effort to restore world trade by international economic readjustments," the new President said in his inaugural address, "but the emergency at home cannot wait on that accomplishment." The New Dealers consequently mistrusted the international gold standard as a threat to national programs for recovery. Yet, unlike Hoover, they rejected the steeply protective tariff, favoring instead the system of reciprocal trade agreements, which Hoover assailed in 1932 as "a violation of American principles." The Roosevelt version of economic nationalism was internationalist in trade by 1934, and from the first nationalist in finance.

When the London Economic Conference opened in June 1933, it became evident that the gold bloc, led by France and Italy, was determined to force through an agreement stabilizing foreign exchanges. By now the American government was fully committed to its program of raising commodity prices through reducing the value of the dollar in terms of gold—a policy obviously incompatible with immediate stabilization of the dollar in terms of an international gold standard. Roosevelt declined to subordinate his domestic policy to international stabilization. This view emerged only gradually in the course of the conference. Meanwhile the antics of an odd American delegation had dissipated American influence in London. As the gold bloc continued to press for stabilization, Roosevelt, in what he conceived as an effort to recall the conference to more fruitful topics, sent a testy message scolding the conference for succumbing to the "old fetishes of the so-called international bankers." Though some Englishmen, among them J. M. Keynes, defended Roosevelt, the "bombshell" message precipitated the unsuccessful end of the conference.

During the next several years, the financial policies of the great powers reflected the mutual suspicions that the London Conference had intensified. But in 1936, with the American economy much improved and the dollar again fixed, in practice, in terms of gold, Roosevelt permitted the negotiation of a stabilization agreement with Great Britain and France. The President was moved to that decision also by his hope for closer political relationships with those democratic countries. The new agreement, to which other European democracies soon adhered, called for consultation and cooperation among the treasuries of the signatories to manage the value of their currencies in their common interest.

Liberalizing American trade. Roosevelt made it clear that his opposition to the international gold standard did not mean that he believed in economic self-containment. In March 1934 he asked Congress for authority to enter into commercial agreements with foreign nations and to revise tariff rates in accordance with such agreements up to 50 percent either way. This proposal for the executive negotiation of reciprocal trade agreements raised a storm of opposition, partly because some members of Congress—and the protectionist lobbies—objected to the weakening of the congressional role in tariff-making, partly

I was thirty-six years old when in my maiden address in Congress I pleaded for lower tariffs and fewer trade restrictions. I was sixty-two years old when in 1934 we finally won the right to reduce them.... I never ceased attempting ... to keep alive and advance my economics and peace policy....

In 1929 the United States' share of the world's foreign trade had been 13.8 percent; by 1933 it had fallen to 9.9 percent. All our exports had declined appreciably; some disastrously....

Over and above the economic side ... but closely tied in with it ... hung the political side. To me it seemed virtually impossible to develop friendly relations with other nations in the political sphere so long as we provoked their animosity in the economic sphere. How could we promote peace with them while waging war on them commercially ... following the passage of the ... high-tariff Act [of 1930]....

My associates and I ... agreed that we should try to secure ... bilateral trade agreements....

War did come, despite the trade agreements. But ... war did not break out between the United States and any country with which we had been able to negotiate a trade agreement.

From Cordell Hull, *Memoirs*, 1948.

---

because businessmen feared the new system would result in lower rates. Only two Republicans supported the bill in the House, only three in the Senate. But with Hull's devoted backing, the bill became law in June 1934.

By the end of 1935, reciprocal trade agreements were in effect with fourteen countries; by 1945, with twenty-nine countries. While the program did little in the thirties to relieve the balance-of-payments problem between the United States and foreign countries (indeed debts owed to the United States grew steadily during the thirties), it did display Hull's hope of bringing about a large measure of economic internationalism with attending gains for American trade.

Disarmament. In an effort to compose matters after the breakup of the London Economic Conference, Roosevelt wrote to Ramsay MacDonald, the British prime minister, "I am concerned by events in Germany, for I feel that an insane rush to further armaments in Continental Europe is infinitely more dangerous than any number of squabbles over gold or stabilization or tariffs." From an early point—earlier, indeed, than any European statesman of comparable rank—Roosevelt was convinced that Hitler meant war. Yet, while he saw the approaching horror with clarity, he also saw it with aloofness. This was partly the result of geography, which conferred on the United States the luxury of detachment; partly the result of politics, for Roosevelt had little choice but to defer to the isolationist preferences of the vast major-

ity of the people; partly the result of the depression, which gave the American domestic scene first claim on his attention.

The combination of concern and aloofness produced a basic contradiction in the heart of his foreign policy. Roosevelt addressed himself to two problems: first, how to stop the world drift toward war; and, second, if that drift proved irresistible, how to make sure that the United States would not be involved. Plainly the goals of international peace and national isolation—of world disarmament and American neutrality—were in latent conflict. World disarmament implied American cooperation in a world system. Rigid neutrality implied a systematic reduction of America's international commitments. In 1933 and 1934 the tension between these two ideas complicated the conduct of America's foreign policy.

Disarmament had been a major theme of foreign affairs in the twenties, though efforts to work out formulas for land armaments had proved unsuccessful. A new disarmament conference, beginning in Geneva in 1932, had bogged down because of Germany's demand for equality in armed strength, which was impossible to reconcile with the insistence of other nations, especially France, on having reliable protection against a possible recurrence of German aggression.

The replacement of the Weimar Republic by the Nazi regime gave the German demand for equality an ominous cast. In May 1933 Roosevelt authorized the American representative at Geneva to say that, if a substantial reduction of armaments was effected by international agreement, the United States was prepared to consult with the other states in case of a threat to peace. If the other states identified an aggressor and took measures against aggression, the United States, if it concurred in their judgment, would "refrain from any action tending to defeat such collective effort which these states may thus make to restore peace." In other words, the United States would forgo its traditional insistence on neutral rights, including the freedom of the seas, in the interest of supporting measures of collective security. But, when the Administration asked Congress to pass a resolution authorizing the executive at his discretion to embargo arms shipments to aggressor nations, the Senate Foreign Relations Committee amended the resolution to compel the President to embargo arms shipments to *all* nations involved in a war. This amendment destroyed the original purpose of the resolution, which was to discriminate against aggressors. Its effect would now be to strengthen those who had arms already and to abandon those who had none.

The Administration tried in vain to defeat the amendment. Failing, it dropped the resolution itself, thereby canceling the effect of the American initiative at Geneva. What the President had proposed, the Congress had now disowned. The episode confirmed the skepticism in European chancelleries over the seriousness of American diplomacy.

Even congressional approval of the arms embargo would probably not have saved the Geneva conference. Hitler, hell-bent on rearmament, was committed to a revolt against the entire Versailles system. When Germany walked out of the League in October 1933, land disarmament was dead. And the withdrawal of Japan from the League in 1933 and the Japanese decision in 1934 to terminate the Washington Naval Treaty signaled the end of naval disarmament. By 1934 the hope of averting war through disarmament had gone.

The American government had been prepared to cooperate in the supervision of a disarmed world. It was not prepared to cooperate in keeping the peace at the risk of war in a world intent on rearmament. Since disarmament had failed, the alternative, in the American view, was neutrality.

Relations with Great Britain and the Soviet Union.

The collapse of disarmament was accompanied by a deterioration in American relations with the leading anti-Hitler powers. Roosevelt's bombshell message had exasperated London, and the policies of the British government exasperated Washington. An important faction in the British Cabinet, led by Neville Chamberlain, the chancellor of the exchequer, so

deeply distrusted the United States that in 1934 it seriously considered whether Britain should base its strategy on cooperation with Japan instead of with the United States. In that event, Roosevelt warned the British, the United States would endeavor to link its security with that of Canada, Australia, and New Zealand.

The Japanese themselves soon took care of the problem by presenting the British with rearmament demands so extreme that even the pro-Tokyo Cabinet members had to abandon their policy.

Roosevelt's efforts to establish friendly relations with the Soviet Union were hardly more successful. Support for the recognition of the communist regime had been growing for some time before 1933. Businessmen saw in Russia a market for American surplus production. The renewal of Japanese aggression argued for a normalization of Soviet-American relations

Hitler meant war

Maxim Litvinov and Cordell Hull

as a means of restraining the Japanese. "The world," Cordell Hull told Roosevelt, "is moving into a dangerous period both in Europe and in Asia. Russia could be a great help in stabilizing this situation."

In October 1933 Maxim Litvinov, the Soviet commissar for foreign affairs, came to Washington to work out a set of agreements. In one document Litvinov gave a detailed pledge to refrain from any intervention in American internal affairs—a pledge that covered not only the Soviet government itself but any organizations "under its direct or indirect control." Another memorandum provided what seemed to be a formula for the settlement of Russian debts to the United States. The discussions concluded in the establishment of formal relations between the two governments.

Despite this beginning, relations soon returned to a state of mistrust. The attempt to make the Soviet government live up to its promises on propaganda and debts led to interminable negotiation, recrimination, and frustration. American representatives in Moscow encountered harassment and hostility. Finally, when American communists went to Moscow in July 1935 for the seventh congress of the Comintern, their presence seemed, in the view of the American ambassador, to constitute "a flagrant violation of Litvinov's pledge" and a justification for the severance of diplo-

matic ties. Though the government did not go that far, relations with Soviet Russia reached a new low less than two years after recognition.

Isolationism at Flood Tide

The rout of the internationalists. The breakdown of attempts to strengthen relations with Britain and the Soviet Union coincided with a crystallization of isolationist sentiment in the United States. By the early 1930s, few Americans were prepared to make an all-out defense of Wilson's decision of 1917. "Revisionist" historians had launched a reconsideration of such problems as German "war guilt" and American entry into the war. Their scholarship seemed to reveal the war as a sordid scramble among imperialist powers. If this was so, then the United States had been drawn into the war under false pretenses.

The next question was: Who had drawn the United States in and why? The new disillusion was clinched in 1934 and 1935 by the work of a Senate committee set up under the chairmanship of Gerald P. Nye of North Dakota to investigate the munitions industry. The Nye Committee unearthed a wealth of documentation purporting to show that the United States had been shoved into war when international bankers, especially the House of Morgan, saw no other way to guarantee repayment of the vast credits they had granted to the western Allies. To demonstrate that no President could be trusted with discretionary power in matters of war and peace, Nye charged Wilson with duplicity in pretending to be ignorant of the secret treaties.

The Nye Committee consolidated the isolationist argument. The isolationists could conceive of no world war that would present a moral issue between the antagonists or a strategic threat to American security. They were also convinced that American freedom could not survive participation in another holocaust. America's best contribution to peace and democracy, in their judgment, lay in absolute rejection of the power struggles of Europe and Asia.

Roosevelt was quickly to learn the new power of organized isolationism. In January 1935, a short time after the stunning Democratic victory in the 1934 elections, he sent the Senate a recommendation that the United States join the World Court. "At this period in international relationships," he said, "when every act is of moment to the future of world peace, the United States has an opportunity once more to throw its weight into the scale in favor of peace." Joining the World Court could hardly have been a more innocuous act, but the isolationist bloc staged an extraordinary appeal to public opinion, and an outpouring of protest defeated the resolution. Roosevelt wrote to Henry Stimson, "These are not normal times . . . people are jumpy. . . . This is so in every other country as well as our own. . . . We shall go through a period of non-cooperation in everything . . . for the next year or two."

The design of neutrality. The next problem, as Nye, Arthur Vandenberg, and their Nye Committee colleagues saw it, was to make sure the forces that had brought about American participation in the First World War would never have their way again.

If the United States had been drawn into that war to ensure the repayment of debts owed to American bankers and munitions-makers, then to keep out of war it would be necessary to forbid loans and the export of arms to belligerents. If the United States had been drawn into that war because American ships carried supplies to belligerent nations or because American citizens insisted on traveling on belligerent ships, then to keep out of war such actions should be prohibited. If the United States had been drawn into war by the unneutral decisions of a President with too much discretion in the conduct of foreign policy, then the President should be denied the opportunity to tamper with neutrality.

The Administration, yielding to isolationist pressure, agreed that the President should have authority to prohibit American ships from carrying arms and munitions, to withdraw the protection of the government from Americans traveling on belligerent vessels, and to impose an embargo on arms and loans. But the Administration wanted the President to be able to use these powers at his discretion. The senators, with the image of the perfidious Wilson in their mind, wanted to make it mandatory that he use them against *all* belligerents—which would, of course, nullify American influence in the case of conflict. In the end the Senate passed a mandatory bill, the House a discretionary bill. The resulting compromise of August 31, 1935, contained a mandatory arms embargo but made it good only until March 1, 1936. In other respects—such as American travel on belligerent vessels—the bill gave the President discretion. The Administration decided to accept the measure rather than risk further exacerbation of isolationist sentiment through a veto. On signing the act, Roosevelt warned that "the inflexible provisions . . . might have exactly the opposite effect from that which was intended."

Neutrality on Test

Italy invades Ethiopia. Early in October 1935 Italian troops invaded Ethiopia from Eritrea and Ital-

ian Somaliland. In his message to Congress in January 1936, Roosevelt indicted nations that had the "fantastic conception that they, and they alone, are chosen to fulfill a mission and that all the others among the billion and a half of human beings in the world must and shall learn from them and be subject to them." At the same time, he issued a proclamation of neutrality and invoked the mandatory arms embargo.

The supposition in Washington was that the embargo would hurt Italy more than Ethiopia, since Ethiopia lacked dollars to buy arms in the United States and ships to carry them away. Actually the arms embargo did Italy little initial harm, since it had its own munitions industry. Where the restriction of American exports really could hurt the Italian warmaking capacity was in raw materials, especially in oil. But the Neutrality Act covered only implements of war. Roosevelt accordingly followed up the arms embargo with a call for a voluntary restriction of other exports. This action initiated the experiment in what became known as the "moral embargo."

The moral embargo aroused the protests of the Italian government as well as of American oil companies, and moral suasion did not turn out to be effective. Oil shipments to Italy were 600 percent larger in August and September 1935 than they had been for the same two months in 1934. Nevertheless, the American policy preceded by many weeks any comparable action by the League, and it strengthened the hands of those in Geneva contending for economic sanctions against Italy. The League decision was finally taken in a limited way (not including oil, for example) on November 18, 1935.

When Congress convened in 1936, one of its first tasks was to replace the neutrality resolution of 1935. The Administration tried to increase the presidential role in the management of neutrality, but in the end it seemed simpler to extend the existing act until May 1, 1937, with an amendment banning credits to belligerents. One apparently minor change did increase executive discretion; it was now up to the President to decide that a state of war existed before the act could be invoked.

The outbreak of civil war in Spain on July 17, 1936, deepened Roosevelt's sense of a general European disintegration. In a speech four weeks later, he set forth with earnestness his hatred of war, his commitment to neutrality, and his determination to resist the forces that might draw the United States into another world conflict. His private correspondence reflected a belief that somehow a conference among heads of state might avert the drift to Armageddon; but he found no formula that offered any promise of success and thus took no action.

The attempt of Spanish fascists under General Francisco Franco to overthrow the democratic government of Spain created new problems. The mandatory embargo applied to wars between nations, not to civil wars. Early in January 1937, Congress, with Roosevelt's full support and with but one negative vote in both houses, enacted a resolution aligning the United States with Britain and France in a program of nonintervention and in banning shipments of implements of war to either side in Spain. Neutral in intention, the resolution in fact helped Franco, for he received far more military assistance from Italy and Germany than his opponents received from the Soviet Union.

Then Congress faced once again the question of renewing or rewriting the existing neutrality legislation. The main innovation in the 1937 debate was the so-called cash-and-carry proposal, which provided that, once the President had proclaimed the existence of a state of war, no nonmilitary goods could be shipped to a belligerent until the purchaser acquired full title and took them away itself. The Administration supported this idea in order to head off a drive for an automatic embargo on all goods. Ironically, the amendment would clearly have the unneutral effect of favoring the maritime powers, notably Britain and Japan, and of closing American markets to nations like Germany and China. Nevertheless, Congress adopted the provision by sweeping majorities.

Aggression in the Far East

The problem of China. For many Americans the problems of Europe had come to seem more remote, or at least less America's business, than the problems of the Far East. As far back as the announcement of the Open Door doctrine, the United States had conceived of itself as playing a direct role in the affairs of East Asia. By the First World War Washington had concluded that the great threat to the Open Door would come from Japan. Both the Washington Naval Conference and the Stimson Doctrine were designed to restrain Tokyo's imperial aspirations.

In addition, years of missionary endeavor had given many Americans warm sympathy with China in its struggle for nationhood. Roosevelt, who shared this sympathy, himself endorsed the Stimson Doctrine. Then the Tangku truce of May 1933 suspended hostilities between China and Japan. But in April 1934, Eiji Amau, spokesman for the Japanese foreign office, demanded for Japan a free hand in China and warned the West against coming to China's assistance. Soon Japan denounced the Five-Power Treaty.

Those developments confronted the United States with perplexing problems. Some historians have argued that the American motive was to secure markets and investment outlets in China for American capitalism. But American trade with China was negligible, and American investment there far below British. Similarly, American economic interests in the Philippines yielded to domestic economic interests when Congress in 1934 again enacted legislation providing for the independence of the islands after a period of transition. Japan was the most profitable American market in Asia. Nor was the tendency of the Roosevelt Administration to carry out the desires of the business community ever marked. What concerned Roosevelt was the Japanese challenge to international order—the fear that, if aggression ran on with impunity, the peace system would collapse and war might engulf the United States. The preservation of that system therefore seemed a vital American interest. In addition, an expanding Japan could deny the United States strategic materials, like natural rubber, that were essential to national security and prosperity.

But what could America do? To the State Department, the cornerstone in a containment policy had to be the buildup of the United States navy. So long as America remained weak in Asian waters, Cordell Hull reasoned, any attempt to oppose the Japanese or to help the Chinese would be pinpricks that would serve only to provoke Tokyo unnecessarily. Naval superiority became not only the indispensable condition for a future American policy in East Asia but a powerful argument against present action. Thus the State Department generally opposed proposals to condemn Japan or aid China.

The renewal of Japanese aggression. In the meantime, the Chinese, under the leadership of Chiang Kai-shek (Jiang Jieshi), were making progress toward the unification of their nation. Perhaps wishing to halt the process before it went too far, the Japanese used troop clashes at the Marco Polo Bridge in July 1937 as an excuse for an invasion of China. By the end of the month, Japanese soldiers had seized Peking (Beijing) and Tientsin (Tianjin). The subsequent bombing of Shanghai by Japanese planes and the sack of Nanking (Nanjing) in December horrified Americans. The Chinese retreated to the interior, established their capital at Chungking (Chongqing), and prepared to keep up their resistance.

Popular sympathy in the United States was wholly with the Chinese, but official reaction was cautious. Britain and America warded off Chinese pressure for invocation of the Nine-Power Treaty (see p. 623) and instead allowed the matter to go to the League for perfunctory condemnation. The President, however, displayed his solicitude for the Chinese cause by refusing to proclaim the existence of a state of war between China and Japan. Without such a

Japanese attack Tientsin

proclamation, the arms embargo and the cash-and-carry provision for nonmilitary commodities would not go into effect. Most observers felt that these provisions would hurt China, which had to import implements of war, more than they would Japan, which had ample stockpiles and a productive capacity of its own. Between July and November 1937 the value of licensed munitions shipments to China was $86 million; to Japan, $1.5 million. Moreover, an arms embargo could not cut off what Japan needed most—oil and scrap metal. And cash-and-carry would favor Japan as a solvent customer and naval power.

Awakening the Nation

The quarantine speech. The disintegration of the peace system promised to loose war upon the world—a war contemporaries believed would be vastly more destructive than the war of 1914–18. Moreover, as the peace system collapsed, Nazi Germany might well seize control of the power and re-

sources of Europe. Roosevelt regarded that prospect as a mortal threat to the security of the United States. Fearing the strategic consequences of Nazi expansion, detesting Nazi anti-Semitism and the tyrannical Nazi ideology, American leaders watched Hitler with increasing anxiety. Roosevelt even proposed a personal meeting with Neville Chamberlain, now British prime minister. But Chamberlain had no confidence in the United States—"it is always best and safest," he said in 1937, "to count on nothing from the Americans but words"—and he dedicated himself instead to the hope of making Hitler reasonable through a program of appeasement.

The renewal of warfare in China heightened the sense of international urgency. It also turned Roosevelt's attention to an idea that had been in the back of his mind for many years—the deterrence of aggression by holding over potential aggressors the threat (as he had put it in a "Plan to Preserve World Peace," written for a prize competition in 1923) of "the severance of all trade or financial relations, and the prohibition of all intercourse." Carrying his campaign to alert the nation to the heart of American isolationism, Roosevelt, in a speech at Chicago in October 1937,

F. D. R.: the contagion of war

It seems to be unfortunately true that the epidemic of world lawlessness is spreading.

When an epidemic of physical disease starts to spread, the community approves and joins in a quarantine of the patients in order to protect the health of the community against the spread of the disease....

War is a contagion, whether it be declared or undeclared. It can engulf states and peoples remote from the original scene of hostilities. We are determined to keep out of war, yet we cannot insure ourselves against the disastrous effects of war and the dangers of involvement. We are adopting such measures as will minimize our risk of involvement, but we cannot have complete protection in a world of disorder in which confidence and security have broken down....

Most important of all, the will for peace on the part of peace-loving nations must express itself to the end that nations that may be tempted to violate their agreements and the rights of others will desist from such a course. There must be positive endeavors to preserve peace.

From Franklin D. Roosevelt, Speech at Chicago, October 1937.

declared that "the present reign of terror and international lawlessness" had reached a stage "where the very foundations of civilization are seriously threatened." If aggression continued, he said, "let no one imagine America will escape." In a cryptic passage, he compared "the epidemic of world lawlessness" to an epidemic of physical disease and advocated a "quarantine" to protect the community against the contagion.

Aftermath of the quarantine speech. Roosevelt's main purpose was undoubtedly educational: he wanted to awaken the nation to the dangers of world war. A secondary purpose was very likely to explore the readiness of the American people to support some form of boycott of aggressors—moral, diplomatic, perhaps economic.

In the international sphere, the quarantine speech encouraged the British to call the signatories of the Nine-Power Treaty to a conference at Brussels to deal with the new Sino-Japanese conflict. But first the British sent word to Washington that they could do nothing about imposing sanctions against Japan unless they received "assurance of military support" in the event of Japanese retaliation. Roosevelt declined to give such guarantees; the British declined to act without them; and the Brussels Conference came to nothing.

In the meantime, Under Secretary of State Sumner Welles suggested that Roosevelt follow up his quarantine speech by convening a conference of neutral nations to set forth a peace program based on certain standards of international behavior. But Chamberlain, absorbed in the appeasement policy,

rejected the American initiative on the ground that it ran the danger of "cutting across our efforts here." Winston Churchill later wrote that Chamberlain's decision was "the loss of the last frail chance to save the world from tyranny otherwise than by war."

Within the United States opinion about the quarantine speech was mixed, but the organized reaction was so unfavorable that the President at a press conference seemed to retreat from what he had said. Further, most Americans, while sharing Roosevelt's detestation of dictators, detested war even more. When Japanese planes sank the American gunboat *Panay* in the Yangtze River (Chang Jiang) in December 1937, the nation accepted Japanese apologies and indemnification with relief. Interest was rising in a constitutional amendment offered by Congressman Louis Ludlow of Indiana proposing that declarations of war be subject to popular referendum except in case of invasion. The country, moreover, was sinking into an economic recession, and the Administration needed congressional support for its new recovery program. The quarantine idea, vague enough at best, now perished between American reluctance and British indifference.

The Road to War

The end of appeasement. In 1936 German troops moved into the Rhineland. In March 1938 Germany invaded and annexed Austria. Roosevelt invited thirty-two countries to set up a joint committee to facilitate the emigration of persecuted Jews from Germany and Austria, but neither the United States nor any other nation was willing to provide an adequate asylum. The President did arrange for some 15,000 refugees on visitors permits to remain in the United States, but he did not combat congressional and public opinion that opposed any relaxation of the immigration quotas. Among the Jews who reached America were eminent scholars in every field of learning who made striking contributions not only to scientific endeavor but also to national culture.

In the months after he swallowed Austria, Hitler began to use the plight of the German minority in the

Aggressions leading to the Second World War in Europe

Rushing toward climax: Hitler in Czechoslovakia, 1939

Sudetenland as a pretext for demands on the government of Czechoslovakia.

As the Czech crisis deepened in September, Chamberlain requested a personal conference with Hitler. There followed a series of meetings attended by Hitler and Chamberlain, and ultimately Prime Minister Daladier of France and Mussolini. No representatives of Czechoslovakia were present. In the interval between the talks at Godesberg (September 23) and those at Munich (September 29), when it seemed as if Chamberlain was standing firm against Hitler, Roosevelt sent him an encouraging cable ("GOOD MAN") and brought pressure on Hitler to resume negotiations. But at the Munich meeting—where the Soviet Union was excluded, to the dismay of the Kremlin—the democratic powers swallowed Hitler's terms. Czechoslovakia had no choice other than to acquiesce bitterly in the German annexation of the Sudetenland.

The first reaction in the United States was one of relief: the appeasement policy seemed to have averted war. But soon people began to compute the price of appeasement: not just the establishment of German hegemony in Central Europe, but the incentive offered everywhere to intimidation and aggression.

Rearmament. During the 1920s the regular army had fallen well below the size authorized by the National Defense Act of 1920 and the navy below the levels permitted by the various international agreements. When Roosevelt came into office in 1933, the army ranked seventeenth in the world in active strength. From the start of his Administration, he had tried to rebuild American military and naval power. Thus the Public Works Administration constructed cruisers and aircraft-carriers; and in 1935 Congress authorized the army to increase its enlisted strength. In a message to Congress in January 1938 Roosevelt called for larger defense appropriations. In May Congress passed the Naval Expansion Act. In the months after Munich, Roosevelt requested further increases in the defense budget and encouraged British and French purchasing missions to place defense orders in the United States.

In other respects Roosevelt began to tighten his ship in preparation for storms ahead. Following the failure of his "purge" in 1938 (see p. 694), he moved toward a tacit political truce, moderating his liberal objectives in the hope of gaining support for his foreign and defense policies. He also gathered support in the American hemisphere. In December 1938 in the Declaration of Lima, the American republics announced their collective determination to resist fascist threats to peace.

The Neutrality Act remained the greatest obstacle to a positive policy. In 1939, as the Munich settlement seemed to be growing increasingly unstable, Roosevelt considered how he might modify the neutrality system in order to make American aid available to democratic nations. Hitler's invasion of Czechoslovakia on March 15, 1939, persuaded even Neville Chamberlain of the bankruptcy of appeasement. The State Department denounced Germany's "wanton lawlessness," and the Administration stepped up its campaign for the modification of the arms embargo. As Cordell Hull put it, the law "plays into the hands of those nations which have taken the lead in building up their fighting power. It works directly against the interests of the peace-loving nations." But isolationist senators, confident there would be no war in 1939, insisted that the matter be laid over to the next session of Congress.

In Europe events rushed toward climax. The invasion of Czechoslovakia was followed by the German occupation of Memel (March 23), the collapse of the Spanish Republic (March 28), and the Italian invasion of Albania (April 7). Through the summer Hitler carried on a war of nerves against Poland, using a German minority in Danzig as his tool. In the meantime his emissaries were secretly negotiating a nonaggression pact with the Soviet Union. On August 23 the German-Russian pact was signed in Moscow. The next day Britain and Poland signed a pact of mutual assistance. On September 1 Germany attacked Poland. Two days later Britain and France declared war on Germany. The Second World War was under way.

America and the War

First reactions. "When peace has been broken anywhere," Roosevelt said in a fireside chat on the evening of September 3, 1939, 'the peace of all countries everywhere is in danger." He reaffirmed his determination "to use every effort" to keep war out of America. But, in marked contrast to Wilson's appeal in 1914 that his countrymen be "neutral in fact as well as in name," he added that he could not ask that "every American remain neutral in thought. . . . Even a neutral cannot be asked to close his mind or his conscience." When he issued the proclamation of neutrality, he also indicated that he would call Congress into special session in order to repeal the arms embargo.

The isolationist leaders in the Senate, backed by former President Hoover and by such national figures as Colonel Charles A. Lindbergh, as well as by the American Communist party (following the Soviet-Nazi pact), declared that Roosevelt's course was leading straight to war. The opposition was strong enough to compel the Administration to accept restrictive compromises in exchange for the elimination of the embargo. The neutrality-revision bill then passed Congress, and the President signed it on November 4, 1939. The law placed the arms trade on a cash-and-carry basis. Where the previous legislation had favored Germany, with its well-established war industries, the new law enabled Britain and France to buy war materials in the United States so long as they were willing to pay cash and to carry their purchases away in their own ships.

Meanwhile the Nazi air force and Panzer divisions had subdued Poland in a three-week campaign. The French and British had been able to do little to create a diversion on the western front, and the war settled into an aspect of apparent quiescence that won it the derisive name of "the phony war." While opinion polls showed an overwhelming public preference in America for the western Allies against Germany (in October 1939, 62 percent of the population favored all possible aid to the Allies short of war), less than 30 percent favored American entry into the war even if Britain and France were in danger of defeat.

American emotions were perhaps more engaged when the Soviet Union, having advanced into eastern Poland in September, moved into the small Baltic republics of Latvia, Estonia, and Lithuania in October and invaded Finland in late November. The American people, remembering Finnish punctiliousness in the payment of war debts, grew indignant over the onslaught on the "gallant little Finns." Roosevelt sharply condemned "this dreadful rape." Isolationists, however, were alert not to let emotion over Finland drag the nation closer toward war. The Administration's cautious program of aid to Finland encountered strong opposition in Congress and had hardly gone into effect when the Winter War came to an end in March 1940.

Blitzkrieg. Hitler was already preparing the blow that he hoped would break the will of his western antagonists. On April 9, 1940, Germany attacked Denmark and Norway. An Anglo-French attempt to land forces in Norway miscarried, and by the end of the month Norwegian resistance was broken. Popular discontent in Britain over the Chamberlain government now forced Chamberlain to resign, and Winston Churchill, who had long criticized the appeasement policy and, after the outbreak of war, had served as first lord of the admiralty, became prime minister.

A savage air war: London in flames

Chamberlain was in the course of resigning on May 10 when Nazi mechanized divisions invaded the Netherlands, Belgium, and Luxembourg. In a week they were thrusting deep into northern France. The British and French were unable to cope with the speed of the German attack. The main part of the British forces retreated to Dunkirk, where they were evacuated, along with some French forces, across the English Channel by a heroic flotilla of small boats conjured up from British ports. In a few days Italy, joining the war, invaded France from the south. "The hand that held the dagger," Roosevelt said grimly, "has struck it into the back of its neighbor." Soon Paris fell, Marshal Pétain became head of the French government, and on June 22 France and Germany signed an armistice at Compiègne. The next day, from London, General Charles de Gaulle, then an obscure and lonely figure, pledged continued French resistance.

The success of the Nazi blitzkrieg had a stunning effect on American opinion. Citing "the almost incredible events of the past two weeks," Roosevelt asked Congress for more than a billion dollars in additional defense appropriations. He called in particular for the annual production of fifty thousand warplanes. He also set up a National Defense Advisory Commission to plan defense production. And he began to consider how he could aid Britain, now standing alone against the Berlin-Rome Axis. Churchill's rise to power ended the glumness that had marked Anglo-American relations during the Chamberlain period. Roosevelt, who had for some months exchanged letters with the new prime minister, recognized him as a man of congenial temperament and stature. When Churchill offered his own people nothing but "blood, toil, tears and sweat," when he prom-

ised to "wage war by sea, land and air, with all our might and with all the strength that God can give us," he made a profound appeal to the American imagination.

But Britain needed more than sympathy. On May 15 Churchill sent Roosevelt a long list of specific requirements, including old destroyers, new aircraft, and materials of war. For the moment Washington could do little, partly because of America's own defense needs, partly (as in the case of the destroyers) because Roosevelt feared that congressional assent would not be forthcoming. After Dunkirk the American government did scrape together small arms and ammunition for the British to use in the desperate eventuality of a German invasion. But the problems of American policy were now further complicated by the approach of the 1940 presidential campaign.

The Election of 1940

The third term. The struggle between isolationists and interventionists cut across party lines. Roosevelt found some of the most effective supporters of his foreign policy in the ranks of internationalist Republicans—a fact he acknowledged in June 1940, when he appointed Henry L. Stimson of New York as Secretary of War and Frank Knox of Illinois as Secretary of the Navy. However, the basic sentiment of the Republican party, especially in Congress, was isolationist. When the Republicans gathered in Philadelphia to select a presidential candidate, they read Stimson and Knox out of the party and prepared to choose between two candidates, Senator Robert A. Taft of Ohio and Thomas E. Dewey of New York, both identified with isolationism though neither held the rigid views of Senator Nye.

The Republican regulars did not allow for the enthusiasm with which a group of internationalists rallied support for a dark-horse candidate, Wendell L. Willkie of Indiana. Willkie, an affable and articulate businessman, had magnetic qualities of personality that justified the title of "the rich man's Roosevelt." As president of Commonwealth & Southern, a leading public-utilities holding company, Willkie had won attention as an antagonist of the New Deal during the fight over the Tennessee Valley Authority. Actually he had been a Democrat himself most of his life; his personal views and values were on the liberal side; and, most critically of all in 1940, he sympathized with the Roosevelt policy of aid to Great Britain. To general astonishment, the Willkie forces staged a blitzkrieg of their own at Philadelphia, and the former Democrat emerged as the Republican candidate.

As for the Democrats, Roosevelt had failed, whether through design or negligence, to develop an heir apparent. For many months ardent New Dealers had demanded that he stand himself for a third term. Conservative Democrats, led by Vice President Garner and Postmaster General Farley, sought to organize opposition on the ground that a third term would violate a sacred American tradition. But the international urgencies made Roosevelt seem to most Democrats the indispensable candidate. The Democratic convention accordingly renominated him at Chicago in July, though it swallowed hard at his insistence on Henry A. Wallace, the Secretary of Agriculture, for Vice President.

Foreign policy and the campaign. While Americans concerned themselves with presidential politics, the German Luftwaffe launched a savage air war against England. The Royal Air Force put up a magnificent defense in what became known as the Battle of Britain. But if Britain hoped to repulse an anticipated German invasion—as well as maintain its own lines of supply—it needed immediate reinforcement of its battered destroyer fleet. Churchill, renewing his request for American destroyers, cabled Roosevelt on July 31, "I must tell you that in the long history of the world this is a thing to do *now*."

Though the United States had over-age destroyers to spare, the Naval Appropriations Act required prior approval of the Chief of Naval Operations before they could be released. Moreover, Roosevelt feared the political repercussions in a campaign in which he was already under attack for unneutral acts. But he was persuaded that he could legally release the destroyers without amending the law; he consulted his cabinet and congressional leaders; and he received assurances that Willkie, the Republican candidate, would not oppose the transaction. Accordingly, on September 2 the United States by executive agreement transferred fifty destroyers to Britain in exchange for ninety-nine-year leases of bases in Newfoundland and the Caribbean.

Willkie's support of conscription also enabled the Administration to obtain a Selective Service Act in August. Still, though Willkie's internationalism minimized the role of foreign policy in the campaign, it did not altogether eliminate peace and war as an issue. Indeed, as the campaign wore on, the Republican candidate, rattled both by his own inexperience and by discordant counsel among his advisers, assailed Roosevelt's foreign policy more and more extravagantly in terms that he would later dismiss as "campaign oratory." Soon he predicted that Roosevelt, if elected, would have the nation in war by April 1941. By the end of the campaign Roosevelt was himself assuring American parents: "I have said this before, but I shall say it again and again and again: Your boys are not going to be sent into any foreign wars."

The election showed that Roosevelt still retained the national confidence. He received 27 million popu-

Wendell Willkie: magnetic qualities

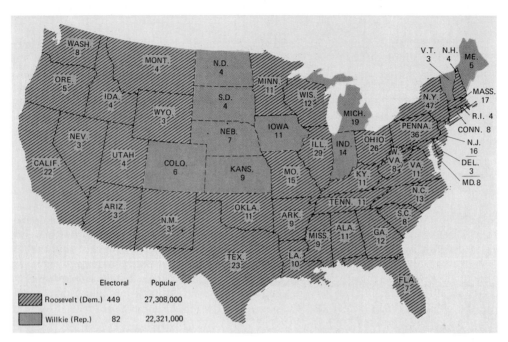

	Electoral	Popular
Roosevelt (Dem.)	449	27,308,000
Willkie (Rep.)	82	22,321,000

The election of 1940

lar votes against 22 million for Willkie; the Electoral College margin was 449 to 82. But he received only 54.8 percent of the vote as against 60.8 percent in 1936, and more than ever before he needed his pluralities in the cities. Because of the equivocal way in which both candidates had presented the foreign issues—had, indeed, somewhat misrepresented their own convictions—the election did not serve either to clarify public thinking or to produce a setting for future action.

Aid Short of War

The Lend-Lease Act. Through 1940 Britain had been able to get the goods it needed under the system of cash-and-carry. But, as Churchill urged on Roosevelt in December, both features of the system were in peril—"cash" because Britain's supply of American dollars was nearing exhaustion, "carry" because of the effectiveness of the German submarine campaign against British shipping.

"The thing to do," Roosevelt now told Secretary of the Treasury Morgenthau, "is to get away from a dollar sign. I don't want to put the thing in terms of dollars or loans." As he explained to his press conference, if a neighbor's house was on fire, you would not waste time arguing about the cost of the hose; you would put the fire out and get the hose back afterward. Why not say to England, "We will give you the guns and the ships you need, provided that when the war is over you will return to us in kind the guns and ships we have loaned to you"?

In January 1941 the Administration introduced the so-called lend-lease bill to carry out Roosevelt's intention. The measure authorized the President to sell, transfer, exchange, lend, lease, or otherwise dispose of war equipment and other commodities to the "government of any country whose defense the President deems vital to the defense of the United States." So sweeping a proposal aroused bitter isolationist opposition. "The lend-lease-give program," said Senator Burton K. Wheeler, "is the New Deal's triple A foreign policy; it will plow under every fourth American boy." Senators Taft and Vandenberg feared that Congress, if it passed the bill, would surrender much of its constitutional authority over foreign policy. Among those who testified against the bill were Charles A. Lindbergh, Charles A. Beard, the historian, and Joseph P. Kennedy, the former ambassador to England; Wendell Willkie led a parade of witnesses in its favor. But public sentiment strongly supported the proposal. Assured of biannual review of lend-lease appropriations, Congress passed the bill. It became law on March 11, 1941. "Through this legislation," Roosevelt said, "our country has determined to do its full part in creating an adequate arsenal of democracy."

The Battle of the Atlantic. The Lend-Lease Act decisively committed the economic power of the United States to the support of Britain. It also implied, as its opponents had predicted, at least a partial commitment of American naval power; for, if the United States deemed aid to Britain vital to American security, then clearly the United States had better make sure that goods intended for Britain actually arrived there. Shortly after the passage of lend-lease, the Ger-

McDonnell-Douglas factory: one arsenal of democracy

Strikes in defense industries, some of them instigated by communists, further kept the country from living up to its full responsibility as the "arsenal of democracy." Some positive step seemed necessary to galvanize America and to reassure Britain. On May 27, 1941, the President in a speech to the nation proclaimed "that an unlimited national emergency exists and requires the strengthening of our defense to the extreme limit of our national power."

Roosevelt's proclamation called for preparing American defenses to repel any attack on the Western Hemisphere. To that end, in July by executive agreement he dispatched American troops to Iceland, outside the hemisphere. Had the Nazis reached Iceland first, he argued, they would have threatened the flow of munitions to England, a matter of policy Congress had approved in the Lend-Lease Act. Senator Robert Taft disagreed. The President, he said, had no constitutional right to send troops to Iceland without congressional approval, for there had been no attack upon the United States, nor was there a threat of an attack. Though only one senator supported Taft's protest, the President was stretching his authority at least to its limits and in so doing moving American forces to the very edge of the war.

mans joined the challenge by extending the North Atlantic war zone westward to the coast of Greenland. As German submarines and destroyers sank increasing numbers of British ships, Roosevelt sought means for protecting the Atlantic lifeline and strengthening the defenses of the Western Hemisphere. In April 1941 he concluded an executive agreement with the Danish government-in-exile to send American troops to Greenland, a part of the Western Hemisphere, and he extended to that area American naval and air patrols. Those moves lessened but did not resolve the problem of the Atlantic lifeline.

Unlimited national emergency. Roosevelt's policy of aid to Great Britain was not limited only by the fear of an adverse public reaction. The President himself apparently cherished the hope, which many around him had abandoned by the spring of 1941, that Hitler might be defeated without direct American military involvement.

Yet Britain's situation seemed to be growing steadily worse. In the United States itself the attitude of business as usual impeded full mobilization of the economy for defense production. The Office of Production Management had succeeded the National Defense Advisory Commission in January 1941, but the new agency lacked adequate authority over allocations and priorities. Many businessmen were disinclined to convert their facilities to defense needs.

Isolationism's Last Stand

The great debate. The slow unfolding of American policy had been accompanied by an intensification of public debate. In 1940 the Committee to Defend America by Aiding the Allies was established under

The U.S.-British destroyer-bases agreement, 1940

Threat and Promise, 1941.

Every realist knows that the democratic way of life is ... being directly assailed in every part of the world.... This assault has blotted out the whole pattern of democratic life in an appalling number of independent nations, great and small. The assailants are still on the march....

The future and safety of our country and our democracy are overwhelmingly involved in events far beyond our borders.... No realistic American can expect from a dictator's peace international generosity, or return to true independence, or world disarmament, or freedom ... or even good business....

The need of the moment is that our action and our policy should be devoted primarily—almost exclusively—to meeting this foreign peril. For all our domestic problems are now a part of the great emergency....

In the future days, which we seek to make secure, we look forward to a world founded upon four essential human freedoms.

The first is freedom of speech and expression—everywhere in the world.

The second is freedom of every person to worship God in his own way—everywhere in the world.

The third is freedom from want—which ... means economic understandings which will secure to every nation a healthy peacetime life for its inhabitants—everywhere in the world.

The fourth is freedom from fear—which ... means a world-wide reduction of armaments to such a point and in such a thorough fashion that no nation will be in a position to commit an act of physical aggression against any neighbor—everywhere in the world.

Franklin D. Roosevelt, State of the Union Message to Congress, January 1941.

the chairmanship of the Kansas editor William Allen White to argue the moderate interventionist position. In 1941 the Fight for Freedom Committee contended for American entry into the war. On the other side, the America First Committee argued that Hitler's victory would not menace American security. Each side took its case to the public through newspaper advertisements, radio broadcasts, and mass meetings.

The resulting debate became more bitter even than the arguments of the thirties over the New Deal. It was, in addition, unpredictable, cutting across political, economic, and geographical lines. Isolationists were to be found in all parts of the country, in all social classes, and in all political parties. Still, to a considerable degree, isolationism as a political force represented the conservative Republican wing of the business community, with special strength in the Middle West. Progressives like Burton K. Wheeler, Socialists like Norman Thomas, and the communists also criticized Roosevelt's policies. The German-American Bund and the fringe of pro-Nazi groups in America endorsed the isolationist position.

The isolationist dilemma. Most Americans remained uncertainly in the middle of the violent debate. "I am 100 percent plus against our participation in this criminal war," wrote Josephus Daniels, the old

Wilsonian, once Roosevelt's chief as Secretary of the Navy in the First World War, now ambassador to Mexico, "but, of course, I trust that Europe will be delivered from totalitarian governments and the scourge of force." This was the isolationist dilemma: at some point, the two sentiments were bound to collide.

An analysis of votes in Congress during these years shows, not a rigid isolationist-interventionist division, but a large middle bloc trying to steer a course between the two extremes. Most members of Congress, like most Americans, wished that all-out support of Britain short of war would somehow bring British victory without American participation. In providing Britain such support, they edged steadily toward involvement. Yet involvement was not their purpose; it was rather the last resort they earnestly hoped to avoid. Men like Henry L. Stimson, Harold L. Ickes, and the members of the Fight for Freedom Committee felt that Roosevelt himself, by refusing to call for an American declaration of war, was engaged in self-delusion. Still, the President's policy of hoping for the best while preparing for the worst expressed the predominant sense of the electorate in 1941. Had he been more forthright about the risks he took, he might have appeared less duplicitous to his opponents. He might also in so doing have heightened the fears of Americans, lost their support, and thus constrained his ability to combat the terror that was threatening the world.

Hitler widens the war. After the Soviet Union attacked Finland, Roosevelt had condemned Stalin's regime as "a dictatorship as absolute as any other dictatorship in the world." Nonetheless, American diplomats, noting growing evidence of tension between Germany and Russia, told a skeptical Kremlin in the winter of 1940–41 that a German attack might be in the making. Stalin remained impervious to warnings. When Hitler, despairing of an early defeat of Britain, decided to eliminate the potential threat of Russia by a sudden blow, the Soviet regime was taken by surprise. The Nazi invasion of the U.S.S.R. on June 22, 1941, brought the European war into a new phase.

Winston Churchill had long since decided that, in such an eventuality, he would offer Russia full British support. "I have only one purpose," he said, "the destruction of Hitler. . . . If Hitler invaded Hell, I would make at least a favorable reference to the Devil in the House of Commons." Roosevelt was ready to accept this policy. Despite warnings that Russia could not be expected to hold out against the Nazi onslaughts, he sent Harry Hopkins to Moscow in July. Hopkins' relatively optimistic report confirmed Churchill and Roosevelt in their decision to do what they could to stiffen Soviet resistance.

Most Americans supported this decision. The American communists, of course, rapidly called off their antiwar agitation and became passionate proponents of national defense. From an isolationist viewpoint, however, Hitler's new embroilment strengthened the case against American participation.

The Atlantic Charter. In August, Roosevelt and Churchill met on warships off Argentia on the coast of Newfoundland. While Roosevelt avoided military commitments, he did agree with Churchill on "certain common principles in the national policies of their respective countries on which they base their hopes for a better future for the world." In the Atlantic Charter, Britain and the United States disclaimed territorial aggrandizement, affirmed the right of all peoples to choose their own form of government and to express freely their wishes concerning territorial changes (though Churchill excepted the peoples within the British Empire), assured all states equal access to trade and raw materials ("with due respect to their existing obligations"), proposed collaboration among all nations in the economic field, and promised "after the final destruction of the Nazi tyranny" the disarmament of all aggressor nations "pending the establishment of a wider and permanent system of general security."

By the time of the conference American destroyers were escorting convoys as far as Iceland, leaving the British navy to conduct them the rest of the way. The question of what American ships should do if they encountered a German raider was left unanswered until a U-boat fired on the destroyer *Greer* early in September. Though the President did not so inform the American people, the *Greer* had provoked the attack. Saying the time had come for "active defense," Roosevelt instructed the navy to "shoot on sight" any Axis ships in the American neutrality zone. In October the Germans badly damaged one American destroyer and sank another, the *Reuben James*, with considerable loss of life. In November Congress revised the Neutrality Act to allow merchantmen to carry arms and to proceed to British ports. Roosevelt had consulted Congress about that measure, but he had not told the whole truth. To have done so, he feared, would have risked too much, for the House of Representatives had renewed the Selective Service Act by a margin of only one vote. Accord-

The first summit: Argentia, 1941

ingly the President had been disingenuous, as he knew, but in what he believed was a commanding cause.

Both the Argentia meeting and the new Atlantic policy goaded the isolationists into ever more impassioned attacks on the Administration. In an angry speech at Des Moines, Iowa, in September, Charles A. Lindbergh declared that "the three most important groups who have been pressing this country toward war are the British, the Jewish and the Roosevelt administration." Most isolationists disowned Lindbergh's anti-Semitism, but the course of the war and of the American role in it was rapidly diminishing the range of maneuver between the Nazis and their enemies.

Thunder in the East

The Japanese dilemma. Despite the Japanese occupation of coastal China in 1937 and the failure of the Brussels Conference (see p. 714), the Chiang Kaishek (Jiang Jieshi) government and the Chinese communists under Mao Tse-tung (Mao Zedong) had kept up stalwart resistance. The Chinese plight increasingly enlisted the sympathy of the United States and Britain. Though both governments were reluctant to provoke Japanese retaliation, they began in 1938 to seek ways to get financial assistance to China.

The Japanese response was less explosive than the State Department had predicted. One reason for this restraint was the extent to which the Japanese war effort had itself become dependent on the United States. In 1938, for example, the United States supplied Japan with 90 percent of its metal scrap, 91 percent of its copper, and 66 percent of its oil. This trade confronted Washington with embarrassing problems. It was sanctioned by the Japanese-American commercial treaty of 1911, and the commodities involved were beyond the reach of existing neutrality legislation. To call for a "moral" embargo of the sort used in the Italo-Ethiopian conflict would penalize China as well as Japan. Its hands thus tied, the United States was left in the position of fueling a war machine of which it profoundly disapproved. In an effort to regain freedom of action, Washington informed Tokyo in July 1939 of its intention to terminate the commercial treaty, though, it added in January 1940, it would not for the time being disturb the existing trade.

Then the Nazi successes in Europe transformed the situation. The expansionists in Tokyo felt their long-awaited opportunity had come to seize the colonial empires of France and the Netherlands, even perhaps of Britain. The relatively moderate government was overthrown. In its place came a tough government, dominated by the military and dedicated to the achievement of a "new order in Greater East Asia." In September Japan joined Germany and Italy in the Tripartite Pact. The Axis now extended to Asia.

The American response. The American response was an embargo on essential materials, especially aviation gasoline and scrap metal. Since this action could be justified in terms of America's own defense needs, it did not have the flavor of an open affront to Japan. Behind the scenes, American representatives took part in staff discussions with British and Dutch officials to consider plans for the defense of the western Pacific in case a Japanese attack forced the United States into war.

Roosevelt, however, was primarily concerned with the crisis in Europe. He therefore wished to stave off a showdown with Japan. Accordingly 1941 was marked by long, intricate, and repetitious discussions between the two countries. In June the German invasion of the Soviet Union relieved Japan of its anxieties about a possible attack from Siberia. In mid-July 1941 Japanese troops invaded southern Indochina and occupied Saigon. Roosevelt told the Japanese ambassador that if Japan withdrew from Indochina he would secure its neutralization and assure Japan access to its raw materials. If Japan persisted in its course, and especially if it moved into the Dutch East Indies, the United States would help the Dutch and probably cut off oil exports to Japan. When Japan did not reply, Roosevelt on July 26 froze Japanese assets in the United States and a few days later embargoed oil shipments.

These actions brought about a reappraisal in Tokyo. Prime Minister Fumimaro Konoye, a moderate, in August proposed a meeting with Roosevelt. Japan, Konoye's foreign minister promised, would withdraw its troops from Indochina as soon as the "China incident" was settled, would not expand southward or make war on the Soviet Union unless attacked, and would not feel bound by the Tripartite Pact to go to war if the United States became engaged in a defensive war with Germany. Though Roosevelt considered those terms favorable as a basis for peace in the Pacific, Hull insisted on an agreement about China, which he viewed as the major issue, before any conference took place between the President and the prime minister. The Secretary of State and his advisers made the territorial integrity of China the crux of their diplomacy partly out of long habit and conviction, and partly in the false belief that Japan would in no event attack the United States. Persuaded by their belief, Roosevelt in his reply to Konoye on September 3 made China the key to negotiations. That was unacceptable to the Japanese war party. Late

Pearl Harbor, December 7, 1941

in September Konoye tried again, only to be rebuffed as before by Hull's demand for a prior agreement on China. Had Hull done otherwise, he would have agreed at least for the near future to giving Japan a free hand in China.

There was to be no turning back from that breakdown of diplomacy. As Roosevelt had long recognized, the first interest of the United States lay in preventing Nazi domination of Europe and Great Britain. Pursuit of that interest entailed avoiding, or at the least postponing, war with Japan. On that account the question of China might have been left until after the end of the European war. There was, however, no assurance that Konoye could have continued to restrain the Japanese army, which any concessions might have emboldened, as Roosevelt and Churchill agreed. Japan, moreover, had no right to dominion in China, and the Chinese resistance did evoke a natural American sympathy. But the timing of Hull's advice to Roosevelt, and the adamancy of both the American and Japanese positions on China, eliminated the last chance for a Pacific armistice, however transitory.

The Rising Sun over the Pacific. In mid-October the militants in the Japanese cabinet forced Konoye's resignation. Though his successor, General Hideki Tojo, was a leader of the war party, debate continued until November 5. The army then agreed to a last effort at accommodation with the United States provided that the emperor approve plans for an immediate attack if negotiations failed. Earlier the Japanese leaders had defined their minimum demands to include the abandonment of China by the United States

and the restoration of normal commercial relations, with renewed delivery of oil and scrap metal. Now Tojo told Admiral Kichisabura Nomura, Japanese ambassador, that other matters would be negotiable but that Japan could never yield on the question of China.

By decoding secret Japanese messages, the Americans had been able to follow some of the Japanese moves. Officials in Washington realized that a decisive moment was approaching. Late in November American forces in the Pacific, including those in Hawaii, were sent the first of a number of alerts ordering them onto a war footing. Everyone expected attack, but the conviction was absolute that the Japanese would move toward the south. In Washington, Cordell Hull continued to meet with Japanese representatives. On December 6 Roosevelt sent a final appeal to the emperor.

In the meantime, a striking force of Japanese aircraft carriers had left the Kuriles on November 26 and was making its way toward Pearl Harbor. On December 7, 1941, while discussions continued in Washington, the Japanese launched a devastating attack on the fleet and air force in Hawaii. An epoch in American history had come to an end.

"In the past few years—and, most violently, in the past few days—we have learned a terrible lesson," said Franklin Roosevelt two days later. "We must begin the great task that is before us by abandoning once and for all the illusion that we can ever again isolate ourselves from the rest of humanity." He added, "We are going to win the war, and we are going to win the peace that follows."

Thunder in the East **725**

Suggestions for Reading

THE MAKING OF AMERICAN FOREIGN POLICY

R. Dallek, *Franklin D. Roosevelt and American Foreign Policy, 1932–1945** (1979), provides a judicious account of its subject. S. Adler, *The Uncertain Giant: American Foreign Policy Between the Wars* (1966), and R. A. Divine, *The Reluctant Belligerent: American Entry into World War II** (1965), cover the main events of the period. For a cogent transatlantic view, see Jean-Baptiste Duroselle, *From Wilson to Roosevelt: Foreign Policy of the United States, 1913–1945* (1963). J. E. Wiltz, *From Isolation to War, 1931–1941** (1968), provides an incisive discussion of leading issues. R. E. Osgood, *Ideals and Self-Interest in America's Foreign Relations** (1953), offers a stimulating analytical framework from which to view American foreign policy. See also G. F. Kennan, *American Diplomacy, 1900–1950** (1951), and W. Lippmann, *U.S. Foreign Policy: Shield of the Republic* (1943).

For Roosevelt's first term, the raw material of foreign affairs can be conveniently found in E. B. Nixon, ed., *Franklin D. Roosevelt and Foreign Affairs*, 3 vols. (1969). F. Freidel, *Franklin D. Roosevelt: Launching the New Deal** (1973), covers the London Economic Conference. M. Tate, *The United States and Armaments* (1948), describes the frustrations of disarmament in the years between the wars. The story from 1937 to Pearl Harbor is splendidly recorded in two magisterial volumes by W. L. Langer and S. E. Gleason, *The Challenge to Isolation* (1952) and *The Undeclared War* (1953). 1941 is well covered in J. M. Burns, *Roosevelt: The Soldier of Freedom** (1970). For military aspects, see M. S. Watson, *Chief of Staff: Prewar Plans and Preparations* (1950). On intelligence problems, the outstanding work is R. Wohlstetter, *Pearl Harbor** (1962).

Cordell Hull, *Memoirs*, 2 vols. (1948), supplies the view from the office of the Secretary of State. It may be supplemented by J. W. Pratt, *Cordell Hull*, 2 vols. (1964). S. Welles, *A Time for Decision* (1964), and H. Feis, *Seen From E. A.: Three International Episodes** (1947), amplify the State Department view. For H. L. Stimson, there are three works: his own book with M. Bundy, *On Active Service in Peace and War* (1948); a perceptive biography by E. E. Morison, *Turmoil and Tradition* (1960); and a prosecutor's brief by R. N. Current, *Secretary Stimson* (1954). R. E. Sherwood, *Roosevelt and Hopkins* (1948, rev. ed., 1950), is vivid and penetrating; and the second volume of J. M. Blum, *From the Morgenthau Diaries: Years of Urgency* (1965), is valuable for the years before Pearl Harbor.

Two waves of revisionism have washed over these years. The old isolationist school can be consulted in two books by C. A. Beard—*American Foreign Policy in the Making, 1932–1940* (1946) and *President Roosevelt and the Coming of War, 1941* (1948). C. C. Tansill sums up the isolationist case in *Back Door to War* (1952). A recent restatement of isolationist ideas is in B. Russett, *No Clear and Present Danger** (1972). In *Roosevelt: From Munich to Pearl Harbor* (1950), B. Rauch provides a careful rebuttal. The contemporary school of revisionism, committed to the thesis that American foreign policy has always been the expression of the imperialist necessities of American capitalism, is represented in L. C. Gardner, *Economic Aspects of New Deal Diplomacy* (1964), and in the relevant chapters of W. A. Williams, *The Tragedy of American Diplomacy** (1959; rev. ed., 1962).

THE POLITICS OF FOREIGN POLICY

S. Adler, *The Isolationist Impulse* (1957); M. Jonas, *Isolationism in America, 1935–1941* (1966); and S. Lubell, *The Future of American Politics* (1952), consider the sources of isolationism. F. Waldrop, *McCormick of Chicago* (1966), is an illuminating essay on the isolationist mood. J. K. Nelson, *The Peace Prophets: American Pacifist Thought, 1919–1941* (1967), discusses the peace movement. Congressional reactions to foreign affairs can be traced in F. L. Israel, *Nevada's Key Pittman* (1963); M. C. McKenna, *Borah* (1961); B. K. Wheeler, *Yankee from the West* (1962); and W. S. Cole, *Senator Gerald P. Nye and American Foreign Relations* (1962). See also J. E. Wiltz, *In Search of Peace: the Senate Munitions Inquiry, 1934–1936* (1963); for the neutrality debate, R. A. Divine, *The Illusion of Neutrality* (1962); and for Willkie, D. B. Johnson, *The Republican Party and Wendell Willkie* (1960).

The angry controversy of 1939–41 is well covered in W. Johnson, *The Battle Against Isolationism* (1944); M. L. Chadwin, *The Hawks of World War II* (1968; in paperback as *The Warhawks: American Interventionists before Pearl Harbor*); and W. S. Cole, *America First: The Battle Against Intervention* (1953). The musings of a leading isolationist can be followed in C. A. Lindbergh, *Wartime Journals* (1970).

EUROPE

J. W. Gantenbein, *Documentary Background of World War II* (1948), lives up to its title. For interpretations, K. Eubank, *The Origins of World War II** (1969), sums up the accepted view; and A. J. P. Taylor, *The Origins of the Second World War** (1962), is a stimulating essay in heterodoxy. W. S. Churchill's classic volumes, *The Gathering Storm* (1948) and *Their Finest Hour* (1949), are majestic and indispensable.

A. Bullock, *Hitler: A Study in Tyranny** (1952), is the best biography. Six useful works discuss Nazi Germany and America: H. L. Trefousse, *Germany and American Neutrality* (1951); J. V. Compton, *The Swastika and the Eagle* (1967); A. Frye, *Nazi Germany and the Western Hemisphere, 1933–1941* (1967); A. A. Offner, *American Appeasement: United States Foreign Policy and Germany, 1933–1938** (1969); R. Dallek, *Democrat and Diplomat: The Life of William E. Dodd* (1968); and H. W. Gatzke, *Germany and the United States* (1981). For American relations with the Soviet Union, see R. P. Browder, *The Origins of Soviet-American Diplomacy* (1953); B. Farnsworth, *William C. Bullitt and the Soviet Union* (1967); and E. M. Bennett, *Recognition of Russia: An American Foreign Policy Dilemma* (1970). B. Harris, *The United States and the Italo-Ethiopian Crisis* (1964), displays the American response to the events of 1935; and F. J. Taylor, *The United States and the Spanish Civil War* (1956), and A. Guttmann, *The Wound in the Heart: America and the Spanish Civil War* (1962), consider the problems of 1937–38. Four books throw light on Anglo-American relations at various points: H. Feis, *1933: Characters in Crisis* (1966); W. F. Kimball, *'The Most Unsordid Act': Lend-Lease, 1939–1941* (1969); T. A. Wilson, *The First Summit: Roosevelt and Churchill at Placentia Bay, 1941* (1969); H. D. Hall, *North American Supply* (1955); and the engaging J. P. Lash, *Roosevelt and Churchill* (1976).

FAR EAST

D. Borg, *The United States and the Far Eastern Crisis of 1933–1938* (1964), is a basic work. The Japanese problem is assessed from various angles in H. Feis, *The Road to Pearl Harbor** (1950); D. J. Lu, *From the Marco Polo Bridge to Pearl Harbor: Japan's Entry into World War II* (1961); P. W. Schroeder, *The Axis Alliance and Japanese-American Relations* (1958); C. E. Neu, *The Troubled Encounter: The U.S. and Japan** (1975); R. Butow, *Tojo and the Coming of the War** (1961); and A. Iriye, *Power and Culture: The Japanese-American War** (1981). For American diplomatic reactions, see W. Johnson's rendering of the papers of J. C. Grew, *Turbulent Era: A Diplomatic Record of Forty Years*, 2 vols. (1952), and W. H. Heinrichs, *American Ambassador: Joseph C. Grew and the Development of the United States Diplomatic Tradition* (1967).

LATIN AMERICA

B. Wood, *The Making of the Good Neighbor Policy* (1961), is the best historical account; L. Duggan, *The Americas: Search for Hemispheric Security* (1949), is the testimony of a participant. D. Green, *The Containment of Latin America* (1971), is a revisionist critique of the Good Neighbor policy.

*Available in a paperback edition.

29

THE WORLD IN FLAMES

The bitter wreckage of ships and planes at Pearl Harbor ended the illusion that the United States could be a world power and remain safe from world conflict. In the shocking strike from the placid Hawaiian skies, the Japanese crippled the Pacific fleet, destroyed nearly 200 planes, and killed nearly 2,500 men. The navy lost three times as many men in this single attack as it had lost in the Spanish-American and First World wars combined. Four days after Pearl Harbor, on December 11, 1941, Germany and Italy declared war on the United States and Congress declared war on them. America was now committed to global war.

America Organizes for War

Arms for global war. War brought profound changes to American society. The first problem was to produce the machines and weapons for global warfare. In 1941 military spending had reached a monthly rate of about $2 billion; but only 15 percent of industrial output had gone for military purposes, and businessmen had resisted pressure to shift to war production. Roosevelt now laid down unprecedented objectives for 1942—60,000 planes, 45,000 tanks, 20,000 antiaircraft guns, 8 million tons of shipping—and set up the War Production Board under Donald Nelson to convert the economy to a war basis.

In the first six months of 1942, the government placed over $100 billion in war contracts—more goods on order than the economy had ever produced in a single year. The structure of central control buckled under the strain. An effective priority system was essential, but sometimes more priorities were issued than there were goods to satisfy them. In the confusion the military, who had already gained authority over procurement, demanded control over production. Nelson, backed by the President and Congress, fended off this proposal. In 1943 the WPB's Controlled Materials Plan introduced order into the allocation of critical materials, about which the military continued to have considerable voice.

Roosevelt, in his characteristic style, assigned important areas of authority to other civilian agencies. In December 1942 the War Food Administration assumed direction of the nation's food program. Shortages in oil and rubber brought about the appointment, also outside the WPB, of "czars" with exceptional powers to expedite production. The War Manpower Commission supervised the mobilization of men and women for both civilian and military purposes. And the Office of Scientific Research and Development, under the direction of Dr. Vannevar Bush, conducted scientific and technical mobilization; its scientists and engineers were responsible for

Omaha beachhead, 1944

short-range rockets (especially the "bazooka"), the proximity fuse, and other remarkable gains in military technology.

In 1942 the proportion of the economy committed to war production grew from 15 to 33 percent. By the end of 1943 federal expenditures for goods and services constituted a sum larger than the total output of the economy when Roosevelt took office a decade earlier. The gross national product grew from $99.7 billion in 1940 to $211.9 billion in 1945. The WPB continued to be shaken by feuds, both internal and external. In the interest of efficiency in procurement, the army and navy relied increasingly on big business in the awarding of war contracts. Nelson tried without success to divert a substantial proportion of those contracts to smaller concerns, for which he also attempted to get reconversion privileges in 1944. Convinced that any move toward reconversion was premature, the army and navy persuaded Roosevelt to force Nelson to resign. Still, in one way or another, the WPB had succeeded in guiding the productive energies of the economy to enable America in a surprisingly short time to outproduce all other nations in the world.

The fight for stabilization. This extraordinary feat was a result of the stimulus provided by government spending to the productive talents of American managers and workers. Federal purchases of goods and services rose from $6 billion in 1940 to $89 billion in 1944. Total federal spending during the war years came to over $320 billion—an amount twice as great as the total of all previous federal spending in the history of the republic.

How was this prodigious expenditure to be paid for? The first resort was to a broadening and deepening of the tax structure. By 1944 surtaxes had risen to 94 percent of net income in the highest brackets; and people at every level were paying taxes that would have seemed inconceivable a short time before. Total tax revenues in the war years came to about $130 billion. This was far less than Roosevelt had requested, however, and, as a result, the government was able to meet only about 41 percent of the cost of the war on a pay-as-you-go basis—not enough, though a much larger proportion than during the First World War.

The rest of the defense bill was made up by borrowing. In 1944 alone the excess of expenditures over receipts amounted to more than $50 billion—a figure over twice the total size of the accumulated debt in 1941. By the end of the war the national debt had grown to about $280 billion, nearly six times as large as it had been when bombs fell on Pearl Harbor. The budgetary deficits so loudly bewailed in New Deal days now seemed negligible compared with the deficit

spending of war. An incidental effect was to support the Keynesian argument that public spending would end the depression: unemployment rapidly vanished in 1941 and 1942, and Congress abolished old New Deal agencies like the Works Progress Administration. The problem became, not to find jobs for people, but to find people for jobs.

The tremendous increase in public spending released strong inflationary pressures. The shift from civilian to war production reduced the quantity of goods available for purchase just as the quantity of money jingling in people's pockets was increasing. By 1944, for example, the production of civilian automobiles, of washing machines and other consumer durables, of nondefense housing and the like had virtually come to an end. Unless prices were to soar out of sight, means had to be found to hold the volume of spendable money down to the volume of available goods.

One recourse was to fiscal policy. Taxation was an obvious means of reducing the supply of spendable money in people's hands. The war-bond drive was another way by which the government sought to persuade people to put their money away instead of using it to bid up prices; nearly $100 billion worth of the various series of war bonds were sold in these years. But it was evident from an early point that indirect measures would not be enough to eliminate the "inflationary gap"—the gap, that is, between too few goods and too much money. As early as August 1941 Roosevelt had accordingly established the Office of Price Administration under the direction of Leon Henderson, a hard-driving New Deal economist.

Waiting for rationing coupons

Nisei internees: victims of hysteria

Price control presented one of the toughest problems of war administration. Every economic interest wanted rigid policing of the other fellow's prices but tended to regard attempts to police its own prices as subversive of the free-enterprise system. In April 1942 the OPA imposed a general price freeze, joining to this a system by which necessities of life in short supply—meat, gasoline, tires—were rationed to the consumers through an allotment of coupons. The farm bloc, however, succeeded in gaining exceptions for agricultural prices; and the increase in the cost of food brought about demands for wage increases. The War Labor Board, set up in January 1942, sought to meet this problem by the Little Steel formula of July, permitting wage increases to keep pace with the 15 percent rise in the cost of living since January 1941. In September Roosevelt requested new authority to stabilize the cost of living, including farm prices and wages. The Stabilization Act of 1942 established the Office of Economic Stabilization under the direction of former Supreme Court Justice James F. Byrnes.

Special interests nevertheless continued unabashed guerrilla warfare against price control in their own sectors. The farm bloc was unrelenting in its demand that exceptions be made for itself. John L. Lewis led the United Mine Workers in a fight against the Little Steel formula; for a time in 1943 the government was forced to seize and operate the coal mines. Henderson, who had affronted Congress by the unquenchable zeal of his war against inflation, had been forced to resign in December 1942. But a "hold-the-line" order in April 1943, followed by a campaign in May to "roll back" food prices, helped bring the price level to a plateau by mid-1943. For the rest of the war the OPA, under the able direction of Chester Bowles, was able to maintain substantial price stability in spite of the development of some "black markets" in which rationed goods were sold expensively and illegally. From October 1942 to the end of the Pacific war, consumers' prices rose only 8.7 percent. For all its unpopularity, especially among businessmen, politicians, and farm leaders, the OPA was one of the war's successes.

The problem remained of concerting the efforts of various agencies dealing with production and stabilization. In May 1943 Roosevelt set up the Office of War Mobilization and put Byrnes in charge. Employing his judicial and political skill to intervene when operating agencies disagreed, Byrnes did an effective job in pulling together the infinitely ramified strands of America's domestic war effort.

The conception of the war power under the American Constitution rests ... on basic political principles.... The chief architects of the conception were men of affairs who had participated in war....

Soldiers must answer for their decisions to the nation's system of law.... It is essential to every democratic value ... that official action, taken in the name of war power, should be held to standards of responsibility.... The courts ... should not ... declare such problems to be beyond the reach of judicial review.... Surely the right answer to bad law is good law, rather than no law at all....

The Japanese [relocation] ... program rests on ... propositions of the utmost potential menace:

1. Protective custody ... is a permitted form of imprisonment....

2. Political opinion, not criminal acts, may contain enough danger to justify such imprisonment.

3. Men, women, and children of a given racial group, both Americans and resident aliens, can be presumed to possess the kind of dangerous ideas which require their imprisonment.

4. In time of war ... the military ... can decide what political opinions require imprisonment, and which groups are infected with them.

5. The decision of the military can be carried out without indictment, trial, examination, jury ... counsel for the defense ... or any of the other safeguards of the Bill of Rights....

A great principle was never lost so casually.

Eugene V. Rostow, "Our Worst War Time Mistake," in *Harpers*, September 1945.

The people behind the lines. The attack on Pearl Harbor produced a surge of national unity. Though various groups of Americans remained suspicious of Great Britain or of the Soviet Union, and others were reluctant to contemplate postwar involvements in world affairs, the isolationist-interventionist debate receded. Throughout the war popular confidence in the government remained high. Nevertheless, like any period of war, this was a time of upheaval and anxiety.

To combat the threat of enemy activity within the United States, Roosevelt gave new authority to the Federal Bureau of Investigation, including the power to tap wires in national security cases. Under the astute direction and relentless self-advertisement of J. Edgar Hoover, the FBI had already established itself in congressional and public opinion. Its new mandate encouraged it to widen its investigations into the beliefs as well as the deeds of Americans. But the years 1941–45 were not marred by the widespread assaults on civil freedom that had characterized the years 1917–20 (see pp. 605, 619). Perhaps because they were not perceived to constitute a real threat to the nation, German-Americans and Italian-Americans were not subjected to jingoistic harassment, though for a year the government restricted the movement of unnaturalized Italian immigrants. In contrast, the tragic exception to this general tolerance was the fate of the over one hundred thousand Japanese-Americans, immigrants and citizens alike, who were brutally removed from their homes along the Pacific Coast and relocated in internment camps in the interior—an act of national hysteria wholly unjustified.

Of native Americans suspected of sympathy for fascism, some had their publications—for example, Father Coughlin's *Social Justice*—denied the mails. Toward the end of the war, an effort to convict a number of American fascists in a mass sedition trial miscarried. In the meantime, the Department of Justice had taken effective steps against Nazi agents and organizations. So far as is known, no acts of enemy sabotage were committed in the United States during the war. In the main, Attorney General Francis Biddle strove with success to maintain an atmosphere of moderation.

If war meant anxiety, it also meant opportunity. It uprooted people from familiar settings, exposed them to new experience, changed the direction of their lives. The rise in output and employment was accompanied by a tremendous increase in real income, partly from the prevalence of overtime pay for workers. Wartime tax policies strengthened the tendency toward income redistribution that had begun under the New Deal. The wealthiest 5 percent of

Americans had received 30 percent in 1929 and 24 percent in 1941; by 1944 their share was down to 20.7 percent.

After the long years of depression, both workers and the middle class savored the prosperity of the war years. They spent freely for available consumer goods and saved with the expectation of buying refrigerators and radios, and especially automobiles and houses, after the war. Facilities for housing, transportation, schooling, and recreation were critically short in communities impacted by war industries, particularly in the rapidly growing cities of the South, the Southwest, and the West Coast. Those shortages intensified yearnings for a comfortable tomorrow, yearnings shared by men and women in the armed services. For the duration, most civilians, though irritated by rationing, lived better lives than they had for more than a decade.

Between 1941 and 1945 shortages of labor brought some 6.5 million women, most of them middle-aged and married, into the working force. Except for the rare feminists, they did not much question conventional attitudes toward women's roles or protest against the disparity between men's and women's wages or the lack of day-care centers for the children of working mothers. Some women war-workers did not intend to remain on the job after the war, though many of them either did not leave or soon returned. Most took satisfaction in their contributions to wartime tasks, a point the federal government stressed. They were also pleased by their new income. Supplementing their husbands' earnings, that income gave their families, often for the first time, access to the necessities and some of the comforts of a middle-class standard of living.

Ultimately the demand for labor also provided new opportunities for blacks, though throughout the war they received much less than equal treatment. Their resulting resentments fostered an unprecedented and often effective militancy. During the defense boom before Pearl Harbor, blacks were, as ever, the last hired. Many remained unemployed. Those who found jobs ordinarily received low wages, small chance for promotion, and often no chance to join self-consciously segregated labor unions. Worse, the army and navy persisted in the segregation of the armed forces, consigned most blacks to menial tasks, and with few exceptions denied blacks training for commissions or for élite service like that of the air corps. "A jim crow army," as one critic said, "cannot fight for a free world." So persuaded, the head of the Brotherhood of Sleeping Car Porters, A. Philip Randolph, one of the great black leaders of the century, organized the Negro March on Washington Committee, which planned to recruit thousands of blacks for a rally at the Lincoln Memorial in the spring of 1941

to demand equal rights to work and the desegregation of the armed forces. Roosevelt persuaded Randolph to call off the march in return for Executive Order 8802 of June 1941, which made it national policy to forbid discrimination in employment in defense industries. Roosevelt also appointed the Fair Employment Practices Committee to enforce that policy by investigating complaints and taking steps to redress grievances.

The FEPC, detested though it was in the South, lacked the authority to fulfill its mission. Though war industries did hire blacks, Mexican-Americans, and other minorities, discrimination in wages and seniority remained the rule in spite of efforts of the FEPC to combat it. The War and Navy Departments, moreover, took only token steps toward desegregation in the services. Consequently Randolph kept alive his March on Washington Movement with its black membership and its commitment to mass, nonviolent protest. Ghandian nonviolent techniques became the tactics of newer organizations, most notably the Congress on Racial Equality (CORE), which included whites among its members and successfully employed sit-ins during the war to desegregate various Northern restaurants, theaters, and skating rinks. By 1945 CORE was planning freedom rides to desegregate public transportation in the South.

The movement of thousands of black workers to industrial centers, south and north, provoked the hostility of many prejudiced whites who objected to black neighbors and even more to their competition

War workers

Black power: 1942

We know that our fate is tied up with the fate of the democratic way of life And so, out of the depths of our hearts, a cry goes up for the triumph of the United Nations. But we would not be honest with ourselves were we to stop with a call for a victory of arms alone.... Unless this war sounds the death knell to the old Anglo-American empire systems, the hapless story of which is one of exploitation for the profit and power of a monopoly capitalist economy, it will have been fought in vain. Our aim then must not only be to defeat nazism, fascism, and militarism on the battlefield but to win the peace, for democracy, for freedom and the Brotherhood of Man without regard to his pigmentation, land of his birth or the God of his fathers....

While the March on Washington Movement may find it advisable to form a citizens committee of friendly white citizens to give moral support ... it does not imply that these white citizens ... should be taken into the March on Washington Movement as members. The essential value of an all-Negro movement such as the March on Washington is that it helps to create faith by Negroes in Negroes. It develops a sense of self-reliance with Negroes depending on Negroes in vital matters. It helps to break down the slave psychology and inferiority-complex in Negroes which comes and is nourished with Negroes relying on white people for direction and support. This inevitably happens in mixed organizations that are supposed to be in the interest of the Negro.

From A. Philip Randolph, Keynote Address to the Policy Conference of the March on Washington Movement, September 1942.

for jobs, housing, and schooling. Episodes of racial violence visited a dozen cities and culminated in 1943 in riots involving attacks on Mexican-Americans in Los Angeles and on blacks in New York and most grimly in Detroit. There in June over thirty people, white and black, died during two days of guerrilla fighting that ceased only with the intervention of the National Guard. Continuing evidence of white racism, official and private, discouraged blacks and damped but did not dispel the new militancy. The achievements of the FEPC, inadequate though they were, raised hopes for the future, as still more did the occasional victories of nonviolent protest. Even the head of the moderate NAACP foresaw that only continuing protest—"a rising wind," as he put it—would fasten public policy to the cause of civil rights.

Early politics of the war. Political developments after Pearl Harbor quickly refuted the isolationist prediction that war must doom democracy and free discussion. In Congress the dominating conservative coalition of Republicans and Southern Democrats seized the opportunity to liquidate New Deal agencies that appeared to have lost their function. On the other hand, Congress also provided responsible counsel on many aspects of the war effort—most notably in the Senate War Investigating Committee, which, under the able chairmanship of Harry S Truman of Missouri, exposed waste and confusion in the defense

Detroit, 1943: two days of guerilla fighting

effort and made many valuable recommendations to the executive.

Relations with Congress presented Roosevelt with difficult problems. The 1942 congressional election took place in a time when military defeats had yet to be offset by any striking victories, and in an atmosphere suffused with wartime irritations, especially over the OPA's efforts to hold prices and rents down. It resulted in striking Republican gains—ten seats in the Senate, forty-seven in the House. This outcome confirmed the conservative complexion of the Congress, increased Roosevelt's difficulties in dealing with that body, and filled the Republicans with high hopes for the presidential election of 1944.

The War in Europe

Beat Hitler first. The manifold activities at home, however, provided only the backdrop for the essential problem of war—victory over the enemy. For the United States there were two enemies—the Japanese, advancing rapidly into Southeast Asia in the weeks after Pearl Harbor; and the European Axis, now engaged in savage warfare on the Russian front and presumably preparing an eventual invasion of England. The immediate problem for the United States was whether to throw its military might against Germany or against Japan.

American military planners had already concluded by March 1941 that, if the United States entered the war, American strategy must be to beat Hitler first. There were several reasons for this decision. For one thing, Germany, with its command of most of the western coast of Europe and its access to the Atlantic, presented a direct threat to the Western Hemisphere; there was particular concern over Axis penetration of Latin America. For another, Germany seemed far more likely than Japan to achieve some revolutionary breakthrough in military technology. In addition, Great Britain was fully engaged in fighting the Axis, while in the Far East, China was both less active in its resistance to Japan and less accessible to outside support.

The Nazi attack on the Soviet Union in June 1941, far from reversing the Europe-first argument, was considered to reinforce it; for the Russo-German war increased both the chance of defeating Germany and the urgency of doing so before Germany conquered Russia. Nor did the Japanese attack on Pearl Harbor shake the American decision. When Winston Churchill came to Washington in December 1941, he found complete agreement on his proposition that "the defeat of Germany, entailing a collapse, will leave Japan exposed to overwhelming force, whereas the defeat of Japan would not by any means bring the World War to an end."

Diverging strategies in Europe. The agreement between the United States and Britain on beating Germany first was not matched, however, by agreement on the best way of doing it. The British strategy—reflecting the memory of the bitter trench warfare of the First World War, with which Americans had limited experience—was to postpone direct assault on Germany until a combination of naval blockade, aerial bombing, psychological warfare, and military attack on the Axis periphery had sufficiently weakened Germany's capacity to resist.

Where the British strategy was to attack the enemy where he was weakest, the American was to attack the enemy where he was strongest. From the American viewpoint, the Churchill plan of "pecking at the periphery" would waste resources without winning victory. As Roosevelt used to observe when Churchill advocated a landing at one or another European point remote from Germany, "All right, but where do we go from there?" The American Joint Chiefs of Staff, ably led by General George C. Marshall, felt that only a massive thrust across the English Channel and France into the heart of Germany would achieve victory. In their view—a view generally shared by Roosevelt—all Anglo-American efforts should be concentrated on establishing a second front in France.

Detour to North Africa. The Soviet Union, in desperate need of relief from the hammer blows of the German army and air force, brought strong pressure for a second front in 1942. Though the British accepted a cross-Channel invasion in principle, they continued to object in practice. They felt that the Americans underestimated the difficulties of amphibious landings on fortified coasts; they regarded American troops as untried; and they doubted whether the American economy could quickly achieve the production levels necessary to sustain a great invasion. There were particularly ominous shortages in landing craft and in modern tanks. Accordingly, when the American Joint Chiefs submitted in the spring of 1942 a plan for the invasion of France later that year, the British turned it down.

Still, something had to be done in 1942, if only to reassure the hard-pressed and bitterly disappointed Russians. Churchill consequently proposed an invasion of North Africa. The American Joint Chiefs felt that a North African diversion, by committing Anglo-American forces to a Mediterranean campaign as well as by preempting necessary men and materiel, would delay the invasion of France, perhaps until

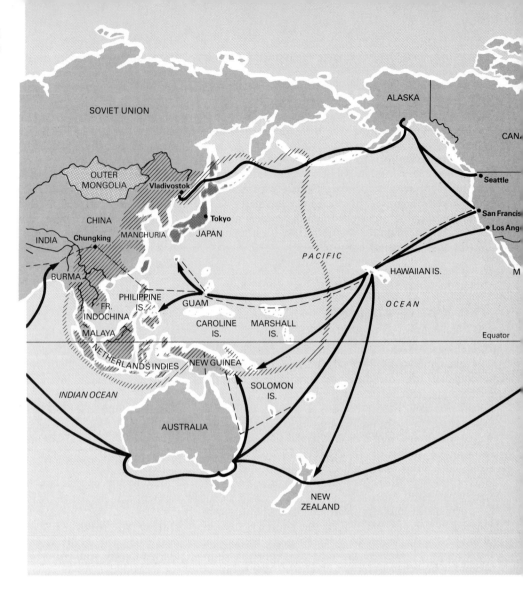

1944. But Roosevelt accepted Churchill's argument
that an invasion of North Africa in 1942 could be a
preliminary to a cross-Channel attack in 1943. In July
the decision was made to invade North Africa in the
autumn. The operation was placed under the command of General Dwight D. Eisenhower.

On November 8, 1942, Anglo-American forces
disembarked at Casablanca in Morocco and at Oran
and Algiers in Algeria. The landings achieved tactical
surprise. Within short order, local resistance came to
an end. But military success raised political problems.
The collaborationist regime of Marshal Pétain, established at Vichy and in control of unoccupied southern France, exercised nominal authority in North
Africa. The United States, which had maintained

diplomatic relations with the Vichy government, had
some hope of winning the support of pro-Vichy officials and military leaders in Algeria and Morocco.
Roosevelt and Churchill supposed that General
Charles de Gaulle, commander of the Free French in
London, would be unacceptable to the North African
French, who had sworn oaths of loyalty to Pétain. But
the Americans believed that General Henri Giraud,
who had recently escaped from a German prison
camp, would be exempt from de Gaulle's unpopularity.

But Giraud, as a condition for cooperation, at first
demanded supreme command of the invasion for
himself. The situation was further complicated by the
presence in Algiers of Admiral Jean François Darlan, a

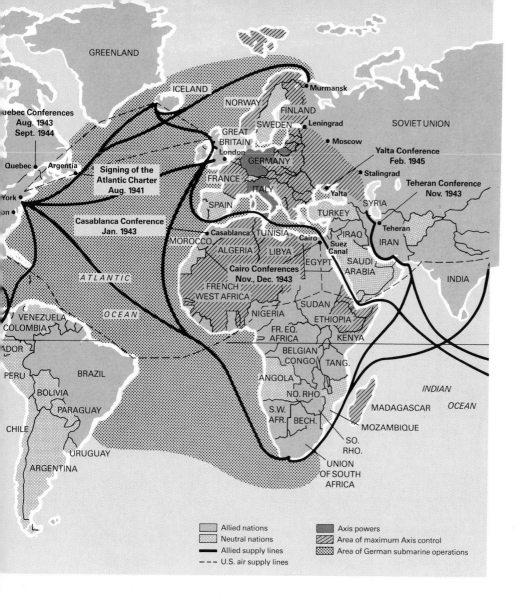

Allied nations	Axis powers
Neutral nations	Area of maximum Axis control
Allied supply lines	Area of German submarine operations
U.S. air supply lines	

prominent French collaborationist and Pétain's successor-designate. Darlan proved as ready to collaborate with the Americans in 1942 as he had been with the Germans in 1940. On November 11 he signed an armistice agreement and Eisenhower recognized him as *de facto* political chief in North Africa—an action that provoked a storm of criticism in England and the United States from those who feared that it inaugurated a policy of making deals with fascists. Roosevelt defended Eisenhower's action as "a temporary expedient, justified solely by the stress of battle." The Darlan deal accelerated the Anglo-American military success in Algeria and Morocco, and Darlan's assassination on December 24 spared Roosevelt and Churchill political embarrassment. But they offended de Gaulle again by

giving much of Darlan's authority to Giraud, whose prestige in North Africa turned out to be overrated.

In the meantime, Hitler, after ordering the occupation of Vichy France, rushed German troops by sea and air to Tunisia. Eisenhower promptly advanced into Tunisia from the west, while the British Eighth Army, under the command of General Bernard Montgomery, entered from Tripoli to the east. The Anglo-American forces encountered the brilliant generalship of Field Marshal Rommel, who came to be known as the Desert Fox. Nonetheless, the Anglo-American vise closed inexorably. On May 12, 1943, the Axis troops surrendered. The British and Americans had captured or destroyed fifteen Axis divisions, had regained the Mediterranean for their shipping,

The defeat of the Axis, 1942–45

Axis Powers at the outbreak of war

Greatest area of Axis military power

Allies

– – – Heaviest Allied Bombing

⋯⋯⋯ Inside limit of U-Boat operations

✦ SINKING OF
THE "BISMARCK"

FINLAND

NORWAY

SWEDEN

ESTONIA

LATVIA

LITHUANIA

R U S S I A

Volga R.

Stalingrad

1942

Moscow

Leningrad

1943

1941

Don R.

1943

Dnieper R.

1944

EAST PRUSSIA

Danzig

Königsberg

Vistula R. Warsaw

1945

P O L A N D

Oder R.

1945

Berlin

Potsdam

Prague

CZECHOSLOVAKIA

Vienna

AUSTRIA

HUNGARY

Budapest

1944

1944

ROMANIA

Bucharest

Danube R.

BULGARIA

Sofia

YUGOSLAVIA

Belgrade

ALBANIA

GREECE

Athens

BLACK SEA

T U R K E Y

Ankara

Sevastopol

Yalta

AEGEAN SEA

CRETE

CYPRUS

SYRIA

PALESTINE

TRANS JORDAN

RED SEA

Suez Canal

Nile R.

EGYPT

El Alamein

1942

Tobruk

1943

LIBYA

MEDITERRANEAN SEA

MALTA

SICILY

Palermo

1943

Tunis

Bizerte

TUNISIA

1943

ALGERIA

Algiers

Oran

1942

FRENCH MOROCCO

Casablanca

1942

Tangier

Gibraltar

SPAIN

PORTUGAL

Tagus R.

Ebro R.

SARDINIA

CORSICA

1944

ITALY

Rome

Anzio

Monte Cassino

Salerno

Florence

Po R.

1944

ADRIATIC SEA

Trieste

Nice

Marseilles

Vichy

1944

SWITZ.

Border of Vichy France

Maginot Line

Rhine R.

Stuttgart

Munich

Berchtesgaden

Frankfort

RUHR

Cologne

Trier

Reims

Compiègne

Paris

Seine R.

Loire R.

F R A N C E

BASTOGNE

1945

BELG.

Brussels

Dunkirk

Dieppe

NORMANDY

ENGLISH CHANNEL

1944

NETH.

Hamburg

Elbe R.

Torgau

G E R M A N Y

DENMARK

BALTIC SEA

GREAT BRITAIN

London

Coventry

IRELAND

NORTH SEA

A T L A N T I C   O C E A N

0   300
MILES

THE DEFEAT OF GERMANY

WESTERN FRONT			EASTERN FRONT
		January 20, 1942	Russian counteroffensive begins, reaches Kharkov May 12
		June 28, 1942	German summer offensive begins. Reaches Stalingrad Aug. 22
British stop German African drive at El Alamein	June 29, 1942		
British offensive begins with victory at El Alamein; Tobruk falls Nov. 13, Bengasi Nov. 20	November 4, 1942		
U.S. and British landings in North Africa. French sign armistice Nov. 11	November 8, 1942		
		November 19, 1942	Russian counteroffensive begins at Stalingrad
British take Tripoli	January 24, 1943	January 18, 1943	Russians raise siege at Leningrad
		February 2, 1943	Germans surrender at Stalingrad
		February 14, 1943	Russians take Rostov, followed by Kharkov Feb. 16, Rzhev Mar. 9
U.S. and British lines meet in North Africa	April 7, 1943		
British take Tunis, Americans take Bizerte	May 7, 1943		
Surrender of Axis in North Africa	May 13, 1943		
Invasion of Sicily, completed August 17	July 10, 1943		
Resignation of Mussolini	July 25, 1943		
		August 4, 1943	Russians reverse German offensive and take Orel and Belgurod
British troops invade Italy	September 3, 1943		
Unconditional surrender of Italy	September 8, 1943		
Americans invade Salerno. Allied advance begins, crosses Volturno River Oct. 14, reaches Sangro River Dec. 25	September 9, 1943		
		September 25, 1943	Russian advance takes Smolensk, moves on to Kiev Nov. 7, enters Poland Jan. 3, 1944
Landing at Anzio	January 22, 1944		
		January 29, 1944	Moscow-Leningrad area clear of German forces
		April 10, 1944	Russians take Odessa
		May 9, 1944	Russians take Sevastopol
Cassino falls after two month battle	May 18, 1944		
Liberation of Rome	June 4, 1944		
Allied invasion of Normandy	June 6, 1944		
		June 23, 1944	Russians begin summer offensive south of Leningrad
Cherbourg captured	June 27, 1944		
Caen falls	July 9, 1944		
American "Break Out" at St. Lo	July 25, 1944		
British take Florence, Italy	August 12, 1944		
Allies invade southern France	August 15, 1944		
Liberation of Paris	August 25, 1944		
Liberation of Brussels and Antwerp	September 4, 1944		
		September 8, 1944	Surrender of Bulgaria
Liberation of Luxembourg	September 11, 1944		
American forces enter Germany	September 12, 1944		
		September 22, 1944	Russians take Tallinn
		October 20, 1944	Russians enter East Prussia; seize Belgrade, Yugoslavia
Americans take Aachen, followed by Metz, Nov. 22, Strasbourg, Nov. 23	October 21, 1944		
German counteroffensive and Battle of the Bulge until Dec. 26	December 16, 1944		
		December 29, 1944	Russians take Budapest, Hungary
		January 12, 1945	Russians advance in Poland, Warsaw falls Jan. 17, Lodz Jan. 19. Russians at Oder River Jan. 23
British offensive in Holland	February 8, 1945		
Americans cross Saar River	February 22, 1945		
Fall of Cologne and Düsseldorf. Americans capture Remagen Bridge across Rhine	March 7, 1945		
Americans reach Elbe River	April 11, 1945		
		April 13, 1945	Russians begin drive to Berlin, enter Apr. 24
Americans take Nuremberg	April 21, 1945		
Americans meet Russians at Torgau	April 25, 1945	April 25, 1945	Russians meet Americans at Torgau
		May 2, 1945	Berlin falls
Unconditional surrender of Germany. May 8 end of war in Europe	May 7, 1945		

and had thereby laid open to attack what Churchill called the "soft underbelly" of the Axis.

The Mediterranean or France? "All right, but where do we go from there?" Roosevelt had asked. As the Joint Chiefs of Staff had feared, the British advocated moving on into Sicily and Italy in order to maintain the initiative in the Mediterranean. The Americans reluctantly accepted this logic. The result was the invasion of Sicily in July and of Italy in September. When Mussolini fell from his dictatorial seat in July, Eisenhower, with the approval of Roosevelt and Churchill, reorganized a new Italian government under Field Marshal Pietro Badoglio and the reigning king, both fascists. As part of that deal, Badoglio surrendered in September, though by that time German troops controlled southern Italy, where they put up dogged resistance. The Italian front soon was marked by bitter and bloody fighting. When Allied progress up the spine of Italy was stopped at Monte Cassino early in 1944, an attempt was made to circumvent the enemy by amphibious landings at Anzio near Rome late in January. But for many weeks Allied troops could not break out of the Anzio beachhead, and Rome itself did not fall for another four months. In the end, the Italian campaign—especially beyond Rome—cost more and achieved less than its proponents had expected.

In the meantime, argument continued over the invasion of France. The British service chiefs still wanted to delay Overlord (the code name for the cross-Channel operation) for the sake of new adventures in the Mediterranean. But the American Joint Chiefs, with Soviet backing, insisted on a firm commitment to a second front in France. Postponement had already soured the Soviet temper, for the Russians were bearing the brunt of the fighting against the Nazis and counted on Roosevelt's promise of a cross-channel invasion in 1943. At the end of November 1943, Churchill finally consented to May 1944 as a target date.

The actual invasion did not take place until June 6. The Germans, deceived by elaborate stratagems, did not expect a sole attack in Normandy. The Allied forces were thus able to consolidate their position and fan out for movement along a larger front. On July 25 General George Patton's Third Army broke through into Brittany. The war in France now developed extraordinary mobility. American and British divisions raced toward Paris, which was liberated on August 25; and by September 13 Allied forces had penetrated deep into Belgium and crossed the German frontier at Aachen.

These developments, on top of the long-sustained Anglo-American air offensive against Germany, made Hitler's situation more desperate every day. From 1942, when the British and American air forces took substantial command of the air, Germany had been subjected to a series of devastating air raids. Though they were less effective than their advocates claimed at the time, by the autumn of 1944, Allied air attacks—which by the end of the war amounted to 1.5 million bomber sorties and 2.7 million tons of bombs dropped—were exerting a heavy toll on German production (most essentially, of fighter aircraft), and rail and road transportation. The raids also destroyed German cities with inevitable cruelty and ultimately damaged German civilian morale.

In addition, a Soviet offensive, timed to coincide with the Anglo-American landings in France, was driving the Germans back in the east. Indeed, on D-day there were 199 German divisions on the eastern front as against 86 in the west and south. The Russians, who suffered enormous losses throughout the war, seemed to most Germans to be their most fearful enemies. As morale dropped even among high-ranking German officers, an attempt on Hitler's life on July 20, 1944, provided heartening evidence of resistance within the *Reich*.

General Montgomery, the top British commander in the west, now urged Eisenhower to concentrate all Allied resources on ending the war by a single decisive thrust into Germany. Eisenhower, looking at Allied port and trucking facilities, concluded that logistic support was lacking for the Montgomery plan. Accordingly, in a controversial decision, he settled instead for a "broad-front" strategy of building up strength along the entire western front in preparation for a general advance into Germany.

St. Malo, France, August 1944

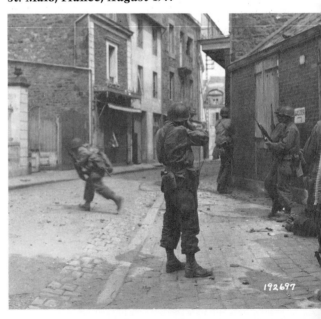

192697

Southern France or the Ljublana Gap? A final argument over strategy remained. The Americans had long wished to follow up the invasion of Normandy with troop landings in southern France; Eisenhower regarded this as essential to the invasion of Germany. The British wanted to switch the whole operation to the east and mount instead an invasion through Trieste and the Ljublana Gap of Yugoslavia toward Vienna.

This debate gave rise to the subsequent myth that Churchill, wishing to forestall the Soviet advance into eastern Europe, favored a Balkan invasion rather than a second front in France. Actually Churchill's Mediterranean strategy of 1942–43 was based on military considerations. Churchill never advocated an invasion of the Balkans, as an alternative to the second front or otherwise. The proposed attack through the Ljublana Gap in 1944—the "stab in the Adriatic armpit," as Churchill called it—would have left most of the Balkans untouched.

By 1944, it is true, Churchill was becoming increasingly concerned over the spread of Soviet power, and a definite object of the Ljublana plan was to beat the Russians to Vienna. The Americans rejected the proposal, partly because of the logistic difficulties presented by an Istrian campaign, partly because Roosevelt expected to be able to resolve any postwar political difficulties with the Soviet Union. And so the invasion of southern France took place according to schedule on August 15, 1944. With the fresh Allied advance up the Rhone Valley, the iron ring around Germany was drawing tight.

The War in the Pacific

Holding the line. Though the European theater of war had priority, the United States and Great Britain did not neglect the Far East. Pearl Harbor had marked only the beginning of a period of exultant Japanese aggression. "For three months after the Pearl Harbor attack," Admiral Samuel Eliot Morison has written, "the Pacific was practically a Japanese lake." One after another the bastions of western empire fell to the Japanese: Guam, Wake Island, and Hong Kong in December 1941; Singapore in February 1942; Java in March; and, after the terrible holding action on Bataan, the Philippines in May. Japanese forces were moving into Burma and threatening advances as far to the west as India and to the south as Australia. Japanese politicians were looking forward to the formation of the Greater East Asia Co-Prosperity Sphere, where Japan would mobilize the power of East Asia behind a wall of air and naval defense.

The Allied forces in the Pacific felt themselves the stepchildren of the war. Still, even when they believed themselves starved for supplies, their situation was by no means hopeless. The Japanese had failed to destroy a single aircraft carrier at Pearl Harbor; and the American carrier striking force was not only able to secure the South Pacific supply line between Hawaii and Australia but could conduct sporadic harassments of the enemy (including an air raid on Tokyo in April 1942).

Moreover, the Japanese themselves, instead of pausing for consolidation, struck out on ambitious new programs of conquest in the spring of 1942. Japanese political leaders hoped to extend the sway of the emperor by isolating and perhaps invading Australia; and Admiral Yamamoto, the chief Japanese sea lord, wished to force the American Pacific Fleet into a final engagement before it had a chance to recoup the losses of Pearl Harbor. In May 1942, therefore, the Japanese occupied Tulagi in the Solomon Islands and launched a naval expedition across the Coral Sea toward Port Moresby in Papua, New Guinea. But an American carrier task force intercepted the Japanese ships, and, in an extraordinary battle of carrier-based aircraft, the Americans turned back the enemy. This was the first sea battle in history in which the ships involved exchanged no shots—indeed, did not even come within sight of one another.

The Battle of the Coral Sea marked the high point of Japanese advances in the south. Yamamoto now shifted his operations to the north-central Pacific. A month later, the bulk of the Japanese navy—some two hundred ships—headed toward Midway Island and the western Aleutians. But the Americans, having broken the Japanese code, could anticipate enemy intentions. There followed the decisive naval battle of the war, in which the American fleets, brilliantly led by Admirals Raymond A. Spruance and Frank J. Fletcher, destroyed four Japanese aircraft-carriers and many other ships and forced the enemy into disorderly retreat. The Japanese never again had sufficient naval air strength to take the long-range offensive.

The road to Tokyo. The threat to communications from Hawaii to Australia remained, however, so long as the Japanese held bases in the Solomons and the Bismarcks. Moreover, the Bismarck Barrier, a chain of small islands, gave the Japanese a powerful defense block athwart the road to Tokyo. Intelligence reports that the Japanese were building an airstrip on the island of Guadalcanal in the Solomons precipitated American action in August 1942. There followed six months of grueling combat in the steaming, fetid jungles of Guadalcanal and in the serene waters around the island. By February 1943 the Japanese abandoned Guadalcanal.

The Second World War in the Pacific

SIBERIA (U. S. S. R.)

Russians 1945

OUTER MONGOLIA

MANCHURIA 1931

KOREA

CHINA

Dairen
Peking
Tientsin
Yenan Nanking
"The Hump" Chungking
Stilwell Road
Burma Road Kunming
1943
BURMA
INDIA
Rangoon
THAILAND

Hiroshima
Nagasaki
Tokyo
JAPAN
SHANTUNG PEN.
Shanghai
1937
OKINAWA
FORMOSA
Hong Kong
FR. INDO CHINA
1942

SAKHALIN
KURILE IS.
1942

ALASKA

ALEUTIAN IS.
1943

PACIFIC OCEAN

1942   Midway I.
June 3–6, 1942

Attack on Pearl Harbor
Dec. 7, 1941

HAWAIIAN IS.

IWO JIMA
GUAM
ENIWETOK
WAKE I.
Nimitz
MARSHALL IS.
CAROLINE IS.
KWAJALEIN   1944
1941–42   TARAWA
GILBERT IS.
1943

PHILIPPINE IS.
LUZON
LEYTE
MacArthur
1944-45
1943
1942

Malay Pen.
SINGAPORE
BORNEO
MINDANAO
SUMATRA
1942
CELEBES
JAVA
NETHERLANDS INDIES

NEW GUINEA
PORT MORESBY

BISMARCK BARRIER
SOLOMON IS.
GUADALCANAL
1942

1942
Coral Sea
May 4–8, 1942
1942

NEW CALEDONIA

INDIAN OCEAN

AUSTRALIA

NEW ZEALAND

⇦ Japanese advances
⬅ Allied advances
←--- Allied air operations

Yanks in the Solomon Islands, June 1943

In January 1943 the Joint Chiefs, noting that only 15 percent of Allied resources was applied to the Pacific, argued for enough additional strength to permit the launching of an offensive. The British acquiesced, stipulating only that Pacific operations should be kept within such limits as would not handicap the war against Germany. The American planners—for the Pacific war was accepted as essentially an American responsibility—now considered the question of the best route to Tokyo.

If European strategy was a compromise between diverging American and British views, Pacific strategy was a compromise between the diverging views of the American army and navy. General Douglas MacArthur, who had been American commander in the Philippines and had been evacuated to Australia early in 1942 to take command of the army in the South Pacific, argued forcefully for an advance from the South Pacific through New Guinea to the Philippines and then to Japan. Admiral Chester Nimitz, on behalf of the navy, contended for an advance through the central Pacific to Formosa, the Chinese coast, and

THE DEFEAT OF JAPAN

ISLAND WARFARE The South Pacific: MacArthur		ISLAND WARFARE The Central Pacific: Nimitz
Marines land on Guadalcanal, campaign to control Solomon Islands begins. Feb. 9, 1943, Japanese abandon Guadalcanal	August 7, 1942	
Counteroffensive at Papua begins reconquest of New Guinea, completed Sept. 16, 1943	January 23, 1943	
Landings at Rendova, New Georgia	June 30, 1943	
Landings at Bougainville, Northern Solomons. Solomons secure by end of year	November 1, 1943	
	November 21, 1943	Landings at Tarawa and Makin Islands begin battle for the Gilbert Islands and campaign for the Central Pacific. Tarawa secure November 24
	January 31, 1944	Invasion of Marshall Islands. Roi and Namur fall Feb. 3, Kwajalein Feb. 6, Eniwetok Feb. 22
Invasion of Admiralty Islands. Secure Mar. 25	March 1, 1944	
Conquests of air base, Hollandia, Dutch New Guinea	April 22, 1944	
	June 15, 1944	Invasion of Saipan, Marianas Islands. Secure July 9. Air raids of superfortresses against Japan from Saipan begin November 24
	July 21, 1944	Invasion of Guam, Marianas Islands. Secure Aug. 9
Invasion of Morotai	September 15, 1944	
	September 15, 1944	Invasion of Peleliu, Palaus Islands. Islands secure Nov. 25
Invasion of Leyte, Philippine Islands	October 29, 1944	
Invasion of Mindoro, Philippine Islands	December 15, 1944	
Invasion of Luzon, Philippine Islands. Fall of Manila Feb. 25	January 9, 1945	
	February 17, 1945	Invasion of Iwo Jima. Secure March 17
	April 1, 1945	Invasion of Okinawa. Secure June 21
	August 6, 1945	Hiroshima. Soviet Union enters war Aug. 8. Nagasaki Aug. 9
	August 10, 1945	Japanese offer of surrender

thence to Japan. MacArthur protested that this would be a gravely mistaken diversion of limited resources. But the navy responded persuasively that a single axis of advance would allow the Japanese to concentrate their defensive action. In the end the Joint Chiefs in Washington decided on parallel offensives along both routes.

The invention of new tactical techniques facilitated the American offensive. In March 1943, in the Battle of the Bismarck Sea, General George Kenney's bombers destroyed a Japanese troop convoy headed for New Guinea—an action that dissuaded the Japanese thereafter from attempting to move large bodies of troops within range of Allied air power. Knowing that the Japanese would not risk large-scale reinforcement, American forces could simply bypass the stronger Japanese bases. This "leapfrogging" technique became the basic pattern of the American counteroffensive.

By March 1944 Nimitz' forces had leapfrogged at Tarawa and Kwajalein, and MacArthur's forces had broken the Bismarck Barrier. Nimitz was now moving into the Marianas; in June the Pacific Fleet under Admiral Spruance smashed the Japanese navy again in the Battle of the Philippine Sea; MacArthur continued to press along the northwest coast of New Guinea toward the Philippines (see map, p. 742). The time was approaching for a final decision about the road to Tokyo.

Luzon or Formosa? MacArthur insisted on the recapture of the Philippines, and especially of Luzon, as the indispensable preliminary. He invoked not only strategic arguments—that Luzon would be a safer staging area for invasion than Formosa (Taiwan)—but political and emotional arguments. Was the President willing, the general asked, "to accept responsibility for breaking a solemn promise to eighteen million Christian Filipinos that the Americans would return?" (The promise had been MacArthur's.) Admirals King and Nimitz advocated leapfrogging part or all of the Philippines in the interest of an immediate attack on Formosa. In a conference at Pearl Harbor in July 1944, Roosevelt leaned toward the MacArthur view but did

General Douglas MacArthur at Leyte Gulf

not settle the question in MacArthur's favor until early October.

Once given the signal, MacArthur lost no time. On October 20 he disembarked on the beach at Leyte, saying, "People of the Philippines: I have returned." A few days later, in the Battle of Leyte Gulf, the American navy in the Philippines completed the destruction of Japanese naval striking power; in number of ships engaged, this was the greatest naval battle of all history. MacArthur's troops meanwhile pressed on toward Manila, while Nimitz' forces were making their way toward Japan from the central Pacific. Japan itself was now under a stern naval blockade and ever more devastating air attacks.

The riddle of China. Washington had hoped that China could play a leading role in the war against Japan. Indeed, through the war, Roosevelt, despite Churchill's skepticism, persisted in treating China as if it were a major power. However, the Nationalist regime of Chiang Kai-shek (Jiang Jieshi)—driven into the interior, cut off from sources of supply, exhausted by four years of war, and demoralized by inflation, intrigue, and graft—was increasingly incapable of serious action.

Keeping China in the war nevertheless remained a major American objective. In 1941 and 1942 the Chinese government, now established in Chungking (Chongqing), received a trickle of supplies flown over the "hump" of the Himalayas from India. Then in 1943 an assortment of Chinese, Indian, and American troops, under the command of General Joseph W. Stilwell, began to construct a road and pipeline across northern Burma to Kunming. Soon Stilwell was sent to Chungking (Chongqing) as commander of the American forces in China, with orders to maximize the Chinese contribution to the war against Japan. But, where Stilwell saw only one enemy, he discovered that Chiang Kai-shek (Jiang Jieshi) saw a second—the increasingly powerful Chinese communists, spreading out from their base in Yenan (Yanan).

Seeking particularly to mobilize the poverty-stricken and land-hungry peasants, the communists won respect, even among Westerners, as an embodiment of reform, austerity, and discipline. War sharpened the contrast between the self-indulgence of Chungking (Chongqing) and the dedication of Yenan (Yanan). Chiang (Jiang) himself seemed to be paying less and less attention to Japan in his preoccupation with the threat of Mao Tse-tung (Mao Zedong) and his Eighth Route Army. By 1944 four hundred thousand Nationalist troops had been diverted to check the spread of communist influence. Stilwell, eager to get as many Chinese divisions as possible—whatever their politics—into action against the Japanese, soon came to consider Chiang (Jiang) a main obstacle to the fulfillment of his mission.

In June 1944 the Fourteenth Air Force began to attack Japan from Chinese airstrips. This action provoked the Japanese into counterattacking the bomber bases and renewing their offensive against Chungking (Chongqing). Now the difficulties between Stilwell and Chiang (Jiang) came to a head. A brave, narrow, intense man, Stilwell was devoid of diplomatic skill and baffled by the unfathomable depths of Chinese politics. When the Joint Chiefs recommended that the Chinese army be placed under Stilwell's command, Chiang (Jiang) instead demanded his dismissal. Roosevelt complied. The military potential of China was disappearing in the swirl of Chinese civil discord.

The Fourth Term

Politics as usual. The congressional elections of 1942 brought into office the most conservative Congress Washington had known for a decade. Congressional refusal in the spring of 1943 to continue the National Resources Planning Board was a symbolic rejection of the whole idea of New Deal planning. Passage in June of the Smith-Connally Act over Roosevelt's veto bestowed on a reluctant government new powers to crack down on trade unions in labor disputes. Congress liquidated the National Youth Administration, harassed the Farm Security Administration, and sought in a variety of ways to curtail social programs and expenditures.

Roosevelt himself gave ground before the conservative attack. In a press conference in December 1943 he explained that the New Deal had come into existence because the United States was suffering from a grave internal disorder. But in December 1941 the patient had been in a bad external smashup. "Old Dr. New Deal . . . knew a great deal about internal medicine, but nothing about surgery. So he got his partner, who was an orthopedic surgeon, Dr. Win-the-War, to take care of this fellow who had been in this bad accident." Roosevelt went on to praise the ministrations of Dr. New Deal but added, "At the present time, obviously, the principal emphasis, the overwhelming first emphasis should be on winning the war."

The occupation of the White House by Dr. Win-the-War had already engendered a certain disenchantment in the American liberal community. Though Roosevelt retained the essential confidence of liberals, he was no longer articulating their day-to-day hopes. Many of them had been upset by his wartime

suspension of antitrust proceedings, by his relationships with Darlan and Badoglio, by his tepid policies toward civil rights, and by his hesitation in locating areas of asylum for the Jewish population of Europe that the Nazis were systematically murdering. In their frustration, the President's liberal critics listened to other voices. They found consolation in particular in Vice President Henry Wallace, with his celebration of "the century of the common man," and, more surprisingly, in Wendell Willkie, the Republican presidential candidate of 1940 (see p. 719). In the years after his defeat, Willkie had shown himself a political leader generous in disposition and courageous in utterance. Increasingly he was a champion of civil rights and a critic of big business. His book *One World*, published in 1943 after his trip as a presidential emissary to Britain, the Soviet Union, the Middle East, and China seemed to sum up the best aspirations of American liberal internationalism.

The campaign of 1944. As the titular leader of the Republican party, Willkie retained hopes of a second presidential nomination in 1944. But his liberal and internationalist tendencies, on top of a chronic political maladroitness, had estranged most of the leaders of his party. After suffering a bad defeat in the Wisconsin presidential primary in April, he withdrew from the race. Thomas E. Dewey, who had been elected governor of New York in 1942, was now emerging as the favored Republican contender. A young man—he had just passed his forty-second birthday—he had already gained a reputation for executive efficiency and vigor. The Republican convention, meeting in Chicago at the end of June, promptly nominated Dewey on the first ballot. To balance Dewey's growing inclinations toward liberalism and internationalism, Governor John W. Bricker of Ohio, a conservative isolationist, was named for second place.

The Democrats renominated Roosevelt without suffering the trauma of 1940. "For myself, I do not want to run," he wrote the chairman of the Democratic National Committee in July. "All that is within me cries to go back to my home on the Hudson. . . . But as a good soldier . . . I will accept and serve." The struggle was over the vice-presidential nomination. Wallace, with the ardent support of the labor-liberal wing of the party, sought renomination. But the Democratic South and the urban bosses opposed him, and, though Roosevelt said he "personally" would vote for Wallace if a delegate, he did not insist on Wallace's renomination. For a time Roosevelt leaned toward James F. Byrnes. When Ed Flynn of New York and Sidney Hillman of the Amalgamated Clothing Workers vetoed Byrnes, Roosevelt said he would be "very glad to run" with either Senator Harry S Truman of

Renomination, 1944

Missouri or Justice William O. Douglas of the Supreme Court. The contest narrowed down to Truman and Wallace, and Truman, with Roosevelt's private support, won on the third ballot.

The campaign was overshadowed by the war. The initial restraint of Dewey's speeches failed to stir the electorate. He stepped up the harshness of his attack, implying a connection between Roosevelt and communism, but his main achievement was to force Roosevelt himself into the arena. An uproariously successful speech by Roosevelt before the Teamsters Union in Washington on September 23 showed that the old campaigner had lost none of his magic. In October he sought to meet doubts about his health by riding around New York City all day in an open car through pouring rain. In the meantime, he spoke with eloquence about the need for internationalism in the postwar world and for a postwar economic bill of rights with federal guarantees to education, employment, and expanded social security. On November 7

Roosevelt received 25.6 million popular and 432 electoral votes as against 22 million and 99 for Dewey. The Democrats lost one seat in the Senate, gained twenty in the House, and captured five governorships. The election, though the closest of his triumphs, was a categorical confirmation of Roosevelt as America's chosen leader for the peace.

The Diplomacy of Coalition

The question of war aims. Even before Pearl Harbor Roosevelt had outlined his broad ideas on the postwar settlement. In his message to Congress on January 6, 1941, he said that the United States looked forward to a world founded upon "four essential human freedoms—freedom of speech and expression, freedom of worship, freedom from want, freedom from fear." In August of the same year, the Atlantic Charter (see p. 723) further particularized the American conception of the postwar world, laying stress on national self-determination, equal access to trade and raw materials, and a lasting peace to be achieved through a permanent system of general security. On January 1, 1942, twenty-six nations (led by the United States, Britain, the Soviet Union, and China) signed a joint declaration subscribing to the Atlantic Charter, pledging their full resources to victory, promising not to make a separate peace, and dedicating themselves to "defend life, liberty, independence, and religious freedom, and to preserve human rights and justice in their own lands as well as in other lands." Roosevelt called this a "declaration by United Nations," and his phrase was employed thereafter to describe the grand alliance.

In practice, three of the United Nations—the United States, Britain, and the Soviet Union—were more important than the rest. The United States and Britain, with common traditions and interests, had little difficulty in establishing partnership. Roosevelt and Churchill regarded each other with mutual respect and delight and were almost immediately on intimate terms. The formation of the Anglo-American Combined Chiefs of Staff in December 1941 guaranteed close military coordination; combined boards were subsequently set up in other fields. Friction, of course, was not entirely eliminated. There were persistent differences over European strategy, and Churchill quickly made it clear that he had no intention of applying the Atlantic Charter to British possessions. "We mean to hold our own," he said. "I have not become the King's First Minister in order to preside over the liquidation of the British Empire." Nonetheless, disagreements were held within a framework of reciprocal confidence.

> *The economic bill of rights as embodied in the President's message to Congress ... is:*
>
> *The right to a useful and remunerative job ... ;*
>
> *The right to earn enough to provide adequate food and clothing and recreation;*
>
> *The right of every farmer ... and his family to a decent living;*
>
> *The right of every business man ... to trade in an atmosphere of freedom from unfair competition ... ;*
>
> *The right of every family to a decent home;*
>
> *The right to adequate medical care and the opportunity to achieve and enjoy good health;*
>
> *The right to adequate protection from the economic fears of old age, sickness, accidents and unemployment;*
>
> *The right to a good education....*
>
> *To assure the full realization of this right to a useful and remunerative job, an adequate program must provide America with sixty million productive jobs....*
>
> *This will require large outlays of money which should be raised through normal investment channels. But while private capital should finance this expansive program, the Government should recognize its responsibility for sharing part of any special ... risk of loss attached to such financing.*

An Economic Bill of Rights

Henry A. Wallace as quoted in *The New York Times*, **January 26, 1945.**

With regard to the postwar world, Churchill, though by instinct a balance-of-power man, was prepared to go a considerable distance with Roosevelt's version of the United Nations as one keystone of a peace system. In Wilsonian rhetoric, Roosevelt declared that peace must "spell the end of the system of unilateral action, the exclusive alliances, the spheres of influence, the balances of power, and all the other expedients that have been tried for centuries—and have always failed." A reversion to those principles, he held, would create the conditions for future wars; it would also mean the repudiation of the Atlantic Charter, the Four Freedoms, and the values for which the war had presumably been fought. Roosevelt expected the four great powers—the United States, the United Kingdom, the Soviet Union, and China—to work in concert to keep the peace. He also viewed the United States as the dominant influence in the Americas. Indeed whatever his rhetoric, he continued to understand the importance of power in international politics. Still, he recognized that all nations had an interest in all the affairs of the globe, and all would therefore deserve representation in a postwar international organization. As he saw it, moreover, international prosperity was to be assured by the reduction of barriers to an expanding world trade.

The Russians viewed the world primarily in terms of spheres of influence and balances of power. They placed little confidence in the United Nations. Their physical safety, as they read their bitter histori-

cal experience, demanded the absolute guarantee that all states along the Russian border in eastern Europe should have "friendly governments," by which they meant governments reliably subservient to Moscow and based upon socialist principles. They had no intention of allowing other states a role in eastern Europe. In 1939 the Soviet-Nazi pact had enabled Russia to begin to fulfill part of what it considered its security requirements through the acquisition of the Baltic states, Karelian Finland, and eastern Poland. In November 1940 Moscow had pressed further demands on Hitler—a free hand in Finland, predominance in Romania and Bulgaria, bases in the Dardanelles. After the German attack, Stalin hoped to gain from the West what Hitler had not dared yield him.

These were traditional Russian objectives not dependent on ideology. But ideology intensified the possibilities of discord. The Soviet view, grounded in the Marxist-Leninist analysis of history, excluded the idea of long-term peace between communist and capitalist states. The very existence of the United States as the citadel of capitalism was, by definition, a threat to the security of the Soviet Union. While short-term accommodations with capitalism might be undertaken for tactical reasons, such arrangements would at best be an armed truce. But Stalin was not necessarily the helpless prisoner of this ideology. He saw himself less as the disciple of Marx and Lenin than as their fellow prophet. Sensing that Stalin was the only force capable of overcoming Stalinism, Roosevelt placed great emphasis on his personal relations with the Soviet leader.

So long, however, as Russian survival depended on the establishment of a second front, Moscow's purposes, whether strategic or ideological, were muted. Thus the Soviet government adhered to the Atlantic Charter (though with a reservation about adapting its principles to "the circumstances, needs, and historic peculiarities of particular countries") and acquiesced in the British refusal, under American pressure, to recognize the Soviet conquest of the Baltic republics. But Stalin's basic hope, as expressed in a proposal to Britain at the end of 1941, was for a straight sphere-of-influence deal.

The early wartime conferences. It soon became evident that the diplomacy of coalition required not only constant communication among the nations but periodic face-to-face meetings among their leaders. Thus Churchill followed his Washington visit in December 1941–January 1942 with a visit to Moscow in August, where he explained to an angry Stalin the reasons for the postponement of the second front ("Now they know the worst," he wrote Roosevelt, "and having made their protest are entirely friendly; this in spite of the fact that this is their most anxious and agonizing time").

The successes in North Africa at the end of 1942 opened a new phase of the war and emphasized the need for a conference among all three leaders. Stalin, however, felt that he could not leave the Soviet Union; so Roosevelt and Churchill met with their staffs at Casablanca on the Atlantic coast of Morocco in January 1943. The Casablanca Conference laid plans for future military action in the Mediterranean. Roosevelt and Churchill also sought, with little success, to unite the anti-Vichy French by bringing about a reconciliation between General de Gaulle and General Giraud. The main contribution of Casablanca, however, was the doctrine of "unconditional surrender."

By unconditional surrender Roosevelt meant no more than the surrender by Axis governments without conditions—that is, without assurance of the survival of the political leadership that had brought on the war. "It does not mean," he explained at Casablanca, "the destruction of the population of Germany, Italy, or Japan, but it does mean the destruction of the philosophies in those countries which are based on conquest and the subjugation of other people." Unconditional surrender was not a last-minute improvisation. It had been discussed in the State Department since the preceding spring and had been raised with Churchill (who, in turn, raised it with the British War Cabinet) before the press conference at which it was announced. The doctrine was designed

Roosevelt and Churchill, North Africa, 1943

partly to overcome misgivings generated by the Anglo-American willingness to deal with Darlan but even more to prevent Hitler from breaking up the Allied coalition by playing off one side against the other. The fear that the Soviet Union might seek a separate peace with Germany haunted British and American policy-makers in 1942–43, and unconditional surrender seemed the best insurance against such an eventuality.

Critics subsequently claimed that unconditional surrender stiffened Axis resistance and prolonged the war. This argument is not easy to substantiate with regard to the European war. Unconditional surrender had little effect in delaying the Italian surrender. In the case of Germany, no one seems to have been deterred from surrendering who would have surrendered otherwise, and up to the last moment such Nazi leaders as Goering and Himmler were sure they could work out their own deals with the Allies. An associated argument that unconditional surrender played into the hands of the communists by creating a power vacuum in central Europe seems odd in view of the fact that Stalin tried hard in 1944 to persuade Roosevelt and Churchill to modify the doctrine.

From Big Two to Big Three. Roosevelt and Churchill met again in Washington in May 1943, and in Quebec in August. Both meetings dealt mainly with Anglo-American military questions. The Soviet

Union still remained outside the conference circuit until October, when Cordell Hull and Anthony Eden journeyed to Moscow to pave the way for a meeting of the Big Three.

Relations between the Soviet Union and its western allies were now somewhat ambivalent. On the one hand, a temporary recession of ideology was evident when Stalin, in order to rally his people against the invader, replaced the appeal of Marxism with that of nationalism. "We are under no illusions that they are fighting for us," he once observed to Averell Harriman, the American ambassador. "They are fighting for Mother Russia." In May 1943 the Comintern, the instrumentality of communist revolution, was dissolved.

On the other hand, shadows of future problems were casting themselves ahead, especially in the liberated nations. The Soviet Union protested its exclusion from the Allied Control Commission for Italy. It had made clear its disinclination to relinquish the part of Poland it had seized in 1939, and in April 1943 it broke off relations with the Polish government-in-exile in London because the Poles asked the International Red Cross to investigate German charges, probably accurate, that the Russians had massacred several thousand Polish officers at Katyn. In Yugoslavia, the communist partisans, led by Marshal Tito, were already in conflict with a monarchist resistance movement of Chetniks led by General Mihailovich. A similar feud between communist and noncommunist guerrillas divided the resistance movement in Greece. Further, Roosevelt, at Churchill's instigation, had decided to keep secret Anglo-American development of certain weapons, of which the most important was the atomic bomb, then still far from completion though as the President knew, Stalin had obtained some general information about it. That secrecy reflected an uncertainty about Soviet intentions, a reservation about postwar cooperation, of which Stalin was aware. He harbored similar reservations himself, as well as persistent resentment about the postponement of the second front in France.

But such events remained in the background when the foreign secretaries met in October. Molotov, the Soviet foreign secretary, went agreeably along with a statement of pieties advocated by Hull and soon issued as the Declaration of Moscow. This included affirmation of "the necessity of establishing at the earliest practicable date a general international organization . . . for the maintenance of international peace." The Moscow Conference also established the European Advisory Commission to plan for German collapse.

The next step was the long-delayed meeting of the three leaders, arranged for Teheran in late November. This was preceded by a separate conference in Cairo where Roosevelt and Churchill met with Chiang Kai-shek (Jiang Jieshi); Stalin did not take part because Russia was not in the Far Eastern war. The Cairo Declaration promised to strip Japan of its conquests, to free Korea, and to return Manchuria and Taiwan to China. The Teheran meeting concentrated on military problems, including an Anglo-American commitment to a cross-Channel invasion within six months. The meeting also considered the future of Germany, problems in eastern Europe and the Far East, and the shape of the postwar peace system. "We came here with hope and determination," the three leaders wrote in the Declaration of Teheran. "We leave here, friends in fact, in spirit and in purpose."

Postwar planning. More progress was made in defining the structure of the future international organization when the Allies held a series of meetings at Dumbarton Oaks in Washington in August–September 1944. But the creation of broad frameworks for postwar collaboration did not solve the concrete problems of the postwar settlement. The fate of Germany posed especially perplexing questions. All members of the Big Three had played at one time or another with notions of German dismemberment; this approach seemed to prevail as late as Teheran. But when the European Advisory Commission took over, dismemberment receded into the background. The EAC concentrated instead on determining the zones of Allied occupation. In the end, Britain took the northwestern zone, America the southwestern, and Russia the eastern. Berlin, though situated in the Soviet zone, was to be jointly held; the question of access to Berlin was left, on military advice, to the commanders in the field.

As for the German economy, the most drastic proposals came from the United States Treasury Department in August 1944. Secretary Morgenthau urged both territorial transfers and partition; in addition, he recommended the dismantling of German heavy industry and the transformation of Germany into an agricultural state. For a moment Roosevelt fell in with the Morgenthau plan. Even Churchill accepted it briefly during the second Quebec Conference in September, partly in the hope of securing postwar economic aid in exchange. But in a few weeks this scheme dropped by the wayside, though its emphasis on a Spartan treatment of occupied Germany remained American doctrine.

Growing doubts about Soviet policy compounded the uncertainty over the future. The Polish question was more acute than ever. Churchill, in an effort to restore the position of the Polish government-in-exile in London, had been urging that government to accept Soviet territorial demands, including the Curzon line to the east and (in compensation) the Oder-Neisse line to the west (see map, p. 766); in November 1944 the British government pledged support for the Oder-Neisse line even if the United States refused to go along. But Stalin, who saw Poland as "the corridor for attack on Russia," considered the Polish question as "one of life and death" and refused to accept the London regime. In August the Polish Home Army, whose affiliations were with London, set off a revolt against the Germans in Warsaw. The Red Army, a few miles outside the city, declined to aid the uprising; the Soviet Union would not even permit planes carrying supplies to Warsaw from the west to land on Russian soil. This seemed a calculated attempt to destroy noncommunist Poles. In addition, the Soviet Union was setting up a group of procommunists in Lublin as the nucleus of a postwar Polish government. And, citing the Anglo-American example in Italy, the Russians, after the surrender of Bulgaria, denied the western Allies any role in the Bulgarian Control Commission.

In October Churchill paid another visit to Moscow. His effort to bring about a reconciliation between the London and Lublin Poles failed; but he and Stalin agreed on a scheme for southeastern Europe, according to which in the period after liberation Britain would recognize Russia's predominant interest in Romania, Bulgaria, and Hungary, and Russia would recognize Britain's predominant interest in Greece, with Yugoslavia split fifty-fifty. Roosevelt went along with this only as a temporary wartime arrangement, but Stalin and perhaps Churchill too probably expected it to register postwar realities.

Yalta, 1945: hopeful assumption soon to be falsified

Triumph and Tragedy

The Big Three at Yalta. Roosevelt's reelection in November 1944 found the Allied forces pressing hard down the last mile to victory. But bloodshed was far from over. With Eisenhower's forces deployed along the length of the Siegfried line, the Germans saw an opportunity in December 1944 to launch an attack in the Ardennes Forest. The desperate German offensive resulted in some early breakthroughs, but the Americans held at Bastogne, and, after weeks of severe fight-

**The Polish
question: F. D. R.**

From a reply from Franklin D. Roosevelt to Joseph Stalin, December 31, 1944.

ing, the Battle of the Bulge came to an end in January. On the other side of the world, the Japanese continued their resistance. Manila was not liberated until February 1945; and the forces of Admiral Nimitz coming in from the central Pacific had to fight every step of the way before they could gain such islands to the south of Japan as Iwo Jima (in February) and Okinawa (in April).

The approach of victory did not simplify the political problems of the triumphant coalition. In December communist resistance groups revolted against the British-backed provisional government of newly liberated Greece. Though Stalin, respecting the October agreement, made no objection to Churchill's military intervention in Greece, the fact that local communists had taken such initiative seemed a poor omen. The Polish tangle showed no signs of unraveling. The fate of Germany remained undecided. The future of eastern Europe and the Far East was still swathed in obscurity. The persistence of these problems argued for another meeting of the Big Three. They met in a conference at Yalta in the Crimea in February 1945.

Some of the decisions taken at Yalta pertained to Europe. The most critical of these had to do with the liberated nations of eastern Europe. Roosevelt and Churchill rejected Stalin's proposal that they accept the Lublin government in Poland. Instead, the three leaders agreed on a reorganization of the Polish government to include leaders from abroad—this provisional government to be "pledged to the holding of free and unfettered elections as soon as possible." For liberated Europe in general, the conference promised "interim governmental authorities broadly representative of all democratic elements in the population and pledged to the earliest possible establishment through free elections of governments responsive to the will of the people." With regard to Germany, the conference postponed decisions on dismemberment and on future frontiers, endorsed the EAC provisions for zonal occupation (adding a zone for France) and for an Allied Control Council, and evaded a Soviet demand of $20 billion for German reparations while conceding the figure as a "basis for discussion."

The Yalta discussions also dealt with the Far East, where the American Joint Chiefs were eager to secure from Stalin a precise commitment about entering the war. While Stalin had said vaguely in 1943 that the Soviet Union would declare war on Japan after the defeat of Germany, some feared that Russia would let the United States undertake a costly invasion of Japan and then move into Manchuria and China at the last minute to reap the benefits of victory. Moreover, the military estimated that the invasion of Japan, scheduled for the spring of 1946, might cost over a million casualties to American forces alone—another reason for desiring early Soviet participation. In secret discussions with Roosevelt, Stalin agreed to declare war on Japan within two or three months after the surrender of Germany on condition that the Kurile Islands and southern Sakhalin be restored to Russia and that the commercial interest of the Soviet Union in Dairen (Lüda) and its rail communications be recognized. When Roosevelt obtained the assent of Chiang Kai-shek (Jiang Jieshi) to these measures, the Soviet Union would agree "that China shall retain full sovereignty in Manchuria" and would conclude a treaty of friendship and alliance with the Chiang Kai-shek (Jiang Jieshi) government.

A third topic at Yalta was the organization of the United Nations. Here the Soviet Union accepted American proposals on voting procedure that it had opposed at Dumbarton Oaks and agreed that a United Nations conference should be called at San Francisco in April to prepare the charter for a permanent organization. With British support, the Russians also secured votes in the General Assembly for Byelorussia and the Ukraine. Roosevelt attached great importance to the apparent Soviet willingness to collaborate in a structure of international order. He doubtless also supposed that the deliberations of the United Nations, especially among the great powers, would provide the means of remedying the omissions or errors or ambiguities of the various summit conferences.

Roosevelt and Churchill returned from Yalta well satisfied. They expected Stalin, as Churchill put it, "to live in honourable friendship and equality with the Western democracies." During the war the Soviet government had discharged its military commitments with commendable promptitude. The Yalta agreements, however, represented the first experiment in postwar political collaboration. Here, as Churchill himself later wrote, "Our hopeful assumptions were soon to be falsified. Still, they were the only ones possible at the time."

After the war right-wing critics wrote that Roosevelt and Churchill had perpetrated a "betrayal" at Yalta, selling eastern Europe and China "down the river" in a vain effort to "appease" Stalin. The Yalta text makes it hard to sustain such charges. Had the agreements been kept, eastern Europe would have had freely elected democratic governments and Chiang Kai-shek (Jiang Jieshi) would have been confirmed in control of China and Manchuria. Stalin later abandoned his Yalta pledges in order to achieve his purposes. The Soviet Union, moreover, gained no territory as a result of Yalta (except the Kurile Islands) that was not already, or about to be, under Soviet domination as a result of military operations—and such operations could have been checked only by countervailing force from the West.

In more recent years left-wing critics have made opposite charges: that Stalin conceded more at Yalta than did Roosevelt and Churchill, and that behind American policy was an aggressive determination to dominate the world, promote counterrevolution and, in particular, make eastern Europe and the Far East safe for American capitalism. Again the Yalta documents fail to sustain such charges. Roosevelt remarked at Yalta that "two years would be the limit"

for keeping American troops in Europe; and the evidence suggests that the western Allies would have been wholly satisfied with an eastern Europe composed of nations friendly to Russia and (in the words of a State Department analysis) "in favor of far-reaching economic and social reforms, but not, however, in favor of a left-wing totalitarian regime to achieve these reforms."

All in all, military realities at the time set the terms of the agreements at Yalta. Roosevelt let those realities take precedence over political considerations. Short of preparing for a war against the Soviet Union, he had no other choice. And as he saw it, American interests then lay essentially in speeding victory in Europe and Asia. Like Churchill, he could depend only on hopeful assumptions about the future of eastern Europe.

Victory in Europe. For the Soviet Union, cooperation with noncommunists had been a response to the rise of Nazism. The Yalta Conference, taking place in the shadow of the Ardennes counteroffensive, reflected the still dangerous Nazi military threat. But the picture began to alter rapidly. A fortnight after Yalta, the United States Ninth Army had reached the Rhine at Düsseldorf. With the end of the war in sight, the Soviet need for wartime cooperation was disappearing: it was now time to begin the postwar struggle for eastern Europe. Within a few weeks the Soviet Union took swift action in Romania and Poland to frustrate the Yalta pledges of political freedom. Stalin himself opened up a political offensive against the West, charging that the United States and Britain were engaged in separate peace negotiations with Germany, as indeed some of their agents secretly were in Switzerland. Roosevelt replied with indignation that he deeply resented these "vile misrepresentations."

At the end of March 1945 Roosevelt cabled Churchill that he was "watching with anxiety and concern the development of the Soviet attitude." This attitude portended danger not only for immediate issues, but for "future world cooperation." The President sent stern warnings to the Soviet leader and on April 6 told Churchill, "We must not permit anybody to entertain a false impression that we are afraid. Our Armies will in a very few days be in a position that will permit us to become 'tougher' than has heretofore appeared advantageous to the war effort." But Roosevelt, worn out by long years of terrible responsibility, was reaching the end. On April 12 he died of a massive cerebral hemorrhage, as truly a casualty of war as any man who died in battle.

These ominous political developments put military problems in a new context. As the Anglo-American armies plunged ahead into Germany, Churchill argued in March and April that they should race the

Americans and Russians, Torgau, Germany, April 1945

Russians to Berlin. "From a political standpoint," he said, "we should march as far east into Germany as possible." But General Eisenhower replied, "I regard it as militarily unsound . . . to make Berlin a major objective." The imperative consideration, in the view of the American Joint Chiefs, was the destruction of the German armed forces; and this, Eisenhower believed (incorrectly, as it turned out), required the pursuit of the remaining German troops to a supposed last stand in the south.

A month later, Churchill renewed his pleading, this time in connection with Prague. He proposed that Allied forces remain as far east as they could until Soviet Russia clarified its intentions with regard to Poland and Germany. Harry S Truman, who had succeeded to the American Presidency, hesitated at suggestions for deeper American involvement in central Europe, partly because of a fear of prejudicing future Soviet cooperation with the United Nations, partly because of the need for redeploying American troops to the Pacific. He accordingly treated the problem as a tactical one to be decided by the commander in the field. Eisenhower, for his part, declined to abandon strictly military criteria in the absence of orders from above. Though he could have put American troops into Prague far in advance of the Red Army, he refused to do so. It is by no means clear that Churchill's plan would have basically changed the postwar balance in Europe. But it seems evident that the American generals, as General Omar Bradley later wrote, "looked naïvely on this British inclination to complicate the war with political foresight and non-military objectives."

By now events in Europe were rushing to climax. Hitler's thousand-year *Reich*, racked by months of Allied bombing and now overrun by Allied armies from both west and east, was falling to pieces. The German dictator himself took refuge in his bunker in Berlin and on April 30 committed suicide. On May 3 the process of piecemeal German surrender began, with a ceremony of unconditional surrender at Eisenhower's headquarters in Rheims on May 7, and a sur-

Victory in Europe: an outburst of joy

The development of nuclear power not only constitutes an important addition to the technological and military power of the United States, but creates grave political and economic problems for the future of this country.

Nuclear bombs cannot possibly remain a "secret weapon" at the exclusive disposal of this country for more than a few years. The scientific facts on which their construction is based are well known to scientists of other countries. Unless an effective international control of nuclear explosives is instituted, a race for nuclear armaments is certain to ensue following the first revelation of our possession of nuclear weapons to the world. Within ten years other countries may have nuclear bombs.... In the war to which such an armaments race is likely to lead, the United States, with its agglomeration of population and industry in comparatively few metropolitan districts, will be at a disadvantage compared to nations whose population and industry are scattered over large areas.

We believe that these considerations make the use of nuclear bombs for an early unannounced attack against Japan inadvisable. If the United States were to be the first to release this new means of indiscriminate destruction upon mankind, we would sacrifice public support throughout the world, precipitate the race for armaments, and prejudice the possibility of reaching international agreement on the future control of such weapons.

From the Committee on Social and Political Implications, Report to the Secretary of War, June 1945.

render to the Russians in Berlin the next day. As Churchill later wrote, the end of hostilities was "the signal for the greatest outburst of joy in the history of mankind." He added somberly that he himself moved amid cheering crowds "with an aching heart and a mind oppressed by forebodings."

Victory in the Far East. While the European war was coming to its troubled end, American forces continued to make steady progress in the Pacific. But Japanese resistance grew every day more fanatical. The use of kamikaze suicide planes and the last-ditch fighting in Iwo Jima and Okinawa seemed to confirm the horrendous American estimates of casualties to be expected in an invasion of the homeland. Within civilian Japan, though, sensible people recognized that the war was irretrievably lost.

In the meantime, an extraordinary new factor entered into American calculations. In 1939 the scientist Albert Einstein had called Roosevelt's attention to the possibility of using atomic energy for military purposes. In the next years the government sponsored a secret $2 billion operation known as the Manhattan Project to attempt the building of an atomic bomb. A brilliant group of physicists, working under the direction of J. Robert Oppenheimer in Los Alamos, New Mexico, steadily broke down the incredibly complex scientific and technological problems involved in the production of the weapon. On April 25, 1945, Secretary of War Stimson could tell President Truman,

"Within four months we shall in all probability have completed the most terrible weapon ever known in human history, one bomb of which could destroy a whole city."

The next question was how and when this frightful weapon should be employed. Roosevelt seems never to have doubted that, once available, the bomb would be dropped. The momentum of wartime atomic policy militated to that conclusion. On June 1 a special committee recommended to Truman that the bomb be used against Japan as soon as possible. Many Manhattan Project scientists, aware of the ghastly character of the weapon, opposed this recommendation, favoring a preliminary demonstration to the world in a desert or on a barren island. But this course was rejected, partly because of the fear that the bomb might not go off, partly because only two bombs would be available by August and it seemed essential to reserve them for direct military use.

Within Japan, a new government was looking for a way out. In July it requested Soviet mediation to bring the war to an end, though it added, "So long as the enemy demands unconditional surrender, we will fight as one man." Moscow was cold to this request while Stalin departed for a new Big Three meeting at Potsdam, near Berlin. At the same time, the American government, following the Japanese peace explorations through decoded cable intercepts, came to the conclusion that the best way to hasten the end of the war would be to issue a solemn plea to the Japanese to

The atomic bomb: the President's view

surrender before it was too late. This warning was embodied somewhat cryptically in a declaration issued at Potsdam by Truman and Clement Attlee, who had succeeded Churchill as British prime minister, urging the Japanese to give up or face "the utter devastation of the Japanese homeland." The Japanese government was inclined to accept this ultimatum, but the military leaders angrily disagreed. On July 28 the Japanese prime minister, in a statement designed for domestic consumption, pronounced the Potsdam Declaration "unworthy of public notice."

Truman had already been informed while at Potsdam that the first bomb test in New Mexico on July 16 had been a triumphant success. The rejection of the Potsdam Declaration now convinced him that the militarists were in control of Tokyo and that there was no point in delaying the use of the bomb against Japan. Some of the President's advisers, Secretary of State Byrnes particularly, believed that the use of the bomb would enhance the American position in negotiations with the Soviet Union. For Truman, that possibility was at most a secondary consideration, though he did decide neither to consult Stalin about the bomb nor to offer him, any more than Roosevelt had, any broad scientific information about the nature of the weapon. Primarily Truman was moved by his interpretation of Japanese political and military conditions. On his orders, on August 6, in a blinding flash of heat and horror, the first atomic bomb fell on Hiroshima, killing nearly one hundred thousand people, fatally injuring another hundred thousand through blast or radiation, and reducing the city to rubble.

Even after this appalling blow the Japanese military vetoed the civilian desire to accept the Potsdam Declaration. Two days after Hiroshima, the Red Army invaded Manchuria and, on the third day, with no word from Tokyo, the American air command, operating on earlier orders, dropped a second bomb on Nagasaki. In Tokyo the military still objected to unconditional surrender. It required the personal intervention of the emperor to overcome their opposition. With Japanese acceptance of Potsdam conditioned on the preservation of the imperial prerogatives, the act of surrender took place on September 2, 1945.

The decision to drop the atomic bomb was the most tragic in the long course of American history. Perhaps only so drastic a step would have achieved unconditional surrender so rapidly. On the other hand, thoughtful observers have wondered whether the American government, with Japan essentially beaten and on the verge of capitulation, had exhausted all the possible alternatives before at last having recourse to the bomb—whether there were not resources of negotiation or demonstration that, even at the cost of prolonging the war, should have been first attempted, with the bomb held in reserve as a weapon of last resort. Here perhaps prior atomic policy, and, still more, the doctrine of unconditional surrender had terrible consequences. Certainly, though the bomb terminated the war, it also placed the United States for many years in an ambiguous position before the world as the only nation to have employed so horrible a weapon.

Victory thus came—but in a way that converted triumph into tragedy. The Second World War ended.

More than 25 million persons, soldiers and civilians, had died during the five years. Sixteen million Americans—more than 10 percent of the population—had been under arms; total casualties amounted to over a million, with nearly three hundred thousand deaths in battle. Now, in the autumn of 1945, the world stood on the threshold of a new epoch in history—an epoch incalculably rich in hazards and potentialities. With apprehensive steps, humanity was entering the atomic age.

Suggestions for Reading

THE SECOND WORLD WAR: THE HOME FRONT

R. E. Sherwood, *Roosevelt and Hopkins* (1948, rev. ed., 1950), remains the most vivid account of Roosevelt as a war-leader; it should be supplemented by J. M. Burns' valuable study, *Roosevelt: The Soldier of Freedom** (1970). For war mobilization, see the Bureau of the Budget, *The United States at War* (1946); E. Janeway, *The Struggle for Survival* (1951); and H. M. Somers, *Presidential Agency: OWMR* (1950); on price control, L. V. Chandler, *Inflation in the United States, 1940–1948* (1951); C. Bowles, *Promises to Keep* (1971); and, for the penetrating reflections of a leading controller, J. K. Galbraith, *Theory of Price Control** (1952). The mobilization of science and technology is incisively depicted in J. P. Baxter, III, *Scientists Against Time** (1946); on mobilization of manpower, see G. Flynn, *The Mess in Washington* (1979); R. G. Hewlett and O. E. Anderson, Jr., *The New World* (1962), is authoritative on the development of the atomic bomb. Volume III of J. M. Blum, *From the Morgenthau Diaries: Years of War, 1941–1945* (1967), throws light on a variety of issues that concerned the Treasury.

For American society in wartime, see J. M. Blum, *V Was For Victory** (1976), which also deals with politics; R. Polenberg, *War and Society: The United States, 1941–1945** (1972); R. Polenberg, ed., *America at War: The Home Front, 1941–1945* (1968); and R. Lingeman, *Don't You Know There's a War On* (1970). Also illuminating is A. W. Winkler, *The Politics of Propaganda: The Office of War Information, 1942–1945* (1978). Francis Biddle provides thoughtful discussion of the civil-liberties problems he faced as Attorney General in *Democratic Thinking and the War* (1944) and in his distinguished memoir *In Brief Authority* (1962). On the Japanese-Americans, there are several good studies of which a recent and trenchant one is R. Daniels, *Concentration Camps* (1971). L. S. Wittner, *Rebels Against War: The American Peace Movement, 1946–1960** (1969), is excellent on its subject. For black Americans, see H. Garfinkel, *When Negroes March** (1959); L. Ruchames, *Race, Jobs and Politics: The Story of FEPC* (1953); R. M. Dalfiume, *Desegregation of the United States Armed Forces* (1969); A. Meier and E. Rudwick, *CORE** (1973); and the magisterial study by G. Myrdal, *An American Dilemma* (1944 rev. ed., 1962). On women, the best study is that of Chafe, previously cited. On wartime politics, besides various studies cited above, see the excellent study of the Republicans in E. Barnard, *Wendell Willkie: Fighter for Freedom** (1966), and the analysis of Democratic dissenters in J. M. Blum, ed., *The Price of Vision: The Diary of Henry A. Wallace, 1942–1946* (1973).

THE SECOND WORLD WAR: MILITARY OPERATIONS

A. R. Buchanan, *The United States and World War II*, 2 vols. (1964), is a survey. For able analyses of American strategy, see S. E. Morison, *Strategy and Compromise* (1958); L. Morton, *Strategy and Command* (1962); K. R. Greenfield, ed., *Command Decisions* (1959); K. R. Greenfield, *American Strategy in World War II: A Reconsideration** (1963); and R. F. Wrigley, *Eisenhower's Lieutenants* (1981). The role of the American services is intensively portrayed in three multivolume series: Office of the Chief of Military History, *The United States Army in World War II*; S. E. Morison, *History of United States Naval Operations in World War II* (summarized in *The Two-Ocean War*, 1963); and W. F. Craven and J. L. Cate, *The Army Air Forces in World War II*, 7 vols. (1949–58). There is indispensable background in the six volumes of W. S. Churchill, *The Second World War* (1948–53); in two volumes on the Secretary of War: H. L. Stimson and McGeorge Bundy, *On Active Service in Peace and War* (1948), and E. E. Morison, *Turmoil and Tradition* (1960); and in the biography of the Chief of Staff, F. C. Pogue, *George C. Marshall*, 3 vols. (1963–73). Among the formidable number of American war memoirs, the most useful on the European theater are those of Dwight D. Eisenhower, Omar Bradley, H. H. Arnold, W. Bedell Smith, and Mark Clark; on the Pacific theater, those of Douglas MacArthur, Joseph Stilwell, Claire Chennault, Albert Wedemeyer, Courtney Whitney, Robert Eichelberger, W. F. Halsey, George C. Kenney, Walter Kreuger, and, as recounted by Walter Whitehill, Ernest J. King.

For the American military role in Europe, C. B. MacDonald, *The Mighty Endeavor: American Armed Forces in the European Theater in World War II* (1969), offers a comprehensive account. For strategic debates in Europe, see C. Wilmot, *The Struggle for Europe* (1952); S. E. Ambrose, *The Supreme Commander: The War Years of General Dwight D. Eisenhower* (1970); M. Howard, *The Mediterranean Strategy in the Second World War* (1968); and two volumes by T. Higgins: *Winston Churchill and the Second Front, 1940–1943* (1957) and *Soft Underbelly: The Anglo-American Controversy Over the Italian Campaign, 1939–1945* (1968). J. Toland, *The Last Hundred Days* (1966), and C. Ryan, *The Last Battle* (1966), cover the fall of Germany. For the Pacific war, see J. Toland, *The Rising Sun: The Decline and Fall of the Japanese Empire** (1970); B. Tuchman, *Stilwell and the American Experience in China, 1911–1945** (1971); T. H. White and A. Jacoby, *Thunder Out of China** (1946); J. Hersey, *Hiroshima** (1946); W. S. Schoenberger, *Decisions of Destiny* (1970); W. Manchester, *MacArthur* (1979); and various volumes in the Army history, especially those by Louis Morton, C. F. Romanus, and Riley Sunderland.

The GI's view of the war is candidly portrayed in the gritty newspaper reporting of Ernie Pyle, *Here is Your War* (1943) and *Brave Men* (1944), and the sardonic cartoons of Bill Mauldin, *Up Front* (1945). See also the *New Yorker Book of War Pieces* (1947), and such novels as Norman Mailer, *The Naked and the Dead** (1948); James Jones, *From Here to Eternity** (1951); William Styron, *The Long March** (1952); and Joseph Heller, *Catch-22** (1961). S. A. Stouffer et al., *The American Soldier,** 2 vols. (1949), contains important sociological data.

THE SECOND WORLD WAR: DIPLOMACY
J. L. Snell, *Illusion and Necessity: The Diplomacy of Global War* (1963); G. Smith, *American Diplomacy During the Second World War* (1965); and especially R. Dallek, *Franklin D. Roosevelt and American Foreign Policy, 1932–1945** (1979), are useful surveys. The volumes of H. Feis—*The China Tangle* (1953), *Churchill, Roosevelt, Stalin** (1957, 2nd ed., 1967), *The Atomic Bomb and the End of World War II* (rev. ed., 1966)—provide brilliant coverage of diplomatic questions. Two books by R. A. Divine, *Roosevelt and World War II** (1969) and *Second Chance: The Triumph of Internationalism in America** (1967), deal with war and postwar issues. For revisionist views of American policy, see S. Ambrose, *Rise to Globalism** (1971), and G. Kolko, *The Politics of War: The World and United States Foreign Policy, 1943–1945* (1969). On the question of the Anglo-American invasion of Europe, see M. Stoler, *The Politics of the Second Front* (1977). On Yalta, E. R. Stettinius, *Roosevelt and the Russians—The Yalta Conference* (1949), defends Administration policy, W. H. Chamberlin, *America's Second Crusade** (1950), attacks it from the right, and D. S. Clemens, *Yalta* (1970), questions it from the left. On relations with Russia, see W. H. McNeill, *America, Britain and Russia* (1953); J. L. Gaddis, *The United States and the Origins of the Cold War** (1972); A. Ulam, *Expansion and Coexistence** (1968); J. R. Deane, *The Strange Alliance* (1953); P. E. Mosely, *The Kremlin and World Politics* (1960); M. Herz, *Beginnings of the Cold War* (1966); G. C. Herring, *Aid to Russia, 1941–1946** (1973); W. A. Harriman, *America and Russia in a Changing World* (1971); and D. Yergin, *Shattered Peace** (1977). On relations with France, see W. L. Langer, *Our Vichy Gamble* (1947), and M. Viorst, *Hostile Allies* (1965). On China, see Tang Tsou, *America's Failure in China, 1941–1950** (1963). On atomic diplomacy, see R. G. Hewlett and O. E. Anderson, *The New World* (1962), and M. J. Sherwin, *A World Destroyed: The Atomic Bomb and the Grand Alliance** (1975).

Particularly useful memoirs are Cordell Hull, *Memoirs*, 2 vols. (1948); W. D. Leahy, *I Was There* (1950); J. F. Byrnes, *Speaking Frankly* (1974) and *All in One Lifetime* (1958); Sumner Welles, *The Time for Decision* (1944) and *Seven Decisions That Shaped History* (1951); R. D. Murphy, *Diplomat Among Warriors* (1964); J. C. Grew, *Turbulent Era: A Diplomatic Record of Forty Years*, 2 vols. (1952); G. F. Kennan, *Memoirs 1925–1950* (1967); and A. Harriman and E. Abel, *Special Envoy to Churchill and Stalin* (1975). Indispensable glimpses of American policy from foreign perspectives can be found in the memoirs or diaries of Winston Churchill, Charles de Gaulle, Joseph Goebbels, Albert Speer, Galeazzo Ciano, Milovan Djilas, Ivan Maisky, Lord Avon (Anthony Eden), Lord Halifax, Lord Montgomery, Harold Macmillan, Lord Alexander, Lord Tedder, Sir Frederick Morgan, Sir John Slessor, Sir Alexander Cadogan, Harold Nicolson, Lord Casey, and Sir Robert Menzies.

*Available in a paperback edition.

1945–
1984
THE
NATIONAL
EXPERIENCE

America entered the postwar age feeling the elation and bearing the burden of superpowership. Isolation, in the classic sense of "no entangling alliances," was dead. The invention of nuclear weapons confronted humanity with the possibility of extinction. For the first time since the early republic, foreign affairs became an abiding national preoccupation.

Hope for a better world after the defeat of Nazism soon gave way to fear of a new totalitarian assault on the democratic nations. No doubt Stalin's purposes were initially defensive. Still, given Stalin's suspicions of friend and foe alike, no one can tell how far his apprehension about Soviet security would have led him to project Soviet power had he not encountered western resistance. The Truman Doctrine, the Marshall Plan, and the North Atlantic Treaty Organization successfully contained Soviet ambitions in Europe.

The invasion of South Korea in 1950 opened a new phase of the Cold War. Now containment became a global policy. The United States assumed responsibility for places less stable, less democratic, and less defensible militarily than the nations of Western Europe. This new globalism stimulated an indiscriminate anticommunism, based not, as it had been in the 1940s on tangible threats to national security, but on an abstract and doctrinaire obsession with communism as a metaphysical evil. Anticommunism as a secular faith, with Secretary of State John Foster Dulles and Senator Joe McCarthy as its prophets, reached an apogee during the Korean War. With the end of that war and the tranquilizing influence of President Eisenhower, the anticommunist fever abated for a generation.

The standards of human rights piously affirmed by the United States when condemning despotism abroad prompted minorities at home to demand justice for themselves. The struggle of black Americans for their constitutional rights gathered new force. The 1954 Supreme Court decision forbidding segregation in public schools gave the struggle the blessing of the Constitution. Though the path was long, tortuous, and often bloody, the civil-rights movement persevered. Its example inspired other revolts against discrimination in American society, the most significant of which was the movement for women's liberation.

After the Eisenhower interlude, Presidents Kennedy and Johnson renewed the Roosevelt-Truman reform impulse, especially in racial justice and in the war against poverty. Presidential activism had less happy consequences in foreign policy. Though Kennedy learned from early mistakes and labored hard to temper the Cold War, Johnson plunged into the Americanization of a long-running civil war in Vietnam. As half a million troops wrought appalling destruction without bringing the war to an end, more and more Americans at home turned against what they came to see as a senseless, even immoral, conflict. The Vietnam War, along with the horrifying assassinations of John Kennedy, of his brother Robert, and of Martin Luther King, Jr., the three leaders of the sixties with the strongest appeal to American idealism, helped persuade an impassioned minority of young Americans that American society itself was irremediably corrupt and hopeless.

The reaction against this sometimes hysterical protest brought to the Presidency in 1968 Richard Nixon, a politician counted on by his Republican supporters to enforce middle-class values. In foreign affairs Nixon, once a famous red-hunter, showed realism and initiative in improving relations with Russia and China. At home his deep personal insecurity and morbid suspicions set off a fanatic and eventually criminal drive to revenge himself against fancied "enemies." The result was the Watergate scandal, followed by Nixon's resignation to escape impeachment.

Emotions subsided under his successor, Gerald Ford. Jimmy Carter, the Democrat elected President in 1976, combined good intentions with irresolute policy and performance. In 1980 the electorate turned to Ronald Reagan, a conservative Republican dedicated in domestic policy to the reduction of the role of government and in foreign policy to the revival of crusading anticommunism and to the restoration of American world dominance. Reagan's assault on the welfare state excited controversy at home, while abroad Soviet-American relations sank to a new low. In the meantime, the superpowers continued to build and deploy nuclear weapons, and forebodings intensified around the planet about the possible end of the human race.

30
THE COLD WAR

The United States emerged from the Second World War a relatively unified, powerful, and confident nation. Victory gave Americans an uncritical pride in the productivity of their economy, in the prowess of their armed forces, in the rectitude of their motives, and in the strength of their liberal ideals.

The Americans of 1945 did not suppose, as many of their parents had in 1918, that victory permitted retreat from international responsibility. But they had differing conceptions of America's world role. Some hoped to use American power to build a lasting structure of world peace. Some sought new outlets for an ebullient American capitalism. Some, like former Vice President Henry Wallace, called for "the century of the common man." Some, like the magazine publisher Henry R. Luce, dreamed imperially of "the American Century." Problems remained at home: in particular, to prevent a repetition of the economic depression, the political hysteria, and the social complacency that followed the First World War.

Truman Takes Over

The new President. "I feel as though the moon and all the stars and all the planets have fallen on me," Harry S Truman told newspapermen on the April day in 1945 when he heard the report of Roosevelt's death.

"Please, boys, give me your prayers. I need them very much." A back-bencher from Missouri who had barely retained his own seat in the Senate four and a half years before, he had to fill the mighty place of the man who had dominated the affairs of the United States and the world for a dozen years.

On the record Truman seemed a Missouri courthouse politician, a beneficiary of the notorious Pendergast machine in Kansas City, a Democratic wheel horse in the Senate, an old-time political pro whose chief attribute was loyalty to his organization and his President. On the other hand, those who knew him valued the spontaneous decency that had led him to fight the Ku Klux Klan at the height of its power in Missouri, the courage in adversity that had enabled him to hold his Senate seat in 1940, and the concern for popular welfare he had displayed throughout his public career. As wartime chairman of the Senate Committee to Investigate the National Defense Program, he had discharged a delicate job with intelligence and responsibility. He kept on his desk a motto from Mark Twain: "Always do right. This will gratify some people, & astonish the rest." No one could tell what the chemistry of the Presidency would do with this strange mixture of human elements.

Initial impressions were not encouraging. In his fourth week as President, Truman casually signed an order that abruptly stopped the delivery of goods under the lend-lease program. The sudden termina-

762   **South Korea: to the front for limited objectives**

tion of lend-lease deliveries caused resentment and misunderstanding abroad. "This experience brought home to me," Truman subsequently wrote, "not only that I had to know exactly where I was going but also that I had to know that my basic policies were being carried out. It I had read that order, as I should have, the incident would not have occurred. But the best time to learn that lesson was right at the beginning of my duties as President."

The candor, the humility, and the cockiness were all characteristic. Though he never totally divested himself of a tendency to shoot from the hip, Truman gradually developed authority in his new role. His wide knowledge of history gave him a vigorous sense of the dignity of the Presidency. He worked hard. He accepted responsibility: he used to say of the presidential desk, "The buck stops here." He reconstructed the Cabinet, gradually transforming a Roosevelt Administration into a Truman Administration. Winston Churchill, meeting him at Potsdam in July 1945, was impressed by "his gay, precise, sparkling manner and obvious power of decision."

Experiment in World Order

The postwar atmosphere. This power of decision was almost immediately put to the test. For war had left the international order in a condition of acute derangement. With the Axis states vanquished, the European Allies battered and exhausted, the colonial empires in dissolution, and the underdeveloped world in tumult, great gaping holes appeared in the structure of world power. And war had also left only two states—the United States and the Soviet Union—with the political dynamism, ideological confidence, and military force to flow into these vacuums of power. The war had accustomed both states, moreover, to thinking and acting on a world scale.

The war's end thus saw a geopolitical rivalry between America and Russia as well as a clear-cut difference over the principles on which the peace should be organized—whether in terms of great-power spheres-of-influence or United Nations universalism (see p. 746). And the factor that transformed this structural conflict into something akin to a religious war and began to give it apocalyptic overtones was the apparently irreconcilable ideological disagreement between the two superpowers. With the prewar world in pieces, America and Russia appeared in 1945 as the first truly global powers in the history of the human race, exerting their influence everywhere around the planet, encountering no serious opposition anywhere, except from each other—each, as Tocqueville had prophesied

in *Democracy in America* a century earlier, seemingly "marked out by the will of Heaven to sway the destinies of half the globe."

Launching the United Nations. Nevertheless war had bound the victors together in coalition, and the Dumbarton Oaks conference of 1944 had laid down the main lines for a postwar structure. On April 29, 1945, representatives of fifty nations met at San Francisco to create a permanent United Nations organization.

The UN Charter, essentially an American product, was in the direct line of descent from the Covenant of the League of Nations. Of the UN organs, the General Assembly and the Security Council had the widest authority. The Assembly was the legislative body, though its powers were limited to discussion and recommendation. The Security Council was the action agency assigned, in the language of the charter, "the primary responsibility for the maintenance of international peace and security."

The Security Council consisted of five permanent members—the United States, Britain, Russia, France, and China—with six further members (after 1966, ten) elected by the General Assembly. The charter gave the Council authority to settle international disputes by peaceful means—through investigation or mediation or whatever method seemed suitable. If

United Nations Building, New York City

such methods failed, Chapter 7 of the charter authorized the Council to take appropriate measures against any state that broke the peace. If necessary, it might use armed force supplied by the member states. However, the charter also limited the Security Council's authority to invoke these powers—especially by giving each permanent member a veto. Neither the United States nor the Soviet Union would have joined the UN without this means of protecting its interests. By 1984 the Soviet Union had used the veto 115 times, the United States 37 times.

Collective effort. Surrounding the UN was a constellation of subsidiary agencies, among which the United Nations Relief and Rehabilitation Administration had particularly urgent responsibilities. Established in 1943 to bring food, clothing, medicine, and other supplies to liberated countries, UNRRA disbursed $2.7 billion over the next five years combating hunger and other ravages of war. Its director and many of its workers were American, and the United States contributed nearly three-quarters of its financial support.

While UNRRA tackled the immediate crisis, the western Allies, meeting in July 1944 at Bretton Woods, New Hampshire, planned a long-term international economic framework. Bretton Woods led to the establishment of two institutions: the International Monetary Fund, designed to create a world monetary system based on fixed exchange rates; and the International Bank for Reconstruction and Development (better known as the World Bank), designed to supply capital for investment and trade in underdeveloped areas. The Soviet Union, regarding these institutions as the instruments of international capitalism, declined to participate.

It did, however, join other specialized UN agencies—the Food and Agricultural Organization, the International Trade Organization, the World Health Organization, and the International Labor Organization (taken over from the League). In addition, the newly organized United Nations Educational, Scientific, and Cultural Organization (UNESCO) fostered international efforts to raise cultural standards and promote intellectual exchange.

The Cold War Begins

The coalition in trouble. The United Nations could not abolish profound disagreements in interest and ideology. These disagreements, held in check during the war by common opposition to Hitler, found new nourishment in postwar difficulties.

For Stalin the overriding concern remained the security of the Soviet Union. Determined to safeguard Soviet frontiers by keeping eastern Europe under Soviet control, he may well have construed the Yalta agreement in terms of his sphere-of-influence deal with Churchill at Moscow four months before (see p. 750). In addition, he doubtless expected that the free elections promised at Yalta would produce pro-Soviet regimes. But events soon made it clear that he had overestimated Soviet popularity in eastern Europe and underestimated western concern over the extension of Soviet power into central Europe. When after Yalta Stalin moved to excluded non-communists from the Polish government, the new American President, only a few weeks in office, conveyed his disapproval in salty language to V. M. Molotov, the Soviet foreign minister. In May 1945 Truman sent Harry Hopkins to Moscow to make it clear that Truman was carrying forward Roosevelt's policies, to emphasize that Poland had become the "symbol" of the ability of Russia and the West to work out their problems, and to warn that "if present trends continued unchecked, the entire structure of world cooperation . . . would be destroyed." As Churchill later described the mood in the summer of 1945, "The agreements and understandings at Yalta, such as they were, had already been broken or brushed aside by the triumphant Kremlin. New perils, perhaps as terrible as those we had surmounted, loomed and glared upon the torn and harassed world."

It was in this atmosphere that Truman, Stalin, and Churchill (superseded in mid-conference by Attlee) met at Potsdam outside Berlin at the end of July. Of all the power vacuums created by the war, the most vital was in the heart of Europe. The western powers acquiesced in a temporary Polish occupation of Germany up to the Oder-Neisse line, with the final territorial settlement to be reserved for the peace conference. The west, concerned by Soviet "looting" of German industry, refused the Soviet demand for the reparations Moscow believed had been promised at Yalta. In the end the Russians resentfully accepted a compromise. Zones of military occupation were confirmed, with each nation—America, Britain, France, and Russia—supreme in its own zone and each also participating in an Allied Control Council responsible for matters affecting Germany as a whole.

While the Potsdam Conference marked a retreat from the punitive proposals considered a year earlier at Quebec, the American occupation authorities at first imposed severe political and economic measures on Germany. American troops were forbidden to "fraternize" with Germans. An International Military Tribunal established at American instigation tried twenty-two top Nazis in Nürnberg from November 1945 to October 1946; nineteen were convicted of war crimes, and twelve were sentenced to death. Though condemned by some as "victors' justice," the Nürnberg and later trials compiled a mass of evidence documenting the brutality of Nazi rule.

The curtain falls. Potsdam was the last meeting between Stalin and the western leaders. Suspicions now grew apace on both sides. The Administration was at first uncertain in its response. Secretary of State James F. Byrnes, an indefatigable negotiator, had no great faith in the Russians but thought agreement possible on specific issues. Secretary of Commerce Henry A. Wallace argued that the Russians should be given the benefit of the doubt. In 1947 the National Security Act established a unified defense establishment, creating a Secretary of Defense, a National Security Council, and a Central Intelligence Agency. Secretary of Defense James V. Forrestal, persuaded that the Russians were bent on world conquest, advocated a hard line.

Contention over Iran in the winter of 1945–46 deepened Truman's mistrust of the Soviet Union. At the wartime Teheran conference, the Big Three had agreed to respect the territorial integrity of Iran. After the war, Britain and America withdrew their forces; the Russians did not. A brief crisis ended when American pressure forced Soviet withdrawal in May 1946.

The unleashed power of the atom intensified mutal distrust. In June 1946 Bernard Baruch, as American delegate to the UN Atomic Energy Commission, proposed that all nuclear technology, civil and military, be placed under UN control. The Baruch plan envisaged an International Atomic Development Authority, exempt from the great-power veto, owning and operating nuclear materials and facilities and punishing violators of its rules. While ostensibly evenhanded in its approach, the plan, as the Russians noted, placed authority in an international agency under American domination. They were accordingly unwilling to surrender their veto or to accept inspection within the Soviet Union. The chance of international control was thus lost, and the future of nuclear weapons remained in national hands.

In eastern Europe, when the Communist party won only 17 percent of the vote in the Hungarian election of November 1945, Stalin moved to consolidate the Soviet position. In an important speech on February 9, 1946, he declared that the capitalist system rendered war inevitable. On March 5, Churchill, speaking at Fulton, Missouri, with Truman beside him on the platform, responded by warning against the "expansive tendencies" of the Soviet Union. "From Stettin in the Baltic to Trieste in the Adriatic," he said, "an iron curtain has descended across the Continent." How should the West meet the Russian challenge? "I am convinced that there is nothing they admire so much as strength, and there is nothing for which they have less respect than weakness, especially military weakness."

Hope of a peace treaty settling the future of Germany vanished. The occupation zones now evolved into *de facto* partition. Each side softened its German policy and began to sponsor revival in its own zone. In 1949 the German Federal Republic was established in the west, the German Democratic Republic in the east.

As for the Axis satellites, the Council of Foreign Ministers set up at Potsdam carried forward the task of drawing up peace treaties. In December 1946 Byrnes and the Russians concluded treaties with Italy, Bulgaria, Hungary, Romania, and Finland. By these treaties the western powers acquiesced in Soviet control of eastern Europe. In tacit exchange, the Soviet Union acquiesced in American control of occupied Japan.

The Truman Doctrine. Early in 1947, Byrnes resigned, and Truman appointed General George C. Marshall in his place. Marshall's unique national eminence helped remove the discussion of foreign policy from a partisan context. So too did the collaboration in a "bipartisan" foreign policy of Arthur H. Vandenberg, a Republican senator from Michigan, whose prewar record as an isolationist gave his views special weight among conservatives.

In the meantime communist pressure was mounting against Greece and Turkey; and early in 1947, Great Britain, in acute economic straits itself, notified Washington that in five weeks it must end financial support to a Greek government besieged by

The partition of Germany and Austria

DENMARK SWEDEN U.S.S.R.

EAST PRUSSIA

U.S. and Br.

NETH.

POLAND

Berlin

(Joint occupation by four powers)

GERMANY

Odor R.

Neisse R.

CZECHOSLOVAKIA

FRANCE

Vienna

SWITZ. AUSTRIA HUNGARY

ITALY YUGOSLAVIA

☐ Occupied by U.S.   ☐ Occupied by U.S.S.R.
☐ Occupied by France ☐ Transferred to Poland
☐ Occupied by Gr. Britain

The Soviet challenge

communist guerrillas receiving support from Marshal Tito, the Communist leader of Yugoslavia. Though Stalin had not instigated the Greek uprising and regarded it with dubiety, these facts were not known in the West, which supposed that the collapse of Greece would embolden Moscow to move against Italy and France.

Truman accordingly decided that America must take up the burden. Recalling the hard fight for a loan to Britain itself a year before, Truman feared that a conventional request for aid to Greece and Turkey would not pass the Congress. Accepting Vandenberg's judgment that he had to scare the hell out of the country, he went to Capitol Hill in person to urge what soon became known as the Truman Doctrine. "I believe," Truman said, "that it must be the policy of the United States to support free peoples who are resisting attempted subjugation by armed minorities or outside pressures." Some, within the Administration and without, flinched at open-ended language going far beyond the immediate problem. But Congress responded to presidential evangelism and in May 1947 passed a bill granting $400 million in aid to Greece and Turkey over the next fifteen months. Though the subsequent collapse of the Greek insurgency was due as much to Tito's break with Stalin in 1948 as to American assistance, the apparent efficacy of the Truman Doctrine in its initial application strengthened belief in both America's ability and its obligation to serve as guardian of freedom throughout the world.

The containment policy. As the Russians hardened their grip on eastern Europe, Ambassador Averell Harriman warned from Moscow that they

could use their zone, not just to secure their own frontiers, but as a springboard from which to dominate central and western Europe, now lying economi-

General Douglas MacArthur and Emperor Hirohito, 1945

Soviet-American relations: a dissenting view

We are reckoning with a force which cannot be handled successfully by a 'Get tough with Russia' policy. 'Getting tough' never bought anything real and lasting—whether for schoolyard bullies or businessmen or world powers. The tougher we get, the tougher the Russians will get.... I believe that we can get cooperation once Russia understands that our primary objective is neither saving the British Empire nor purchasing oil in the Near East with the lives of American soldiers....

On our part, we should recognize that we have no more business in the political affairs of Eastern Europe than Russia has in the political affairs of Latin America, Western Europe and the United States. We may not like what Russia does in Eastern Europe. Her type of land reform, industrial expropriation, and suppression of basic liberties offends the great majority of the people of the United States. But whether we like it or not the Russians will try to socialize their sphere of influence just as we try to democratize our sphere of influence.... We cannot permit the door to be closed against our trade in Eastern Europe any more than we can in China. But at the same time we have to recognize that the Balkans are closer to Russia than to us—and that Russia cannot permit either England or the United States to dominate the politics of that area.... Under friendly peaceful competition the Russian world and the American world will gradually become more alike. The Russians will be forced to grant more and more of the personal freedoms; and we shall become more and more absorbed with the problems of social-economic justice.

From Henry A. Wallace, Speech at Madison Square Garden, September 12, 1946.

cally prostrate and politically vulnerable before them. Stalin's instrumentality, some supposed, would be the obedient Communist parties of France, Italy, and Germany through which he might, without Russian military action, promote the Stalinization of the continent and thereby succeed where Hitler had failed in wielding the whole force of Europe by a single hand.

The American return to Europe under the Truman Doctrine was the first application of an evolving philosophy. The most extended statement was made by George F. Kennan, a member of the foreign service with long experience of the Soviet Union. Writing anonymously in *Foreign Affairs* in July 1947, Kennan argued that Soviet communism was like "a fluid stream which moves constantly, wherever it is permitted to move, toward a given goal." American policy, Kennan proposed, must be that of "the firm and vigilant containment of Russian expansive tendencies." The purpose of containment was not to enter the Russian sphere or overthrow the Soviet regime but rather to block the Soviet effort to flow into "every nook and cranny available to it in the basin of the world." In time this would force a measure of circumspection on the Kremlin and "promote tendencies which must eventually find their outlet in either the break-up or the gradual mellowing of Soviet power."

The containment idea provoked heated debate in the United States. On the right, traditional isolationists, led by Senator Robert A. Taft of Ohio, doubted America's financial or moral capacity to sustain an activist international policy. In the center, commentators like Walter Lippmann feared that the containment psychology would lead people to see the Soviet Union as primarily a military threat to be met by military means and involve the United States beyond its sphere of direct and vital interest. On the left, Americans unwilling to surrender the idea of the innocence or moderation of Stalin denounced the policy as aggressive and provocative. This group found a spokesman in Henry Wallace, whom Truman fired in 1946 after Wallace publicly attacked the new directions of policy.

The Marshall Plan. The Truman Doctrine was an emergency effort to shore up crumbling positions in Greece and Turkey. It had been made necessary by the hard-pressed economic condition of Britain. Britain's plight was symptomatic of the plight of all western Europe. European city-dwellers were living on less than 2,000 calories a day. The cradle of Western civilization seemed to Winston Churchill in 1947 "a rubble heap, a charnel house, a breeding ground for pestilence and hate." "The patient is sinking," said Secretary Marshall, "while the doctors deliberate."

In an address at the Harvard commencement on June 5, 1947, Marshall called on the European coun-

The Marshall Plan

From George C. Marshall, Commencement Speech at Harvard University, 1947.

tries themselves to draw up a plan for European recovery. "This is the business of the Europeans. . . . The role of this country should consist of friendly aid in the drafting of a European program and of later support. . . . The program should be a joint one, agreed to by a number, if not all, of European nations." Marshall added, significantly, "Our policy is directed not against any country or doctrine but against hunger, poverty, desperation, and chaos."

This was the proposal that, as British Foreign Secretary Ernest Bevin later told Parliament, he "grabbed . . . with both hands." Within three weeks, representatives of European states, west and east, assembled in Paris. The prospect of east European participation faded, however, when the Russians denounced the plan as American economic imperialism and pulled out of the meeting, taking their satellites with them. A pro-Soviet coup in Czechoslovakia in February 1948—itself conceivably an overreaction to the Marshall Plan—completed the division of Europe. It also smoothed the way for the passage of the plan by the American Congress in March.

The sixteen remaining states (including Turkey) now began integrated economic planning through the Organization of European Economic Cooperation. With generous contributions by the United States—$12.5 billion in four years—the Marshall Plan countries by 1951 raised their industrial output 40 percent over 1938. The stimulus provided by the Marshall Plan and the OEEC led to further experiments in European integration—especially the European Coal and Steel Community (1952) and the European Economic Community, better known as the Common Market, established by the Rome Treaties in 1957.

The dramatic economic recovery reduced the political threat of communism and set western Europe on the road to independence in world affairs.

The division of Europe. In response to the Truman Doctrine and Marshall Plan, the Soviet Union completed the consolidation of control in eastern Europe.

The Marshall Plan: wheat for Greece

**Berlin airlift:
it broke the blockade**

In 1947 Moscow set up the Cominform to replace the prewar Comintern as the mechanism by which the Soviet Union managed foreign Communist parties. In 1949 it organized the Council for Mutual Economic Assistance (COMECON) to assure Soviet economic domination of the satellites.

In addition, Stalin systematically extinguished political dissent in eastern Europe through staged trials, forced confessions, and executions. At first the Soviet purge concentrated on socialist and peasant politicians; but by 1949 it swept through the Communist parties themselves, liquidating leaders suspected of inadequate loyalty to Moscow, such as Laszlo Rajk in Hungary, Traicho Kostov in Bulgaria, and Rudolf Slansky in Czechoslovakia. Yugoslavia, which owed its liberation to its own efforts rather than to the Red Army, was relatively inaccessible to Soviet power. Here Tito's independent course soon led to his excommunication by Moscow.

In the spring of 1948 the Soviet Union confronted the West with a new challenge when it cut off West Berlin by blockading all highway, river, and rail traffic into the former German capital. The evident purpose was to force the western powers out of Berlin. The western answer was to supply West Berlin through an airlift. When it became apparent that even winter could not halt the airlift and that a western counter-blockade was hurting East Germany, Moscow developed second thoughts. On May 12, 1949—321 days after the start of the airlift—the Russians ended the blockade.

The Berlin crisis, following so closely on the communist coup in Czechoslovakia, convinced many western Europeans of the need for a regional defense arrangement. Truman agreed that only "an inclusive security system" could dispel the fear that the Soviet Union might overrun western Europe. On April 4, 1949, the North Atlantic nations established an alliance in which (in the language of Article 5 of the final pact) "an armed attack against one or more of them in Europe or North America shall be considered an attack against them all." Article 11, however, provided that the treaty was to be carried out by the signatories "in accordance with their respective constitutional processes," which presumably meant, in the American case, that Congress would have to authorize an American response. The original members of the North Atlantic Treaty Organization (NATO) were the United States, Britain, France, Italy, Belgium, the Netherlands, Denmark, Norway, Portugal, Luxembourg, Iceland, and Canada. Later they were joined by Greece, Turkey, West Germany, and Spain. In 1955, after the admission of West Germany to NATO, Moscow established a counterpart military organization under the Warsaw Pact.

The occupation of Japan. In Japan, where the United States had a free hand in occupation policy, General Douglas MacArthur, the supreme allied commander, had ordered a series of political and economic purges, culminating in the trial and punishment of Japanese wartime officials under standards more stringent than at Nürnberg. At the same time he sought to transform the vanquished country into a model western democracy. A new constitution, adopted under American direction in 1946, renounced war as a sovereign right, adding that "land, sea and air forces, as well as other war potential, will never be maintained." The *zaibatsu*, the great family trusts, were threatened with dissolution; trade unions were encouraged; women were given the vote; land was redistributed among the peasants; the educational system was reorganized; and Shinto was abolished as the state religion.

But increasing apprehension about the Soviet Union soon raised the question whether a disarmed Japan would not leave a dangerous power vacuum in the Far East. A peace treaty, finally negotiated in 1951, registered the altered American attitude. The treaty terminated the occupation, conceded to Japan "the inherent right of individual or collective self-defense," and opened the way for American troops and installations to remain through bilateral agreement.

MacArthur's democratization of Japan was an apparent success. But one dubious result was to increase the confidence of Americans in their capacity to build and rebuild nations around the world.

Why the Cold War?

The historical controversy. The postwar antagonism, known by 1947 as the Cold War, was, according to the official Anglo-American thesis, the necessary western response to an unprovoked course of expansion by Soviet communism.

To American eyes, the Russian course portended a new phase in the world struggle between democracy and totalitarianism, with communism inheriting the mantle just relinquished by fascism. Communism in the forties did not, save in China, imply—as it might in later years—popular movements determined to reclaim political and economic independence for their nations. For most Americans, communism meant Stalinism, the system that ruled Soviet Russia, a system correctly seen as not only extraordinarily cruel and repressive at home but in secure command of most Communist parties through the world. Stalinism was also seen, perhaps less correctly, as inherently aggressive and insatiable. This impression was understandable, however, when a Soviet official like Maxim Litvinov, foreign minister in the 1930s and later ambassador to Washington, well known to the West as a champion of collective security, privately warned western friends against appeasement. If the West acceded to current Soviet demands, he said in 1946, "it would be faced, after a more or less short time, with the next series of demands."

In later years the official thesis fell under attack, especially in the United States. The "revisionist" critique took many forms, but predominant arguments were that America was more the postwar aggressor than Russia; that the American government systematically whipped up anticommunist emotions in order to cloak its real intentions, which were to establish economic hegemony throughout the world; and that (in the view, at least, of the more extreme revisionists) Washington had no choice but to seek an "open door" for American trade and investment because American capitalism had to expand in order to survive.

One part of the revisionist critique had lasting influence—that is, its insistence on looking at the postwar situation from the Soviet as well as the western viewpoint. For the Soviet Union had suffered greater losses in the war than any other nation. The western interest in eastern Europe could have been honestly perceived in Moscow as a threat to Soviet security. In retrospect, it seems probable that Moscow was not intent on military aggression or dedicated, as a practical goal, to "world conquest." Stalin, cautious and opportunistic, carefully refrained from committing the Red Army outside his own sphere of vital interest. While not forgoing the pleasures and benefits of intrigue and subversion in other parts of the world, he was prepared, in exchange for a free hand in the Soviet sphere, to concede American and Britain free hands in their spheres, including the freedom to suppress communist movements. He was even perhaps prepared to place China and Greece within the western sphere.

The "open door" interpretation of American policy has stood up less well. It is hard, for example, to explain American interest in eastern Europe by a supposed quest for markets, investment outlets, and raw materials. While Washington certainly worked for a freely trading world—against, among other things, the high-tariff predilections of much of American business—it was not this desire that prompted objections to Soviet policy in eastern Europe, where the American economic stake was negligible. Moreover, some of the most ardent proponents of trade expansion argued that accommodation with Russia, not confrontation, was the surest way to find outlets for American goods. So Henry Wallace both championed the "open door" policy and opposed the policy of "containment."

The postwar American military posture was hardly that of a nation bent on world empire. No government in modern history had conducted so swift a demobilization of its conventional military force; nor had any electorate so unitedly demanded it. Even as Soviet-American relations grew worse, the United States cut back its armed forces until they were almost an eighth of their wartime size. Though revisionist historians subsequently argued that American policy-makers had seen the atomic bomb as the means of controlling the postwar world, Washington in fact made no sustained attempt to practice nuclear diplomacy against the Soviet Union, ignoring those, like the British philosopher Bertrand Russell, who urged the threat of the bomb to compel the Russians to good behavior.

Nor were American leaders in the forties obsessively anticommunist. In China, for example, Truman worked for a coalition between Chiang Kai-shek (Jiang Jieshi) and Mao Tse-tung (Mao Zedong), and communism in Yugoslavia was not an obstacle to American aid after Tito's break with Stalin. Nor did Washington dismiss the Soviet point about "friendly" regimes along the Russian border. The western powers would have been satisfied had the Russians settled for the Finnish pattern throughout eastern Europe—that is, permitting internal freedoms so long as foreign policy was acceptable to Moscow.

The fundamental issue, as the Truman Administration saw it, lay not between capitalism and revolution but between democracy and Stalinism. In western Europe democratic socialist leaders—Clement Attlee and Ernest Bevin in England, Leon Blum in France, Ernst Reuter and Willy Brandt in West Germany—were in the forefront of opposition to the spread of Stalinism. These men had no interest in an open door for American capitalism; they had a profound interest in the future of democratic socialism. Observing the dismal fate of democratic socialists in eastern Europe, they concluded that they would meet the same fate if postwar chaos brought communism to power in their own countries. For a time, indeed, they regarded Washington's response to the Stalinist threat as naively slow.

The Cold War soon became an intricate, interlocking, reciprocal process, involving authentic differences in principle, real and supposed clashes of interest, and a wide range of misunderstanding and misperception. Each superpower believed with passion that its own safety as well as world peace depended on the success of its peculiar conception of world order. Each superpower, in pursuing its own clearly expressed and ardently cherished principles, only confirmed the fear of the other that it was bent on aggression. Soviet behavior in eastern Europe, Iran, and Berlin and the activity of Communist parties elsewhere seemed to confirm the western notion of an expansive Soviet Union. American postwar policy, especially in its expressions of concern about eastern Europe, assumed a threatening aspect for the Russians. Each superpower persevered in corroborating the fears of the other. Together they proceeded to deepen the Cold War.

Confusion on the Home Front

The process of reconversion. In domestic policy Truman was a down-the-line New Dealer. His message to Congress on September 6, 1945, was his answer to the question (as he later wrote) of whether "the progress of the New Deal [was] to be halted in the aftermath of war as decisively as the progress of Woodrow Wilson's New Freedom had been halted after the first World War." Truman saw himself as both the continuator and the consolidator of Roosevelt's brilliant improvisations. A man of orderly administrative habits, he tried to systematize the Presidency and to rationalize the recently expanded government.

At the same time, he was faced with the problem of reconverting the nation's economy from war to peace. Predictions of 8 or 10 million unemployed had been common in 1945. But the economy showed far more resilience than anyone expected. Between 1945 and 1946 government purchases of goods and services declined by a sum equal to almost one-quarter of the gross national product. This decline, according to theorists, should have brought in its wake a disastrous fall in the national output and a rise in unemployment. But the gross national product declined only slightly in the same period, and employment actually increased by 3 million.

This achievement was due in great part to the pent-up demand for consumer goods after the deprivations of the war years. It was also due to sensible government policy. The Servicemen's Readjustment Act of 1944, better known as the G.I. Bill of Rights, was a remarkably creative law by which the federal government offered veterans four years of college education as well as vocational training and medical care. The Employment Act of 1946 established the Council of Economic Advisers and charged the federal government with responsibility for maintaining a high level of economic activity.

Inflation rather than depression was the greater threat. With the war over, the nation was chafing more than ever under price and wage controls. Businessmen evaded the system through black markets; labor, seeking wage increases after years of wartime denial, went out on strike. When a railroad strike paralyzed the economy in the spring of 1946, Truman asked Congress for power to draft strikers into the army—a request that even conservatives deemed intemperate and that the Senate rejected. Congress subsequently extended the OPA but so weakened its authority that Truman vetoed the bill. There followed an interval in July 1946 with no controls at all, during which time prices shot up almost 25 percent. When Congress passed another bill a few weeks later, it was too late to put back the lid. Supply soon caught up

To strengthen the right to equality of opportunity, the President's Committee recommends:

1. In general:

The elimination of segregation, based on race, color, creed, or national origin, from American life.

The separate but equal doctrine has failed in three important respects. First, it is inconsistent with the fundamental equalitarianism of the American way of life in that it marks groups with the brand of inferior status. Secondly, where it has been followed, the results have been separate and unequal facilities for minority peoples. Finally, it has kept people apart despite incontrovertible evidence that an environment favorable to civil rights is fostered whenever groups are permitted to live and work together. There is no adequate defense of segregation.... We believe that federal funds, supplied by taxpayers all over the nation, must not be used to support or perpetuate the pattern of segregation in education, public housing, public health services, or other public services and facilities.... A federal Fair Employment Practice Act prohibiting discrimination in private employment should provide both educational machinery and legal sanctions for enforcement purposes.

From the President's Committee on Civil Rights, *To Secure These Rights,* **1947.**

with demand, however, and the average annual inflation rate for the five years after the removal of controls was 6 percent.

The election of 1946. As the midterm congressional election approached, Truman seemed to have lost control of the economic and political situation. Republicans asked, "Had enough?" "To err is Truman" became a popular joke. To no one's surprise, the Republicans carried both houses of Congress for the first time since 1928. The new Eightieth Congress proved a bulwark of conservatism. Its dominant figure was Robert A. Taft of Ohio, son of the former President and a senator of inexhaustible energy, knowledge, and self-confidence. His admirers regarded him as the epitome of old-fashioned American wisdom; his critics said he had the best mind in Washington until he made it up.

Taft had long been concerned with ending what he regarded as the privileged position created for organized labor by the Wagner Act of 1935. The Taft-Hartley bill as amended outlawed the closed shop but permitted a measure of union security through the "union shop" (that is, a contract requiring workers to join the union after being hired—as distinct from the closed shop, which demands that they join before being hired). However, its Section 14B legalized so-called right-to-work laws by which states could forbid the requirement of union membership as a condition of employment. It also provided for a cooling-off period before resort to strikes. Labor leaders denounced the law extravagantly as a "slave labor" measure, and

Truman vetoed it. But in early 1947 Congress passed the Taft-Hartley bill over his veto.

The conservatives also passed in 1947 a constitutional amendment forbidding presidential third terms—a belated act of vengeance against Franklin D. Roosevelt. The Twenty-second Amendment was ratified by the required thirty-six states in February 1951.

Truman fights back. As the 1948 presidential election approached, Truman concluded that his only hope for reelection lay in the militant advocacy of a liberal program. In early 1948 he bombarded Congress with a series of reform proposals. Much of this was a reaffirmation of New Deal objectives, but in the field of racial justice he broke new ground.

Though reared according to the Southern customs of a border state, Truman was a man of humane instinct. He was also aware of the considerable change in the mood of black America wrought by the New Deal and the war. In 1946 he appointed a President's Committee on Civil Rights. A year later the committee recommended a permanent civil rights commission, a mandatory FEPC, antilynching and anti-poll-tax laws, and a strengthening of civil-rights statutes and enforcement machinery. In an eloquent message on February 2, 1948, Truman made these proposals part of his program. This attempt to realize the promises of the Declaration of Independence for all Americans, regardless of race or color, was Truman's boldest initiative in the domestic field.

The civil-rights proposals alienated the conservative Democrats of the South. Liberals were dismayed by the elimination of New Deal personalities, like Harold Ickes and Francis Biddle, from the Administration Old-line Democratic bosses though the President was sure to be beaten. As the Democratic convention drew near, a "dump-Truman" movement gained momentum. The anti-Truman forces were unable to agree on an alternative, however, and in the end Truman won renomination with little difficulty.

The 1948 campaign. The Republicans had once again nominated Governor Thomas E. Dewey of New York. Dewey campaigned with the complacent confidence of a man who could not lose. Republican optimism swelled even further when a communist-manipulated Progressive party nominated Henry A. Wallace for the Presidency and when diehard Southern Democrats formed the States Rights Democratic party (better known as the Dixiecrats) and nominated Strom Thurmond of South Carolina.

Only Truman thought he could win. He began a "give 'em hell" campaign across the country, telling audiences at every whistlestop that the record of the "do-nothing, good-for-nothing" Republican Eightieth

Truman in 1948: 356 speeches

Congress proved the worthlessness of Republican campaign promises. A fall in the price of corn and hogs alarmed the farmers. The Dixiecrat revolt confirmed liberals and blacks in their Democratic allegiance, while the Wallace movement eliminated communism as an issue between the major parties and kept Catholics in the Democratic camp. Neither Dewey's personality nor his campaign roused enthusiasm. Truman, on the other hand, emerged as a pungent orator, an indomitable fighter, and—in contrast to his opponent—an intensely *human* being. Shouting crowds greeted Truman's appearances with the joyful cry, "Pour it on, Harry." By election day he had traveled 31,700 miles and had delivered 356 speeches.

Public-opinion polls forecast a sure Republican victory. The Chicago *Tribune* put out an election extra announcing Dewey as the next President. But Truman received 24.1 million popular votes against 22 million for Dewey, and 303 electoral votes against 189. Thurmond carried four states (South Carolina, Mississippi, Alabama, and Louisiana) and polled 1.2 million votes. Wallace also polled 1.2 million votes but carried no states. In addition, the Democrats captured both houses of Congress. Truman, who ran behind the Democratic ticket, owed his victory to the vitality of the Roosevelt coalition as well as to his own efforts.

Second Term

Return to frustration. "We have rejected the discredited theory that the fortunes of the nation should be in the hands of a privileged few," Truman said in January 1949. "Instead, we believe that our economic system should rest on a democratic foundation and that wealth should be created for the benefit of all. The recent election shows that the American people are in favor of this kind of society." His state-of-the-union message was a ringing summons to a new era of social reform. "Every segment of our population and every individual," he concluded, "has a right to expect from his government a fair deal."

But his Fair Deal roused strong opposition. Secretary of Agriculture Charles F. Brannan's plan to support farm income rather than prices and Federal Security Administrator Oscar Ewing's proposal for national health insurance were condemned as "socialistic." Congress refused to repeal the Taft-Hartley Act and rejected Truman's requests for federal aid to education and for middle-income housing. A Senate filibuster killed the FEPC. On the other hand, though thwarted in his legislative program for civil rights, Truman through executive action ended segregation within the government and the armed services.

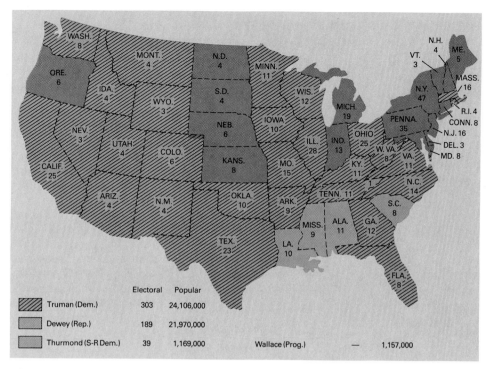

	Electoral	Popular
Truman (Dem.)	303	24,106,000
Dewey (Rep.)	189	21,970,000
Thurmond (S-R Dem.)	39	1,169,000
Wallace (Prog.)	—	1,157,000

The election of 1948

The developing world. A "revolution of rising expectations" had been sweeping through the Third World ever since the war. Underdeveloped countries, stridently nationalist in mood, were shaking off the political and economic bonds of western empire and demanding independence, growth, and modernization.

In listing points in his inaugural address in 1949, Truman placed particular emphasis on Point Four—"a bold new program" to offer technical assistance to developing countries. The war against world poverty, Truman said, "is the only war we seek." The Point Four program received limited funding, however, and had only modest impact. Foreign policy under the masterful direction of the new Secretary of State, the urbane and imperious Dean Acheson, remained resolutely oriented toward Europe. Though the United States welcomed independence in India (1946) and in Indonesia (1949), elsewhere, as in the case of the French and Indochina, it subordinated theoretical anticolonial sentiments to the imperial nostalgia of NATO allies.

The Truman administration showed little concern for Latin America and Africa. Economic interests (oil) and domestic political pressures led to a more active role in the Near East. Historically the Americans most involved there had been missionaries, educators, and archaeologists. Strategically and economically the United States had regarded the Middle East, as the region began to be called during the Second World War, as an Anglo-French preserve. But war

weakened Anglo-French control, opening the area to American and Soviet penetration as well as to the gathering force of Arab nationalism.

American interest centered especially in the country long known to pilgrims as the Holy Land and ruled since 1922 by Britain under a League of Nations mandate. Jews in America and elsewhere had not forgotten the Balfour Declaration of 1917 pledging British sympathy for "the establishment in Palestine of a National Home for the Jewish people." Nazi anti-Semitism had meanwhile won Zionism wide support among non-Jews in America and Europe.

The Balfour Declaration, however, had its ambiguities. Arabs stressed the proviso that "nothing shall be done which may prejudice the civil and religious rights of existing non-Jewish communities in Palestine." While the Arab League, formed in 1945, vowed undying opposition to a Jewish national state, Jewish underground bands, led by Menachem Begin and Yitzhak Shamir, waged a campaign of terror against the British. Efforts to resolve the problem through partition failed. In May 1948 Britain terminated its mandate. Jews proclaimed the republic of Israel with the veteran Zionist Chaim Weizmann as president.

In Washington the defense establishment, seeking access to the vast Middle Eastern oil reserves, favored a pro-Arab policy. So did American oil companies. But Truman, moved by humanitarian and also by political considerations, promptly recognized the new state over the vehement opposition of his national security advisers. The Arab League's invasion of

The birth of Israel, 1948: celebration in Washington

Israel was successfully repelled in 1948–49. Israel now began a robust but perennially hazardous existence.

The China conundrum. The most conspicuous communist gain in the Third World was not the result of premeditated Soviet design. Stalin seems to have believed nearly as firmly as the United States in the capacity of the Nationalist regime of Chiang Kai-shek (Jiang Jieshi) to organize China. Both superpowers underestimated the revolutionary drives in China— the ancient resentments against foreign domination, the pent-up demand for agrarian reform, the growing revulsion against the corruption and autocracy of the Kuomintang (Guomindang), and the skill and tenacity with which the Chinese communists under Mao Tse-tung (Mao Zedong) exploited these discontents.

After the war Washington began by favoring a coalition between the Nationalists and the Communists. The new American ambassador to China, General Patrick J. Hurley, took enthusiastic personal charge of this effort. When a disenchanted Hurley re-

signed in November 1945, Truman appointed General George C. Marshall to continue his work. But the Nationalists believed that they could win a civil war; the communists were committed by ideology to domination. In January 1947 Marshall abandoned his mission, blaming its failure on both the reactionaries in the Kuomintang (Guomindang) and the communists.

The Nationalists soon overextended themselves. The communists, welded by quasi-religious conviction and helped by the increasing popular hatred of the Nationalist government, started to win victories. With each victory they captured more arms and attracted more deserters. In 1947 Truman sent General Albert Wedemeyer to China on a fact-finding tour. "The only basis on which national Chinese resistance to Soviet aims can be revitalized," Wedemeyer reported, "is through the presently corrupt, reactionary and inefficient Chinese National government." Therefore the United States should aid that government. But "until drastic political and economic reforms are undertaken United States aid cannot accomplish its purpose."

Chiang (Jiang) made no serious attempt at reform. Washington resolutely opposed proposals that would have entangled the United States in the fighting. By January 1949 the Nationalist armies had abandoned Peking (Beijing) and Tientsin (Tianjin). Shanghai fell in May, Canton (Guangzhou) in October. By the end of the year, the Nationalist regime had fled to the island of Formosa (Taiwan).

The collapse of Chiang (Jiang) provoked a bitter political debate in the United States. Some contended that anti-Nationalist prejudice—if not outright treason—in the State Department caused the "loss of China." But, as Wedemeyer explained the Nationalist defeat, it was "lack of spirit, primarily lack of spirit. It was not lack of equipment. In my judgment they could have defended the Yangtze (Chang Jiang) with broomsticks if they had the will to do it."

Truman and Acheson prepared to recognize the communist regime in the hope of encouraging Titoism in the Far East. "The Russians will turn out to be the 'foreign devils' in China," Truman wrote Vandenberg in 1949, "and that situation will help establish a Chinese Government that we can recognize and support." The American government put out a white paper placing the blame on Chiang (Jiang), pronounced Taiwan part of mainland China, and declared American neutrality. Recognition was delayed in the hope of getting the communist regime to accept specified international obligations. But the Chinese proved difficult; and in the United States congressional and public opinion, stirred up by the well-financed, pro-Chiang (Jiang) "China Lobby," and soon by the Korean War, made recognition of Red China an unmentionable issue.

Chinese communists entering Shanghai, 1949

Limited War

The end of nuclear monopoly. If the rhetoric of the Truman Doctrine seemed to call for global containment of communism, Truman himself did not construe the doctrine in any such crusading way, applying it neither to China nor to eastern Europe. Even with regard to Russia, he made amiable public reference to Stalin in 1948 as "Uncle Joe." In 1949 he seemed to view the contest with the Soviet Union without alarm. The forward drive of communism in Europe had been stopped, in Berlin as well as in western Europe. In China the policy was to "let the dust settle."

All this encouraged the President to continue to clamp down on the defense budget. In 1947–50, national-security expenditures averaged only $13 billion a year. By 1949 the army was down to ten active divisions. The capacity to fight small wars had dwindled. Deterrence rested on the idea of a retaliatory air-atomic strike against the Soviet Union. If war broke out, it seemed that Washington faced the choice either of doing nothing or of blowing up the world. Observers feared that this situation might invite communist aggression in some marginal area where the United States would not wish to respond by atomic war and lacked the means to respond otherwise.

Then in September 1949 evidence reached Washington that an atomic explosion had occurred in the Soviet Union. With one stroke the Russians had not only broken the atomic monopoly but had proved to the world their own technological capacity. The era of American invincibility had come to an end.

In response, Truman concluded a bitter argument among his scientific advisers by directing the Atomic Energy Commission to proceed with the construction of a hydrogen bomb, a weapon even more fearful than the atomic bomb. At the same time, he instructed the National Security Council to undertake a basic reappraisal of America's strategic position. The result, a document known as NSC 68 (April 1950), accelerated a shift from a political to a military definition of the Cold War. Postulating a Soviet "design for world domination," NSC 68 called both for a rapid build-up in nuclear weapons and for enlarged capacity to fight conventional wars. Then a new development reinforced the thesis that air-atomic power would not by itself assure American security and helped NSC 68 gain presidential approval in September.

War in Korea. When American and Soviet troops entered Korea after the collapse of Japan in 1945, they had accepted the thirty-eighth parallel as a military dividing line. Time and the Cold War converted the military demarcation into a political frontier. In 1948

Americans in Korea: war for a limited goal

the Russians set up a People's Democratic Republic in North Korea, while the Americans recognized the Republic of South Korea. In June 1949 Soviet and American forces withdrew from Korea. The position of South Korea in the American security system was not altogether clear. Both General Douglas MacArthur and Secretary of State Acheson declared that it lay outside the American defense perimeter in the Pacific. Should an attack occur, Acheson said, "The initial reliance must be on the people attacked to resist it and then upon the commitments of the entire civilized world under the Charter of the United Nations."

At just this time Kim Il-sung, the communist dictator of North Korea, came to Moscow to seek Stalin's support for a North Korean invasion of South Korea. Misled perhaps by the MacArthur and Acheson statements, misled too perhaps by Kim's confidence that the South Koreans would welcome the North Koreans as liberators, Stalin gave Kim a green light. On June 25, 1950, North Korean troops crossed the thirty-eighth parallel in a surprise invasion.

Truman faced what he later recalled as his toughest decision. In retrospect it appears that Stalin may only have acquiesced in a project that Kim wished for internal Korean reasons and that seemed to involve minimal risks for the Soviet Union. But Truman wrongly saw the invasion as primarily a Soviet effort to test the American will. If the United States did not react in Korea, he believed, the Russians would sponsor similar thrusts elsewhere; and the result might be a third world war. And indeed, even if Stalin had not instigated the invasion, no one can tell how he would have interpreted an American failure to respond.

Without hesitation, Truman committed American forces under General MacArthur to the defense of South Korea. At the same time he brought the matter before the United Nations Security Council. The absence of the Soviet delegate, who was boycotting the Security Council in pique over its refusal to seat Communist China, made it possible for the UN to endorse the American intervention. Truman rejected proposals that he ask Congress for a joint resolution authorizing the commitment of the American troops to combat. His reliance instead on dubious theories of inherent presidential power dangerously enlarged the freedom of future Presidents to take the nation into war.

The original UN intention in South Korea was simply to repel the North Korean invasion. At first the communists drove the UN troops—made up of ROK (Republic of Korea) forces and American troops, soon to be reinforced by a smattering of units from other nations, especially Great Britain and Turkey—back to the southeastern corner of the peninsula. But on September 15, in a daring move, MacArthur landed an amphibious force at Inchon behind the enemy lines. By September 27 the UN forces were in Seoul, and by October 1 they had recovered almost all of Korea below the thirty-eighth parallel.

MacArthur at Inchon

Crossing the thirty-eighth parallel. Mac-Arthur's brilliant generalship now raised the question whether the UN forces should pursue the enemy into North Korea. Despite warnings from Peking (Beijng) that crossing the thirty-eighth parallel might provoke Chinese intervention, the UN General Assembly at Washington's instigation reaffirmed that the goal was "the establishment of a unified, independent, and democratic Korea," and authorized UN forces on October 7 to move north.

On October 15, 1950, Truman and MacArthur met at Wake Island. When the President asked the General about the chances of Chinese or Soviet intervention in Korea, MacArthur replied, "Very little. . . . If the Chinese tried to get down to Pyongyang there would be the greatest slaughter." He added that he believed all enemy resistance would end by Thanksgiving. Superbly confident, MacArthur ignored cautions from Washington and deployed his forces in a thin line across North Korea. On November 24 he declared that his final drive to end the war was "now approaching its decisive effort." Two days later, a Chinese communist army drove a wedge through the central sector. The UN forces retreated in disarray two-thirds of the way down the peninsula.

Relations between MacArthur and Washington, not easy in victory, became prickly in defeat. Years of proconsulship had charged a naturally proud and flamboyant personality with a conviction of independent authority. In a barrage of public statements after his November defeat MacArthur suggested that the blame lay, not in his own faulty intelligence or tactics, but in the Washington decision to limit the war to Korea and to forbid attack on Chinese bases in Manchuria. This "privileged sanctuary," he said in one message, was "an enormous handicap, without precedent in military history." On December 6 Truman ordered MacArthur to clear all subsequent statements with Washington.

No substitute for victory? The tension between MacArthur and Truman reflected fundamental disagreement over the purpose of the war. MacArthur believed that the United States must pursue the Korean conflict to a victorious conclusion. If this required an escalation of the war—the bombing of Manchurian bases, the blockade and nuclear bombing of China, the entry of the Nationalist Chinese—then so be it. "In war there is no substitute for victory."

The Administration, on the other hand, saw the conflict as a limited war for limited objectives. If Manchuria was a privileged sanctuary, so were Okinawa and Japan. To commit American military strength to the mainland of Asia might abandon Europe to Soviet aggression. To transform a limited war into a general war against Communist China would be, in General Omar Bradley's phrase, to fight "the wrong war, at the wrong place, at the wrong time, and with the wrong enemy."

The Administration was content to achieve the original objective of its intervention—the integrity of South Korea. A reversal of military fortunes now gave hope that this limited goal could be won. General Matthew B. Ridgway, who had taken command of the Eighth Army in December, began to recover the initiative. By March most of South Korea was once again free of communists, and Ridgway's troops were pressing on the thirty-eighth parallel. The Administration called for a diplomatic settlement. But a defiant MacArthur statement demanding enemy surrender killed the President's move toward negotiation. "By this act," Truman later said, "MacArthur left me no choice—I could no longer tolerate his insubordination." In April, when Congressman Joseph Martin of Massachusetts, the Republican leader in the House, produced a new and provocative MacArthur letter, Truman relieved MacArthur of his command.

Truman's decision caused an outburst of public indignation. Senator Joseph McCarthy of Wisconsin ascribed MacArthur's recall to the machinations of a White House clique besotted by "bourbon and benedictine." Senator William Jenner of Indiana declared, "This country today is in the hands of a secret inner coterie which is directed by agents of the Soviet

The shifting front in Korea

Union." The fever reached its pitch on April 19 when MacArthur, returning to the United States for the first time in fourteen years, addressed a joint session of Congress. He concluded with a reference to a barracks-room ballad popular in his youth "which proclaimed most proudly that 'old soldiers never die; they just fade away.'"

There followed an extraordinary inquiry by the Senate Foreign Relations and Armed Services committees into the circumstances of MacArthur's dismissal. Beginning on May 3, MacArthur, Acheson, Marshall, Bradley, and other military and civilian leaders underwent a congressional interrogation that, in time, canvassed the most basic problems of global strategy. This ventilation of the issues dispelled much of the turbulence. The Administration persuaded most of the country that the President and the Joint Chiefs, having the global interests of the country in view, were justified in overruling MacArthur's recommendations. Truman rode out the storm; and MacArthur in due course began to fade away.

The Korean War: Repercussions

Could the Cold War have been avoided? By now the Cold War was in full swing. In retrospect it seems probable that each of the superpowers in these years was acting more on defensive grounds and on local considerations than the other realized. Neither nation had a master plan for world dominion. Yet who could be certain that Soviet aims would have remained local and limited had the West not developed counterpolicies? Acheson wrote twenty years after, "A school of academic criticism has concluded that we overreacted to Stalin, which in turn caused him to overreact to policies of the United States. This may be true. Fortunately, perhaps, these authors were not called upon to analyze a situation in which the United States had not taken the action which it did take."

The Marxist-Leninist analysis required Soviet leaders to believe that the mere existence of a capitalist power was by definition a threat to their own survival. Could the democracies really have relied on the self-restraint of a dicatator portrayed by his closest associates as increasingly paranoid if there had been no western resistance—no Truman Doctrine, no Marshall Plan, no NATO, no rearmament, no response to the Berlin blockade or to the invasion of South Korea? Had the democracies not rallied, would not Moscow have had an irresistible temptation to keep moving, always in the name of Soviet security? There thus seems even in retrospect an awful inevitability about

the Cold War. Given the international power disequilibrium, the ideological antagonism, and the mutual misperceptions, no one should be surprised at what ensued. The real surprise would have been if there had been no Cold War.

The globalization of containment. Though the limitations imposed on the Korean War showed that the defense of western Europe remained the top American priority, the fact that the war was fought at all expressed the growing American belief that Soviet expansion, if blocked in the main theater, would break out in secondary theaters. Interpreting the North Korean invasion as part of a worldwide communist offensive, Truman proceeded to batten down hatches all around the world. Korea thus transformed containment from a selective European policy into a general global policy.

The image of an aggressive Russia commanding a highly centralized world communist movement—an image neither new, nor, in the age of Stalin, altogether false—now fastened itself dogmatically on the American mind. The new China, for example, began to be perceived simply as an extension of Soviet power. Three days after the North Korean attack, Truman canceled the policy of neutrality in the Chinese civil war, declared that the seizure of Taiwan by "communist forces" would threaten American security in the Pacific, and ordered the Seventh Fleet to prevent a mainland attack on the island (and also to prevent a Nationalist attack on the mainland). By 1951 Assistant Secretary of State Dean Rusk could speak of the Mao regime as a "colonial Russian government—a Slavic Manchukuo."

The nationalist uprising against French control in Indochina was incorporated into the larger pattern. Roosevelt had opposed the restoration of Indochina to French rule, favoring instead an international trusteeship to prepare Indochina for independence. This wise suggestion was forgotten after his death, and the return of the French colonial government produced dogged resistance on the part of Ho Chi Minh and the so-called Viet Minh. Ho was a nationalist as well as a communist; and the Viet Minh were seen by most Indochinese as a movement for national independence. Washington had paid little attention to the fighting in Indochina until the fall of mainland China. After Korea the State Department, condemning Ho as "an agent of world communism," pronounced the French role in Indochina "an integral part of the world-wide resistance by the Free Nations to Communist attempts at conquest."

In the United States, the Korean War brought about a quick reversal of the policy of military retrenchment. National-defense expenditures rapidly increased from 4 percent of the gross national product in 1948, to above 13 percent by 1953. Two years after the attack on South Korea, the nation had 3.6 million men under arms—an increase of nearly 2.2 million. The Soviet problem was seen more and more in military terms. With American financial backing, Britain and France launched rearmament programs, and in September 1950 Acheson persuaded his European allies to go along with a measure of rearmament in Germany. In 1951 NATO forces were integrated under the command of General Eisenhower. Truman's decision to send four additional American divisions to Europe set off an impassioned but inconclusive "Great Debate" in which conservative legislators, led by Taft, challenged Truman's conviction that he had the power to take that step without congressional authorization.

Domestic repercussions. The Korean War had widespread domestic impact. Defense spending revived inflationary impulses in the economy until the imposition of direct controls in January 1951 stabilized prices. Unlike Roosevelt, who had sought when possible to act on the basis of congressional statute, Truman embraced an enlarged view of inherent presidential prerogative. Fearing in April 1952 that a na-

tionwide steel strike would stop the flow of arms to the troops in Korea, he directed the government to seize and operate the steel mills, defending this action as an exercise of the emergency powers of the President. But the Supreme Court, in the notable case of *Youngstown Steel & Tube Co.* v. *Sawyer*, rejected the presidential thesis, at least in its immediate application.

It was easier to contain the economic than the psychological consequences of Korea. With the intensification of the Cold War, many Americans demanded to know why the nation they deemed so powerful and so safe in 1945 should now, five years later, appear in deadly peril. Some, resenting the complexity of history, found a satisfactory answer by tracing all troubles to the workings of the communist conspiracy—unsleeping, omnipresent, and diabolically cunning. Unquestionably there had been communist penetration of the American government, the labor movement, and the intellectual community. Disclosures of communist espionage in Canada and Britain, especially the theft of atomic secrets by the Soviet spies Klaus Fuchs and Allan Nunn May, increased public apprehension. The denunciation in 1948 by Whittaker Chambers, an ex-communist, of Alger Hiss,

The policy of neutrality canceled: the Seventh Fleet in Taiwan

a former State Department official, as a fellow communist spy and Hiss's conviction for perjury in 1950 caused further alarm. If Hiss, a man of apparently unimpeachable respectability, was a Soviet agent, who might not be? The Administration compounded its troubles when Truman called the Hiss affair a "red herring" and Acheson, after Hiss's conviction, said, "I do not intend to turn my back on Alger Hiss." In 1951, Julius and Ethel Rosenberg were charged as atomic spies and later executed on the ground of espionage in wartime.

Early recognizing the gravity of the problem and at the same time hoping to keep public reaction under control, Truman in 1947 had set up a federal loyalty program. "Disloyal and subversive elements must be removed from the employ of government," Truman said. "We must not, however, permit employees of the Federal government to be labelled as disloyal . . . when no valid basis exists for arriving at such a conclusion." Despite these injunctions, the loyalty program—as a consequence of overzealous investigators, ignorant or malicious informers, and apprehensive loyalty boards—began to assume a drastic and promiscuous character. By December 1952, 6.6 million people had been checked for security. No cases of espionage were uncovered by the investigations. "It was not realized at first," Acheson later wrote, "how dangerous was the practice of secret evidence and secret informers, how alien to all our conceptions of justice and the rights of the citizen. . . . Experience proved again how soon good men become callous in the use of bad practices."

The government also initiated prosecutions against top communist leaders under the Smith Act of 1940, which prohibited groups from conspiring to advocate the violent overthrow of the government. Throughout the country, citizens anxious to protect their communities against the dread infection sometimes, in ardor or panic, failed to distinguish between disloyalty and traditional American radicalism or mere dissent. Then in February 1950 a little-known senator from Wisconsin, Joseph R. McCarthy, gave a speech in Wheeling, West Virginia. "I have here in my hand a list," he said—a list of communists in the State Department; whether he said there were 205 or 81 or 57 or "a lot" of communists (and this was a question around which much controversy would revolve) was in the end less important than his insistence that these communists were "known to the Secretary of State" and were "still working and making policy." With this speech, a remarkable figure began a brief but lurid career on the national stage.

The rise of McCarthyism. McCarthy's charges prompted an astonished Senate to appoint a subcommittee under Senator Millard Tydings of Maryland to look into his allegations. After weeks of hearings, the Tydings Committee declared that McCarthy had worked a "fraud and a hoax." Yet, for all the apparent failure of McCarthy's charges, the hearings also revealed the facility, agility, and lack of scruple with which he operated. His characteristic weapon was what the journalist Richard Rovere called the "multiple untruth"—a statement so complicated, flexible, and grandiose in its mendacity as almost to defy rational refutation. To this McCarthy added unlimited impudence, an instinct for demagoguery, and an unmatched skill in alley-fighting. If the Tydings Committee thought it had disciplined McCarthy, it was wrong. In the election of 1950, McCarthy's intervention in Maryland, marked by a broad hint that Tydings, a conservative Democrat whom Roosevelt had tried in vain to purge in 1938, was procommunist, brought about Tydings' defeat. From that moment, the Wisconsin senator became a formidable figure in the Senate.

The Korean War meanwhile wrought a significant change in the public atmosphere. It created a climate that transformed McCarthy's crusade from an eccentric sideshow into a popular movement. If communists were killing American boys in Korea, why should communists be given the benefit of the doubt in the United States? Though Truman's loyalty program had in some respects overridden traditional safeguards of civil freedom, it did not go nearly far enough for McCarthy and his followers. In September 1950, Congress passed the McCarran Internal Security Act, establishing a Subversive Activities Control Board to follow communist activities in the United States and denying admission to the country of anyone who had once been a member of a totalitarian organization.* Congress passed the bill over Truman's veto.

The spectacle of McCarthyism infuriated the President. He told the American Legion:

Slander, lies, character assassination—these things are a threat to every single citizen everywhere in this country. When even one American—who has done nothing wrong—is forced by fear to shut his mind and close his mouth, then all Americans are in peril. It is the job of all of us—of every American who loves his country and his freedom—to rise up and put a stop to this terrible business.

---

*A second McCarran Act, also passed over Truman's veto, was the Immigration and Nationality Act of 1952. While this bill finally abolished the Asian-exclusion provisions of 1924, it retained the national-origins quota system, which discriminated in favor of immigrants from northern and western Europe and which critics condemned as a form of racism built into federal law. It also required that foreigners visiting the United States go through so complicated a system of loyalty checks that many came to feel that the United States regarded them as potential criminals.

The 1952 Election

Truman in retreat. But the backwash of the Korean War gave McCarthy an eager audience. The Administration and its leading officials—especially Secretary of State Acheson—fell under unsparing attack as communist sympathizers. The Republicans scored impressive gains in the congressional elections of 1950 and looked forward with increasing confidence to 1952.

Their confidence grew with revelations of corruption in the Reconstruction Finance Corporation and the Bureau of Internal Revenue. The disclosures of 1951–52 called attention to the decline that had taken place in the governmental service from the relatively incorruptible thirties—a decline brought about in part because Truman's scorn for the "professional liberal" had driven many of the old New Dealers from government to be replaced by party hacks. When the facts got out, moreover, Truman constrained by loyalty to old political associates, seemed grudging in his response. All this strengthened the idea of a "mess in Washington" and a growing national conviction that the Democratic party had been in power too long.

The campaign of 1952. Robert A. Taft's triumphant reelection to the Senate in 1950 made him the leading contender for the Republican nomination. But the powerful Eastern wing of the party, regarding the Ohio senator as too isolationist, turned to General Dwight D. Eisenhower. At the convention in July the Eisenhower supporters outmaneuvered their opposition in a battle over contested delegates. Eisenhower was nominated on the first ballot. Senator Richard M. Nixon of California, who had played an important part in the exposure of Alger Hiss, became his running mate.

After Truman withdrew from the Democratic contest, the convention drafted Governor Adlai Stevenson of Illinois. Though Stevenson had served in the Navy Department during the war and thereafter at the UN, he was little known to voters outside his home state. In the next three months, carrying out his pledge to "talk sense to the American people," he established himself as a brilliant, literate, and eloquent candidate.

In fact, Eisenhower and Stevenson were not dissimilar in their moderation on domestic issues and their internationalism in foreign policy. They differed, however, on their attitude toward McCarthyism; and the Republican campaign, based on the themes of "Korea, communism, and corruption," magnified the differences. Nixon, a more experienced

**The nominees:
Chicago, 1952**

From the beginning we will bring into government men and women to whom low public morals are unthinkable. Thus, we will not only drive wrong-doers and their cronies out of government. We will make sure that they do not get into government in the first place....

Then we will begin to move forward. With that accomplished, we will make these our objectives, our immediate aims for the government of the United States:

First, to save: That means an administration which knows how to practice the wiser spending of less of the people's money;

Second, to streamline: That means an administration which knows how to make government the more efficient servant of the people;

Third, to decentralize: That means an administration which is determined effectively to bring government close to the people. It means, also, faith in the people to act more wisely in their own behalf than can a bureaucrat removed a thousand miles from the scene of action.

Fourth, to unify: That means an administration able to make the whole government a joint, cooperative enterprise for the whole people's benefit.

From Dwight D. Eisenhower, Campaign Address at St. Louis, September 1952.

Eisenhower in 1952: a personal triumph

campaigner than Eisenhower, referred to the Democratic candidate as "Adlai the appeaser . . . who got a Ph.D. from Dean Acheson's College of Cowardly Communist Containment." "I further charge," Nixon added, "that Mr. Truman, Dean Acheson and other administration officials for political reasons covered up this Communist Conspiracy and attempted to halt its exposure." Intellectual supporters of Stevenson were derided as "eggheads."

The campaign was interrupted by a revelation that Nixon had been a beneficiary of a fund collected on his behalf by California businessmen. For a moment, Eisenhower considered asking Nixon to retire from the ticket. But a histrionic television speech in an autobiographical vein saved the vice presidential candidate. When Eisenhower, late in the campaign, declared his intention to go to Korea if elected, he clinched his victory. The popular vote showed 33.9 million for Eisenhower, 27.3 million for Stevenson; the margin in the Electoral College was 442 to 89. Though Eisenhower's election was more a personal than a party triumph, twenty years of Democratic rule had come to an end.

The presidential reputation of Harry S Truman has improved over the years. "There are two Trumans," the mordant commentator Elmer Davis said at the time, "the White House Truman and the courthouse Truman. He does the big things right, and the little things wrong." In 1952 the little things were on the minds of voters. In retrospect the big things seem more important. Even some of the big things, like the abuse of the loyalty program, the sweeping language of

Government has three duties.

Stevenson: *a new day*

First, government is an umpire, denying special privilege, ensuring equal rights, restraining monopoly and greed and bigotry....

Second, government has the duty of creating an economic climate in which creative men can take risks and reap rewards, so that our economic life will have a continuous flow of fresh ideas and fresh leadership; and, of course, it means the building of solid defenses against the greatest threat to that flow—depression....

Third, government has the duty of helping the people develop their country.

The Federal Government made the Louisiana Purchase, and on that land a nation grew to greatness. No private corporation would have built Grand Coulee Dam, yet in the Grand Coulee country people are building their homes and establishing their private business, and farmers are converting desert into garden....

We take our stand upon the fundamental principle that the role of government is, to sum up, just this: To remove the roadblocks put in the way of the people by nature and by greedy men; to release the energies of the people, so that free men may work the miracles of the future as they have worked the miracles of the past.

From Adlai E. Stevenson, Campaign Address at St. Louis, October 1952.

the Truman Doctrine and the claims to inherent presidential war-making power, remain questionable. The use of the atomic bomb, though arguably justified in the circumstances, was a tragic decision. Still Truman did many very big things right—the defense of western Europe against Stalinism, the Marshall Plan, NATO, the relief of General MacArthur, civil rights; he kept alive the spirit of liberal democracy at home and responsible internationalism abroad; and the memory of this brave, doughty, unpretentious, peppery, forever candid man has grown in popular affection.

The election of 1952

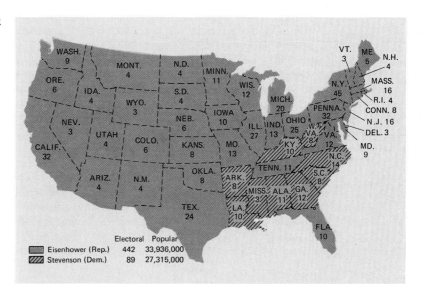

	Electoral	Popular
Eisenhower (Rep.)	442	33,936,000
Stevenson (Dem.)	89	27,315,000

Suggestions for Reading

TRUMAN AND HIS POLICIES

Truman's *Memoirs*, 2 vols. (1955–56) are pungent and controversial. Two readable volumes by R. J. Donovan—*Conflict and Crisis** (1977) and *Tumultuous Years** (1982)—provide the best narrative account of the Truman Presidency. A. L. Hamby, *Beyond the New Deal: Harry S. Truman and American Liberalism** (1973), is an excellent analytical study. R. H. Ferrell, *Harry S. Truman and the Modern American Presidency** (1983), pays particular attention to foreign policy.

FOREIGN AFFAIRS

For general foreign policy, Seyom Brown, *The Faces of Power: Constancy and Change in United States Foreign Policy from Truman to Reagan** (1983), is cogent and judicious. Lawrence Freedman, *The Evolution of Nuclear Strategy** (1981), is incisive and sophisticated. Gregg Herken, *The Winning Weapon: The Atomic Bomb in the Cold War, 1945–50** (1980), describes the impact of the bomb on the wartime alliance.

For the Cold War, W. H. McNeill, *America, Britain and Russia* (1951), and Herbert Feis, *Churchill, Roosevelt, Stalin** (1957), remain fundamental works. J. L. Gaddis's two books—*The United States and the Origins of the Cold War** (1972) and *Strategies of Containment** (1981)—are intelligent and dispassionate; Gaddis with T. H. Etzold, eds., *Containment: Documents on American Policy and Strategy** (1978), is a useful compilation. The revisionist argument is conveniently summarized in T. G. Paterson, *On Every Front: The Making of the Cold War** (1979). D. S. McClellan, *Dean Acheson: The State Department Years* (1976), portrays a major architect of United States policy. Dean Acheson, *Present at the Creation* (1969), is a formidable and stylish memoir. W. A. Harriman (and Elie Abel), *Special Envoy to Churchill and Stalin, 1941–1946* (1975), is indispensable. James F. Byrnes, Charles E. Bohlen, Lucius Clay, James Forrestal, G. F. Kennan, A. H. Vandenberg have left important memoirs and diaries; for dissenting views, see J. M. Blum, ed., *The Price of Victory: The Diary of Henry A. Wallace, 1942–1946* (1973).

Victor Rothwell, *Britain and the Cold War, 1941–1947* (1982) offers a British perspective, and C. S. Maier, ed., *The Origins of the Cold War and Contemporary Europe** (1978) discusses European implications. Vojtech Mastny, *Russia's Road to the Cold War** (1979), is a persuasive reconstruction, while Strobe Talbott, ed., *Khrushchev Remembers*, 2 vols. (1970–74), is fascinating.

For the Cold War in other areas, see B. R. Kuniholm, *The Origins of the Cold War in the Near East** (1980); Yonosuke Nagai and Akira Iriye, eds, *The Origins of the Cold War in Asia* (1977); Russell Buhite, *Soviet-American Relations in Asia, 1945–1954* (1982); Dorothy Borg and Waldo Heinrichs, eds., *Uncertain Years: Chinese-American Relations, 1947–1950* (1980); and R. M. Blum, *Drawing the Line: The Origin of the American Containment Policy in East Asia* (1982). E. J. Kahn, Jr., *The China Hands* (1975) tells the shaming story of the State Department's Far Eastern experts. C. M. Dobbs, *The Unwanted Symbol: American Foreign Policy, The Cold War, and Korea, 1945–1950* (1981), argues that Washington misperceived an essentially local conflict. J. C. Goulden, *Korea, the Untold Story of the War** (1982), describes the war itself. MacArthur is discussed admiringly in Douglas MacArthur, *Reminiscences* (1964), sympathetically in William Manchester, *American Caesar** (1978), and coolly in R. H. Rovere and Arthur Schlesinger, Jr., *The General and the President* (1951; reissued as *The Truman-MacArthur Controversy*, 1965).

DOMESTIC ISSUES

Samuel Lubell, *The Future of American Politics* (1952), is an illuminating analysis of political currents. J. T. Patterson, *Mr. Republican: A Biography of Robert A. Taft* (1972), and R. N. Smith, *Thomas E. Dewey and His Times* (1982), portray two influential Republican leaders. On economic questions, E. S. Flash, Jr., *Economic Advice and Presidential Leadership* (1965), discusses the Council of Economic Advisers; C. D. Goodwin, ed., *Exhortation and Controls: The Search for a Wage–Price Policy, 1945–1961** (1975), concentrates on anti-inflation policies; and Herbert Stein, *Presidential Economics: The Making of Economic Policy from Roosevelt to Reagan* (1984), provides a conservative evaluation. For Truman and civil rights see, D. R. McCoy and R. T. Ruetten, *Quest and Response* (1973).

Earl Latham, *The Communist Controversy in Washington** (1966), is a sober guide. R. H. Rovere, *Senator Joe McCarthy** (1959) is a brilliant essay; there are scholarly biographies by T. C. Reeves and by D. M. Oshinsky. Larger repercussions are covered analytically in J. P. Diggins, *Up from Communism* (1975) and more tendentiously in David Caute, *The Great Fear* (1978). For anti-Stalinist liberalism, see Reinhold Niebuhr, *The Children of Light and the Children of Darkness** (1944) and *The Irony of American History* (1952), and Arthur Schlesinger, Jr., *The Vital Center* (1949); for a critique, Christopher Lasch, *The New Radicalism in America* (1965).

* Available in a paperback edition.

31
CONSOLIDATION AND CONFLICT

In the years since 1929 the American people had experienced the worst depression in their history, the worst hot war, the worst Cold War, the worst limited war. Since 1933 they had followed Presidents who believed strongly in affirmative government and vigorous action. But a nation's capacity for crisis and crusades is limited. Just as the first two decades of the twentieth century—the activist decades dominated by Theodore Roosevelt and Woodrow Wilson—left the people with a yearning for normalcy, so the high-tension thirties and forties produced a fresh desire for respite. The new quest for normalcy, though, took place in stormier times and within the frameworks established by depression and war.

The Eisenhower Mood

The new President. President Dwight D. Eisenhower embodied the popular mood. Sixty-two years old on his inauguration, he was already a national hero, beloved by his countrymen. After quiet years in the peacetime army, Eisenhower had been one of that group of remarkable military men who emerged during the Second World War. His service as supreme commander of the Allied Forces in Europe was followed by a postwar tour of duty as Chief of Staff. President of Columbia University in 1948, he returned to

Europe as supreme commander of NATO in 1951. He resigned this post to seek the Republican nomination in 1952.

People weary of the "mess in Washington" and wanting an end to the controversies of the New Deal era saw him as the man to heal the nation's wounds. His appointed role, wrote the influential columnist Walter Lippmann, was "that of the restorer of order and peace after an age of violence and faction." His experience, his famous geniality, and his expressed dislike of politics recommended him as national conciliator.

Actually his surface affability concealed a vigorous concern with large issues, cold and shrewd judgment, a hot temper, much craftiness, and a dazzling instinct for self-preservation. His nonpolitical pose was his major political weapon. In fact, politics had few tougher training schools than the Army, and Eisenhower was an expert. Coolly recognizing that he was far more popular than the Republican party, he did not propose to risk national influence by coming on as a partisan leader.

He cultivated the impression that he was a warm-hearted man above the battle who did not always know what his own administration was doing. He posed as an opponent of strong presidential leadership, affirming his wish to redress the balance between executive and legislative branches after the excesses of the Roosevelt years. He encouraged the idea that, within the executive branch, he deferred to Secretary

An ambitious road program

of State John Foster Dulles in foreign affairs and to White House chief of staff Governor Sherman Adams in domestic affairs. He was not, he assured everyone, the desk-pounding sort of President. He exploited his reputation for rambling imprecision in press conferences. Anticipating a question on a tough issue, he once told his press secretary, "Don't worry, Jim, if that question comes, I'll just confuse them."

Eisenhower wanted the press and the opposition to underestimate him. In fact, he deployed his subordinates to draw enemy fire and was firmly in charge whenever he wished to be, which was a good deal more often than many supposed at the time. "He was a far more complex and devious man than most people realized," his Vice President Richard Nixon later said of him, characteristically adding, "and in the best sense of those words."

Eisenhower economics. In domestic policy Eisenhower offered the nation what he called "modern Republicanism." This meant in practice an acceptance of the New Deal tempered by a determination to reduce public spending and the activity of the federal government. Actually Eisenhower had little interest in domestic matters and, though he had no wish to dismantle the New Deal, was in some respects more con-

servative than Robert A. Taft, the most powerful Republican in the Senate.

His Cabinet was dominated by Secretary of the Treasury George M. Humphrey, an Ohio businessman who reinforced deeply conservative views with a strong personality. When the new Secretary of Defense, Charles E. Wilson of General Motors, was asked whether he foresaw a conflict between his business and official commitments, he replied, "I cannot conceive of one because for years I thought what was good for our country was good for General Motors, and *vice versa.*" The Secretary of the Interior, Douglas McKay of Oregon, summed up the general attitude when he said, "We're here in the saddle as an Administration representing business and industry."

The death in July 1953 of Senator Taft, who was in his way a Tory reformer, removed what might have been a constructive influence on Eisenhower's domestic policy. Thereafter the Administration stalled on social questions. It concentrated instead, without great success, on fiscal conservatism. No Administration was more responsive to the business community, but "business confidence" turned out, as so often, to be irrelevant to economic health. Preferring recession to the supposed inflationary risks of public spending, the Administration did little to combat downturns in

1953–54, 1957–58, and 1960–61. The average annual rate of economic growth slowed from 4.3 percent in the last six Truman years to 2.5 percent in the Eisenhower years. For all his concern with balancing the budget, Eisenhower achieved a surplus less than half the time and produced in 1959 the largest peacetime deficit to that point in American history.

His most influential domestic initiative was the Interstate Highway Act of 1956, which he proudly described as the "most ambitious road program by any nation in all history." This law authorized the federal government to pay 90 percent of the construction costs of interstate highways. The result was to commit the nation more than ever to the individually owned automobile. Great freeways carried the middle class and their shops and services into the suburbs, leaving the city to the poor and the minorities. Pollution, environmental damage and petroleum consumption in-

creased, while public mass transport, especially the railroads, deteriorated. The automobile continued to remold American life much as railroads had done a century earlier.

The interstate highway program was the great exception to Eisenhower's general dislike of federal intervention. He feared "statism" and proposed to transfer federal functions either to state and local governments or to private enterprise. But in 1960 the size and structure of the federal government were much what they had been in 1952.

McCarthy: zenith. In 1951 Joe McCarthy had denounced General Marshall as part of "a conspiracy so immense and an infamy so black as to dwarf any previous venture in the history of man." During the 1952 campaign, to avoid offending McCarthy, Eisenhower deleted a paragraph of praise for Marshall from a speech delivered in Wisconsin. This action foreshadowed the President's reluctance to engage himself personally in the McCarthy issue. As he later put it, "I will not get in the gutter with *that* guy." The Wisconsin senator, agile and unscrupulous as ever, took full advantage of the Administration's indulgence. Before 1953 only the bully of the Senate, he now began, as chairman of the Senate Committee on Government Operations, to swagger without challenge through the executive branch in pursuit of alleged communists and fellow travelers.

A main target was the State Department. Determined to propitiate the right wing, Secretary of State Dulles was ready to collaborate with McCarthy and even to anticipate his demands. Veteran diplomats whose political reporting aroused McCarthy's ire were drummed from the service. A McCarthy disciple was appointed chief of State Department personnel. The Secretary ordered State Department libraries abroad to remove books by "authors who obviously follow the Communist line or participate in Communist front organizations." The thrillers of Dashiell Hammett, *The Selected Works of Tom Paine*, and even Whittaker Chambers' *Witness* were banned; a number of proscribed books were actually burned. By June 1953 the panic had spread so widely that the President himself intervened to arrest it. "Don't join the book burners," he said. "Don't think you are going to conceal faults by concealing evidence that they ever existed."

The panic did not abate. Many Americans now looked to the FBI as the bastion of national freedom and turned J. Edgar Hoover, the bureau's able but increasingly weird director, into a national hero. Posses of road-company McCarthys sprang up across the land. What began as an effort to guard the national security became a heresy hunt employing guilt by association, loyalty oaths, testimony of secret informers, blacklists, interrogation and intimidation by legislative committees. In the 1954 campaign Vice President Nixon boasted of the number of "security risks" who had been driven from government. One notable victim was the great physicist Dr. J. Robert Oppenheimer, the father of the atomic bomb but subsequently an opponent of the hydrogen bomb. Oppenheimer's security clearance was withdrawn in 1953 because of ancient left-wing associations well known to security officers a decade before, when Oppenheimer was heading the Manhattan Project. A review board declared that the Oppenheimer case "demonstrated that the Government can search . . . the soul of an individual whose relationship to his Government is in question." It added that national security "in times of peril must be absolute."

Thoughtful people began to wonder whether such ideas as these might not be the most subversive of all. George Kennan said that "absolute security" was an unattainable and self-devouring end—that its frenzied pursuit would lead only to absolute tyranny. Judge Learned Hand summed up the feelings of many Americans:

I believe that that community is already in process of dissolution where each man begins to eye his neighbor as a possible enemy, where nonconformity with the accepted creed, political as well as religious, is a mark of disaffection; where denunciation, without specification or backing, takes the place of evidence.

McCarthy: decline. The Korean War had given McCarthy his opportunity for influence, and the end of that war in July 1953 brought about his decline. As war frustrations receded, McCarthyism began to lose its emotional base. By now, in his increasingly erratic course, McCarthy had become embroiled with the army, launching a sensational, if unproductive, search for communists and spies at Fort Monmouth, New Jersey. Goaded beyond endurance, the army finally fought back. The denouement took place in a series of televised hearings from April 22 to June 17, 1954.

The Army-McCarthy hearings were a compelling spectacle, marked by vivid and sharply etched personalities and passages of passion and conflict. They commanded a fascinated audience, amounting at times to 20 million people. Viewers trained through long exposure to TV westerns to distinguish between good and bad guys had little trouble deciding to which category McCarthy belonged. After thirty-five days of the grating voice, the sarcastic condescension, the irrelevant interruption ("point of order, Mr. Chairman, point of order"), and the unsupported accusation, McCarthy effectively achieved his own destruction. The spell was at last broken. On December 2, 1954, the Senate censured McCarthy by a sixty-seven to twenty-two vote. The Wisconsin senator was finished. His death in 1957 merely ratified his political demise.

Eisenhower welcomed McCarthy's downfall, and admirers later discerned his "hidden hand" in the result. But the President's refusal to make the public case against McCarthyism wasted an opportunity to reaffirm the great traditions of civil freedom and due process that the Wisconsin senator had so effectively damaged. The impact of McCarthyism should not be exaggerated. Many Americans denounced the senator and his works with courage and impunity. He left, however, a heritage—not only in the broken lives of those he attacked but, paradoxically, in a greatly enhanced conception of presidential prerogative. When McCarthy demanded access to Department of Defense files, Eisenhower in May 1954 claimed "an uncontrolled discretion" to refuse information anywhere in the executive branch. This was the most absolute assertion of the presidential right to withhold information from Congress ever uttered to that point. Because of the detestation of McCarthy, right-minded people generally applauded the Eisenhower theory. But this theory, which acquired in 1957 the name of "executive privilege," ushered in an extraordinary time of executive denial. In its remaining years, the

Eisenhower Administration rejected more congressional requests, often entirely reasonable, for information than Presidents had done in the first century of American history.

The battle of desegregation. The gravest domestic issue lay in the field of race relations. The struggle to assure blacks their full rights as American citizens had gathered momentum during and after the Second World War. Though most of Truman's civil-rights program was rejected by Congress, his fight for that program established civil rights as a national issue.

Thwarted in Congress, the champions of racial justice turned to the courts. The Supreme Court, once chary of taking on cases involving rights of blacks, started doing so after the war. The early decisions reflected the Fabian tactics of the Court under Chief Justice Fred M. Vinson of Kentucky (1946–53). The Vinson Court sought to work toward equal rights within the inherited legal framework—that is, by accepting the *Plessy* v. *Ferguson* doctrine (see p. 419) of "separate but equal," construing it literally, and rejecting separate facilities when they were not in full and exact fact equal.

Beginning in 1952, attorneys for the National Association for the Advancement of Colored People (NAACP) argued before the Supreme Court against state laws requiring the segregation of children in public education. On May 17, 1954, in the case of *Brown* v. *Board of Education of Topeka*, the Court, speaking through Earl Warren, the new Chief Justice, responded with a unanimous decision reversing *Plessy* v. *Ferguson* and interpreting the Fourteenth Amendment as outlawing racial discrimination in public schools. "We conclude," the Court said, "that in the field of public education, the doctrine of 'separate but equal' has no place. Separate educational facilities are inherently unequal." A year later, the Court called on school authorities to submit plans for desegregation and gave local federal courts the responsibility of deciding whether the plans constituted "good faith compliance." The Court concluded by ordering action "with all deliberate speed."

The border states moved toward compliance. But in South Carolina, Georgia, Alabama, and Mississippi, resistance began to harden, especially after the spread in 1955–56 of the militantly segregationist White Citizens' Councils and a 1956 manifesto by Southern members of Congress, condemning the decision. Some Southern states passed laws to frustrate the Supreme Court ruling. A favorite device was to divert state funds to what might be passed off technically as a private school system. Extreme segregationists revived the pre-Civil War doctrine of nullification under the more mellifluous name of "interposition."

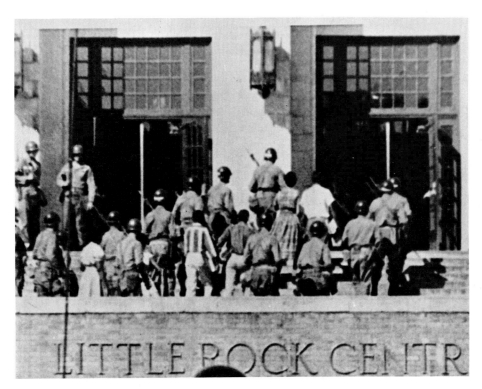

Little Rock, 1957: separate but equal had no place

LITTLE ROCK CENTR

Crisis in Little Rock. Eisenhower declined to endorse the *Brown* decision and remained skeptical about government efforts to promote civil rights: "It is difficult through law and through force to change a man's heart." Southern resistance reached a climax in 1957 in Little Rock, Arkansas, when Governor Orval Faubus tried to deny nine black students enrollment in the Central High School. Faubus's open challenge compelled the President to defend the Supreme Court. When the black boys and girls sought to enter Central High School, they were mobbed by angry whites. On September 24, 1957, Eisenhower sent federal troops into Little Rock. Order was restored, and black children entered the school.

In the meantime, Congress was finally taking action on behalf of racial justice. The Civil Rights Act of 1957, the first of its kind since Reconstruction, authorized the Department of Justice to seek injunctions on behalf of black voting rights. A second act, in 1960, provided for the appointment of federal referees to safeguard voting rights. For its part, the Warren Court extended the principle of the *Brown* case to new fields, striking down segregation over the next years in interstate commerce, in public buildings, in airports and interstate bus terminals, in parks and other public recreational facilities. Both Congress and the Court, by concentrating on segregation as embodied in law, left untouched the wide and bitter realm of *de facto* discrimination; but at the same time, by accepting

and, in the Court's case, declaring the moral necessity of equality, they were changing the values of American society.

Blacks themselves were increasingly in the forefront of the struggle. Lawyers like Thurgood Marshall of the NAACP argued the constitutional cases. In December 1955, the blacks of Montgomery, Alabama, under the inspiration of a young minister, Dr. Martin Luther King, Jr., boycotted the city's segregated bus system. King, who was strongly influenced by Thoreau and Gandhi, counseled his followers to avoid provocation and to confront "physical force with an even stronger force, namely, soul force." The boycott, reinforced by suits in the federal courts, achieved the desegregation of the bus system in a year. Nonviolent resistance was widely used in the winter of 1959–60 to challenge the refusal to serve blacks at Southern lunch counters. The rapid spread of "sit-in" demonstrations through the South and the support they evoked in the North and among moderate Southern whites testified to the rising moral force of the protest against segregation. If only limited progress was made in school desegregation and in assuring the right to vote, vast progress was made in gaining acceptance for the moral case against discrimination. The rather pallid Southern filibuster against a civil-rights bill in 1960 was marked by the fact that, with one or two exceptions, no one tried any longer even to argue the philosophy of white supremacy.

794 *Consolidation and Conflict*

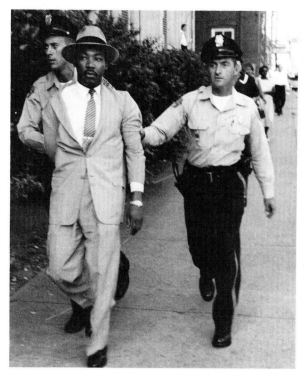

Martin Luther King, Jr.: inspiration in Montgomery

The Warren Court. Eisenhower later regretted his appointment of Earl Warren. The former Republican governor of California turned out to have a spacious view of the Constitution; and his humane approach received support and elaboration from three other distinguished Eisenhower appointees—John M. Harlan, Potter Stewart, and, most consistently, William J. Brennan—as well as from hold-overs from the Roosevelt Court, Hugo Black, Felix Frankfurter, and William O. Douglas.

In addition to its initiatives in the field of racial justice, the Warren Court, especially in the 1956–57 term, sought to mend the holes McCarthyism had made in the fabric of civil freedom. The *Watkins* and *Sweezy* cases, with their condemnation of exposure "for the sake of exposure," restricted legislative investigations to questions deemed pertinent to a legislative objective. The *Yates* case construed the Smith Act of 1940 as distinguishing between "the statement of an idea which may prompt its hearers to take unlawful action, and advocacy that such action be taken." The *Jencks* case required that Federal Bureau of Investigation reports, if used by the prosecution in a criminal trial, be made available to the defense. These decisions stirred up passing furor and led to right-wing rage at the Court. In the longer run their impact was less drastic than civil libertarians hoped or than the heirs of McCarthy feared.

Thoughtful critics felt at times that the activism of the Warren Court was carrying the judiciary into decisions that properly belonged to legislative or executive processes. Defenders replied that legislative and executive inertia had created a vacuum of power, which, if not filled by the Supreme Court, would have severely strained the bonds of social order.

The second term. As a national hero, above politics, Eisenhower enjoyed a popularity far exceeding that of his party. In 1954, the Democrats took control of both the House and the Senate. In spite of a coronary thrombosis in 1955 and ileitis in 1956, Eisenhower decided to run for reelection. "Some of my medical advisers," he said, "believe that adverse effects on my health will be less in the Presidency than in any other position I might hold." Most voters accepted with sympathy his need for a more carefully regulated life, made affectionate jokes about his long hours on the golf course, and accorded him undiminished confidence. Though Eisenhower several times suggested to Nixon that he might prefer a Cabinet post, the Vice President ignored the hint and secured his own renomination.

The Democrats, over the brief opposition of Harry Truman, renominated Adlai Stevenson, whose penetrating comment on national issues had kept him in the forefront among the party leaders. Estes Kefauver of Tennessee, who had been Stevenson's chief rival till shortly before the convention, received the vice-presidential nomination over John F. Kennedy of Massachusetts. Eisenhower won decisively, carrying the popular vote by 35.6 to 26 million and the Electoral College by 457 to 73. The Democrats, who had regained control of Congress in 1954, slightly increased their majorities in both houses.

If Eisenhower's first term had seen the end of both the Korean War and McCarthyism—if, indeed, only a Republican could perhaps have presided so tranquilly over the liquidation of those angry issues—his second term proved less successful. The Administration's reluctance to move swiftly against 7.5 percent unemployment in 1958 damaged confidence, and its claim to moral rectitude was tarnished in a series of scandals. These scandals forced the resignation of the Secretary of the Air Force, the chairman of the Republican National Committee, the chairman of the Interstate Commerce Commission, the General Services Administrator, the Public Buildings Administrator, a number of lesser officials, and, finally, in September 1958, Sherman Adams, the Assistant to the President.

The 1958 elections brought a Democratic landslide. The Democratic majority in the House—282 to 153—was the largest since 1936. In addition, the Democrats gained a 62 to 34 majority in the Senate. But the Democratic sweep had little effect on the President's conservative policies. The departure of the moderate Adams, ironically, gave Eisenhower's more conservative inclinations free play. His posture in domestic affairs remained to the end one of dogged defense of the budget.

The American People in the Fifties

A homogenized society? Worn out by twenty years of crisis, many Americans sought respite from public issues. They wanted security rather than adventure, comfort rather than challenge. Society preferred those who lacked rough edges, eschewed eccentricity, and played the company game. In a training film circulated by a leading chemical firm, the sound track said, as the camera panned over men in white coats at a Monsanto laboratory, "No geniuses here; just a bunch of average Americans working together." More and more people were spending their whole lives in organizations—their days in great corporations, their nights in great suburban enclaves. By 1960 the suburban population had increased nearly 50 percent in a decade and almost equaled that of the central cities. Both corporation and suburb appeared to foster a pervasive, benign, and invincible conformity. America had be-

come, it was said, a case of the bland leading the bland.

The compelling medium of television advanced the process of homogenization. Originally developed in the 1930s, television went on the market in the late forties. In 1950, 3.2 million Americans owned sets; in 1960, 50 million. By 1960 more households had television than had running water or indoor toilets. Programming was dominated by three large networks and a collection of advertising agencies. The result dismayed thoughtful viewers. Edward R. Murrow, who himself did much to elevate the medium, wrote, "Television in the main is being used to distract, delude, amuse and insulate."

Most striking of all was the hold the mood of quiescence seemed to have on the young. Older generations, recalling their springtimes of revolt—cultural in the twenties, political in the thirties—looked with incredulity on this "uncommitted generation" composed of prudent young men and women who shunned risk and subordinated everything to a steady job, a house in the suburbs, and a company retirement plan—a generation apparently fearful of politics, mistrustful of ideas, incurious about society, desperate about personal security.

Even the church threatened to become an instrument of the new acquiescence. Though religious sta-

The compelling medium: to distract and amuse

tistics are notoriously unreliable, it appears that in the second quarter of the century church membership grew twice as fast as population. This religiosity was conspicuously indifferent, however, to historical religion. Eighty percent of those responding to one public opinion poll claimed they regarded the Bible as the revealed word of God, but only 35 percent could name the four Gospels and over half could not name one. Belief was deemed good in general. As Eisenhower said, "Our government makes no sense unless it is founded in a deeply felt religious faith—and I don't care what it is." Religion became a part of "belonging," a convenient way to establish social identity.

In place of the austere intellectual structure of the traditional faiths, the best-selling religious books of the period purveyed a "cult of reassurance"—Rabbi Joshua Loth Liebmann's *Peace of Mind* (1946), Bishop Fulton J. Sheen's *Peace of Soul* (1949), the Reverend Norman Vincent Peale's *The Power of Positive Thinking* (1952). These and other books portrayed God as the man upstairs, someone up there watching over me, the everlasting source of protection and comfort. The nondoctrinal faith seemed designed to guarantee success for the individual in his professional career and victory for the nation in its struggle against atheistic communism.

Stirrings under the surface. Yet the break between decades is never sharp, and under the complacent surface of the fifties other tendencies were at work. The religious community, for example, did not watch the outburst of popular religiosity with unqualified enthusiasm. The "neo-orthodoxy" of Reinhold Niebuhr, especially as formulated in *The Nature and Destiny of Man* (1941, 1943), had profound influence among believers and nonbelievers alike as a majestic restatement of traditional Christian insights. Where the cult of reassurance identified faith with middle-class values, the Niebuhrians insisted on the independence of Christian faith from the official culture. Where one used faith to sanction the status quo, the other urged the church to reestablish transcendent norms. Niebuhr himself sharply criticized the notion that public avowals demonstrated authentic belief. "The greatest corruption of all," he wrote, "is a corrupt religion." He agreed that religion could produce peace of soul, but not the peace of positive thoughts or of self-congratulation; true religion aimed rather at the "peace of God which passeth all understanding." "That peace passes understanding," added Niebuhr, "precisely because it is a peace with pain in it." The object of faith was to induce not contentment but contrition, not complacency but repentance.

The intellectual community weighed the decade and found it smug and torpid. Novelists and social critics portrayed American conformism in such books as David Riesman's *The Lonely Crowd* (1952), Sloan Wilson's *The Man in the Gray Flannel Suit* (1955), and W. H. Whyte, Jr.'s, *The Organization Man* (1956). In *The Affluent Society* (1958), J. K. Galbraith persuasively questioned the "conventional wisdom" that put forward the maximization of economic growth as the answer to all problems, pointing out that in America this had produced a combination of private opulence and public squalor and had notably failed to eradicate poverty.

As the rise of the "lost generation" had expressed a rejection of Babbittry by the youth of the 1920s, so the rise of the "beat generation" expressed a dissent by the youth of the fifties from the ethos of affluence. The rebels of the fifties were more chaotic and pitiful than their lighthearted and talented predecessors. Hipsters and beatniks admired "cool cats" like James Dean and Marlon Brando, and lost no opportunity to exhibit their biting contempt for the "squares" of the world. Sympathetic observers saw in these "antiheroes" a brave attempt to reject the suffocating embrace of a conformist society. Others dismissed them as "rebels without a cause," dedicated to an aimless flight from responsibility. As the beat novelist Jack Kerouac put it in an exchange between two characters in *On The Road* (1957), "We gotta go and never stop going till we get there." "Where we going, man?" "I don't know, but we gotta go."

James Dean: one cool cat

Republican Foreign Policy

Ending the Korean War. In foreign affairs the general in the White House hoped to be a man of peace. Fulfilling his 1952 campaign pledge, he had visited Korea in the interval between his election and the inauguration. Cease-fire negotiations, initiated in July 1951, continued to drag on, however, as did hostilities; indeed, some of the heaviest fighting of the war took place around Porkchop Hill in the Chorwon area in July 1953.

The sticking-point was whether, and how, prisoners of war should be repatriated. Many of the North Koreans and Chinese in United Nations hands had made clear that they did not want to return to their homelands. United Nations negotiators accordingly rejected communist insistence on compulsory repatriation. In the spring of 1953, exasperated by the deadlock, Eisenhower decided to signal the communists "that, in the absence of satisfactory progress, we intended to move decisively without inhibition in our use of weapons, and would no longer be responsible for confining hostilities to the Korean Peninsula." Whether because of this threat of nuclear war, or because the death of Stalin in March 1953 had given new flexibility to Soviet policy, the North Koreans now accepted voluntary repatriation. An armistice was concluded at Panmunjom on July 27, 1953.

The armistice provided for a demilitarized zone and called for a political conference to settle the future of Korea. But the conference was never held, and in subsequent years each side repeatedly charged the other with violations of the armistice. The United States signed a mutual-defense treaty with South Korea in 1954 and kept an uncertain hand in South Korean affairs. The increasingly capricious actions of President Syngman Rhee caused widespread protest both in South Korea and in Washington, culminating in his overthrow in April 1960 and the establishment in 1961 of a new—and eventually, more dictatorial—government under General Park Chung Hee.

The Korean War had lasted three years and one month. During that time 33,629 Americans had lost their lives in battle, along with about 3,000 from other UN countries and about 50,000 South Koreans. Total communist battle casualties were estimated at 1.5 million. For all the frustration the war produced at home, it had stopped aggression in Korea, briefly strengthened the authority of the United Nations, and shown the communist world that the democratic nations were prepared to meet military challenge. It had also accustomed the nation to the idea of war on presidential initiative and to the belief that American military force was effective on the Asian mainland.

Eisenhower and Dulles. Ending the Korean War marked a first success for Eisenhower as a man of peace. His pacific instincts and pragmatic temper, however, were somewhat at odds with the ideological militancy of his party and especially of his Secretary of State. The grandson of one Secretary of State (John Foster) and nephew of another (Robert Lansing), John Foster Dulles had begun his diplomatic career as his grandfather's secretary at the Hague Conference of 1907. An isolationist in the thirties, he emerged by 1944 as the leading Republican spokesman on foreign affairs. By profession a lawyer and by avocation a Presbyterian layman, Dulles united a talent for close legal argument with a penchant for righteous moralism. Critics found him tricky and sanctimonious. One British foreign secretary, Herbert Morrison, spoke of his "duplicity," and another, Harold Macmillan, questioned his "intellectual integrity."

Though identified with many aspects of the Truman-Acheson foreign policy, Dulles had turned against that policy as the 1952 election drew near. Dismissing containment as "negative, futile and immoral," he called for a new policy of "liberation." The mere statement by the United States "that it wants

John Foster Dulles: a penchant for moralism

American missiles in Germany

and expects liberation to occur would change, in an electrifying way, the mood of the captive peoples."

In this mood Eisenhower cancelled Truman's 1950 order to neutralize the Straits of Formosa, thereby "unleashing" Chiang Kai-shek (Jiang Jieshi) for presumed reconquest of the mainland. However, Nationalist forces were in effect released by a mutual-security pact in 1955. American inaction in face of anti-Soviet upheavals in East Germany in 1953 and Hungary in 1956 ended talk of "liberation" and "rollback." The Administration continued to insist it was reversing the Truman-Acheson policies. "Isn't it wonderful," said Vice President Nixon in 1954, "finally to have a Secretary of State who isn't taken in by the Communists, who stands up to them?" But observers were more impressed by continuities than reversals. Dulles's tone was more moralistic and ideological than Acheson's and his proposals were more belligerent; but his militancy was offset by Eisenhower's caution and optimism. Underneath the rhetoric, containment was quietly reinstated as American policy.

The President and his Secretary of State differed in their attitudes toward negotiation. Where Dulles thought a gain for one side must be a loss for the other, Eisenhower sought opportunities for mutual gain. "The hard and uncompromising line that the United States took toward Soviet Russia and Red China between 1953 and the early months of 1959," Sherman Adams later wrote, "was more a Dulles line than an Eisenhower one." Still the difference should not be exaggerated. Eisenhower fully accepted the premises of the Cold War and saw value in the tough-cop, nice-cop routine. Dulle's truculent preachments had their uses both in intimidating the Russians and in reserving for the President himself the benign role of guardian of the peace.

Massive retaliation. If containment was reinstated, it was containment with a difference. After the Soviet Union developed the atomic bomb, the Truman administration had concluded that American nuclear supremacy could not last and therefore supplied no basis for long-term strategy. Containment, so NSC 68 argued, required increased conventional capabilities. An administration used to the idea of public spending thought the economy could bear the added cost. But Eisenhower considered fiscal conservatism essential to economic health and therefore wanted a course that would simultaneously restrain Soviet aggression and the defense budget. He found the answer by 1954 in making nuclear weapons the center of American strategy.

Despite the fact that Truman had dropped the atomic bomb and approved the hydrogen bomb, he regarded the nuclear weapon with dismay: "This isn't a military weapon. . . . We have to treat this differently from rifles and cannon." Eisenhower, on the other hand, saw "no distinction between conventional weapons and atomic weapons" (as he told Winston Churchill, again British prime minister, in 1953). "I see no reason," he said publicly in 1955, "why they shouldn't be used just exactly as you would use a bullet or anything else." In this conviction he readily employed the threat of nuclear war (termed "nuclear blackmail" when employed by the Russians) in Korea and elsewhere.

Reliance on conventional means for containment, moreover, enabled the Soviet Union to take initiatives at times and places of its choosing. In 1954 Dulles proclaimed the "new look" in American strategy based "primarily upon a great capacity to retaliate, instantly, by means and at places of our choosing." "Rather than let the Communists nibble us to death all over the world in little wars," said Nixon, "we would rely in the future primarily on our massive mobile retaliatory power."

Eisenhower thus moved from Truman's defensive interpretation of containment to the offensive concept of "massive retaliation" and from Truman's balanced forces to major reliance on nuclear weapons. The "new look" expected to deter aggression by instilling uncertainty in the mind of the enemy as to what the United States might do when provoked, with nuclear attack on the Soviet Union now a possible response. The "necessary art," Dulles said, was "the ability to get to the verge without getting into war. . . . If you are scared to go to the brink, you are lost." Success depended on Moscow's believing that Washington would actually drop the bomb—a premise bound to become more problematic as Soviet nuclear strength continued to grow.

Eisenhower and Russia. Eisenhower had a genuine desire for conciliation and peace. The death of Stalin gave new opportunity to western diplomacy as well as new outlets both to energies of normalization stirring within the Soviet Union and to energies of nationalism spreading elsewhere in the communist empire. Anticipating a less rigid Soviet leadership, Churchill argued for a summit meeting. But Dulles, forever fearful that a reduction in Soviet-American tension would relax the western guard, opposed the idea. In 1953–54 the West may well have lost a chance to test significant new Soviet proposals, especially regarding the neutralization of Germany.

By early 1955 Churchill finally persuaded Dulles to drop his opposition. When the Soviet Union, after a decade's stalemate, agreed to sign an Austrian peace treaty in May, omens for the Big Four meeting at Geneva seemed auspicious. Eisenhower, for all his nonchalance about nuclear weapons, acknowledged future perils. "We are rapidly getting to the point," he wrote the next year, "that no war can be won." At Geneva in July he set forth a creative "Open Skies" plan, proposing that the two superpowers exchange blueprints of military establishments and permit mutual aerial photographic overflights. A system of continuous reciprocal monitoring, Eisenhower argued, could reassure each superpower against surprise attack. The Russians rejected this promising idea, however, because they saw Open Skies as an American espionage scheme, because they insisted that inspection be accompanied by arms reduction and no doubt because they thought Open Skies would cancel the relative intelligence advantage they enjoyed over an open society like the United States.

Europe, North Africa, and the Middle East

In August 1960, the CIA took steps to enlist members of the criminal underworld with gambling syndicate contacts to aid in assassinating Castro.... [Richard] Bissell and [Sheffield] Edwards testified that they were certain that both [Allen W.] Dulles and his Deputy General [C. P.] Cabell were aware of and authorized the initial phase of the assassination plot involving underworld figures. They acknowledged, however, that Dulles and Cabell were not told about the plot until after the underworld figures had been contacted.... [John] McCone testified that he did not know about or authorize the plots. [Richard] Helms, Bissell and [William] Harvey all testified that they did not tell McCone of the assassination effort either when McCone assumed the position of DCI [Director of Central Intelligence] in November 1961 or at any time thereafter until August 1963 when Helms gave McCone a memorandum from which McCone concluded that the operation with underworld figures prior to the Bay of Pigs had involved assassination. The Inspector General's Report states that Harvey received Helms' approval not to brief McCone when the assassination efforts were resumed in 1962.... On May 7, 1962, Edwards and the CIA's General Counsel, Lawrence Houston, briefed Attorney General Robert Kennedy on the operation involving underworld figures, describing it as terminated.... Two plans to assassinate Castro were explored by Task Force W, the CIA section then concerned with covert Cuban operations, in early 1963.

From *Alleged Assassination Plots Involving Foreign Leaders*, an interim report of the Senate Select Committee on Intelligence Activities (94th Congress, 1st Session), November 20, 1975.

Supplementing massive retaliation. The problem of small local wars remained. Here Dulles proposed to replace American conventional forces by a network of allies recruited through bilateral military assistance programs and in some parts of the world through collective military pacts. So in 1954 the Americans set up the Southeast Asia Treaty Organization (SEATO), bringing three Asian states (Thailand, Pakistan, and the Philippines) together with the United States, Britain, France, Australia, and New Zealand. SEATO's provisions were less stringent than those of NATO, calling only for consultation among the signatories in case of communist subversion and for action by each state "in accordance with its constitutional processes" in case of armed attack. In the Middle East Dulles induced the British to create a regional defense organization under the Baghdad Pact of 1955 (CENTO—the Central Treaty Organization). Condemning neutralism as "immoral," Dulles hoped to force all nations to choose sides in the Cold War. Critics, feeling that Dulles had undue faith in the capacity of military pacts to stabilize underdeveloped areas, referred acidly to his "pactomania."

For direct American intervention abroad, the Eisenhower Administration turned from conventional armed force to the Central Intelligence Agency. Established in 1947, the CIA under Truman had concentrated on helping democratic (including socialist) parties, trade unions, and newspapers in western Europe and on espionage in eastern Europe and the Soviet Union. In the 1950s CIA "covert action"—that is, the attempt by clandestine means to alter policies and governments in other countries—grew ambitious and aggressive.

The fact that CIA director Allen W. Dulles was the Secretary of State's brother gave the agency unusual freedom of initiative. The CIA began not just to support friends but to subvert foes—helping to overthrow governments regarded as procommunist in Iran (1953) and Guatemala (1954), failing to do so in Indonesia (1958), helping to install supposedly prowestern governments in Egypt (1954) and Laos (1959), organizing an expedition of Cuban refugees against the Fidel Castro regime (1960), even plotting the assassination of Castro (with the collaboration, incredibly, of American gangsters) and of the procommunist Congolese leader Patrice Lumumba (1960). By 1957 the CIA devoted more than 50 percent of its personnel and more than 80 percent of its budget to "covert action."

Eisenhower's own Board of Consultants on Foreign Intelligence Activities repeatedly warned him against CIA meddling in the internal affairs of other countries. As early as 1956 Robert Lovett, a former Secretary of Defense, and David Bruce, a distinguished diplomat, pleaded for reconsideration of "the long-range wisdom of activities that have entailed our virtual abandonment of the international 'golden rule,' and which, if successful to the degree claimed for them, are responsible in a great measure for stirring up the turmoil and raising the doubts about us that exist in many countries of the world. . . . Where will we be tomorrow?'' Where indeed? But Eisenhower consistently ignored his board's recommendations. CIA activity fed the American government's conviction both of its ability and its right to decide the destiny of other nations.

Institutionalizing the Cold War. Seeing the godless communist conspiracy as both evil in itself and the source of all the world's troubles, Dulles absolutized the philosophy of the Cold War. His rigid views took root in a group of government agencies—the State Department (which he purged of active dissenters), the Defense Department, the National Security Council, the CIA—all of which developed vested institutional interests in the idea of a militarily expansionist Soviet Union. The Cold War conferred power, appropriations, and public influence on these agencies; and, by the natural law of bureaucracies, their stake in the conflict steadily increased.

The Cold War had long since been institutionalized in the Soviet Union, where the Russians were already equipped with a dogma of inevitable conflict and, through its network of communist parties, with the means of local intervention. Stalin's death, after harsh and obscure feuds among Soviet leaders, concluded in the victory of N. S. Khrushchev by 1957–58. Khrushchev, an impulsive man with a plunger's instinct, replaced Stalin's Cold War of position by a Cold War of movement.

On both sides there now arose a propensity to perceive local conflicts in global terms, political conflicts in moral terms, and relative differences in absolute terms. Each side saw humanity as divided between forces of light and forces of darkness. Each assumed that the opposing bloc was under the organized and unified control of the other. Washington supposed that what was then called the free world should reshape itself on the American model, Moscow that the communist world should reshape itself on the Russian model.

Nationalism and the Superpowers

Nationalism versus the Cold War. Containment had begun in Europe, where it was a reasonable response to the struggle between democracy and Stalinism. In its extended form after Korea, it now presupposed a world consumed, as Europe had been, by this struggle. And indeed, for a decade after 1945, America and Russia managed to bestride the globe as superpow-

Ho Chi Minh

ers, working to consolidate their positions around the planet—America through its pacts, Russia through its parties.

But European concepts of the Cold War did not apply to regions increasingly convulsed by demands for political and economic independence against colonial or neocolonial control. In most cases the new nationalist states had no great interest in the conflict between America and Russia except as they could exploit it for their own purposes. As the superpowers tried to enlist developing countries on one side or the other in their Cold War, the new states tended to respond by playing off one superpower against the other and using the Cold War as a means of getting aid for themselves. Despite pretenses and alliances, the new states—even, it developed, those that pronounced themselves communist—responded in the end to their own national interests.

Crisis in east Asia. By the early fifties, the United States was paying 80 percent of the cost of the French war against Ho Chi Minh and the Viet Minh. The French position, however, had grown desperate. In March 1954, with substantial French forces under siege in the valley of Dienbienphu in western Tonkin, Paris asked Washington for armed intervention.

Eisenhower told a press conference that Indochina was of ''transcendent'' concern; ''you have a row of dominoes set up, you knock over the first one. . . . You could have the beginning of a disintegration that would have the most profound influences.'' Dulles now advocated the use of nuclear weapons to raise the siege of Dienbienphu. Vice President Nixon suggested the possibility of ''putting American boys in." But leading senators, among them Lyndon B. Johnson and John F. Kennedy, were skeptical. General Matthew B. Ridgway, now Army Chief of Staff, was vigorously opposed. So was Winston Churchill. "What we are being asked to do," Churchill said, "is assist in misleading the Congress into approving a military operation which would be in itself ineffective, and might well bring the world to the verge of major war." Eisenhower decided against military intervention.

Dienbienphu fell, after fifty-six days, on May 7. Four days later Eisenhower informed Paris that he would seek authority from Congress to send troops to Indochina if the French would make political concessions to anticommunist nationalists. Soon, however, Pierre Mendès-France came to power in Paris pledged to end the war in a month. In the next weeks negotiations at Geneva produced a provisional settlement. The Geneva Accords provided for the temporary partition of Vietnam at the seventeenth parallel—this to be a "military demarcation line" and "not in any way [to] be interpreted as constituting a political or territorial boundary"—with reunification to come through elections scheduled for July 1956. The Accords also limited the size of foreign military missions in Vietnam.

Washington had watched the negotiations with grim disapproval, and the National Security Council pronounced the result a "disaster . . . a major forward stride of Communism which may lead to the loss of Southeast Asia." After setting up SEATO, the Administration now gave special assistance to South Vietnam and its new premier, Ngo Dinh Diem, a devout Catholic and stubborn nationalist whose strength of purpose had impressed many Americans, liberal and conservative, during his American stay in 1950–53. In 1955 Diem rejected the elections provided for in the Geneva Accords. Soon he deposed Emperor Bao Dai, the French puppet, and, as president of the new Republic of Vietnam, moved to revive the economy, suppress political opposition, and confirm his personal control. The discontent aroused by Diem's increasingly arbitrary regime gave Vietnamese communists a new chance to seize power. In 1958 a communist-nationalist movement called the National Liberation Front or, more popularly, the Viet Cong, began guerrilla warfare against Diem. This development alarmed Washington. "The loss of South Vietnam," said Eisenhower on April 4, 1959, "would set in motion a crumbling process that could, as it progressed, have grave consequences for us."

In neighboring Laos, the military crisis was more acute and American intervention more active. The Pathet Lao, a communist-led guerrilla movement, was roaming the countryside; and the United States in 1958 vetoed the effort of Prince Souvanna Phouma to establish a neutral Laos under a coalition government with Pathet Lao participation. In 1959 the CIA installed a prowestern government in Vientiane. Regarding the upper Mekong Valley as the gateway to Southeast Asia, the United States put nearly $300 million

French troops at Dienbienphu

into Laos between the period of the Geneva Accords and the end of 1960—more aid per capita than it sent to any other country.

Eisenhower discerned (incorrectly) Chinese Communist intervention in Indochina, and in any event the Administration regarded Communist China as a wholly-owned subsidiary of the Soviet Union. After his unleashing, Chiang Kai-shek (Jiang Jieshi) had put troops on the offshore islands of Quemoy (Jinman) and Matsu (Mazu) in the Straits of Formosa. When the Chinese Communists started bombing the islands in late 1954, Eisenhower persuaded Congress in January 1955 to pass the Formosa Resolution, authorizing the President to use armed force "as he deems necessary" to defend Formosa (Taiwan) and the neighboring Pescadores islands.

The bombings subsided, and in the next years Chiang (Jiang) sent a hundred thousand Nationalist troops to the offshore islands. Heavy communist bombardment resumed in August 1958. Though Eisenhower was irritated by the reinforcement of the offshore islands, he saw no alternative but to convince Peking (Beijing) that the United States would intervene, "perhaps using nuclear weapons," if the communists attempted an invasion. After three months the shelling tapered off. Under American pressure Chiang (Jiang) eventually reduced the size of his forces on the islands.

Nationalism in the Middle East. Conflicting concerns—about Soviet expansion, about Arab oil, and about the survival of Israel—had thrust the United States into the Middle Eastern cauldron. The first two factors shaped American policy in 1951 when Mohammed Mossadegh, the prime minister of Iran, nationalized British oil holdings and challenged the authority of the shah, Mohammed Reza Pahlavi, who soon fled the country. Truman, regarding Mossadegh as an honest if exasperating nationalist, attempted mediation lest Iran's quarrel with the British encourage Soviet intervention. The quarrel dragged on, and in 1953 Eisenhower, who regarded Mossadegh as a communist tool, decided to overthrow him and restore the shah—a program carried through in August 1953 in a coup organized by a CIA agent (who happened to be a grandson of Theodore Roosevelt). Thereafter America succeeded Britain as Iran's western patron.

The center of Arab nationalism was the new regime in Egypt, installed by revolution in 1952 and, after 1954, under the purposeful leadership of Colonel Gamal Abdel Nasser. Moscow established relations with Nasser, sent Egypt arms, and proposed to subsidize the construction of a great dam at Aswan on the Nile. Washington at first offered western financing for the dam. Then in July 1956 Dulles, annoyed by

Gamal Abdel Nasser, Arab nationalist

Nasser's dalliance with the Russians, withdrew the American offer just as Egypt was about to accept it. Nasser retaliated by nationalizing the Suez Canal.

Britain and France regarded Nasser's seizure of the canal as a threat to western Europe's vital supplies of oil. Moreover, Sir Anthony Eden, now British prime minister, saw Nasser in the image of Hitler and believed that appeasement would only inflame his ambitions. Israel feared that Egyptian rearmament would permanently alter the balance of power in the Middle East. In October, British and French officials met secretly with Israeli leaders in France. On October 29, Israel attacked Egypt. Two days later Britain and France entered the war against Egypt on the patently spurious excuse of trying to localize the conflict. Ironically, one result of the Anglo-French intervention was to save Egyptian forces from probable defeat by the Israelis.

Washington, which had not been consulted by the plotters, roundly disowned the Suez expedition and threatened to deny financial support to the faltering British pound. It also initiated action in the

United Nations—backed by the Soviet Union and opposed by Britain and France—to condemn Israel as the aggressor. On November 6 Eden ordered a cease-fire. While the rigid American line in the UN resulted in the rescue of Nasser without rebuke for Egyptian harassment of Israel, the Anglo-French adventure was nonetheless ill-conceived and ill-prepared, and Dulles was right in supposing that gunboat imperialism was obsolescent.

Still, despite the power of Arab nationalism, Dulles persisted in regarding Soviet penetration as the essential problem. "The existing vacuum in the Middle East," Eisenhower told Congress in January 1957, "must be filled by the United States before it is filled by Russia. . . . Considering Russia's announced purpose of dominating the world, it is easy to understand its hope of dominating the Middle East." Eisenhower asked Congress to declare a vital American interest in preventing such domination and to authorize the commitment of American forces to aid Middle Eastern nations "requesting such aid, against overt armed aggression from any nation controlled by International Communism." Congress by joint resolution passed the so-called Eisenhower Doctrine in March 1957. In July 1958 Eisenhower landed fourteen thousand troops to protect a prowestern government in Lebanon.

Nationalism in Latin America. Latin America too was swept by nationalist ferment after the Second

Fidel Castro: romantic Marxist

World War. The resulting revolutions sometimes (as in Argentina) took authoritarian, sometimes (as in Venezuela) democratic, forms. Then toward the end of the forties a counterrevolutionary reaction set in. By 1954 thirteen Latin American presidents were military men. Now a new surge of protest arose against dictatorships, bringing the overthrow of, among others, Perón of Argentina in 1955, Pérez Jiménez of Venezuela in 1958, Batista of Cuba in 1959, and Trujillo of the Dominican Republic in 1961.

Through this ebb and flow, Washington, insofar as it thought about the hemisphere at all, tried to fit it into the framework of the Cold War. Franklin D. Roosevelt's Good Neighbor ideals were neglected. The Truman Administration concentrated on a program of inter-American military cooperation. In 1954 Eisenhower's CIA overthrew the democratic Arbenz government in Guatemala, which the administration regarded as hostile to the United Fruit Company and vulnerable to Marxism. The result for Guatemala was a long series of right-wing military regimes. Throughout the hemisphere, the administration showed a weakness for authoritarian governments. Nixon, visiting Cuba, praised the "competence and stability" of the Batista dictatorship. When in 1958 Nixon visited Peru and Venezuela after dictators personally decorated by Eisenhower had been thrown out, he was stoned and spat upon.

Batista fled Cuba in 1959, and Latin Americans welcomed a new revolutionary government led by a bearded, cigar-smoking leader, the flamboyant and audacious Fidel Castro. Castro initiated a long-needed program of social and agrarian reform. But he combined this program with terror equal to that of his predecessor. A romantic Marxist nationalist rather than a disciplined communist, Castro needed the United States as his enemy and therefore rebuffed conciliatory American gestures. For its part, Washington grew obsessed with the expropriation of American property in Cuba. Despite his excesses, Castro became for a moment a hero through much of the hemisphere.

The Cuban revolution altered Washington's indifference to Latin American demands for economic development and national self-assertion. When President Kubitschek of Brazil proposed "Operation Pan America" and an Inter-American Development Bank in 1957, Washington had shown no interest; but by 1960 the Administration was ready to offer "a broad new social development program for Latin America" based on the Inter-American Development Bank—a program endorsed by the Organization of American States in the Act of Bogotá in September 1960.

In time, surrounded increasingly by communists and lashed by the intensities of his own turbulent personality, Castro led Cuba into the Soviet camp.

Fearful of a Soviet satellite in the Western Hemisphere, Eisenhower in March 1960 agreed to a CIA proposal to arm and train a force of Cuban exiles for use against the Cuban regime. On its own the CIA began planning to assassinate Castro. When Castro ordered the United States to cut its embassy to eleven persons, the Eisenhower Administration broke relations in January 1961.

The United States and the Soviet Union

Khrushchev the adventurer. The Soviet Union, seeing in anti-colonialism and revolution a potent means of reducing western power, met the challenge of Third World nationalism with relish. Communism, Moscow assured underdeveloped countries, offered the best road to modernization. This claim acquired momentary plausibility from unexpected Soviet technological breakthroughs—the hydrogen bomb in 1953; *Sputnik*; the first earth satellite, and the first intercontinental ballistic missile (ICBM) in 1957; the first moon satellite in 1959; and the first man in space in 1961.

The ebullient Khrushchev, now securely in command, proceeded to transform the defensive Cold War of Stalin into a more far-flung and aggressive contest. His speeches were boastful and belligerent, and the launching of *Sputnik* seemed to verify his horrendous claims about Soviet ICBM superiority. He liked to tell small countries how many "rockets" would be required to destroy them, and he did not hesitate (as in 1956 against Britain and France over Suez and later against the United States over Cuba) to threaten war. He greatly increased Soviet activity in the Middle East, Southeast Asia, Latin America, and Africa and appeared eager to exploit every western vulnerability. Hoping perhaps to end up with a denuclearized Germany, he reopened the Berlin question in November 1958, threatening a termination of allied rights in West Berlin.

The launching of *Sputnik* caused great alarm in the United States. The Gaither Report to the National Security Council in 1957 predicted an imminent time of danger when the Soviet Union would possess more missiles than the United States. "There is no dispute about the missile gap," Henry Kissinger wrote as late as 1961. Democrats assailed the Administration for letting the nation fall behind in nuclear striking power. Educators demanded increased national investment in the sciences. Though the Pentagon welcomed the "missile gap" as an argument for more military spending, Eisenhower himself was skeptical. He did not want further to unbalance the budget. Moreover, photographic reconnaissance of Soviet territory by a high-altitude CIA aircraft, the U-2, while limited in its coverage, failed to confirm the fearsome predictions.

In fact, Eisenhower was right. The Soviet Union had postponed its ICBM buildup pending technological improvements. Khrushchev, having rejected Open Skies, was able to deceive the west about Soviet nuclear strength and to threaten with missiles he did not have.

Khrushchev the coexister. Khrushchev was more complicated than he first appeared. With his famous "secret speech" denouncing the crimes of Stalin at the Twentieth Party Congress in 1956, he launched the "de-Stalinization" process and started a movement toward normalization in Soviet society. In world affairs he proclaimed the gospel of "peaceful coexistence," amending the Leninist doctrine of the inevitability of war. In the nuclear age, he said, the conflict between capitalism and communism would be decided by peaceful competition between social systems.

Soviet as well as western leaders were increasingly impressed by the incalculable perils presented by nuclear weapons—by the fact, for example, that a single plane could deliver more destructive power than all the planes in all the air forces delivered during the Second World War. Also the problem of radioactive fallout had come sharply to the world's attention in 1954, when both the United States and the Soviet Union tested large-yield nuclear weapons in the atmosphere. As scientists analyzed the effects of radioactive contamination on the bones, blood, and germ plasm of humans, concern mounted over nuclear testing. In March 1958 the Soviet Union suspended testing, and the United States and Britain followed suit in October (while Russia briefly resumed).

Khrushchev's very truculence may have been an attempt to force the west to accept the Soviet Union and détente. It was also an attempt to head off Communist China, which regarded "peaceful coexistence" as a betrayal of world revolution and which might soon challenge Russia for leadership of the international communist movement. Sino-Soviet relations began to deteriorate in 1958—a development unknown to the State Department, which persisted for another half-dozen years in talking about the "Sino-Soviet bloc."

Exasperated by Khrushchev's inflammatory language and worldwide meddling, the West did not appreciate his more pacific purposes. Moreover, if

Camp David, 1959: Eisenhower and Khrushchev

Khrushchev could secure "peaceful coexistence" (from which he always rigorously excluded ideological coexistence), he confidently predicted the withering away of capitalism and the triumph of communism by peaceful means. That is what he meant when he told the western democracies, "We will bury you"—not that the communists would kill their adversaries but that they would outlive them.

His policy thus bounded back and forth between belligerence and conciliation. Early in 1959 Khrushchev grew conciliatory again; and the West in March accepted a summit meeting in principle. Even Secretary of State Dulles, now ravaged by cancer, acquiesced in the drift toward negotiation. In April Dulles resigned, to be replaced by Christian A. Herter; five weeks later Dulles was dead. Though a foreign ministers' meeting in Geneva in May resulted in a deadlock over Berlin, the movement toward the summit continued. In the summer of 1959 Nixon visited Russia, and in September Khrushchev himself visited the United States. The Khrushchev tour, marked by a series of picturesque incidents, including a visit to Disneyland, reached its climax in private talks between Khrushchev and Eisenhower at Camp David, in Maryland. The United States agreed to a summit meeting, and Khrushchev agreed to drop his deadline on Berlin.

The dark year. The summit meeting was scheduled for Paris on May 16, 1960. Then on May 5 Khrushchev announced the shooting down of an American plane over the Soviet Union. Washington promptly said that the plane had innocently strayed from course on a meteorological flight. On May 7 Khrushchev gleefully sprang his trap. The pilot was alive, he said, and had confessed that he was engaged in espionage. Khrushchev added, "I am quite willing to grant that the President knew nothing about the plane."

At this point the Administration owned up to the act of espionage. Secretary Herter argued that the United States was morally entitled to conduct U-2 flights in order to protect the "free world" from surprise attack. Herter and, soon, Nixon implied that the flights would continue. Eisenhower, rejecting Khrushchev's proffered escape clause, accepted full responsibility. Khrushchev now came to Paris demanding that Eisenhower apologize for the flights and punish those responsible. Eisenhower rejected these demands, and the summit collapsed.

End of the Eisenhower Era

The election of 1960. Voters faced the election of 1960 in a troubled state of mind. After the U-2 fiasco, the request of the Japanese government that, in view

Nixon and Kennedy, 1960: TV, a political innovation

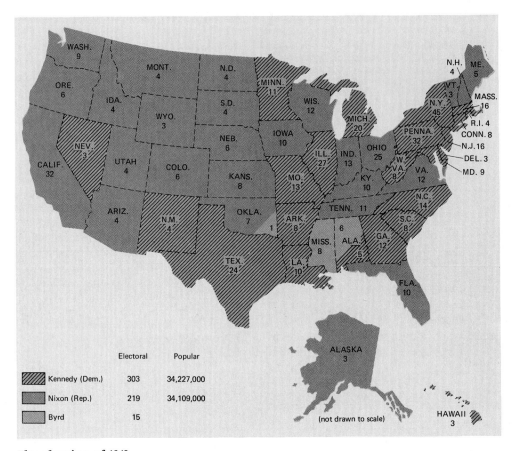

The election of 1960

of anti-American riots in Tokyo, Eisenhower cancel a scheduled presidential visit provided further evidence of a decline in American influence. Within the United States, the rise of unemployment to over 6 percent caused further problems for the Republicans.

Vice President Nixon won the Republican nomination with Henry Cabot Lodge of Massachusetts as his running mate. The Democrats turned to Senator John F. Kennedy of Massachusetts, who had eliminated Senator Hubert Humphrey of Minnesota in crucial primaries. The Democratic Senate leader, Lyndon B. Johnson, who ran second to Kennedy in the convention, accepted the vice-presidential nomination.

New states, 1959

The conjunction of an immense military establishment and a large arms industry is new in the American experience. The total influence—economic, political, even spiritual—is felt in every city, every State house, every office of the Federal government. We recognize the imperative need for this development. Yet we must not fail to comprehend its grave implications. Our toil, resources and livelihood are all involved; so is the very structure of our society.

In the councils of government, we must guard against the acquisition of unwarranted influence, whether sought or unsought, by the military-industrial complex. The potential for the disastrous rise of misplaced power exists and will persist. We must never let the weight of this combination endanger our liberties or democratic processes. We should take nothing for granted....

Akin to, and largely responsible for the sweeping changes in our industrial-military posture, has been the technological revolution during recent decades.... The prospect of domination of the nation's scholars by Federal employment, project allocations, and the power of money is ever present—and is gravely to be regarded. Yet, in holding scientific research and discovery in respect, as we should, we must also be alert to the equal and opposite danger that public policy could itself become the captive of a scientific-technological élite.

From Dwight D. Eisenhower, Farewell Address, January 17, 1961.

Eisenhower's farewell address

The 1960 campaign was marked by an innovation in American politics—a series of television debates in which the two candidates responded to questions put to them by newspaper reporters. Kennedy's poise and command in these confrontations countered the Republican argument that he was too young and inexperienced for the Presidency. The campaign itself revolved around the question of America's condition as a nation. The United States, Kennedy contended, was falling behind both in the world competition with communism and in meeting its own goals of economic growth and social progress. The process of decline could be reversed only by a "supreme national effort" under strong presidential leadership to "get the country moving again"—a "New Frontier."

The popular vote was the closest since 1888. With the admission of Alaska (January 3, 1959) and Hawaii (August 21, 1959), there were now fifty states in the Union. Kennedy's popular margin was only 119,057 out of 68.3 million votes; taking into account the votes for splinter-party candidates, he was a minority victor. The margin in the Electoral College was more decisive—303 for Kennedy to 219 for Nixon (with 15 Southern votes for Senator Harry F. Byrd of Virginia).

The Eisenhower record. Like Washington and Jackson, Eisenhower left behind a testament for the American people in the form of a farewell address. Speaking with unaccustomed directness, he said that public policy could become "the captive of a scientific-technological élite" and warned against "the acquisition of unwarranted influence, whether sought or unsought, by the military-industrial complex." Though these had not been themes of his own Administration, they identified salient problems of the future.

Eisenhower's most decisive achievement was simply to acquiesce in—and thereby legitimize—the changes Franklin Roosevelt had wrought in American society. In domestic affairs he did little to tackle emerging problems of racial justice, of the cities, of the environment, of resources and energy, at a time when these problems were still relatively manageable.

In foreign policy, he bequeathed a runaway CIA and declining influence in the world. On the day before inauguration, he told Kennedy that the United States should be ready "to intervene unilaterally" in Laos, which he described as the key to Southeast Asia. As for the Cuban exiles under CIA training, he recommended that "this effort be continued and accelerated."

Yet, for all the bellicosity of this valedictory counsel, his own Administration had been a rare interlude of peace in an age of continuous war. Whether through good luck or good management or a combination of both, the American government concluded one war and began no others during the Eisenhower Presidency. The people would remember the man of war as a man of peace, and historians eventually discovered that the apparently genial and passive general had been, behind the mask, a President of force and cunning.

Suggestions for Reading

EISENHOWER AND HIS POLICIES

Eisenhower's memoirs—*The White House Years*, vol. 2 *Mandate for Change* (1963) and vol. 3 *Waging Peace* (1965)—are instructive but formal; the more authentic voice is to be found in R. H. Ferrell, ed., *The Eisenhower Diaries* (1961). The most thorough biography is S. E. Ambrose, *Eisenhower*, 2 vols. (1983–84); Peter Lyon, *Eisenhower: Portrait of the Hero* (1974), is lively; and Herbert Parmet, *Eisenhower and the American Crusades* (1972), and C. C. Alexander, *Holding the Line: The Eisenhower Era, 1952–1961** (1975), are useful studies. F. I. Greenstein, *The Hidden-Hand Presidency** (1982), makes the case for Eisenhower's covert leadership skills. Sherman Adams, W. B. Ewald, Jr., Emmet Hughes and Arthur Larson have written revealing memoirs of the Eisenhower Presidency; see also R. M. Nixon, *Six Crises* (1962).

FOREIGN AFFAIRS

In addition to the works by Brown and Freedman cited in the previous chapter, see Stanley Hoffmann's brilliant essay *Gulliver's Troubles; Or the Setting of American Foreign Policy* (1968). R. A. Divine, *Eisenhower and the Cold War** (1981), is useful but uncritical and omits Eisenhower's use of the CIA: for which see Harry Rositzke, *The CIA's Secret Operations* (1977), B. W. Cook, *The Declassified Eisenhower* (1981); and, for the Guatemala case, S. C. Schlesinger and Stephen Kinzer, *Bitter Fruit: The Untold Story of the American Coup in Guatemala** (1982). Townsend Hoopes, *The Devil and John Foster Dulles* (1973), is an able critical biography; R. W. Pruessen, *John Foster Dulles: The Road to Power* (1982), is more sympathetic. B. I. Kaufman, *Trade and Aid: Eisenhower's Foreign Policy, 1953–1961* (1982), is an excellent treatment of economic aspects. R. H. Fifield, *Americans in Southeast Asia: The Roots of Commitment* (1973), sets the Vietnam scene, and R. B. Smith, *International History of the Vietnam War*, 2 vols. (1984–   ), gives the global context. Donald Neff, *Warriors at Suez: Eisenhower Takes America into the Middle East** (1981), is useful. Peter Grose, *Israel and the Mind of America* (1984), surveys American attitudes and policies. Milton Eisenhower, *The Wine Is Bitter* (1963), discusses the awakening of the Eisenhower Administration to Latin American problems; and P. W. Bonsal, *Cuba, Castro and the United States* (1971), is an authoritative account by the American ambassador to Cuba in 1959–60.

DOMESTIC ISSUES

P. A. Carter, *Another Part of the Fifties* (1983) is a lively and opinionated survey of politics and culture. In addition to the works by Flash, Goodwin, and Stein mentioned in Chapter 30, J. L. Sundquist, *Politics and Policy: The Eisenhower, Kennedy, and Johnson Years** (1968), provides a cogent review of public policy. Samuel Lubell, *The Revolt of the Moderate* (1956), is a searching contemporaneous diagnosis of the electorate. J. B. Martin, *Adlai Stevenson,**2 vols. (1976–77), is a first-rate biography. T. H. White offers a memorable picture of the 1960 election in *The Making of the President, 1960** (1961).

On McCarthyism at high noon and at twilight, see, in addition to works mentioned in Chapter 30, J. A. Wechsler, *The Age of Suspicion* (1953), P. M. Stern, *The Oppenheimer Case* (1969), and Stanley Kutler, *The American Inquisition** (1982). W. L. O'Neill, *A Better World: The Great Schism: Stalinism and the American Intellectuals** (1982) and M. S. McAuliffe, *Crisis on the Left: Cold War Politics and American Liberals* (1978), offer diverging pictures of the arguments within the liberal community.

Harvard Sitkoff, *The Struggle for Black Equality, 1954–1980** (1981), is an able survey. Richard Kluger, *Simple Justice** (1975), is a rich account of the school desegregation decision of 1954; Anthony Lewis, *Portrait of a Decade* (1964), and J. H. Wilkinson III, *From Brown to Bakke: The Supreme Court and School Integration, 1954–1978** (1979), describe the aftermath. M. L. King, Jr., *Stride Toward Freedom* (1958), is a central document in the black revolution; August Meier, et al, eds, *Black Protest Thought in the 20th Century* (2nd ed., 1971), is a valuable anthology; Harold Cruse, *The Crisis of the Negro Intellectual** (1967), is perceptive if erratic. Bernard Schwartz, *Super Chief: Earl Warren and His Supreme Court** (1983), is the standard biography, and R. H. Saylor, B. B. Boyer, and R. E. Gooding, Jr., eds, *The Warren Court: A Critical Analysis** (1969) is informed and sympathetic. A. M. Bickel, *The Supreme Court and Idea of Progress** (1970), enters a thoughtful dissent.

For appraisals of American society, Eric Larrabee, *The Self-Conscious Society* (1960), is a useful review. The more enduring works include J. K. Galbraith, *American Capitalism: The Concept of Countervailing Power** (1952) and *The Affluent Society** (1958) (both reissued in revised editions); David Riesman et al., *The Lonely Crowd** (1952); W. H. Whyte, Jr., *The Organization Man** (1956); David Potter, *People of Plenty** (1954); and, for an eclectic view, Max Lerner, *America As a Civilization** (1957). The values of the business community are discussed in F. X. Sutton et al., *The American Business Creed* (1956). C. W. Mills offers a radical analysis in *White Collar** (1951) and *The Power Elite** (1956). For the impact of the mass media, see D. J. Boorstin, *The Image** (1962). On the religious boom, see Will Herberg, *Protestant-Catholic-Jew** (2nd ed., 1960), and W. L. Miller, *Piety Along the Potomac: Notes on Politics and Morals in the Fifties* (1964). Bruce Cook, *The Beat Generation** (1971), is an effective account.

*Available in a paperback edition.

32

REFORM AND REVOLT

John F. Kennedy, forty-three years old on his inauguration, was the youngest man and the first Roman Catholic elected to the American Presidency as well as the first President born in the twentieth century. Scion of a numerous, spirited, and wealthy Irish-American family, a Harvard graduate and war hero, he was elected after the war to the House of Representatives and in 1952 to the Senate. His book *Profiles in Courage* received the Pulitzer Prize for biography in 1957. Handsome in appearance and graceful in manner, cool, lucid, and ironic in play of mind—he once described himself as an "idealist without illusions"—activist in temperament and purpose, he had an affirmative view of the Presidency and a high sense of America's national and world responsibilities. He was proficient in the game of politics, but he also hoped, in the manner of Wilson and Roosevelt, to tap resources of idealism he felt had been too long repressed in American society. He attracted and sought out men and women of ideas; intellectuals and academics now entered government in unprecedented numbers.

The Thousand Days

Kennedy and the Cold War. Though a child of the Cold War, the new President saw it not as a religious but as a geopolitical conflict. Still, in those terms, the Cold War seemed active enough, especially after a militant speech delivered by Khrushchev on January 6, 1961, two weeks before Kennedy's inauguration. The Soviet leader exultantly predicted the irresistible triumph of communism, especially—in passages that alarmed Washington—through Soviet support for "national liberation wars" in the Third World. Asia, Africa, and Latin America, Khrushchev said, were "the most important centers of revolutionary struggle against imperialism."

Khrushchev's bellicosity was probably intended less as a provocation to the United States than as part of a complex maneuver involving China. For he also took occasion to reaffirm his rejection of nuclear war and his belief in "peaceful coexistence"—views that Communist China continued to oppose. By insisting on them in an otherwise truculent context, Khrushchev may have been trying to show the communist movement that nuclear coexistence was not incompatible with revolution in the Third World. Perhaps he thought militancy would bemuse the Chinese, while softer words would gratify the West. Inevitably Peking (Beijing) and Washington read only the passages written for the other.

Kennedy responded grandiloquently in his inaugural address: "Let every nation know, whether it wishes us well or ill, that we shall pay any price, bear any burden, meet any hardship, support any friend, oppose any foe, in order to assure the survival and the success of liberty." The irony was that both leaders

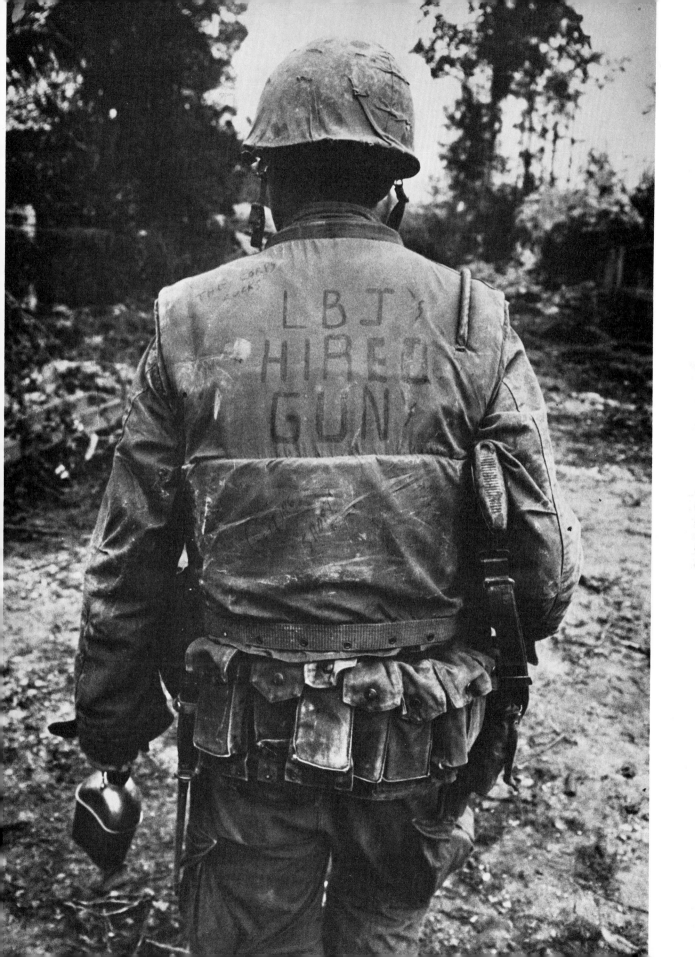

wanted to escape from the arms race. While Khrushchev was twisting and turning in his hope of diminishing the risk of nuclear catastrophe without losing ground to China, Kennedy believed that a third world war would mean the end of civilization. His inaugural address went on to condemn the arms race, asked to "bring the absolute power to destroy other nations under the absolute control of all nations," and declared: "Let us never negotiate out of fear. But let us never fear to negotiate."

The world of diversity. Dean Rusk, the new Secretary of State, held tenacious Cold War views. Adlai Stevenson, now ambassador to the United Nations, was moving beyond his Cold War positions of the fifties. Kennedy himself, despite his inaugural extravagance, had an acute sense of the limitations of American power. Later in 1961 he called on the American people to "face the fact that the United States is neither omnipotent nor omniscient—that we are only 6 percent of the world's population—that we cannot impose our will upon the other 94 percent of mankind—that we cannot right every wrong or reverse each adversity—and that therefore there cannot be an American solution to every world problem."

Kennedy thus had no illusions about the feasibility of a *pax Americana*. But, if he did not think there could be an American solution to every world problem, he did not think there could be a Russian solution either. His broad idea, which he set forth to Khrushchev in a meeting in Vienna in June 1961, was that each superpower should abstain from initiatives that, by upsetting the rough balance into which the postwar world had settled, might invite miscalculation and compel reaction by the other. In the longer run, his vision was of what he called a "world of diversity"—a world of nations various in institutions and creeds, "where, within a framework of international cooperation, every country can solve its own problems according to its own traditions and ideals."

In his view, the "revolution of national independence" was the source and guarantee of the world of diversity. Communism could be one element in this pluralistic world, but diversity, he argued, was ultimately incompatible with the communist belief that all societies went through the same stages and all

Khrushchev and Kennedy, Vienna, 1961: a "world of diversity"

What kind of peace do we seek? Not a Pax Americana enforced on the world by American weapons of war. Not the peace of the grave or the security of the slave. I am talking about genuine peace.... Some say that it is useless to speak of world peace or world law or world disarmament—and that it will be useless until the leaders of the Soviet Union adopt a more enlightened attitude. I hope they do. I believe we can help them do it. But I also believe that we must reexamine our own attitude—as individuals and as a Nation—for our attitude is as essential as theirs.... World peace, like community peace, does not require that each man love his neighbor—it requires only that they live together in mutual tolerance, submitting their disputes to a just and peaceful settlement. And history teaches us that enmities between nations, as between individuals, do not last forever. However fixed our likes and dislikes may seem, the tide of time and events will often bring surprising changes in the relations between nations and neighbors....

It is sad to read these Soviet statements—to realize the extent of the gulf between us. But it is also a warning—a warning to the American people not to fall into the same trap as the Soviets, not to see only a distorted and desperate view of the other side, not to see conflict as inevitable, accommodation as impossible, and communication as nothing more than an exchange of threats. No government or social system is so evil that its people must be considered as lacking in virtue.... We are both caught up in a vicious and dangerous cycle in which suspicion on one side breeds suspicion on the other, and new weapons beget counterweapons.... If we cannot now end our differences, at least we can help make the world safe for diversity. For, in the final analysis, our most basic common link is that we all inhabit this small planet. We all breathe the same air. We all cherish our children's future. And we are all mortal.

From John F. Kennedy, Speech at American University, Washington, D.C., June 10, 1963.

roads had a single destination. "The great currents of history," he said, "are carrying the world away from the monolithic and toward the pluralist idea." In a speech at the American University in June 1963 he summed up his policy in a conscious revision of Wilson's famous line: "If we cannot now end our differences, at least we can help make the world safe for diversity."

Struggle for the Third World. Given the nuclear stalemate, Kennedy agreed with Khrushchev that the Third World had become the main battleground between democracy and communism. As senator he had rejected Dulles' aphorism that neutralism was "immoral." As President, he affirmed the new Administration's sympathy with states struggling for nationhood outside the framework of the Cold War.

Kennedy's purpose was to encourage the developing countries of Africa, Asia, and Latin America to use democratic methods in their quest for independence and growth. An increasing share of American foreign aid now went to modernize economies rather than to build armies. The Peace Corps—an undertaking especially close to Kennedy's heart—channeled the idealism of individual Americans into face-to-face cooperation in the developing countries. Kennedy himself sought close relations with nationalist leaders, a course pursued with special success in black Africa.

There remained the problem of protecting the fragile democratization process against communist disruption—the problem spotlighted by Khrushchev's fervent espousal of national-liberation wars. The American view was that, the nuclear standoff having reduced the threat of general war, the great danger to world peace would come if local crises in the Third World led on to Soviet-American confrontation. To prevent this, it seemed necessary to persuade Moscow to abandon the national-liberation-war strategy. The search for ways of frustrating Soviet attempts to exploit insurgencies in the Third World became a Washington obsession.

The initial answer was thought to lie in teaching countries under attack the techniques of "counterinsurgency." On Kennedy's personal insistence, counterinsurgency doctrine was propounded, counterinsurgency schools were established, and elite counterinsurgency units, like the Green Berets, were organized. The theory was that counterinsurgency would operate within a context of social reform. But the political component did not take root, and the counterinsurgency mystique primarily nourished the American belief in the capacity and right to intervene in foreign lands. It brought out the worst in the over-confident activism of the New Frontier: the faith that American energy and technology could solve everything; the "when in doubt, do something" approach to policy; the officious pragmatism that could quickly degenerate into cynical manipulation.

Latin America: crisis and hope. It also provided a new outlet for the energies of the CIA. The potential conflict between the constructive and aggressive sides of Kennedy's Third World policy became manifest early in the new Administration. Kennedy had inherited from Eisenhower the force of anti-Castro Cubans trained and equipped by the CIA. Confronted with the choice of disbanding this group or permitting it to try an invasion of their homeland, Kennedy let the expedition go ahead.

On April 17, 1961, about twelve hundred Cubans landed at the Bahia de Cochinas (Bay of Pigs), on the southern coast of Cuba. The American hand could not be concealed. After three days the invasion collapsed. To the world, and to many Americans, the Bay of Pigs was an indefensible exercise in intervention. Refusing escalation, Kennedy spurned proposals that he send in the marines and took full responsibility for the fiasco, remarking wryly that victory had a hundred fathers but defeat was an orphan.

In the longer run, he pursued a policy directed toward Cuba's economic and diplomatic isolation. The CIA developed a program of covert action designed to encourage resistance and sabotage in Cuba. It even continued to plot the assassination of Castro, though with the usual non-success. Those in charge of this project did not disclose it to John McCone, who became CIA director after the Bay of Pigs, nor, so far as is known, to Kennedy himself. The CIA pin-pricks had little effect, except to irritate Castro, who continued to incite guerrilla action against democratic regimes in Latin America, especially Venezuela.

Kennedy's main reliance, however, was on the Alliance for Progress, a program designed to use United States aid to advance economic development and democratic reform through the hemisphere. "Those who make peaceful revolution impossible," Kennedy told the Latin American diplomatic corps, "will make violent revolution inevitable"; and the Alliance insisted, to the dismay of both North American business and Latin American oligarchies, on economic planning and structural change within a democratic framework. At a conference at Punta del Este, Uruguay, in August 1961 the Latin American states, except for Cuba, subscribed to the goals of the Alliance. Castro himself called the Alliance "a politically wise concept put forth to hold back the time of revolution . . . a very intelligent strategy."

The Alliance was accompanied by a determined effort to reinforce progressive democracy in Latin America. When an army coup nullified the results of a presidential election in Peru in 1962, Kennedy suspended relations until the military junta pledged new

Kennedy in Mexico City: a dramatic visit

elections. His dramatically successful visits to Venezuela, Colombia, Mexico, and Central America enabled the United States for a moment to recover its popularity of Good Neighbor days. No President since Roosevelt had shown such interest in the hemisphere.

Trouble in Southeast Asia. Another troubling inheritance was the crisis in Laos. Kennedy, who felt in general that the United States was "overcommitted" in Southeast Asia, felt in particular that neither superpower had enough at stake in Laos to justify armed confrontation. He consequently rejected Eisenhower's counsel of unilateral American military intervention. Instead he sought neutralization under the leadership of Prince Souvanna Phouma.

Khrushchev concurred at Vienna, and in 1962 the superpowers agreed on a neutralist coalition including representatives of the prowestern faction and of the communist Pathet Lao. True neutrality was not, however, achieved. North Vietnam continued to send men and supplies to the Viet Cong in South Vietnam via the Ho Chi Minh trails in southeastern Laos and maintained a military presence in Laos to protect the infiltration effort. In response, a CIA mission aided the Souvanna Phouma government. When Pathet Lao ministers withdrew from the coalition in 1963, the Pathet Lao insurgency resumed in the northeast. The result was *de facto* partition.

In South Vietnam, the situation appeared militarily more manageable. In the spring of 1961 Vice President Johnson, on a visit to Saigon, pronounced Diem the Churchill of South Asia; and said on his return, "We must decide whether to help these countries to the best of our ability or throw in the towel in the area and pull back our defenses to San Francisco." Kennedy sent a small force of Green Berets to instruct the South Vietnamese army in the black arts of counterinsurgency, thereby breaching the Geneva Accords of 1955 (see p. 803). Despite the great numerical superiority of the South Vietnamese forces—250,000 in November 1961 against 15,000 Viet Cong—the situation of the Saigon government grew worse. That same month a presidential mission, headed by General Maxwell Taylor, recommended the dispatch of an American combat force—perhaps 10,000 men—and urged air strikes against the "ultimate source of aggression" in North Vietnam.

Kennedy rejected these recommendations. Sending in troops, he remarked, was "like taking a drink. The effect wears off, and you have to take another." Nevertheless, while declining to commit American combat units, he feared that the "loss" of Vietnam would have adverse political consequences at home and abroad and accepted the theory that the assignment of American military "advisers" would stiffen South Vietnamese resistance. By 1962 American helicopters and personnel were taking a limited part in the fighting. At the same time, aware that lack of popular support was a central cause of Diem's difficulties, Kennedy urged the regime to enlarge its base by political and economic reform. Diem, profoundly authoritarian by temperament, disdained such advice.

Deeper into the quagmire. The Viet Cong continued to gain, and Buddhist protests against the Saigon government in the spring of 1963 demonstrated Diem's failure to unite his people. Diem's brother Ngo Dinh Nhu urged him on to further repression. Kennedy intensified pressure on Diem to get rid of his brother and reform his regime.

Henry Cabot Lodge, sent to Saigon in August as American ambassador to carry out this policy, was confronted by new outrages against the Buddhists. Dissident Vietnamese generals soon received assurance that, if there was a coup, a new regime would receive American support. In October, with Lodge's knowledge, the generals prepared for a coup. On November 1 they overthrew and murdered Diem and Nhu—whom Lodge had arranged to fly out of the country—and South Vietnam moved into a new phase of turmoil.

Kennedy never fully clarified his views on Vietnam. On the one hand, he accepted the domino theory; "for us to withdraw," he said in July 1963, ". . . would mean a collapse not only of South Vietnam but of Southeast Asia." While regarding the United States as overcommitted in Southeast Asia, Kennedy felt that, the commitment having been made, America could not let South Vietnam fall cheaply to the communists. He increased the number of American advisers to 16,732 by the end of 1963, though only 73 died in combat in these years.

On the other hand, his memory of the French failure a decade before convinced him that a "white man's war" would only rally Vietnamese nationalism against the alien presence. He rigorously opposed the dispatch of American combat units, American bombers, and any total commitment to the salvation of South Vietnam. "In the final analysis," he said of the people of South Vietnam in September 1963, "it is their war. They are the ones who have to win it or lose it. We can help them, we can give them equipment, we can send our men out there as advisers, but they have to win it, the people of Vietnam."

In July 1962 he had ordered the Pentagon to prepare a plan for American disengagement by the end of 1965. In October 1963 he announced the first troop withdrawal, enjoining his Secretary of Defense that this meant "all the helicopter pilots too." He confided to Mike Mansfield, the Senate majority leader, that his goal was total withdrawal; "but I can't do it until 1965—after I'm reelected." Still by failing to proclaim this intention, lest the prospect of an American pull-out undermine the Saigon government, and by enlarging the American role, Kennedy complicated the problems of subsequent disengagement. And his development of limited-war capabilities made large-scale military intervention possible.

From "massive retaliation" to "flexible response." Confronted by Khrushchev's Cold War of movement, Kennedy felt that the "massive retaliation" strategy of relying on nuclear weapons to deter local as well as general war increased the risk of nuclear holocaust. Secretary of Defense Robert S. McNamara, a professor turned industrial manager, therefore began the diversification of American military force so that the level of reaction could be graduated to meet the level of threat—a shift in strategic doctrine to "flexible response." This shift implied an increase in the American capability for conventional war. It was designed primarily to enable the West to respond to Soviet aggression in Europe without immediate resort to nuclear weapons. The fateful side-effect was to create forces that could be used in limited "brushfire" wars elsewhere in the world.

Moreover, Kennedy was imprisoned by the "missile gap" illusion he had himself expounded during his campaign. He therefore yielded to Pentagon pressure and in the spring of 1961 requested not only more conventional force but more long-range nuclear missiles. When new reconnaissance satellites disproved the "missile gap," the American buildup was already under way.

The buildup had baleful consequences. It was more than American security demanded; it ended any hope of freezing the rival missile forces at lower levels; and it sent the wrong message to Moscow, compelling Khrushchev to worry about his own missile gap. In September 1961 the Soviet Union began an extensive series of tests in the atmosphere, exploding in October a device nearly three thousand times more powerful than the bomb dropped on Hiroshima.

The Kennedy-McNamara hope was to achieve a "stable balance of terror" by moving toward a situation in which both superpowers would have sufficient deterrent strength to absorb a surprise first strike and retain the ability to retaliate. Rejecting proposals that the United States aim for a first-strike capability, McNamara argued that overwhelming superiority on one side might tempt the other to launch a preemptive strike in a time of crisis. The best way to avoid nuclear war, he contended, was for each superpower to have a "secure second-strike capability"—an idea he hoped to persuade the Russians to accept, thereby introducing rationality and limitation into the arms race. This was the doctrine of "mutual assured destruction" (whose acronym MAD gave great pleasure to its opponents). Privately McNamara recommended to Kennedy and later to Lyndon Johnson that "they never initiate, under any circumstances, the use of nuclear weapons. I believe they accepted my recommendations." Unlike Eisenhower, neither Kennedy nor Johnson ever threatened non-retaliatory nuclear strikes.

For the longer run, Kennedy wanted to stop the arms race altogether. Speaking before the United Nations in 1961, he presented a plan for general and complete disarmament. "The risks inherent in disarmament," he said, "pale in comparison to the risks inherent in an unlimited arms race. . . . Mankind must put an end to war—or war will put an end to mankind." The appeal fell on deaf ears. With reluctance, Kennedy himself resumed atmospheric testing in April 1962. So the two superpowers, still in the lockstep of the Cold War, proceeded to intensify the arms race.

Kennedy and Khrushchev. The Vienna meeting in June 1961 had not been a success. Perhaps misled by the Bay of Pigs into seeing Kennedy as irresolute, Khrushchev brusquely rejected Kennedy's proposal of a global standstill and adopted an intransigent, even bullying, attitude on most questions.

For Moscow, Germany remained a critical issue, the more so because of the rising flow of refugees—now thirty thousand a month—from East Germany into West Berlin. Khrushchev told Kennedy that he planned to conclude with East Germany a peace treaty that would extinguish western rights in West Berlin. Kennedy replied that so drastic an alteration in the world balance of power was unacceptable. Khrushchev said, if America wanted war over Berlin, there was nothing the Soviet Union could do about it; he would sign the treaty by December 31. Kennedy commented, "It will be a cold winter."

Returning to the United States, Kennedy requested a further increase in the defense budget, called out 150,000 reservists, and announced a program, which set off an ugly outburst of near-panic and which he soon regretted, of fallout shelters for protection against nuclear attack. Though these measures, especially the last, soon came to seem an overreaction, all of them, including the last, may have persuaded Khrushchev that he could not solve the Berlin question by intimidation. In addition, Kennedy, acknowledging Russia's security interests in eastern Europe, declared his readiness to work out arrangements "to meet these concerns." On August 13 the East Germans erected the Berlin Wall, thereby stopping the

Soviet missiles in Cuba

refugee flow. Khrushchev postponed his treaty deadline in October; and the Berlin crisis, for a moment so frightening to the world, subsided.

In western Europe, Kennedy hoped for steady movement toward unification, particularly through the admission of Great Britain to the European Economic Community (see p. 769). To this end, he secured the passage in September 1962 of the Trade Expansion Act, creating authority to negotiate tariff reductions up to 50 percent for the purpose of bargaining with an enlarged Common Market. But Kennedy's so-called grand design for Europe was frustrated by President de Gaulle's veto of British membership—an action that deferred British entry until 1972. In the meantime, the "Kennedy Round" of tariff negotiations led to significant reductions of barriers to world trade.

The missile crisis. Khrushchev by no means abandoned his goal of driving the West out of Berlin. In the summer of 1962, carrying his Cold War of movement to its ultimate audacity, he decided, over Castro's initial objection, to establish nuclear missile bases in Cuba. The Russians had never before placed their missiles in any other country. If successful, the operations would not only protect Cuba from American

invasion—the objective later alleged by Khrushchev (though this could have been more simply achieved by stationing Soviet troops on the island)—but would give Russia a potent bargaining counter when it chose to reopen the Berlin question. Moreover, by making shorter-range missiles effective against American targets, it would increase Soviet nuclear first-strike capacity against American targets by half. And it would deal America a shattering political blow by showing the Soviet capacity to penetrate the American sphere of influence. "Our missiles," Khrushchev later declared in his memoirs, "would have equalized . . . 'the balance of power.'"

Washington had not objected to Russian supply of defensive weapons to Cuba; but Kennedy warned in September 1962 that, if there was evidence of "significant offensive capability either in Cuban hands or under Soviet direction . . . the gravest issues would arise." Khrushchev repeatedly denied publicly and privately that he had any such intention. Nor did Washington consider such recklessness likely. Then, on October 14, a U-2 overflight found conclusive evidence that Khrushchev had lied.

Kennedy's decision was that, one way or another, the Soviet nuclear missiles had to be removed from Cuba. Critics have suggested that he should have accepted them without protest. After all the Americans had their Jupiter missiles in Turkey. Moreover, the United States would still retain nuclear superiority even after the Cuban buildup. But Kennedy regarded Soviet missile bases in Cuba as "a deliberately provocative and unjustified change in the status quo." If the United States were to accept so gross an intrusion into what the Russians, themselves so preternaturally sensitive to spheres of interest, had previously respected as the American zone, this, he feared, might embolden Khrushchev to acts that would make the third world war inescapable.

For six days Kennedy and a small group of advisers debated behind locked doors how best to get the missiles out. One faction, led by Dean Acheson and the Joint Chiefs of Staff, advocated the destruction of the bases by surprise air attack. The other, led by Attorney General Robert F. Kennedy, the President's brother, and Secretary of Defense McNamara, sharply opposed this course on moral grounds—as a Pearl Harbor in reverse against a small country—and on practical grounds—because it might kill Russians at the missile sites and force the Soviet Union into drastic retaliation. Naval blockade, this group argued, would both show the American determination to get the missiles out and allow Moscow time to pull back. Kennedy announced his course in the first public disclosure of the crisis on October 22—to establish a naval quarantine against further shipments; to demand the dismantling of the bases and the removal of the missiles; and to warn that any nuclear attack launched from Cuba would be regarded "as an attack by the Soviet Union on the United States, requiring a full retaliatory response upon the Soviet Union."

The days that followed were more tense than any since the Second World War. Moscow continued to deny the presence of nuclear weapons until, in a dramatic moment before the United Nations, Ambassador Adlai Stevenson confronted the Soviet delegate with blown-up aerial photographs of the nuclear installations. Meanwhile work was continuing day and night to make the bases operational. An American invasion force was massing in Florida. Soviet ships, presumably carrying more missiles, were drawing near the island. Kennedy kept the interception line close to Cuba to give Khrushchev maximum time for reflection. Finally, after indescribable suspense, Soviet ships began to turn back. "We're eyeball to eyeball," said Dean Rusk, "and I think the other fellow just blinked."

It remained for negotiation to complete the resolution of the crisis. On October 26 Kennedy received a long, passionate letter from Khrushchev dilating on the horror of nuclear war and offering to remove the missiles and send no more if the United States would end the quarantine and agree not to invade Cuba. But on the following morning there arrived a second letter from Khrushchev, harder in tone and proposing an entirely different trade: the Soviet missiles in Cuba for the American missiles in Turkey; a Soviet guarantee of Turkish integrity for an American guarantee of Cuban integrity. Robert Kennedy now recommended that his brother ignore the second letter and respond to the first. The President followed this advice. Robert Kennedy took the American restatement of the first Khrushchev proposal to the Soviet ambassador, who then asked about the Turkish missiles. The Attorney General replied that, while this could be no *quid pro quo*, "it was our judgment that, within a short time after this crisis was over, those missiles would be gone." The next day, October 28, a favorable reply came from Khrushchev.

Khrushchev's bluff had failed. In short order the bases were dismantled and the missiles on their way home. Castro's resistance, however, made it impossible to establish the UN inspection to which Khrushchev had agreed, and the United States never formally completed the reciprocal pledge not to invade Cuba. But in substance the deal went into effect anyway. U-2 overflights, which the Russian antiaircraft batteries made no attempt to stop, took the place of UN inspection; the Jupiter missiles left Turkey; and the United States, which had no intention of invading Cuba in any case, soon ended hit-and-run raids by Cuban refugees from American territory. In the autumn of 1963 Kennedy initiated secret explorations looking toward a normalization of relations with Cuba.

Détente: 1963. The American success—Kennedy forbade gloating and refused to claim a triumph—was the result of Kennedy's combination of toughness and restraint and of his careful deployment of power. He hoped he had made to Khrushchev the point he had tried to make in Vienna—that neither side dare tamper carelessly with the complex and explosive international equilibrium.

The missile crisis, by forcing both Kennedy and Khrushchev to stare down the nuclear abyss, now brought them into *de facto* alliance against their own national security bureaucracies. "One of the ironic things," Kennedy observed, ". . . is that Mr. Khrushchev and I occupy approximately the same political positions inside our governments. He would like to prevent a nuclear war but is under severe pressure from his hard-line crowd, which interprets every move in that direction as appeasement. I've got similar problems. . . . The hard-liners in the Soviet Union and the United States feed on one another."

Kennedy now renewed his quest for a test-ban treaty. "I am haunted," he said in March 1963, "by the feeling that by 1970, unless we are successful, there may be ten nuclear powers instead of four, and by 1975 fifteen or twenty." Negotiations bogged down during the spring. In an effort to break the deadlock, Kennedy, in his notable speech at American University in June 1963, called on Americans as well as Russians to rethink the Cold War: "We must reexamine our own attitude—as individuals and as a Nation—for our attitude is as essential as theirs." He rejected the "holy war" ideology: "No government or social system is so evil that its people must be considered as lacking in virtue." Both sides, he said, were "caught up in a vicious and dangerous cycle in which suspicion on one side breeds suspicion on the other, and new weapons beget counterweapons."

The establishment in June 1963 of the "Hot Line," a direct teletype link between the White House and the Kremlin, was a significant attempt to break the cycle by reducing the risk of conflict through misunderstanding or miscalculation. Kennedy's next hope was for a ban on all nuclear testing. But the Joint Chiefs of Staff claimed that a ban on underground tests could not be verified without at least 7 annual on-site inspections of earth shocks. The Russians would not accept more than 3. Kennedy would have compromised at 5, but he feared that military opposition would doom the treaty in the Senate. In July the United States, the Soviet Union, and Britain agreed in Moscow to a limited ban, outlawing tests in self-policing environments—in the atmosphere, in outer space, and under water. "Yesterday a shaft of light," Kennedy said, "cut into the darkness." The Joint Chiefs conditioned support for the treaty on continuation of underground testing. With this proviso, the Senate ratified the treaty in September by a vote of 80–19. The failure to achieve a comprehensive test ban lost a great opportunity to stop the development of ever more appalling weapons. Still the partial test ban, though France and China declined to sign, represented the most significant formal step toward arms control since the onset of the Cold War.

Space. The competition between the superpowers produced at least one benign by-product. In April 1961 the Russians put the first man, Yuri Gagarin, into space orbit. On May 25, 1961, Kennedy declared that the United States "should commit itself to achieving the goal, before this decade is out, of landing a man on the moon and returning him safely to earth." The idea was greeted with disapproval by those who thought the money should be spent in meeting human needs on earth and with skepticism by those who doubted whether the project was feasible.

Nonetheless, Kennedy pushed ahead. In February 1962 John Glenn became the first American to enter space orbit; and National Aeronautic and Space Administration (NASA) scientists in the Apollo program were already hard at work breaking down the

Apollo 11: man on the moon

technical problems of a moonshot. Six months before the deadline, on July 16, 1969, the moonship *Apollo* 11 was launched from Cape Kennedy, Florida. On July 20 Captain Neil A. Armstrong became the first man to walk on the moon.

Beating Russia to the moon was not Kennedy's main interest. Indeed, he suggested at Vienna in 1961 and again at the UN in 1963 that the Americans and the Russians go to the moon together. He was responding rather to the newest of new frontiers, to the ultimate challenge and mystery of space itself. "Why, some say, the moon? . . . The great British explorer George Mallory, who was to die on Mount Everest, was asked why did he want to climb it, and he said, 'Because it is there.' Well, space is there, and . . . the moon and planets are there, and new hopes for knowledge and peace are there." Kennedy's sense of history was surely right. When all else about the twentieth century is forgotten, it may still be remembered as the century when man first burst his terrestrial bonds and began the endless voyage, beyond planet and galaxy, into the illimitable dark.

The New Frontier. Kennedy's campaign appeal in 1960 had been to get the country moving again. He meant this in a large sense, hoping to lead an intellectual breakaway from the stagnation of the Eisenhower years. He meant it too in an immediate economic sense. Inheriting 7 percent unemployment from his predecessor, he responded with a set of expansionist policies: an investment tax credit, liberalization of tax depreciation allowances, worker training programs, and finally general tax reduction, enacted in 1964. During the Kennedy years economic growth averaged 5.6 percent, and unemployment was brought down to 5.7 percent.

Inflation was meanwhile held at 1.3 percent, in part because of "wage-price guideposts" designed to keep wage increases within the limits of advances in productivity. This early form of what came later to be known as "incomes policy" rested on the perception that increased productivity was the only way to increase wages without increasing prices. United States Steel's cavalier rejection of the guideposts led to the steel battle of 1962. When U.S. Steel raised its prices after the Administration had persuaded the union to accept a noninflationary wage contract, Kennedy exploded in cold anger—"My father always told me that all businessmen were sons-of-bitches, but I never believed it till now"—and forced the corporation to retract its action.

While general fiscal stimulus increased aggregate output and employment, it did not reach into pockets of localized and "structural" poverty. Income tax reduction, for example, was of little help for people too poor to pay income taxes. In 1960 one out of every five Americans was living in poverty (as officially defined). Kennedy recognized that the poor of the sixties, unlike the ambitious immigrants of the nineties or the angry unemployed of the thirties, were largely a demoralized and inarticulate minority who in many cases had inherited their poverty and accepted it as a permanent condition. He attacked the "culture of poverty" through the Area Redevelopment Act of 1961 and through programs directed at Appalachia, an eleven-state region stretching from Pennsylvania to Alabama and centering in eastern Kentucky and West Virginia. In 1963 he decided that, if the forgotten Americans were to be helped, tax reduction required a counterpart in the form of a comprehensive war on poverty.

Kennedy was more successful in economic management than in social reform. Elected by an exceptionally narrow popular margin, he was confronted in Congress by the powerful coalition of Republicans and Southern Democrats that had dominated domestic policy since 1938. He could do some things, like government support of the arts, through executive orders; but major proposals—federal aid to education,

medical care for the aged (Medicare), a Department of Urban Affairs—required statutes and were blocked by the conservative coalition. Kennedy instead dramatized his proposals through presidential messages and speeches, thereby pressing the process of public education that, he expected, would assure enactment in his second term.

The black revolution. Kennedy's most signal domestic achievement lay in the field of racial justice. Congressional opposition compelled him to concentrate at first on executive rather than legislative action. Challenged by "freedom riders" defying Jim Crow in interstate bus terminals, Attorney General Robert Kennedy found ways to end segregation in interstate transportation. In October 1962 the President sent federal troops into Oxford, Mississippi in order to protect James Meredith, a black student, in the right, assured him by the courts, to attend the University of Mississippi. The Administration worked to secure blacks the right to vote and appointed an unprecedented number to higher office.

But Kennedy still underestimated the moral dynamism of the civil-rights cause. "This Administration," said Martin Luther King, Jr., "has outstripped all previous ones in the breadth of its civil rights activity. Yet the movement, instead of breaking out into the open plains of progress, remains constricted and confined." To the left of King's Southern Christian Leadership Conference rose more militant organizations—the Congress of Racial Equality (CORE) and the Student Nonviolent Coordinating Committee (SNCC). As black discontent grew, so too did Southern resistance. In April 1963, when King began a campaign to end discrimination in shops, restaurants, and

Washington, D.C., 1963: "I have a dream"

employment in Birmingham, Alabama, Police Commissioner Eugene "Bull" Connor harassed King's marchers with firehoses, electric cattle prods, and growling police dogs.

The Birmingham episode caused a surge of indignation throughout the nation. Then, in June, Governor George Wallace of Alabama personally tried to block the admission of two black students to the state university, but he folded under federal pressure. That night Kennedy went on television to pronounce the civil-rights question "a moral issue . . . as old as the scriptures and . . . as clear as the American Constitution," and to commit the nation to the proposition "that race has no place in American life or law." With this speech he launched a fight for new and more sweeping civil-rights legislation.

In August Dr. King led a quarter of a million people, black and white, on a great march in front of the Lincoln Memorial in Washington, where they listened to King's moving eloquence ("I have a dream") and sang the old Baptist hymn the civil-rights movement had made its own, "We Shall Overcome." "In the process of gaining our rightful place," King said at the Lincoln Memorial, "we must not be guilty of wrongful deeds. Let us not seek to satisfy our thirst for freedom by drinking from the cup of bitterness and hatred."

But in the same year black novelist James Baldwin, in his bitter warning to white America, *The Fire Next Time*, wrote that the black American "no longer believes in the good faith of white Americans."

Kennedy and America. On November 22, 1963, while riding with his wife in an open car through Dallas, Texas, Kennedy was shot and killed. His murder sent a wave of incredulity, shame, and grief across the United States and around the planet.

In the next decades his place in history became a subject of contention. Revisionists portrayed him as a rigid and embattled Cold Warrior; Khrushchev disagreed, writing that Kennedy "understood better than Eisenhower that an improvement in relations was the only rational course." Some dismissed his leadership in domestic affairs as too much style and too little substance; others, noting his narrow margins in Congress, valued the educational impact of his dramatization of major issues.

On balance it may be said that Kennedy inherited tough problems at home and abroad and had little enough time and parliamentary leverage to do as much about them as he keenly wished. His brief days in the White House were days of steady growth. He made mistakes but candidly acknowledged them and always learned from them. He had confidence in human reason and hope for human nature. His contagious optimism gave his countrymen the sense that,

with sufficient intelligence, steadfastness, and good will, the nation could meet its responsibilities. His directness and openness of mind, his faith in reasoned discussion, his ironic, often self-mocking, wit, and his generous vision of American possibility broke the crust that had settled over the country in the 1950s. His irreverence toward conventional ideas and institutions provoked a discharge of critical energy throughout American society reminiscent of the Progressive period and the New Deal. He came to be loved in the black community and was the only President since Roosevelt with anything to say to the young. In other lands he was seen as a carrier of American idealism and a friend of humanity. For a moment he made politics seem in truth (in a phrase he cherished from John Buchan's *Pilgrim's Way*) "the greatest and most honorable adventure."

Kennedy's funeral: a wave of grief and shame

The Johnson Years

The Great Society. The Presidency now descended to a political leader of an older generation, Lyndon Baines Johnson. A Texan, fifty-five years old, Johnson had come to the Vice Presidency from twenty-three years in Congress, ending as Democratic leader of the Senate. No President since Polk had had such impressive legislative experience. He was also the first President from a Southern state since Andrew Johnson a century before. A New Dealer who had become more conservative in his middle years, he retained an authentic concern for the poor and, though a Southerner, for black America. His admirers rejoiced in the power of his formidable personality, the sincerity of his social concern, and the resourcefulness with which he pursued his purposes; others found him egotistical, secretive, devious, and vindictive.

In the national shock after Dallas the new President took over his responsibilities with firmness and strength. He appointed a commission under Chief Justice Warren to investigate the assassination. The commission reported in 1964 that the murderer was a rootless and embittered former communist named Lee Harvey Oswald. Critics later challenged both the commission's procedures and its conclusions.

Johnson made clear his determination to continue his predecessor's policies and (unlike Truman in 1945) his predecessor's Cabinet. His experience and inclination led him toward the field of domestic affairs. Both tax-reduction and civil-rights bills were on their way to enactment at the time of Kennedy's death, and the rush of national remorse assured them quick passage. The tax cut, injecting $12 billion into the economy, speeded economic growth. The Civil Rights Act of 1964 prohibited discrimination in the use of federal funds and in places of public accommodation and established an Equal Employment Opportunity Commission.

Seeking a distinctive name for his domestic program, Johnson in May 1964 called for a Great Society—"a place where the city of man serves not only the needs of the body and the demands of commerce but the desire for beauty and the hunger for community." The Great Society incorporated and soon extended Kennedy's New Frontier, especially with the passage of the Economic Opportunity Act of 1964, which carried into legislation Kennedy's vision of a war on poverty.

The election of 1964

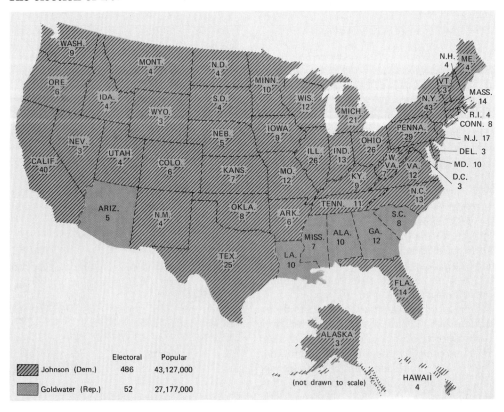

	Electoral	Popular
Johnson (Dem.)	486	43,127,000
Goldwater (Rep.)	52	27,177,000

The Great Society provided the central issue of the 1964 presidential campaign. Johnson selected the veteran liberal Senator Hubert Humphrey of Minnesota as his running mate. The Republicans nominated Senator Barry Goldwater of Arizona, a likable businessman with inflexibly conservative views. Convinced that the danger to freedom came from government, Goldwater had proposed in *The Conscience of a Conservative* (1960) that the graduated income tax be abolished. He also urged the sale of the TVA, questioned the social-security system, and advocated the bombing of North Vietnam. Though Goldwater's personal dash and his campaign slogan—"In your heart you know he's right"—evoked passionate enthusiasm among his followers, many voters were disturbed by the spirit that led him, in accepting the Republican nomination, to proclaim: "Extremism in the defense of liberty is no vice."

The Johnson-Humphrey ticket won 61.1 percent of the popular vote and carried all but six states—the most decisive presidential triumph since 1936. Victory brought thirty-seven Northern Democrats to the House of Representatives—enough to assure, for the first time since 1938, a working progressive majority. This enabled Johnson in 1965–66 to compile the most impressive record of domestic legislation in a single session for thirty years.

Long-sought bills for federal aid to education and for medical care to the old (Medicare) and to the poor (Medicaid) were at last enacted. Responding belatedly to the crisis of the cities, Congress passed low-income housing laws, a rent-supplement program, and the Model Cities Act, under which federal block grants encouraged cities to plan their own future. The Voting Rights Act of 1965 outlawed remaining barriers to the right to vote and empowered the national government to register those whom the states refused to put on the voting list. In an executive order of September 24, 1965, Johnson instituted the "affirmative action" policy, requiring federal contractors and institutions receiving federal assistance to make special efforts to employ women and non-whites. Congress also liberalized the immigration laws, abolishing the national origins quota of 1924; institutionalized Kennedy's experiments in federal support for the arts in the National Foundation on the Arts and Humanities Act; established public broadcasting; gave the government authority to set safety standards for automobiles and highways; and created two new federal departments—Housing and Urban Development (to which Johnson appointed Robert C. Weaver, the first black to serve in the Cabinet) and Transportation.

Among Great Society programs the most original was the war on poverty, conducted by the Office of Economic Opportunity. Headed by Sargent Shriver, Kennedy's brother-in-law and former head of the Peace Corps, OEO included a Job Corps for dropouts from the educational system; a Neighborhood Youth Corps for unemployed teenagers; the Volunteers in Service to America (VISTA), in effect a domestic Peace Corps; a Head Start program for young children; an Upward Bound program to send bright children to college; and, in its most controversial feature, a Community Action program designed to secure the "maximum feasible participation" of the poor in planning and running the antipoverty effort. A venture so unprecedented could not avoid experiment and confusion. Local politicians particularly saw Community

Action as a threat to their own prerogatives, and other critics felt that OEO gave professionals in the social-welfare field undue opportunity to impose their own ideas on the helpless poor.

Between 1964 and 1970 federal spending for health, education, welfare services, and income maintenance tripled. One signficant result was to alter the composition of the federal budget. The "defense shift" of 1948–53 had created a pattern by which government spending held at about 28 to 29 percent of the gross national product, nondefense spending at about 15 percent, and defense spending at about 9 to 10 percent. With the "welfare shift" of the sixties total government spending rose to about 33 percent of the gross national product, with nondefense spending rising to about 25 percent and defense spending declining to about 6 to 7 percent.

Much of the "welfare shift" benefited people over sixty-five, especially through social security and Medicare. Only a small share went to experimental Great Society programs that, oversold and underfunded, were perhaps too readily dismissed as failures. The reform effort produced no significant change in the distribution of income. But the number of Americans below the poverty line declined by nearly half in the ten years after 1959, and the poor, the old, and the blacks were better off. Though much criticized in later years, Johnson's Great Society represented the culmination of New Deal liberalism in its effort to reverse patterns of privation and inequality in American economic life.

Foreign policy: Latin America.

As time went on, however, Johnson's increasing absorption in foreign affairs diverted his attention from domestic problems. Abroad as at home Johnson initially promised to continue Kennedy's policies. But in foreign policy he quickly introduced modifications. Latin American policy was soon reshaped to make it more acceptable both to North American business and to right-wing governments south of the border. While continuing economic assistance, Johnson liquidated the two distinctive goals of the Alliance for Progress—structural change and political democratization. Thus Washington welcomed the military coup that established military dictatorship in Brazil in 1964.

The reversion to older ways received its most spectacular expression in Johnson's response to civil war in the Dominican Republic in 1965. Claiming that a popular revolution against a conservative regime had been taken over by "a band of communist conspirators," Johnson, without consulting the Organization of American States, sent 22,289 marines to the Dominican Republic. The size, the unilateral character, and the impetuosity of American intervention revived in Latin America the mistrust that Roosevelt's Good Neighbor policy and Kennedy's Alliance for Progress had striven to dispel.

Vietnam: the war Americanized.

The most intractable item in Johnson's inheritance was the war in Indochina. For the public, Vietnam was still a marginal issue. Johnson barely mentioned it in his January 1964 state-of-the-union address and gave it little more than a hundred words a year later. This lack of public emphasis, however, was due less to presidential indifference than to a desire to manage the situation without congressional interference.

For the overthrow of Diem had failed to bring stability. Concerned over the growing strength of the Viet Cong, now presumed to number nearly one hundred thousand, Johnson cancelled Kennedy's disengagement plan and laid on the "A-34" program of clandestine hit-and-run military operations against North Vietnam. When South Vietnamese commandoes under A-34 raided two islands in the Gulf of Tonkin at the end of July, North Vietnamese PT boats, pursuing the raiders, encountered the destroyer *Maddox* on electronic intelligence patrol and fired on it on August 2. Two days later another American destroyer was reported under attack in the gulf. Though subsequent investigations raised the greatest doubt about the second report, the Administration ordered retaliatory air strikes against North Vietnamese targets, and sent Congress the Southeast Asia resolution authorizing the President to "take all necessary steps, including the use of armed force" to assist South Vietnam and prevent aggression. To popular applause the Senate passed the Tonkin Gulf resolution, as it was promptly known, by a vote of 88 to 2, the House by 416 to 0.

In the presidential campaign Johnson condemned Goldwater for his advocacy of escalation. But early in 1965 Washington was persuaded that South Vietnam was on the verge of collapse. Something, it was felt, had to be done to save the situation; and a Viet Cong mortar attack killing American advisers at Pleiku in February provided a pretext. Johnson instantly ordered reprisal bombing against northern targets. This in March swelled into the Rolling Thunder campaign of systematic air war against North Vietnam. In April he threw American combat units, for the first time, into offensive action.

Up to this point, Hanoi's main role had been to infiltrate men into South Vietnam—4,400 to 7,400 in 1964, according to American estimates, and mostly native southerners. Now, in response to American escalation, units of the North Vietnamese regular army began for the first time to appear in South Vietnam. In June General William C. Westmoreland, the American commander in Saigon, requested the dispatch of 200,000 American troops. Johnson replied: "We will meet his needs." With the sending of American bombers into North Vietnam and American combat units into South Vietnam, the Indochina War entered a new and fatal phase. By the end of 1965 there were 184,300 American troops in Vietnam.

The Johnson rationale. The immediate reason for the Americanization of the war was to restore morale in Saigon by displaying American determination to stay the course. A second reason was the hope that bombing would break the will of the North Vietnamese and induce them to order the National Liberation Front to call off the war. Though the experience of the Second World War and of Korea had demonstrated the limitations of strategic bombing, Johnson simply could not conceive that, if pounded long enough, North Vietnam would not have a breaking-point. Some historians argue that the consistent American objective for twenty-five years was to prevent a communist takeover of South Vietnam, not to achieve military victory. While this was true much of the time, Johnson was undoubtedly sincere in his confidence that, if American power were applied, the problem could be solved. In this spirit he exhorted the troops to "nail that coonskin to the wall."

He further believed that bombing, if it could not altogether stop infiltration into South Vietnam, would at least make the cost prohibitive. Since most infiltration took place along the Ho Chi Minh trail network, American planes began in 1964 to carry out bombing missions against North Vietnamese units in Laos, where the CIA had already organized an army of Meo tribesmen to prevent the Pathet Lao and the North Vietnamese from overrunning the Plaine des Jarres. A secret war in Laos thus developed alongside the open war in Vietnam.

The larger reason for the Americanization of the war lay in the assumption, inherited from previous Administrations and not reexamined now, that the defense of South Vietnam from communist takeover was vital to the security of the United States. Johnson felt that concessions to communism in Indochina would encourage communist aggression first in South Asia and eventually all along the frontiers of freedom. "Ike has made a promise," he would say. "I have to keep it." Keeping American commitments in Vietnam thus became a test of American will and credibility everywhere. "We learned from Hitler at Munich," said Johnson, "that success only feeds the appetite of aggression. . . . To withdraw from one battlefield means only to prepare for the next."

Since it was hard to see in Ho Chi Minh and North Vietnam a threat comparable to that presented by Hitler at Munich, the Administration contended that the "free world" was confronted by a premeditated plan of Chinese expansion, of which the NLF and North Vietnam were only the spearhead. "Over this war, and all Asia," said Johnson, "is another reality: the deepening shadow of Communist China. . . . The contest in Vietnam is part of a wider pattern of aggressive purpose." Vice President Humphrey added in 1967, "The threat to world peace is militant, aggressive Asian communism, with its headquarters in Peking, China."

The American effort also had a positive goal. The experience of military occupation after the Second World War had given Americans undue faith in their talent for "nation-building." Johnson, the old New Dealer, talked about TVAs on the Mekong. Humphrey saw "a tremendous opening here for realizing the dream of the Great Society in the great area of Asia, not just here at home." Social evangelism thus provided further justification for the American adventure.

Nor did Johnson see the war as reason for hostility toward the Soviet Union; rather, he believed that, if the problem of national-liberation wars could be solved in Vietnam, relations with the Soviet Union would be stabilized. In October 1964 Khrushchev had been replaced by the collective leadership of L. I. Brezhnev (who in time became the dominant partner) and A. N. Kosygin. Johnson, seeking to thaw the Cold War, announced a policy of "bridge-building" to eastern Europe. In 1966 he joined with the Soviet Union in supporting a UN treaty providing for the peaceful uses of outer space. In 1967 he secured the ratification of a consular convention with Russia and met with Kosygin in Glassboro, New Jersey. In 1968 he concluded with Russia and fifty other nations a treaty on the nonproliferation of nuclear weapons.

"Hawks" and "doves." Despite an endless series of optimistic assurances from General Westmoreland, the Americanization of the war did not produce the expected results. The number of American troops steadily grew—385,300 by the end of 1966; 485,600 by the end of 1967; 538,300 by the end of 1968—but Westmoreland's "meatgrinder" strategy of victory through "attrition" made no progress against the capacity of the NLF and the North Vietnamese, benefiting from the 10 to 1 ratio of guerrilla war, to replenish their losses and match every escalation. In the mean-

time, American casualties also grew: deaths in combat rose from 1,369 in 1965 to 5,008 in 1966, 9,378 in 1967, and 14,592 in 1968.

The bombing increased too. By the end of 1968 American planes had dropped 3.2 million tons of explosives on this hapless land (as against a total of 2 million tons on all fronts in the Second World War and 635,000 tons in the Korean War). The result was a country gutted and devastated by bombs, burned by napalm, turned into a wasteland by chemical defoliation, a land of ruin and wreck. "It became necessary to destroy the town to save it," said an American major standing in the rubble of Ben Tre; and for more and more Americans this summed up the ghastly logic of the American intervention. The technological war was too gross to cope with guerrilla warfare: it was like trying to weed a garden with a bulldozer. Bombing failed to stop the movement of troops and supplies; instead of breaking the spirit of the enemy, it succeeded, if anything, in hardening Hanoi's will. In August 1967, McNamara, who had developed grave doubts about the war and had become the main proponent of negotiation within the Administration, told the Senate Armed Services Committee that air power had failed.

Johnson nevertheless escalated the bombing, though never enough to suit the Joint Chiefs of Staff. Fearing that too drastic action might bring China into the war, Johnson also imposed political restrictions on military tactics. Negotiating efforts punctuated the process of escalation, most notably during the thirty-seven-day bombing pause of December 1964–January 1965. American proposals always included the preservation of the Saigon regime and the withdrawal of North Vietnamese forces prior to American withdrawal. From the viewpoint of Hanoi and the National Liberation Front, such terms meant defeat.

Within the United States escalation received enthusiastic support from "hawks" in Congress and the country. But, as the national debate intensified, "doves" spoke out with increasing passion. In the Senate, doubts about the war found effective lodgment in the Foreign Relations Committee, whose chairman, J. William Fulbright, became a caustic and increasingly influential critic. Soon Robert Kennedy, now senator from New York, added a powerful voice. In February 1966 Kennedy proposed that the NLF be admitted "to a share of power and responsibility" in a coalition government as the only way to end the war. Vice President Humphrey replied that this would be like putting "a fox in the chicken coop; soon there wouldn't be any chickens left"; and the debate sharpened. As dove senators, joined by foreign-policy experts like Walter Lippmann, George F. Kennan, and Hans Morgenthau, enlarged the attack on the war, Johnson denounced the opposition as "nervous Nellies" ready to "turn on their own leaders, and their country, and on our fighting men."

In the spring of 1967 Lippmann wrote that the Indochina War had become "the most unpopular war in American history." Antiwar protests exploded in major cities, culminating on October 21, 1967, when 200,000 people led by noted literary figures like Nor-

man Mailer and Robert Lowell marched on the Pentagon. Johnson himself could no longer appear safely in public, except on military installations. Though the campuses had generally supported escalation, the restriction of educational deferments early in 1968 confronted college students with the reality of the war. "L.B.J., L.B.J.," students chanted, "How Many Kids Did You Kill Today?" Never before in American history were so many young men declaring conscientious objection, burning draft cards, or fleeing abroad to avoid military service. "Hell No, We Won't Go." Many more, accepting what they saw as their democratic obligation, brought antiwar convictions with them into the army. Middle-class parents, oblivious as long as the war swept up only poor whites and poor blacks, began to wonder whether Vietnam was worth the sacrifice of their own sons.

Johnson's domestic hopes were a casualty of his increasing absorption in Vietnam. The mounting cost of the war argued against expansion of domestic programs. The very phrase Great Society disappeared from the President's lexicon.

A Decade of Upheaval

Women in revolt. The antiwar agitation was only one expression of a volatile and passionate time. The social criticism of the Kennedy years and the example of the civil-rights movement had stimulated a mood of

The new feminism

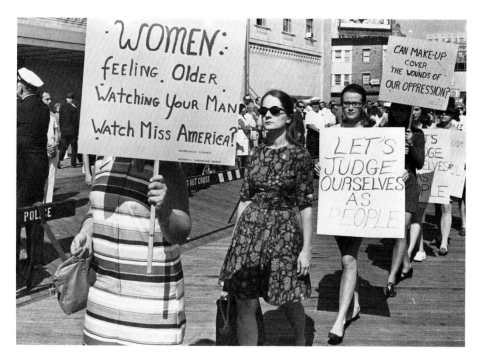

The American always ostentatiously ignored sex, and American history mentioned hardly the name of a woman.... American art, like the American language and American education, was as far as possible sexless.... [Yet] in every city, town, and farm-house were myriads of new types—or type-writers—telephone and telegraph-girls, shop-clerks, factory-hands, running into millions on millions, and, as classes, unknown to themselves as to historians.... All these new women had been created since 1840; all were to show their meaning before 1940.

The Education of Henry Adams (1918).

We, men, and women who hereby constitute ourselves as the National Organization for Women, believe that the time has come for a new movement toward true equality for all women in America, and toward a fully equal partnership of the sexes, as part of the world-wide revolution of human rights now taking place within and beyond our national borders....

WE REJECT the current assumption that a man must carry the sole burden of supporting himself, his wife, and family, and that a woman is automatically entitled to lifelong support by a man upon her marriage, or that marriage, home and family are primarily woman's world and responsibility—hers, to dominate—his to support. We believe that a true partnership between the sexes demands a different concept of marriage, an equitable sharing of the responsibilities of home and children and of the economic burdens of their support....

IN THE INTERESTS OF THE HUMAN DIGNITY OF WOMEN, we will protest, and endeavor to change, the false image of women now prevalent in the mass media, and in the texts, ceremonies, laws, and practices of the major social institutions. Such images perpetuate contempt for women by society and by women for themselves.... WE BELIEVE THAT women will do most to create a new image of women by acting now, and by speaking out in behalf of their own equality, freedom, and human dignity—not in pleas for special privilege, nor in enmity toward men, who are also victims of the current, half-equality between the sexes—but in an active, self-respective partnership with men.

From the National Organization for Women, Statement of Purpose, 1966.

rebellion. Students, blue-collar workers, convicts, homosexuals began to reject the roles in which society had cast them—roles that, they believed, demeaned their status and falsified their identity. Most striking of all was the revolt of the only minority that, in fact, constituted a majority of Americans—women, who, outnumbered by men as late as 1945, exceeded the male population by 5.5 million in 1970.

Earlier feminist pressure had improved the legal position of women and given them the vote. To the American male the notion that women still saw themselves in a state of subjection came as a shock. Philip Wylie's popular polemic *Generation of Vipers* (1942) had portrayed the American man as systematically castrated by his women, from mother to teacher to wife to daughter, and pronounced "momism" the

curse of American life. In comic strips Maggie forever chased Jiggs with her rolling-pin.

Yet all indexes showed women mired in social and economic inferiority. The "feminine mystique" defined a women as husband's wife, children's mother, family's faithful servant, never as a person in her own right. When women struck out on their own, most professions (except for elementary-school teaching, nursing, library work, and prostitution) resisted them. Shirley Chisholm, the first black congresswomen, said she endured more discrimination as a woman than as a black. Women constituted more than 51 percent of the population in 1970 but only 9 percent of the full professors on university faculties, 7.6 percent of the doctors, and 2.8 percent of the lawyers. The average earnings of a woman college graduate were less than those of a man with four years of high school.

In some respects the position of women had been getting worse. The early feminist movement had stimulated able women to seek careers. The example of Eleanor Roosevelt and Frances Perkins in the thirties, the participation of women in the Second World War as WACs and WAVEs and as workers in munitions plants—all this had strengthened the image of the self-reliant woman. But in the forties and fifties the tide had turned, as the tide had turned against the blacks after Reconstruction. The proportion of women undergraduates declined from 47 percent in 1920 to 31 percent in 1950; their median earnings relative to similarly employed men were declining; in 1971 the percentage of women in managerial and proprietorial jobs was lower than in 1960. A Commission on the Status of Women, established by Kennedy in 1962, fully documented the proposition that women were second-class citizens.

It was against this background that Betty Friedan in her influential book *The Feminine Mystique* (1963) called on women to recognize what society was doing to them and to demand equal rights and opportunities. Finding even the civil-rights groups and the New Left dominated by "male chauvinism"—"the

Malcolm X: an eloquent voice

only position for women in SNCC," said the black militant Stokely Carmichael in 1964, "is prone"— Friedan and others established the National Organization for Women (NOW) in 1966. The recruiting instrument for women's liberation was the "consciousness-raising" group, where women met in "rap sessions" to reflect on their lives. Courses in women's studies, widely instituted in these years, provided historical background. Such activity raised the consciousness of many men too, startled to discover the manifold ways in which male condescension and female subordination were built into the structure and language of society.

The black revolution turns left. In the black community the center of agitation was shifting from the South to the North. In 1910 only 9 percent of blacks lived outside the South and only 27 percent in urban areas. By 1970 47 percent lived outside the South and 70 percent in urban areas.

Where Southern blacks sought the removal of legal and political barriers, Northern blacks, who nominally possessed the freedoms provided by the new civil-rights legislation, wanted equal social and economic opportunity. Where Southern blacks were responsive to religious traditions and accustomed to daily relations with whites, Northern blacks were less involved in the old-time religion and, shut off in ghettos, were more hostile toward whites. Though Martin Luther King, Jr., remained the preeminent black leader, he proved less effective in Chicago than in Birmingham.

Despair in the ghettos produced challenges to King's ideals of nonviolence and an integrated society. A movement known as the Black Muslims gathered strength. Its leader was Elijah Muhammad, its most eloquent voice Malcolm X, and its program one of black separatism, self-discipline, and self-defense. Breaking with the Muslims in 1964, Malcolm X called for "a working unity among all peoples, black as well as white." He had hardly embarked in new directions, however, before he was murdered in February 1965, apparently as an aftermath of the feud with the Muslims. His powerful *Autobiography* (1965) became a central document of black nationalism.

Events strengthened the nationalist mood. In August 1965 riots in Watts, California, eventually suppressed by the National Guard, resulted in thirty-four deaths. In 1966 National Guardsmen put down riots in Chicago. In 1967 riots swept through the black sections of Tampa, Cincinnati, Atlanta, and New Brunswick, New Jersey, and broke out with desperate force in Detroit and Newark. These developments both encouraged and expressed a growing radicalization of the urban black—a radicalization symbolized in the

The case for violence

There has always existed in the Black colony of Afro-America a fundamental difference over which tactics from the broad spectrum of alternatives Black people should employ in their struggle for national liberation. One side of this difference contends that Black people ... must employ no tactic that will anger the oppressor whites. This view holds that Black people constitute a hopeless minority and that salvation for Black people lies in developing brotherly relations....

On the other side of the difference, we find that the point of departure is the principle that the oppressor has no rights that the oppressed is bound to respect. Kill the slavemaster, destroy him utterly, move against him with implacable fortitude. Break his oppressive power by any means necessary.... The heirs of Malcolm have picked up the gun and, taking first things first, are moving to expose the endorsed leaders for the Black masses to see them for what they are and always have been. The choice offered by the heirs of Malcolm is to repudiate the oppressor ... or face a merciless, speedy and most timely execution for treason.

From Huey P. Newton, "In Defense of Self Defense," The Black Panther, July 3, 1967.

---

summer of 1966 when Stokely Carmichael of SNCC raised the standard of "black power."

Black power. Black power could imply simply a demand for black regrouping and self-reliance as part of the transition to eventual integration on an equal basis. Integration on any other basis, it was contended, would mean surrender to white values. In this sense black power was an affirmation of racial and cultural pride. Black became beautiful; blacks threw away hair-straighteners and rejoiced in the Afro; soul music and soul food became badges not of shame but of identity; black studies programs became common in universities. Black power, said Dr. King, was a "call to manhood."

But, as expounded by black nationalists, it meant permanent racial separation, even retaliatory vengeance against the "honky." Blacks, Carmichael said in 1968, must become "the executioners of our executioners." In this more drastic mood, slogans of the King period—"We Shall Overcome"—gave way to more bitter phrases—"Burn, Baby, Burn."

The older black leaders condemned separatism and violence as self-defeating. As King wrote of the new militancy, "In advocating violence it is imitating the worst, the most brutal, and the most uncivilized value of American life." He added, "There is no salvation for the Negro through isolation. . . . The black man needs the white man and the white man needs the black man."

The emergence of black power constituted an unmistakable warning to white America. Lyndon Johnson, appropriating for himself the slogan "We Shall Overcome," pressed the fight for civil-rights legis-

lation, securing the passage of an open-housing law in 1968. He appointed Thurgood Marshall as the first black Justice to the Supreme Court. A presidential Commission on Civil Disorders, set up during the riots of 1967 under the chairmanship of Governor Otto Kerner of Illinois, concluded somberly: "Our nation is moving toward two societies, one black, one white—separate but unequal."

A few weeks later Martin Luther King, Jr. was assassinated in Memphis. Riots exploded in ghetto

Detroit, 1967

Probably the most destructive feature of Black Power is its unconscious and often conscious call for retaliatory violence.... The problem with hatred and violence is that they intensify the fears of the white majority, and leave them less ashamed of their prejudices toward Negroes. In the guilt and confusion confronting our society, violence only adds to the chaos. It deepens the brutality of the oppressor and increases the bitterness of the oppressed. Violence is the antithesis of creativity and wholeness. It destroys community and makes brotherhood impossible....

The ultimate weakness of violence is that it is a descending spiral, begetting the very thing it seeks to destroy. Instead of diminishing evil, it multiplies it. Through violence you may murder the liar, but you cannot murder the lie, nor establish the truth. Through violence you may murder the hater, but you do not murder hate. In fact, violence merely increases hate. So it goes. Returning violence for violence multiplies violence, adding deeper darkness to a night already devoid of stars. Darkness cannot drive out darkness; only light can do that. Hate cannot drive out hate; only love can do that.

From Martin Luther King, Jr., *Where Do We Go from Here: Chaos or Community?*, 1967.

after ghetto across the land, resulting in forty-three deaths, thirty-five hundred injuries, and twenty-seven thousand arrests. The subsequent murder of Robert Kennedy, the one white leader in whom black Americans believed, intensified hopelessness. But this mood was still more a warning than a broad reality. Polls in 1969 showed that the majority of black Americans continued to feel that they could win equality without violence and to accept the ideal of a multiracial society.

Revolt on the campus. The campuses, silent during the fifties, were stirred into purposeful activity by the New Frontier. The Peace Corps, VISTA, and civil-rights projects like "Freedom Summer" in Mississippi in 1964 were only the most dramatic form of the new commitment. But after John Kennedy's murder in 1963 and the Americanization of the Indochina War in 1965 youthful idealism took a new turn.

Tension between generations was hardly novel, but it now assumed unprecedentedly doctrinaire

Revolt on the campus: Cornell, 1969

forms, as in the motto popularized in demonstrations at the University of California in 1964: "You can't trust anyone over thirty." The militant young saw the older generation as the instrumentality of a corrupt society controlled by great bureaucracies of government and business. In its influential Port Huron statement (1962), Students for a Democratic Society denounced élitism and centralization and raised the standard of "participatory democracy." Against dehumanizing bureaucracy they cried: "Don't bend, fold, spindle or mutilate!" Against Vietnam: "Make love, not war."

The university, as the first large organization the young encountered, became a prime target in their revolt against the world of structures. More young men and women were going to college than ever before; total enrollment rose from 3.8 million in 1960 to 8.5 million in 1970. What university presidents hailed as the "multiversity," many students saw as a callously impersonal assembly line of higher education. As the war continued to escalate, radical students, with mounting rage, assailed academic collaboration with military effort—the Reserve Officers Training Corps, recruiting on campuses by CIA or by companies manufacturing tools of war like napalm, research financed by the Pentagon or CIA. As undergraduate defiance and provocation increased, university authorities began to call in the local police. In 1968–69 four thousand students were arrested. Where police violence went out of control—as at Columbia University and the Democratic convention in 1968 and at Harvard in 1969—student radicalization intensified.

The New Left. Violence begot violence. In 1967, the SDS national secretary announced, "We are working to build a guerrilla force in an urban environment." Characteristic of the new mood was the SDS's Weatherman faction (so-called because of the Bob Dylan lyric, "You don't need a weatherman to know which way the wind blows"). Seeing American (or, as they preferred to put it, Amerikan) society as irretrievably corrupt, they concluded that the only way to deal with an inherently destructive apparatus was to destroy it.

An ideology emerged to justify violence. In his book *One Dimensional Man* (1964), the philosopher Herbert Marcuse joined insights from Marx and Freud to argue that the welfare state had integrated the working class into capitalism and disqualified it as an agency of revolutionary change. Though Marcuse was not himself a man of violence, he argued for the suppression of ideas he considered antisocial and affirmed "a 'natural right' of resistance for oppressed and overpowered minorities. . . . If they use violence, they do not start a new chain of violence but try to break an established one. . . . No third person, and

least of all the educator and intellectual, has the right to preach them abstention."

One function of violence in New Left ideology was to "unmask" the "Establishment" by provoking it into acts of violent retaliation. Some of the time, however, the Establishment, whether because of bad conscience or Machiavellian ingenuity, employed a subtler tactic denounced by the militants as "co-optation"—the tactic of disarming dissent by absorbing it. Thus revolutionaries appeared on television talk shows and commanded large lecture fees. But government also showed itself capable of more drastic action. Policemen beat up long-haired demonstrators; the FBI sent agents, who also sometimes turned out to be *provocateurs*, into New Left groups; and the Department of Justice made recurrent efforts to indict and imprison New Left leaders. This produced a series of celebrated trials: in 1968, the trial of Dr. Benjamin Spock and three others for conspiring to encourage draft resistants to violate the Selective Service Act; in 1969–70, the prolonged and raucous trial of seven New

Haight-Ashbury, 1970

Woodstock, 1969: youth counterculture

Left leaders for crossing state lines with the intent to incite violence at the 1968 Democratic convention; and a number of trials of black militants.

The hippie scene. Not all the disaffected young took the path of political activism. Some responded rather by dropping out of society. These defectors followed trails marked out by the beatniks of the fifties.

Disdaining ties, jackets, and socks, affecting long hair, beards, and beads, spurning the adult world as "uptight" and "plastic," the "hippies" congregated in the Haight-Ashbury district of San Francisco or the Sunset Strip of Los Angeles or New York's East Village. Some called themselves "flower children," in part because of their custom of offering flowers to cops and other persecutors, and celebrated their rites, not in the teach-ins or sit-ins of the activists, but in "be-ins" or "love-ins." Some joined together in "communes" weirdly reminiscent of the communitarian enthusiasm in nineteenth-century America. By 1970 over two hundred communes involved perhaps forty thousand people, mostly under the age of thirty.

Do your own thing, drop out, turn on—these were the principles of the hippie ethos. Above all, the hippie mystique relied on drugs. During the nineteenth century in America, narcotics had been sold freely; before the Pure Food and Drug Act of 1906 (see p. 563), popular patent medicines often had a narcotic base. In 1914 the Federal Narcotics Bureau estimated that one in every four hundred Americans was an addict. The Harrison Act of that year was the first of a series of federal attempts to regulate narcotics, one result of which was to give the underworld control of the drug traffic.

For those trying to blow their minds and open wide what Aldous Huxley called in an influential book *The Doors of Perception* (1954), marijuana ("pot" or "grass") was the most common drug. Others turned to stronger hallucinogens, notably lysergic acid diethylamide (LSD or "acid") and mescaline; others to amphetamines, especially methedrine ("pep pills" or "speed"). LSD "highs" sometimes produced "good trips," with extraordinary heightening of perceptions of sound, color, and motion; they also produced "bad trips" and chemical changes leading to panic, prolonged depression, psychosis, and suicide.

Rise of the counterculture. Out of New Left activism, the hippie movement, the communes, the drug trips, the rock music, there emerged what was known from within as "the Movement" and from without as the "counterculture."

Music played a vital role in the formation of the counterculture. English groups, especially the Beatles

First is the danger of futility, the belief there is nothing one man or one woman can do against the enormous array of the world's ills—against misery and ignorance, injustice and violence.... Few will have the greatness to bend history itself; but each of us can work to change a small portion of events, and in the total of all those acts will be written the history of this generation.

It is from numberless diverse acts of courage and belief that human history is shaped. Each time a man stands up for an ideal, or acts to improve the lot of others, or strikes out against injustice, he sends a tiny ripple of hope, and crossing each other from a million different centers of energy and daring those ripples build a current which can sweep down the mightiest walls of oppression and resistance.

Robert F. Kennedy in Cape Town, South Africa, June 6, 1966.

and later the Rolling Stones, registered the trajectory of the young—from the communal "We All Live in a Yellow Submarine" through the psychedelic "Lucy in the Sky with Diamonds" to Mick Jagger's sinister "Sympathy for the Devil." Bob Dylan was the generation's American bard, singing his poignant and evocative songs—first social conscience and then folk rock—about drugs, race, sex, life, and memory.

If Marcuse was the influential ideologist for the political rebellion, Norman Mailer was, initially at least, the most eloquent exponent of the cultural rebellion. A gifted writer and bravura personality, Mailer had first won attention with his novel on the Second World War, *The Naked and the Dead* (1948). His 1957 essay "The White Negro" mythologized the "hipster" (from which the word "hippie" subsequently came) as an existential sub-hero, surviving in a death-haunted society by setting out on "that uncharted journey with the rebellious imperatives of the self." Mailer foresaw the "underground revolution" of the sixties; but by the time it arrived he had moved on to other things. Too many aspects of "straight" society, from the Kennedys to the moonshot, fascinated him; and, as a man who relished audiences and influence, he became almost a member of the Establishment himself.

After an astonishingly short period, the millennial hope of young Americans in the late sixties and early seventies simply evaporated. It came to seem, even to veterans of the Movement, an exotic memory. Sociologists and historians were hard put to account for this short and sharp season of unrest. Some placed emphasis on the extraordinary population increase in the sixties of persons between the ages of fourteen and twenty-four, the children of the postwar baby boom. In the seventy years between 1890 and 1960 that age group had increased by only 12.5 million. In the single decade of the 1960s, it grew by a fantastic 13.8 million. So unprecedented an enlargement in the youth popu-

lation created for a giddy moment a vivid youth consciousness, a separate youth culture, even perhaps, as the young felt themselves increasingly oppressed, a youth class. The demographic explosion coincided, moreover, with authentic social conflicts, especially over war and race.

Still only a minority of the young entered the counterculture. Most went about the business of growing up without notable alienation or protest. The end of the Indochina War and the rise of unemployment in the early seventies hastened the decline of the rebel young. Moreover, as the rate of population growth slowed after the mid-fifties, the fourteen-to-twenty-four group became a smaller and more manageable injection into society.

Nonetheless, the revolt left its mark. It compelled many people over thirty to acknowledge the gap between their professed ideals and the lives they actually lived. It helped force issues to the top of the national agenda—not only war and race but the role of women, the protection of the environment, the functions of education, the implications of a runaway technology, the significance of community and self-hood. For all its transience and excess, the youth rebellion of the sixties contributed to a fundamental reappraisal of American values.

The social fabric unravels. As the decade came to an end, the idyl—the Age of Aquarius—was turning sour. In the cities the flower people gave way to a new, tough breed, the "street people," priding themselves on "ripping off" (stealing), "trashing" (vandalism), "gang bangs" (mass rape), and promiscuous violence. Even worse were roving motorcycle gangs, like the sadistic Hell's Angels in California. In August 1969 the atrocious murder of the actress Sharon Tate and six others at the order of Charles Manson by three women members of Manson's hippie "family," though it was briefly glorified by the Weathermen and by some in

Despite the long years of support and vast expenditure of lives and funds, the United States in the end abandoned South Vietnam. There is no other way to put it.... After introduction of American combat troops into South Vietnam in 1965, the war still might have been ended within a few years, except for the ill-considered policy of graduated response against North Vietnam. Bomb a little, stop it a while to give the enemy a chance to cry uncle, then bomb a little bit more but never enough to really hurt. That was no way to win. Yet even with the handicap of graduated response, the war still could have been brought to a favorable end following defeat of the enemy's Tet offensive in 1968. The United States had in South Vietnam at that time the finest military force—though not the largest—ever assembled. Had President Johnson provided reinforcements, and had he authorized the operations I had planned in Laos and Cambodia and north of the DMZ, along with intensified bombing and the mining of Haiphong Harbor, the North Vietnamese would have broken. But that was not to be. Press and television had created an aura not of victory but of defeat, and timid officials in Washington listened more to the media than to their own representatives on the scene.

From General William C. Westmoreland, *A Soldier Reports,* **1976.**

the drug culture, forced many in the new generation to confront, as one put it, "the pig in ourselves, the childish, egotistical, selfish irresponsibility."

The decade that had begun in exhilaration and hope was dissolving into bitterness and hate. "Before my term is ended," Kennedy had said in 1961, "we shall have to test anew whether a nation organized and governed such as ours can endure. The outcome is by no means certain." Convinced that the inequalities in American society were a source of danger to American life, Kennedy tried to get America moving toward his New Frontier, carrying the poor and nonwhites with him. He was murdered. After his death his brother Robert made himself the champion of the outcasts and victims of American life. He was murdered. Martin Luther King, Jr. was the eloquent advocate of nonviolence. He was murdered. Some Americans regarded these murders as aberrations. Others began to lose faith in a society that destroyed the three men of the decade who seemed most to embody American idealism.

Still others, shocked by the panorama of epithets, marches, burnings, riots, shootings, bombings, became incensed over the new "permissive society" with its liberated women, militant blacks, and angry youth. The counter-culture in its turn provoked a moralistic counter-revolution dedicated to the reinstatement of social discipline. Phyllis Schlafly celebrated the values of old-fashioned feminity against the heresies of women's liberation. George Wallace, now moving onto the national scene, denounced "pointy-head intellectuals" and affirmed local sovereignty against federally enforced equal rights.

The Warren Court became a particular target. In *Gideon* v. *Wainwright* (1963), the Court, overruling its own previous decisions, freed a defendant on the ground that he had been denied counsel in a state court. Even more infuriating to the radical right were decisions in *Escobedo* v. *Illinois* and *Miranda* v. *Arizona* (1964) reversing state criminal convictions on the ground that the defendants had been denied counsel during police interrogations and had not been advised by the police of their constitutional rights. Conservatives assailed these judicial affirmations of the rights of the accused as the "coddling" of criminals.

The 1968 election. The emotions behind the conservative counter-revolution gathered force as the presidential election approached. In the meantime, war continued in Vietnam, and the Administration persisted in discerning light at the end of the tunnel.

"I see progress as I travel all over Vietnam," said General Westmoreland in November 1967. ". . . The enemy's hopes are bankrupt." In February 1968, during the Tet holiday, the lunar New Year, a massive enemy offensive took American and South Vietnamese forces by surprise, convulsed thirty provincial capitals, and even penetrated the American Embassy in Saigon. While the North Vietnamese failed to achieve their maximum objectives and suffered grievous losses in the process, the Tet offensive destroyed what remained of the Johnson Administration's credibility on Vietnam.

Westmoreland's reaction was to escalate further; and the Joint Chiefs' February request for 206,000 additional troops produced a showdown within the

Administration. Johnson, exasperated by McNamara's opposition to escalation, had shifted him to the World Bank; but the new Secretary of Defense, Clark Clifford, once a hawk, had begun to question the war when a 1967 mission disclosed to him that pro-American Asian states saw much less at stake in Indochina than Washington did. Now in the Pentagon, Clifford concluded that further escalation was futile.

The Tet offensive intensified domestic criticism of the war. "Are we like the God of the Old Testament," Robert Kennedy asked, "that can decide, in Washington, D.C., what cities, what towns, what hamlets in Vietnam are going to be destroyed?" Antiwar activists, having failed to persuade Kennedy to oppose Johnson, turned to another senatorial dove, Eugene McCarthy of Minnesota. A man of enigmatic and mis-

chievous intelligence, McCarthy, followed by a virtual "children's crusade," campaigned masterfully against Johnson and the war in the New Hampshire primary in March. The Tet offensive, McCarthy's strength in New Hampshire, and Kennedy's entry into the contest for Democratic nomination increased the pressure on Johnson. Faced by defeat in the impending Wisconsin primary, Johnson on March 31 withdrew from the presidential contest.

Humphrey became the Administration candidate. Once a liberal leader, Humphrey was now identified with Johnson and the war and did nothing to diminish this identification. Kennedy and McCarthy, on the other hand, generated crusading enthusiasm among their followers—Kennedy among the poor, the blacks, the Hispanic-Americans, McCarthy among

Robert F. Kennedy: arousing enthusiasm

The election of 1968

Richard M. Nixon, 1968: an astonishing comeback

suburbanites and independent voters, both among the young and the intellectuals. Their combined vote in a succession of primaries expressed a widespread repudiation of the Johnson Administration within his own party. However, on June 6, the night of his victory in the California primary, Kennedy was murdered by a Palestinian Arab who resented the senator's sympathy for Israel. The nation, appalled at the assassination of a second Kennedy within five years, mourned the death of a man many believed the most brilliant and creative among the national leaders.

After Kennedy's death Humphrey had no serious opposition. Protest against the war policy erupted, however, in shocking scenes at the Democratic convention in Chicago in August, when local police in a frenzy of violence clubbed hundreds of antiwar agitators. Senator Edmund Muskie of Maine received the vice-presidential nomination. In the meantime, Richard M. Nixon, completing an astonishing political comeback, won the Republican nomination and picked Governor Spiro T. Agnew of Maryland, the first suburban politician to rise to national prominence, as his running mate.

Nixon, who in past years had been more hawkish than the Administration, pledged that "new leadership will end the war." In domestic policy he presented himself as a champion of "law and order." Humphrey came out from under the shadow of the unpopular Johnson Presidency too slowly to rouse the enthusiasm of the Kennedy-McCarthy wing of the party. The most picturesque candidate, running on the American Independent party ticket, was George Wallace, who threatened for a time to do well not only in the South but among blue-collar workers in the North. In October, however, when organized labor threw itself into the contest, the working-class vote moved back to the Democrats.

The vote cast—73.2 million—was the largest in American history, but it included only 60.6 percent of the eligible electorate (as against 61.7 percent in 1964 and 64 in 1960). Nixon received 31.8 million votes as against 31.3 million for Humphrey and 9.9 million for Wallace. With only 43.4 percent of the total, he became a minority president. The margins were greater in the Electoral College: 301 for Nixon, 191 for Humphrey, and 46, all in the Deep South, for Wallace. The Democrats carried both houses of Congress, which made Nixon the first President since Zachary Taylor whose party on his election did not control at least one chamber.

Lyndon Johnson left the White House an unlamented President. Yet history may judge his Great Society a serious effort to overcome the tensions and inequities produced by social and technological change. The irony of his Presidency was that he sacrificed domestic policy, a field in which his knowledge was great and his instinct sure, to foreign policy, where his knowledge was scant and his instinct simplistic.

Suggestions for Reading

KENNEDY AND JOHNSON

Herbert Parmet's two volumes—*Jack: The Struggles of John F. Kennedy* (1980) and *JFK: The Presidency of John F. Kennedy** (1983)—are documented and evenhandedly critical. Two comprehensive accounts by participants written shortly after Kennedy's death are T. C. Sorensen, *Kennedy* (1965), and Arthur Schlesinger, Jr., *A Thousand Days** (1965); the latter is supplemented in Schlesinger, *Robert Kennedy and His Times** (1978). Henry Fairlie, *The Kennedy Promise* (1972), is a thoughtful polemic. L. J. Paper, *The Promise and the Performance: The Leadership of John F. Kennedy** (1975), offers a political scientist's view. Valuable memoirs from the Kennedy Administration include Pierre Salinger, *With Kennedy* (1966); K. P. O'Donnell and D. F. Powers with Joseph W. McCarthy, *"Johnny, We Hardly Knew Ye"** (1972); Lawrence F. O'Brien, *No Final Victories* (1974); and J. K. Galbraith, *A Life in Our Times** (1981). William Manchester, *Death of a President** (1967), provides a sometimes powerful, sometimes lurid, account of the assassination, and G. R. Blakey and R. N. Billings, *The Plot to Kill the President* (1981), is a reasoned dissent from the Warren Commission report.

For Johnson, his own memoir, *The Vantage Point* (1971), is formal but useful. Doris Kearns, *Lyndon Johnson and the American Dream** (1976), is an absorbing psychological analysis; George Reedy, *Lyndon B. Johnson, A Memoir* (1982), is a brilliant portrait by a close associate; E. F. Goldman, *The Tragedy of Lyndon Johnson* (1969), is the assessment by an historian who served briefly in Johnson's White House; and Robert Caro, *The Years of Lyndon Johnson: The Path to Power* (1982), is the first volume of an exhaustive and prosecutorial biography. Harry McPherson, *A Political Education* (1972), and Jack Valenti, *A Very Human President* (1975), are sympathetic accounts by Johnson associates. Hubert Humphrey, *The Education of a Public Man* (1976), is the autobiography of Johnson's Vice President.

FOREIGN AFFAIRS

For Kennedy's foreign policy, in addition to Brown, Freedman, and Hoffmann, cited in previous chapters and Sorensen and Schlesinger above, there is wide-ranging coverage in W. W. Rostow, *The Diffusion of Power* (1972), and useful observations in Roger Hilsman, *To Move a Nation** (1967); Chester Bowles, *Promises to Keep** (1971); W. I. Attwood, *The Reds and the Blacks* (1967); and George Ball, *The Past Has Another Pattern** (1982). W. I. Cohen, *Dean Rusk* (1980), is sympathetic and informative. On the missile crisis, R. F. Kennedy, *Thirteen Days** (1969) is indispensable testimony from a participant; G. T. Allison, *Essence of Decision** (1971), is an astute analysis. Norman Cousins, *The Improbable Triumvirate** (1972), is a fascinating account by a Kennedy emissary of the quest for détente in 1963. R. D. Mahoney, *JFK: Ordeal in Africa* (1984), is well researched and written.

D. S. Blaufarb, *The Counterinsurgency Era* (1977), is a good history of a bad idea. Louise FitzSimons, *The Kennedy Doctrine* (1972), and R. J. Walton, *Cold War and Counter-Revolution* (1972), depict Kennedy as an unreconstructed Cold Warrior.

On Vietnam, Stanley Karnow, *Vietnam: A History* (1984), is massive and dispassionate. Frances Fitz-Gerald, *Fire in the Lake** (1972) illuminates the clash of cultures. David Halberstam, *The Best and the Brightest** (1972), is a lively indictment. L. H. Gelb with R. K. Betts, *The Irony of Vietnam: The System Worked** (1979), argues that American leaders never expected to "win" the war. Guenter Lewy, *America in Vietnam** (1978), is a retrospective defense; H. G. Summers, Jr., *On Strategy: A Critical Analysis of the Vietnam War** (1983), second-guesses the conduct of the war. Among the two hundred (by 1984) novels about Vietnam, see especially Tim O'Brien, *Going After Cacciato** (1978); Philip Caputo, *A Rumor of War** (1977); Michael Herr, *Dispatches** (1977); and Robert Stone, *Dog Soldiers** (1974). Three films—Ted Post's *Go Tell the Spartans* (1978), Michael Cimino's *The Deer Hunter* (1978), and Francis Ford Coppola's *Apocalypse Now* (1979)—offer unforgettable images of the fighting.

SOCIETY IN FERMENT

W. L. O'Neill, *Coming Apart: An Informal History of America in the 1960's** (1971), is perceptive but uneven. Michael Harrington, *The Other America** (1963), helped set off the war on poverty, and J. T. Patterson, *America's Struggle Against Poverty, 1900–1980** (1981), puts that war in historical perspective. J. E. Schwarz, *America's Hidden Success* (1983), is a scholar's positive assessment of the Kennedy–Johnson social policy; Charles Murray, *Losing Ground** (1984), is sharply critical.

On civil rights, Carl Brauer, *John F. Kennedy and the Second Reconstruction** (1977), is an able scholarly account. The course of the black revolution can be traced in James Baldwin, *The Fire Next Time** (1963); Malcolm X, *Autobiography** (1965); Eldridge Cleaver, *Soul on Ice** (1967); Stokely Carmichael and C. V. Hamilton, Jr., *Black Power** (1967); and M. L. King, Jr., *Where Do We Go From Here: Chaos or Community?** (1967) S. B. Oates, *Let the Trumpet Sound: The Life of Martin Luther King, Jr.** (1982), is thorough and sympathetic.

On the stirrings among the young, Alexander Klein, ed., *Natural Enemies: Youth and the Clash of Generations* (1970), is a collection of documents, and Margaret Mead, *Culture and Commitment** (1970), a sagacious analysis. For women's liberation, see W. H. Chafe, *The American Woman, Her Changing Social, Economic and Political Roles, 1920–1970** (1974) and *Women and Equality** (1977); and G. G. Yates, *What Women Want: The Ideas of the Movement** (1975). Betty Friedan, *The Feminine Mystique** (1963), is a basic document, and Robin Morgan, ed., *Sisterhood Is Powerful** (1970), and Judith Hole and Ellen Levine, eds., *Rebirth of Feminism** (1972), are useful anthologies. For an anti-feminist statement, see Phyllis Schlafly, *The Power of the Positive Woman** (1977).

Ronald Berman, *America in the Sixties** (1968) is a thoughtful survey of intellectual developments from a conservative viewpoint; Morris Dickstein, *Gates of Eden: American Culture in the Sixties** (1977), is acute and more sympathetic. G. O. Larson, *The Reluctant Patron: The United States Government and the Arts, 1943–1965** (1983), describes the evolution of a national arts policy. On the counterculture, Norman Mailer, *Advertisements for Myself** (1959) and *The Presidential Papers** (1963), are essential introductions. Irwin Unger, *The Movement** (1974), and E. J. Bacciocco, Jr., *The New Left in America* (1974), are scholarly studies. Mike Nichols's film *The Graduate* (1967) portrays the more amiable side of the youth rebellion; and two later films—John Sayles's *The Return of the Secaucus Seven* (1980) and Lawrence Kasdan's *The Big Chill* (1984)—provide bittersweet retrospectives. David Musto, *The American Disease* (1973), tells the history of drugs in America. Peter Clecak, *America's Quest for the Ideal Self: Dissent and Fulfillment in the 60s and 70s* (1984), and Christopher Lasch, *The Culture of Narcissism** (1979), reflect on the meaning of the times.

For the 1968 election, see T. H. White, *The Making of a President 1968* (1969); Lewis Chester, et al., *An American Melodrama* (1969); Eugene McCarthy, *The Year of the People* (1968); and Jeremy Larner, *Nobody Knows: Reflections on the McCarthy Campaign of 1968* (1970).

*Available in a paperback edition.

33

THE PRESIDENCY REBUKED AND RESTORED

The man who became President in January 1969 was the antithesis of the rebel mood of the sixties. Fifty-six years old on his inauguration, Richard Milhous Nixon came from a lower-middle-class Quaker family in California, where a frugal upbringing had instilled traditional virtues of work, discipline, and ambition. Receiving a law degree in 1937, he served in the navy during the Second World War and entered politics thereafter, gaining election to the House of Representatives in 1946 and to the Senate in 1950. His diligence as a member of a House investigating committee helped break the case of Alger Hiss, and anticommunism was the issue with which he was most identified in his early career. His alacrity in dispensing accusations of disloyalty outraged his political opponents, who called him Tricky Dick, but Republicans admired him as an intelligent lawyer and a good party man.

Elected Vice President in 1952, Nixon did not enjoy easy relations with Eisenhower but served him faithfully. After his defeat by Kennedy in 1960, Nixon was defeated again in 1962 for the governorship of California; and his career was supposed over. "You won't have Nixon to kick around any more," he told the press. But, with dogged perseverance, he rebuilt his position. Lonely and solemn as a young man, he appeared fluent and affable in middle age. Sympathizers saw him as the embodiment of middle-class values in a degenerate time. Critics found him defensive, righteous, and shifty.

From Confrontation to Negotiation

Once more into the quagmire. Foreign affairs were Nixon's consuming interest and, in his view of himself, his field of main expertise. His first Secretary of State, William P. Rogers, had been Attorney General during the Eisenhower Administration; but the dominating influence was Henry A. Kissinger, a Harvard intellectual who had come to the United States from Germany as a boy in 1938 and was an accomplished diplomatic historian as well as an astute analyst of strategic problems. Nixon and Kissinger shared the view that, as the new President said in 1970, "The postwar period in international relations has ended." The era of overwhelming American military and economic superiority was over. The problem now was to adjust commitments to the emerging limits of power.

The Indochina War remained the nation's most anguishing international concern. Nixon and Kissinger hoped for American disengagement but believed that this had to be achieved "honorably." "Our defeat and humiliation in South Vietnam," Nixon said in November 1969, "without question would promote recklessness in the councils of those great powers who have not abandoned their goals of world conquest." The point, said Kissinger, was "to withdraw as an expression of policy and not as a collapse."

Nixon began by "winding down" American participation through a steady policy of "Vietnamization"—the replacement of American by South Viet-

Nixon and Kissinger: central control of foreign policy

namese troops. In April 1969 there were 543,000 American soldiers in Vietnam; by the summer of 1972, there were 50,000. While troop withdrawals proceeded, Kissinger made thirteen secret trips to France for peace talks with the North Vietnamese. Ho Chi Minh died in September 1969; but neither his successors in Hanoi nor the National Liberation Front in South Vietnam were prepared to abandon the objective of thirty years: the control of South Vietnam. The American proposals, varying in detail, all called for the concurrent withdrawal of American and North Vietnamese forces from South Vietnam, and all involved a favored position for the regime in Saigon, now headed by General Nguyen Van Thieu. Indeed, at times, the American proposals appeared subject to Thieu's veto. The objectives remained irreconcilable.

Widening the war. Vietnamization also required measures to reinforce Saigon. Nixon hailed Thieu as one of the four or five greatest political leaders of the world. Further strengthening of Thieu's regime soon demanded, in Nixon's judgment, extraordinary military measures—measures long urged by the Joint Chiefs of Staff, rejected by Johnson, and designed to destroy the North Vietnamese buildup in Cambodia and Laos.

For nearly twenty years the wily Prince Sihanouk had managed through artful dodging to preserve the neutrality of Cambodia. In the middle sixties Hanoi had begun to set up staging areas in Cambodia for attacks on South Vietnam. Early in 1969 Nixon initiated secret B-52 raids over Cambodia—thirty-five hundred in the next fourteen months, concealed from Congress by a system of false bombing reports. In March 1970 Sihanouk was overthrown by a prowest-ern coup headed by General Lon Nol. On April 30 Nixon announced an American incursion into Cambodia to "clean out major enemy sanctuaries." If, said Nixon, "the world's most powerful nation . . . acts like a pitiful, helpless giant . . . all other nations will be on notice that despite its overwhelming power the United States when a real crisis comes will be found wanting."

The invasion of Cambodia set off the most widespread and intense college protests in American history, involving 1.5 million students and half of America's twenty-five hundred campuses. On May 4, 1970, four students were killed and ten wounded by National Guardsmen at Kent State University in Ohio; Nixon, who a few days before had described student agitators as "bums," observed sententiously, "When dissent turns to violence, it invites tragedy." On May 14 police killed two black youths and wounded twelve at Jackson State College in Mississippi.

The Cambodian episode also produced strong reactions on Capitol Hill. For some time legislators had been restive over the loss to the executive of the constitutional power to declare war. The dispatch of American troops into Cambodia now raised the constitutional issue in acute form. Congress, hoping to reclaim lost powers, repealed the Tonkin Gulf resolution (see p. 826) and debated a variety of proposals to cut off funds for the further prosecution of the war. The publication by the *New York Times* and other journals in June 1971 of the so-called Pentagon Papers, made available by a former Pentagon official named Daniel Ellsberg, strengthened the antiwar mood by

Kent State University, May 4, 1970

documenting concealments and deceptions that had accompanied earlier stages of the war.

At the same time, television was bringing the savagery of the "living-room war" into millions of American homes every night. People watched with growing discomfort as the tiny screen showed Vietnamese children horribly burned by American napalm or Americans systematically setting fire to Vietnamese villages. The disclosure that American soldiers had massacred more than a hundred unarmed Vietnamese civilians at My Lai in March 1968 made war atrocities a national issue. My Lai forced Americans suddenly to wonder whether the United States had not brutalized itself in Vietnam. Many concluded that the means employed and the destruction wrought had grown out of all proportion to the interests involved and the goals sought. In 1971 public opinion polls reported that 65 percent of respondents believed it "morally wrong" for Americans to be fighting in Vietnam, though 1972 polls showed that a majority still supported Nixon's position that South Vietnam should not fall under communist control.

Disgust with the war was seeping into the army itself. By 1970 soldiers in Vietnam were wearing peace symbols and refusing to go into combat. The use of marijuana was general; and, according to estimates, 10 to 15 percent of the troops were addicted to heroin. "Fragging"—the use of fragmentation grenades to kill unpopular officers—was not unknown. In the United States, underground newspapers and antiwar coffee houses ventilated G.I. discontent. Amnesty for draft dodgers and deserters became an increasingly popular issue. Military morale and discipline were probably worse than at any point in American history. The incipient demoralization of the army strengthened the spreading determination to get out of the war.

Indochina dénouement. But the war went on. As American ground strength declined, Nixon relied increasingly on air and naval power to persuade Hanoi to lower its price for peace. By the end of 1971 his Administration had dropped 3.3 million tons of bombs on South Vietnam, Laos, Cambodia, and, toward the end, North Vietnam—more in three years than the Johnson Administration had dropped in five (and the bombing rate mounted in Nixon's fourth year). Yet aerial terror accomplished no more than it had in the past. When a strong North Vietnamese offensive in the spring of 1972 set back South Vietnamese forces, Nixon, fearing loss of "respect for the office of the President of the United States" on the eve of a scheduled trip to Moscow, retaliated by ordering the air force to widen the bombing of North Vietnam and the navy to mine North Vietnamese harbors. This would be, he said, the "decisive military action to end the war"; and it was required because "an American

defeat in Vietnam would encourage this kind of aggression all over the world . . . in the Mid-East, in Europe, and other areas." Some supposed that intensification of the war would cause the Russians to cancel the summit; but Moscow, fearing that cancellation might throw Washington into the embrace of Peking (Beijing), swallowed hard and digested the new escalation. The war went on.

As the 1972 election approached, the Nixon Administration, determined to neutralize the war as a campaign issue, made a change of decisive significance in the American negotiating position. It finally abandoned its longtime insistence that the withdrawal of American troops from South Vietnam be accompanied by the simultaneous withdrawal of North Vietnamese troops. Had this concession been made in 1969, American disengagement might have taken place then, and more than 15,000 Americans (and many more Vietnamese), killed from 1969 to 1972, would have lived.

In August the withdrawal of American ground combat troops was completed. Nixon also soon offered reconstruction assistance to North Vietnam. For its part, Hanoi dropped its demands for a political settlement in advance of a cease-fire and for the immediate elimination of Thieu. "Peace is at hand," Kissinger announced on October 26. But Thieu declined to come aboard. He thought, not unreasonably, that an agreement that removed American troops while leaving 145,000 North Vietnamese in place in South Vietnam did not bode well for his own future.

After the election Kissinger tried to reshape the agreement to meet some of Thieu's objections. Hanoi resisted the proposed changes. In December the talks broke down. Over Christmas, in one of the most savage acts of a savage war, Nixon ordered the bombing of Hanoi and Haiphong, with B-52s smashing the North Vietnamese cities for twelve days. The ostensible reason was to force concessions from Hanoi. Another purpose was to persuade Thieu to accept the agreement by improving his relative military position and by reminding him of the damage American air power had the capacity to inflict. On January 5, 1973, Nixon secretly promised Thieu that "we will respond with full force should the settlement be violated by North Vietnam." A billion dollars' worth of planes, tanks, and other weapons was rushed to South Vietnam. Thieu remained dubious. But continued American pressure obliged him to accede. The agreement, as signed in Paris on January 23, differed little from the one originally reached in October.

The Paris Accords established a cease-fire and proposed complicated machinery to bring about a political settlement. Given the irreconcilable differences between the two regimes, the machinery was plainly unworkable. Skeptics discerned a cynical policy de-

The Indochina War

signed to provide a "decent interval" between American withdrawal and Thieu's collapse. The last American troops, along with American prisoners-of-war, went at the end of March 1973. Both Vietnamese governments violated the Paris Accords from the start. The "cease-fire war" began. More South Vietnamese soldiers died in 1974 than in 1967. In March 1975 Hanoi launched a major offensive. The American government, asking Congress for emergency military assistance, claimed that failure to go the last mile with Thieu would cause the world to look on the United States as a feeble and perfidious nation. Congress had heard such talk before and was unmoved. At the end of April 1975 Thieu fell in South Vietnam and Lon Nol in Cambodia.

The Indochina War was at last at an end. The aftermath refuted the domino theory that had led the United States into the war. Hanoi's victory, while it established a cruelly repressive communist regime in Vietnam, failed to produce the long-feared coordinated communist control of East Asia. With the American presence removed, the communist states fell to fighting among themselves. In Cambodia, now called Kampuchea, a vicious Marxist regime under Pol Pot brutalized, starved, and murdered hundreds of thousands of Cambodians. In 1978–79 communist Vietnam invaded communist Kampuchea and overthrew Pol Pot. Communist China thereupon invaded communist Vietnam. Communist China (and to some degree the United States) supported Pol Pot. Communist Russia supported Vietnam. Conflicting national interests once again proved more potent than alleged ideological affinities. The dominoes, instead of falling in unison against the west, crashed angrily into one another.

Indochina inquest. The war had killed at least 1.5 million Indochinese and turned a third of the population into refugees. The 6.7 million tons of bombs dropped by American planes left the landscape scarred with craters. Defoliation, undertaken to deprive the Viet Cong of forest cover, affected one-third of the forest area of South Vietnam. President Marcos of the Philippines spoke for many Asians when he said in 1971, "Heaven forbid that the U.S. should duplicate what it has done in South Vietnam if the war should come to our country."

For the United States the Indochina War had lasted longer than any war in its history. It left more Americans dead—fifty-seven thousand—than any war except the Civil War and the two World Wars, and cost more money than any war except the Second World War.

The war devastated an American generation. There were no parades for returning veterans. The country that had carelessly sent soldiers to Vietnam treated them with cruel indifference when they came home. Many of the 2.8 million who served in Vietnam suffered from emotional dislocation; one government-sponsored study reported that nearly 60 percent returned with nightmares, diseases, nervous conditions, and alcohol and drug abuse. On the other extreme were the young men who had acted early on the conviction that so many came to in the end: the war was immoral. The debate whether 570,000 "draft offenders," of whom 30,000 went underground or fled the country, mostly to Canada, should receive amnesty carried the divisions of war into the aftermath. As for the 15 million men of military age who neither fought nor fled, the war had gravely weakened their faith in the judgment and the word of their government.

America's myth of itself as benevolent, wise, and invincible drained away in the jungles of Indochina.

The bitter experience corroded the spirit of self-confidence that had characterized America in 1945. By the early seventies the American people were divided, the economy was in trouble, the armed forces were in discredit, national motives were in doubt, and liberal ideals themselves seemed implicated in the disaster. One result was an intensive examination of the bases of American foreign policy to account for the ghastly consequence.

Most Americans believed that America had extended its power around the planet in order to protect free nations from communist aggression. But the shock of Vietnam put the situation in a chilling new light. In the course of twenty-five years, it now seemed, America had established an empire of its own. It had military commitments to 47 nations; 375 major bases and 3,000 minor facilities in foreign lands; 1 million troops stationed abroad; 2.5 million more troops under arms at home. It had spent more than $1 trillion for its own military programs and $150 billion for foreign aid. American business also controlled more than half of all direct foreign private investment, produced more than half of the world's manufactured products, and consumed a disproportionate quantity of the world's raw materials.

Anatomy of empire. How had this empire arisen? On the left, Vietnam confirmed the tendency to ascribe everything—not only the Indochina War but the Cold War and even American participation in the Second World War—to the supposed quest of American capitalism for world hegemony. It was true that American overseas investments had grown strikingly in the postwar period—from $8.4 billion in 1945 to more than $100 billion by 1973. Though it was hard to argue that America went into Vietnam to gain markets or protect investments, sophisticated exponents of the Open Door thesis contended that, because defeat in Vietnam would jeopardize American markets and investments throughout the Third World, economic interest compelled Washington to a course of ruthless counterrevolution.

Close analysis of the figures showed, however, that the dependence of American capitalism on the underdeveloped world was limited. Two-thirds of American exports went to industrialized rather than to developing countries, and sales to the Third World amounted to about 3 percent of the annual national output. Investment in the Third World represented a declining fraction of total foreign investment—35 percent in 1960 and only 26 percent in 1973. Of Third World investment, 40 percent was in petroleum; with that excluded, only about one-sixth of American overseas investment was in the developing nations, and few American businesses seemed interested in increasing that proportion. In so far as American capitalism depended on the world outside, it depended on markets and investments in developed and not in underdeveloped countries. Nor had American business been, for example, notably eager for escalation in Vietnam.

If not American capitalism, what? No single explanation of the imperial impulse seemed satisfactory. A number of factors converged to lead Americans to appoint themselves custodians of freedom, entitled to intervene freely and righteously around the planet. The American empire, such as it was, resulted from the perversion of initially honorable beliefs: the belief in the necessity of creating an international structure of peace; the belief in America's mission to uplift and save suffering humanity; the belief in America's capacity to rebuild and instruct other nations. The distortion of these beliefs was brought about by the real threat of Stalinist communism—American presence in other lands was mostly at the invitation of governments fearful of the Russians—and then by the rigid form taken by the counterideology of anticommunism.

A special pressure encouraging interventionist policies, above all in Vietnam, was the military establishment. The armed forces had emerged from the Second World War with unprecedented power and status. When the wartime military leaders, most of whom were sober and responsible men, departed the scene, a new group took over, more in the school of MacArthur than of Marshall, professionally persuaded that political problems had military solutions, professionally committed to multiplying threats, appropriations, and weapons, professionally adept at playing upon national desires to appear virile and patriotic. This was not quite Eisenhower's "military-industrial complex." The military establishment was an independent force in its own right, operating according to its institutional aspirations and not at the bidding of business, which by the late sixties had turned predominantly against escalation in Vietnam.

A look at other nations corroborated the proposition that the imperial impulse was not rooted in a specific system of ownership. Every great power, whatever its ideology, had its military machine. Every military machine supposed that national security required the domination of "strategic" weaker states, if only to prevent their domination by some rival power. If, for example, the invasion by the Red Army to overthrow a national-communist regime in Czechoslovakia in 1968 was not imperialism, then the term had no meaning. If it was imperialism, then imperialism was not uniquely rooted in capitalism, nor would the abolition of capitalism end it. It seemed likely that no change in systems of ideology or ownership would reduce the power of the professional military in a time of chronic international crisis.

The decline of the superpowers. After the Second World War, the United States and the Soviet Union, entering the vacuums of power left in the wake of war, had divided and dominated the planet. Each superpower had sought to extend its empire in order to protect itself from the other. But the reign of the superpowers was drawing to a close. Where American and Soviet power had flowed into the vacuums from without, the resurgence of nationalism—in Europe, within the communist world, and in the Third World—was now replenishing these vacuums from within. The reinvigoration of nationalism meant growing opposition to the United States in the western bloc, growing opposition to the Soviet Union in the communist bloc, and growing opposition to both in the Third World. The consequence was to place limits on the power of the two countries. Tocqueville's celebrated forecast—America and Russia, each "marked out by the will of Heaven to sway the destinies of half the globe"—had in the end an exceedingly short run.

In addition, the fragmentation of the communist world by nationalism altered the nature of the problem that communism presented to the United States. The intensifying quarrel between Russia and China meant the end of any single center of authority in the communist movement and hence the end of a unified communist ideology and discipline. In the age of Stalin communist parties everywhere had responded to the directives of Moscow. Now the rise of "polycentrism" set communist states free to pursue national policies. It could no longer be assumed that the extension of communism meant the automatic extension of Soviet, or Chinese, power.

As the threat of monolithic communism thus receded, Vietnam emphasized the limits of American power. For a season Americans began to conclude that not everything that happened in the world was of equal concern to the United States; that in an age of local upheaval and savagery many terrible things would take place that the United States lacked the power to prevent or the wisdom to cure; and that

Washington could not be the permanent guarantor of stability on a turbulent planet.

Responding to the new mood, Nixon in July 1969 promulgated what he thereafter termed the Nixon Doctrine. The "central thesis," Nixon said in 1970, was that "the United States will participate in the defense and development of allies and friends, but cannot—and will not—conceive *all* the plans, design *all* the programs, execute *all* the decisions and undertake *all* the defense of the free nations of the world. We will help where it will make a real difference and is considered in our interest." Even in such cases, he added, the nations directly threatened had the "primary responsibility" of providing the manpower for their own defense.

Rapprochement with communist powers. Though Nixon himself had been a zealous Cold Warrior who had condemned Kennedy and Johnson as inadequately militant in their Cuba and Vietnam policies, he was also a realist. As President, he began to liberate himself from the ideological obsessions of the Dulles years. Kissinger, the student of Metternich and Bismarck, reinforced a geopolitical view. Security, as Nixon saw it, demanded no longer the rollback of communism but rather the reestablishment of the classical balance of power. "It will be a safer world and a better world," he said in 1971, "if we have a strong, healthy United States, Europe, Soviet Union, China, Japan—each balancing the other, not playing one against the other, an even balance."

An era of negotiation: Nixon and Mao

His boldest step in the pursuit of the balance-of-power design was his reversal of American policy toward the Chinese People's Republic. After the Korean War domestic political pressures had frozen successive Administrations into a posture of grim nonrecognition of the Peking (Beijing) regime. The excesses of the Cultural Revolution of 1966–68 seemed to verify the theory that Maoism represented the ultimate in communist fanaticism. However, China and the Soviet Union had each come to fear the rival communist state more than the common capitalist adversary. When Russia stationed nearly fifty divisions along its Chinese frontier, Mao Tse-tung (Mao Zedong) and Chou En-lai (Zhou Enlai) evidently decided they must take steps to block a Soviet-American alliance against China. Washington was responsive, and a mission by Kissinger to Peking (Beijing) in July 1971 was followed by an extraordinary presidential trip to China in early 1972. Nixon stayed in China for nearly a week—a longer state visit than any President had ever made to a foreign nation. On February 27, he signed a declaration saying that Taiwan, where Chiang Kai-shek (Jiang Jieshi) still ruled, was legally part of mainland China, that American forces would eventually withdraw from Taiwan, and that the island's future was to be settled by the Chinese themselves.

As for the relationship between the United States and the Soviet Union, this, Nixon said, was moving "from an era of confrontation to an era of negotiation." Progress was made toward defining the status quo in Europe. The ratification in May 1972 of treaties by West Germany with Russia and Poland opened the way to the territorial settlement the wartime coalition had failed to conclude after the Second World War. A quadripartite agreement on the status of West Berlin gave promise of ending what had been for twenty-five years a situation of danger between the Soviet Union and the West. A European Security Conference, long proposed by the Soviet Union and finally held in Helsinki in August 1975, ratified Europe's postwar borders. "Basket Three" of the Helsinki Agreement gave new international status to human rights. At the same time, responding to Russia's need for modern technology, the Administration encouraged Soviet-American trade and even undertook to seek most-favored-nation tariff status (that is, the extension of tariff concessions made to other countries) for the Soviet Union.

Through this network of relationships—diplomatic, economic, and commercial—joined together and made mutually dependent by the concept of "linkage," Kissinger hoped to "give the Soviets a stake in international equilibrium." Détente, combined with the Chinese connection, would continue containment in a new form and make up for the relative decline in American military power.

The arms race. In the 1960s the Soviet Union had drastically expanded its production of land-based intercontinental ballistic missiles (ICBMs). By 1972, it had 50 percent more missile-launchers than the United States. But the United States retained a more than two-to-one superiority in warheads, and American security rested not only on ICBMs but on submarine-based missiles (the Polaris-Poseidon system) and on the strategic bombing force—three independent systems, each capable of inflicting deadly damage even after a Soviet first strike, and one at least, the sea-based deterrent, invulnerable to Soviet attack. With the Soviet Union now in a comparable state of assured retaliatory capacity, it seemed absurd for the two powers, each with the ability to incinerate the other, to continue piling overkill on overkill.

A first series of Strategic Arms Limitation Talks (SALT-I) began in 1969 and concluded with a Nixon-Brezhnev meeting in Moscow in 1972. The resulting treaty limited the deployment of defensive anti-ballistic missile (ABM) systems, which, from the viewpoint of "mutual assured destruction" (MAD), were destabilizing because they could provide an incentive to first strikes. In addition, an interim agreement on offensive systems required both countries to stop building ICBM launchers (which the United States had no intention of doing anyway). The effect was to trade the Soviet lead in ICBMs for the American lead in technology and bombers, thereby balancing Soviet quantitative superiority against American qualitative superiority.

SALT-I was based on the MAD conception of nuclear stand-off (or what the Nixon Administration called nuclear "sufficiency"). "What in the name of God is strategic superiority?" cried Henry Kissinger, who became Secretary of State in 1973 (in an outburst he later retracted). "What is the significance of it, politically, militarily, operationally, at these levels of numbers? What can you do with it?" While SALT-I produced no reductions, it set in motion a process that offered hope for reduction in the future.

However, discontent was rising within the Administration over MAD. Some critics wanted to reestablish American strategic superiority. Others argued that the threat of reciprocal mass slaughter was barbarous and that it lacked credibility as a deterrent. Technological improvements gave missiles new accuracy and precision; and James Schlesinger, who became Secretary of Defense in 1973, favored a widening of nuclear "options" with special attention both to "counterforce"—attacks on military installations and missile sites—and to tactical weapons. Critics questioned Schlesinger's idea of controlled and limited nuclear war and detected in counterforce the potentiality for a first-strike capability. MAD may have been mad, but to many the alternative seemed even madder.

In the meantime, both superpowers continued to develop weapons systems not covered in SALT-I. In 1969 Nixon, over congressional opposition, made the fatal decision to introduce the Multiple Independently-targeted Re-entry Vehicle (MIRV), which, because it packed several missiles in a single warhead, immensely complicated problems of verification and ushered in a new and more uncontrollable phase of the arms race. (In 1974 Kissinger said, "I wish I had thought through the implications of a MIRVed world.") For its part, the Soviet Union MIRVed its ICBMs, built the Backfire supersonic bomber, and strove in other ways to enlarge its already formidable counterforce power and to add qualitative improvement to quantitative superiority. Technology was the perpetual enemy of stability; and the qualitative arms race was subverting the quantitative limits imposed by SALT-I. Improvement in the delivery and accuracy of smaller warheads made possible the abandonment of huge megatonnage hydrogen weapons and the slight reduction of the nuclear stockpile from a high point of about 32,000 in 1967.

SALT talks continued. An agreement reached at Vladivostok in December 1974 set ICBM and MIRV ceilings at levels so high they became goals, not limitations. The nuclear arms race rushed on.

Beyond the superpowers. Kissinger's theory was that détente could work only if the Soviet Union and the United States respected each other's spheres of influence. He saw the Soviet Union as a status quo power for which revolution beyond the Soviet zone was a temptation, not a necessity—a temptation from which the Kremlin would quickly recede when the United States refused to act "like a pitiful, helpless giant" and showed the "will" to defend what Russia would accept as legitimate American interests. He therefore saw no incompatibility between seeking an accommodation with Moscow and reacting vigorously against communist activities elsewhere. In so doing, the Nixon Administration displayed what critics regarded as a fondness toward regimes of the authoritarian right.

In Europe Nixon so sedulously identified Washington with right-wing dictatorships in Greece and Portugal that, when the inevitable political upheavals took place, democratic regimes came to power with anti-American predispositions. In the case of Portugal, Kissinger threatened the provisional government with diplomatic and economic isolation for its inclusion of communists and displayed unwarranted pessimism about the nation's political future. He also overreacted to the transient phenomenon of Eurocommunism,

seeing democratic professions by western communist parties as evidence not of political weakness, but of tactical cunning.

In Asia the Nixon Administration ignored Pakistan's brutal repression of the Bangladesh independence movement and, despite public avowals of neutrality, gave secret instructions to "tilt" American power toward Pakistan during its war with India in 1971. In Africa the Administration tilted toward white regimes—not only South Africa and Rhodesia but Portuguese colonial regimes in Angola and Mozambique. Portugal's departure from Angola in 1975 left the newly independent state torn between rival guerrilla forces, one side backed by the Soviet Union, the other by South Africa, China, and the United States. Kissinger approved large-scale covert intervention by the CIA, overriding warnings from the State Department that the result would be even larger counterescalation by the Russians. The introduction of 10,000 Cuban troops soon assured victory for the side favored by Moscow. In 1976 Congress prohibited further CIA covert action in Angola without express congressional approval. Belatedly recognizing that a successful African policy required a measure of support in black Africa, Kissinger now reversed course and endorsed black majority rule.

In Latin America Nixon, commending the military dictatorship in Brazil, observed wishfully, "As Brazil goes so will go the rest of that Latin American continent." The election of a Marxist regime headed by Salvador Allende in Chile in 1970 produced special excitement in Washington. Before the election Kissinger had directed the CIA to take covert action against Allende's candidacy. After the election he authorized the CIA to spend $8 million to "destabilize" the new government. Allende strove in the main to preserve constitutional processes; but he had received only 36 percent of the vote, and his economic policy was neither well managed nor perhaps acceptable to the Chilean majority. In the end his regime might have fallen anyway. But Washington, reinforcing the CIA by a credit squeeze and other economic measures, contributed to Allende's downfall and probable murder in a military coup in 1973.

The succeeding military regime under General Augusto Pinochet shocked the world by its policies of repression and torture. Yet it remained a favorite of Washington, receiving more than twice as much bilateral economic assistance in 1975 as the next-largest Latin American recipient of United States aid. In Kissinger's view, a Pinochet regime, because it did not upset the existing balance of force, would be better for détente than a regime inclined to the other side. This was the Soviet theory of détente too, as Moscow had shown in Czechoslovakia and elsewhere.

The theory that every Marxist victory in the Third World was an addition to Soviet power denied the reality of polycentrism and made Washington an arsenal of counterrevolution. In a deeper sense, Washington's support of authoritarian regimes for short-run diplomatic purposes ignored the human values involved. Such a policy damaged what had been historically America's most precious international asset—the bond that was felt to run between the United States and ordinary people around the planet.

Middle Eastern cockpit. The Middle East continued to present perplexing questions. The Soviet Union was increasing its influence among the Arab states in pursuit of historic Russian ambitions in the area. The United States had a deep moral interest in Israel and a strong—if conflicting—economic interest in Arab oil. Both Russian and American concerns were superimposed on a world torn by indigenous hatreds with a life and potency of their own.

To oppose Soviet aspirations in the Persian Gulf area, Nixon looked to the shah of Iran. In the Kennedy-Johnson years, American relations with Iran had been distant. Visiting Teheran in May 1972, Nixon now asked the shah to become the "protector" of American interests in the Gulf area. In exchange the shah received, along with certain political assurances, the unrestricted right to buy the most advanced American weapons. United States arms sales to Iran, which had totaled $1.2 billion over the twenty-two years since 1950, increased almost sixteenfold to a total of $19.5 billion from 1972 to 1979. Though the shah was in his way a modernizer, he was increasingly possessed by delusions of grandeur; he was surrounded by sycophants and thieves; and his secret police systematically tortured and killed his opponents. Nonetheless he appeared for the moment in firm charge of his country.

In the Near East, the Arab states remained unreconciled to the existence of Israel. In June 1967 Israel, responding to the Egyptian blockade of the port of Elath on the Gulf of Aqaba, launched a surprise attack on Egypt and won a smashing victory in the Six Days War. After the war Israel retained possession of territories deemed essential to defense against future Arab attack—the Sinai Peninsula against Egypt and the Golan Heights against Syria as well as the Gaza Strip and the West Bank of the Jordan River. In November 1967 the UN Security Council passed Resolution 242 calling for "withdrawal of Israeli forces from territories occupied in the recent conflict" (though not necessarily, it was noted, from *all* such territories) and for the "acknowledgment" of the sovereignty and independence of all states in the area.

The package deal thus outlined was not achieved, the Arab states refusing to recognize Israel, Israel refusing to abandon the territory won in 1967. The bitterness of the Palestinian refugees—Arabs expelled from Israel—added another explosive element, especially after the formation of the Palestine Liberation Organization and more extreme terrorist groups, mostly operating out of the small kingdom of Jordan. In 1970 King Hussein of Jordan attacked the Palestinian guerrillas, whereupon Syria, with presumed Soviet support, invaded Jordan. The threat of Israeli and U.S. counterintervention forced Syria to withdraw.

The death of Nasser in September 1970 brought Anwar el-Sadat into power in Cairo and in 1972 the expulsion of 10,000 Soviet military advisers. A precarious peace, punctuated by Arab raids and Israeli reprisals, prevailed until October 5, 1973. Then, on Yom Kippur, the Jewish holy day of atonement, Egypt and Syria struck at Israel. Caught by surprise, Israeli forces reeled under the blow. The Egyptians were fighting with advanced Soviet weapons, and the United States at once rushed arms to Israel. After ten days of Israeli disarray, a counterattack cut off the Egyptian Third Army in the Sinai. There followed a series of still unfathomed events. On the night of October 24 Nixon put American nuclear forces on worldwide alert—a most unusual step. The ostensible reason was to counter an alleged Soviet threat to intervene militarily on behalf of Egypt, though it was later questioned whether available intelligence confirmed such a Soviet intention. Israeli officials subsequently claimed that the alert was accompanied by warnings that, if Israel did not spare the Egyptian force and conclude the war, it would have to fight on alone. The American purpose was to bring a stalemate and preserve the American position as Middle East mediator.

A powerful new factor, suddenly introduced into the Middle East equation, argued against the United States' taking a drastic anti-Arab position. In 1960 Venezuela had persuaded the oil-producing states of the Middle East to join in forming the Organization of Petroleum Exporting Countries (OPEC). The original point of OPEC was to concert policies in order to defend national economies against the manipulation of the world market by western oil companies. On October 19, 1973, OPEC, now controlled by an Arab majority, imposed a ban on oil exports to the United States and western Europe in retaliation for American support of Israel. It also quadrupled the price of Middle Eastern oil. These actions represented a historic reversal in the balance of power between the industrialized nations and the Third World. For centuries access to vital raw materials has been a particular motive for western imperialism. OPEC showed that possession of raw materials, which once placed underdeveloped countries at the mercy of the West, now placed the West at their mercy.

The October War thus altered the situation in the Middle East in two salient respects: it shattered the belief in Israel's military invincibility, and it demonstrated western vulnerability in face of Arab use of oil as a political weapon. Both American interests—Israel and oil—called more urgently than ever for a political settlement. This became Kissinger's major objective in 1974–75. Relying on a strong personal relationship with Sadat as well as on the traditional American influence in Israel, he visited the Middle East on an average of one out of every six weeks. His "shuttle diplomacy" sought to bring Israel and Egypt step by step toward a resolution of outstanding issues. At the same time, he tried to reduce Soviet influence by systematically excluding Moscow from his Middle Eastern negotiations. In September 1975 an interim agreement on the Sinai provided for partial Israeli troop withdrawal in exchange for an American commitment to supply Israel with advanced arms and aircraft and not to negotiate with the Palestine Liberation Organization so long as the PLO refused to recognize Israel's right to exist. The Middle East demonstrated Kissinger's virtuoso qualities as a negotiator—his intelligence, resourcefulness, perseverance, and stamina.

Debate over détente. At first the Nixon-Kissinger policy of rapprochement with China and Russia encountered little resistance at home. Nixon's anticommunist credentials facilitated the process. Observers wryly noted the irony of the old Red-hunter exchanging unctuous toasts with Chou En-lai (Zhou Enlai) and Brezhnev. Even conservatives confined themselves to stoical warnings.

Moreover, "détente" responded to concrete interests of both superpowers—the prevention of nuclear war; the containment of military budgets; Soviet apprehension about China and need for western technology; American acknowledgment of the disappearance of a monolithic communist threat; the intensifying claims in both countries of internal problems. But the Administration, cherishing a meaningless 12-point agreement on "Basic Principles" signed by Nixon and Brezhnev on May 29, 1972, oversold détente as an international cure-all.

In fact, where détente had reality, it was as the expression of stability in the equilibrium of power; it was the recognition of situations that had already come into existence. It was, in short, the consequence rather than the cause of stabilization. It therefore applied primarily to Europe. In parts of the world where power relationships were in flux, détente was a wistful hope. In the Middle East, Africa, East Asia, instability had deep historic roots and was far beyond the joint capacity of the Soviet Union and the United States to control even if they should agree on policy.

The very concept of détente was ambiguous. In Soviet eyes détente meant only a series of specific and limited agreements. It did not imply a broad guarantee of the status quo nor exclude Soviet support of national-liberation movements. So Moscow happily pursued its Cold War of movement in Africa and elsewhere. For its part, the Administration was unable to make good on all its assurances to Moscow. Thus Soviet restrictions on the migration of Jews led in 1973–74 to the denial by the American Congress of most-favored-nation status and to the passage of the Jackson Amendment, an attempt to condition commercial concessions on changes in Soviet emigration policy. American interference in what Moscow regarded as an internal question drove the Kremlin to cancel the Soviet-American trade agreement of 1972.

When détente failed to live up to unrealistic expectations, disenchantment set in. Critics were especially disturbed by what they regarded as a decay in American military power. By 1975 defense expenditures were less in constant dollars than they had been at any time since before the Korean War. Defense spending dropped dramatically from 49 percent of federal outlays in Eisenhower's last year to 29 percent in Nixon's last year. The budget for strategic forces was about one-third in real terms what it had been at the end of the Eisenhower Administration. If Russia achieved a war-winning capability, critics believed, this would demoralize the West and allow Soviet power to expand through nuclear blackmail.

On the issue of human rights critics were joined by liberals who favored arms control but were outraged by the treatment accorded such Soviet dissenters as the physicist Andrei Sakharov and the novelist Aleksandr Solzhenitsyn. Solzhenitsyn's visit to the United States in 1975 dramatized the problem of Soviet repression. Many Americans saw a dismal preview of the costs of détente in President Ford's refusal to invite him to the White House lest the Kremlin take offense. Nor did the Soviet Union comply with Basket Three of the Helsinki Agreement and its pledges to increase the flow of people, information, and ideas across the Iron Curtain.

By 1976 the bloom went off détente. Many people agreed when the French journalist André Fontaine defined détente as simply "the Cold War pursued by other means—and sometimes by the same."

For some years Kissinger had enjoyed virtual immunity as the architect of American foreign policy. His wit, insouciance, and proficiency seized the national imagination. He beguiled Congress. Polls regularly reported him at the top of the list of most-admired Americans. By the mid-1970s opinion had

I continue to maintain, as in 1945, that on ideology there is no prospect of compromise between the Kremlin and ourselves, but that we must find ways to settle as many areas of conflict as possible in order to live together on this small planet without war. I have constantly believed that internal pressures by the Russian people and the influence of world opinion would lead in time to some relaxation in the Soviet system, and that greater respect for human rights would gradually develop. This has certainly been happening, though unevenly and far too slowly. I heartily approve the policy of détente…. I decry those who contend that any relaxation of tensions must inevitably benefit the Russians, to our disadvantage. It seems to me we have no choice. In this nuclear age, war is unthinkable. Our interest is bound to be served by relieving tensions as much as we can, by working for what I have called 'competitive coexistence.' I for one do not fear the competition.

From W. Averell Harriman (with Elie Abel), *Special Envoy to Churchill and Stalin,* **1941–1946, 1975.**

The only morality they recognize is what will further their cause: meaning they reserve unto themselves the right to commit any crime, to lie, to cheat…. They are the focus of evil in the modern world.

From Ronald Reagan, speech, January 29, 1981, March 8, 1983.

The superpowers often behave like two heavily armed blind men feeling their way around a room, each believing himself in mortal peril from the other whom he assumes to have perfect vision…. Each tends to ascribe to the other side a consistency, foresight and coherence that its own experience belies. Of course, over time even two blind men can do enormous damage to each other, not to speak of the room.

From Henry A. Kissinger, *White House Years,* **1979.**

grown more skeptical. His addiction to ambiguity and secrecy had become self-defeating. In addition, his policy alarmed conservatives by its pursuit of détente and liberals by its intervention in countries outside the realm of direct American interest. Yet together Nixon and Kissinger, an odd couple indeed, had relieved American foreign policy of burdening taboos, shifted national attention from ideology to geopolitics, and adapted American policy to far-reaching changes in the structure of international relationships. In particular, Kissinger's aplomb, tactical flexibility,

and genius for self-exculpatory explanation (as in his fascinating memoirs) made him the most arresting Secretary of State since Dean Acheson.

Decline and Fall

Nixon and the economy. For Nixon domestic policy was admittedly secondary to foreign policy. "I've always thought this country could run itself domestic-ally without a President," he said in 1968. "All you need is a competent cabinet to run the country at home." His disposition was to mistrust the national government, to relax federal regulation, and to give free rein to business enterprise.

His most urgent economic problem was the inflation generated by the Indochina War. In 1970 the consumer price index was 16 percent higher than in 1967 and prices were still rising. In the tradition of economic orthodoxy, Nixon at first supposed that restrictive monetary policy would bring inflation under control. He denounced "jawboning" (official admonitions against price or wage increases) and price-wage guidelines, as developed in the Kennedy years. Instead he called for tight money and high interest rates.

The immediate effect of what he termed his "game plan" was to produce the first recession in a decade. But inflation did not stop. From January 1969 to August 1971, while unemployment rose from 3.5 to 6 percent, the cost of living increased by an astonishing 14.5 percent. Furthermore, inflation was overpricing American exports and weakening the dollar abroad. In 1971 the balance-of-payments deficit reached the record figure of $29.6 billion. There was, in addition, for the first time since 1893, a deficit in the balance of trade; imports exceeded exports by almost $3 billion.

"I will not take this nation down the road of wage and price controls," Nixon said in June 1970, "however politically expedient that may seem." But as "stagflation"—the combination of stagnation and inflation—persisted, Nixon jettisoned his game plan. Fortified by the appointment of a Texas Democrat, John B. Connally, as Secretary of the Treasury, Nixon declared himeslf a Keynesian in the summer of 1971 and on August 15 announced a startling reversal of economic course: a ninety-day price-wage freeze (Phase 1) to be followed in November by Phase 2, a system of wage and price controls. Inflation promptly subsided for 1971 and 1972. In his August announcement Nixon also suspended the convertibility of dollars into gold, thereby making American goods more competitive in world markets. This was followed in December by the formal devaluation of the dollar. These measures meant the end of the international monetary system set up at Bretton Woods (see p. 765) based on the convertibility of the dollar into gold and resulted in a new system of floating exchange rates.

Social policy. The liberal tide of the Kennedy-Johnson years was not yet spent and, despite Nixon's conservative inclinations, shaped much domestic legislation in his first term. Health maintenance organizations, student loan programs, low-income housing, the arts and humanities—all received increased federal support. In 1969–70 Congress laid

down a national environmental policy, establishing the Environmental Protection Agency (EPA) to combat the pollution of air and water. The Occupational Safety and Health Act of 1970 required employers engaged in interstate commerce to furnish working conditions free of hazards to life and health and set up the Occupational Safety and Health Administration (OSHA) to enforce industrial safety standards. Businesspeople criticized both EPA and OSHA for meddlesome regulation and increased production costs. But the two new agencies materially improved the nation's air and water and the safety of the workplace.

The welfare system, partly federal and partly local in character, posed difficult problems, stemming from the remarkable population growth in the postwar years. The war boom had reversed the decline in the birth rate that had occurred during the depression, while medical advances—penicillin and other antibiotics, anti-polio vaccines, new surgical techniques—reduced the death rate. Population, which had grown by only 9 million in the thirties, grew by 18 million in the forties and by 27 million in the fifties—an increase in this last decade almost equal to the country's total population a century earlier. The result by the late sixties was a flood of workers swamping an already overcrowded labor market. From 1947 to 1970 the labor force increased by 25 million, more than 40 percent.

One consequence was an enormous expansion of relief rolls, especially in the category of Aid to Families with Dependent Children (AFDC). The number of persons on welfare doubled from 1961 to 1972. Unemployment, induced by Nixon's high-interest policy, swelled the rolls by nearly 30 percent in 1970 alone. Of those receiving welfare in 1971, more than half were children, one sixth were old people, one tenth were blind or otherwise disabled. AFDC benefits went mostly to household headed by females. Less than 1 percent of the recipients were employable males. Widely condemned for fraud and waste, the system also was believed to drive employed fathers from the household so that their families could qualify for public assistance.

Nixon's initial answer was a bold proposal to replace AFDC by a Family Assistance Program. FAP was a path-breaking concept, but its provision for a guaranteed minimum income antagonized conservatives, while a "work requirement" alienated liberals. After passing the House in 1970, the FAP failed in the Senate and thereafter was dropped from Nixon's agenda. The Administration now approached the welfare problem in other ways. In 1972 Congress raised social security payments by 20 percent and added cost-of-living "indexing" to compensate for inflation. It also liberalized eligibility and benefits in the food-stamp program, a New Deal innovation revived in the Kennedy years.

My fears about the American leadership classes had been confirmed and deepened by what I had seen and experienced during my first four years as President. In politics, academics, and the arts, and even in the business community and the churches, there was a successful and fashionable negativism which, in my judgment, reflected an underlying loss of will....

At the beginning of my second term, Congress, the bureaucracy, and the media were still working in concert to maintain the ideas and ideology of the traditional Eastern liberal establishment that had come down to 1973 through the New Deal, the New Frontier, and the Great Society. Now I planned to give expression to the more conservative values and beliefs of the New Majority throughout the country and use my power to put some teeth into my New American Revolution.

As I noted in my diary, "This is going to be quite a shock to the establishment, but it is the only way, and probably the last time, that we can get government under control before it gets so big that it submerges the individual completely and destroys the dynamism which makes the American system what it is."

From Richard M. Nixon, *The Memoirs of Richard Nixon* (1978).

By 1975 food stamp enrollment approached 20 million, and the program cost $5 billion a year. In 1973 Congress passed the Comprehensive Employment and Training Act. The nationwide CETA system made government in effect an employer of last resort by providing public service jobs as well as job training for the unemployed.

With exceptions like CETA, the Nixon social policy represented a shift from a "service strategy"—the attempt to help the poor through specialized service programs—to an "income strategy"—helping the poor by giving them cash or some cash equivalent, such as food stamps. The services strategy was considered to imply that government and the welfare professional knew best what was good for the poor. The income strategy supposedly gave the poor greater freedom to make their own choices. Though critics felt that cash transfers to poor families would not alleviate such structural problems as education, job training, housing, and transportation, the underlying philosophy had wide appeal. By 1975 income-support programs claimed nearly one third of the federal budget.

Nixon's social policy represented to a degree an extension of the New Frontier and the Great Society. As in foreign policy and in his 1971 resort to incomes policy, he permitted pragmatism to overcome ideology. "Don't you realize," his aide John D. Ehrlichman said to his economic adviser Arthur Burns, "the President doesn't have a philosophy?"

The New Federalism. Still, if Nixon lacked conservative principles, he retained conservative instincts. In the longer run, his hope was to reduce the role of the national government. During the 1968 campaign he talked of the need to "re-establish the sense of community" that he felt had been undermined by the centralizing approach of the New Frontier and the Great Society. "After a third of a century of power flowing from the people and the States to Washington," he said in August 1969, "it is time for a New Federalism in which power, funds, and responsibility will flow from Washington to the States and to the people."

In order to equip local government to assume federal functions, Nixon promoted an idea that had originated in the Jackson Administration (see p. 229) and received modern form in the Johnson Administration—the distribution of federal revenues to the states. "Revenue-sharing" meant federal aid to state and local authorities through "no-strings" money grants rather than through grants to special categories, like the elderly or the disabled. The State and Local Fiscal Assistance Act of 1972 provided for the distribution of $30 billion in unrestricted funds to states and localities over the next five years.

Critics doubted that state and local units were more honest and efficient than the national government. They also contended that "no-strings" revenue-sharing discriminated against the cities, the poor, and the minorities—all beneficiaries of the now-diminished categorical grant-in-aid programs. Categorical grants were plainly better adapted than block grants to the carrying-out of national social priorities. Still, revenue-sharing won support, especially from financially hard-pressed local governments, because of its flexibility, and it was applauded by citizens who considered the national government too remote and unmanageable. In the end, revenue-sharing was the notable achievement of Nixon's New Federalism.

Concentration of presidential power. In pushing his policies, Nixon faced the fact of Democratic control in both houses of Congress. The congressional majority had priorities of its own and the capacity to forward them by legislation, especially through the appropriations power. Confronted by statutes that conflicted with his own priorities, Nixon increasingly responded by refusing to spend funds voted by Congress.

Impoundment, as this practice was called, had a minor status in law and custom. Previous Presidents had used it, however, to effect savings or to stretch out the spending of funds, not to set aside the expressed will of Congress. Nixon not only impounded far more money than any of his predecessors—by 1973, his impoundments affected more than a hundred federal programs and reached the level of $15 billion—but used impoundment to nullify laws passed by the legislative branch and even claimed this power as a constitutional right. The courts later rejected this claim and ordered the release of impounded funds.

Nixon also expanded the unconditional theory of executive privilege set forth in the Eisenhower Administration. Kennedy and Johnson had returned to the traditional and restricted view of the President's power to withhold information from Congress. But Nixon claimed presidential denial as an inherent and unreviewable constitutional right. His Attorneys General asserted on his behalf that Congress had no power to compel testimony over presidential objection from any one of the 2.5 million employees in the executive branch.

In addition to concentrating power in the executive branch at the expense of Congress, he sought to concentrate power in the White House at the expense of the executive departments. Where Franklin D. Roosevelt had fought the Second World War with no more than a dozen special assistants, Nixon by 1972 had forty-eight—the largest White House staff in history. Nixon and his White House aides, especially H. R. Haldeman and John Ehrlichman, had not only a general determination, with which other Presidents could have sympathized, to make the executive bureaucracy responsive to presidential purpose but a specific mistrust of the civil service as Democratic and hostile. They soon began to fear that even members of the Cabinet were becoming the prisoners of their civil servants. Cabinet meetings became infrequent, and Cabinet members found it increasingly difficult to gain access to Nixon. In time the more independent-minded among them departed.

The "great silent majority." "I felt," Nixon wrote in his memoirs, "that the Silent Majority of Americans, with its roots mainly in the Midwest, the West, and the South, had simply never been encouraged to give the Eastern liberal elite a run for its money for control of the nation's key institutions." In Nixon's view, the solid average American, harassed by government, crime, inflation, taxes, riots, drugs, pornography, welfare chiselers, and uppity blacks, represented the foundation of a future conservative majority. "I was anxious," he recalled, "to defend the 'square' virtues"—law-and-order, the flag, and opposition to drugs, abortion and the permissive society. While Nixon's margin over Humphrey in 1968 had been exceedingly narrow, if George Wallace's 13.5 percent could be added to Nixon's 43.4 percent, Nixon would be unbeatable in 1972.

The great bulk of the electorate, it was pointed out, was unyoung, unpoor, and unblack. In particular, there seemed an unprecedented chance to make the South into a Republican stronghold. This led to the "Southern strategy"—a slowdown on civil rights under the policy of "benign neglect"; attacks on the busing of pupils as a means of achieving school integration; a rhetorical barrage against welfare, crime, the media of opinion, and the intellectual community. That strategy had the further advantage of prying away from the Democrats white blue-collar families in the North who felt threatened by racial adjustments demanded of them at a distance by upper-class liberals.

Vice President Agnew emerged as a particularly arresting spokesman for law and order. His gaudy rhetoric (antiwar protesters, he said, were "an effete corps of impudent snobs") and addiction to alliteration ("the nattering nabobs of negativism") won him a devoted national audience. "It is time for the preponderant majority, the responsible citizens of this country, to assert their rights," Agnew said in 1969. "If, in challenging, we polarize the American people, I say it is time for a positive polarization." Agnew concentrated his attack on television and the press, demanding in somewhat menacing terms that they be "made more responsive to the views of the nation."

The antiwar demonstrations of 1969–70, and especially the outbursts following the Kent State shootings, encouraged Nixon to pursue a strategy of confrontation, confident that the majority of voters were fed up with protest and violence. This policy roused doubts among his own appointees: Secretary of the Interior Walter J. Hickel wrote Nixon that his Administration appeared "to lack appropriate concern for the attitude of a great mass of Americans—our young people." Nevertheless Nixon made law and order the central theme of the 1970 midterm election. This appeal failed. The Republicans lost nine seats in the House and eleven governorships but gained two seats in the Senate.

The reconstitution of the Supreme Court was an important element in the strategy. Nixon, who during his campaign had blamed the Warren Court for encouraging crime, now took advantage of vacancies to appoint justices more to his liking. The retirement of Warren in 1968 enabled him to designate Warren Burger, a conservative, as the new Chief Justice. Nixon's next two appointments, both federal judges from the South, were rejected by the Senate, the first because of conflict of interests, the second because of intellectual mediocrity. Subsequently three less vulnerable nominees were approved.

The Burger Court was markedly more conservative than the Warren Court, especially in its tendency to restrict news media in the gathering of information and to decide criminal law cases in favor of the police and prosecution rather than the defendant. But Burger lacked Warren's skill in massing the Court, and the intellectual leader of the conservatives, William Rehnquist, was too extreme to carry many of his brethren with him. For a time, the Burger Court left the Warren inheritance more intact than the conservatives had hoped or liberals feared. While qualifying the *Miranda* rule, which Nixon had particularly denounced in the campaign, it refused opportunities to reverse it. It sustained the cause of school desegregation, approving mandatory busing in *Swann* v. *Charlotte-Mecklenburg* (1971). Some decisions greatly dismayed the right—the Pentagon Papers case (*New York Times* v. *United States*, 1971), in which the Court ruled against prior restraint of the rights of publication; *Furman* v. *Georgia* (1972), in which it outlawed mandatory capital punishment statutes; and, most striking of all *Roe* v. *Wade* (1973), in which it upset state laws prohibiting abortion.

The 1972 election. As 1972 approached, the front-runner for the Democratic nomination was Senator Edmund Muskie of Maine. But Senator George McGovern of South Dakota, a Second World War hero and former professor of history, ardently liberal in his outlook and an early opponent of the Indochina War, succeeded in uniting the Robert Kennedy and Eugene McCarthy forces of 1968. Benefiting by reforms in the delegate-selection process brought about by a Democratic party commission he himself had chaired, McGovern won first-ballot nomination at the Democratic convention in July. Senator Thomas Eagleton of Missouri, his choice as running mate, retired from the ticket after failing to disclose to McGovern a history of psychiatric treatment. His replacement was Sargent Shriver of Maryland, former head of Kennedy's Peace

McGovern and Shriver: off stride

Corps and Johnson's war on poverty and later ambassador to Paris. In August the Republicans renominated Nixon and Agnew.

Thrown off stride by the Eagleton affair, McGovern never recovered momentum. In addition, his proposal during the primaries of his own version of a guaranteed minimum income won him a reputation for radicalism. Republicans denounced him as the champion of "acid, abortion and amnesty." Determined to win over those who had voted for Wallace in 1968, Republican campaigners played astutely upon racial and cultural nerves. The success of the "Southern strategy" was guaranteed when Wallace, disabled in an assassination attempt in May, decided not to field a party of his own. Then Kissinger's claim twelve days before the election that peace was at hand in Vietnam neutralized McGovern's strongest issue. Nor did the Twenty-sixth Amendment, ratified in 1971 and lowering the voting age to eighteen, help the Democrats as much as they had expected.

Nixon sailed to an impressive victory, losing only Massachusetts and the District of Columbia. While the turnout of eligible voters continued to decline, falling to 55.4 percent, he polled 46 million votes against 28.5 million for McGovern, winning the largest proportion (60.8 percent) of the popular vote since 1964 and the largest margin in the Electoral College (520 to 17) since 1936. However, the Democrats added two to their Senate majority and retained control of the House. As in the 1950s, the voters balanced a Republican President with a Democratic Congress.

Watergate. On the night of June 17, 1972, five men, equipped with cameras and electronic bugging devices, had been arrested in the offices of the Democratic National Committee in the Watergate building in Washington. The burglars gave false names, but one, James McCord, was soon identified as chief of security for the Committee to Re-elect the President. The Committee's chairman, John Mitchell, a Nixon intimate who had resigned as Attorney General to run his campaign, promptly denied any involvement on the part of the organization (soon known popularly as CREEP). The incident had little impact on the presidential election. McGovern called the Nixon Administration "the most corrupt" in American history. Few voters listened.

It is not clear whether Nixon knew in advance about the break-in. There can be no doubt, however, that the atmosphere he created in the White House stimulated those around him to lawless action. Underneath his conventional exterior Nixon was a man of agitated and compulsive emotion. "There was another side to him," John Ehrlichman said later, "like the flat, dark side of the moon." He saw life as a battlefield and believed that the nation was swarming with personal enemies bent on his destruction. He was, wrote Jeb Stuart Magruder, CREEP's deputy director, "absolutely paranoid about criticism." The campus riots after Cambodia in 1970, along with the Weathermen and the Black Panthers, fed this paranoia. When John Dean became White House counsel in July 1970, he found, he later said, "a climate of excessive concern

over the political impact of demonstrators, excessive concern over leaks, an insatiable appetite for political intelligence, all coupled with a do-it-yourself White House staff, regardless of the law." Musing about his enemies, Nixon told the White House hatchet man, Charles Colson, "One day we'll get them—we'll get them on the ground where we want them. And we'll stick our heels in, step on them hard and twist, right, Chuck?"

That spirit generated the Enemies List, circulated with the injunction to "use the available Federal machinery to screw our political enemies." In 1970 T. C. Huston, a White House aide, drew up a plan, adopted by Nixon, authorizing, in the name of national security, burglary, electronic surveillance, mail interception, and other practices forbidden by law. J. Edgar Hoover's protest compelled Nixon to rescind his order; but in 1971 Nixon, unsettled by Daniel Ellsberg's release of the Pentagon Papers, set up a secret White House unit known as "the plumbers" to effectuate the Huston plan. The plumbers soon burgled the office of Ellsberg's psychiatrist, forged official cables in an effort to implicate John F. Kennedy in the assassination of Ngo Dinh Diem, wiretapped foreign embassies, and engaged in other edifying activities. This was again done in the name of "national security"—words that, as Egil Krogh, a top plumber, later said "served to

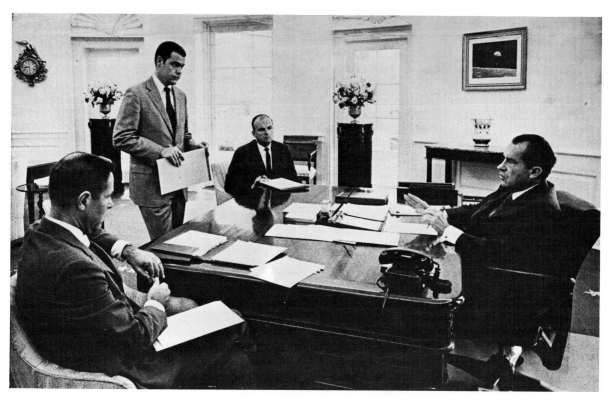

Nixon and staff: one of the most corrupt in American history

block critical analysis. . . . Freedom of the President to pursue his planned course was the ultimate national security objective."

In the winter of 1971–72 polls showed Nixon trailing Muskie and roused concern in the White House about the forthcoming election. The plumbers now moved into domestic politics and helped organize a campaign of "dirty tricks" designed to bring Muskie into disrepute. Early in 1972 G. Gordon Liddy, a plumber who became general counsel of CREEP, outlined larger plans of espionage and sabotage to Mitchell. In May the Democratic headquarters were entered for the first time; bugs were planted on telephones, and documents were copied. All was going well until the night of June 17.

The cover-up. Whether or not Nixon knew of the Watergate entry in advance, he knew about it immediately afterward. In February 1971 he had installed microphones in the White House to record all presidential conversations, and the tapes subsequently provided evidence of Nixon's response to Watergate. On June 20 he held a long conversation with Haldeman, of which eighteen and a half minutes were mysteriously erased from the tape. On June 23 Haldeman observed to him, "We're back in the problem area because the FBI is out of control." Nixon told him to tell the FBI, "Don't go any further into this case, period!" The reasons, he made clear, were political; the pretext would be national security.

The cover-up had begun. Incriminating documents were systematically destroyed. But there were problems. Neither the FBI—though Hoover, who died in May, was replaced by a complaisant political appointee—nor the CIA proved as pliable as the White House hoped. The cover-up strategy relied increasingly on two main elements—bribes and lies. Several hundred thousand dollars were raised to buy the silence of the Watergate defendants and the attendant plumbers. Everyone who knew the truth, from Nixon down, denied publicly and privately that Watergate was anything more than a personal adventure by those caught in the act. "Under my direction," Nixon told a press conference in August, "counsel to the President, Mr. Dean, has conducted an investigation. . . . I can say categorically that his investigation indicates that no one in the White House staff, no one in this Administration, presently employed, was involved in this very bizarre incident." Dean had made no such investigation or report.

In September a federal grand jury indicted the five Watergate burglars and two of the plumbers. Nixon congratulated Dean on the fact that the indictments had gone no further. He added, "I want the most comprehensive notes on all of those that had tried to do us in. . . . They are asking for it and they are going to get it. . . . We have not used the power in the first four years, as you know. We have never used it. We haven't used the Bureau and we haven't used the Justice Department, but things are going to change now."

Things indeed were going to change. In January 1973 the Watergate trial began before Judge John J. Sirica. On February 2 Sirica said he was "not satisfied" that the full story had been disclosed and called for further investigation. On February 7 the Senate voted to establish a select committee to inquire into charges of corruption in the 1972 election. The chairman was Senator Sam Ervin of North Carolina. Robert Woodward and Carl Bernstein, two young reporters on the *Washington Post*, were meanwhile beginning to uncover sources in the executive branch, especially a mysterious and knowledgeable figure whom they identified only as Deep Throat.

Impeachment. "We have a cancer—within—close to the Presidency, that's growing," John Dean told Nixon on March 21. "It's growing daily. It's compounding." Two days later James McCord broke the ranks of the Watergate group, saying there had been perjury in the trial and political pressure on the defendants to plead guilty and remain silent. The conspiracy was unraveling. The problem now, as Nixon, Haldeman, and Ehrlichman saw it, was whom to throw to the wolves. One candidate was Jeb Stuart Magruder. Another was the acting director of the FBI; "let him twist slowly, slowly in the wind," said Ehrlichman. Another, so Dean came to believe, was Dean himself. Another was John Mitchell; "he's the big enchilada," said Ehrlichman. In April Dean and Magruder, fearing that they were being set up as fall guys, followed McCord's example and turned state's evidence. On April 30 Haldeman and Ehrlichman were thrown to the wolves. As for Nixon, his resolve was still, in the language of the tapes, to "tough it out."

On May 17 the Ervin Committee began public hearings, carried by television to an enraptured nation. At the same time, Elliot Richardson, up for confirmation as Attorney General, agreed under senatorial pressure to appoint an independent special prosecutor. He named Professor Archibald Cox of the Harvard Law School, Kennedy's solicitor general. Both Ervin and Cox now pressed their somewhat competitive inquiries. Dean's testimony before the Ervin Committee in June was especially precise and effective. Then in July the committee learned for the first time of the existence of the tapes. There began a struggle—Nixon, on the one hand; Ervin and Cox, on the other—for access to the tapes. Nixon, in his own words, stonewalled, claiming executive privilege first for his staff, later for the tapes and himself. Privately

P—*We are all in it together. This is a war. We take a few shots and it will be over. We will give them a few shots and it will be over. Don't worry. I wouldn't want to be on the other side right now.... I want the most comprehensive notes on all those who tried to do us in. They didn't have to do it. If we had had a very close election, and they were playing the other side I would understand this. No—they were doing this quite deliberately and they are asking for it and they are going to get it. We have not used the power in this first four years as you know. We have never used it. We have not used the Bureau and we have not used the Justice Department but things are going to change now. And they are either going to do it right or go.*

D—*What an exciting prospect.*

P—*Thanks. It has to be done. We have been (adjective deleted) fools for us to come into this election campaign and not do anything with regard to the Democratic Senators who are running, et cetera. And who the hell are they after? They are after us. It is absolutely ridiculous. It is not going to be that way any more.*

From a conversation in the White House between Richard Nixon and John Dean, September 15, 1972.

The Nixon White House

---

he denied, as to Elliot Richardson and other Republican leaders, knowledge or complicity, while publicly he put out a succession of statements, each admitting a little more than the one before.

In the meantime, another issue arose to assail the beleaguered Administration. Investigations by the federal attorney in Maryland concluded that Spiro T. Agnew had received bribes as governor of Maryland and subsequently as Vice President. Though Nixon said in August, "My confidence in his integrity has not been shaken," the evidence was compelling. In October, Agnew resigned his position and confessed to falsifying his income tax returns. He was fined $10,000 and put on probation for three years. In exchange, the other charges were dropped. Acting under the Twenty-fifth Amendment, which had been ratified in 1967, Nixon appointed a new Vice President, Gerald Ford, the minority leader of the House. After Agnew resigned, Nixon said to Richardson, "Now that that's over, we can get rid of Cox."

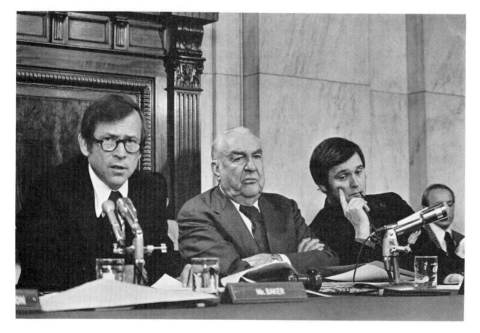

Ervin Committee: they reached an enraptured nation

Cox, in his pursuit of the tapes, was pressing too close. When the Court of Appeals required that Nixon turn over nine tapes to Judge Sirica, Nixon refused to comply. Nixon then ordered Richardson to fire Cox. Richardson declined to do so and resigned, as did his Deputy Attorney General. The ranking official left in the Justice Department carried out Nixon's order. The "Saturday night massacre" produced a "firestorm" of national protest, with nearly a half million telegrams inundating the White House in the next week. Newspapers and magazines called for Nixon's resignation. Impeachment resolutions were introduced in the House of Representatives. Under the explosion of public indignation, Nixon yielded the nine tapes.

It was the beginning of the end. More and more of the lesser Watergate actors were indicted. New issues emerged. Nixon, it developed, had paid only $792 in federal income tax in 1970, $878 in 1971; his claim for tax deductions on his vice-presidential papers had been illegally backdated to escape the provisions of a new tax law, and he owed the government nearly half a million dollars. Millions of federal dollars had been dubiously spent on the improvement of his houses in San Clemente, California, and Key Biscayne, Florida. It was another Nixon first. No previous chief executive had ever tried to make himself rich out of the Presidency.

In December the House Judiciary Committee began an inquiry to determine whether there were grounds for impeachment. The committee immediately confronted a constitutional question. The Founding Fathers had regarded impeachment, in Madison's words, as a means of defending the community against "the incapacity, negligence or perfidy of the chief Magistrate." Hamilton had written in *The Federalist* No. 65 that it applied to "those offences which proceed from the misconduct of public men, or, in other words, from the abuse or violation of some public trust. They are of a nature which may with peculiar propriety be denominated POLITICAL." Impeachment in the original view did not require the breaking of any particular law. However, officials confronted by the threat of impeachment had always argued that impeachment applied only to violations of specific criminal statutes.

Nixon, hopeful that no statutory crime could be proved against him, continued to stonewall. "I'm not a crook," he cried in November. There was more talk of executive privilege and of defending the institution of the Presidency. In March 1974 a federal grand jury indicted Mitchell, Haldeman, Ehrlichman, Colson, and three others. Nixon was named as a "co-conspirator," unindicted because of prosecutorial doubts whether a President could be brought to trial. As Leon Jaworski, the new special prosecutor, subpoenaed more tapes, Nixon decided to anticipate the inevitable

and release the tapes himself. It was a fatal miscalculation. The reaction was worse than to the Saturday night massacre. The tapes displayed Nixon as mean-spirited, indecisive, bigoted, amoral, and—even with a multitude of "expletives deleted" from the transcript—foul-mouthed. The demand for resignation, even among Republicans, rose to a new crescendo.

In mid-July, after weeks of hearings, the House Judiciary Committee voted three articles of impeachment, charging Nixon with obstruction of justice in the Watergate case, with abuse of presidential power in a number of specified respects, and with unconstitutionally defying its subpoenas. Six Republicans joined with the Democratic majority in passing the first article, seven on the second, two on the third.

In the meantime, the Supreme Court had ruled in *U.S.* v. *Nixon* (1974) that Nixon must turn over tapes that might contain evidence of crime. Transcripts of his meetings with Haldeman six days after the break-in left no doubt that he had planned the cover-up. This was at last the "smoking pistol" required to still all doubts. Four Republicans on the Judiciary Committee who had voted against impeachment reversed their positions. Senator Goldwater said that Nixon could count on no more than fifteen votes in the Senate. Four days later, on August 9, Nixon resigned—the first President to do so in the history of the republic. History would not forget Watergate. But it would remember Nixon too for the sense of international strategy that led him to seek new directions in world affairs.

The Imperial Presidency. Resignation left the exact degree of Nixon's guilt undetermined. But the Watergate inquiries did prove that Nixon's Administration was indeed the most corrupt in American history. More than forty members of the Administration underwent criminal prosecution, led by those particular champions of law and order, Agnew and Mitchell. A Vice President, two Cabinet members, a dozen members of the White House staff, and nearly fifteen others scattered through the executive branch pleaded guilty or were convicted after trial.

The principle was established that even the President was not above the law and the Constitution. Most Americans welcomed Nixon's resignation not alone with relief but with a measure of self-congratulation. In the end, it was said, the system had worked. Others took less satisfaction in the result. If Nixon had kept no tapes, or if he had burned them, or if there had not been in the right place at the right time a senator like Ervin, a judge like Sirica, a newspaper like the *Washington Post*, Nixon and his associates might well have survived. It seemed a very near thing.

Yet, as Ervin subsequently reflected, "One of the great advantages of the three separate branches of gov-

In his conduct of the office of President of the United States, Richard M. Nixon, in violation of his constitutional oath faithfully to execute the office of President of the United States ... and in violation of his constitutional duty to take care that the laws be faithfully executed, has prevented, obstructed, and impeded the administration of justice.... Richard M. Nixon, using the powers of his high office, engaged personally and through his subordinates and agents in a course of conduct or plan designed to delay, impede, and obstruct the investigation of such unlawful entry; to cover up, conceal and protect those responsible; and to conceal the existence and scope of other unlawful covert activities.... In all of this, Richard M. Nixon has acted in a manner contrary to his trust as President and subversive of constitutional government, to the great prejudice of the cause of law and justice and to the manifest injury of the people of the United States.

    Wherefore Richard M. Nixon, by such conduct, warrants impeachment and trial, and removal from office.

Article II

    Using the powers of the office of President of the United States, Richard M. Nixon ... has repeatedly engaged in conduct violating the constitutional rights of citizens, impairing the due and proper administration of justice in the conduct of lawful inquiries, or contravening the laws governing agencies of the executive branch....

    Wherefore, Richard M. Nixon, by such conduct, warrants impeachment and trial, and removal from office.

Article III

    In his conduct of the office of President of the United States, Richard M. Nixon ... has failed without lawful cause or excuse to produce papers and things, as directed by duly authorized subpoenas ... and willfully disobeyed such subpoenas ... thereby assuming for himself functions and judgments necessary to the exercise of the sole power of impeachment vested by the Constitution in the House of Representatives....

    Wherefore, Richard M. Nixon, by such conduct, warrants impeachment and trial, and removal from office.

From the House of Representatives Committee on the Judiciary, August 4, 1974.

The House Judiciary Committee: three articles of impeachment

Resignation of an imperial President

ernment is that it's difficult to corrupt all three at the same time." A new interest developed in the problem of presidential power and accountability. The separation of powers had worked well enough through American history to restrain presidential aggrandizement in domestic affairs. But foreign affairs, as Vietnam had already demonstrated, constituted the grave weakness in the original system of accountability. Confronted by presidential initiatives abroad, Congress had come to lack confidence in its information and judgment and was happy to abdicate responsibility to the executive. This was especially the case after the Second World War because the last period of sustained congressional intervention in foreign policy, from the rejection of the Treaty of Versailles to the rigid neutrality legislation of the 1930s, had given Congress itself a severe institutional inferiority complex. International crisis had thus opened the great breach in the system of accountability.

Nixon's particular innovation was to take the powers that had flowed to the Presidency to meet foreign threats, real or imagined, and try to project them for his own purposes at home. "My reading of history taught me," he later wrote, "that when all the leadership institutions of a nation become paralyzed by self-doubt and second thoughts, that nation cannot long survive unless those institutions are reformed, replaced, or circumvented. In my second term I was prepared to adopt whichever of these three methods—or whichever combination of them—was necessary."

Since the growth of presidential power had been in the longer run as much a consequence of congressional abdication as of presidential usurpation, Congress had a major role to play in containing the Imperial Presidency, as it came to be known, and restoring the balance of the Constitution. The Vietnam experience had drawn attention to the expropriation by the Presidency of the war-making power confided by the Constitution to Congress. In 1973 Congress passed a War Powers Act that, on the one hand, gave the President for the first time explicit authority to go to war in certain specified circumstances but on the other required the termination of hostilities within ninety days unless Congress explicitly authorized their continuation. The ambiguity of the statute left unresolved the question whether the act enlarged or restricted a President's power to go to war on his own.

In domestic affairs, Congress passed in 1974 the Congressional Budget and Impoundment Control Act. This law instituted procedures to prevent the unlimited impoundment policies of the Nixon era. It also established a legislative budget process comparable to the one Congress had given the President in the Budget and Accounting Act of 1921 (see p. 624). In the same year Congress passed the Federal Election Campaign Act providing for partial federal financing of presidential campaigns and seeking to limit the role of private money in elections. In *Buckley* v. *Valeo* (1976), the Supreme Court sustained the public financing provisions but, by equating money with speech under the First Amendment, removed limits on personal spending.

Watergate further stimulated a new determination to open up the workings of government. States passed "sunshine laws" designed to increase citizen access to governmental decisions. Political candidates were called on to disclose the sources of their income. A national Freedom of Information Act, passed by Congress in 1966, acquired new vitality. The spotlight even penetrated into what had been the most secretive and sacrosanct agencies of government—the CIA and the FBI. Congressional investigations in 1975–76 revealed extraordinary abuses of power by both agencies—not only the CIA assassination and covert action projects but the FBI's use of *agents provocateurs*, burglaries, wiretapping, mail intercepts, and even J. Edgar Hoover's incredible effort to drive Martin Luther King, Jr., to suicide. The public reaction to these revelations dethroned Hoover posthumously from his long reign as a national hero and produced demands for congressional oversight over the intelligence community.

The Presidency Restored

A Ford, not a Lincoln. Gerald R. Ford, the new President, was sixty-one years old. A Republican wheelhorse, he had served a quarter-century in the House

Gerald R. Ford and Nelson Rockefeller, February 1974

"I am a Ford, not a Lincoln," he had said disarmingly after being sworn in as Vice President; and, after being sworn in as President, "I am acutely aware that you have not elected me as your President by your ballots." Complying with the Twenty-fifth Amendment, he named Governor Nelson Rockefeller of New York as his Vice President. This meant that for the first time in American history both the President and the Vice President had come to office and power not, like all their predecessors, through election but through appointment—a result unintended by the drafters of the Twenty-fifth Amendment seven years before and disconcerting to those who valued the provision in the Constitution (Article II, Section 1) stipulating that the President and Vice President were to "be elected."

A people whose nerves had been worn ragged by Nixon's deceit and mystification found the new President's candor and accessibility initially reassuring. Then, thirty days after he took office, Ford stunned the nation by granting Nixon a "full, free and absolute pardon" for all crimes he committed against the United States during his Presidency. Ford's concern was that a public trial of the disgraced former President would have a divisive effect. His purpose, he explained, was "to heal the wounds throughout the United States."

without ever achieving consideration in any Republican convention as a candidate for President or even for Vice President. Democrats underrated him. He was "so dumb," Lyndon Johnson used to say, "that he can't walk and chew gum at the same time." But even Democrats liked him as an honest, open, even-tempered politician unaccustomed to converting political disagreements into personal enmities.

The effect was the opposite. Most Americans were outraged by the double standard that punished those who had executed Nixon's wishes but spared Nixon himself. Ford seemed to have espoused the principle, dubious in a democracy, that the greater the power the less the accountability. Even many who did

Recession, 1975: the worst in nearly forty years

not wish to put the ex-President behind bars felt that pardon would have been more appropriate after the evidence of Nixon's misdeeds had been clearly established in court and recorded for history. In one stroke Ford inflicted a wound on his Administration from which it never recovered.

Inflation. Nixon's abandonment of price and wage controls after the 1972 election had led to a rapid renewal of inflation—from 3.4 percent in 1971–72 to nearly 9 percent in 1973 and over 12 percent in 1974. The value of the dollar continued to fall—from $1 in 1940 to 50 cents in 1957, 40 cents when Nixon came to office and 25 cents in 1976.

The Ford Administration, ideologically opposed to controls, resorted to the orthodox panacea and tried to combat inflation by slowing down the economy. The result in 1974–75 was the worst recession in nearly forty years. National output had its sharpest decline since the end of war production in 1945–46. Unemployment rose to nearly 9 percent of the labor force—8.25 million people—by mid-1975. By 1976 recession brought the inflation rate down to 4.8 percent, though at painful human cost.

The energy shock. OPEC's price increases and oil embargo of October 1973 had extensive domestic re-

percussions. American economic growth had been based in large part on cheap energy. But signficant changes had taken place in the pattern of energy production. In the 1870s 90 percent of American energy came from sustainable sources, like water power. A century later more than 90 percent came from nonrenewable mineral sources—44 percent from petroleum, 32 percent from natural gas, 18 percent from coal. Moreover, domestic coal production had begun to decline after 1947, domestic oil extraction after 1970, domestic natural gas production after 1974. Estimates of untapped domestic reserves of mineral fuels began to decline too.

In the meantime, demand continued to grow. By the 1970s the United States, with 6 percent of the world's population, was consuming one-third of the world's energy. The increased reliance on oil was accompanied by an increased reliance on imports. Though the United States remained for many years the world's top oil producer, oil imports rose from 8 percent of demand in 1950 to 39 percent in 1976. A steadily increasing proportion of imported oil came from the Middle East—about 30 percent by the early 1970s. Here seven western oil companies—"the Seven Sisters"—had long dominated the field. As OPEC became more aggressive on behalf of the producing countries, the major oil companies, which, despite the

OPEC meeting, 1973: increasingly aggressive

nationalization of their local interests, were still involved in the oil fields because of long-term management contracts and guaranteed access to the oil, became the machinery for maintaining the OPEC cartel—once masters, now servants.

As early as 1952, the Materials Policy Commission, headed by William S. Paley, had warned the Truman Administration of the "extraordinarily rapid rate at which we are utilizing our materials and energy resources." Such warnings, repeated from time to time over a generation, had been ignored in the enthusiasm for economic growth. The oil embargo at last dramatized the resources issue. For a few months, pumps went empty at filling stations, cars queued up for gasoline, speed limits were reduced, conservation measures encouraged.

Energy was now squarely on the national agenda. The Ford Administration favored "deregulation" of oil prices on the theory that higher prices would reduce consumption and that higher profits would encourage production. Many Democrats felt that decontrol would swell oil company profits at the expense of the consumer. Everyone agreed, however, on the need to lower domestic demand through measures of energy conservation. Everyone agreed too on the importance of developing alternative sources of energy. The Energy Policy and Conservation Act of 1975 affirmed these objectives.

The Presidency survives. During the Watergate crisis some had feared that the exposure of Nixon would damage the Presidency as an institution. The aftermath showed the Presidency to be relatively inde-structible. Despite his stigma of illegitimacy as an unelected President, despite his lack of appetite for power and adulation, despite his shaky position in his own party and in the country, Ford drew strength from the continuing authority of the office. When the Democrats greatly increased their congressional majorities in 1974, Ford responded by using the veto power with almost unprecedented freedom, vetoing more public bills in his first months than any President had vetoed in so short a period. Few of his vetoes were overridden.

Presidential authority remained real, if diminished, in foreign affairs. While Ford, following the example of Truman (with whom he liked to compare himself) rather than that of Lyndon Johnson, reconstructed his Cabinet with some promptitude, he retained Kissinger as Secretary of State, thereby ensuring continuity in foreign policy. When Cambodian communists seized an unarmed American ship, the *Mayagüez*, in May 1975, Ford retaliated by ordering air strikes and sending in the marines. Congress joined in the general applause, though Ford had merely informed legislators of his action, rather than consulting them in the spirit of the War Powers Act. Skeptics noted that more marines were killed in the affair than sailors rescued.

The 1976 election. Ford beat back a strong challenge from Ronald Reagan, a former Hollywood actor, a popular governor of California and now the hero of the Republican right, to take his party's nomination. The President's desire to propitiate conservative Republicans had led him to abandon Nelson Rockefeller, and his vice presidential candidate, selected to cheer the Reaganites, was Senator Robert Dole of Kansas. For the Democrats James Earl Carter, Jr., who preferred to style himself Jimmy, a former governor of Georgia almost unknown to the nation, emerged as candidate from a series of arduous primaries. He chose the liberal Senator Walter F. Mondale of Minnesota as his running mate.

The campaign was unenlightening. Neither candidate distinguished himself in a series of three debates. Carter, a man of sharp intelligence but enigmatic views, rested his case more on moralistic reassurance—"I'll never lie to you," he promised his audiences—than on clarity in policy. Condemning Washington's "horrible, bloated bureaucracy," pledg-

ing "a government that is as good and honest and decent . . . and as filled with love as are the American people," Carter sought support as a political outsider who would restore integrity to government.

Each candidate, in accepting $22 million of federal money for the fall campaign, renounced private-fund raising. Ford cut down Carter's early lead, but Carter won the popular vote by 40.3 million to 38.5 million and the Electoral College by 297 to 241. Voter turnout continued to decline—from 55.4 percent in 1972 to 53.3 percent in 1976. In its revulsion against the abuse of government power by "insiders," the electorate turned to a classic "outsider," rejecting an honest and likable but pedestrian President.

Suggestions for Reading

NIXON AND FORD

RN: The Memoirs of Richard Nixon* (1978) is a good deal more revealing, sometimes inadvertently so, than *A Time to Heal: The Autobiography of Gerald Ford* (1979). Nixon biographers have been (understandably) tempted into unverifiable psychoanalytic speculation; but, this aside, F. M. Brodie, *Richard Nixon: The Shaping of His Character** (1980), contains useful information, and Garry Wills, *Nixon Agonistes** (1970), is arresting portraiture. Jules Witcover describes Nixon's political comeback in *The Resurrection of Richard Nixon* (1970). White House associates offer testimony in H. R.

Haldeman, *The Ends of Power** (1978); John Dean, *Blind Ambition: The White House Years** (1976); William Safire, *Before the Fall* (1975); John Ehrlichman, *Witness to Power: The Nixon Years** (1982), as well as in his novel *The Company** (1976); and Raymond Price, *With Nixon* (1977). Spiro T. Agnew justifies himself in *Go Quietly . . . or Else* (1980). R. T. Hartmann, *Palace Politics: An Inside Account of the Ford Years* (1980), is lively and candid.

On public policy, A. J. Reichley, *Conservatives in an Age of Change: The Nixon and Ford Administrations** (1981), is discerning and readable. Nixon's domestic efforts are considered in D. P. Moynihan, *The Politics of a Guaranteed Income** (1973) and *Coping* (1973); R. P. Nathan, *The Plot That Failed** (1975); V. J. and Vee Burke, *Nixon's Good Deed: Welfare Reform** (1976); and Martin Anderson, *Welfare* (1978). P. R. Dommel, *The Politics of Revenue Sharing* (1974), discusses Nixon's New Federalism. For economic policy, see previously cited works by Goodwin and Stein; also A. R. Weber, *In Pursuit of Price Stability** (1973), and Arthur Burns, *Reflections of an Economic Policy-Maker** (1978). F. V. Malek, *Washington's Hidden Tragedy: The Failure to Make Government Work* (1978), offers a conservative assessment. D. E. Kash and R. W. Rycroft, *U.S. Energy Policy: Crisis and Complacency* (1984), recounts the evolution of energy policy since 1973.

As for the politics of the Nixon–Ford years, Samuel Lubell, *The Hidden Crisis in American Politics** (1970), and David Broder, *The Party's Over** (1972), are useful contemporaneous diagnoses; W. D. Burnham, *Critical Elections and the Mainsprings of American Politics** (1970), is a searching study by a political scientist. T. H. White, *The Making of a President 1972** (1973), covers the 1972 election. George McGovern, in his memoir *Grassroots* (1977), and Gary Hart, McGovern's campaign manager, in *Right from the Start: A Chronicle of the McGovern Campaign* (1973), present the Democratic view.

FOREIGN AFFAIRS

The memoirs by Henry Kissinger—*White House Years** (1979) and *Years of Upheaval* (1982)—are formidable, fascinating, flawed, and fundamental. S. M. Hersh, *The Price of Power: Kissinger in the Nixon White House** (1983), is a prosecutor's brief. Stanley Hoffmann, *Primacy or World Order** (1978) and *Dead Ends* (1984), are stimulating commentaries. A. E. Goodman, *The Lost Peace: America's Search for a Negotiated Settlement of the Vietnam War* (1978), and A. R. Isaacs, *Without Honor: Defeat in Vietnam and Cambodia* (1983), describe the last days of the Indochina War. On the Middle East, see W. B. Quandt, *Decade of Decision: American Foreign Policy Toward the Arab-Israeli Conflict, 1967–1976** (1978).

On nuclear strategy, in addition to work previously cited by Freedman, see Fred Kaplan, *The Wizards of Armageddon* (1983), and John Newhouse, *Cold Dawn: The Story of SALT* (1973).

CRISIS OF THE PRESIDENCY

Arthur Schlesinger, Jr., *The Imperial Presidency** (1973), portrays the growth of presidential power. T. E. Cronin, *The State of the Presidency** (2nd ed., 1980), and R. M. Pious, *The American Presidency** (1979), ably set forth recent thought about the Presidency. T. H. White, *Breach of Faith** (1975); Anthony Lukas, *Nightmare* (1976); and Jonathan Schell, *The Time of Illusion** (1976), are vivid surveys of Watergate and its aftermath. Carl Bernstein and Robert Woodward pursue the Watergate story in *All the President's Men** (1974), and Nixon's last days in the White House in *The Final Days** (1975). Leon Jaworski, *The Right and the Power** (1976), and Samuel Ervin, *The Whole Truth: The Watergate Conspiracy* (1980), sum up the case against Nixon. The growth of secrecy and deception in government are portrayed in David Wise, *The Politics of Lying** (1973), and Frank Donner, *The Age of Surveillance** (1980). For the Nixon Supreme Court, see Vincent Blasi, *The Burger Court: The Counterrevolution That Wasn't* (1983).

*Available in a paperback edition.

34

TIDES OF CONSERVATISM

Jimmy Carter, the thirty-ninth President, was fifty-two years old, a native of Georgia, a graduate of Annapolis, a nuclear engineer who had moved on to peanut farming and processing, and a "born again" Baptist of ostentatious piety. His political career had been limited to service in the Georgia legislature and a single term as governor. He was the first President elected from the deep South since Zachary Taylor, the first fundamentalist to run for the Presidency since William Jennings Bryan, the first ex-governor to win since Franklin Roosevelt, and the first successful businessman (unless Herbert Hoover be so regarded) to occupy the White House in American history. His lack of Washington experience was initially regarded, in light of Watergate, as a recommendation; and his election was taken to mark the liquidation of vexing issues—not only Watergate but, in view of his pledge to pardon draft resisters, the Indochina War and, in view of his accent and origin, even the Civil War.

From Negotiation to Confrontation

Carter and foreign affairs. Carter came to the Presidency with little background in world affairs. His main preparation for international relations had come from his association with the Trilateral Commission, a private group founded in 1973, composed of bankers and professors from North America, western Europe, and Japan, and dedicated to strengthening political and economic relationships in the noncommunist world.

From his commission acquaintances Carter plucked Cyrus Vance, a New York lawyer with long government experience, to serve as Secretary of State and Zbigniew Brzezinski, a political scientist and Soviet expert as special assistant for national security. Vance and Brzezinski differed however, in their approach to the Soviet Union. Vance was moderate and conciliatory by temperament, while Brzezinski, a native of Poland who came to America in 1953, wished to confront the Russians at every turn. Carter himself, inclining at times toward Vance and at times toward Brzezinski, left an impression of irresolution and vacillation. As Hamilton Jordan, the President's chief aide, said to Brzezinski, "Who the hell knows whether the President will not veer in some direction tomorrow or the day after tomorrow."

Human rights. In his inaugural address Carter struck what became his Administration's distinctive note in foreign policy. "We can never be indifferent to the fate of freedom elsewhere," he said. ". . . Our commitment to human rights must be absolute."

For forty years "human rights" had been emerging as an international purpose—implied in Roose-

870

velt's Four Freedoms (1941), proclaimed in the United Nations Charter (1945) and the Universal Declaration of Human Rights (1948), most recently embodied in Basket Three of the Helsinki Agreement (1975). It had also won increasing support in the United States. In the early 1970s Congress, rebelling against Kissinger's *Realpolitik*, began to force human rights standards on the executive, forbidding American aid to countries that engaged "in a consistent pattern of gross violations of internationally recognized human rights." Carter now seized on the issue both out of personal conviction and in order to give American foreign policy a moral content it had lacked in the Nixon-Ford years. It seemed a perfect unifying principle, gratifying both Cold Warriors, who wanted to indict the communist world, and idealists, who saw human rights as the only basis for lasting peace.

The human rights campaign proved, however, easier to announce than to execute. Advocates of détente argued that human-rights pressure jeopardized relations with the Soviet Union. Cold Warriors alleged that it undermined stalwart anti-communist allies, like Iran and Nicaragua. Carter himself was soon found visiting authoritarian nations, selling them arms, and saluting their leaders. This led to further charges of hypocrisy and double standards.

Yet inconsistency was inherent in the situation. In the nature of foreign affairs, human rights could be only one of several contending interests, competing against strategic, political, and economic claims on national policy. By establishing a Bureau of Human Rights in the State Department, Carter institutionalized the human-rights role in American foreign policy. For all its contradictions, the human-rights campaign helped restore the broken link between America and ordinary people around the world. It placed human rights on the world's agenda—and on the world's conscience.

The Middle East. Carter at first favored removing the perennially baffling problem of Israel and the Arab states to a Geneva conference, which would necessarily have included the Soviet Union and the Palestine Liberation Organization. Evidently fearful that decisions would be taken out of their hands, Anwar el-Sadat of Egypt and Menachem Begin, the former terrorist who had become Israeli prime minister in May 1977, acted on their own. In November 1977 Sadat undertook a spectacular personal mission to Israel, offering diplomatic recognition in exchange for the return of Arab territories occupied by Israel in 1967. Begin, a conservative nationalist, was ready to yield the Sinai peninsula but neither the Gaza Strip directly to the north nor the West Bank of the River Jordan; nor would he give ground on the question of political status for the Palestinians—a question that Kissinger

Camp David, 1978: Sadat, Carter, and Begin

America ... has abstained from interference in the concerns of others, even when conflict has been for principles to which she clings, as to the last vital drop that visits the heart.... Wherever the standard of freedom and Independence has been or shall be unfurled, there will her heart, her benedictions and her prayers be. But she goes not abroad, in search of monsters to destroy. She is the well-wisher to the freedom and independence of all. She is the champion and vindicator only of her own.

From John Quincy Adams, July 4, 1821.

Ordinarily it is very much wiser and more useful for us to concern ourselves with striving for our own moral and material betterment here at home than to concern ourselves with trying to better the condition of things in other nations. We have plenty of sins of our own to war against, and under ordinary circumstances we can do more for the general uplifting of humanity by striving with heart and soul to put a stop to civic corruption, to brutal lawlessness and violent race prejudices here at home than by passing resolutions about wrong-doing elsewhere.

From Theodore Roosevelt, December 6, 1904.

Because we are free we can never be indifferent to the fate of freedom elsewhere. Our moral sense dictates a clearcut preference for those societies which share with us an abiding respect for individual human rights.... Our commitment to human rights must be absolute.... Ours was the first society openly to define itself in terms of both spirituality and of human liberty. It is that unique self-definition which ... imposes on us a special obligation—to take on those moral duties which, when assumed, seem invariably to be in our own best interests.

From Jimmy Carter, January 20, 1977.

had carefully avoided but that Carter as well as Sadat believed vital to any lasting settlement.

In venturing his peace initiative, Sadat had risked his own life as well as Egypt's position in the Arab world. He became for a season a popular favorite in the United States, while Begin's rigidity lost Israel a measure of American sympathy. When peace talks stalled, Carter called the two leaders to Camp David in Maryland in September 1978.

After a fortnight of delicate and difficult negotiation, Carter persuaded Begin and Sadat to sign a "Framework for Peace in the Middle East." The Camp David accords, which Carter nailed down during a trip to the Middle East the following March, resulted in Egypt's agreement to a peace treaty with Israel ending thirty years of war in exchange for Israel's return of the Sinai to Egypt. The provisions for the West Bank and the Gaza Strip were more ambiguous, envisaging a five-year transitional period during which the Palestinians would receive self-rule and "autonomy" while

Israel retained basic control. Israel, Egypt, Jordan, and "representatives of the Palestinian people" would meanwhile settle the final status of the areas. Ambiguity was inescapable because Sadat needed Palestinian self-determination to justify his deal with Israel in the Arab world while Begin regarded a Palestinian state as a mortal threat. The agreements represented a triumph of intensive personal diplomacy for Carter, but explosive problems remained to darken the future.

American dependence on Middle Eastern oil argued powerfully for the continuing effort to resolve the quarrel between Israel and the Arab world. In the meantime, Washington cultivated its relations with Saudi Arabia, and Carter continued the Nixon policy of regarding the shah of Iran as the American protector in the Persian Gulf region. Visiting Teheran at the end of 1977, Carter congratulated the shah on "the admiration and love which your people give to you." This was gross misjudgment. The shah's megalomania, the corruption of his entourage, the savagery of

**Ayatollah Khomeini:
Arab fanatic**

his secret police had turned his country against him, from the Islamic right to the Marxist left. Vance and Brzezinski, who for once had agreed on Arab-Israeli issues, disagreed over Iran, Brzezinski arguing for a military coup in support of the shah, Vance urging that the United States divorce itself from the shah and arrange a transition government. As Carter dithered in Washington, spreading disaffection forced the shah to flee Iran in January 1979. A theocratic regime, sharply opposed to materialism, modernization, and the twentieth century, took over under the leadership of an aged religious fanatic, the Ayatollah Ruholla Khomeini.

Carter had declined to abandon the shah until the very end. Warned thereafter by the American embassy in Teheran that admitting the shah to the United States would provoke retaliation against American diplomats, Carter nevertheless admitted him for medical treatment in October 1979. A few days later armed students seized the embassy and held fifty Americans hostage, creating a deep and prolonged crisis between the two countries. A rescue attempt by American commandos in 1980 proved a dismal failure and precipitated the resignation of Secretary of State Vance in protest both against the action and against the new directions of American policy.

The Third World. The appointment as ambassador to the United Nations of Andrew Young, a black minister and congressman who had been a lieutenant of Martin Luther King, expressed Carter's interest in improving American relations with the Third World. While Young was not always discreet in utterance, his

intelligence and fluency so bemused the developing countries that the United States slipped away from its position in the Nixon years as the favorite target of Third World hostility. This was a notable accomplishment when more than two-thirds of UN members were new or underdeveloped states.

Young was especially influential in shaping African policy, persuading Carter that communism could not establish a permanent presence in Africa and that alienating the black African "front-line" leaders would only push them into the arms of the Russians. The emergence of Nigeria as America's second largest supplier of foreign oil reinforced the tilt toward black Africa. The Israeli lobby forced Young's resignation in 1979 for failing to report secret talks with a PLO representative.

Latin America lacked an equivalent lobby and suffered consequent neglect. Though Carter was the first Spanish-speaking President, he attended to the Western Hemisphere only at moments of crisis. His main achievement was to gain, after a surprisingly close fight, Senate ratification of treaties providing for the transfer of the Panama Canal to Panama by the year 2000. In the wake of the retreat from Vietnam, the relinquishment of the Canal pricked chauvinistic sensitivities; one senator said irritably, "We stole it fair and square." The result, however, was to terminate a grievance that had long rankled in Latin American breasts and had generated much ill feeling toward the colossus of the north.

Poverty continued to bedevil the Third World despite brave UN talk of a "new international economic order." The gap between poor and rich nations widened. At current growth rates, per capita income in non-oil-producing regions of Asia, Africa, and Latin America was unlikely to reach $200 a year by 2000. After thirty years of effort and experiment, no one knew the answer. Skeptics now believed that foreign aid, so long the liberal panacea, tended to enrich native oligarchies and to undercut the disciplines essential for economic development. The mild ideals of the American Revolution were not easily exportable to peoples brutalized by the miseries of history. But communism provided no better answer, having failed after half a century even to assure basic food supply in the Soviet Union itself. The World Bank, directed by Robert McNamara, became the last citadel of the old crusade against world poverty: after helping destroy one poor country, McNamara was now spending his days trying to save the rest. The "North-South dialogue" went on but to growing and mutual exasperation. The future of the Third World looked uncertain and turbulent.

Vicissitudes of détente.

The Soviet relationship was still the primary issue. Carter began with high hopes. America, he said in May 1977, was at last free of "inordinate fear of communism." His goal was to reduce the chances of nuclear war by completing a SALT-II treaty with the Soviet Union. His policy, however, wobbled between Vance's hopes—and those of Edmund Muskie, who succeeded him as Secretary of State in 1980—and Brzezinski's fears.

SALT-II negotiations progressed in the last Ford years. In March 1977, soon after assuming office, Carter shocked the Russians by submitting new proposals that departed from the Vladivostok Accord (see p. 851) and that were, in the Soviet view, excessively one-sided. This action, accompanied by Carter's public support of Soviet dissidents, excited Soviet mistrust and set back negotiations for a year or more. Carter's decision in December 1978 to establish full diplomatic relations with China increased Soviet displeasure, especially after Brzezinski, over Vance's opposition, pressed for a "security relationship." But the SALT negotiators persevered, and in June 1979 agreement was finally reached in Vienna, Carter and Brezhnev kissing each other in celebration at the Hofburg Palace.

SALT-II, while proposing equal limits on Soviet and American strategic forces, provided no reductions. "With each new agreement," said Senator Daniel Patrick Moynihan, "the nuclear forces on both sides have increased." And the continuing Soviet missile build-up had raised doubts whether Moscow accepted assured destruction as a strategic doctrine and fears that it was bent instead on attaining the nuclear lead. When SALT-II went to the Senate in June 1979, opponents claimed that the treaty would con-

firm Soviet superiority, that it was negotiated from a position of American military weakness, and that crucial provisions were unverifiable. Strategic theologians revived the "missile gap" thesis of twenty years before in the form of a "window of vulnerability" through which, it was asserted, Soviet missiles could wipe out American land-based ICBMs. The window of vulnerability turned out to be as mythical as the missile gap, but, as in the case of the missle gap, damage was done. Moscow's deployment of mobile SS-20 missiles in eastern Europe, however, was not a myth; and it led in December 1979 to the "two-track" decision by NATO, according to which the United States would deploy 572 Pershing II and cruise missiles in western Europe to offset the SS-20s and also pursue arms limitation talks with Moscow.

In the same December, the Red Army entered Afghanistan. Actually the Russians had dominated Afghanistan since a pro-Moscow coup in April 1978. But the failure of the Marxist regime to suppress Moslem insurgency prompted Moscow to install a new regime and send in Russian troops. "This action of the Soviets," Carter said, "has made a more drastic change in my own opinion of what the Soviets' ultimate goals are than anything they've done in the previous time I've been in office." He called the Russian occupation

Celebration in Vienna, 1979: Carter and Brezhnev

of Afghanistan" a stepping stone to their possible control over much of the world's oil supplies" and the gravest threat to world peace since 1945.

Carter thereupon postponed SALT-II, increased defense spending, imposed an embargo on grain sales to Russia and superseded the "Nixon Doctrine" of 1969 (see p. 849) with a "Carter Doctrine" for Southwest Asia. Defining the Persian Gulf region as within the zone of American vital interest, he declared that the United States would repel an assault on that area "by any means necessary—including military force." Critics doubted whether the Soviet invasion of Afghanistan was, as Carter suggested, the first step in the unfolding of a master plan, seeing it rather as an *ad hoc* attempt to forestall a hostile regime on the Russian frontier. They also doubted that the United States could singlehandedly defend the Persian Gulf by conventional means, criticized the failure to consult Persian Gulf states or European allies before promulgating the Carter Doctrine, and condemned the Doctrine as probably unenforceable except by nuclear war.

The once pacific Carter had already become the first President since the Second World War to raise defense spending for three straight years in peacetime. Now Brzezinski and Secretary of Defense Harold Brown persuaded him to move away from the assured destruction doctrine toward a counterforce strategy. In September 1979 Carter approved the MX, an accurate but vulnerable multiple-warhead missile known

in the trade as a "use it or lose it" (first-strike) weapon. On July 25, 1980, he signed Presidential Directive No. 59, which emphasized flexibility in nuclear target selection and called for the capacity to wage limited and protracted nuclear war. Critics feared that this codification of the "countervailing strategy," with its first-strike potentialities, could only give new and horrible stimulus to the nuclear arms race.

Dilemmas of the Economic Order

Carter and domestic policy. Though Carter had run as a quasi-populist candidate, the relish with which he attacked "big government" portended significant departures from New Deal orthodoxy. As his close friend and first budget director, Bert Lance, put it, "He campaigns liberal, but he governs conservative."

To a degree, Carter also appointed liberal. He named three women to his cabinet. More women, blacks, and Hispanic-Americans received federal jobs and judgeships than ever before. His appointments gave regulatory commissions new zeal in protecting the environment, the workplace, the consumer, and highway safety. He instituted the first comprehensive civil-service reform in many years and used his Vice

President, Walter F. Mondale, more successfully than any previous President as a partner in his Administration. In 1977 he persuaded Congress to create a Department of Energy and in 1979 to divide the Department of Health, Education and Welfare into two new departments—the Department of Education and the Department of Health and Human Services.

But on central economic issues, he was the most conservative Democratic President since Grover Cleveland. "One of my major goals," Carter said in 1977, "is to free the American people from the burden of over-regulation." De-regulation—of the airlines, trucking, railroads, banks—became a major Carter cause. Federal spending on social programs reached its height in 1976 and declined thereafter, as a percentage both of the federal budget and of the gross national product (GNP). In his 1978 state-of-the-union message, he expressly repudiated the philosophy of affirmative government.

Revolt against government.
In his dismissal of affirmative government, Carter was responsive to a conservative swing in the country. The liberalism of the sixties had finally exhausted itself in the post-Watergate reforms. But it left in its wake a mass of government social programs and of health, safety, environmental, and equal-opportunity regulations. In addition, there had been a relentless increase in "entitlements," as federal payments to individuals were now known. Social security and Medicare accounted for almost half the entitlements bill; unemployment insurance, farm price supports, military and civil-service pensions, food stamps, student loans, and smaller programs made up the rest. Because entitlement payments were determined, not by statutory dollar ceilings, but by the number meeting eligibility standards, costs were hard to control. With the number of people over 65 growing 50 percent from 16.5 million in 1960 to 24.2 million in 1980, and with social security and other benefits now indexed to keep pace with inflation, entitlement payments exploded. By 1980 they had more than doubled as a percentage of GNP since 1960 and now consumed 46 percent of the federal budget.

A spreading antigovernment mood found dramatic expression in 1978 when California voters by nearly two-to-one approved Proposition 13, limiting property taxes in the state. A national movement arose in support of a constitutional amendment requiring a balanced budget. The enforcement of civil rights through busing and affirmative action also excited resentment. The Supreme Court in the *Bakke* case (1978) ruled that affirmative action in university admissions was not unconstitutional in principle, but that the use of numerical quotas in the particular case was. The Court decision legalizing abortion brought

into being an intensely emotional "right to life" movement; supporters of abortion counterorganized under the banner of "freedom of choice." The feeling spread that government was arbitrary, intrusive, and remote; that government intervention was making problems worse rather than better; that regulation, spending, taxes, and deficits had become an intolerable drain on the economy; and that the inexorable growth of government had to be stopped in its tracks.

In fact, the idea of an inexorable growth was something of an illusion. In 1960 the federal workforce consisted of 2.4 million. By 1980, while the nation grew by 50 million, the federal force grew by only 500,000. The proportion of the total labor force employed by the federal government actually declined from 3.7 to 3 percent. Moreover, defense and the postal service accounted in 1980 for almost three-fifths of federal workers. Where expansion had taken place, it was in state and local government. There the workforce more than doubled between 1960 and 1980, accounting in 1980 for over 80 percent of all government employment. Nor had the tax burden increased dramatically. During these years, effective corporate income-tax rates fell, property taxes as a percent of personal income stayed about the same, and combined federal and state income taxes rose only from 11 to 13 percent of personal income.

Yet acute problems remained, and in a conservative period the national government became a convenient scapegoat. Still, at the same time, Americans also by strong majorities favored specific forms of government intervention, such as national health insurance, government as the employer of last resort, and price and wage controls.

Inflation.
This last preference expressed growing discontent over the failure of conventional remedies to contain inflation. Prices more than doubled during the seventies. Inflation, reduced by the 1974–75 recession to 5.8 percent, resumed in 1977. Carter, when exhortation failed, resorted, like Ford, to slowing down the economy, rather than, like Nixon, to controls. In 1979 he appointed Paul Volcker, an advocate of monetary restriction, as chairman of the Federal Reserve Board. Tight money produced recession and 7.8 percent unemployment in 1980. This time inflation persisted—13.5 percent in 1980, which meant nearly 40 percent in the four Carter years.

Controversy mounted about the cause and cure of inflation. Where inflation during the Second World War and the Korean and Indochina Wars was clearly associated with an excess of demand over supply, inflation in the 1970s grew in the face of abundant supply. Monetarists believe that remedy lay in controlling the growth of the money stock. Others blamed inflation on government spending and saw the remedy in

**The "reserve army of the unemployed":
squeezing inflation out of the system?**

1873, 1907, 1929) had kept the price level down. In the 1930s the New Deal erected an array of built-in economic stabilizers to secure the economy against periodic collapse. By the 1980s there had been no major depression for half a century. But, in seeking to make the economy depression-proof, the New Deal may also have made it inflation-prone. In addition, economic concentration permitted strong sellers (big unions as well as big business) to ignore the law of supply and demand and to collaborate in raising prices and wages by administrative agreement.

Inflationary tendencies had recently been reinforced, moreover, by a disturbing decline in productivity; for increased productivity was the only way higher wages could be absorbed without forcing up prices. Productivity—average output per man-hour of work—had risen about 3 percent annually in the first twenty postwar years. In the 1970s it fell below 1 percent a year.

Whatever set off inflation at particular times, it appeared beyond question the malady to which the postwar economic organism most readily and habitually succumbed. By this view, just as depression had expressed a structural crisis in the economic order half a century earlier, so inflation expressed a structural crisis in the contemporary order—and the conventional wisdom seemed as bankrupt before inflation in 1980 as it had been before depression in 1930. To continue the stop-and-go cycle of combating inflation by recession and then combating recession by inflation seemed intolerable. Those who did not think that inflation would fade away therefore called for price stabilization through incomes policy—more particularly by establishing a public interest in price and wage decisions in areas of economic concentration where prices and wages did not respond to the play of market forces.

INFLATION: THE PURCHASING POWER OF THE DOLLAR DECLINES

	value of the dollar	consumer price index (1967 = 100)
1940	$1.00	42.0
1945	.77	53.9
1950	.58	72.1
1955	.52	80.2
1960	.47	88.7
1965	.44	94.5
1970	.36	116.3
1975	.26	161.2
1980	.17	246.8
1982	.14	287.1

From *Statistical Abstract of the United States 1982–1983.*

balanced budgets. History, however, showed no predictable relation between inflation and government deficits. In 1920, inflation had accompanied a budgetary surplus; in 1931–33, sharp deflation had accompanied deficits. Indeed, deficits had been chronic since 1929, but inflation had not been; most recently, in 1974–76, inflation had receded despite large deficits. In any event, monetary and fiscal stringency could reduce inflation only by producing recession and mass unemployment. "The 'reserve army of the unemployed,'" one economist commented, "will eventually squeeze inflation out of the system—if it doesn't trigger a social revolution first."

Others argued that the problem was structural more than it was fiscal and monetary, that the postwar economy itself had an inherent propensity toward inflation. For, through most of American history, major depressions every twenty years or so (1819, 1837, 1857,

Energy. Despite presidential exhortations and congressional statutes, Americans continued through the 1970s to increase both their consumption and their importation of oil. By 1979 the United States was importing 43 percent of its annual supply—nearly four times as much as in 1970. In the meantime, though domestic oil prices rose nearly 200 percent, domestic production declined. By 1979 it had dropped 10 percent from its peak in 1970.

In April 1977 Carter submitted a comprehensive energy plan that he described as the "moral equivalent of war." Presidential follow-up, however, was feeble; the complex proposals bogged down in Congress; and the program faded away, to be remembered acronymically as MEOW. Two years later the cut-off of Iranian oil after the fall of the shah produced a temporary gasoline shortage reminiscent of 1974, with angry lines at filling stations and Americans screaming at their fellow citizens and, on occasions, shooting them. In response, Congress deregulated the price of domestic crude oil. and imposed a "windfall" profits tax.

Analysts concluded that the prospect for major increases in domestic energy supplies from the four conventional sources—oil, natural gas, coal, and nuclear energy—was bleak. In the case of oil, which supplied about 50 percent of the energy used each year, and natural gas, which supplied about 25 percent, there were geological limits on expansion. Coal, with its indefinite reserves, supplied about 19 percent, but its exploitation raised difficult health, safety, and environmental problems.

Seventy-two nuclear plants in operation in 1979 accounted for about 13 percent of electricity production and about 4 percent of total energy consumption. But a frightening accident that year at the Three Mile Island nuclear plant near Harrisburg, Pennsylvania—an accident coincidentally portrayed in the contemporaneous film *The China Syndrome*—led to anxious debate about future reliance on nuclear energy. Antinuclear demonstrators shouted "Hell No, We Won't Glow," and legislators called for circumspection in subsequent nuclear energy policy.

In the short run, the best hope lay in conservation policies reducing the flow of energy into heating, air conditioning, industry, and transportation. For a people whose lives were organized around the automobile, severe adjustments lay ahead. Americans owned two-fifths of all the cars in use in the world; in 1980 there were 156 million registered cars in the United States. But the "gas-guzzling" automobile of the past was on its way out, and engineers hoped to increase gasoline mileage to 50 miles per gallon by the 1990s. Doubling gas mileage would cut oil imports by nearly 50 percent. There was revived interest too in mass transport.

For the longer run, Carter asked Congress to set up a federal corporation commissioned to spend $88 billion for the creation of a synthetic fuel industry by the 1990s, extracting gasoline from shale oil, tar sands, and coal. He also gave support to solar energy—the conversion of sunlight to energy or heat through photovoltaic cells. Through the "solar transition" it was hoped to derive 20 percent of energy needs from the sun by 2000.

National malaise? "Why have we not been able to get together as a nation to resolve our serious energy problem?" Carter asked the American people in a televised speech in July 1979. To answer that question Carter invited 130 Americans—some famous, some not—to Camp David over a ten-day period to tell him what he was doing wrong. His conclusion was that the trouble lay in a "crisis of the American spirit." The people, he believed, had lost "confidence in the future."

Against Carter's theory that a national malaise was the cause of the ineffectuality of his Presidency others believed that the ineffectuality of his Presidency was the cause of the national malaise. Americans, critics said, had lost confidence, not in their country, but in its leadership. Indeed, Carter's approval rating had sunk to 26 percent in the polls. Though a man of high intelligence, it was the intelligence of an engineer rather than that of a political leader; and, like the earlier engineer in the White

Three Mile Island: symbol for circumspection

House, Herbert Hoover, Carter had evident difficulty in adjusting himself to the tasks of education and persuasion essential to the political process. Moreover, he conveyed no broad sense of the direction in which he wanted to take the country. "Carter believes fifty things," the author of his early presidential messages later recalled, "but no one thing. He holds explicit, thorough positions on every issue under the sun, but he has no large view of relations between them." Lacking any central theme, the Carter Administration was alone among Democratic administrations of the century in failing to gain a popular label (New Freedom, New Deal, Fair Deal, New Frontier, Great Society), the effort to launch "New Foundations" proving a dismal flop.

The 1980 election. In October Senator Edward Kennedy of Massachusetts, who for some time had been leading Carter in the polls, emerged as a challenger for the Democratic nomination. Once a declared candidate himself, however, Kennedy too began to drop in the polls. An accident at Chappaquiddick in Massachusetts in 1969 resulting in the death of a young woman left questions in many people's minds; others regarded Kennedy as too liberal; and, most important

of all, the crises in Iran and Afghanistan led people to rally behind the President at a time of national emergency.

Citing the American hostages in Iran, Carter refused to leave Washington for the primaries but nevertheless won a series of victories. Though Kennedy carried several large states toward the end and gave the campaign's most memorable speech at the Democratic convention, the Carter–Mondale ticket was renominated by a comfortable margin. The Republicans in the meantime turned to Ronald Reagan, movie actor, two-term governor of California, and for a dozen years the favorite of the party's right wing. Reagan selected as his running mate his main challenger in the primaries, George Bush of Texas, a former congressman, party chairman, diplomat, and CIA director, who represented more moderate Republicans.

Some voters, dismayed by the choice between Carter and Reagan, found an alternative in John Anderson, a liberal Republican congressman from Illinois, who ran on an independent ticket. The campaign, the longest and most expensive in history, dealt in slogans and television commercials rather than substance and soon wearied the electorate. Carter's attempt to portray Reagan as a warmonger, racist, and

Republican victors, 1980

Return of the hostages

extremist compromised his own appeal as a presumed decent man and was effectively countered by Reagan's serene geniality in their single television debate.

Only 53.9 percent of those eligible voted on election day, continuing the steady decline in turnout since 1960. Reagan's 44 million votes constituted 50.8 percent of the popular vote and only 27 percent of the voting-age population. Carter received 41 percent of the vote (35.5 million) and Anderson 7 percent (5.7 million). Reagan, however, won a decisive victory in the electoral college, carrying 44 states and accumulating 489 electoral votes to Carter's 49. The Republicans also captured the Senate for the first time since 1952. The so-called Moral Majority, composed of fervent evangelical Christians, contributed to the defeat of a number of liberal Democrats, including the 1972 presidential candidate George McGovern.

Carter was the main issue, and the voters decided emphatically against continuing him in office. Yet he won respect as a man for hard work and high principle; and, though his policies lacked a unifying vision, his emphasis on human rights was a salutary reaffirmation on the American heritage. On his last day in office, he succeeded in negotiating the release of the hostages in Iran after 444 days of detention, thereby relieving his successor of a humiliating international burden.

The Reagan Counter-Revolution

Reagan in the White House. The new President was the oldest man (70 shortly after his inauguration), the first actor, the first labor leader (he had been president of the Screen Actors Guild), and the first divorced man to be elected President. As a young man, he cast his first four presidential votes for Franklin Roosevelt; but later he moved far to the right. Years in Hollywood had not divested him of an image of America as the small-town idyl remembered from his childhood in Illinois and portrayed on the *Saturday Evening Post* covers of Norman Rockwell; and he preached old-time values of individualism, self-help, and upward mobility. Entering politics in the 1960s, he proved a relatively successful governor of California. An accomplished speaker, he radiated affability, optimism, and, despite his age, boyish charm.

Reagan worked much less hard than Carter and was far less in command of information and analysis. But he was far more in command of broad policy. Where Carter had the mind of an engineer, Reagan had the outlook of an ideologue. His Presidency had the unifying themes that Carter's lacked, and he left no doubt about the direction in which he wished to move the country. His mind was anecdotal rather than analytical; and his ideological bent was tempered by a capacity for practical accomodation. He understood, as his predecessor had not, that politics is ultimately an educational process. With his charm, elo-

President Reagan: a genius for simplicity

quence, and genius for simplification, he was dubbed "the Great Communicator." Though no student of public affairs, Reagan set the course of his Administration and surrounded himself with competent colleagues to work out the details. He transformed the terms of national debate, and, reviving the strong Presidency, ended doubts that had arisen in the 1970s about the executive's ability to lead the nation.

Reaganomics.

"Government is not the solution to our problem," Reagan said in his inaugural address. "Government is the problem." Reaganism at home rested on two propositions: that government was the root of evil, and that, once government was "off the people's backs," national problems would solve themselves. Reagan saw it as his mission to reverse the malign direction of the national life, to shrink the national government, and to turn the economy over to private enterprise.

As a candidate, Reagan promised an economic policy that would simultaneously dismantle government regulation, reduce social spending, repair American defenses, end inflation, and balance the budget—a mix derided by George Bush during the primaries (in a phrase later repented) as "voodoo economics." In pursuing these objectives, the new Administration drew on economic ideas developed during the seventies in right-wing "think-tanks," in conservative intellectual journals, and among younger Republicans in Congress.

Reaganomics had three, if divergent, theoretical components. Reaganites agreed in regarding the unregulated market place as the means of salvation but disagreed on the tactics of economic policy. "Supply-side" economics argued that a cut in top tax rates would give the rich increased incentive to work, save, and invest. This would stimulate the economy as a whole, and the tax cuts would pay for themselves through increased revenues. "Supply side," as David Stockman, Reagan's first budget director, said, "is 'trickle-down' theory"—the theory of the Coolidge era that, if you help the few at the top, benefits will trickle down to the rest; or, as more coarsely stated, that, if you feed the horses more oats, the sparrows will eat better. Its congressional advocates were Representative Jack Kemp of New York and Senator William Roth of Delaware, sponsors of the Kemp–Roth bill, and its theory came from the economist Arthur Laffer and the financial journalist Jude Wanniski.

"Monetarism," with the Nobel Prize economist Milton Friedman as high priest, saw the control of the monetary stock as the key and wished in particular through tight money to wring inflation out of the economy. Like supply-siders, monetarists did not worry unduly about deficits. But some Republicans,

especially in Congress, remained faithful to the party's budget-balancing orthodoxy.

The mingling of these somewhat discordant doctrines produced a policy that in 1981 combined a massive tax cut to stimulate the economy with high interest rates to restrain inflation. In the tug-of-war between a soft fiscal policy and a hard monetary policy, monetary policy scored the first victory, throwing the economy in the next year into the worst collapse since the 1930s, unemployment rising to nearly 11 percent.

In the meantime, Reagan, hoping to keep his pledge of a balanced budget by 1984, cut back on government domestic spending (except social security and Medicare) by nearly 10 percent. But these cutbacks were more than offset by the tax reduction of $131 billion and the $92 billion increase in military spending by 1985. Moreover, with excessively high interest rates, the increase in interest payments on the national debt exceeded the cuts in health, education, welfare, and social programs. At the same time, recession reduced tax revenues and increased entitlement claims (as for unemployment compensation). The results were deficits of $111 billion in 1982 and $195 billion in 1983—more in the second year than all the Carter deficits combined and the largest deficit in American history. The national debt, accumulated from the start of the republic, was $551 billion at the end of the Ford Administration. It grew by an additional $670 billion in the first four Reagan years.

The unprecedented deficit had one ironic consequence. It pulled the economy out of the recession of 1982–83—an old-fashioned, Keynesian, demand-side recovery. A further irony was to hear Democrats righteously denounce deficits while Reaganites casually dismissed them. Still another irony was that the apparatus of social protection erected during the New Deal enabled Reagan to ride out the highest unemployment since the Great Depression.

Shrinking government.

Reagan used the deficit to force reductions in social programs. "We can lecture our children about extravagance until we run out of voice and breath," he said. "Or we can cut their extravagance by simply reducing their allowance." But the most costly entitlement programs—social security, Medicare, civil-service and veterans' pensions—had middle-class constituencies and were deemed politically untouchable. Given this fact, given the increase in military spending and the uncontrollable service charges on the national debt, the prospect was one of growing deficits for years to come, with a "structural deficit" that would survive even full employment.

In the meantime, the available target for budget-cutting, in the Administration's view, lay in programs

The liberal party is a party which believes that, as new conditions and problems arise beyond the power of men and women to meet as individuals, it becomes the duty of the Government itself to find new remedies with which to meet them. The liberal party insists that the Government has the definite duty to use all its power and resources to meet new social problems with new social controls—to insure to the average person the right to his own economic and political life, liberty, and the pursuit of happiness.

From Franklin D. Roosevelt, June 16, 1941.

Statements are made labelling the Federal Government an outsider, an intruder, an adversary.... The people of this [TVA] area know that the United States Government is not a stranger or not an enemy. It is the people of fifty states joining in a national effort.... Only a great national effort by a great people working together can explore the mysteries of space, harvest the products at the bottom of the ocean, and mobilize the human, natural, and material resources of our lands.

From John F. Kennedy, May 18, 1963.

Government cannot solve our problems. It can't set our goals. It cannot define our vision. Government cannot eliminate poverty, or provide a bountiful economy, or reduce inflation, or save our cities, or cure illiteracy, or provide energy.

From Jimmy Carter, January 19, 1978.

Government is not the solution to our problem. Government is the problem.

From Ronald Reagan, January 20, 1981.

Modern Presidents on the role of government

---

requiring a "mean test"—proof of need. Though means-tested entitlements—welfare, food stamps, child nutrition, and the like—consumed only 18 percent of the total expenditures for income security, they had the weakest lobbies behind them and suffered nearly 60 percent of the 1981 cuts. Reductions in benefit payments were greatest for households with incomes under $10,000.

Reagan proposed to keep a "safety net" for the "truly needy"—those who, because of age, disability, or illness, were unemployable. But he disliked income supplements for workers. His reductions therefore fell with particular force on the "working poor," now in many cases deprived of food stamps, employment training, welfare benefits, Medicaid, and reduced-price school lunches for their children. "In order to succeed," wrote George Gilder, a prominent Reaganite theoretician, "the poor need most of all the spur of their poverty." Critics, reflecting on the simultaneous tax reductions for the rich, concluded that, in the Reaganite view, the poor needed the spur of poverty and the rich the spur of wealth.

Reagan also wished to transfer social programs to the states—a more determined New Federalism than Nixon's a decade before. In 1981 seventy-seven categorical programs were consolidated into nine block grants. But his 1982 proposal that the states take over welfare, food stamps and education, transportation and social-service programs in exchange for the federal assumption of Medicaid got nowhere. Critics argued that "devolution" would weaken national standards, increase disparities among states and abandon the historic commitment to equitable treatment for all citizens. State governors, already hard pressed financially, resisted what they regarded as the dumping of national responsibilities on local authority. Still the New Federalism addressed real problems, if the sorting out of the several responsibilities of national, state, and local government plainly required further thought.

The Reagan Counter-Revolution **883**

Deregulation. Along with the reduction and devolution of social programs, Reagan sought to retract the regulatory apparatus of government. The Administration pursued this goal in a variety of ways—by cutting regulatory budgets, by diluting or abolishing regulations, by relaxing enforcement, by staffing regulatory agencies with representatives of the industries to be regulated. The head of OSHA, for example, came from a company that had been repeatedly cited for safety violations. Under his direction the number of OSHA inspections and penalties rapidly declined. The new access given industry resulted in systematic-weakening of safeguards in food and drugs, highway safety, nursing homes, and other areas.

Deregulation had special impact on the environment and resources. The sabotage of environmental standards in Reagan's EPA became such a scandal that Congress in 1983 forced the Administration to bring in new leadership. Reagan's first Secretary of the Interior, James Watt, had emerged from the Sagebrush Rebellion, a movement of mineowners and ranchers seeking to rid the west of federal supervision of public lands. The transfer of public property and resources to private control, Watt argued, was essential to promote economic development and to strengthen national security. Reversing the policies of Theodore Roosevelt, he tried to sell up to 35 million acres of public land, opened the continental shelf to offshore oil and gas drilling, encouraged timber-cutting in the national forests, offered public land to coal companies, accelerated the spread of strip-mining and reduced safety inspection of coal mines. Though he enjoyed Reagan's full support, Watt's doctrinaire commitment to the cause of "privatization" and his tasteless cracks about environmentalists (whom he compared to Nazis), liberals (whom he distinguished from real Americans), Indians, Jews, cripples, and the Beach Boys finally led to his resignation in 1983.

Reagan also hoped to devolve regulatory functions from Washington to the states. "Take just one area," he observed of the federal government. "In 1978, there were 35 programs for pollution alone." Critics doubted that the substitution of 50 separate state antipollution programs would mean a diminution of bureaucracy. Even businesspeople feared a "50-headed hydra." Critics also feared that state regulation would be inadequate for national problems and that the absence of uniform national rules would invite competition in lowered standards among states seeking to woo business.

Supporters claimed that deregulation was revitalizing industries like transportation, telecommunications, banking, oil drilling, and coal mining. Critics contended that deregulation had begun a dangerous unravelling of the network of health, safety, and environmental protections built up over decades. Conser-vationists feared in particular that privatization of public lands would lead to "sod-busting"—overgrazing and overplanting—and soil erosion, and create a new dustbowl. Consumers were exasperated by the abandonment of unprofitable but convenient air routes and by the complications following the break-up of the American Telephone and Telegraph Company monopoly. Polls showed decisive majorities in favor of stringent standards for air and water, for safety on the highways and in the workplace.

Consequences of Reaganomics. The policy of cutting taxes for the rich and social programs for the poor led to significant changes in the pattern of income distribution. The nonpartisan Urban Institute reported in 1984 that Reagan policies had resulted in a $25 million transfer in disposable income from the less well-off to the richest fifth of Americans. Disposable income rose by 8.7 percent for the top fifth on the income scale, while the bottom fifth suffered an almost 8 percent drop, with their benefits reduced and their taxes increased (because of regressive social security, payroll, and sales taxes). The number whose cash income fell below the poverty line rose from 29.3 million in 1980 to 35.3 million in 1983—more than one out of every seven Americans, and the highest proportion since Johnson's war on poverty began in 1965. Of the new 5 million poor, 40 percent were under 18. Poverty was especially high among blacks—more than one out of three; blacks accounted for 12 percent of the population but 28 percent of the nation's poor.

The vulnerability of black America was heightened by the Administration's policy of deregulating civil rights. The Reaganites had long opposed affirmative action and mandatory busing as means of achieving integration. In office, they relaxed civil rights enforcement, reversed civil-rights rulings of earlier administrations, and even attempted to give tax exemption to schools practicing segregation. In 1984 the Administration captured control of the Civil Rights Commission, hitherto the government's main claimant agency for racial justice. Where the Second Reconstruction of the 1960s was based on the idea of integrating American society, observed the civil-rights leader Vernon Jordan, "The Reagan counter-revolution is based on re-segregating society."

Reaganites argued that their policies would in the longer run revive American self-reliance and release the productive energies of the country. Critics noted the socially discriminatory effects of the reduction of government services. For the rich had their own automobiles; the poor had to rely on public transit. The rich sent their children to private schools; the poor had to rely on public education. Occupational safety and health regulations protected poor men in factories, not rich men in offices. The rich could buy books and pictures; the poor needed public libraries and museums. The rich had their own recreational facilities; the poor depended on public playgrounds, public parks, public swimming pools. As the eminent political philosopher Doonesbury said, "No one suffers but the poor, and they're used to it."

Dilemmas of conservatism. Conservatism, like liberalism, was a house with many mansions, and Reagan, like Franklin Roosevelt half a century before, presided over a jostling coalition. In its broad outlines, the Reaganite ideology represented a return to the Social Darwinism and laissez-faire of a century earlier. Reagan's economic policy generally reflected the interests of affluent businesspeople and professionals. But much of the crusading zeal behind Reaganism came from small-town and rural conservatives, sometimes referred to as populists, and from the evangelical religious groups gathered together in the Moral Majority. Though establishment conservatism and neopopulism shared the general faith in unfettered private enterprise, their concerns diverged on other issues.

The economic conservatives wanted to reduce government regulation and taxes. They had little interest in prosecuting abortion or homosexuality or in legalizing prayer in public schools. The evangelical moralists wanted to ban liberated women, abortion, adultery, homosexuality, pot, sexual candor, and Darwin. Where libertarian conservatives wanted government to leave people alone, the moralists wanted government to police private behavior. "They want to get government off our backs," observed a critic, "and put it in our beds."

Fundamentalist preachers like Jerry Falwell used television to acquire mass followings and large treasuries. Jesse Helms of North Carolina was their effective spokesman in the Senate. Reagan handled the divergence in his ranks with political skill, making ideological speeches to the zealots while keeping social issues on the legislative "back burner" and retaining a capacity for accommodation as political necessity demanded. His policies, irksome as they were to liberals, did not always satisfy the radical right. Some rightists even denounced him for selling out. Others echoed the cry of Secretary of the Interior Watt: "Let Reagan be Reagan." Republican strategists consoled themselves with the thought that the far right had no place to go.

Reagan and the world. In foreign affairs, Reagan was an unabashed American nationalist. Though (or perhaps because) he had fought the Second World War on the film lots of Hollywood, he wore his patriotism on his sleeve; men who had risked their lives in combat, like Truman, Eisenhower, Kennedy, Johnson, Ford, and McGovern, felt less need to make a public production of their devotion to the republic. No President since Wilson had expressed so ardently the idea of "American exceptionalism"—the idea that the United States was exempt from the historic laws and interests that conditioned other countries. Seeing America as a chosen nation, Reagan had no doubt about its inherent moral superiority over lesser breeds.

Animated by this faith, he saw world affairs less in geopolitical terms, as a contest shaped by national interest and the balance of power, than in moralistic terms, as a contest between good and evil. The Soviet Union, Reagan said in 1982, is an "evil empire . . . the focus of evil in the modern world." The world struggle is "between right and wrong and good and evil." When evil is loose in the world, "we are enjoined by scripture and the Lord Jesus to oppose it with all our might." The communists erect lying and cheating into a philosophy and are exclusively responsible for the world's manifold ills. "Let us not delude ourselves," he said. "The Soviet Union underlies all the unrest that is going on. If they weren't engaged in this game of dominos, there wouldn't be any hot spots in the world."

Ideology thus portrayed the Soviet Union as a fanatic monolith, immune to historical vicissitude and change, carrying out with implacable cunning a master plan of world conquest. In practice—often to the dismay of his rightwing followers—Reagan showed a capacity to foresake ideology if confronted by domestic political interests (as when he abandoned the embargo on grain sales to Russia instituted by Carter after the invasion of Afghanistan), or by the resistance of allies (as when he abandoned opposition to a pipeline supplying western Europe with natural gas from the Soviet Union), or by geopolitical necessity (as when he abandoned all-out support for anti-communist Taiwan in favor of closer relations with communist China). But, despite occasional concessions to practicality, the ideological framework remained intact.

Convinced that the American people were fed up with weakness and humiliation, the Reagan Administration proposed to reverse the supposed decay in America's world position by a crusade of military, economic, and psychological renewal, based on patriotic pride, on increased defense spending, on the extension abroad of private enterprise, and on the intensification of political, economic, and military pressures against the Soviet Union.

Proving American resolve: Central America. If the Soviet Union was the main source of the world's troubles, it seemed urgent to check Soviet power at every point along the periphery. Thus Reagan's first Secretary of State, the highstrung General Alexander Haig, began by calling urgent attention to the Soviet threat to Central America, especially in Nicaragua and El Salvador.

Turbulence in Central America had deep historic roots. For generations, greedy oligarchies supported by the military, by North American corporations, and by Washington, had oppressed and exploited landless laborers. In the 1920s a nationalist insurrection led by General Augusto Cesar Sandino had led to the occupation of Nicaragua by the United States Marines (see p. 644). In El Salvador a conservative government had killed 30,000 peasants in crushing an uprising in 1932. Then, after the Second World War, economic development and population growth brought into existence through much of Central America a new middle class aspiring to democratic liberties. Washington had mixed reactions. In 1954 Eisenhower used the CIA to overthrow a democratic government in Guatemala (see p. 805). But the democratic hope, encouraged by Kennedy's Alliance for Progress, could not be suppressed.

In July 1979 a popular insurrection in Nicaragua threw out the dictatorship of the Somoza family, which had looted the country for forty years. The revolution, led by radical Sandinistas, showed Marxist leanings and received arms from Castro and from the Soviet bloc. The Sandinista victory encouraged revolutionaries in El Salvador and Guatemala. The situation was particularly tense in El Salvador, where a military coup in October 1979 brought in young officers pledged to free the country from domination by the "fourteen families." Rightwing officers, however, joined the oligarchy to block land reform, and by 1980 civil war had broken out.

In Nicaragua, the Carter Administration, after failing to moderate and rescue the Somoza regime, tried in 1980 to come to terms with the Sandinistas. In El Salvador Carter gave conditional support to the October coup. When the new regime moved to the right and began to murder its opponents, Carter suspended aid in the hope of strengthening moderates remaining in the regime. Then, persuaded that communist countries were sending arms via Nicaragua to the rebels in El Salvador, he resumed military aid at the end of his term.

Nicaragua: celebrating the revolution

Our situation invites and our interests prompt us to aim at an ascendant in the system of American affairs.

From Alexander Hamilton, *Federalist*, No. 11.

I candidly confess, that I have ever looked on Cuba as the most interesting addition which could ever be made to our system of States.

From Thomas Jefferson to James Monroe, October 24, 1823.

To-day the United States is practically sovereign on this continent, and its fiat is law upon the subjects to which it confines its interposition.... Its infinite resources combined with its isolated position render it master of the situation.

From Secretary of State Richard Olney to T. F. Bayard, July 20, 1895.

We, the citizens of all the American republics, are, I think, at the threshold of a new era.... We are entering a new era in accepting the plan that no one of our nations must hereafter exploit a neighbor nation at the expense of that neighbor.

From Franklin D. Roosevelt in Cartagena, Colombia, July 10, 1934.

Social reforms are at the heart of the Alliance for Progress. They are the preconditions to economic modernization. And they are the instrument by which we assure the poor and hungry—the worker and the campesino—his full participation in the benefits of our development and in the human dignity which is the purpose of all free societies.... Those who make peaceful revolution impossible will make violent revolution inevitable.

From John F. Kennedy, March 13, 1962.

The goal of the professional guerrilla movements in Central America is as simple as it is sinister—to destabilize the entire region from the Panama Canal to Mexico.... I do not believe that a majority of the Congress or the country is prepared to stand by passively while the people of Central America are delivered to totalitarianism and we ourselves are left vulnerable to new dangers.

From Ronald Reagan, April 27, 1983.

During the 1980 campaign Reagan had denounced Carter's human-rights policy for "de-stabilizing" Nicaragua and El Salvador; and his election greatly cheered the right throughout Central America. Secretary Haig quickly argued that the United States had to reestablish its global credibility by "drawing the line" against "communist aggression" in Central America. Nicaragua (population 2.9 million) was deemed a major threat. In November 1981 Reagan directed the CIA to arm and organize Nicaraguan exiles, soon known as "Contras," to attack the Sandinistas. The aim was ostensibly to stop arms shipments to El Salvador, and Congress in 1982 forbade the use of covert funds to overthrow the regime.

The replacement of Haig as Secretary of State by George Shultz in June 1982 did not alter policy. As American intervention increased, the Nicaragua regime moved to the left and the El Salvador regime to the right. By 1983 in El Salvador rightwing "death squads," tolerated if not encouraged by the regime,

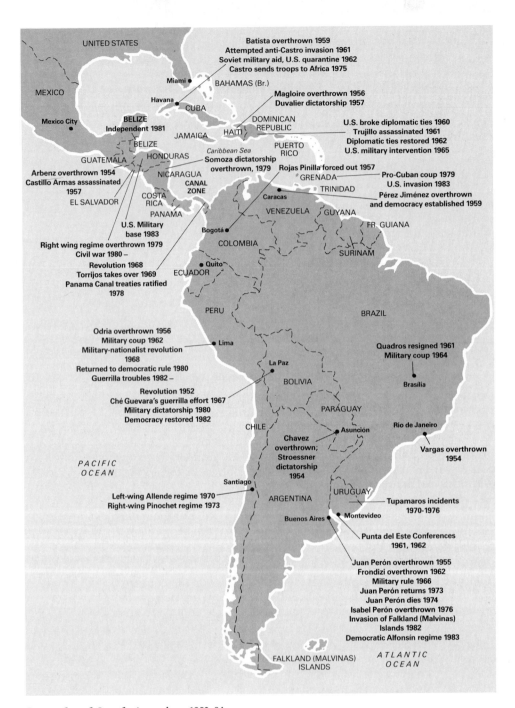

Central and South America, 1952–84

The map shows the following annotations:

UNITED STATES

MEXICO

Mexico City

BELIZE — Independent 1981

Miami

Havana

CUBA
- Batista overthrown 1959
- Attempted anti-Castro invasion 1961
- Soviet military aid, U.S. quarantine 1962
- Castro sends troops to Africa 1975

BAHAMAS (Br.)

HAITI
- Magloire overthrown 1956
- Duvalier dictatorship 1957

DOMINICAN REPUBLIC
- U.S. broke diplomatic ties 1960
- Trujillo assassinated 1961
- Diplomatic ties restored 1962
- U.S. military intervention 1965

JAMAICA

BELIZE

GUATEMALA
- Arbenz overthrown 1954
- Castillo Armas assassinated 1957

HONDURAS

Caribbean Sea

NICARAGUA — Somoza dictatorship overthrown, 1979

EL SALVADOR — Right wing regime overthrown 1979 / Civil war 1980–

COSTA RICA

PANAMA
- U.S. Military base 1983
- Revolution 1968
- Torrijos takes over 1969
- Panama Canal treaties ratified 1978

CANAL ZONE

PUERTO RICO

Rojas Pinilla forced out 1957

GRENADA
- Pro-Cuban coup 1979
- U.S. invasion 1983

TRINIDAD

Pérez Jiménez overthrown and democracy established 1959

Caracas

VENEZUELA

GUYANA

FR. GUIANA

Bogotá

COLOMBIA

SURINAM

Quito

ECUADOR

PERU
- Odria overthrown 1956
- Military coup 1962
- Military-nationalist revolution 1968
- Returned to democratic rule 1980
- Guerrilla troubles 1982–

Lima

BRAZIL

Quadros resigned 1961 / Military coup 1964

Brasília

BOLIVIA
- Revolution 1952
- Ché Guevara's guerrilla effort 1967
- Military dictatorship 1980
- Democracy restored 1982

La Paz

PARÁGUAY

Asunción

Chavez overthrown; Stroessner dictatorship 1954

Río de Janeiro

Vargas overthrown 1954

CHILE
- Left-wing Allende regime 1970
- Right-wing Pinochet regime 1973

Santiago

URUGUAY
- Tupamaros incidents 1970–1976
- Punta del Este Conferences 1961, 1962

Montevideo

ARGENTINA

Buenos Aires
- Juan Perón overthrown 1955
- Frondizi overthrown 1962
- Military rule 1966
- Juan Perón returns 1973
- Juan Perón dies 1974
- Isabel Perón overthrown 1976
- Invasion of Falkland (Malvinas) Islands 1982
- Democratic Alfonsín regime 1983

PACIFIC OCEAN

ATLANTIC OCEAN

FALKLAND (MALVINAS) ISLANDS

tortured and assassinated oppositionists with impunity. Honduras had now become an American military base and trembled on the edge of war with Nicaragua. By the end of 1983 in Central America 110,000 people had died and a million were displaced in countries with a total population of 18 million.

Frustrated at the stalemate in Central America, the United States took advantage of political turmoil on the former British colony of Grenada in the Caribbean to launch a surprise attack in October 1983. The attack on an island of 110,000 with no army, navy, or air force was, not surprisingly, successful. It was greeted with applause by the Grenadans, by neighboring Caribbean islands, and by most Americans, and it led Cuba and Nicaragua to behave for a season with circumspection. Critics, at home and especially abroad, questioned the use of military action as a weapon of first resort and the example Washington was setting to the world. "If you are going to pronounce a new law that, wherever communism reigns against the will of the people," said Prime Minister Margaret Thatcher of Britain, ". . . the United States shall enter, then we are going to have really terrible wars in the world."

Some felt the compulsion to view every development through the prism of the Cold War distorted the reality of a world teeming with problems and hostilities of its own. The Administrations' preoccupation with "Marxism," some believed, diverted attention from more important hemisphere problems, such as the external debt of Latin American countries which amounted to $330 billion in the early 1980s. In Central America, critics argued, Washington should back Mexico, Venezuela, Colombia, and Panama—the so-called Contadora group—in the search for a negotiated solution.

Reagan replied by emphasizing the danger posed by "those who aren't just aiming at El Salvador but, I think, are aiming at the whole of Central . . . and, I'm sure, eventually North America." If the Marxists succeeded, he said, "Our credibility would collapse, our alliances would crumble, and the safety of our homeland would be in jeopardy. . . . If we cannot act decisively so close to home, who will believe us anywhere?"

The Third World. In the Middle East too the Administration regarded the Soviet Union as the overriding danger. Secretary Haig hoped to unite the warring countries in what he called "a consensus of strategic concerns" directed against Russia. Unfortunately Arabs and Israeli feared each other more than they feared Moscow. As the American ambassador to Saudi Arabia put it (for which he was dismissed), if the people in a region "do not share your perception, what good is it?"

In the meantime, little progress had been made in resolving the ambiguities of the Camp David Agreement. Though Begin, dominant in Israel until his resignation in late 1983, returned the Sinai to Egypt on schedule in April 1982, he denied the Palestinians the "autonomy" they thought they had been promised on the West Bank and Gaza Strip and expanded Israeli settlements with the evident purpose of eventual annexation. In Egypt the assassination of Sadat in October 1981, more mourned abroad than at home, brought Hosni Mubarak as his successor and a new concern with internal problems. Hoping to get the peace process back on track, Reagan in an intelligent speech in September 1982 argued for a freeze on settlements and the independence of the West Bank "in association with Jordan." Begin rejected the proposal, and the tangle deepened.

Israel had already invaded Lebanon in June 1982 in order to destroy Palestine Liberation Organization bases. In August U.S. Marines entered Lebanon to supervise the PLO withdrawal, returning the next month after Christian Phalangists with tacit Israeli consent had carried out a shocking massacre of Palestinians in refugee camps. In 1983 the Marines lost their neutral role. Their mission now was to sustain the minority Maronite (Christian) government under Amin Gemayel, especially against Syrian attempts to reclaim northern Lebanon. An outrageous attack on Marine barracks in October 1983 exposed the vulnerability of the small American contingent, and in early 1984 Reagan withdrew the Marines.

For the Third World in general, Reagan saw private investment as the key to economic growth and spoke lyrically about "the magic of the market." The United Nations was now a main Third World forum. Poor countries had three-quarters of the voting strength in the General Assembly; nearly a fifth of the

U. S. Marines leaving Lebanon, 1984

UN's 158 members (over three times the number in 1945) were "microstates" with populations of less than 400,000. Here Ambassador Jeanne Kirkpatrick, an informed and articulate political scientist, adopted a policy of challenge and confrontation. "The UN is against us," she said on one occasion, and, regarding it as an instrument for the extension rather than the resolution of conflict, she cast 14 of the total of 36 vetoes by the United States.

Critics contended that the confrontationist strategy had isolated the United States within the organization. While agreeing that Third World shrillness was exasperating, they insisted that the UN remained the indispensable point of contact with the developing world and the only place where global problems—food, population, energy, inflation, environment, development assistance, drugs—could be collectively considered. But Kirkpatrick enjoyed Reagan's full support, and her style won the acclaim of American nationalists.

The Soviet Union. The Soviet Union remained the supreme concern, and Reagan was determined to restore the United States to a position of military primacy. Undeterred by the finding of his own Scowcroft Commission in 1983 that the "window of vulnerability" for American ICBMs was greatly exaggerated, the Administration set in motion the largest military build-up in American history. National defense spending rose from $160 billion in 1981 to $274 billion in 1984 with further steady increases projected up to $464 billion in 1989—a total of nearly $3 trillion for the decade.

The Administration justified the build-up by claiming that the United States had fallen behind the Soviet Union in military power. This claim was much disputed, critics contending that, while Russians led in some categories, America led in others, and that the result was a fragile balance—the Soviet advantage in ICBMs balanced by the American advantage in submarine-based forces and in strategic aircraft. When asked at a congressional hearing whether he would trade places with his Soviet counterpart, General John Vessey, chairman of the Joint Chiefs of Staff, replied, "Not on your life."

The Administration sought especially to enlarge American nuclear striking power, particularly with the MX missile, now rebaptized in Orwellian style Peacekeeper. Reagan's decision to place the MX in vulnerable Minuteman silos represented, as critics saw it, a further move toward "counterforce" and a first-strike strategy. In 1983–84 the Pershing II missiles began to be deployed in West Germany, a five minute lob to the Soviet Union. In the meantime, National Security Decision Directive 13 set forth plans to enable the United States to "prevail" in a "protracted" nuclear war. By 1984 the stockpile contained 26,000 nuclear weapons and was scheduled to double in the next ten years.

Pentagon officials insisted that nuclear war would not be all that devastating. "If there are enough shovels to go around," said the peppy assistant secretary in charge of civil defense, "everybody's going to make it," the shovels being required to dig holes in the ground, to be covered by a couple of doors and three feet of dirt; "it's the dirt that does it." The Federal Emergency Management Agency eased the pain with straight-faced plans for the evacuation of cities—6.5 million people to be transported out of New York by automobile in 3.3 days to "host areas" in the hinterland. In March 1983 Reagan proposed a ballistic missile defense system in space, an idea dismissed as technological fantasy by many scientists and dubbed the "Star Wars" plan in tribute to the popular space movie. Would the empire strike back?

The emphasis on "war-fighting" led some to fear that the Administration regarded nuclear weapons as usable and nuclear wars as winnable. Some in the Administration argued for the MX as a "bargaining chip" in arms-control negotiations. Others may have believed that an unlimited arms race offered a good way of doing the Soviet Union in. Either the Russians would try to keep up, which would wreck their economy, or they would fail to keep up, which would leave America the decisive military advantage. For its part, the Administration denied war-fighting intent and, along with the Soviet Union, observed the terms of the unratified SALT-II agreement. It also made periodic arms-control proposals, mostly aimed at the Soviet ICBM force and all rejected by Moscow.

Brezhnev died in November 1982 and was succeeded by Yuri Z. Andropov, former head of the KGB, the Soviet intelligence organization. During 1983 Soviet-American relations grew steadily worse. Some in the West blamed the attempted assassination of the Pope in July on the KGB. No one could doubt that the Russians, whether knowingly or not, shot down a Korean civilian airliner flying across Soviet territory, killing 269 people—a "crime against humanity," Reagan said. Andropov, in poor health, disappeared from the scene for long intervals. The war of words grew bitter and strident. By the end of the year the Soviet Union had walked out of all arms-control negotiations. The arms race rushed on.

The fear of nuclear holocaust stirred people to protest across the world, though not very much behind the Iron Curtain. In the United States a mass movement urged a mutual and verifiable freeze on the production, testing, and deployment of nuclear weapons. The "nuclear freeze," embodied in a resolution introduced in Congress by Senators Edward Kennedy and Mark Hatfield, had the backing of veteran diplomats like Averell Harriman and Henry Cabot Lodge as well as, according to polls, of 80 percent of Americans. Robert McNamara, George F. Kennan, and McGeorge Bundy advocated a "no-first-use" declaration by the United States and a comprehensive test-ban agreement with the Soviet Union. Kennan called for an immediate 50-percent reduction in American and Soviet nuclear stockpiles. Senator Henry Jackson proposed joint Soviet-American crisis centers in which each superpower could read the other's radar screens, thereby reducing the possibility of accidental war.

Observers noted that the Reagan foreign policy, while belligerent in language, was often circumspect in action. Yet language had its power too. Using the presidential pulpit with great skill (and with assists from the Kremlin), Reagan succeeded in carrying much American opinion back to the "holy war" of John Foster Dulles, though his Administration architects of American postwar policy. Neither could be accused of cherishing illusions about Soviet Russia.

Now they joined in condemning the confrontationist policies of the Reagan Administration. Neither could see objective reasons justifying the frightening impasse. "If present developments in nuclear arms and United States-Soviet relations are permitted to continue," said Harriman in 1984, "we could face not the risk but the reality of nuclear war." The deterioration of relations, said Kennan, has "the unfailing characteristics, of a march toward war—that, and nothing else." The state of political relations combined with nuclear arms presents "a shadow greater than any that has ever before darkened the face of Western civilization."

Such somber warnings at home and abroad, coinciding with the death of Andropov (who was replaced by a Brezhnev protege, Konstantin U. Chernenko) and with the impending presidential election, led Reagan in 1984 to tone down his rhetoric and profess more conciliatory attitudes toward the Soviet Union.

Cycles of American politics. The Reagan Administration represented the culmination of a conservative tide sweeping through American politics since the early 1970s. Though there were manifest differences between Carter and Reagan, much of Reaganism had its roots in the Carter years: deregulation and the attack on affirmative government in domestic policy, increased arms spending, counterforce, and moralism in foreign policy.

History reminded Americans of an inherent cyclical rhythm in their politics, a continuing alternation between liberalism and conservatism, between public action and private interest. As a nation, America regularly went through seasons of action, passion, idealism, reform, and affirmative government, until the country was worn out. Then people longed for respite and entered into seasons of exhaustion, drift, cynicism, hedonism, and negative government. So the progressive decades at the start of the twentieth century—the decades of Theodore Roosevelt and Woodrow Wilson—were followed by the conservative twenties; the progressive thirties and forties—the decades of Franklin Roosevelt and Harry Truman—by the conservative fifties; the progressive sixties—the decade of Kennedy and Johnson—by the conservative seventies and eighties. Two things regularly happened in the conservative periods: rest recharged the national batteries, and the neglected problems became acute and threatened to become unmanageable. In the twentieth century, historians noted, it had been roughly a thirty-year cycle from one time of progressivism to another: Theodore Roosevelt in 1901, Franklin Roosevelt in 1933, John Kennedy in 1961.

avoided anything like McCarthyism. The hard line, some said, was working. It had redressed the picture of American weakness, restored the nuclear balance in Europe, dissipated communist doubts about American readiness to use military force, and increased international respect for American power. Critics charged that Reagan's abandonment of diplomacy and negotiation had frightened America's allies, increased international distrust in American leadership, galvanized the Soviet bloc, and given new impetus to the nuclear arms race.

The two men with the longest involvement on either side in Soviet-American relations watched the rising tension with special concern. Averell Harriman had first visited the Soviet Union in the 1920s, served as Franklin Roosevelt's wartime ambassador to Moscow, warned after the war of Soviet aggressive purposes, and negotiated the limited test-ban treaty of 1962. George Kennan had helped open the American embassy in Moscow in 1934, had formulated the containment theory after the war (see p. 768), and later served as ambassador to Moscow. Both men had been

Suggestions for Reading

CARTER AND REAGAN

For Carter, his pre-presidential memoir *Why Not the Best** (1975), is followed by his record of his Presidency, *Keeping Faith** (1982). The best biography is Betty Glad, *Jimmy Carter, In Search of the Great White House* (1980). Reagan's pre-presidential memoir, also with a question mark, is *Where's the Rest of Me?* (1965), with R. G. Hubler. The best biography is Lou Cannon, *Reagan* (1982). Ronnie Dugger's *On Reagan: The Man and His Presidency* (1983) has valuable material on Reagan's ideological development. Robert Dallek, *Ronald Reagan: The Politics of Symbolism* (1984), mingles historical insight with psychoanalytical speculation. L. I. Barrett, *Gambling With History: Reagan in the White House** (1984), is an objective account by a White House correspondent.

FOREIGN AFFAIRS

Cyrus Vance's gentlemanly *Hard Choices: Critical Years in American Foreign Policy* (1983), and Zbigniew Brzezinski's pugnacious *Power and Principle: Memoirs of a National Security Adviser* (1983), present diverging views of foreign policy in the Carter years. Harold Brown adds the testimony of the Secretary of Defense in *Thinking About National Security* (1982). Alexander Haig defends his record as Secretary of State in *Caveat: Realism, Reagan and Foreign Policy* (1984).

K. A. Oye, et al., eds., *Eagle Entangled**, is a collecton of essays about aspects of Carter's foreign policy; the same team produced a mid-course assessment of Reagan's foreign policy in *Eagle Defiant** (1983). D. P. Calleo, *The Imperious Economy** (1982), is an excellent analysis of international economic perplexities. On Central America, Walter LaFeber, *Inevitable Revolutions: The United States in Central America* (1983), provides indispensable historical background, and R. S. Leiken, ed., *Central America: Anatomy of Conflict* (1984), ably analyzes current issues. On Iran, see Barry Rubin, *Paved with Good Intentions: The American Experience and Iran** (1980).

On nuclear issues, Solly Zuckerman, *Nuclear Illusion and Reality** (1982), is a lucid and authoritative summation by a leading British defense scientist. The essay "Launch on Warning" in D. P. Moynihan, *Loyalties* (1984), discusses the implications of the shift in nuclear doctrine to counterforce. Robert Scheer, *With Enough Shovels: Reagan, Bush and Nuclear War** (1982), reports the views of Reagan Administration officials. Strobe Talbott, *Endgame* (1979) and *Deadly Gambit* (1984) illuminates arms control negotiations. James Fallows, *National Defense** (1983), is an informed critique of the military procurement process.

DOMESTIC ISSUES

J. A. Califano, Jr., *Governing America** (1981), is an analytical cabinet memoir by Carter's Secretary of Health, Education and Welfare. L. C. Thurow, *The Zero-Sum Society** (1980), is an influential liberal analysis of economic issues. William Simon, *A Time for Truth** (1978); Milton and Rose Friedman, *Free to Choose** (1979); and George Gilder, *Wealth and Poverty* (1981), present the economic ideology behind the Reagan counter-revolution; and P. C. Roberts, *The Supply-Side Revolution* (1984), is an insider's story of Washington policy-making. Herbert Stein, *Presidential Economics* (1984), offers a more skeptical conservative view; and T. B. Edsall, *The New Politics of Inequality* (1984), is a cogent indictment. The deregulation movement is described in S. J. and Martin Tolchin, *Dismantling America: The Rush to Deregulate* (1983); for conservation issues, Jonathan Lash, et al., *Season of Spoils* (1984).

Peter Steinfels, *The Neoconservatives* (1979), analyzes the conservative revival. The future of American politics is provocatively considered in W. D. Burnham, *The Current Crisis in American Politics** (1982); Kevin Phillips, *Post-Conservative America** (1982); and J. M. Burns, *The Power to Lead: The Crisis of the American Presidency* (1984). J. S. Saloma, *Ominous Politics** (1984), is a useful survey of conservative political movements. Elizabeth Drew, *Politics and Money* (1983), discusses the ways in which money distorts the political process.

*Available in a paperback edition.

35

INTO THE
THIRD CENTURY

The year 1976 marked the two hundredth anniversary of the Declaration of Independence, and 1987 the two hundredth anniversary of the Constitution. America is still a youngish nation. If one counts American history by generations, eight span the entire national experience; if by lifetimes, three will do it. Justice Oliver Wendell Holmes, who died just before his ninety-fourth birthday in 1935, told his last secretary, who was still living half a century later, "Always remember that you have spoken to a man who once spoke to a veteran of the American Revolution." In 1982, the Veterans Administration sent pension checks to some fifty Civil War widows.

The New Society

Profile of a population. Midway in the next to last decade of the 20th century, the population of the United States was approaching 235 million. This would have disappointed Abraham Lincoln, who in 1862 had forecast 252 million by 1930. Still, the total had more than quadrupled in a century and more than doubled since 1920. But the postwar baby boom was followed by the most rapid sustained decrease in the nation's fertility rate—the number of births

among women in the child-bearing years—in American history. The rate of population growth between 1970 and 1980 was, except for the depression decade (1930–40), the lowest in the national record. Demography, a notably fallible science, predicted that the population would reach a peak of 309 million by 2050 and then start to decline.

Why had Americans decided to bring fewer children into the world? Women were marrying later. More women had jobs. Parents wondered about the future of children in an age of local and nuclear violence. The invention of new birth control methods, especially the pill, and the spread of vasectomies and other sterilization procedures gave couples new control over the size of their families. So too did the legalization of abortion; legal abortions rose from 18,000 in 1968 (though no one knew how many illegal abortions were taking place) to 1.6 million in 1980. The large family of the fifties fell out of fashion. The two-children family became the new ideal.

The new family was markedly less stable. Beginning with California in 1970, all states (except Illinois and South Dakota) had by 1982 passed some form of "no-fault" divorce, enabling either partner to divorce without having to prove traditional grounds or win the other's consent. In 1930, there had been 1.6 divorces for every thousand Americans; by 1980, the figure had risen to 5.2. A growing number of house-

**America:
a Chosen
Nation?**

For we must consider that we shall be a city upon a hill. The eyes of all people are upon us, so that if we shall deal falsely with our God in this work we have undertaken, and so cause Him to withdraw His present help from us, we shall be made a story and a byword through the world.

From John Winthrop "A Model of Christian Charity" (1630).

Have we not already seen enough of the fallacy and extravagance of those idle theories which have amused us with promises of an exemption from the imperfections, weaknesses, and evils incident to society in every shape? Is it not time to awake from the deceitful dream of a golden age, and to adopt as a practical maxim for the direction of our political conduct that we, as well as the other inhabitants of the globe, are yet remote from the happy empire of perfect wisdom and perfect virtue?

From Alexander Hamilton, *Federalist* No. 6.

We Americans are the peculiar, chosen people—the Israel of our time; we bear the ark of the liberties of the world.... God has predestinated, mankind expects, great things from our race; and great things we feel in our soul. The rest of the nations must soon be in our rear.... Long enough have we been sceptics with regard to ourselves, and doubted whether, indeed, the political Messiah had come. But he has come in us.

From Herman Melville, *White-Jacket* (1850).

Angelic impulses and predatory lusts divide our heart exactly as they divide the heart of other countries.

From William James, November 28, 1903.

The heart of this people is pure. The heart of this people is true.... America is the only idealistic nation in the world.

From Woodrow Wilson, September 8, 1919.

Nations, as individuals, who are completely innocent in their own esteem, are insufferable in their human contacts.... [We must never forget] the depth of evil to which individuals and communities may sink, particularly when they try to play the role of God to history.

From Reinhold Niebuhr, *The Irony of American History* (1952).

Call it mysticism if you will, but I believe God had a divine purpose in placing this land between the two great oceans to be found by those who had a special love of freedom.

From Ronald Reagan, March 31, 1976.

holds, especially among the young, were formed and dissolved without legal ceremony. In 1980 over 18 percent of births were to unmarried mothers; in 1960 the proportion had been 5 percent. One out of every five American children now lived in single-parent homes, more than 80 percent headed by women. The number of such families had increased by an astonishing 69 percent during the 1970s. Barely 20 percent of new households during the 1970s were formed by married couples.

The decline in the birth rate changed the age composition of the people. Between 1970 and 1980, the number of children under 15 declined by 6.5 million. People over 65, 4 percent of the population in 1900, were approaching 12 percent in the 1980s and were expected to reach 22 percent by 2030. The generation of the baby boom—one-third of the population in 1980 was born between 1946 and 1964—was passing through the decades like a pig through a python. Having supplied the basis for the youthful unrest of the sixties, it promised to have different social impact as its members became middle-aged and settled, even more different after 2010 when they would become a large claimant group of old folks. People already spoke of "the graying of America." Groups like the Gray Panthers pressed the claims of the elderly, whether to postpone the retirement age or to increase old-age benefits. Federal spending for the old, which had accounted for 2 percent of the budget in 1940, accounted for 27 percent by the early 1980s.

A baby born in 1985 could expect to live 75 years as against 47 for a baby born in 1900. Indeed, people 85 and over were the fastest growing age group in the 1980s. The increase in life expectancy resulted from new medical techniques and improved health services. Deaths due to heart disease, for example, declined by a quarter from 1970 to 1983. The share of gross national product spent on health more than doubled in the quarter century after 1960. Some thought a disproportionate amount of medical spending went to high-technology care for the very old and dying at a time when infant mortality was far higher in the United States than in Sweden or Japan. Among blacks the infant mortality rate was the highest than in any western industrialized country.

Immigration. Of the population increase in the 1970s, about 40 percent was due to immigration. The annual rate had increased from an average of 85,000 in the 1940s to over 400,000 in the 1970s—higher than in any decade since the first of the century. The composition of the new arrivals changed dramatically as a result of the Immigration and Nationality Act of 1965. That act abolished the discriminatory national-origins quota system (see p. 637) and established needed skills and the reuniting of families as the criteria for admission.

One unexpected consequence was a rapid increase in the number of Asian immigrants from about 7 percent of the total in 1965 to over 40 percent fifteen years later. Another 40 percent came from Latin America and the Caribbean. In 1965 Canada, Mexico, and Great Britain had been the leading sources. In

The graying of America

1980, Mexico, Vietnam, and the Philippines headed the list. Normal immigration was supplemented by the admission of refugees fleeing oppression in Vietnam, Cambodia, Cuba, and Haiti.

In 1976 amendments to the 1965 act limited immigration from the Western Hemisphere to an annual 20,000 visas per country. This change increased the influx of people entering the country illegally. "Wetbacks," fording the Rio Grande from Mexico to provide cheap agricultural labor for Texas and California, were an old problem, but the new wave of illegals came also from the Caribbean and from South America. Estimates of the number of "undocumented" aliens in the United States by 1985 ranged from four to eight million. Though it was charged that illegals were taking jobs away from citizens, evidence suggested that they performed menial tasks rejected by native workers and thereby filled a vacuum in the labor market. Their illegal status, however, exposed them to cruel exploitation in city sweatshops and as rural slaves and caused them to shun public facilities designed to protect and educate the poor.

For the first time in half a century immigration was emerging again as a significant factor in American life. The proportion of Americans who were white and of European ancestry—the basic ethnic stock since colonial days—was steadily declining. It was no longer uncommon to hear Korean spoken on the streets of New York, Arabic in Detroit, Hindi in Los Angeles, and Spanish everywhere. By the early 1980s more than 10 percent of the population spoke a language other than English at home.

Concern about immigration led in the early 1980s to the introduction of the controversial Immigration Reform and Control (Simpson-Mazzoli) bill, proposing amnesty for aliens who had entered the country before a certain date and penalties for employers who knowingly hired illegals. It also proposed an annual limit of 425,000 new immigrants (not counting refugees). The purpose of reform in the 1960s had been nondiscrimination. In the 1980s the purpose had become the restriction of unplanned immigration.

Where the people lived.

Americans, while still a wandering folk, wandered less: where 20 percent had changed residence in 1960, less than 17 percent did so twenty years later. The most striking population shift after the Second World War was to the so-called "sunbelt," the states below the 37th parallel from Virginia across to southern California—a shift encouraged by the invention of air-conditioning. In 1964 California surpassed New York to become the most populous state. Almost 90 percent of population growth in the seventies took place outside the Northeast and Midwest. If those trends continued, 60 percent of the people would live in the sunbelt by 2000.

Money was also moving from the North into the sunbelt, with its advantages in energy sources, raw materials, lower taxes and wages, bracing air, and wide-open spaces. And the population shift had evident political implications. Between the Civil War and the Second World War, only two men born outside the Northeast (including Ohio) lived in the White House. Of the eight Presidents after 1945, only one came from the Northeast. Each new census gave the South and West further weight in the House of Representatives and the Electoral College.

Whether the sunbelt would operate as a political unit remained, however, unclear. Despite the anti-government rhetoric cherished by the politicos of the region, economic growth along the southern rim depended heavily on federal funds. The South and West, for example, received twice as much of the defense dollar as the Northeast and Midwest. The reliance on the federal government, along with the pluralizing effects of industrial growth and urbanization, might leave sunbelt politics with patterns little different from those of the rest of the country.

Ordeal of the city.

For the first time since the early 1800s, rural areas were growing faster than metropolitan areas. The number of Americans living on the countryside or in towns under 2,500 increased 11 percent in the 1970s. Cities were also losing population to suburbs. By 1980 nearly 45 percent of Americans lived in suburbs as against less than 30 percent in central cities. New York, Philadelphia, Detroit, and other major cities actually shrank in population. The mystique of suburbia—ranch houses, picture windows, green lawns, swimming pools, station wagons, shopping malls, high-technology parks—exerted potent appeal.

In fact, the city of 1980 was by most standards a better, cleaner, and safer place to live than the city of 1900. Jacob Riis (see p. 480) found 300,000 people per square mile in New York at the turn of the century. Few cities eighty years later showed a concentration of more than 75,000 per square mile. Substandard housing declined in these years from 50 to about 15 percent of the total stock. Factories caused far less pollution; the automobile liberated city streets from horse droppings; city government was less corrupt.

But the immigrant ghettos of 1900 had been bearable because they were thought to be temporary. As soon as families saved enough money, they moved on—a process accelerated by automobiles and freeways. The subsequent flight to the suburbs eroded the self-sufficiency of the American city. The city of 1900 financed its services out of its own resources. This was no longer the case by 1980. The migrants were beyond the reach of the city's taxing power; and the traditional remedy—annexing the surrounding areas—

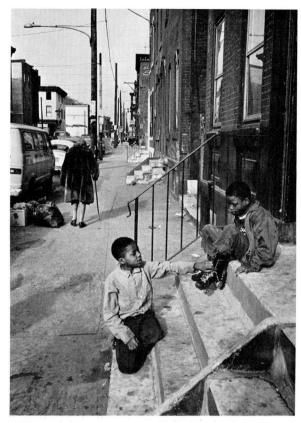

Philadelphia ghetto: a permanent home?

failed before suburban insistence on self-rule. The new city-dwellers, replacing the old middle class, were tax consumers rather than tax producers.

Populated more and more by the poor, the elderly, the brown, and the black, cities had fewer resources on which to draw at the very time that the need for public facilities became more urgent. For the black and the brown, the ghetto was likely to be not a temporary but a permanent home. Education consumed nearly a fifth of municipal budgets and remained the most hopeful means of social conciliation and improvement. But inner-city schools tended to be overcrowded and underequipped. *De facto* segregation and chaotic family life undermined educational motivation. The drop-out rate was three times as high among black high-school students as among white. Many schools were demoralized by defeatism and paralyzed by drug addiction and random violence.

"Crime in the streets" became a political issue; and, though many who invoked the phrase used it as a code word with which to incite emotion against blacks, the rise in crime was sharp and disquieting. Crimes were characteristically committed by males between eighteen and twenty-four, generally poor, often drug addicts. The rate was naturally highest

where poverty, drugs, discrimination, and unemployment converged: the ghetto. And, though some tried to suggest that violent crime was a form of race war committed by blacks against whites, the victims themselves, except in robberies, were typically young, poor, and black.

Beyond street crime there lay the murky underworld of organized crime. Whether or not the Mafia existed as the closely organized, centrally controlled criminal secret society sentimentally portrayed in the popular film *The Godfather* (1972), no one could doubt the existence of interstate criminal syndicates, sometimes working together in loose confederation, sometimes waging savage war against one another, spreading corruption and fear into the business community, the labor movement, and local government.

Criminals, organized or unorganized, indulged themselves increasingly in murders, two-thirds of which were committed with guns. More than 150 million firearms were in American households, of which 55 million were handguns, easily concealed in hip pockets. Two hundred thirty million Americans comfortably outstripped all other modern democratic peoples in rates of homicide, assault, rape, and robbery, providing about fifty times as many gun murders each year as did England, Japan, and West Germany with the same combined population. Pressure for effective federal gun control, arising after the assassinations of the sixties, was regularly frustrated by the impassioned lobbying of the National Rifle Association.

Crime was the ultimate expression of urban disorganization. And the troubles of Metropolis were compounded by the fact that it had begun to give way to Megalopolis. Cities wandered aimlessly into the surrounding countryside, generating suburbs and then exurbs, sprawling across municipal and even state frontiers, creating vast ungovernable urban regions, stretching from Boston to Washington, from Pittsburgh through Chicago to Milwaukee, from San Diego to San Francisco.

The urban crisis of the sixties had been one of riot and upheaval. Though this subsided in the seventies, it was quickly replaced by a new crisis—the crisis of municipal finance. The fiscal plight of the cities was dramatized in 1975 when the greatest of them all, New York City, came very close to financial default. New York's problems arose partly from local circumstance—an improvident borrowing policy, heavy pension commitments to city employees, and an inordinately heavy welfare burden. The crisis resulted too from the fact that New York was a national city, taking in poor citizens from other parts of the United States, thereby reducing tensions and taxes in Southern states and in Puerto Rico.

The decline of urban self-sufficiency argued for a national urban strategy. The Supreme Court decision

Gentrification in Boston

on legislative apportionment in *Baker* v. *Carr* (1962) gave cities more equitable representation in state legislatures, heretofore dominated by rural counties. The establishment in 1965 of the Department of Housing and Urban Development created a base for national action. Vital elements in a national policy included the federalization of welfare, federal guarantees for municipal bonds, and a revision of revenue-sharing to meet specific urban needs. Such a policy confronted, however, the mistrust of cities that had been an abiding prejudice since the time of Jefferson.

In the longer run, the falling birth rate promised some alleviation of urban distress. Moreover, suburban homogeneity crumbled under the increasing migration; and as urban problems—high taxes, pollution, drugs, crime—spread into the suburbs, there were signs of disenchantment with suburbia, even hints of a return flow to the metropolis. By 1980 the process of "gentrification"—rehabilitation of old low-income neighborhoods by upper-income newcomers—was visible in a number of cities. The future of the American city, though clouded, seemed far from hopeless.

How the people worked. The composition of the labor force continued to change. White-collar and service workers had first outnumbered blue-collar workers in the 1950s; thirty years later, there were twice as many. Only a third of American workers were in manufacturing. With the rise of highly mechanized, highly capitalized agriculture after 1940, the proportion of farm workers declined even more—from 30 to 2.7 percent of the workforce.

These changes reflected massive shifts in the structure of the economy. Most striking of all was the decline in heavy industry, once the glory of the American economy—a decline that led observers to speak melodramatically of the "twilight of smokestack America" and even of the "deindustrialization of America." An international redivision of labor was giving the comparative advantage in steel, automobiles, farm machinery, chemicals, rubber, textiles, apparel, and shoes to Third World countries. American steelmakers, for example, had failed to modernize their plants; nearly a tenth of steel was still produced in open-hearth furnaces. Countries with more efficient machinery and lower labor costs now had the competitive upper hand. Automotive production declined from 13 million vehicles in 1978 to 7 million in 1982. As plants closed in Detroit, Akron, Youngstown, Buffalo, the industrial heartland was a scene of stagnation and decay.

The country's growing dependence on the world economy increased its industrial vulnerability. In 1960, the total value of exports and imports amounted to less than 10 percent of the gross national product; by 1983 trade accounted for more than 25 percent. But the policy of combatting inflation by raising interest rates resulted in an overvalued dollar, overpriced exports and the loss of foreign markets. In the early 1980s the United States experienced the largest merchandise trade deficit in its history, with manufactured exports dropping by 20 percent and jobs in manufacturing decreasing by 2 million. A predictable consequence was a rising clamor for tariff protection, quotas, and other means of defending American industries.

The great increase in employment in the 1970s came in services and in retail trades. Eating and drinking places, health services, and business services accounted for more than 40 percent of the new private jobs created between 1973 and 1980. By the end of the

Fast-food: dead-end job

decade the increase in fast-food employment was greater than the total employment in the once thriving industries of automobile and steel. Because trade unions found it difficult to organize the new sectors, union membership declined from 35 percent of nonagricultural workers in 1954 to less than 20 percent in the 1980s. This meant that four out of five members of the nonfarm labor force did not belong to unions.

The impression of economic decline was reinforced by evidences of serious decay in the "infrastructure" of the economy—highways, railroads, bridges, harbors, canals, dams, tunnels, water and sewage systems. According to one estimate, for example, two out of every five bridges in the country were unsafe and required repair or replacement.

One question for the future was whether the free market could rescue America's industrial base, restore American competitiveness in world markets, and renew the nation's infrastructure; or whether economic revival would not require a more purposeful national action. "We cannot become a nation of short-order cooks and saleswomen," said Felix Rohatyn, a New York banker with impressive insights into the economic dilemma. He and others called for one or another form of "industrial policy," designed to bring government, industry and labor together in partnership to overcome the nation's economic troubles. Opponents feared that government intervention would only make matters worse. Supporters pointed

to the success story of American agriculture, the sector of the economy with the highest productivity growth and the greatest competitive advantage in world trade—and also the sector that had experienced the highest degree of federal regulation, research and educational subsidy, price guarantees, crop insurance and other forms of government assistance and control.

Women in the new society. Women in America continued to widen their numerical lead over men. By the mid-1980s there were nearly 8 million more females than males. And barriers to women continued to fall. In 1950 a third of the female population was in the labor force, by the 1980s more than half. In 1970 women took only 8 percent of medical degrees, by 1980 23 percent. A third of all law-school graduates were women, from 5 percent in 1970; 10 percent of engineering graduates, from 1 percent in 1970. In 1980 women held almost a third of executive and managerial jobs as against less than a fifth ten years earlier. Six million women earned more than their husbands. Thirty-five percent of women were in college as against 34 percent of men. Men were increasingly prepared to take a larger share in child rearing and household tasks; many, noting that "Mr." as a title did not betray marital status, were willing to accept "Ms" as a substitute for both "Miss" and "Mrs." Women sat on the Supreme Court and sailed in outer space. Few male sanctuaries remained. Even West Point and Annapolis surrendered. And Geraldine Ferraro of New York received the 1984 Democratic nomination for Vice President.

But progress toward equality brought problems. The incidence among women of stress ailments—alcoholism, drug addiction, heart disease, and nicotine-induced lung cancer—was on the increase. And discrimination remained. Though 6 million more women than men voted in 1980, less than 5 percent of Congress was female, and only one state governor. Women who held full-time jobs in 1983 received only two-thirds the pay of their male counterparts. Wages of white women entering the job market lagged farther behind the wages of comparable white men in 1980 than in 1970. In a lifetime, according to the Census Bureau, a man would probably earn twice as much as a woman with the same education. While more women held traditional male jobs, a "female ghetto" survived. More than 90 percent of typists, receptionists, nurses, bank tellers, and telephone operators were women. Moreover, women were so large a proportion of the poor that sociologists talked about the "feminization of poverty." By the early 1980s, nearly half the 7.5 million households living in poverty were headed by women, as against a quarter twenty years before.

The women's movement suffered acute disappointment in the failure to secure ratification of the Equal Rights Amendment. This amendment, first submitted by Alice Paul's National Women's Party in 1923, proposed to write into the Constitution the rule that "equality of rights under the law shall not be denied or abridged by the United States or by any state on account of sex." In earlier years, many women leaders, including Eleanor Roosevelt, Frances Perkins,

Mary McLeod Bethune, and Carrie Chapman Catt, had opposed ERA on the ground that it would divest women of hard-won protective social legislation. But, when the Civil Rights Act of 1964 outlawed protective legislation based on gender, many previous opponents now endorsed ERA. In 1972 Congress passed ERA, providing a seven-year deadline for ratification by the states. Though polls showed two-thirds of the population in support, a powerful anti-ERA campaign conjured up such fears as that women would be sent into combat and that separate toilet facilities would be abolished. ERA, said Phyllis Schlafly, was "a total assault on the family, marriage, and children." By 1979 only 35 out of the necessary 38 states had ratified, and five of these voted to rescind. The extension of the deadline to 1982 was of no avail.

The National Organization of Women now decided to concentrate on electing women to Congress and state legislatures. While the number of women state legislators had trebled from 1969 to 1981, they were still only 12 percent of the total. In 1984 there were only twenty-four women in the House of Representatives, only two in the Senate. But ERA, abortion, Reagan's *macho* foreign policy, and his patronizing attitude on women's issues had created a "gender gap"—a measurable difference in the way in which women and men saw issues and supported candidates. A new issue, designed to combat economic inequities, was "comparable worth"—a concept that, going beyond equal pay for equal work, called for equal pay for different jobs of comparable value.

The ideological reconsideration of the role of women continued. Women's liberation had generated forms of revolutionary feminism ascribing racism, imperialism, and other evils to male supremacy. Militants saw marriage as a hell where the husband was a rapist, the wife a prostitute, the baby a trap, and the family a prison. As an interim measure, they proposed "marriage contracts" defining reciprocal obligations. Some moved on to attack the "nuclear family" itself, hoping to replace it by an extended family structure with children raised collectively. Some advocated lesbianism as the only true feminist commitment.

Militant feminists provided ammunition for the Phyllis Schlaflys who wished to reaffirm woman's subordinate role. The militants also provoked women's liberation leaders to reformulate their goals. In *The Second Stage* (1981) Betty Friedan urged her sex "to discuss feminist denial of the importance of the family, of women's own needs to give and get love and nurture, tenderloving care." Friedan now called on women to see men, not as foes, but as fellow victims of a dehumanized society. Many women again followed Friedan's lead in seeking to combine the hope of equality with a realistic recognition of sexual differences.

Clerical workers: a "female ghetto"

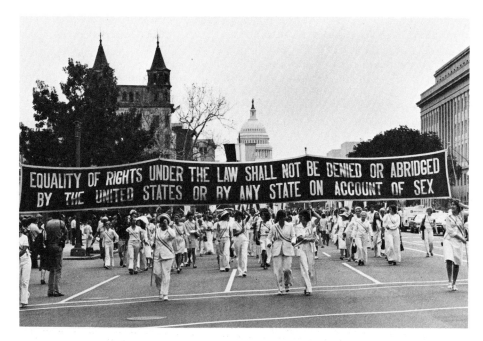

In twenty years the women's movement had wrought deep and probably irreversible changes in women's lives—and men's. The movement had indeed raised the consciousness of American society, had greatly increased male sensitivity to female frustrations and humiliations, and had encouraged in women new convictions of self-reliance and entitlement.

The rise of ethnicity. Women's liberation was only one expression of a broad drive of submerged groups for identity and justice. Other movements followed ethnic lines. The old theory had been that the United States was a "melting pot" where many nationalities fused into one: *e pluribus unum.* But after the Second World War representatives of so-called "ethnic" groups began to see the melting pot as a symbol of cultural imperialism, designed to force a diverse and polyglot society into a white Anglo-Saxon Protestant (WASP) mold. (The word "ethnic" applied properly to any group whose members claimed a common origin but came by the 1970s to refer particularly to immigrants from southern and eastern Europe, especially Poles, Italians, Greeks, and Slavs.)

In practice, ethnicity implied a reassertion of ancestral traditions and values against the dominant WASP culture. Where an older generation had discarded nationality traits in the quest for Americanization, the new generation formed "antidefamation" leagues to combat anti-Semitism, Polish jokes, or the idea that all Italians were members of the Mafia. Writers, saluting the "unmeltable ethnics," drew the portrait of neighborhoods based on nationality, populated by hard-working, unassuming, patriotic people. Social scientists measured "antiethnic" discrimination in American institutions. Thus one study showed that, while Italians, Poles, blacks, and Latins made up over one-third of Chicago's population, they constituted less than one-twenty-fifth of the directors and officers in Chicago's major corporations.

Politics, along with sport, entertainment, and crime, had provided historic means for ethnic advance. However, the ethnic role in politics was marked by conflicts between each established group and the next wave: the Anglo-Saxons versus the Irish; the Irish versus the Italians; the Italians versus the east Europeans; the other white ethnics versus the Jews; all white ethnics versus the browns and the blacks.

The last tension became especially acute as a result of the civil-rights revolution. Low-income whites were not against equal rights in principle; but they were against equal rights at the expense of their children, their neighborhoods, their jobs, and their safety in the streets. Many felt that the national government was intervening on behalf of blacks as it had never done for them and that black gains were taking place at their own expense. Rightwing politicians played astutely on this tension. It also to some degree divided the old New Deal coalition. Low-income whites talked bitterly about "limousine liberals" who fled to the suburbs and left them to face the day-to-day consequences of racial change.

Black America. By the early 1980s 27 million blacks accounted for 12 percent of the American people. During the 1970s, black population increased faster than population as a whole. And, for the first time in decades, the proportion of blacks living in the central cities declined. Many were moving to the suburbs, while more blacks were returning to the South than leaving it, succumbing like whites to the economic lure of the sunbelt.

The position of black Americans had improved radically since the civil-rights revolution. Talk of "white supremacy" vanished. Mandatory legal segregation was abolished, access to public accommodations assured. In 1960, only half as many blacks as whites finished high school; by 1980, four-fifths as many. Blacks now attended colleges in almost the same proportion as whites relative to population totals, and the proportion of those taking degrees had quadrupled since 1960. The proportion of blacks owning their homes increased twice as fast as whites. The representation of blacks in professional and administrative occupations doubled. In the 1970s, the real income of black husband-wife families actually rose more than that of similar white families. 1983 saw the first black astronaut in space and the first black Miss America.

The most striking gain of all—because it accelerated every other dimension of racial progress—came in politics. The Voting Rights Act of 1965 delivered a massive enfranchisement of southern blacks. Of the more than 5,000 elected black officials in 1983, half held office in the South. Even a onetime militant segregationist like George Wallace now crowned a black homecoming queen at the very university that, a decade earlier, he had sworn to deny to black students.

Rev. Jesse Jackson: spokesman for an underclass

Throughout the land blacks registered and voted as never before. By the mid-1980s, Washington, Chicago, Los Angeles, Philadelphia, Detroit, Atlanta, New Orleans, Birmingham, Richmond, Newark, and Spokane had elected black mayors. Urban politics was finally doing for blacks what it had long done for immigrants: providing a means of incorporation into a previously alien political system. One consequence was a reduction of the violence that had marked black protest in the 1960s. In 1984 the candidacy for the Democratic nomination of Jesse Jackson, who united the evangelical zeal of a black preacher with the professional skill of a black politician, gave a potent stimulus to black political action.

Despite the gains, blacks remained predominantly at the lower end of the economic scale. Racial barriers were falling far faster for middle-class than for lower-class blacks. Some observers now perceived two increasingly distinct classes—the educated affluent and the uneducated poor. Middle-class blacks had unprecedented opportunities for professional and managerial careers, while working-class blacks often sank into an "underclass" that trapped them in a web of poverty from which it was almost impossible to escape. The gap in average incomes between whites and blacks was as wide in 1983 as in 1960. The unemployment rate for blacks in the 1980s was twice as high as for whites; among teenage blacks, four or five times as high. Nearly half of all black families were headed by women without husbands—more than twice as large a proportion as in 1960—and half these families had incomes below the poverty line. In New York, blacks accounted for two-thirds of the arrests for violent offenses, also for two-thirds of the prison population, also for the majority of the victims of crime. This situation persuaded some that race *per se* was of declining significance and the black underclass was the victim not of prejudice but of poverty. Others insisted that blacks were still imprisoned in a legacy of institutionalized racism so deeply imbedded that it defied both national legislation and individual good will. It indeed appeared that the analogy between black immigrants to the cities and their European predecessors was invalid. White immigrants had survived squalid ghettos because with time and success they knew they could move into better neighborhoods. Racial prejudice restricted the escape-valve of mobility for blacks. The policies that had absorbed white immigrants did not work for black Americans. The long-run hope lay in new policies that would break entrenched residential patterns and open outer areas to black residents—and in the will to justice in American society.

White America since the 1960s had consistently favored nondiscrimination and equal opportunity (voting rights, public accommodations, affirmative action) but had been more dubious about what it saw as special privileges for blacks (quotas, mandatory busing). The Reagan Administration, by removing the federal government from the struggle for racial justice, deepened black pessimism. Political action now loomed as the most promising remedy.

Hispanic Americans. The fastest growing minority were the Hispanic Americans. During the 1970s Hispanics increased by 60 percent, the result both of immigration, legal and illegal, and of a high birth rate. Some demographers expected Hispanics to overtake blacks as the nation's predominant minority in the early twenty-first century.

Of the 15 to 18 million Hispanics by 1980—the illegals made statistical precision difficult—about 60 percent were Mexican, 15 percent Puerto Rican, 7 percent Cuban. The rest came mostly from the Caribbean and South America. The Mexicans lived in the main in the Southwest, the Puerto Ricans in the Northeast, the Cubans in Florida. Income levels averaged slightly higher than blacks; educational levels, with the linguistic handicap, somewhat lower.

Spanish-speaking enclaves had survived in New Mexico for nearly five centuries, and for many decades Mexicans had entered the United States to satisfy the need for cheap agricultural labor. But it was not till after the Second World War that the Mexican-Americans, who in the sixties called themselves proudly

Cesar Chavez

"Chicanos," began to act as a conscious minority. Pride in their history and traditions facilitated the quest for identity. In California, Cesar Chavez and his United Farm Workers improved the wages and working conditions of migrant farm-laborers. In New Mexico, Reies López Tijerina tried to reclaim land grants that "Anglos" had long since wangled from the original owners. In Texas, José Angel Gutiérrez formed a political party, *La Raza Unida.*

The Puerto Rican population on the mainland rose by 55 percent in the sixties, with more than three-fifths living in New York City. Unlike the other Hispanics, they were American citizens. The brilliant musical show *West Side Story* (1957), adapting the Romeo and Juliet theme to "rumbles" between Puerto Rican and white street gangs, won a sympathetic hearing for problems in the larger community. In 1970 New York elected its first Puerto Rican congressman.

The Puerto Ricans of New York had political rivalries with the blacks as well as problems among themselves. With recession in the United States, the tide of migration began to flow back to Puerto Rico; but returning natives encountered economic difficulties there. They also encountered contention between the Puerto Rican majority, who wished to remain part of the United States as a commonwealth or even to acquire statehood, and a passionate minority that demanded Puerto Rican independence. In 1950 Puerto Rican nationalists had tried to kill President Truman. In later years they carried out intermittent terrorist activities on the mainland.

By the 1980s Hispanic-Americans were emerging as a political force, electing a governor in New Mexico and mayors in Denver, San Antonio, Miami, Tampa, and Santa Fe. Mexicans and Puerto Ricans tended to be Democrats, Cubans Republicans. Unlike the European immigrants of the nineteenth century or the Asian immigrants of the late twentieth century, Hispanics were less eager to learn English and follow the traditional path of assimilation into American life. Their distinctive interest lay in promoting bilingualism in education, in manpower training, and on the ballot. Others feared that bilingualism represented an abandonment of the historic creed of assimilation, that it handicapped newcomers by delaying their induction into English and that it threatened to fragment the country into linguistic ghettos. A common language, many believed, was an essential bond of cohesion in an increasingly disparate society.

Indians. The oldest and truest Americans, the Indians, were no longer the vanishing Americans. As a result of public-health improvements, Indian birth rates were about double those of the nation as a whole. Indian population grew from 343,000 in 1950 to 1.4 million in 1980. Half lived in the West and a quarter in

Red power *We, the first Americans, come to the Congress of the United States that you give us the chance to try to solve what you call the Indian problem. You have had two hundred years and you have not succeeded by your standards. It is clear that you have not succeeded in ours.... We ask you, as the representatives of the people of the United States, to serve as our representatives too—to help us see that assurances do not become empty promises. And, if necessary, to enact legislation which will create such a process where Indians can really shape government policy and control their own lives and destinies....*

The present [congressional] committees have pushed for termination, and have fostered on Congress seemingly neutral and technical legislation, under the guise of Indian expertise, which has taken away our land, our water rights, our mineral resources and handed them over to the white man. You have been duped—as we have been duped. These committees have created a monstrous bureaucracy insensitive to Indians which trembles and cringes before them.... We know you are highly conscious of your national obligations when you deliberate on such problems as the war in Viet Nam. We know that you have even taken those obligations seriously enough to go to Viet Nam in order to personally inform yourself on how the Executive carries out the commitments of the United States. We ask that you do no less at home—for the United States has made older and more sacred commitments to the people who have occupied these shores for twenty-five thousand years.... In essence, we ask the restoration of what you claimed at the founding of your nation— the inalienable right to pursue happiness.

From the American Indian Task Force, Statement to Congress, November 12, 1969.

the South. Over half lived on reservations; most of the rest lived in cities. Wherever they lived, they were the poorest of the poor, at the end of the line in employment, income, education, health, and life expectancy. The suicide rate among Indians was twice that of the rest of the population.

National policy toward the Indians continued to vacillate between the goals of autonomy and assimilation. The effort begun under the New Deal by John Collier to encourage "a self-governing self-determination" and to revitalize tribal government was rejected by Congress after the Second World War. The new policy, crystallized in a congressional resolution of 1953, had the ultimate goal of "termination"—that is, liquidating the reservation system, dismantling the tribes, removing special federal protection and services, and hoping that Indians could somehow fend for themselves as individuals in white society. The Bureau of Indian Affairs in Washington continued to be a white agency governing reservation Indians according to highly paternalistic principles.

The Kennedy Administration arrested the termination process and began to move toward self-determination. But a great deal was at stake—55 million acres of Indian lands with water, timber, grass, and minerals—and white interests, working through the congressional Interior Committees and the Bureau of In-

dian Affairs, were determined to deny Indians control of their territory. Then in 1970 the Nixon Administration asked Congress to repeal the termination resolution of 1953 and proclaimed "self-determination without termination" as the new national policy. The Indians were to assume control of their own affairs, and the national government, acting as trustee, would protect their land and resources. Nixon followed this by setting in process the Indianization of the Indian Bureau; by 1974 more than 60 percent of the Bureau's employees had Indian forebears.

However, Congress failed to pass enabling legislation; and, in so far as the executive branch executed the new policy, the effect was to give power to tribal governments dominated in some cases by leaders who were in collusion with white interests. Indian activists, inspired in part by the black example, meanwhile formed nationalist organizations and denounced the reservation leaders as "Uncle Tomahawks." The National Congress of American Indians (NCAI), founded during the Second World War (in which twenty-five thousand Indians had served in the armed forces), became more aggressive; and the American Indian Movement (AIM), formed by militant urban Indians in 1968, raised the standard of "red power." The violent occupation of the Indian Bureau in Washington in 1972, the invasion the next year of the village of Wounded Knee, South Dakota, scene of the infamous massacre of 1890 (see p. 438), and other acts of terrorism soon, however, discredited the militants.

Indians now increasingly turned to the courts to sue for the restoration of their lost land and water, mineral, and fishing rights, generally on the plea that treaties had been violated and that the transfer of such rights to whites had not received the congressional approval required by the Nonintercourse Act of 1790. In South Dakota the Sioux Nation won compensation for the white man's seizure of the Black Hills. The state of Maine agreed to settle land claims made by the Passamaquoddy and Penobscot tribes.

The Reagan Administration, determined to take government off the Indians' backs too, sought sharp cuts in federal assistance to Indian tribes. "If you want an example of the failures of socialism," said Secretary of the Interior Watt, "don't go to Russia. Come to America, and see the American Indian reservations." Though the Administration proclaimed its devotion to Indian self-government, Indian leaders feared a return to the policy of termination.

A number of books—notably *Custer Died for Your Sins* (1969) by Vine Deloria, Jr., a Standing Rock Sioux, and Dee Brown's *Bury My Heart at Wounded Knee* (1971)—brought the Indian case to an increasingly sympathetic public. For decades the only good Indians in Hollywood had been dead ones; but now films like *Little Big Man* (1970) and *Billy Jack* (1971) displayed Indians as victims rather than villains. Though the future for Native Americans, as many now termed themselves, remained uncertain, the Indi-

ans had succeeded remarkably in changing popular attitudes.

Tribulations of the permissive society. The counter-cultural revolution of the 1960s had challenged the conformist social patterns of the 1950s in the name of the gospel of personal self-fulfillment. This gospel continued in slightly different form in the 1970s. However much the hippie-Weatherman culture of the sixties and the consumer-*Playboy* culture of the seventies differed in political attitudes, they agreed in regarding what one writer termed the "quest for the ideal self" as the supreme aim of life. "Getting in touch with your emotions" and "finding yourself" were key phrases. *How To Be Your Own Best Friend* and *Looking Out For #1* were best-selling books. Hedonism became so preoccupying in the seventies as to produce the description "the Me decade" and learned books about *The Culture of Narcissism.*

But things were changing. The baby-boom generation was growing older; the young revolutionaries, at last over the fatal age of thirty, dropped back into the bourgeois routine. The prosperity of the sixties gave way to economic uncertainty and stern competition in the job market. It became a time to reappraise values. In this process of sorting out, the new society absorbed some of the changes wrought by the permissive society and repudiated others in the name of a new gospel of social discipline.

The counter-culture survived in "laid-back" attitudes toward dress, language, and sexual freedom. Men, once the sober species, continued after the six-

**The New Left
grows older**

When in doubt, burn. *Fire is the revolutionary's god. Fire is instant theater. No words can match fire. / Politicians only notice poverty when the ghettos burn. / The burning of the first draft card caused earth tremors under the Pentagon. / Burn the flag. Burn churches. / Burn, burn, burn.... / Amerika is falling apart: the alternative is revolution or catastrophe. / The revolution has replaced the church as the country's moral authority.*

From Jerry Rubin, *Do It!*, 1970.

I saw us move out of youth-oriented yippie consciousness to think of ourselves as parents, adults, mature men. I had always feared aging ... But I actually enjoy getting older. I have become happier. At 37 I feel better than I have at any other time in my life. I want to be politically active again—but not at the expense of my happiness and health. I do not want to be in a crazy movement that psychologically drains its people.

From Jerry Rubin, *Growing (Up) at 37*, 1976.

Politics and rebellion distinguished the 60s. The search for the self characterized the spirit of the 70s. Money and financial interest will capture the passion of the 80s.... If I am going to have any effect on my society in the next 40 years, I must develop the power that only control of money can bring.... Welcome, Wall Street, here I come!

From Jerry Rubin, "Guess Who's Coming to Wall Street," *New York Times*, July 30, 1980.

---

ties to sport beards, blue jeans, and cowboy boots. Slacks became the casual dress of women from dowagers to hookers. Old inhibitions and reticences disappeared, apparently for good. Where Clark Gable as Rhett Butler had shocked the movie audiences of 1939 by telling Scarlett O'Hara, "Frankly, my dear, I don't give a damn," four-letter Anglo-Saxon monosyllables became common not only in movies but in living rooms. "Soft-core" pornography flourished in the cinemas and the magazine-racks. The question of "hard-core" pornography remained in suspense as a result of an erratic series of Supreme Court decisions.

The new tolerance extended to what had been historically the most sensitive of all problems for Americans—sex. The objective study of sexuality had gained impetus from two works by the biologist Alfred Kinsey: *Sexual Behavior in the Human Male* (1948) and *Sexual Behavior in the Human Female* (1953). The sexual act itself received unrelenting scrutiny from William Masters and Virginia Johnson in *Human Sexual Response* (1968). While sociologists doubted that changes in sexual practices had been all that great, there was plainly a vast change in public attitudes. "Co-habitation" no longer raised eyebrows. Ninety-five percent of males and over 80 percent of females between eighteen and twenty-four acknowledged premarital intercourse. Married couples sometimes indulged in "swinging"—group intercourse

with other couples. Oral sex and other less conventional forms of sexual expression became common.

Homosexuals, male and female, came "out of the closet." Appropriating the word "gay," they organized in defense of their civil rights, persuading the American Psychiatric Association in 1973 to stop listing homosexuality as a psychiatric disorder. Members of Congress confessed to homosexuality, and in some states "gay rights" groups became forces in politics. Homosexual themes became so aggressive in the arts that one observer complained, "The love that dare not speak its name just won't shut up these days."

Drugs were another inheritance from the counter-culture. Though LSD fell out of fashion, marijuana smoking remained routine in many circles. Heroin was now the lower-class addiction, while cocaine became the favorite of the affluent professional. In 1984 it was estimated that 22 million Americans had used cocaine and that 5–6 million used it regularly. Drugs were a big business for organized crime—the estimated $30 billion annual revenues for cocaine would place it seventh among America's top 500 corporations. Efforts to stop the flow of drugs from Colombia, Pakistan, and other nations were of small avail.

Revival of traditional values. While the commitment of the 1960s to freedom of individual choice remained alive in the 1980s, the appeal for discipline gathered new strength. This appeal was reflected in the impressive growth in number and wealth of the evangelicals and fundamentalists—those Protestant sects emphasizing personal conversion, the inerrancy of Scripture and absolutist moralism. Encouraged by the election of a "twice-born" President in 1976 and of a President in 1980 responsive to the Moral Majority, the evangelicals intensified their condemnation of sinful society. The spread of genital herpes and of AIDS (acquired immune deficiency syndrome) was interpreted as divine judgment on sexual promiscuity.

The new mood extended far beyond the Moral Majority. Dismay over crime, drugs, and drink was widespread. States began to raise the drinking age, to crack down on drunken drivers, to impose mandatory sentences for criminals, to restrict bail and parole. Cultural vigilantes censored textbooks, libraries, and school reading assignments. Polls showed that college students in the 1980s, unlike their counterparts in the sixties and seventies and more in the style of students in the fifties, favored the death penalty, questioned abortion on demand and (perhaps because of genital herpes and AIDS) shrank from casual sex.

There was particular concern about the restoration of standards in education. The 1980 census reported that, for the first time in history, a majority of persons in every state had completed four years of high school. College enrollment trebled between 1960 and 1980. But there was increasing dissatisfaction with the results. The popularity of "soft" subjects in the curriculum, declining scores in achievement tests, the absence of discipline in public schools, the persistence of functional illiteracy (23 million adults according to a 1983 report)—all led to demands for greater emphasis on grammar, mathematics, science, and other "core subjects," and for "minimum-competency" requirements for promotion and graduation.

The public school system, according to President Reagan, "began to deteriorate when the federal government started interfering with education." Accordingly he called for cutbacks in federal spending for education and in federal student loans. His main initiatives were to propose prayers for public schools and tuition tax credits for private schools. Critics observed that the public schools doubtless needed prayer but also would benefit from more tangible attention. Tuition tax credits, in their view, could only be a grievous blow against the system of public education on which most Americans still depended. They called instead for increased federal activity to undertake a national literacy campaign, to train and reward teachers in "core" subjects, and in various ways to prod and assist localities to improve the quality of education available to all children.

The electronic media. Formal education through the printed word had to compete more than ever with informal education through the moving image. The movies remained America's most distinctive art. Where the American contribution to the world's literature, music, painting, sculpture had been marginal, film, without the American contribution, would be inconceivable. And the motion picture had always been the people's art. Even during the depression 60 percent of Americans went to the movies every week. But television brought average weekly attendance down to 22 percent by 1960. Production declined. Cinemas closed. Hollywood went to work for the home screen.

Then in the 1970s came a film revival, welling from the bottom up, manifest in campus groups, film societies, bookshops. The movies, having resigned the mass audience to television, found new life in specialized audiences, small theaters, and pictures made on location. Directors like Robert Altman (*M*A*S*H*, 1970; *Nashville*, 1975), Stanley Kubrick (*2001: A*

Space Odyssey, 1969; *A Clockwork Orange, 1971*), Sidney Lumet (*Dog Day Afternoon*, 1975; *Network*, 1976), Woody Allen (*Annie Hall*, 1977; *Zelig*, 1983), Francis Ford Coppola (*The Godfather*, 1972; *Apocalypse Now*, 1979) used the new artistic freedom to explore with sharp and original eye areas of the contemporary scene and the contemporary psyche.

Television, the high-pressure offspring of film and radio, superseded movies as the great leisure-time occupation and newspapers as the source of much of the people's news. More Americans had television sets in 1980 than had modern plumbing, and their sets were turned on an average of seven hours a day. Most television time was expended on soap opera, sports, quiz shows, "sitcoms" (contrived situation comedies), and advertising. Some went to news programs and investigative reports, often of high quality, to discussions and documentaries, and to the dramatization, often more boldly than in the movies, of social questions like racial bigotry (as in Norman Lear's popular show "All In the Family"), adultery, divorce, homosexuality, incest, child abuse.

Defenders of the new medium argued that television extended people's horizons, told them more about current affairs than their local newspapers, and prepared them for a world of danger and violence. Others were especially concerned about television's impact on children. Educators pointed out that, between the ages of 6 and 18, the average child spent 13,000 hours in school and 16,000 hours before the tiny screen. Critics contended that television shortened children's attention span, reduced their linguistic facility and reading ability, enfeebled their sense of reality, habituated them to violence, and nourished the belief that problems were readily resolvable, often by a gunshot (the "Gunsmoke" ethic).

Television was obviously here to stay. Its ultimate impact depended in part on whether it became entirely subservient to advertisers and market forces, or whether, as in Great Britain, a national effort would be made to raise standards. During the 1970s, the Federal Communications Commission had tried to improve children's programming; but the Reagan Administration's deregulation policy led to a marked worsening of "kidvid" in the 1980s. There was now diminished federal support for the Public Broadcasting Service and other forms of educational broadcasting and for National Public Radio. But there were also signs that the national love affair with commercial television was waning. A 1983 survey by the National Association of Broadcasters, an industry group, suggested that viewers were watching television less, were critical of its addiction to violence and sex, and considered it less vital in their lives than they had in a previous survey in 1977.

Literature and art. Despite the lure of television, adult Americans at least seemed to be reading as much as ever. Fifty thousand books were published in 1983 as against 11,000 in 1950. Book sales *per capita* among adults of reading age rose from 2.75 in 1970 to 4.9 in 1980. The continuing expansion of the paperback market, with half a billion sold each year, brought books within everyone's reach.

On lower literary levels, romantic tales ("gothics") vied with science fiction and sex melodrama for the attention of escapists. Serious writers in the years after the Second World War, moving beyond the social art of the depression years, tended to be private, somewhat withdrawn from the problems of society, deeply involved in individual quests for personal identity and meaning. These quests often took place in strongly rendered regional or ethnic contexts. Thus the tradition of Southern writing, intensified and elaborated by Faulkner in the twenties and thirties, was continued in the postwar years by Robert Penn Warren of Tennessee, notably in *All the King's Men* (1946), his novel about Huey Long's Louisiana, and by writers of the next generation—William Styron of Virginia, whose *Confessions of Nat Turner* (1967) was the attempt of a Southern white to come to a reckoning with the historical fact of slavery; Walker Percy of Mississippi and the exquisite women writers Eudora Welty of Mississippi and Flannery O'Connor of Georgia.

In the North the WASP novel of manners, perfected by James and Howells, exemplified in the prewar generation by the astute satire of J. P. Marquand and the sardonic realism of James Gould Cozzens, was still alive. But the age of Anglo-Saxon dominance was receding; brilliant younger writers like John Cheever and John Updike now portrayed the suburban WASP at bay in an increasingly heterogeneous and bewildering society. Gore Vidal's series of historic novels—*Burr* (1973), *1876* (1976), *Lincoln* (1984)—cast a cold eye on the nineteenth century past, while the non-WASP E. L. Doctorow drew a radical bead on more recent history in his vivid novels *The Book of Daniel* (1971) and *Ragtime* (1975).

Ethnicity became as potent a theme in fiction as in sociology. Following the path broken by James T. Farrell in the thirties, Edwin O'Connor (*The Last Hurrah*, 1956) and J. F. Powers recorded further phases in the assimilation of the Irish into American life. Mario Puzo dealt with the Italian-Americans in *The Dark Arena* (1955) and in his best seller *The Godfather* (1969). Richard Wright's *Native Son* (1940) was a powerful portrayal of the fate of the American black; and Ralph Ellison's *Invisible Man* (1952), one of the distinguished novels of the period, displayed in forceful terms the struggle of the black for visibility in

American society. Alice Walker and Toni Morrison gave poignant insights into the ordeal of black women. James Baldwin in a series of books played upon the agony of two minorities—blacks and homosexuals.

The postwar years also saw the emergence of a gifted generation of Jewish novelists. Coming from a traditional culture, afflicted by historical and contemporary woes, the best writers in this school not only offered vivid annotations of Jewish-American life but spoke in some sense for all minorities in the quest for self-understanding. Philip Roth in *Goodbye, Columbus* (1959), *Portnoy's Complaint* (1969), and his Nathan Zuckerman trilogy combined a merciless novelist's eye with sharp comic and mimetic instincts. Bernard Malamud fabulized Jewish urban life in a series of piquant fantasies. J. D. Salinger's tales about the Glass family, especially in *Franny and Zooey* (1961), explored the possibilities of mysticism and sainthood in an affluent society. In *The Catcher in the Rye* (1951) Salinger also portrayed an adolescent crisis of identity—Huck Finn at an Eastern prep school—in terms that spoke arrestingly to a whole generation. And two other Jewish writers, Saul Bellow and Norman Mailer, transcended their cultural base to deal in large terms with the incoherence and anguish of contemporary life.

No American novelist dealt more searchingly with contemporary man than Bellow in such novels as *The Adventures of Augie March* (1953), *Seize the Day* (1954), *Herzog* (1964), and *Humboldt's Gift* (1975). He was the artist of the dialectic between inner consciousness and external society—the predicament of "civilized people" of whom his character Herzog said, "What they love is an imaginary human situation invented by their own genius and which they believe is the only true and the only human reality." But, where Bellow looked on the ravages of modernity with increasing distaste, his younger and less finished contemporary Mailer plunged truculently into the swirl around him.

War veteran, novelist, poet, journalist, film director and actor, political aspirant, pugilist, male chauvinist, showman, public personality, the spoiled and symptomatic talent of his time, Mailer saw art as, above all, the precipitate of minority experience. Though some critics believed Mailer more comfortable in his nonfiction, like *The Armies of the Night* (1968) and *Of a Fire on the Moon* (1970), his highly charged reporting was of a piece with the vision of the American experience conveyed brilliantly in his novel *Why Are We in Vietnam?* (1967). The tension between rationality and irrationality, between the public act and the underground emotion, fascinated him; and though he himself wondered whether his "vision, for lack of some cultivation in the middle, was not too

compulsively ready for the apocalyptic," no writer took on more cheerfully the existential risks of American art.

For many writers, the key to chaos lay in the abandonment of realism, a literary mode that could not survive, they believed, the collapse of a coherent world view. Such writers resorted to forms of fabulation, in which mental constructs replaced the workaday world, thereby, it was thought, creating a reality closer to the truth than realism could ever provide. This writing was anti-rational, mythological, often magical, sometimes apocalyptic, always hostile to the technological cosmology. The satiric fantasies of Kurt Vonnegut, Jr.; the cabalistic hallucinations of Donald Barthelme; the exuberant, savage anarchism of Joseph Heller's *Catch-22* (1961); the wild, quasi-scientific despair of Thomas Pynchon's *Gravity's Rainbow* (1973); the lurid allegory of John Irving's *The World According to Garp* (1978)—all paid tribute through dislocation, parody, and mysticism to an increasingly incomprehensible universe. Mailer's *Ancient Evenings* (1983), saturated in the rites and rituals of old Egypt, was a far cry from the gritty naturalism of *The Naked and the Dead* (1948). "Is the spiritual air poisoned beyond repair?" Mailer asked. "Is there no saving reaction in it. . . . I expect that we're going to have odd convulsions, surrealistic events, that terrorism will increase. . . . There may be a vast potential out there. I don't see the way yet. There is a thinning of the mist, but no light."

The cultural vibrations ran through poetry, where Robert Lowell in *Life Studies* (1959) and *For the Union Dead* (1964) registered the impact of an incoherent age on the Puritan sensibility, and where Sylvia Plath expressed the terror of women in a world of treacherous men. The best drama of the period, Eugene O'Neill's *A Long Day's Journey into Night*, was produced in 1956 but written fifteen years before. Arthur Miller revived the social drama in strong and somber plays like *Death of a Salesman* (1949); and such dramas as Tennessee Williams' *A Streetcar Named Desire* (1947) and Edward Albee's *Who's Afraid of Virginia Woolf?* (1962) concentrated with brilliant if cold effect on the pathology of modern life. In due course new currents struck the drama when the "theater of the absurd" of Ionesco and the "theater of cruelty" of Artaud came from Europe to stimulate American playwrights off Broadway, if not on.

Other arts were affected by the tendencies toward anarchy and nihilism. In painting, abstract expressionism superseded for a season the representational art of an earlier time. Jackson Pollock, who had died little known in 1956, was now taken up as the forerunner of an attempt to give the tensions of contemporary culture their objective correlative in color and design. In

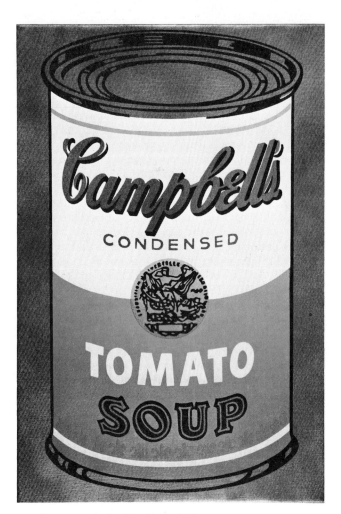

Pop art: Andy Warhol, 1965

the sixties "pop art" sought to discover artistic significance in the commercial artifacts of the consumer culture.

The development of a public arts policy represented a significant change in the position of the arts in American society. The WPA arts projects under the New Deal had given writers (like Bellow, Cheever, and Ellison) and painters (like Pollock, Philip Guston, and Willem de Kooning) employment as part of the relief program. The National Endowments for the Arts and Humanities established in the 1960s acquired sufficient congressional and popular support by the 1980s to survive the Reagan Administration's attempts to cut their budgets. After the opening of New York's Lincoln Center in 1962, cultural and performing arts centers, headed by the Kennedy Center in Washington, spread across the land. By 1983 some 2000 such centers housed arts organizations, decentralized cultural life, and made the arts accessible to millions of people. This striking development emphasized the extent to which the arts had become a vital and approved part of American life.

The Velocity of History

The law of acceleration. The salient fact of the modern age was the increasing instability generated by the cumulative momentum of science and technology. Henry Adams had been the first American historian to note the ever-quickening acceleration in the velocity of history. "The world did not [just] double or treble its movement between 1800 and 1900," he wrote in "The Rule of Phase Applied to History" (1909), "but, measured by any standard known to science—by horsepower, calories, volts, mass in any shape—the tension and vibration and volume and so-called progression of society were fully a thousand times greater in 1900 than in 1800." And the pace of change, urged ever onward by the self-generating processes of scientific inquiry, exploded in the twentieth century when, it was noted, of all the scientists who had ever lived in the history of the planet, 90 percent were alive and active.

The acceleration of change was a major factor in the energy crisis with industrial expansion devouring increasing quantities of oil, coal, and natural gas. By the early 1980s the combination of worldwide recession with conservation measures had lowered the consumption of oil, creating the appearance of an international oil glut. By 1983 only 5 percent of oil supplies to the United States came from Arab OPEC countries, as against 17 percent a decade earlier, and OPEC itself was no longer the unified and aggressive organization it had been. But experts declined to exclude the possibility of future oil shortages and shocks.

In any event, the price of energy was five times higher than a decade before, and the energy future remained clouded. Nuclear energy, once seen as the key to the world's energy dilemma, was regarded with mounting dubiety. Nuclear plants turned out to be more expensive and less safe than anticipated; the radiation risks after the near meltdown at Three Mile Island turned out to be higher than originally supposed. The disposal of radioactive wastes raised difficult problems; no one wanted to live in the vicinity of underground nuclear dumps. An emotional lobby of environmentalists and others campaigned against nuclear energy. Even though 87 nuclear plants were cancelled between 1975 and 1983, still 77 nuclear plants in 1983 produced 13 percent of the nation's electricity; and nuclear energy, under proper safeguards, was bound to have a role in the future.

The law of acceleration also contributed to an incipient ecological crisis. Unbridled expansion had produced pollution of water and air, erosion of the soil, disturbance of the balance of nature, and disruption of the self-replenishing cycle that for eons had sustained life on earth. America the beautiful was

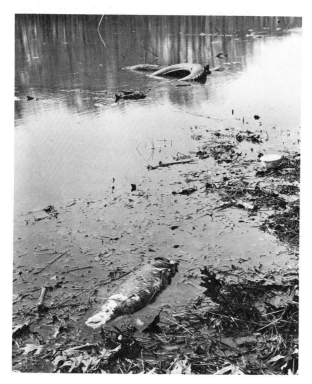

Pollution: America the beautiful?

marked, not by alabaster cities and fruited plains, but by black oil slicks smearing the beaches; by rivers and lakes filled with sewage, industrial wastes, phosphates, and detergents; by towns enveloped in smog spewed forth by automobile exhausts, factory chimneys, and burning dumps; by the destruction through the use of pesticides of the relationship among plants, animals, and the natural environment. Most ludicrous of all was the possibility that fluorocarbon gases discharged from aerosol spray cans would breach the shield of ozone that protected the earth from ultraviolet radiation. If this prediction came true—much scientific evidence supported it—then, someone observed, the world would perish neither with a bang nor a whimper but with a "psssst."

The electronic society. Henry Adams had predicted in particular that his law of acceleration would carry the world from what he called the Mechanical Phase into the Electric Phase, "the sharpest change of direction, taken at the highest rate of speed, ever effected by the human mind."

The dream of a machine that would instantaneously solve intricate mathematical problems had a long history, but it was not till 1946 at the University of Pennsylvania that the first electronic digital computer was built. It weighed thirty tons, occupied the space of a two-car garage, and cost nearly $10 million. In 1948 Bell Laboratories developed the transistor, a

small, solid-state device that made possible the use of integrated circuits. The computer grew still smaller, swifter, and cheaper with the development in 1959 of semiconductor packages imprinting transistor devices on a piece of silicon. The process of "miniaturization" eventually made it possible to imprint 100,000 transistors on a thin silicon wafer. "In three decades," someone observed, "a whole roomful of vacuum tubes and other components has been reduced to the size of a cornflake." The "microchip" became the pivot of the electronic revolution.

No invention since the steam engine promised so many drastic changes. By incorporating intelligence and memory in machines, the computer brought about a revolution in "data processing"—the storage, retrieval, and analysis of information. People now spoke of the "information society," in which national strength depended less on the goods manufactured than on the information produced and processed. The new machines, by controlling a multiplicity of variables, made possible calculations that no human brain could have performed, any more than the human eye could have seen cellular structure before the invention of the microscope. Moreover, the microchip was inexpensive, easy to produce, low in its energy needs, and capable of an infinite variety of application.

The microchip revolution was predominantly an American creation, though by the 1980s Japan was mounting a serious challenge in supercomputers and was far ahead in robotics. Microelectronics were already transforming basic aspects of American life. Electronic calculators and watches were widespread; the home computer and the word processor were in increasing use; offices and factories were beginning to be more completely automated; telecommunications, employing optical fibers and satellites, flashed information across the country and the world; engineers, doctors, bankers, economists, teachers, and students relied increasingly on computers; children congregated in video-game arcades; the invasion of privacy by two-way cable systems and electronic information banks seemed a growing threat; robots were on the march. And new generations of electronic monsters loomed ahead: machines that could walk, talk, see . . . reason?

Consequences of high technology. The microchip brought problems as well as benefits. For the first time in modern history, technological innovation threatened to destroy more jobs than it created. From 1980 to 1983, the "high technology" sector generated less than half the jobs lost in manufacturing. Though the labor force was now growing more slowly, and though unemployment could be relieved for a time by sharing work through reduction of hours and by federal employment of the jobless to rebuild the

School for the "information society"

cian and the voter, interceding for each on behalf of the other and providing the links that held the party system together. Electronic innovations were now severing those links and bypassing the traditional political structure. Television presented the politicians directly to the voter; computerized public opinion polls presented the voter directly to the politician; and the mediating agencies were withering away.

As voters increasingly made their own judgments on the basis of what they themselves saw on the tiny screen, party loyalties, once as sacred as religious affiliations, lost their grip. Beginning in the fifties, voters began to use both parties for their own purposes, thus balancing off a Republican President with a Democratic Congress. Not only ticket-splitting but nonvoting increased. The proportion of voters describing themselves as "independent" grew strikingly. The "independent" party was twice as large as the Republican party and almost as large as the Democrats. Among young voters independents outnumbered Democrats. The political analyst Samuel Lubell saw "a war of the voters against the party system." Some observers expected a trend toward multiple parties and minority victors; others even began to speculate about a "politics without parties." Whether or not the two-party system was in dissolution, no one could deny that it was in crisis.

High technology held out the possibility either of the extreme centralization or decentralization of society. Some feared that the new electronic instruments signalled the rise of an intrusive and authoritarian "computer state." Others predicted that work, education, religion, even shopping would be increasingly concentrated in the home, now become the "electronic cottage," and feared that the family computer terminal would intensify the isolation and alienation of mass society.

Nor could anyone predict the ultimate impact on the human consciousness. The computer, as a machine committed to logic, might strengthen rational and analytic tendencies. On the other hand, the computer's qualities of instantaneity, and collectivity, everything descending on us from everywhere all at once, might carry the contemporary sensibility itself into a stage of profound dissocation. The Canadian Marshall McLuhan saw incalculable consequences in the shift from a typographical to an electronic culture. Where Marx had located the motive force of history in changes in the means of production, McLuhan located it in changes in the means of communication.

The sensibility created by the print media, he argued, had given experience a frame and viewed it in sequence and from a distance. The print culture's qualities were logic, precision, specialization, individualism. But in the electronic age, "The contained, the

nation's infrastructure, the prospect of high levels of future employment seemed inescapable.

Moreover, high technology created two kinds of jobs: well-paid jobs for skilled engineers and programmers; poorly paid, tedious jobs for unskilled and semiskilled operatives and clerks. This development, along with the rise in dead-end jobs in fast-foods and other service industries, led alarmists to write about the "declining middle" of the American work force. Some even foresaw the "disappearance of the middle class."

This prospective polarization of the labor force had ominous political implications. At the same time, the electronic revolution was eroding the traditional structure of American politics. For a century a cluster of agencies—the political machine, the farm organization, the trade union, the chamber of commerce, the ethnic federation—had mediated between the politidistinct, the separate—our western legacy—are being replaced by the flowing, the unified, the fused." The multiform ways of seeing and experiencing opened by the new modes of communication promised to alter the very reflexes of psychological reaction and expectation. Where the print culture had programmed the mind in a one-at-a-time, step-by-step way, the electronic culture undermined linear processes of thought, replacing one-at-a-time by all-at-once. Though the terms of McLuhan's argument were extravagant and McLuhan himself soon fell out of fashion, there remained the possibility that, beneath the hyperbole and the showmanship, he was onto a significant and fertile truth.

Genetic engineering. The winds of acceleration blew through all the sciences. Molecular biology in particular now thrust forward into the very bases of human life. The discovery in 1953 of the double-helix structure of deoxyribonucleic acid (DNA), for which the American James D. Watson and two Englishmen received the Nobel Prize in 1962, showed scientists how the genetic code of life was organized, how it might be deciphered, how it could even be manipulated.

With surprising speed, scientists learned how to sever and splice genes, how to induce cellular organisms to manufacture complex proteins, how to manufacture artificial genes in the test tube. "Recombinant DNA"—the combining of genes into new substances—promised not only the cure of genetic diseases but genetic transplantation, test-tube babies, and "cloning"—that is, the production of genetically identical copies of individual human beings. By 1984 $2.5 billion was invested in more than a hundred companies in the growing biotechnology industry.

Scientists also saw the possibility of remolding the human mind through drugs, psychosurgery (brain operations designed to modify behavior), electrochemical controls, and the system of behavioral conditioning and reinforcement set forth by the psychologist B. F. Skinner. Within a generation science had begun to devise the means not only to blow up the world but to transform reproduction, consciousness, intellect, behavior, and the very genetic nature of human beings.

These developments opened frightening vistas of manipulation by white-coated Dr. Strangeloves or Dr. Moreaus. Scientists themselves worried about the consequences of their discoveries. James D. Watson proposed in 1971 a pause in experimentation with human cell fusion and embryos. "If we do not think about the matter now, the possibility of our having a free choice will one day suddenly be gone." Federal guidelines for recombinant DNA research were imposed in 1975.

But, as the belief grew that benefits were certain and risks speculative, the guidelines were relaxed in the 1980s.

The endless frontier. The most spectacular expression of the onward thrust of science and technology came in man's escape from gravity and wondrous leap into space. The manned landing on the moon (1969) was followed by the dispatch of unmanned spacecraft to far reaches of the solar system. In 1976 Viking 1 and 2 transmitted photographs and scientific data from Mars back to earth. In 1979 Voyagers 1 and 2 flew past Jupiter, photographed its great moons, and streaked on to Saturn. In 1983 Pioneer 10 became the first man-made object to leave the solar system and sail on forever in the great void of interstellar space. In the late 1980s Galileo will orbit in space around Jupiter and send a probe into the very atmosphere of the giant planet. Such missions greatly enlarged scientific knowledge about the formation of planets and the geology of the solar system.

The government's emphasis in the Reagan years shifted, however, from space science to the military and commercial exploitation of space. The success of the space shuttle, a reusable manned rocket, led in the early 1980s to proposals for a permanent space station, a project favored by private industry but opposed by many scientists as a misguided diversion from serious space exploration.

The adventure of space and the possibility of life elsewhere in the galaxy continued to seize the popular imagination. Science fiction was never more popular; and films like Stanley Kubrick's haunting *2001: A Space Odyssey*, George Lucas's *Star Wars* trilogy, and Steven Spielberg's *Close Encounters of the Third Kind* (1977) and *E.T.* (1982) broke box-office records. Credulous people believed that UFOs (unidentified flying objects) were conducting an alien surveillance of the troubled earth.

As the space probes went forward, the question grew ever more insistent whether earthlings were alone in the universe. Pioneer 10, in case it might be intercepted by sentient beings in distant galaxies, carried a plaque displaying images of a nude man and woman and a diagram of the solar system. Scientists devised more systematic means to communicate with other intelligences in the cosmos. In 1971 American radio astronomers, physicists, biologists, and cryptographers joined colleagues from the Soviet Union and other nations at Byurakan Astrophysical Observatory in Soviet Armenia for the world's first Conference on Communication with Extra-Terrestrial Intelligence. In 1976 NASA set up its Search for Extra-Terrestrial Intelligence (SETI) program. With every passing year, scientists around the world watched and

If extraterrestrial civilizations are ever discovered, the affect on human scientific and technological capabilities will be immense, and the discovery can positively influence the whole future of Man.... Why should an advanced society wish to expend the effort to communicate such information to a backward, emerging, novice civilization like our own? I can imagine that they are motivated by benevolence; that during their emerging phases, they were themselves helped along by such messages and that this is a tradition worthy of continuance.... I do not believe that there is any significant danger from the receipt of such a message, providing the most elementary cautions are adhered to.

From Carl Sagan, *The Cosmic Connection*, 1973.

A thousand, or ten thousand, years of evolutionary difference is just nothing on cosmic scales; and the chances that we could come across another civilization in the Universe at approximately the same level of development—and with which we could effect some kind of intellectual understanding—are, therefore, vanishingly small. And such being the case, what gain ... could we hope to derive from contacts with hypothetical civilisations which are likely to be removed, not thousands, but millions or hundred millions of years from our level? Certainly the risks entailed in such an encounter would vastly exceed any possible interest—let alone benefit; and could easily prove fatal. Therefore, should we ever hear that "space-phone" ringing in the form of observational evidence which may admit of no other explanation, for God's sake let us not answer; but rather make ourselves as inconspicuous as we can to avoid attracting attention.

From Professor Zdenek Kopal, University of Manchester, quoted in the London *Telegraph*, March 3, 1972.

The pessimists assume that once a civilisation has opened the Pandora Box of nuclear reactions it will, sooner rather than later, eliminate itself; the optimists believe that a few pinches of SALT may suffice to prevent this. My own cherished belief is that those species in the galaxy which are mentally unstable biological misfits (as homo sap. seems to be) will choose the first alternative; while the sane, good and beautiful will survive. Thanks to this process of natural selection, the baddies perish and the universe is inhabited by goodies, all over the starry sky. It is a comforting thought, and not quite as silly as it may seem.

From Arthur Koestler, "Horizons in Space," *Encounter*, October 1979.

listened ever more urgently for signals from the sky, wondering what nature of being might be on similar watch on unknown planets, what forms of intelligence, perhaps immeasurably superior forms, might exist in the cold reaches of galactic space.

Into the future. As Henry Adams's law of acceleration had predicted, the onward surge of science and technology was drastically speeding the rate of historical change. The first rockets were launched during the Second World War; a quarter century later men rocketed to the moon. The first electronic computer was built in 1946; thirty-five years later scientists were working on fifth-generation computers. The double helix was unveiled in 1953; thirty years later, biotechnology threatened to remake humankind. The first atomic bomb was dropped in 1945; forty years later the world shuddered under the possibility of nuclear holocaust.

Humanity was subjected in the last half of the twentieth century to a series of incredible shocks, each of which by itself would have taken decades to

Adventure in space

digest and control. All the shocks accelerated the velocity of history; the nuclear shock threatened the end of history.

The arms race rushed on. The chances of nuclear war through accident or miscalculation or madness multiplied. According to the Joint Chiefs of Staff in 1982, the worldwide count of intercontinental nuclear weapons had gone up 200 percent in the preceding decade, explosive power some 30 percent, and hard-target-kill potential 200 percent. By 1984 nearly 50,000 nuclear warheads were in existence, most with de-

structive power ten or twenty times greater than the bomb dropped on Hiroshima. Official estimates forecast that more than thirty countries would be able to produce nuclear weapons by the year 2000. A large-scale nuclear war would kill from 300 million to a billion people outright. The whirling clouds of dust and soot generated by the multiple detonation of nuclear weapons would blot out the sun and bring about "nuclear winter," leaving the survivors of the awful blast to freeze or starve to death. The prospect, unless nuclear weaponry were to be brought under control,

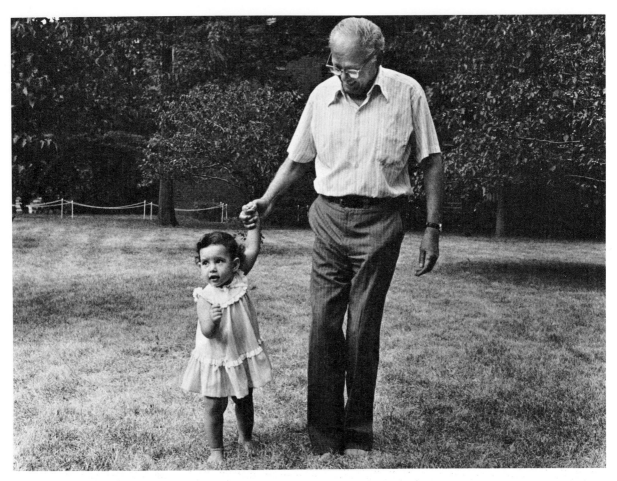

The old and the new stand side by side

was nothing less than the extinction of the human race.

Let us leave the last gloomy word to Henry Adams. "Man has mounted science, and is now run away with," he wrote to his brother Charles Francis Adams, Jr., on April 11, 1862, a few days after the Battle of Shiloh, while the *Monitor* and the *Merri-mack* were maneuvering around Newport News. "I firmly believe that before many centuries more, science will be the master of man. The engines he will have invented will be beyond his strength to control. Some day science shall have the existence of mankind in its power, and the human race commit suicide by blowing up the world."

Suggestions for Reading

THE SOCIETY

J. K. Galbraith, *The New Industrial State** (1967) and *Economics and the Public Purpose** (1973), reflect on the economic structure of industrial society. Daniel Bell, *The Cultural Contradictions of Capitalism** (1976), examines cultural implications. Clark Kerr, *The Future of Industrial Societies* (1984), peers into the shadows ahead.

Barry Bluestone and Bennett Harrison, *The Deindustrialization of America** (1982), is pessimistic about the American economy. Robert Kuttner, *The Economic Illusion* (1984), discusses the future of the labor force. G. C. Fite, *American Farmers: The New Minority* (1981), ably shows how success proved the farmer's undoing. O. L. Graham, *Toward a Planned Society** (1976), records the evolution of the planning ethos. Felix Rohatyn, *The Twenty-Year Century* (1984), R. A. Muller, *Revitalizing America* (1980), and Robert Reich, *The Next American Frontier** (1983), discuss industrial policy.

L. Y. Jones, *Great Expectations** (1980), reflects on the baby boom generation. For the graying of America, see W. A. Achenbaum, *Old Age in the New Land: The American Experience Since 1970** (1978); *Shades of Gray** (1983); and Stephen Crystal, *America's Old Age Crisis** (1982). Betty Friedan, *The Second Stage** (1981), points to new directions for liberated women. J. M. Kreps, *Women and the American Economy** (1976), and Caroline Bird, *The Two-Paycheck Marriage: How Women at Work are Changing Life in America** (1979), focus on women's economic role. Morton Hunt, *Sexual Behavior in the 1970s* (1974), updates Kinsey; and Paul Robinson, *The Modernization of Sex* (1976), is a stimulating review of changing mores. John D'Emilio, *Sexual Politics, Sexual Communities: The Making of a Homosexual Minority in the United States* (1983), describes the emergence of homosexuals. Harvey Cox, *Religion in the Secular City* (1983), assesses new religious tendencies. Paul Starr, *The Social Transformation of American Medicine** (1983), is an impressive study.

John Crewdson, *The Tarnished Door* (1983), surveys immigration problems. P. S. J. Cafferty and William McReady, eds., *Hispanics in the United States: A New Social Agenda** (1984), is a valuable introduction. E. D. Baltzell, *The Protestant Establishment** (1964), depicts the WASP at bay. On the ethnicity vogue, see Michael Novak, *The Rise of the Unmeltable Ethnics* (1972), and for a useful corrective, Orlando Patterson, *Ethnic Chauvinism* (1977). On black Americans, in addition to works by Sitkoff and Wilkinson cited in previous chapters, see W. J. Wilson, *The Declining Significance of Race: Blacks and Changing Institutions** (1978); and, for a conservative view, see Thomas Sowell, *Ethnic America** (1982), and *Civil Rights: Rhetoric or Reality?* (1984). Works on the American Indian include, A. M. Josephy, ed., *Red Power** (1971), and A. M. Josephy, *Now That the Buffalo's Gone: A Study of Today's American Indians* (1982).

CULTURE
D. J. Czitrom, *Media and the American Mind** (1982), is a pioneering inquiry. Marshall McLuhan's eccentric but suggestive ideas can be traced in *The Gutenberg Galaxy** (1962), *Understanding Media** (1964), and *The Medium is the Message* (1967). V. C. Ferkiss, *Technological Man* (1969), and Alvin Toffler, *Future Shock** (1970) and *The Third Wave** (1980), speculate about the consequences of the increased velocity of history.

David Halberstam, *The Powers That Be** (1979), is a lively account of the media. The impact of film is ably discussed in Robert Sklar, *Movie-Made America** (1975), and Garth Jowett, *Film: The Democratic Art* (1976). Diane Ravitch, *The Troubled Crusade: American Education 1945–1980* (1983), is an intelligent critical account. Tony Tanner, *City of Words: American Fiction 1950–1970* (1971), and Warner Berthoff, *A Literature Without Qualities: American Writing Since 1945* (1979), are sensitive and rewarding. Frederick Karl, *American Fictions: 1940–1980* (1984), is a defense and explication of literary modernism. Alfred Kazin, *Bright Book of Life** (1973), is a discussion by a leading critic of novelists from Hemingway to Mailer. Grant Webster, *The Republic of Letters* (1979), is a history of postwar literary opinion.

THINGS TO COME
Robert Stobaugh and Daniel Yergin, eds., *Energy Future** (3rd ed., 1983), and Daniel Yergin, et al, *Global Insecurity: A Strategy for Energy and Economic Renewal** (1983), consider energy problems. J. N. Shurkin, *Engines of the Mind: A History of the Computer* (1984), recounts the evolution of the new technology; J. D. Bolter, *Turing's Man: Western Culture in the Computer Age* (1984), and Sherry Turkle, *The Second Self* (1984), attempt to assess the computer's impact on culture and society. Tom Wolfe, *The Right Stuff** (1979), describes the first astronauts. Gerard O'Neill, *The Hight Frontier** (1977), considers the possibility of human colonies in space. The case for the existence of other beings in the universe is analyzed in Philip Morrison, et al, eds., *The Search for Extraterrestrial Intelligence* (1977); Carl Sagan and I. S. Shklovsky, *Intelligent Life in the Universe** (1968); and Sagan, *The Cosmic Connection** (1973). Jonathan Schell, *The Fate of the Earth** (1982), is an eloquent meditation on the possibility of human extinction.

*Available in a paperback edition.

Appendix A

The Declaration of Independence
The Constitution of the United States of America
Admission of States
Population of the United States

The Declaration of Independence*

THE UNANIMOUS DECLARATION OF THE THIRTEEN UNITED STATES OF AMERICA,

WHEN in the Course of human events it becomes necessary for one people to dissolve the political bands which have connected them with another, and to assume among the Powers of the earth, the separate and equal station to which the Laws of Nature and of Nature's God entitle them, a decent respect to the opinions of mankind requires that they should declare the causes which impel them to the separation.

We hold these truths to be self-evident, that all men are created equal, that they are endowed by their Creator with certain unalienable Rights, that among these are Life, Liberty and the pursuit of Happiness. That to secure these rights, Governments are instituted among Men, deriving their just Powers from the consent of the governed. That whenever any Form of Government becomes destructive of these ends, it is the Right of the People to alter or to abolish it, and to institute new Government, laying its foundation on such principles and organizing its Powers in such form, as to them shall seem most likely to effect their Safety and Happiness. Prudence, indeed, will dictate that Governments long established should not be changed for light and transient causes; and accordingly all experience hath shewn, that mankind are more disposed to suffer, while evils are sufferable, than to right themselves by abolishing the forms to which they are accustomed. But when a long train of abuses and usurpations, pursuing invariably the same Object evinces a design to reduce them under absolute Despotism, it is their right, it is their duty, to throw off such Government, and to provide new Guards for their future security. Such has been the patient sufferance of these Colonies; and such is now the necessity which constrains them to alter their former Systems of Government. The history of the present King of Great Britain is a history of repeated injuries and usurpations, all having in direct object the establishment of an absolute

Tyranny over these States. To prove this, let Facts be submitted to a candid world.

He has refused his Assent to Laws, the most wholesome and necessary for the public good.

He has forbidden his Governors to pass Laws of immediate and pressing importance, unless suspended in their operation till his Assent should be obtained; and when so suspended, he has utterly neglected to attend to them.

He has refused to pass other Laws for the accommodation of large districts of people, unless those people would relinquish the right of Representation in the Legislature, a right inestimable to them and formidable to tyrants only.

He has called together legislative bodies at places unusual, uncomfortable, and distant from the depository of their Public Records, for the sole Purpose of fatiguing them into compliance with his measures.

He has dissolved Representative Houses repeatedly, for opposing with manly firmness his invasions on the rights of the People.

He has refused for a long time, after such dissolutions, to cause others to be elected; whereby the Legislative Powers, incapable of Annihilation, have returned to the People at large for their exercise; the State remaining in the mean time exposed to all the dangers of invasion from without, and convulsions within.

He has endeavoured to prevent the Population of these States; for that purpose obstructing the Laws for Naturalization of Foreigners; refusing to pass others to encourage their migrations hither, and raising the conditions of new Appropriations of Lands.

He has obstructed the Administration of Justice, by refusing his Assent to Laws for establishing Judiciary Powers.

He has made Judges dependent on his Will alone, for the tenure of their offices, and the amount and payment of their salaries.

He has erected a multitude of New Offices, and sent

*Reprinted from the facsimile of the engrossed copy in the National Archives. The original spelling, capitalization, and punctuation have been retained. Paragraphing has been added.

hither swarms of Officers to harrass our People, and eat out their substance.

He has kept among us, in times of peace, Standing Armies without the Consent of our legislatures.

He has affected to render the Military independent of and superior to the Civil Power.

He has combined with others to subject us to a jurisdiction foreign to our constitution, and unacknowledged by our laws; giving his Assent to their Acts of pretended Legislation:

For Quartering large bodies of armed troops among us:

For protecting them, by a mock Trial, from Punishment for any Murders which they should commit on the Inhabitants of these States:

For cutting off our Trade with all parts of the world:

For imposing Taxes on us without our Consent:

For depriving us in many cases, of the benefits of Trial by Jury:

For transporting us beyond Seas to be tried for pretended offences:

For abolishing the free System of English Laws in a neighbouring Province, establishing therein an Arbitrary government, and enlarging its Boundaries so as to render it at once an example and fit instrument for introducing the same absolute rule into these Colonies:

For taking away our Charters, abolishing our most valuable Laws, and altering fundamentally the Forms of our Governments:

For suspending our own Legislatures, and declaring themselves invested with Power to legislate for us in all cases whatsoever.

He has abdicated Government here, by declaring us out of his Protection, and waging War against us.

He has plundered our seas, ravaged our Coasts, burnt our towns, and destroyed the lives of our people.

He is at this time transporting large Armies of foreign Mercenaries to compleat the works of death, desolation and tyranny, already begun with circumstances of Cruelty and perfidy scarcely paralleled in the most barbarous ages, and totally unworthy the Head of a civilized nation.

He has constrained our fellow Citizens taken Captive on the high Seas to bear Arms against their Country, to become the executioners of their friends and Brethren, or to fall themselves by their Hands.

He has excited domestic insurrections amongst us, and has endeavoured to bring on the inhabitants of our frontiers, the merciless Indian Savages, whose known rule of warfare, is an undistinguished destruction of all ages, sexes and conditions.

In every stage of these Oppressions We have Petitioned for Redress in the most humble terms: Our repeated Petitions have been answered only by repeated injury. A Prince, whose character is thus marked by every act which may define a Tyrant, is unfit to be the ruler of a free People.

Nor have We been wanting in attentions to our Brittish brethren. We have warned them from time to time of attempts by their legislature to extend an unwarrantable jurisdiction over us. We have reminded them of the circumstances of our emigration and settlement here. We have appealed to their native justice and magnanimity, and we have conjured them by the ties of our common kindred to disavow these usurpations, which, would inevitably interrupt our connections and correspondence. They too have been deaf to the voice of justice and of consanguinity. We must, therefore, acquiesce in the necessity, which denounces our Separation, and hold them, as we hold the rest of mankind, Enemies in War, in Peace Friends.

WE, THEREFORE, the Representatives of the UNITED STATES OF AMERICA, in General Congress, Assembled, appealing to the Supreme Judge of the world for the rectitude of our intentions, do, in the Name, and by Authority of the good People of these Colonies, solemnly publish and declare, That these United Colonies are, and of Right ought to be FREE AND INDEPENDENT STATES; that they are Absolved from all Allegiance to the British Crown, and that all political connection between them and the State of Great Britain, is and ought to be totally dissolved; and that, as Free and Independent States, they have full Power to levy War, conclude Peace, contract Alliances, establish Commerce, and to do all other Acts and Things which Independent States may of right do. And for the support of this Declaration, with a firm reliance on the protection of divine Providence, we mutually pledge to each other our Lives, our Fortunes and our sacred Honor.

The Constitution of the United States of America*

We the People of the United States, in Order to form a more perfect Union, establish Justice, insure domestic Tranquility, provide for the common defence, promote the general Welfare, and secure the Blessings of Liberty to ourselves and our Posterity, do ordain and establish this Constitution for the United States of America.

Article. I.

Section. 1. All legislative Powers herein granted shall be vested in a Congress of the United States, which shall consist of a Senate and House of Representatives.

Section. 2. The House of Representatives shall be composed of Members chosen every second Year by the People of the several States, and the Electors in each State shall have the Qualifications requisite for Electors of the most numerous Branch of the State Legislature.

No Person shall be a Representative who shall not have attained to the Age of twenty five Years, and been seven Years a Citizen of the United States, and who shall not, when elected, be an Inhabitant of that State in which he shall be chosen.

Representatives and direct Taxes† shall be apportioned among the several States which may be included within this Union, according to their respective Numbers, which shall be determined by adding to the whole Number of free Persons, including those bound to Service for a Term of Years, and excluding Indians not taxed, three fifths of all other Persons.‡ The actual Enumeration shall be made within three Years after the first Meeting of the Congress of the United States, and within every subsequent Term of ten Years, in such Manner as they shall by Law direct. The Number of Representatives shall not exceed one for every thirty Thousand, but each State shall have at Least one Representative; and until such enumeration shall be made, the State of New Hampshire shall be entitled to chuse three; Massachusetts eight; Rhode Island and Providence Plantations one; Connecticut five; New York six; New Jersey four; Pennsylvania eight; Delaware one; Maryland six; Virginia ten; North Carolina five; South Carolina five; and Georgia three.

When vacancies happen in the Representation from any State, the Executive Authority thereof shall issue Writs of Election to fill such Vacancies.

The House of Representatives shall chuse their Speaker and other Officers; and shall have the sole Power of Impeachment.

Section. 3. The Senate of the United States shall be composed of two Senators from each State, chosen by the Legislature thereof, for six Years; and each Senator shall have one Vote.*

Immediately after they shall be assembled in Consequence of the first Election, they shall be divided as equally as may be into three Classes. The Seats of the Senators of the first Class shall be vacated at the Expiration of the second Year, of the second Class at the Expiration of the fourth Year, and of the third Class at the Expiration of the sixth Year, so that one third may be chosen every second Year; and if Vacancies happen by Resignation, or otherwise, during the Recess of the Legislature of any State, the Executive thereof may make temporary Appointments until the next Meeting of the Legislature, which shall then fill such Vacancies.†

No Person shall be a Senator who shall not have attained to the Age of thirty Years, and been nine Years a Citizen of the United States, and who shall not, when elected, be an Inhabitant of that State for which he shall be chosen.

The Vice President of the United States shall be President of the Senate, but shall have no Vote, unless they be equally divided.

The Senate shall chuse their other Officers, and also a

---

*From the engrossed copy in the National Archives. Original spelling, capitalization, and punctuation have been retained.
† Modified by the Sixteenth Amendment.
‡ Replaced by the Fourteenth Amendment.

*Superseded by the Seventeenth Amendment.
† Modified by the Seventeenth Amendment.

President pro tempore, in the Absence of the Vice President, or when he shall exercise the Office of President of the United States.

The Senate shall have the sole Power to try all Impeachments. When sitting for that Purpose, they shall be on Oath or Affirmation. When the President of the United States is tried, the Chief Justice shall preside: And no Person shall be convicted without the Concurrence of two thirds of the Members present.

Judgment in Cases of Impeachment shall not extend further than to removal from Office, and disqualification to hold and enjoy any Office of honor, Trust or Profit under the United States: but the Party convicted shall nevertheless be liable and subject to Indictment, Trial, Judgment and Punishment, according to Law.

Section. 4. The Times, Places and Manner of holding Elections for Senators and Representatives, shall be prescribed in each State by the Legislature thereof, but the Congress may at any time by Law make or alter such Regulation, except as to the Places of chusing Senators.

The Congress shall assemble at least once in every Year, and such Meeting shall be on the first Monday in December, unless they shall by Law appoint a different Day.*

Section. 5. Each House shall be the Judge of the Elections, Returns and Qualifications of its own Members, and a Majority of each shall constitute a Quorum to do Business; but a smaller Number may adjourn from day to day, and may be authorized to compel the Attendance of absent Members, in such Manner, and under such Penalties as each House may provide.

Each House may determine the Rules of its Proceedings, punish its Members for disorderly Behaviour, and, with the Concurrence of two thirds, expel a Member.

Each House shall keep a Journal of its Proceedings, and from time to time publish the same, excepting such Parts as may in their Judgment require Secrecy; and the Yeas and Nays of the Members of either House on any question shall, at the Desire of one fifth of those Present, be entered on the Journal.

Neither House, during the Session of Congress, shall, without the Consent of the other, adjourn for more than three days, nor to any other Place than that in which the two Houses shall be sitting.

Section. 6. The Senators and Representatives shall receive a Compensation for their Services, to be ascertained by Law, and paid out of the Treasury of the United States. They shall in all Cases, except Treason, Felony and Breach of the Peace, be privileged from Arrest during their Attendance at the Session of their respective Houses, and in going to and returning from the same; and for any Speech or Debate in either House, they shall not be questioned in any other Place.

No Senator or Representative shall, during the Time for which he was elected, be appointed to any civil Office under the Authority of the United States, which shall have been created, or the Emoluments whereof shall have been encreased during such time; and no Person holding any Office under the United States, shall be a Member of either House during his Continuance in Office.

Section. 7. All Bills for raising Revenue shall originate in the House of Representatives; but the Senate may propose or concur with Amendments as on other Bills.

Every Bill which shall have passed the House of Representatives and the Senate shall, before it become a Law, be presented to the President of the United States; If he approve he shall sign it, but if not he shall return it, with his Objections to that House in which it shall have originated, who shall enter the Objections at large on their Journal, and proceed to reconsider it. If after such Reconsideration two thirds of that House shall agree to pass the Bill, it shall be sent, together with the Objections, to the other House, by which it shall likewise be reconsidered, and if approved by two thirds of that House, it shall become a Law. But in all such Cases the Votes of both Houses shall be determined by yeas and Nays, and the Names of the Persons voting for and against the Bill shall be entered on the Journal of each House respectively. If any Bill shall not be returned by the President within ten Days (Sundays excepted) after it shall have been presented to him, the Same shall be a Law, in like Manner as if he had signed it, unless the Congress by their Adjournment prevent its Return, in which Case it shall not be a Law.

Every Order, Resolution, or Vote to which the Concurrence of the Senate and House of Representatives may be necessary (except on a question of Adjournment) shall be presented to the President of the United States; and before the Same shall take Effect, shall be approved by him, or being disapproved by him shall be repassed by two thirds of the Senate and House of Representatives, according to the Rules and Limitations prescribed in the Case of a Bill.

Section. 8. The Congress shall have Power To lay and collect Taxes, Duties, Imposts and Excises, to pay the Debts and provide for the common Defence and general Welfare of the United States; but all Duties, Imposts and Excises shall be uniform throughout the United States;

To borrow Money on the credit of the United States;

To regulate Commerce with foreign Nations, and among the several States, and with the Indian Tribes;

To establish an uniform Rule of Naturalization, and uniform Laws on the subject of Bankruptcies throughout the United States;

To coin Money, regulate the Value thereof, and of foreign Coin, and fix the Standard of Weights and Measures;

To provide for the Punishment of counterfeiting the Securities and current Coin of the United States;

To establish Post Offices and post Roads;

To promote the Progress of Science and useful Arts, by securing for limited Times to Authors and Inventors the exclusive Right to their respective Writings and Discoveries;

*Superseded by the Twentieth Amendment.

To constitute Tribunals inferior to the supreme Court;

To define and punish Piracies and Felonies committed on the high Seas, and Offences against the Law of Nations;

To declare War, grant Letters of Marque and Reprisal, and make Rules concerning Captures on Land and Water;

To raise and support Armies, but no Appropriation of Money to that Use shall be for a longer Term than two Years;

To provide and maintain a Navy;

To make Rules for the Government and Regulation of the land and naval Forces;

To provide for calling forth the Militia to execute the Laws of the Union, suppress Insurrections and repel Invasions;

To provide for organizing, arming, and disciplining, the Militia, and for governing such Part of them as may be employed in the Service of the United States, reserving to the States respectively, the Appointment of the Officers, and the Authority of training the Militia according to the discipline prescribed by Congress;

To exercise exclusive Legislation in all Cases whatsoever, over such District (not exceeding ten Miles square) as may, by Cession of particular States, and the Acceptance of Congress, become the Seat of the Government of the United States, and to exercise like Authority over all Places purchased by the Consent of the Legislature of the State in which the Same shall be, for the Erection of Forts, Magazines, Arsenals, dock-Yards, and other needful Buildings;—And

To make all Laws which shall be necessary and proper for carrying into Execution the foregoing Powers, and all other Powers vested by this Constitution in the Government of the United States, or in any Department or Officer thereof.

Section. 9. The Migration or Importation of such Persons as any of the States now existing shall think proper to admit, shall not be prohibited by the Congress prior to the Year one thousand eight hundred and eight, but a Tax or duty may be imposed on such Importation, not exceeding ten dollars for each Person.

The Privilege of the Writ of Habeas Corpus shall not be suspended, unless when in Cases of Rebellion or Invasion the public Safety may require it.

No Bill of Attainder or ex post facto Law shall be passed.

No Capitation, or other direct, Tax shall be laid, unless in Proportion to the Census or Enumeration herein before directed to be taken.

No Tax or Duty shall be laid on Articles exported from any State.

No Preference shall be given by any Regulation of Commerce or Revenue to the Ports of one State over those of another: nor shall Vessels bound to, or from, one State, be obliged to enter, clear, or pay Duties in another.

No Money shall be drawn from the Treasury, but in Consequence of Appropriations made by Law, and a regular Statement and Account of the Receipts and Expenditures of all public Money shall be published from time to time.

No Title of Nobility shall be granted by the United States: And no Person holding any Office of Profit or Trust under them, shall, without the Consent of the Congress, accept of any present, Emolument, Office, or Title, of any kind whatever, from any King, Prince, or foreign State.

Section. 10. No State shall enter into any Treaty, Alliance, or Confederation; grant Letters of Marque and Reprisal; coin Money; emit Bills of Credit; make any Thing but gold and silver Coin a Tender in Payment of Debts; pass any Bill of Attainder, ex post facto Law, or Law impairing the Obligation of Contracts, or grant any Title of Nobility.

No State shall, without the Consent of the Congress, lay any Imposts or Duties on Imports or Exports, except what may be absolutely necessary for executing its inspection Laws: and the net Produce of all Duties and Imposts, laid by any State on Imports or Exports, shall be for the Use of the Treasury of the United States; and all such Laws shall be subject to the Revision and Controul of the Congress.

No State shall, without the Consent of Congress, lay any Duty of Tonnage, keep Troops, or Ships of War in time of Peace, enter into any Agreement or Compact with another State, or with a foreign Power, or engage in War, unless actually invaded, or in such imminent Danger as will not admit of delay.

Article. II.

Section. 1. The executive Power shall be vested in a President of the United States of America. He shall hold his Office during the Term of four Years, and, together with the Vice President, chosen for the same Term, be elected, as follows:

Each State shall appoint, in such Manner as the Legislature thereof may direct, a Number of Electors, equal to the whole Number of Senators and Representatives to which the State may be entitled in the Congress: but no Senator or Representative, or Person holding an Office of Trust or Profit under the United States, shall be appointed an Elector.

The Electors shall meet in their respective States, and vote by Ballot for two Persons, of whom one at least shall not be an Inhabitant of the same State with themselves. And they shall make a List of all the Persons voted for, and of the Number of Votes for each; which List they shall sign and certify, and transmit sealed to the Seat of the Government of the United States, directed to the President of the Senate. The President of the Senate shall, in the Presence of the Senate and House of Representatives, open all the Certificates, and the Votes shall then be counted. The Person having the greatest Number of Votes shall be the President, if such Number be a Majority of the whole Number of Electors appointed; and if there be more than one who have such Majority, and have an equal Number of Votes, then the House of Representatives shall immediately chuse by Ballot one of them for President; and if no Person have a Majority, then from the five highest on the List the said House shall in like Manner chuse the President. But in chusing the President, the Votes shall be taken by States, the Representation from each State having one Vote; A quorum for this Purpose shall consist of a Member or Members from two thirds of the States, and a Majority of all the States shall be necessary to a Choice. In every Case, after the Choice of the President, the Person having the greatest Number of Votes of the Electors shall be the Vice President. But if there should remain two or more who have equal Votes, the Senate shall chuse from them by Ballot the Vice President.*

The Congress may determine the Time of chusing the Electors, and the Day on which they shall give their Votes; which Day shall be the same throughout the United States.

No Person except a natural born Citizen, or a Citizen of the United States, at the time of the Adoption of this Constitution, shall be eligible to the Office of President, neither shall any Person be eligible to that Office who shall not have attained to the Age of thirty five Years, and been fourteen Years a Resident within the United States.

In Case of the Removal of the President from Office, or of his Death, Resignation, or Inability to discharge the Powers and Duties of the said Office, the Same shall devolve on the Vice President, and the Congress may by Law provide for the Case of Removal, Death, Resignation or Inability, both of the President and Vice President, declaring what Officer shall then act as President, and such Officer shall act accordingly, until the Disability be removed, or a President shall be elected.†

The President shall, at stated Times, receive for his Services, a Compensation, which shall neither be encreased nor diminished during the Period for which he shall have been elected, and he shall not receive within that Period any other Emolument from the United States, or any of them.

Before he enter on the Execution of his Office, he shall take the following Oath or Affirmation:—''I do solemnly swear (or affirm) that I will faithfully execute the Office of President of the United States, and will to the best of my Ability, preserve, protect and defend the Constitution of the United States.''

Section. 2. The President shall be Commander in Chief of the Army and Navy of the United States, and of the Militia of the several States, when called into the actual Service of the United States; he may require the Opinion, in writing, of the principal Officer in each of the executive Departments, upon any Subject relating to the Duties of their respective Offices, and he shall have Power to grant Reprieves and Pardons for Offences against the United States, except in Cases of Impeachment.

He shall have Power, by and with the Advice and Consent of the Senate, to make Treaties, provided two thirds of the Senators present concur; and he shall nominate, and by and with the Advice and Consent of the Senate, shall appoint Ambassadors, other public Ministers and Consuls, Judges of the supreme Court, and all other Officers of the United States, whose Appointments are not herein otherwise provided for, and which shall be established by Law; but the Congress may by Law vest the Appointment of such inferior Officers, as they think proper, in the President alone, in the Courts of Law, or in the Heads of Departments.

The President shall have Power to fill up all Vacancies that may happen during the Recess of the Senate, by granting Commissions which shall expire at the End of their next Session.

Section. 3. He shall from time to time give to the Congress Information of the State of the Union, and recommend to their Consideration such Measures as he shall judge necessary and expedient; he may, on extraordinary Occasions, convene both Houses, or either of them, and in Case of Disagreement between them, with Respect to the Time of Adjournment, he may adjourn them to such Time as he shall think proper; he shall receive Ambassadors and other public Ministers; he shall take Care that the Laws be faithfully executed, and shall Commission all the Officers of the United States.

Section. 4. The President, Vice President and all civil Officers of the United States, shall be removed from Office on Impeachment for, and Conviction of, Treason, Bribery, or other high Crimes and Misdemeanors.

Article. III.

Section. 1. The judicial Power of the United States, shall be vested in one supreme Court, and in such inferior Courts as the Congress may from time to time ordain and establish. The Judges, both of the supreme and inferior Courts, shall hold their Offices during good Behaviour, and shall, at stated Times, receive for their Services, a Compensation, which shall not be diminished during their Continuance in Office.

Section. 2. The judicial Power shall extend to all Cases, in Law and Equity, arising under this Constitution, the Laws of the United States, and Treaties made, or which shall be made, under their Authority;—to all Cases affecting Ambassadors, other public Ministers and Consuls;—to all Cases of admiralty and maritime Jurisdiction;—to Controversies to which the United States shall be a Party;—to Controversies between two or more States;—between a State and Citizens of another State;*—between Citizens of different States,—between Citizens of the same State

*Superseded by the Twelfth Amendment.
†Modified by the Twenty-fifth Amendment.

*Modified by the Eleventh Amendment.

claiming Lands under Grants of different States, and between a State, or the Citizens thereof, and foreign States, Citizens or Subjects.

In all Cases affecting Ambassadors, other public Ministers and Consuls, and those in which a State shall be Party, the supreme Court shall have original Jurisdiction. In all the other Cases before mentioned, the supreme Court shall have appellate Jurisdiction, both as to Law and Fact, with such Exceptions, and under such Regulations as the Congress shall make.

The Trial of all Crimes, except in Cases of Impeachment, shall be by Jury; and such Trial shall be held in the State where the said Crimes shall have been committed; but when not committed within any State, the Trial shall be at such Place or Places as the Congress may by Law have directed.

Section. 3. Treason against the United States, shall consist only in levying War against them, or in adhering to their Enemies, giving them Aid and Comfort. No Person shall be convicted of Treason unless on the Testimony of two Witnesses to the same overt Act, or on Confession in open Court.

The Congress shall have Power to declare the Punishment of Treason, but no Attainder of Treason shall work Corruption of Blood, or Forfeiture except during the Life of the Person attainted.

Article. IV.

Section. 1. Full Faith and Credit shall be given in each State to the public Acts, Records, and judicial Proceedings of every other State. And the Congress may by general Laws prescribe the Manner in which such Acts, Records and Proceedings shall be proved, and the Effect thereof.

Section. 2. The Citizens of each State shall be entitled to all Privileges and Immunities of Citizens in the several States.

A Person charged in any State with Treason, Felony, or other Crime, who shall flee from Justice, and be found in another State, shall on Demand of the executive Authority of the State from which he fled, be delivered up, to be removed to the State having Jurisdiction of the Crime.

No Person held to Service or Labour in one State, under the Laws thereof, escaping into another, shall, in Consequence of any Law or Regulation therein, be discharged from such Service or Labour, but shall be delivered up on Claim of the Party to whom such Service or Labour may be due.

Section. 3. New States may be admitted by the Congress into this Union; but no new State shall be formed or erected within the Jurisdiction of any other State, nor any State be formed by the Junction of two or more States, or Parts of States, without the Consent of the Legislatures of the States concerned as well as of the Congress.

The Congress shall have Power to dispose of and make all needful Rules and Regulations respecting the Territory or other Property belonging to the United States; and nothing in this Constitution shall be so construed as to Prejudice any Claims of the United States, or of any particular State.

Section. 4. The United States shall guarantee to every State in this Union a Republican Form of Government, and shall protect each of them against Invasion; and on Application of the Legislature, or of the Executive (when the Legislature cannot be convened) against domestic Violence.

Article. V.

The Congress, whenever two thirds of both Houses shall deem it necessary, shall propose Amendments to this Constitution, or, on the Application of the Legislatures of two thirds of the several States, shall call a Convention for proposing Amendments, which, in either Case, shall be valid to all Intents and Purposes, as Part of this Constitution, when ratified by the Legislatures of three fourths of the several States, or by Conventions in three fourths thereof, as the one or the other Mode of Ratification may be proposed by the Congress; Provided that no Amendment which may be made prior to the Year One thousand eight hundred and eight shall in any Manner affect the first and fourth Clauses in the Ninth Section of the first Article; and that no State, without its Consent, shall be deprived of its equal Suffrage in the Senate.

Article. VI.

All Debts contracted and Engagements entered into, before the Adoption of this Constitution, shall be as valid against the United States under this Constitution, as under the Confederation.

This Constitution, and the Laws of the United States which shall be made in Pursuance thereof; and all Treaties made, or which shall be made, under the Authority of the United States, shall be the supreme Law of the Land; and the Judges in every State shall be bound thereby, any Thing in the Constitution or Laws of any State to the Contrary notwithstanding.

The Senators and Representatives before mentioned, and the Members of the several State Legislatures, and all executive and judicial Officers, both of the United States and of the several States, shall be bound by Oath or Affirmation, to support this Constitution; but no religious Test shall ever be required as a Qualification to any Office or public Trust under the United States.

Article. VII.

The Ratification of the Conventions of nine States, shall be sufficient for the Establishment of this Constitution between the States so ratifying the Same.

done in Convention by the Unanimous Consent of the States present the Seventeenth Day of September in the Year of our Lord one thousand seven hundred and Eighty seven and of the Independence of the United States of America the Twelfth. **In witness** whereof We have hereunto subscribed our Names,

Articles in Addition to, and Amendment of, the Constitution of the United States of America, Proposed by Congress, and Ratified by the Legislatures of the Several States, Pursuant to the Fifth Article of the Original Constitution.

Amendment I*

Congress shall make no law respecting an establishment of religion, or prohibiting the free exercise thereof; or abridging the freedom of speech, or of the press; or the right of the people peaceably to assemble, and to petition the Government for a redress of grievances.

Amendment II

A well regulated Militia, being necessary to the security of a free State, the right of the people to keep and bear Arms shall not be infringed.

Amendment III

No Soldier shall, in time of peace, be quartered in any house, without the consent of the Owner, nor in time of war, but in a manner to be prescribed by law.

Amendment IV

The right of the people to be secure in their persons, houses, papers, and effects, against unreasonable searches and seizures, shall not be violated, and no Warrants shall issue, but upon probable cause, supported by Oath or affirmation, and particularly describing the place to be searched, and the persons or things to be seized.

Amendment V

No person shall be held to answer for a capital or otherwise infamous crime, unless on a presentment or indictment of a Grand Jury, except in cases arising in the land or naval forces, or in the Militia, when in actual service in time of War or public danger; nor shall any person be subject for the same offence to be twice put in jeopardy of life or limb; nor shall be compelled in any criminal case to be a witness against himself, nor be deprived of life, liberty, or property, without due process of law; nor shall

private property be taken for public use, without just compensation.

Amendment VI

In all criminal prosecutions, the accused shall enjoy the right to a speedy and public trial, by an impartial jury of the State and district wherein the crime shall have been committed, which district shall have been previously ascertained by law, and to be informed of the nature and cause of the accusation; to be confronted with the witnesses against him; to have compulsory process for obtaining witnesses in his favor, and to have the Assistance of Counsel for his defence.

Amendment VII

In suits at common law, where the value in controversy shall exceed twenty dollars, the right of trial by jury shall be preserved, and no fact tried by a jury, shall be otherwise reexamined in any Court of the United States, than according to the rules of the common law.

Amendment VIII

Excessive bail shall not be required, nor excessive fines imposed, nor cruel and unusual punishments inflicted.

Amendment IX

The enumeration in the Constitution, of certain rights, shall not be construed to deny or disparage others retained by the people.

Amendment X

The powers not delegated to the United States by the Constitution; nor prohibited by it to the States, are reserved to the States respectively, or to the people.

Amendment XI*

The Judicial power of the United States shall not be construed to extend to any suit in law or equity, commenced or prosecuted against one of the United States by Citizens of another State, or by Citizens or Subjects of any Foreign State.

Amendment XII†

The Electors shall meet in their respective States and vote by ballot for President and Vice-President, one of whom, at least, shall not be an inhabitant of the same

*The first ten amendments were passed by Congress September 25, 1789. They were ratified by three-fourths of the states December 15, 1791.

*Passed March 4, 1794. Ratified January 23, 1795.
†Passed December 9, 1803. Ratified June 15, 1804.

State with themselves; they shall name in their ballots the person voted for as President, and in distinct ballots the person voted for as Vice-President, and they shall make distinct lists of all persons voted for as President, and of all persons voted for as Vice-President, and of the number of votes for each, which lists they shall sign and certify, and transmit sealed to the seat of the government of the United States, directed to the President of the Senate;—The President of the Senate shall, in the presence of the Senate and House of Representatives, open all the certificates and the votes shall then be counted;—The person having the greatest number of votes for President, shall be the President, if such number be a majority of the whole number of Electors appointed; and if no person have such majority, then from the persons having the highest numbers not exceeding three on the list of those voted for as President, the House of Representatives shall choose immediately, by ballot, the President. But in choosing the President, the votes shall be taken by states, the representation from each state having one vote; a quorum for this purpose shall consist of a member or members from two-thirds of the states, and a majority of all the states shall be necessary to a choice. And if the House of Representatives shall not choose a President whenever the right of choice shall devolve upon them, before the fourth day of March next following, then the Vice-President shall act as President, as in the case of the death or other constitutional disability of the President.—The person having the greatest number of votes as Vice-President, shall be the Vice-President, if such number be a majority of the whole number of Electors appointed, and if no person have a majority, then from the two highest numbers on the list, the Senate shall choose the Vice-President; a quorum for the purpose shall consist of two-thirds of the whole number of Senators, and a majority of the whole number shall be necessary to a choice. But no person constitutionally ineligible to the office of President shall be eligible to that of Vice-President of the United States.

Amendment XIII*

SECTION 1. Neither slavery nor involuntary servitude, except as a punishment for crime whereof the party shall have been duly convicted, shall exist within the United States, or any place subject to their jurisdiction.

SECTION 2. Congress shall have power to enforce this article by appropriate legislation.

Amendment XIV†

SECTION 1. All persons born or naturalized in the United States, and subject to the jurisdiction thereof, are citizens of the United States and of the State wherein they reside.

No State shall make or enforce any law which shall abridge the privileges or immunities of citizens of the United States; nor shall any State deprive any person of life, liberty, or property, without due process of law; nor deny to any person within its jurisdiction the equal protection of the laws.

SECTION 2. Representatives shall be apportioned among the several States according to their respective numbers, counting the whole number of persons in each State, excluding Indians not taxed. But when the right to vote at any election for the choice of electors for President and Vice-President of the United States, Representatives in Congress, the Executive and Judicial officers of a State, or the members of the Legislature thereof, is denied to any of the male inhabitants of such State, being twenty-one years of age, and citizens of the United States, or in any way abridged, except for participation in rebellion, or other crime, the basis of representation therein shall be reduced in the proportion which the number of such male citizens shall bear to the whole number of male citizens twenty-one years of age in such State.

SECTION 3. No person shall be a Senator or Representative in Congress, or elector of President and Vice-President, or hold any office, civil or military, under the United States, or under any State, who, having previously taken an oath, as a member of Congress, or as an officer of the United States, or as a member of any State legislature, or as an executive or judicial officer of any State, to support the Constitution of the United States, shall have engaged in insurrection or rebellion against the same, or given aid or comfort to the enemies thereof. But Congress may by a vote of two-thirds of each House, remove such disability.

SECTION 4. The validity of the public debt of the United States, authorized by law, including debts incurred for payment of pensions and bounties for services in suppressing insurrection or rebellion, shall not be questioned. But neither the United States nor any State shall assume or pay any debt or obligation incurred in aid of insurrection or rebellion against the United States, or any claim for the loss or emancipation of any slave; but all such debts, obligations, and claims shall be held illegal and void.

SECTION 5. The Congress shall have the power to enforce, by appropriate legislation, the provisions of this article.

Amendment XV*

SECTION 1. The right of citizens of the United States to vote shall not be denied or abridged by the United States or by any State on account of race, color, or previous condition of servitude—

SECTION 2. The Congress shall have power to enforce this article by appropriate legislation.

*Passed January 31, 1865. Ratified December 6, 1865.
†Passed June 13, 1866. Ratified July 9, 1868.

*Passed February 26, 1869. Ratified February 2, 1870.

Amendment XVI*

The Congress shall have power to lay and collect taxes on incomes, from whatever source derived, without apportionment among the several States, and without regard to any census or enumeration.

Amendment XVII†

The Senate of the United States shall be composed of two Senators from each State, elected by the people thereof, for six years; and each Senator shall have one vote. The electors in each State shall have the qualifications requisite for electors of the most numerous branch of the State legislatures.

When vacancies happen in the representation of any State in the Senate, the executive authority of such State shall issue writs of election to fill such vacancies: *Provided,* That the legislature of any State may empower the executive thereof to make temporary appointments until the people fill the vacancies by election as the legislature may direct.

This amendment shall not be so construed as to affect the election or term of any Senator chosen before it becomes valid as part of the Constitution.

Amendment XVIII‡

SECTION 1. After one year from the ratification of this article the manufacture, sale, or transportation of intoxicating liquors within, the importation thereof into, or the exportation thereof from the United States and all territory subject to the jurisdiction thereof for beverage purposes is hereby prohibited.

SECTION 2. The Congress and the several States shall have concurrent power to enforce this article by appropriate legislation.

SECTION 3. This article shall be inoperative unless it shall have been ratified as an amendment to the Constitution by the legislatures of the several States, as provided in the Constitution, within seven years from the date of the submission hereof to the States by the Congress.

Amendment XIX§

The right of citizens of the United States to vote shall not be denied or abridged by the United States or by any State on account of sex.

Congress shall have power to enforce this article by appropriate legislation.

Amendment XX*

SECTION 1. The terms of the President and Vice-President shall end at noon on the 20th day of January, and the terms of Senators and Representatives at noon on the 3d day of January, of the years in which such terms would have ended if this article had not been ratified; and the terms of their successors shall then begin.

SECTION 2. The Congress shall assemble at least once in every year, and such meeting shall begin at noon on the 3d day of January, unless they shall by law appoint a different day.

SECTION 3. If, at the time fixed for the beginning of the term of the President, the President elect shall have died, the Vice-President elect shall become President. If a President shall not have been chosen before the time fixed for the beginning of his term, or if the President elect shall have failed to qualify, then the Vice-President elect shall act as President until a President shall have qualified; and the Congress may by law provide for the case wherein neither a President elect nor a Vice-President elect shall have qualified, declaring who shall then act as President, or the manner in which one who is to act shall be selected, and such person shall act accordingly until a President or Vice-President shall have qualified.

SECTION 4. The Congress may by law provide for the case of the death of any of the persons from whom the House of Representatives may choose a President whenever the right of choice shall have devolved upon them, and for the case of the death of any of the persons from whom the Senate may choose a Vice-President whenever the right of choice shall have devolved upon them.

SECTION 5. Sections 1 and 2 shall take effect on the 15th day of October following the ratification of this article.

SECTION 6. This article shall be inoperative unless it shall have been ratified as an amendment to the Constitution by the legislatures of three-fourths of the several States within seven years from the date of its submission.

Amendment XXI†

SECTION 1. The eighteenth article of amendment to the Constitution of the United States is hereby repealed.

SECTION 2. The transportation or importation into any State, Territory, or possession of the United States for delivery or use therein of intoxicating liquors, in violation of the laws thereof, is hereby prohibited.

SECTION 3. This article shall be inoperative unless it shall have been ratified as an amendment to the Constitution by conventions in the several States, as provided in the Constitution, within seven years from the date of the submission hereof to the States by the Congress.

*Passed July 12, 1909. Ratified February 3, 1913.
†Passed May 13, 1912. Ratified April 8, 1913.
‡Passed December 18, 1917. Ratified January 16, 1919.
§Passed June 4, 1919. Ratified August 18, 1920.

*Passed March 2, 1932. Ratified January 23, 1933.
†Passed February 20, 1933. Ratified December 5, 1933.

Amendment XXII[*]

No person shall be elected to the office of the President more than twice, and no person who has held the office of President, or acted as President, for more than two years of a term to which some other person was elected President shall be elected to the office of the President more than once.

But this Article shall not apply to any person holding the office of President when this Article was proposed by the Congress, and shall not prevent any person who may be holding the office of President, or acting as President, during the term within which this Article becomes operative from holding the office of President or acting as President during the remainder of such term.

Amendment XXIII[†]

SECTION 1. The District constituting the seat of Government of the United States shall appoint in such manner as the Congress may direct:

A number of electors of President and Vice President equal to the whole number of Senators and Representatives in Congress to which the District would be entitled if it were a State, but in no event more than the least populous State; they shall be in addition to those appointed by the States, but they shall be considered, for the purposes of the election of President and Vice President, to be electors appointed by the State; and they shall meet in the District and perform such duties as provided by the twelfth article of amendment.

SECTION 2. The Congress shall have power to enforce this article by appropriate legislation.

Amendment XXIV[‡]

SECTION 1. The right of citizens of the United States to vote in any primary or other election for President or Vice President, or for Senator or Representative in Congress, shall not be denied or abridged by the United States or any State by reason of failure to pay any poll tax or other tax.

SECTION 2. The Congress shall have power to enforce this article by appropriate legislation.

Amendment XXV[§]

SECTION 1. In case of the removal of the President from office or of his death or resignation, the Vice President shall become President.

SECTION 2. Whenever there is a vacancy in the office of the Vice President, the President shall nominate a Vice President who shall take office upon confirmation by a majority vote of both Houses of Congress.

SECTION 3. Whenever the President transmits to the President pro tempore of the Senate and the Speaker of the House of Representatives his written declaration that he is unable to discharge the powers and duties of his office, and until he transmits to them a written declaration to the contrary, such powers and duties shall be discharged by the Vice President as Acting President.

SECTION 4. Whenever the Vice President and a majority of either the principal officers of the executive department or of such other body as Congress may by law provide, transmit to the President pro tempore of the Senate and the Speaker of the House of Representatives their written declaration that the President is unable to discharge the powers and duties of his office, the Vice President shall immediately assume the powers and duties of the office of Acting President.

Thereafter, when the President transmits to the President pro tempore of the Senate and the Speaker of the House of Representatives his written declaration that no inability exists, he shall resume the powers and duties of his office unless the Vice President and a majority of either the principal officers of the executive department or of such other body as Congress may by law provide, transmit within four days to the President pro tempore of the Senate and the Speaker of the House of Representatives their written declaration that the President is unable to discharge the powers and duties of his office. Thereupon Congress shall decide the issue, assembling within forty-eight hours for that purpose if not in session. If the Congress, within twenty-one days after receipt of the latter written declaration, or, if Congress is not in session, within twenty-one days after Congress is required to assemble, determines by two-thirds vote of both Houses that the President is unable to discharge the powers and duties of his office, the Vice President shall continue to discharge the same as Acting President; otherwise, the President shall resume the powers and duties of his office.

Amendment XXVI[*]

SECTION 1. The right of citizens of the United States, who are eighteen years of age or older, to vote shall not be denied or abridged by the United States or by any State on account of age.

SECTION 2. The Congress shall have power to enforce this article by appropriate legislation.

[*]Passed March 12, 1947. Ratified March 1, 1951.
[†]Passed June 16, 1960. Ratified April 3, 1961.
[‡]Passed August 27, 1962. Ratified January 23, 1964.
[§]Passed July 6, 1965. Ratified February 11, 1967.

[*]Passed March 23, 1971. Ratified July 5, 1971.

Admission of States

Order of admission	State	Date of admission	Order of admission	State	Date of admission
1	Delaware	December 7, 1787	26	Michigan	January 26, 1837
2	Pennsylvania	December 12, 1787	27	Florida	March 3, 1845
3	New Jersey	December 18, 1787	28	Texas	December 29, 1845
4	Georgia	January 2, 1788	29	Iowa	December 28, 1846
5	Connecticut	January 9, 1788	30	Wisconsin	May 29, 1848
6	Massachusetts	February 7, 1788	31	California	September 9, 1850
7	Maryland	April 28, 1788	32	Minnesota	May 11, 1858
8	South Carolina	May 23, 1788	33	Oregon	February 14, 1859
9	New Hampshire	June 21, 1788	34	Kansas	January 29, 1861
10	Virginia	June 25, 1788	35	West Virginia	June 20, 1863
11	New York	July 26, 1788	36	Nevada	October 31, 1864
12	North Carolina	November 21, 1789	37	Nebraska	March 1, 1867
13	Rhode Island	May 29, 1790	38	Colorado	August 1, 1876
14	Vermont	March 4, 1791	39	North Dakota	November 2, 1889
15	Kentucky	June 1, 1792	40	South Dakota	November 2, 1889
16	Tennessee	June 1, 1796	41	Montana	November 8, 1889
17	Ohio	March 1, 1803	42	Washington	November 11, 1889
18	Louisiana	April 30, 1812	43	Idaho	July 3, 1890
19	Indiana	December 11, 1816	44	Wyoming	July 10, 1890
20	Mississippi	December 10, 1817	45	Utah	January 4, 1896
21	Illinois	December 3, 1818	46	Oklahoma	November 16, 1907
22	Alabama	December 14, 1819	47	New Mexico	January 6, 1912
23	Maine	March 15, 1820	48	Arizona	February 14, 1912
24	Missouri	August 10, 1821	49	Alaska	January 3, 1959
25	Arkansas	June 15, 1836	50	Hawaii	August 21, 1959

Year	Total population (in thousands)	Number per square mile of land area (continental United States)	Year	Total population (in thousands)	Number per square mile of land area (continental United States)
1790	3,929	4.5	1829	12,565	
1791	4,056		1830	12,901	7.4
1792	4,194		1831	13,321	
1793	4,332		1832	13,742	
1794	4,469		1833	14,162	
1795	4,607		1834	14,582	
1796	4,745		1835	15,003	
1797	4,883		1836	15,423	
1798	5,021		1837	15,843	
1799	5,159		1838	16,264	
1800	5,297	6.1	1839	16,684	
1801	5,486		1840	17,120	9.8
1802	5,679		1841	17,733	
1803	5,872		1842	18,345	
1804	5,065		1843	18,957	
1805	6,258		1844	19,569	
1806	6,451		1845	20,182	
1807	6,644		1846	20,794	
1808	6,838		1847	21,406	
1809	7,031		1848	22,018	
1810	7,224	4.3	1849	22,631	
1811	7,460		1850	23,261	7.9
1812	7,700		1851	24,086	
1813	7,939		1852	24,911	
1814	8,179		1853	25,736	
1815	8,419		1854	26,561	
1816	8,659		1855	27,386	
1817	8,899		1856	28,212	
1818	9,139		1857	29,037	
1819	9,379		1858	29,862	
1820	9,618	5.6	1859	30,687	
1821	9,939		1860	31,513	10.6
1822	10,268		1861	32,351	
1823	10,596		1862	33,188	
1824	10,924		1863	34,026	
1825	11,252		1864	34,863	
1826	11,580		1865	35,701	
1827	11,909		1866	36,538	
1828	12,237		1867	37,376	

Figures are from *Historical Statistics of the United States, Colonial Times to 1957* (1961), pp. 7, 8; *Statistical Abstract of the United States: 1974,* p. 5; Census Bureau for 1974 and 1975.

the United States (1790-1945)

Year	Total population (in thousands)	Number per square mile of land area (continental United States)	Year	Total population (in thousands)*	Number per square mile of land area (continental United States)
1868	38,213		1907	87,000	
1869	39,051		1908	88,709	
1870	39,905	13.4	1909	90,492	
1871	40,938		1910	92,407	31.0
1872	41,972		1911	93,868	
1873	43,006		1912	95,331	
1874	44,040		1913	97,227	
1875	45,073		1914	99,118	
1876	46,107		1915	100,549	
1877	47,141		1916	101,966	
1878	48,174		1917	103,414	
1879	49,208		1918	104,550	
1880	50,262	16.9	1919	105,063	
1881	51,542		1920	106,466	35.6
1882	52,821		1921	108,541	
1883	54,100		1922	110,055	
1884	55,379		1923	111,950	
1885	56,658		1924	114,113	
1886	57,938		1925	115,832	
1887	59,217		1926	117,399	
1888	60,496		1927	119,038	
1889	61,775		1928	120,501	
1890	63,056	21.2	1929	121,770	
1891	64,361		1930	122,775	41.2
1892	65,666		1931	124,040	
1893	66,970		1932	124,840	
1894	68,275		1933	125,579	
1895	69,580		1934	126,374	
1896	70,885		1935	127,250	
1897	72,189		1936	128,053	
1898	73,494		1937	128,825	
1899	74,799		1938	129,825	
1900	76,094	25.6	1939	130,880	
1901	77,585		1940	131,669	44.2
1902	79,160		1941	133,894	
1903	80,632		1942	135,361	
1904	82,165		1943	137,250	
1905	83,820		1944	138,916	
1906	85,437		1945	140,468	

*Figures after 1940 represent total population including Armed Forces abroad, except in official census years.
†Figure includes Alaska and Hawaii.

Population of the United States (1946-1981)

Year	Total population (in thousands)*	Number per square mile of land area (continental United States)	Year	Total population (in thousands)*	Number per square mile of land area (continental United States)
1946	141,936		1964	191,833	
1947	144,698		1965	194,237	
1948	147,208		1966	196,485	
1949	149,767		1967	198,629	
1950	150,697	50.7	1968	200,619	
1951	154,878		1969	202,599	
1952	157,553		1970	203,875	57.5†
1953	160,184		1971	207,045	
1954	163,026		1972	208,842	
1955	165,931		1973	210,396	
1956	168,903		1974	211,894	
1957	171,984		1975	213,631	
1958	174,882		1976	215,152	
1959	177,830		1977	216,880	
1960	178,464	60.1	1978	218,717	
1961	183,672		1979	220,584	
1962	186,504		1980	226,546	64.0
1963	189,197		1981	229,807	

*Figures after 1940 represent total population including Armed Forces abroad, except in official census years.
†Figure includes Alaska and Hawaii.

Appendix B

Presidential Elections
Presidents, Vice Presidents, and Cabinet Members
Justices of the U.S. Supreme Court

Presidential Elections (1789-1840)

Year	Number of states	Candidates	Parties	Popular vote	Electoral vote	Percentage of popular vote
1789	11	GEORGE WASHINGTON	No party designations		69	
		John Adams			34	
		Minor Candidates			35	
1792	15	GEORGE WASHINGTON	No party designations		132	
		John Adams			77	
		George Clinton			50	
		Minor Candidates			5	
1796	16	JOHN ADAMS	Federalist		71	
		Thomas Jefferson	Democratic-Republican		68	
		Thomas Pinckney	Federalist		59	
		Aaron Burr	Democratic-Republican		30	
		Minor Candidates			48	
1800	16	THOMAS JEFFERSON	Democratic-Republican		73	
		Aaron Burr	Democratic-Republican		73	
		John Adams	Federalist		65	
		Charles C. Pinckney	Federalist		64	
		John Jay	Federalist		1	
1804	17	THOMAS JEFFERSON	Democratic-Republican		162	
		Charles C. Pinckney	Federalist		14	
1808	17	JAMES MADISON	Democratic-Republican		122	
		Charles C. Pinckney	Federalist		47	
		George Clinton	Democratic-Republican		6	
1812	18	JAMES MADISON	Democratic-Republican		128	
		DeWitt Clinton	Federalist		89	
1816	19	JAMES MONROE	Democratic-Republican		183	
		Rufus King	Federalist		34	
1820	24	JAMES MONROE	Democratic-Republican		231	
		John Quincy Adams	Independent Republican		1	
1824	24	JOHN QUINCY ADAMS	Democratic-Republican	108,740	84	30.5
		Andrew Jackson	Democratic-Republican	153,544	99	43.1
		William H. Crawford	Democratic-Republican	46,618	41	13.1
		Henry Clay	Democratic-Republican	47,136	37	13.2
1828	24	ANDREW JACKSON	Democratic	647,286	178	56.0
		John Quincy Adams	National Republican	508,064	83	44.0
1832	24	ANDREW JACKSON	Democratic	687,502	219	55.0
		Henry Clay	National Republican	530,189	49	42.4
		William Wirt	Anti-Masonic	33,108	7	2.6
		John Floyd	National Republican		11	
1836	26	MARTIN VAN BUREN	Democratic	765,483	170	50.9
		William H. Harrison	Whig		73	
		Hugh L. White	Whig	739,795	26	49.1
		Daniel Webster	Whig		14	
		W. P. Mangum	Whig		11	
1840	26	WILLIAM H. HARRISON	Whig	1,274,624	234	53.1
		Martin Van Buren	Democratic	1,127,781	60	46.9

Candidates receiving less than 1 percent of the popular vote have been omitted. For that reason the percentage of popular vote given for any election year may not total 100 percent.

Before the passage of the Twelfth Amendment in 1804, the Electoral College voted for two presidential candidates; the runner-up became Vice President. Figures are from *Historical Statistics of the United States, Colonial Times to 1957* (1961), pp. 682–83; and the U.S. Department of Justice.

Presidential Elections (1844-1900)

Year	Number of states	Candidates	Parties	Popular vote	Electoral vote	Percentage of popular vote
1844	26	JAMES K. POLK	Democratic	1,338,464	170	49.6
		Henry Clay	Whig	1,300,097	105	48.1
		James G. Birney	Liberty	62,300		2.3
1848	30	ZACHARY TAYLOR	Whig	1,360,967	163	47.4
		Lewis Cass	Democratic	1,222,342	127	42.5
		Martin Van Buren	Free Soil	291,263		10.1
1852	31	FRANKLIN PIERCE	Democratic	1,601,117	254	50.9
		Winfield Scott	Whig	1,385,453	42	44.1
		John P. Hale	Free Soil	155,825		5.0
1856	31	JAMES BUCHANAN	Democratic	1,832,955	174	45.3
		John C. Frémont	Republican	1,339,932	114	33.1
		Millard Fillmore	American	871,731	8	21.6
1860	33	ABRAHAM LINCOLN	Republican	1,865,593	180	39.8
		Stephen A. Douglas	Democratic	1,382,713	12	29.5
		John C. Breckinridge	Democratic	848,356	72	18.1
		John Bell	Constitutional Union	592,906	39	12.6
1864	36	ABRAHAM LINCOLN	Republican	2,206,938	212	55.0
		George B. McClellan	Democratic	1,803,787	21	45.0
1868	37	ULYSSES S. GRANT	Republican	3,013,421	214	52.7
		Horatio Seymour	Democratic	2,706,829	80	47.3
1872	37	ULYSSES S. GRANT	Republican	3,596,745	286	55.6
		Horace Greeley	Democratic	2,843,446	*	43.9
1876	38	RUTHERFORD B. HAYES	Republican	4,036,572	185	48.0
		Samuel J. Tilden	Democratic	4,284,020	184	51.0
1880	38	JAMES A. GARFIELD	Republican	4,453,295	214	48.5
		Winfield S. Hancock	Democratic	4,414,082	155	48.1
		James B. Weaver	Greenback-Labor	308,578		3.4
1884	38	GROVER CLEVELAND	Democratic	4,879,507	219	48.5
		James G. Blaine	Republican	4,850,293	182	48.2
		Benjamin F. Butler	Greenback-Labor	175,370		1.8
		John P. St. John	Prohibition	150,369		1.5
1888	38	BENJAMIN HARRISON	Republican	5,477,129	233	47.9
		Grover Cleveland	Democratic	5,537,857	168	48.6
		Clinton B. Fisk	Prohibition	249,506		2.2
		Anson J. Streeter	Union Labor	146,935		1.3
1892	44	GROVER CLEVELAND	Democratic	5,555,426	277	46.1
		Benjamin Harrison	Republican	5,182,690	145	43.0
		James B. Weaver	People's	1,029,846	22	8.5
		John Bidwell	Prohibition	264,133		2.2
1896	45	WILLIAM McKINLEY	Republican	7,102,246	271	51.1
		William J. Bryan	Democratic	6,492,559	176	47.7
1900	45	WILLIAM McKINLEY	Republican	7,218,491	292	51.7
		William J. Bryan	Democratic; Populist	6,356,734	155	45.5
		John C. Wooley	Prohibition	208,914		1.5

*Greeley died shortly after the election; the electors supporting him then divided their votes among minor candidates.
Candidates receiving less than 1 percent of the popular vote have been omitted. For that reason the percentage of popular vote given for any election year may not total 100 percent.

Presidential Elections (1904-1932)

Year	Number of states	Candidates	Parties	Popular vote	Electoral vote	Percentage of popular vote
1904	45	THEODORE ROOSEVELT	Republican	7,628,461	336	57.4
		Alton B. Parker	Democratic	5,084,223	140	37.6
		Eugene V. Debs	Socialist	402,283		3.0
		Silas C. Swallow	Prohibition	258,536		1.9
1908	46	WILLIAM H. TAFT	Republican	7,675,320	321	51.6
		William J. Bryan	Democratic	6,412,294	162	43.1
		Eugene V. Debs	Socialist	420,793		2.8
		Eugene W. Chafin	Prohibition	253,840		1.7
1912	48	WOODROW WILSON	Democratic	6,296,547	435	41.9
		Theodore Roosevelt	Progressive	4,118,571	88	27.4
		William H. Taft	Republican	3,486,720	8	23.2
		Eugene V. Debs	Socialist	900,672		6.0
		Eugene W. Chafin	Prohibition	206,275		1.4
1916	48	WOODROW WILSON	Democratic	9,127,695	277	49.4
		Charles E. Hughes	Republican	8,533,507	254	46.2
		A. L. Benson	Socialist	585,113		3.2
		J. Frank Hanly	Prohibition	220,506		1.2
1920	48	WARREN G. HARDING	Republican	16,143,407	404	60.4
		James N. Cox	Democratic	9,130,328	127	34.2
		Eugene V. Debs	Socialist	919,799		3.4
		P. P. Christensen	Farmer-Labor	265,411		1.0
1924	48	CALVIN COOLIDGE	Republican	15,718,211	382	54.0
		John W. Davis	Democratic	8,385,283	136	28.8
		Robert M. La Follette	Progressive	4,831,289	13	16.6
1928	48	HERBERT C. HOOVER	Republican	21,391,993	444	58.2
		Alfred E. Smith	Democratic	15,016,169	87	40.9
1932	48	FRANKLIN D. ROOSEVELT	Democratic	22,809,638	472	57.4
		Herbert C. Hoover	Republican	15,758,901	59	39.7
		Norman Thomas	Socialist	881,951		2.2

Candidates receiving less than 1 percent of the popular vote have been omitted. For that reason the percentage of popular vote given for any election year may not total 100 percent.

Presidential Elections (1936-1980)

Year	Number of states	Candidates	Parties	Popular vote	Electoral vote	Percentage of popular vote
1936	48	FRANKLIN D. ROOSEVELT	Democratic	27,752,869	523	60.8
		Alfred M. Landon	Republican	16,674,665	8	36.5
		William Lemke	Union	882,479		1.9
1940	48	FRANKLIN D. ROOSEVELT	Democratic	27,307,819	449	54.8
		Wendell L. Willkie	Republican	22,321,018	82	44.8
1944	48	FRANKLIN D. ROOSEVELT	Democratic	25,606,585	432	53.5
		Thomas E. Dewey	Republican	22,014,745	99	46.0
1948	48	HARRY S. TRUMAN	Democratic	24,105,812	303	49.5
		Thomas E. Dewey	Republican	21,970,065	189	45.1
		J. Strom Thurmond	States' Rights	1,169,063	39	2.4
		Henry A. Wallace	Progressive	1,157,172		2.4
1952	48	DWIGHT D. EISENHOWER	Republican	33,936,234	442	55.1
		Adlai E. Stevenson	Democratic	27,314,992	89	44.4
1956	48	DWIGHT D. EISENHOWER	Republican	35,590,472	457	57.6
		Adlai E. Stevenson	Democratic	26,022,752	73	42.1
1960	50	JOHN F. KENNEDY	Democratic	34,227,096	303	49.9
		Richard M. Nixon	Republican	34,108,546	219	49.6
1964	50	LYNDON B. JOHNSON	Democratic	43,126,506	486	61.1
		Barry M. Goldwater	Republican	27,176,799	52	38.5
1968	50	RICHARD M. NIXON	Republican	31,785,480	301	43.4
		Hubert H. Humphrey	Democratic	31,275,165	191	42.7
		George C. Wallace	American Independent	9,906,473	46	13.5
1972	50	RICHARD M. NIXON	Republican	47,169,911	520	60.7
		George S. McGovern	Democratic	29,170,383	17	37.5
1976	50	JIMMY CARTER	Democratic	40,827,394	297	50.0
		Gerald R. Ford	Republican	39,145,977	240	47.9
1980	50	RONALD W. REAGAN	Republican	43,899,248	489	50.8
		Jimmy Carter	Democratic	35,481,435	49	41.0
		John B. Anderson	Independent	5,719,437		6.6
		Ed Clark	Libertarian	920,859		1.0

Candidates receiving less than 1 percent of the popular vote have been omitted. For that reason the percentage of popular vote given for any election year may not total 100 percent.

Presidents, Vice Presidents, and Cabinet Members (1789-1841)

President	Vice President	Secretary of State	Secretary of Treasury	Secretary of War
George Washington 1789–97	John Adams 1789–97	Thomas Jefferson 1789–94 Edmund Randolph 1794–95 Timothy Pickering 1795–97	Alexander Hamilton 1789–95 Oliver Wolcott 1795–97	Henry Knox 1789–95 Timothy Pickering 1795–96 James McHenry 1796–97
John Adams 1797–1801	Thomas Jefferson 1797–1801	Timothy Pickering 1797–1800 John Marshall 1800–01	Oliver Wolcott 1797–1801 Samuel Dexter 1801	James McHenry 1797–1800 Samuel Dexter 1800–01
Thomas Jefferson 1801–09	Aaron Burr 1801–05 George Clinton 1805–09	James Madison 1801–09	Samuel Dexter 1801 Albert Gallatin 1801–09	Henry Dearborn 1801–09
James Madison 1809–17	George Clinton 1809–13 Elbridge Gerry 1813–17	Robert Smith 1809–11 James Monroe 1811–17	Albert Gallatin 1809–14 George Campbell 1814 Alexander Dallas 1814–16 William Crawford 1816–17	William Eustis 1809–13 John Armstrong 1813–14 James Monroe 1814–15 William Crawford 1815–17
James Monroe 1817–25	Daniel D. Tompkins 1817–25	John Quincy Adams 1817–25	William Crawford 1817–25	George Graham 1817 John C. Calhoun 1817–25
John Quincy Adams 1825–29	John C. Calhoun 1825–29	Henry Clay 1825–29	Richard Rush 1825–29	James Barbour 1825–28 Peter B. Porter 1828–29
Andrew Jackson 1829–37	John C. Calhoun 1829–33 Martin Van Buren 1833–37	Martin Van Buren 1829–31 Edward Livingston 1831–33 Louis McLane 1833–34 John Forsyth 1834–37	Samuel Ingham 1829–31 Louis McLane 1831–33 William Duane 1833 Roger B. Taney 1833–34 Levi Woodbury 1834–37	John H. Eaton 1829–31 Lewis Cass 1831–37 Benjamin Butler 1837
Martin Van Buren 1837–41	Richard M. Johnson 1837–41	John Forsyth 1837–41	Levi Woodbury 1837–41	Joel R. Poinsett 1837–41

Secretary of Navy	Postmaster General	Attorney General
	Samuel Osgood 1789–91	Edmund Randolph 1789–94
	Timothy Pickering 1791–95	William Bradford 1794–95
	Joseph Habersham 1795–97	Charles Lee 1795–97
Benjamin Stoddert 1798–1801	Joseph Habersham 1797–1801	Charles Lee 1797–1801
Benjamin Stoddert 1801 Robert Smith 1801–09	Joseph Habersham 1801 Gideon Granger 1801–09	Levi Lincoln 1801–05 John Breckinridge 1805-07 Caesar Rodney 1807–09
Paul Hamilton 1809–13 William Jones 1813–14 Benjamin Crowninshield 1814–17	Gideon Granger 1809–14 Return Meigs 1814–17	Caesar Rodney 1809–11 William Pinkney 1811–14 Richard Rush 1814–17
Benjamin Crowninshield 1817–18 Smith Thompson 1818–23 Samuel Southard 1823–25	Return Meigs 1817–23 John McLean 1823–25	Richard Rush 1817 William Wirt 1817–25
Samuel Southard 1825–29	John McLean 1825–29	William Wirt 1825–29
John Branch 1829–31 Levi Woodbury 1831–34 Mahlon Dickerson 1834–37	William Barry 1829–35 Amos Kendall 1835–37	John M. Berrien 1829–31 Roger B. Taney 1831–33 Benjamin Butler 1833–37
Mahlon Dickerson 1837–38 James K. Paulding 1838–41	Amos Kendall 1837–40 John M. Niles 1840–41	Benjamin Butler 1837–38 Felix Grundy 1838–40 Henry D. Gilpin 1840–41

Presidents, Vice Presidents, and Cabinet Members (1841-77)

President	Vice President	Secretary of State	Secretary of Treasury	Secretary of War
William H. Harrison 1841	John Tyler 1841	Daniel Webster 1841	Thomas Ewing 1841	John Bell 1841
John Tyler 1841–45		Daniel Webster 1841–43 Hugh S. Legaré 1843 Abel P. Upshur 1843–44 John C. Calhoun 1844–45	Thomas Ewing 1841 Walter Forward 1841–43 John C. Spencer 1843–44 George M. Bibb 1844–45	John Bell 1841 John C. Spencer 1841–43 James M. Porter 1843–44 William Wilkins 1844–45
James K. Polk 1845–49	George M. Dallas 1845–49	James Buchanan 1845–49	Robert J. Walker 1845–49	William L. Marcy 1845–49
Zachary Taylor 1849–50	Millard Fillmore 1849–50	John M. Clayton 1849–50	William M. Meredith 1849–50	George W. Crawford 1849–50
Millard Fillmore 1850–53		Daniel Webster 1850–52 Edward Everett 1852–53	Thomas Corwin 1850–53	Charles M. Conrad 1850–53
Franklin Pierce 1853–57	William R. King 1853–57	William L. Marcy 1853–57	James Guthrie 1853–57	Jefferson Davis 1853–57
James Buchanan 1857–61	John C. Breckinridge 1857–61	Lewis Cass 1857–60 Jeremiah S. Black 1860–61	Howell Cobb 1857–60 Philip F. Thomas 1860–61 John A. Dix 1861	John B. Floyd 1857–61 Joseph Holt 1861
Abraham Lincoln 1861–65	Hannibal Hamlin 1861–65 Andrew Johnson 1865	William H. Seward 1861–65	Salmon P. Chase 1861–64 William P. Fessenden 1864–65 Hugh McCulloch 1865	Simon Cameron 1861–62 Edwin M. Stanton 1862–65
Andrew Johnson 1865–69		William H. Seward 1865–69	Hugh McCulloch 1865–69	Edwin M. Stanton 1865–67 Ulysses S. Grant 1867–68 John M. Schofield 1868–69
Ulysses S. Grant 1869–77	Schuyler Colfax 1869–73 Henry Wilson 1873–77	Elihu B. Washburne 1869 Hamilton Fish 1869–77	George S. Boutwell 1869–73 William A. Richardson 1873–74 Benjamin H. Bristow 1874–76 Lot M. Morrill 1876–77	John A. Rawlins 1869 William T. Sherman 1869 William W. Belknap 1869–76 Alphonso Taft 1876 James D. Cameron 1876–77

Secretary of Navy	Postmaster General	Attorney General	Secretary of Interior
George E. Badger 1841	Francis Granger 1841	John J. Crittenden 1841	
George E. Badger 1841 Abel P. Upshur 1841–43 David Henshaw 1843–44 Thomas Gilmer 1844 John Y. Mason 1844–45	Francis Granger 1841 Charles A. Wickliffe 1841–45	John J. Crittenden 1841 Hugh S. Legaré 1841–43 John Nelson 1843–45	
George Bancroft 1845–46 John Y. Mason 1846–49	Cave Johnson 1845–49	John Y. Mason 1845–46 Nathan Clifford 1846–48 Isaac Toucey 1848–49	
William B. Preston 1849–50	Jacob Collamer 1849–50	Reverdy Johnson 1849–50	Thomas Ewing 1849–50
William A. Graham 1850–52 John P. Kennedy 1852–53	Nathan K. Hall 1850–52 Sam D. Hubbard 1852–53	John J. Crittenden 1850–53	Thomas McKennan 1850 A. H. H. Stuart 1850–53
James C. Dobbin 1853–57	James Campbell 1853–57	Caleb Cushing 1853–57	Robert McClelland 1853–57
Isaac Toucey 1857–61	Aaron V. Brown 1857–59 Joseph Holt 1859–61 Horatio King 1861	Jeremiah S. Black 1857–60 Edwin M. Stanton 1860–61	Jacob Thompson 1857–61
Gideon Welles 1861–65	Horatio King 1861 Montgomery Blair 1861–64 William Dennison 1864–65	Edward Bates 1861–64 James Speed 1864–65	Caleb B. Smith 1861–63 John P. Usher 1863–65
Gideon Welles 1865–69	William Dennison 1865–66 Alexander Randall 1866–69	James Speed 1865–66 Henry Stanbery 1866–68 William M. Evarts 1868–69	John P. Usher 1865 James Harlan 1865–66 O. H. Browning 1866–69
Adolph E. Borie 1869 George M. Robeson 1869–77	John A. J. Creswell 1869–74 James W. Marshall 1874 Marshall Jewell 1874–76 James N. Tyner 1876–77	Ebenezer R. Hoar 1869–70 Amos T. Akerman 1870–71 G. H. Williams 1871–75 Edwards Pierrepont 1875–76 Alphonso Taft 1876–77	Jacob D. Cox 1869–70 Columbus Delano 1870–75 Zachariah Chandler 1875–77

Presidents, Vice Presidents, and Cabinet Members (1877-1923)

President	Vice President	Secretary of State	Secretary of Treasury	Secretary of War	Secretary of Navy
Rutherford B. Hayes 1877–81	William A. Wheeler 1877–81	William M. Evarts 1877–81	John Sherman 1877–81	George W. McCrary 1877–79 Alexander Ramsey 1879–81	R. W. Thompson 1877–81 Nathan Goff, Jr. 1881
James A. Garfield 1881	Chester A. Arthur 1881	James G. Blaine 1881	William Windom 1881	Robert T. Lincoln 1881	William H. Hunt 1881
Chester A. Arthur 1881–85		F. T. Frelinghuysen 1881–85	Charles J. Folger 1881–84 Walter Q. Gresham 1884 Hugh McCulloch 1884–85	Robert T. Lincoln 1881–85	William E. Chandler 1881–85
Grover Cleveland 1885–89	T. A. Hendricks 1885	Thomas F. Bayard 1885–89	Daniel Manning 1885–87 Charles S. Fairchild 1887–89	William C. Endicott 1885–89	William C. Whitney 1885–89
Benjamin Harrison 1889–93	Levi P. Morton 1889–93	James G. Blaine 1889–92 John W. Foster 1892–93	William Windom 1889–91 Charles Foster 1891–93	Redfield Procter 1889–91 Stephen B. Elkins 1891–93	Benjamin F. Tracy 1889–93
Grover Cleveland 1893–97	Adlai E. Stevenson 1893–97	Walter Q. Gresham 1893–95 Richard Olney 1895–97	John G. Carlisle 1893–97	Daniel S. Lamont 1893–97	Hilary A. Herbert 1893–97
William McKinley 1897–1901	Garret A. Hobart 1897–1901 Theodore Roosevelt 1901	John Sherman 1897–98 William R. Day 1898 John Hay 1898–1901	Lyman J. Gage 1897–1901	Russell A. Alger 1897–99 Elihu Root 1899–1901	John D. Long 1897–1901
Theodore Roosevelt 1901–09	Charles Fairbanks 1905–09	John Hay 1901–05 Elihu Root 1905–09 Robert Bacon 1909	Lyman J. Gage 1901–02 Leslie M. Shaw 1902–07 George B. Cortelyou 1907–09	Elihu Root 1901–04 William H. Taft 1904–08 Luke E. Wright 1908–09	John D. Long 1901–02 William H. Moody 1902–04 Paul Morton 1904–05 Charles J. Bonaparte 1905–06 Victor H. Metcalf 1906–08 T. H. Newberry 1908–09
William H. Taft 1909–13	James S. Sherman 1909–13	Philander C. Knox 1909–13	Franklin MacVeagh 1909–13	Jacob M. Dickinson 1909–11 Henry L. Stimson 1911–13	George von L. Meyer 1909–13
Woodrow Wilson 1913–21	Thomas R. Marshall 1913–21	William J. Bryan 1913–15 Robert Lansing 1915–20 Bainbridge Colby 1920–21	William G. McAdoo 1913–18 Carter Glass 1918–20 David F. Houston 1920–21	Lindley M. Garrison 1913–16 Newton D. Baker 1916–21	Josephus Daniels 1913–21
Warren G. Harding 1921–23	Calvin Coolidge 1921–23	Charles E. Hughes 1921–23	Andrew W. Mellon 1921–23	John W. Weeks 1921–23	Edwin Denby 1921–23

Postmaster General	Attorney General	Secretary of Interior	Secretary of Agriculture	Secretary of Commerce and Labor	
David M. Key 1877–80 Horace Maynard 1880–81	Charles Devens 1877–81	Carl Schurz 1877–81			
Thomas L. James 1881	Wayne MacVeagh 1881	S. J. Kirkwood 1881			
Thomas L. James 1881 Timothy O. Howe 1881–83 Walter Q. Gresham 1883–84 Frank Hatton 1884–85	B. H. Brewster 1881–85	Henry M. Teller 1881–85			
William F. Vilas 1885–88 Don M. Dickinson 1888–89	A. H. Garland 1885–89	L. Q. C. Lamar 1885–88 William F. Vilas 1888–89	Norman J. Colman 1889		
John Wanamaker 1889–93	W. H. H. Miller 1889–93	John W. Noble 1889–93	Jeremiah M. Rusk 1889–93		
Wilson S. Bissel 1893–95 William L. Wilson 1895–97	Richard Olney 1893–95 Judson Harmon 1895–97	Hoke Smith 1893–96 David R. Francis 1896–97	J. Sterling Morton 1893–97		
James A. Gary 1897–98 Charles E. Smith 1898–1901	Joseph McKenna 1897–98 John W. Griggs 1898–1901 Philander C. Knox 1901	Cornelius N. Bliss 1897–98 E. A. Hitchcock 1898–1901	James Wilson 1897–1901		
Charles E. Smith 1901–02 Henry C. Payne 1902–04 Robert J. Wynne 1904–05 George B. Cortelyou 1905–07 George von L. Meyer 1907–09	Philander C. Knox 1901–04 William H. Moody 1904–06 Charles J. Bonaparte 1906–09	E. A. Hitchcock 1901–07 James R. Garfield 1907–09	James Wilson 1901–09	George B. Cortelyou 1903–04 Victor H. Metcalf 1904–06 Oscar S. Straus 1906–09	
Frank H. Hitchcock 1909–13	G. W. Wickersham 1909–13	R. A. Ballinger 1909–11 Walter L. Fisher 1911–13	James Wilson 1909–13	Charles Nagel 1909–13	
				Secretary of Commerce	Secretary of Labor
Albert S. Burleson 1913–21	J. C. McReynolds 1913–14 T. W. Gregory 1914–19 A. Mitchell Palmer 1919–21	Franklin K. Lane 1913–20 John B. Payne 1920–21	David F. Houston 1913–20 E. T. Meredith 1920–21	W. C. Redfield 1913–19 J. W. Alexander 1919–21	William B. Wilson 1913–21
Will H. Hays 1921–22 Hubert Work 1922–23 Harry S. New 1923	H. M. Daugherty 1921–23	Albert B. Fall 1921–23 Hubert Work 1923	Henry C. Wallace 1921–23	Herbert C. Hoover 1921–23	James J. Davis 1921–23

Presidents, Vice Presidents, and Cabinet Members (1923-63)

President	Vice President	Secretary of State	Secretary of Treasury	Secretary of War	Secretary of Navy
Calvin Coolidge 1923–29	Charles G. Dawes 1925–29	Charles E. Hughes 1923–25 Frank B. Kellogg 1925–29	Andrew W. Mellon 1923–29	John W. Weeks 1923–25 Dwight F. Davis 1925–29	Edwin Denby 1923–24 Curtis D. Wilbur 1924–29
Herbert C. Hoover 1929–33	Charles Curtis 1929–33	Henry L. Stimson 1929–33	Andrew W. Mellon 1929–32 Ogden L. Mills 1932–33	James W. Good 1929 Patrick J. Hurley 1929–33	Charles F. Adams 1929–33
Franklin Delano Roosevelt 1933–45	John Nance Garner 1933–41 Henry A. Wallace 1941–45 Harry S Truman 1945	Cordell Hull 1933–44 E. R. Stettinius, Jr. 1944–45	William H. Woodin 1933–34 Henry Morgenthau, Jr. 1934–45	George H. Dern 1933–36 Harry H. Woodring 1936–40 Henry L. Stimson 1940–45	Claude A. Swanson 1933–40 Charles Edison 1940 Frank Knox 1940–44 James V. Forrestal 1944–45
Harry S Truman 1945–53	Alben W. Barkley 1949–53	James F. Byrnes 1945–47 George C. Marshall 1947–49 Dean G. Acheson 1949–53	Fred M. Vinson 1945–46 John W. Snyder 1946–53	Robert P. Patterson 1945–47 Kenneth C. Royall 1947	James V. Forrestal 1945–47
				Secretary of Defense James V. Forrestal 1947–49 Louis A. Johnson 1949–50 George C. Marshall 1950–51 Robert A. Lovett 1951–53	
Dwight D. Eisenhower 1953–61	Richard M. Nixon 1953–61	John Foster Dulles 1953–59 Christian A. Herter 1959–61	George M. Humphrey 1953–57 Robert B. Anderson 1957–61	Charles E. Wilson 1953–57 Neil H. McElroy 1957–61 Thomas S. Gates 1959–61	
John F. Kennedy 1961–63	Lyndon B. Johnson 1961–63	Dean Rusk 1961–63	C. Douglas Dillon 1961–63	Robert S. McNamara 1961–63	

Postmaster General	Attorney General	Secretary of Interior	Secretary of Agriculture	Secretary of Commerce	Secretary of Labor	Secretary of Health, Education and Welfare
Harry S. New 1923–29	H. M. Daugherty 1923–24 Harlan F. Stone 1924–25 John G. Sargent 1925–29	Hubert Work 1923–28 Roy O. West 1928–29	Henry C. Wallace 1923–24 Howard M. Gore 1924–25 W. M. Jardine 1925–29	Herbert C. Hoover 1923–28 William F. Whiting 1928–29	James J. Davis 1923–29	
Walter F. Brown 1929–33	J. D. Mitchell 1929–33	Ray L. Wilbur 1929–33	Arthur M. Hyde 1929–33	Robert P. Lamont 1929–32 Roy D. Chapin 1932–33	James J. Davis 1929–30 William N. Doak 1930–33	
James A. Farley 1933–40 Frank C. Walker 1940–45	H. S. Cummings 1933–39 Frank Murphy 1939–40 Robert Jackson 1940–41 Francis Biddle 1941–45	Harold L. Ickes 1933–45	Henry A. Wallace 1933–40 Claude R. Wickard 1940–45	Daniel C. Roper 1933–39 Harry L. Hopkins 1939–40 Jesse Jones 1940–45 Henry A. Wallace 1945	Frances Perkins 1933–45	
R. E. Hannegan 1945–47 Jesse M. Donaldson 1947–53	Tom C. Clark 1945–49 J. H. McGrath 1949–52 James P. McGranery 1952–53	Harold L. Ickes 1945–46 Julius A. Krug 1946–49 Oscar L. Chapman 1949–53	C. P. Anderson 1945–48 C. F. Brannan 1948–53	W. A. Harriman 1946–48 Charles Sawyer 1948–53	L. B. Schwellenbach 1945–48 Maurice J. Tobin 1948–53	
A. E. Summerfield 1953–61	H. Brownell, Jr. 1953–57 William P. Rogers 1957–61	Douglas McKay 1953–56 Fred Seaton 1956–61	Ezra T. Benson 1953–61	Sinclair Weeks 1953–58 Lewis L. Strauss 1958–61	Martin P. Durkin 1953 James P. Mitchell 1953–61	Oveta Culp Hobby 1953–55 Marion B. Folsom 1955–58 Arthur S. Flemming 1958–61
J. Edward Day 1961–63 John A. Gronouski 1963	Robert F. Kennedy 1961–63	Stewart L. Udall 1961–63	Orville L. Freeman 1961–63	Luther H. Hodges 1961–63	Arthur J. Goldberg 1961–62 W. Willard Wirtz 1962–63	A. H. Ribicoff 1961–62 Anthony J. Celebrezze 1962–63

Presidents, Vice Presidents, and Cabinet Members (1963-77)

President	Vice President	Secretary of State	Secretary of Treasury	Secretary of Defense	Postmaster General*	Attorney General
Lyndon B. Johnson 1963–69	Hubert H. Humphrey 1965–69	Dean Rusk 1963–69	C. Douglas Dillon 1963–65 Henry H. Fowler 1965–68 Joseph W. Barr 1968–69	Robert S. McNamara 1963–68 Clark M. Clifford 1968–69	John A. Gronouski 1963–65 Lawrence F. O'Brien 1965–68 W. Marvin Watson 1968–69	Robert F. Kennedy 1963–65 N. deB. Katzenbach 1965–67 Ramsey Clark 1967–69
Richard M. Nixon 1969–74	Spiro T. Agnew 1969–73 Gerald R. Ford 1973–74	William P. Rogers 1969–73 Henry A. Kissinger 1973–74	David M. Kennedy 1969–70 John B. Connally 1970–72 George P. Shultz 1972–74 William E. Simon 1974	Melvin R. Laird 1969–73 Elliot L. Richardson 1973 James R. Schlesinger 1973–74	Winton M. Blount 1969–71	John M. Mitchell 1969–72 Richard G. Kleindienst 1972–73 Elliot L. Richardson 1973 William B. Saxbe 1974
Gerald R. Ford 1974–77	Nelson A. Rockefeller 1974–77	Henry A. Kissinger 1974–77	William E. Simon 1974–77	James R. Schlesinger 1974–75 Donald H. Rumsfeld 1975–77		William B. Saxbe 1974–75 Edward H. Levi 1975–77

*On July 1, 1971, the Post Office became an independent agency. After that date, the Postmaster General was no longer a member of the Cabinet.

Secretary of Interior	Secretary of Agriculture	Secretary of Commerce	Secretary of Labor	Secretary of Health, Education and Welfare	Secretary of Housing and Urban Development	Secretary of Transportation
Stewart L. Udall 1963–69	Orville L. Freeman 1963–69	Luther H. Hodges 1963–65 John T. Connor 1965–67 Alexander B. Trowbridge 1967–68 C. R. Smith 1968–69	W. Willard Wirtz 1963–69	Anthony J. Celebrezze 1963–65 John W. Gardner 1965–68 Wilbur J. Cohen 1968–69	Robert C. Weaver 1966–68 Robert C. Wood 1968–69	Alan S. Boyd 1966–69
Walter J. Hickel 1969–71 Rogers C. B. Morton 1971–74	Clifford M. Hardin 1969–71 Earl L. Butz 1971–74	Maurice H. Stans 1969–72 Peter G. Peterson 1972 Frederick B. Dent 1972–74	George P. Shultz 1969–70 James D. Hodgson 1970–73 Peter J. Brennan 1973–74	Robert H. Finch 1969–70 Elliot L. Richardson 1970–73 Caspar W. Weinberger 1973–74	George W. Romney 1969–73 James T. Lynn 1973–74	John A. Volpe 1969–73 Claude S. Brinegar 1973–74
Rogers C. B. Morton 1974–75 Stanley K. Hathaway 1975 Thomas D. Kleppe 1975–77	Earl L. Butz 1974–76	Frederick B. Dent 1974–75 Rogers C. B. Morton 1975 Elliot L. Richardson 1975–77	Peter J. Brennan 1974–75 John T. Dunlop 1975–76 W. J. Usery 1976–77	Caspar W. Weinberger 1974–75 Forrest D. Mathews 1975–77	James T. Lynn 1974–75 Carla A. Hills 1975–77	Claude S. Brinegar 1974–75 William T. Coleman 1975–77

Presidents, Vice Presidents, and Cabinet Members (1977-   )

President	Vice President	Secretary of State	Secretary of Treasury	Secretary of Defense	Attorney General	Secretary of Interior
Jimmy Carter 1977–81	Walter F. Mondale 1977–81	Cyrus R. Vance 1977–80 Edmund S. Muskie 1980–81	W. Michael Blumenthal 1977–79 G. William Miller 1979–81	Harold Brown 1977–81	Griffin Bell 1977–79 Benjamin R. Civiletti 1979–81	Cecil D. Andrus 1977–81
Ronald W. Reagan 1981–	George H. Bush 1981–	Alexander M. Haig, Jr. 1981–82 George P. Shultz 1982–	Donald T. Regan 1981–	Caspar W. Weinberger 1981–	William French Smith 1981–	James G. Watt 1981–83 William P. Clark 1983–

Secretary of Agriculture	Secretary of Commerce	Secretary of Labor	Secretary of Health, Education and Welfare		Secretary of Housing and Urban Development	Secretary of Transportation	Secretary of Energy
Robert Bergland 1977–81	Juanita Kreps 1977–81	F. Ray Marshall 1977–81	Joseph Califano 1977–79 Patricia Roberts Harris 1979–80		Patricia Roberts Harris 1977–79 Moon Landrieu 1979–81	Brock Adams 1977–79 Neil E. Goldschmidt 1979–81	James R. Schlesinger 1977–79 Charles W. Duncan, Jr. 1979–81
			Secretary of Health and Human Services	**Secretary of Education**			
			Patricia Roberts Harris 1980–81	Shirley M. Hufstedler 1980–81			
John R. Block 1981–	Malcolm Baldrige 1981–	Raymond J. Donovan 1981–	Richard S. Schweiker 1981–83 Margaret M. Heckler 1983–	Terrel H. Bell 1981–	Samuel R. Pierce, Jr. 1981–	Drew Lewis 1981–83 Elizabeth H. Dole 1983–	James B. Edwards 1981–82 Donald P. Hodel 1982–

Justices of the U.S. Supreme Court

	1789	1790	1792	1794	1796	1798	1800	1802	1804	1806	1808	1810	1812	1814	1816	1818	1820	1822

Appointing President

George Washington 1789–97	John Adams 1797–1801	Thomas Jefferson 1801–09	James Madison 1809–17	James Monroe 1817–25

Chief Justice

John Jay 1789–95

Oliver Ellsworth 1796–1800

John Marshall 1801–35

Associate Justices

William Cushing 1789–1810

James Wilson 1789–98

John Blair, Jr. 1789–96

James Iredell 1790–99

Thomas Johnson 1791–93

William Paterson 1793–1806

Samuel Chase 1796–1811

Bushrod Washington 1798–1829

Alfred Moore 1799–1804

William Johnson 1804–34

Brockholst Livingston 1806–23

Thomas Todd 1807–26

Joseph Story 1811–45

Gabriel Duvall 1812–35

*Presidents serving only partial terms of office.

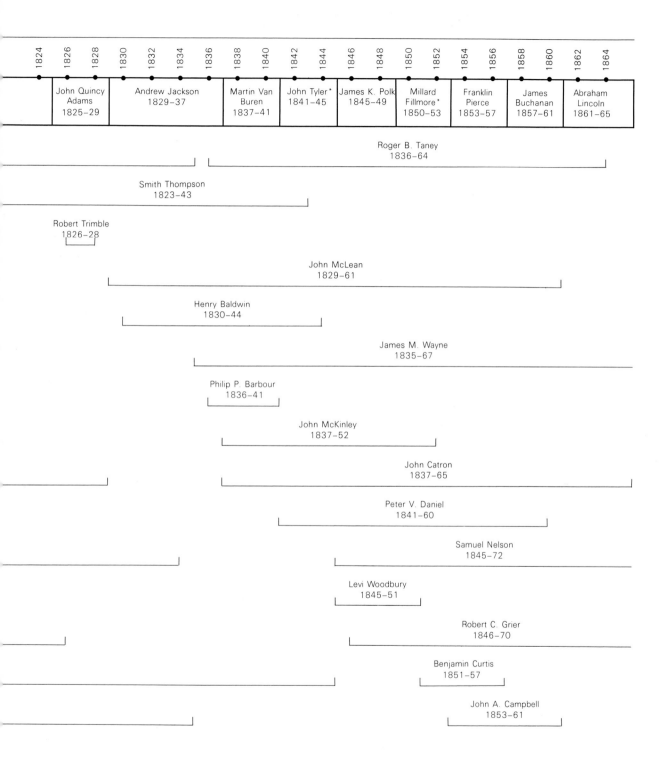

Presidents (1824–1865)

1824 1826 1828 1830 1832 1834 1836 1838 1840 1842 1844 1846 1848 1850 1852 1854 1856 1858 1860 1862 1864

John Quincy Adams 1825–29

Andrew Jackson 1829–37

Martin Van Buren 1837–41

John Tyler* 1841–45

James K. Polk 1845–49

Millard Fillmore* 1850–53

Franklin Pierce 1853–57

James Buchanan 1857–61

Abraham Lincoln 1861–65

Roger B. Taney 1836–64

Smith Thompson 1823–43

Robert Trimble 1826–28

John McLean 1829–61

Henry Baldwin 1830–44

James M. Wayne 1835–67

Philip P. Barbour 1836–41

John McKinley 1837–52

John Catron 1837–65

Peter V. Daniel 1841–60

Samuel Nelson 1845–72

Levi Woodbury 1845–51

Robert C. Grier 1846–70

Benjamin Curtis 1851–57

John A. Campbell 1853–61

Justices of the U.S. Supreme Court (Cont.)

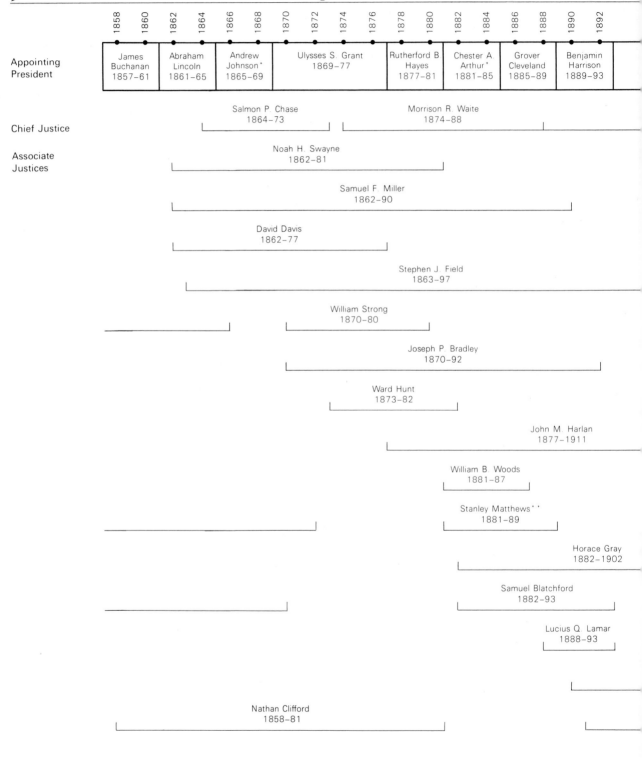

	1858	1860	1862	1864	1866	1868	1870	1872	1874	1876	1878	1880	1882	1884	1886	1888	1890	1892

Appointing President

James Buchanan 1857–61 | Abraham Lincoln 1861–65 | Andrew Johnson* 1865–69 | Ulysses S. Grant 1869–77 | Rutherford B. Hayes 1877–81 | Chester A. Arthur* 1881–85 | Grover Cleveland 1885–89 | Benjamin Harrison 1889–93

Chief Justice

Salmon P. Chase 1864–73
Morrison R. Waite 1874–88

Associate Justices

Noah H. Swayne 1862–81

Samuel F. Miller 1862–90

David Davis 1862–77

Stephen J. Field 1863–97

William Strong 1870–80

Joseph P. Bradley 1870–92

Ward Hunt 1873–82

John M. Harlan 1877–1911

William B. Woods 1881–87

Stanley Matthews** 1881–89

Horace Gray 1882–1902

Samuel Blatchford 1882–93

Lucius Q. Lamar 1888–93

Nathan Clifford 1858–81

*Presidents serving only partial terms of office.
**Appointed by James A. Garfield.

956 *Appendix B*

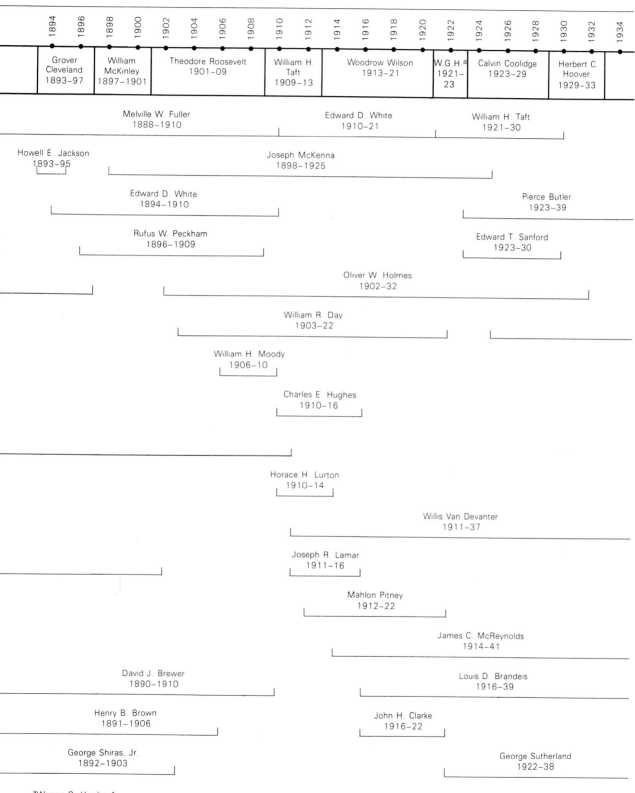

Justices of the U.S. Supreme Court (Cont.)

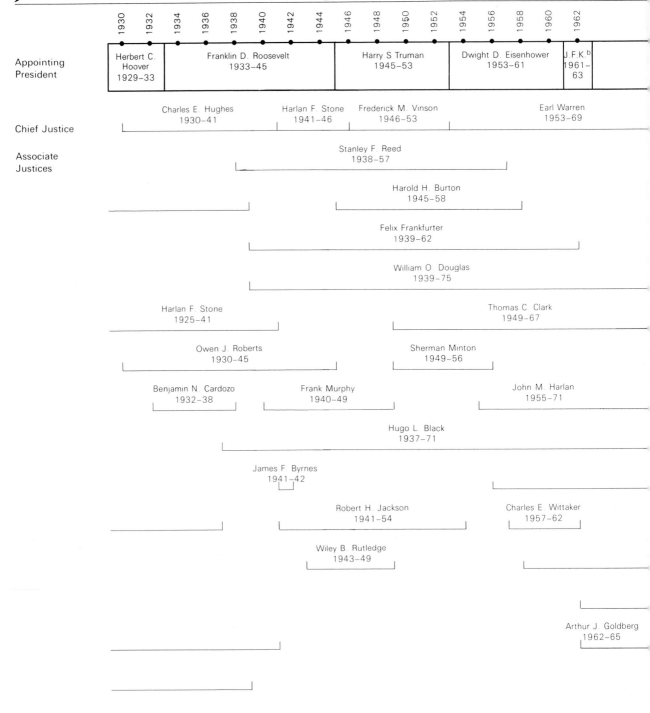

	1930	1932	1934	1936	1938	1940	1942	1944	1946	1948	1950	1952	1954	1956	1958	1960	1962

Appointing President

Herbert C. Hoover 1929–33	Franklin D. Roosevelt 1933–45	Harry S Truman 1945–53	Dwight D. Eisenhower 1953–61	J.F.K.[b] 1961–63

Chief Justice

Charles E. Hughes 1930–41
Harlan F. Stone 1941–46
Frederick M. Vinson 1946–53
Earl Warren 1953–69

Associate Justices

Stanley F. Reed 1938–57

Harold H. Burton 1945–58

Felix Frankfurter 1939–62

William O. Douglas 1939–75

Harlan F. Stone 1925–41

Thomas C. Clark 1949–67

Owen J. Roberts 1930–45

Sherman Minton 1949–56

Benjamin N. Cardozo 1932–38

Frank Murphy 1940–49

John M. Harlan 1955–71

Hugo L. Black 1937–71

James F. Byrnes 1941–42

Robert H. Jackson 1941–54

Charles E. Wittaker 1957–62

Wiley B. Rutledge 1943–49

Arthur J. Goldberg 1962–65

*Presidents serving only partial terms of office.
[b]John F. Kennedy*
  1961–63

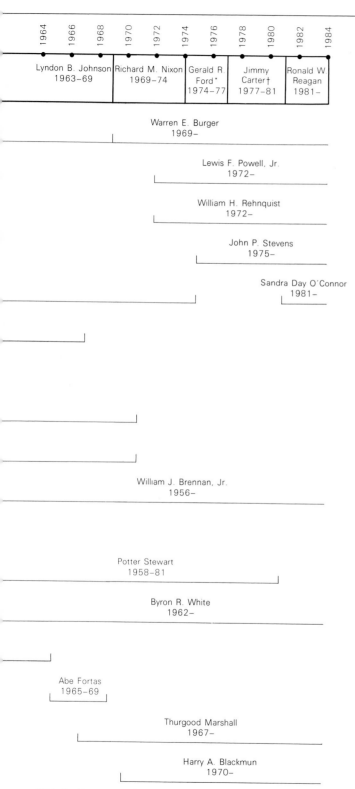

1964 1966 1968 1970 1972 1974 1976 1978 1980 1982 1984

Lyndon B. Johnson
1963–69

Richard M. Nixon
1969–74

Gerald R.
Ford*
1974–77

Jimmy
Carter†
1977–81

Ronald W.
Reagan
1981–

Warren E. Burger
1969–

Lewis F. Powell, Jr.
1972–

William H. Rehnquist
1972–

John P. Stevens
1975–

Sandra Day O'Connor
1981–

William J. Brennan, Jr.
1956–

Potter Stewart
1958–81

Byron R. White
1962–

Abe Fortas
1965–69

Thurgood Marshall
1967–

Harry A. Blackmun
1970–

†Only President to complete his full term of office without appointing a Justice to the Supreme Court.

Appendix B **959**

Picture Credits

Birch, courtesy of the United States Naval Academy

186 Detail, portrait by Francis Alexander, Dartmouth College Museum and Galleries, Hanover, New Hampshire

193 Detail, lithograph by J. H. Bufford, The New-York Historical Society

196 *Conestoga Wagons* by Thomas Birch, 1816, The Shelburne Museum

197 Portrait by Gilbert Stuart, The Metropolitan Museum of Art, bequest of Seth Low, 1929

198 Detail, portrait by Rembrandt Peale, courtesy The Supreme Court of the United States

202 Etching after a drawing by Basil Hall, The New-York Historical Society

204 Lithograph by A. Imbert, The Metropolitan Museum of Art, Harris Brisbane Dick Fund, 1941

206 Cincinnati Public Library; Photo: Fontayne and Porter

207 U.S. Army Military History Institute

210 The Charleston Museum

214 The Merrimack Valley Textile Museum

216 The Merrimack Valley Textile Museum

221 The White House Collection

222 *Pat Lyon at the Forge*, by John Neagle, Brown Brothers

225 Photograph by Philippe Haas, The Metropolitan Museum of Art, gift of I. N. Phelps Stokes, Edward S. Hawes, Alice Mary Hawes, Marion Augusta Hawes, 1937

226 Silk election bandanna, University of Hartford: J. Doyle DeWitt Collection

228 The Bettmann Archive

231 Rare Book Division, The New York Public Library, Astor, Lenox and Tilden Foundations

234 Detail, print by Currier and Ives, Yale University Art Gallery, Mabel Brady Garvan Collection

236 Brown Brothers

237 Detail, engraving after Ralph Earle, Prints Division, The New York Public Library, Astor, Lenox and Tilden Foundations

238 Brown Brothers

240 American Antiquarian Society

242 Library of Congress

243 Lithograph by H. R. Robinson, The New-York Historical Society

245 Indiana Historical Society Library

251 Lithograph by John Hailer, Prints Division, The New York Public Library, Astor, Lenox and Tilden Foundations

253 The Bettmann Archive

255 Watercolor by Jacques Gerard Miller, The New-York Historical Society

256 Portrait by Waldo and Jewett. Allen Memorial Art Museum, Oberlin College, gift of Lewis Tappan

257 Detail, portrait by Washington Allston, Museum of Fine Arts, Boston, William Francis Channing Fund

258 Lithograph by J. Bonnet after C. Autenrieth, Eno Collection #262, Prints Division, The New York Public Library, Astor, Lenox and Tilden Foundations

259 North Carolina State Archives, Albert Barden Photograph Collection

260 The New-York Historical Society

263 Daguerreotype by Southworth and Hawes, The Metropolitan Museum of Art, gift of I. N. Phelps Stokes, Edward S. Hawes, Alice Mary Hawes, Marion Augusta Hawes, 1937

264 Oneida Community, ''The Children's Hour,'' The Bettmann Archive

265 Women's History Archive, Sophia Smith Collection, Smith College, Northampton, Massachusetts

266 Women's History Archive, Sophia Smith Collection, Smith College, Northampton, Massachusetts

267 Women's History Archive, Sophia Smith Collection, Smith College, Northampton, Massachusetts

268 Detail, print by Currier and Ives, Culver Pictures

269 Culver Pictures

270 *J. W. C. Joshua Commanding the Sun to Stand Still*, 1848, Lithograph, Print Division, The New York Public Library, Astor, Lenox and Tilden Foundations

275 California State Library, California Section

279 (*top*) The New-York Historical Society; (*bottom*) Watercolor by A. J. Miller, The Walters Art Gallery

281 Drawing by Hutton, The Henry E. Huntington Library and Art Gallery

282 Library of Congress

283 Utah State Historical Society

287 Lithograph by Bayot after Nebel, Chicago Historical Society

291 Daguerreotype by Southworth and Hawes, The Metropolitan Museum of Art, gift of I. N. Phelps Stokes, Edward S. Hawes, Alice Mary Hawes, Marion Augusta Hawes, 1937

292 Drawing by Audubon, Southwest Museum, Highland Park, Los Angeles

293 Brown Brothers

294 (*top*) The Bettmann Archive; (*bottom*) Daguerreotype by Southworth and Hawes, The Metropolitan Museum of Art, gift of I. N. Phelps Stokes, Edward S. Hawes, Alice Mary Hawes, Marion Augusta Hawes, 1937

295 (*top*) Brown Brothers; (*bottom*) Daguerreotype by Southworth and Hawes, The Metropolitan Museum of Art, gift of I. N. Phelps Stokes, Edward S. Hawes, Alice Mary Hawes, Marion Augusta Hawes, 1937

298 Daguerreotype by Southworth and Hawes, The Metropolitan Museum of Art, gift of I. N. Phelps Stokes, Edward S. Hawes, Alice Mary Hawes, Marion Augusta Hawes, 1937

303 The New-York Historical Society

304 Library of Congress

305 (*top*) Photograph by Mathew Brady, Library of Congress; (*bottom*) Detail, portrait by Eaton, Portrait Collection, Harvard University, gift to Houghton Library by Mrs. Henry K. Metcalf

309 Members of first Japanese Mission to the United States, 1860, Brady Collection. Records of the Office of the Chief Signal Officer (111-B-2325) National Archives

310 The White House

311 The Museum of the City of New York

314 Edmund B. Sullivan Collection, University of Hartford

315 Nebraska Historical Society

318 Courtesy International Harvester Company

319 The Bettmann Archive

321 Brown Brothers

322 American Antiquarian Society

327 Brown Brothers

329 Library of Congress

332 Kansas State Historical Society

334 Library of Congress

335 (*top*) National Archives; (*bottom*) Library of Congress

336 from Blassingame, John W. (ed), *The Frederick Douglass Papers,* Yale University Press, New Haven

337 from Griffith, Cyril E., *The African Dream,* © 1975, Pennsylvania State University Press

340 Library of Congress

341 Library of Congress

342 Library of Congress

345 Library of Congress

348 The Bettmann Archive

349 National Archives

357 Library of Congress

359 Edouard Manet, *Battle of the Kearsage and the Alabama,* The John G. Johnson Collection, The Philadelphia Museum of Art

361 Contrabands at Follers House, Cumberland Landing, Pammekey River, 1862, James E. Taylor Collection, reproduced by permission of The Huntington Library, San Marino, California

362 Chicago Historical Society

363 State Photographic Archives, Strozier Library, Florida State University

364 Louis A. Warren, Lincoln Library and Museum, Ft. Wayne, Indiana

365 Winslow Homer, *The Letter Home,* from Campaign Sketches, 1863. Lithograph. Print Division, The New York Public Library, Astor, Lenox and Tilden Foundations

367 The Mariner's Museum, Newport News, Virginia

369 Alfred G. Waud, *Crossing the Chickahominy.* Plate 110 of Century Collection, reproduced by permission of the American Heritage Society

370 Photograph by Timothy O'Sullivan, Library of Congress

371 Photograph by Mathew Brady, The Bettmann Archive

377 HBJ Collection

378 Photograph by Timothy O'Sullivan, Library of Congress

379 Association of American Railroads

383 National Archives, Records of the Office of the Chief Signal Officer (111-B-4748)

384 (*top*) Photograph by Mathew Brady, Library of Congress; (*bottom*) Cook Collection, Valentine Museum, Richmond, Virginia

389 Library of Congress

390 *Taking the Oath and Drawing Rations,* sculpture after John Rogers, 1866, The Corcoran Gallery of Art, gift of the Honorable Orme Wilson

391 The Metropolitan Museum of Art

392 Library of Congress

393 National Gallery of Art, Washington, D.C.

394 (*top*) Library of Congress; (*bottom*) Valentine Museum, Richmond Virginia

395 (*top*) The National Museum of Art, Smithsonian Institution; (*bottom*) Culver Pictures

396 Library of Congress

401 The Granger Collection

406 Brady/Handy Collection, Library of Congress

407 (*top*) after a photo by Mathew Brady, Library of Congress; (*bottom*) Library of Congress

410 Sophia Smith Collection, Smith College

413 Atlanta Historical Society
414 Ewing Galloway
417 The Granger Collection
420 Library of Congress
421 (top) Photograph by Frances Benjamin Johnson, Library of Congress; (bottom) Brown Brothers
424 Brown Brothers
425 Brown Brothers
427 Birmingham Publishing Company
428 (top) Cook Collection, Valentine Museum, Richmond, Virginia; (bottom) Brown Brothers
429 Library of Congress
433 Photograph by J. C. H. Grabill, Library of Congress
435 Photograph by Alexander Gardner, The Kansas State Historical Society
437 The Bettmann Archive
438 The Bettmann Archive
441 (top) Montana Historical Society; (bottom) Colorado Historical Society
443 Photograph by Erwin Smith, Library of Congress
445 Baker Library, Harvard University
447 Photograph Archives, Division of Library Resources, Oklahoma Historical Society
449 Montana Historical Society
450 Photograph by Solomon Butcher, Library of Congress
453 HBJ Collection
454 Great Northern Railway, St. Paul, Minnesota
458 Photograph by Steichen, The Museum of Modern Art
459 Photograph by Detroit Photographing Company, Library of Congress
463 Photograph by Dickson, Library of Congress
464 Brown Brothers
465 Brown Brothers
467 Photograph by Detroit Photographing Company, Library of Congress
469 Library of Congress
470 AFL-CIO News
475 The Museum of the City of New York
477 Courtesy of A T & T
478 The Bettmann Archive
479 Photograph by Byron, The Museum of the City of New York
481 Photograph by Lewis Hine, Library of Congress
482 Library of Congress
484 The Keystone-Mast Collection, University of California, Riverside
486 The Bettmann Archive
489 Brown Brothers
491 Photoworld, FPG
492 Chicago Architectural Photographing Co.
493 (top) Culver Pictures; (bottom) The Bettmann Archive
494 The Bettmann Archive
499 Library of Congress
502 The Bettmann Archive
505 Library of Congress
506 Brown Brothers
507 Library of Congress
510 Cartoon by Keppler, Prints Division, The New York Public Library, Astor, Lenox and Tilden Foundations
513 Library of Congress
514 Brown Brothers
515 (top) Kansas State Historical Society; (bottom) HBJ Collection
518 Culver Pictures
519 Culver Pictures

520 Library of Congress
521 Library of Congress
525 National Archives
526 Cartoon by J. Keppler, Prints Division, The New York Public Library, Astor, Lenox and Tilden Foundations
528 Brown Brothers
529 The Bettmann Archive
530 The New York Public Library, Astor, Lenox and Tilden Foundations
533 Library of Congress
537 Rockett Collection, Library of Congress
538 The Bettmann Archive
539 The Bettmann Archive
547 The Museum of the City of New York
549 Photograph by Lewis Hine, National Archives
550 Photograph by Lewis Hine, International Museum of Photography, George Eastman House
552 Library of Congress
553 (top) HBJ Collection; (bottom) Brown Brothers
554 Library of Congress
555 (top) Tamiment Library, New York University; (bottom) Library of Congress
553 Brown Brothers
560 Brown Brothers
565 Brown Brothers
567 Mariner's Museum, Newport News, Virginia
569 Underwood and Underwood Collection, The Bettmann Archive
575 Brown Brothers
576 Brown Brothers
578 The Bettmann Archive
579 Culver Pictures
580 (top) HBJ Collection; (bottom) UPI/The Bettmann Archive
582 The Bettmann Archive
584 Culver Pictures
587 Library of Congress
588 Library of Congress
591 National Archives
592 © 1915 by The New York Times Company. Reprinted by permission
594 UPI/The Bettmann Archive
596 Culver Pictures
599 Records of the Office of the Chief Signal Officer (111-SC-94980), National Archives
600 (top) The New-York Historical Society; (bottom) USSC National Archives
601 National Archives
602 National Archives
604 Records of the Office of the Chief Signal Officer (111-SC-35757)
609 March of Time, Life Magazine © Time, Inc.
610 Photo Trends
611 Library of Congress
613 Brown Brothers
617 Boston Globe Photo
618 Photograph by J. Fujita, Chicago Historical Society
619 UPI/The Bettmann Archive
620 UPI/The Bettmann Archive
621 UPI/The Bettmann Archive
624 Culver Pictures
626 Library of Congress
631 Library of Congress
632 National Archives
633 Culver Pictures
634 Culver Pictures
635 University of Louisville Photographic Archive, Caufield and Shook Collection 109089
636 Photoworld, FPG

638 Culver Pictures
639 Gouache by Ben Shahn, The Museum of the City of New York
640 Historical Picture Service
641 State Historical Society of Wisconsin
642 The Bettmann Archive
643 (top, left) Academy of Motion Picture Arts and Sciences, courtesy of United Artists; (top, right) Life, June 3, 1926; (bottom) Brown Brothers
648 Culver Pictures
649 The Bettmann Archive
650 Brown Brothers
651 The Museum of the City of New York
656 UPI/The Bettmann Archive
658 © 1929 by The New York Times Company. Reprinted by permission
660 Reginald Marsh, Bread Line-No One Has Starved, 1932 (Restruck 1969). Etching. Collection of Whitney Museum of American Art. Original plate donated by William Benton
661 Culver Pictures
662 (top) Photograph by Russell Lee/Library of Congress; (bottom) White Angel Breadline, Photograph by Dorothea Lange/Culver Pictures
665 Library of Congress
669 National Archives
671 Wide World Photos
672 Wide World Photos
675 The Bettmann Archive
677 Brown Brothers
678 Wide World Photos
680 Franklin D. Roosevelt Library
682 The National Park Service
685 UPI/The Bettmann Archive
686 (top) Franklin D. Roosevelt Library; (bottom) WPA Photo, National Archives
689 U.S. Department of Agriculture
692 Brown Brothers
694 Wide World Photos
695 Wide World Photos
696 Library of Congress
698 Brown Brothers
700 Stuart Davis, Composition 1935, National Collection of Fine Arts, Smithsonian Institution, transfer from General Services Administration
701 Wide World Photos
705 Imperial War Museum, London
709 Zeitgeschichtliches Bildarchiv Heinrich Hoffmann
710 UPI/The Bettmann Archive
713 Imperial War Museum, London
714 Brown Brothers
715 Wide World Photos
716 Wide World Photos
717 UPI/The Bettmann Archive
718 Wide World Photos
719 Wide World Photos
721 McDonnell-Douglas Corporation
723 Imperial War Museum, London
725 UPI/The Bettmann Archive
729 U.S. Army Photo
730 Photograph by John Vachon, Library of Congress
731 National Archives
733 UPI/The Bettmann Archive
734 (top) Culver Pictures; (bottom) Wide World Photos
740 Pentagon, U.S. Army
742 Department of the Navy, National Archives
744 The Bettmann Archive
746 UPI/The Bettmann Archive

Picture Credits

Index

Boldface numbers refer to maps, charts, or illustrations.

Bridger, James, 280
Brisbane, Albert, 264
Bristow, Benjamin H., 409
British Corn Laws (1846), 308
Brock, Isaac, 183
Brook Farm, 264
Brooks, Preston, 333
Brooks, Van Wyck, 650, 700
Brotherhood of Sleeping Car Porters, 733
Brown, B. Gratz, 408
Brown, Dee, 907
Brown, Harold, 876
Brown, Jacob, 184
Brown, John, 332, 342–43, 344
Brown College, 76
Browne, Robert, 24
Brownlow, William G., 313
Brownson, Orestes, 253
Brown v. Board of Education (1954), 793, 794
Bruce, Blanche K., 406, 408, 410
Bruce, David, 801
Brussels Conference (1937), 714, 724
Bryan, Charles, 641
Bryan, William Jennings, 540, 563, 571, 666, 677; as campaigner, 520–22; and Philippine debate, 537–39; Scopes trial, 640–41; as Secretary of State, 581, 583, 585, 586, 587, 590, 591–93
Bryce, James, 482, 494, 501
Brzezinski, Zbigniew, 870, 874, 875
Buchan, John, 823
Buchanan, James, 285, 297, 306, 307, 333–34; Administration of, 334, 336–37, 338, 339, 343, 346–47
Buckley v. Valeo (1976), 864
Buckner, Simon Bolivar, 366
Budget and Accounting Act (1921), 624, 864
Buell, Don Carlos, 366, 367, 373
Buena Vista, Battle of, 287
Buffalo, 434, 438
Bulgaria, 750, 766
Bulgarian Control Commission, 750
Bulge, Battle of, 751
Bull Moose party. See Progressive party
Bull Run, Battles of: (1861), 360; (1862), **370**
Bulwer, Henry Lytton, 307
Bundy, McGeorge, 891
Bunker Hill. See Breed's Hill
Bureau of Corporations, 561–62
Bureau of Human Rights, 872
Bureau of Internal Revenue, 783
Bureau of Labor, 561–62
Burger, Warren, 858
Burgoyne, John, 104, 115
Burke, Edmund, 102
Burleigh, Charles C., 269
Burleson, Albert S., 583
Burlingame Treaty (1868), 503
Burma, 741
Burnham, Daniel H., 492
Burns, Anthony, 341
Burns, Arthur, 856
Burnside, Ambrose, 373, 380
Burr, Aaron, 156, 163–64, 176
Bush, George, 880, 882
Bush, Vannevar, 728
Business and industry, 319–21, 452–54; competition in, 194, 456–57, 461, 642, 679–80; consolidation, 460–62, 469, 549, 561, 634; and crash of 1929, 658–63; and environmental regulations, 913; factory systems, 212–25, 314, 320, 466–68, 632–35; industrial policy, 901; investments in, 147–48, 149, 319, 426, 632, 636, 647–49, 656–59, 660, 900; management in, 456–58, 459–61, 462–63, 634–35; and New Deal, 679–81,

687–88, 690–91, 700; pricing, 635, 679–80; productivity, 632–36, 660, 878; regulation of, 465, 559, 565, 585, 625, 656; technology in, 403, 454, 459, 632. See also Capitalism; Corporations; Holding Companies; Laissez-faire policy; Tariffs, protective; Trusts; individual industries
Busing, 857, 877
Bute, Earl of, 87, 88, 89
Butler, Andrew P., 333
Butler, Benjamin F., 360, 371
Butler, Edward, 482
Butler, Pierce, 133
Butterfield Overland Mail Company, 317
Byrd, Harry F., 809
Byrnes, James F., 618, 731, 745, 755, 766

Cabinet, the, 144, 150
Cable, George W., 424
Cabot, John, 13, 14, 16
Calhoun, John C., 192, 194–95, 226, 290; and annexation of Texas, 278; and Compromise of 1850, 293–94; and nullification, 234–35, 236; on slavery, 270, 290; as Vice President, 224n, 234–35, 236; and War of 1812, 181
California, 276, 280—82, 285–88, 291–93; anti-Japanese sentiment in, 571, 586, 637; gold rush, 292, 338, 440; Proposition 13, 877; statehood, 295
California Trail, 281
Callahan, E. A., 462
Callender, James T., 163
Calles, Plutarco Elias, 644
Calvert, Cecilius, 29–30
Calvert, George, 29
Calvin, John, 15, 23
Calvinism, 15, 73–74, 252, 254
Cambodia, 844, 845, 846
Cameron, Simon, 348
Camp David, 879; Eisenhower-Khrushchev meeting, 807; Sadat-Begin meeting, 873, 889
Canada, 526, 570, 578, 770; and American Revolution, 113; as English colony, 86–87, 88, 101; and War of 1812, 183–84, 185
Canals, 204–205, 315
Canning, George, 200, 201
Cannon, Joe, 576
Capitalism, 889; and American empire, 848–49; and communism, 747, 771, 780; and democracy, 465, 771; industrial, 216, 225, 464. See also Business and industry; Laissez-faire policy
Capone, Al, 639
Cardozo, Benjamin N., 692
Cardozo, Francis, 406
Caribbean, 6, 35, 87, 152, 289, 306, 524, 526, 529, 537, 567–69, 578, 587; naval bases in, 719. See also Latin America
Carlisle, Lord, 115, 117
Carlyle, Thomas, 253
Carmichael, Stokely, 831, 832
Carnegie, Andrew, 459–60, 464, 485, 537
Carnegie Steel Company, 459–60
Carpetbaggers, 400–401, 406, 414, 416, 422
Carranza, Venustiano, 587–89
Carter, Jimmy, 868; Administration of, 879–81; Camp David meeting, **872;** domestic policy, 876–79; on federal government, 883; foreign policy, 870–76, 886; and human rights, 872, 873, 881
Carter Doctrine, 876
Carteret, Sir George, 39, 40
Cartier, Jacques, 13

Carver, John, 24
Casablanca Conference (1943), 748
Cass, Lewis, 231, 290, 291, 297, 334
Castro, Cipriano, 567
Castro, Fidel, 801, 805–806, 817, 819, 886
Catchings, Waddill, 651
Cathay Company, 16
Cather, Willa, 450
Catherine of Aragon, 15
Catholics. See Roman Catholicism
Catt, Carrie Chapman, 485, 554, 902
Cattle raising, 442–44
Cavalier, Robert, 53
Cavendish, Thomas, 18
Central America. See Caribbean; Latin America
Central Intelligence Agency (CIA), 803, 834; Bay of Pigs, 816; congressional oversight of, 851, 864; covert operations, 801–802, 804, 805, 817, 827, 851; in Latin America, 886, 887; and U-2 flights, 807; and Watergate, 860
Central Treaty Organization (CENTO), 801
Cervera, Pascual, 534, 535
Chalmers, James R., 377
Chamberlain, Mellen, 105
Chamberlain, Neville, 713, 714, 716, 717–18
Chambers, Whittaker, 781, 792
Champlain, Samuel de, 14
Chancellorsville, Battle of, 373–74
Chandler, Alfred D., Jr., 635
Chandler, Zachariah, 502, 503
Channing, William Ellery, 253, 257, 276, 304
Chaplin, Charlie, 642
Charity Organizations Society, 483
Charles I, King of England, 22, 25, 29, 34, 35, 40, 46, 91
Charles II, King of England, 34, 35, 37, 42, 45, 47
Charles River Bridge v. Warren Bridge (1837), 244
Charlestown, 41, 70, 104
Charter of Liberties (1683), 39
Charter of Privileges (1701), 45
Chase, Salmon P., 169, 329, 333, 348, 370, 380, 382; as Chief Justice, 402
Chauncy, Charles, 73, 74, 75
Chautauqua movement, 488
Chavez, Cesar, 905
Cheever, John, 910
Chernenko, Konstantin U., 891
Cherokee Indians, 55, 98, 232, 233
Cheves, Langdon, 181
Cheyenne Indians, 435–36
Chiang Kai-shek, 665, 713, 724, 744–45, 749, 751–52, 772, 776, 799, 804, 850
Child Labor Act (1916), 586
Chile, 851
China, 501, **525,** 551; American imperialism in, 528, 538, 539–40; missionaries in, 527, Open Door Policy, 539–40, 570, 587, 623, 712; U.S. investments in, 578, 586; U.S. trade with, 308, 403, 528, 530, 537, 538, 539–40
China, People's Republic of, 777–78, 799; and Cambodia, 846; Cultural Revolution, 850; détente with, 850, 851, 853, 875, 885; and Formosa Straits, 804; and Korean War, 778–79, 798; and Soviet Union, 799, 804, 806, 812, 849, 851, 853, 875; and Vietnam War, 827, 846
China, Republic of, 587, 623; communists of, 776, **777;** and Japan, 613, 665–66, 712–13; nationalists of, 712, 772, 776, 779, 780; and Second World War, 713, 724, 744–45, 749, 751–52
Chinese Eastern Railway, 665

Chisholm, Shirley, 830
Chisholm v. *Georgia* (1793), 162
Chivington, John M., 435
Choate, Joseph H., 519
Chou En-lai, 850, 853
Chopin, Kate, 424
Chovart, Médart, 54
Christian Scientists, 486
Church: and reform, 485–87; separation of state and, 120–21. *See also* Religion; individual denominations
Churchill, Winston, 764, 765, 768, 799, 800, 803; and Atlantic Charter, 723–24, 746, 748; and Second World War, 714, 717, 718, 719, 723, 725, 734–41, 746–53; at Yalta, 751–52
Church of England, 15, 23, 24, 487. *See also* Anglican Church; Episcopal Church
Church of Jesus Christ of Latter-Day Saints. *See* Mormon Church
Cities, 898–900; antiurbanism, 474, 899–900; black Americans in, 420, 618, 904; financial problems of, 482, 898–99; growth of, 474–81, 549; and machine politics, 481–83; pollution in, 479, 900; population in, 474; and slums, 477, 480, 898–99. *See also* Municipal government; Urban society
Civilian Conservation Corps (CCC), 682
Civil liberties, 269; and McCarthyism, 781; and Supreme Court, 793–94; and Truman, 773–74
Civil rights: for black Americans, 395–96, 407, 409, 420–21, 884; movement in 1960s, 822–23, 832; and Nixon, 857–58; and Truman, 773–74, 793. *See also* Segregation
Civil Rights Acts: of 1866, 396–97, 398, 407; of 1875, 407, 416, 418; of 1957, 794; of 1960, 794; of 1964, 824, 902
Civil Rights Cases (1883), 418
Civil Rights Commission, 884
Civil service: and Jackson, 224, 228; and Nixon, 859; reform, 506, 508, 876. *See also* Spoils system
Civil Service Act (1883), 506
Civil Service Commission, 506, 508
Civil War, 356–85; alignment of states, **358;** black soldiers in, 377–78; border states in, 359–60; campaigns of, 359, 365–69, 372–75, 377–79, 381–84; casualties of, 367, 373, 376, 378; conscription and recruitment for, 363–64, 376; economic consequences of, 369–70, 392; and Emancipation Proclamation, 371–72; and England, 361–62, 372; financing of, 369–70, 404; preparations for, 356–62; slavery issue in, 360–61. *See also* Confederacy; Union
Clark, Champ, 581
Clark, J. Reuben, 663
Clark, James Freeman, 253
Clark, William, 174–75
Classes, social, 202, 216, 481, 483–84, 559–60, 642–44
Clay, Henry, 224, 228, 230, 236, 238–39, 240, 283; American System of, 192–201 passim, 224, 244–45, 284; and Compromise of 1850, 293–97; and Latin American revolutions, 200, 226; and Missouri Compromise, 212; and National Republicans, 220; and Treaty of Ghent, 187–88; and War of 1812, 181, 183, 187–88
Clayton, John M., 307
Clayton Act (1914), 585, 625
Clayton-Bulwer Treaty (1850), 307
Clemenceau, Georges, 609, 611–12
Cleveland, Grover, 507, 520, 526–27, 530, 531, 532, 536; Administration of, 446, 457,

508–509, 516–19; labor policy of, 471; monetary policy of, 516–19
Clifford, Clark, 838
Clinton, De Witt, 182, 204
Clinton, George, 176
Clinton, Henry, 104, 113, 117, 118
Clipper ships, 309–10
Coal mining: and energy crisis, 867, 879; strikes, 562, 617–18
Cobb, Howell, 334
Cody, Bill, 450
Cohens v. *Virginia* (1821), 198
Colbert, Jean Baptiste, 54
Cold War, 777, 828; beginnings of, 765–72; and détente, 820–21; institutionalization of, 780–81, 801–802; and Kennedy, 812–15; and nationalism, 802–806; and nuclear-test-ban treaty, 806, 818, 820–21; and peaceful coexistence, 806, 812
Cole, Nathan, 74
Coleridge, Samuel, 253
Colfax, Schuyler, 404, 405
Colleges and universities, 75–76, 215, 262, 489–91, 834, 909
Colleton, Sir John, 40
Collier, John, 439, 906
Colombia, 568, 587, 889
Colonial life: cities, 68–71; education, 64, 69, 75–76; farms, 66–68, 79; governments, 64–66, 68, 71–72; plantations, 58–65, 79; religion, 65, 68, 72–75; society, 64, 66, 68, 78–79; towns, 65–66, 71, 79
Colonies, American, **28;** assemblies, 51–52, 71–72, 92–94, 101, 105–106, 123; authority of Parliament questioned in, 88, 91–102, 105–108; counties in, 68, 72; defiance in, 39, 45–51, 93–108; England's policies for, 34–52, 82–84, 88, 90–108; militias, 66, 103–105, 110; proprietary, 29–30, 37–42, 43–45, 51; relations with Indians, 9–14, 53–56, 82–85, 89–90, 99; religion, 23–29; during Restoration, 37–45; royal, 39–40, 42, 45, 48, 51–52; taxation in, 49, 52, 82–84, 90–102 *passim;* western policy of, 82–84, 99–100
Colored Farmers' National Alliance and Cooperative Union, 513
Colson, Charles, 859, 862
Columbia College, 76
Columbus, Christopher, 8–10, 12
Comanche Indians, 434, 435
Cominform, 769
Comintern, 710, 749, 769
Commission on Civil Disorder, 832
Commission on the Status of Women, 831
Committee on Civil Rights, 773
Committee on Public Information, 605
Committee to Defend America by Aiding the Allies, 721–22
Committee to Re-elect the President (CREEP), 859, 860
Committees of Correspondence, 99, 101
Commodity Credit Corporation, 513n
Common Market. *See* European Economic Community
Commons, John R., 557, 641, 651
Commonwealth v. *Hunt* (1842), 321
Communes, 835
Communism, 600–602, 607, 616, 619–20, 648, 668, 766, 767, 771, 809; and capitalism, 747, 771, 780; containment of vs. coexistence with, 767–68, 772, 777, 780–81, 799; and Red scare, 619–20, 782, 791–93; resistance to, 765, 766, 771, 777; and uncommitted nations, 802. *See also* Cold War; Soviet Union

Communist Labor party, 618
Communist party, American, 672, 696, 717
Communitarianism, 263–64
Community Action, 825–26
Comprehensive Employment and Training Act (CETA) (1973), 856
Compromise of 1850, 293–98
Computers, 913
Concord, Battle of, 103–104
Confederacy: and amnesty, 391–92; and border states, 359–60; economy and finances of, 358, 360, 370; and Emancipation Proclamation, 371–72; and England, 372, 405; formation of, 345–46; government of, 362; military of, 358, 362–63; and readmission of states, 391–92. *See also* Civil War; Reconstruction; Secession
Confederate States of America, 345–46
Confederation of Industrial Organizations (CIO), 514
Conference for Progressive Political Action, 641
Conference on Communication with Extra-Terrestrial Intelligence (1971), 915
Confiscation Acts: of 1861, 371; of 1862, 371
Congo, 595
Congregationalists, 23–24, 25, 72, 252, 254
Congress, U.S., 133, 145; Billion Dollar, 509–11, 517; and human rights, 872; power of, 198, 502; and Reconstruction, 381, 390, 395–99; representation in, 133, 134, 135; and Vietnam War, 844, 864; Watergate reaction of, 864. *See also* House of Representatives; Senate
Congressional Budget and Impoundment Control Act (1974), 864
Congressional elections of: 1826, 225–26; 1862, 373, 380; 1866, 398; 1874, 409, 414; 1878, 504; 1882, 506; 1888, 509; 1890, 551; 1894, 518; 1910, 577–78; 1914, 585; 1922, 626–41; 1930, 661; 1932, 672; 1934, 684; 1938, 694–95; 1942, 735, 745; 1946, 773; 1950, 783; 1954, 792, 795; 1958, 795–96; 1970, 858; 1974, 867
Congressional Union, 554
Congress of Industrial Organizations (CIO), 555, 693, 697, 698
Congress of Racial Equality (CORE), 733, 822
Conkling, Roscoe, 500, 502, 503, 504
Connally, John B., 855
Connecticut, 28–29, 45, 46, 48–49, 50
Connor, Eugene, 823
Conscription: First World War, 598–600; Second World War, 719; Vietnam War, 834–35
Conservation, 632; and energy crisis, 867, 879; and New Deal, 682–84; and T. Roosevelt, 564, 577
Conservatism, 503–11, 555, 877, 885, 892, 909
Constitution, U.S.: amending of, 134; checks and balances, 133, 135, 146; equality principle, 121–22, 136, 418; opposition to, 135–36; ratification of, 134–36; separation of powers, 133, 144, 157; sovereignty question, 162; strict vs. loose interpretation of, 149, 195; supremacy of, 134; 198–99, 228, 235–36. *See also* Amendments to Constitution; Bill of Rights
Constitutional Convention, 130, 131–34
Constitutional Union party, 344
Continental Army, 105, 110–15, 121
Continental Congress, First, 101–103, 105
Continental Congress, Second, 105–108; under Articles of Confederation, 123–31; lack of enforcement power, 125–28, 129; and Revolutionary War, 110–13, 116–17, 119

Nixon, Richard M., 783–84, 790, 792, 795, 799, 800, 802, 805, 807–809, 839–40; Administration of, 857, 863–64, 867, 906; and China, 850; domestic policy, 854–56, 866; foreign policy, 842, 847, 849–54; impeachment of, 860; New Federalism of, 856–57; pardon of, 862; and silent majority, 857–58; and Supreme Court, 858; and Vietnam War, 842–46; and Watergate, 858–63; White House staff of, 857, **859**
Nixon Doctrine, 849, 876
Nomura, Kichisabura, 725
Nonintercourse Act: of 1790, 907; of 1809, 180
Non-Resistance Society, 263
Norfolk, 70
Normandy: D-Day in, **729,** 740
Norris, Frank, 556
Norris, George, 576, 637, 652, 672, 683
Norsemen, 8, 12
North, Lord, 98, 100–101, 102–103, 106, 119
North, Simeon, 214–15
North, the: abolitionists in, 265–70, 289–99; race prejudice in, 230–31, 268–70, 409, 417, 419. *See also* Trade and commerce; Union
North Africa, 735–40
North American Review, 304
North Atlantic Treaty Organization (NATO), 770, 781, 801, 875
North Carolina, 40–41, 51
North Dakota: statehood, 516
Northern Pacific Railway, 447, 456
Northern Securities Company, 561
Northwest Ordinance (1787), 126–27, 132, 330
Northwest territory, **124,** 126–28, 151–52, 153
Northwestern Alliance, 513
Norway, 446, 717, 770
Nova Scotia, 3, 85
Noyes, John Humphrey, 264
Nuclear energy, 879, 912
Nuclear weapons: arms race in, 853, 876, 890, 917; atom bomb, 754–55; as deterrent, 772, 777, 799–800, 818; hydrogen bomb, 777, 799; nuclear freeze, 891; proliferation of, 777, 818, 828; and SALT, 850–51, 875, 876, 890; and test-ban treaty, 820–21, 892
Nullification, 232–37
Nürnberg, 765–66
Nye, Gerald P., 710–11, 715, 719

Oberlin College, 261, 266
Occupational Health and Safety Act (1970), 855
Occupational Safety and Health Administration (OSHA), 855, 884
O'Connor, Edwin, 910
O'Connor, Flannery, 910
Odets, Clifford, 700
Office of Economic Opportunity (OEO), 826
Office of Economic Stabilization, 731
Office of Price Administration (OPA), 730–31, 735, 772
Office of Production Management, 721
Office of Scientific Research and Development, 728
Office of War Mobilization, 731
Oglethorpe, James, 56
Ohio: statehood, 171
Ohio Company, 84, 99, 124–25, 126
Ohio Life Insurance and Trust Company, 338
Oil industry, 460–62, 622, 879
Oklahoma Territory, 447–48

Oliver, Andrew, 93
Oliver, James, 450
Olmsted, Frederick L., 491, 492
Olney, Richard, 471, 518, 530
O'Mahoney, Joseph C., 690
Oneida Community, 264
O'Neill, Eugene, 911
Onís, Luis de, 189
Open Door Policy, 539–40, 570, 587, 712
Open Skies policy, 800, 806
Opium War, 308
Oppenheimer, J. Robert, 754, 792
Order of the Star Spangled Banner. *See* Know-Nothings
Order of United Americans, 312
Oregon: acquisition of, 283, 284–85; settlement of, 278–81
Oregon Trail, 281
Organization of American States (OAS), 805, 826
Organization for European Economic Cooperation, 769
Organization of Petroleum Exporting Countries (OPEC), 852, 866, 912
Orlando, Vittorio, 609
Orr, James Lawrence, 398
Osceola, Chief, 232
Ostend Manifesto (1854), 306–307, 333–34
Oswald, Lee Harvey, 824
Otis, Harrison Gray, 187
Otis, James, 95
Overman, Lee S., 603

Pacific Telegraph Company, 317
Paine, Thomas, 106, 129–30, 154, 252
Pakenham, Sir Edward, 185
Pakenham, Richard, 285
Pakistan, 801, 851
Palestine, 852
Palestine Liberation Organization (PLO), 852, 853, 872, 874, 889
Paley, William S., 867
Palmer, A. Mitchell, 617, 619–20, 621
Palmerston, Lord, 361–62
Panama, 568, 889
Panama Canal, 307, 568, **569,** 874
Panama Railroad, 310
Panama Treaties (1936), 706
Pan-American Conference (1928), 644
Pan-American Union, 529
Panics of: 1819, 202, 217, 223, 234; 1837, 242, 280, 308; 1857, 338–39; 1873, 408–409, 458; 1893, 458, 516; 1907, 565, 584; 1929, 658, 663
Pare, Thomas Nelson, 424
Paris Accords (1973), 843
Paris Conference. *See* Treaty of Versailles
Park Chung Hee, 798
Parker, Alton B., 563
Parker, Sir Peter, 113
Parker, Theodore, 250, 253–54, 269, 341
Paterson, William, 133
Pathet Lao, 803, 817, 827
Patrons of Husbandry, 512–14
Patterson, James T., 576
Patton, George, 670
Paul, Alice, 554, 902
Paxton boys, 89
Payne-Aldrich Act (1909), 576
Peabody, Sophia and Elizabeth, 253
Peace Corps, 815, 825, 833
Peace of Aix-la-Chapelle (1748), 82
Peace of Amiens (1802), 173

Peace of Paris (1763), 88
Peace of Ryswick (1697), 54
Peacock, Alexander R., 459
Peale, Norman Vincent, 797
Pearl Harbor, 725
Peek, George N., 676
Pemberton, John C., 375
Pendleton, George H., 381, 404, 506
Penn, William, **33,** 41–45
Pennsylvania, 42–45, 68, 85
Pennsylvania College, 76
Pennsylvania Railroad, 456, 458
Pentagon Papers, 844, 858, 859
Pepperell, William, 56
Pepys, Samuel, 42, 43
Pequot Indians, 53
Percy, Walker, 910
Pérez Jiménez, Marcos, 805
Perkins, Frances, 484, 677, 697, 699, 831, 902
Permanent Court of International Justice, 610, 646
Perón, Juan, 805
Perry, B. F., 391
Perry, Matthew C., 309
Perry, Oliver Hazard, 183, 188
Pershing, John J., 600, 608
Peru, 11–12
Pétain, Marshal, 718, 736
Phelps, Dodge & Company, 320
Philadelphia, 70, 71
Philadelphia and Reading Railroad, 458
Philip, Chief, 53
Philippine Islands, **537,** 567, 801; independence, 666; Second World War, 742–44; under U.S., 535–39
Phillips, Wendell, 265, 341, 380
Pickens, F. W., 349–50
Pickering, John, 169
Pickering, Timothy, 158, 163, 175, 187
Pickett, George E., 375, 384
Pickford, Mary, 642
Pierce, Franklin, 297, 306, 307–308, 326, 329, 330, 331–32, 530
Pierrepont, Edwards, 410
Pike, Zebulon, 175
Pilgrims, 24–25
Pinchot, Gifford, 560, 564, 565, 577, 652
Pinckney, Charles Cotesworth, 159, 164, 175, 179, 211
Pinckney, Thomas, 151, 153, 156, 157
Pinckney's Treaty (1795), 153, **154,** 172
Pingree, Hazen, 484, 558
Pinkney, William, 180
Pinochet, Augusto, 851
Piracy, 15–19; on Barbary coast, 129, 177
Pitcairn, John, 104
Pitt, William, 86–87, 88, 93, 96, 102
Pizarro, Francisco, 9
Plantation system, 21, 58–65, 79, 207–209, 317–18
Plath, Sylvia, 911
Platt, Tom, 502, 506, 560
Platt Amendment, 538–39, 706
Plessy v. *Ferguson* (1896), 418, 419, 793
Plumb, Glenn E., 616
Plymouth colony, 24, 48–49
Pocahontas, 19, **20,** 21
Poe, Edgar Allan, 304, 474
Poland, 750, 751, 850
Politics: caucus role in, 223; cycles in, 892; dislike of parties, 157, 166–68, 196; and independents, 914; and laissez-faire, 500–501; machine, 482, 502, 559, 639, 670; and national nominating conventions, 223, 239; origin of parties, 154–55; and party loyalty,

A 4
B 5
C 6
D 7
E 8
F 9
G 0
H 1
I 2
J 3

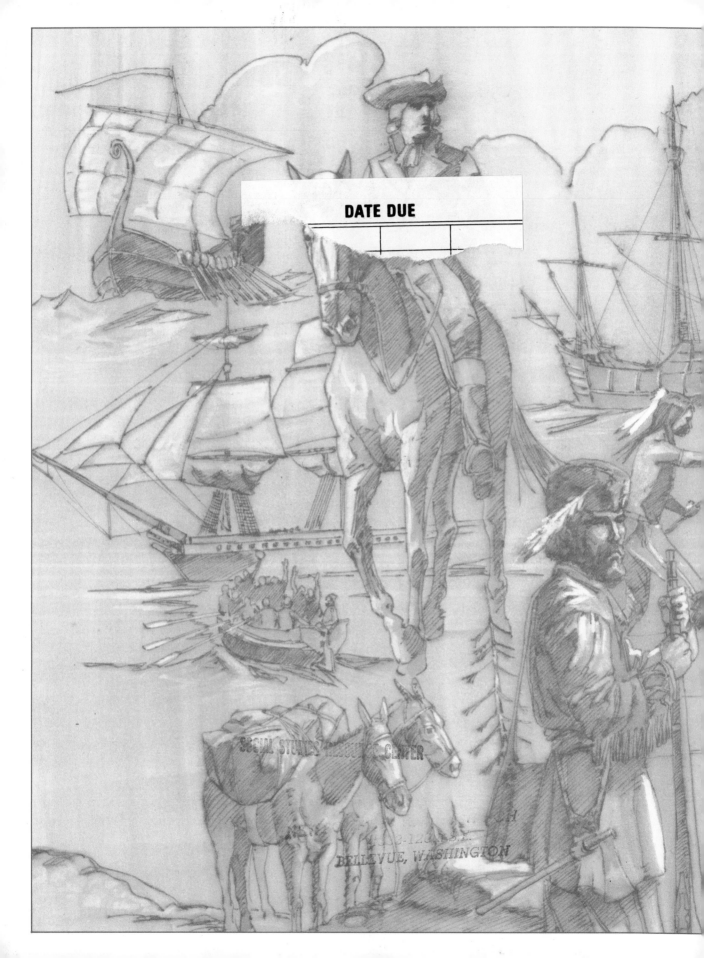

DATE DUE